Family Medicine

Paul M. Paulman • Robert B. Taylor •
Audrey A. Paulman • Laeth S. Nasir
Editors

Family Medicine

Principles and Practice

Eighth Edition

Volume 2

With 198 figures and 357 Tables

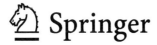 Springer

Editors
Paul M. Paulman
Department of Family Medicine
University of Nebraska Medical Center
Omaha, NE, USA

Robert B. Taylor
Department of Family and Community
Medicine
Eastern Virginia Medical School
Norfolk, VA, USA

Oregon Health Science University
Portland, OR, USA

Audrey A. Paulman
Department of Family Medicine
University of Nebraska Medical Center
Omaha, NE, USA

Laeth S. Nasir
Department of Family Medicine
Creighton University School of Medicine
Omaha, NE, USA

ISBN 978-3-030-54440-9   ISBN 978-3-030-54441-6 (eBook)
ISBN 978-3-030-54442-3 (print and electronic bundle)
https://doi.org/10.1007/978-3-030-54441-6

This Springer imprint is published by the registered company Springer Nature Switzerland AG
The registered company address is: Gewerbestrasse 11, 6330 Cham, Switzerland

"Thanks to all family physicians and others who provide primary care to their patients; without you, there would be no reason to publish this book."

Preface to the Eighth Edition

Family Medicine: Principles and Practice, eighth edition, is designed to provide point of care and reference information for family physicians, mid-level providers, residents, medical and osteopathic students, and all others who provide primary care for patients. The supervising editors from the seventh edition also supervised the production of this volume. The fact that only a few chapters were removed and a few chapters added is yet another tribute to Dr. Robert Taylor's book design as he published the first of this series and continues to serve on the editorial team and provide advice and counsel. Given that this project took place during the COVID-19 pandemic, the addition of a chapter covering pandemics is very timely.

The editors are very grateful to the staff and administrators at Springer and chapter authors who not only provided very good chapter manuscripts but also cared for themselves and their families during this pandemic. My personal thanks to Dr. Audrey Paulman and Dr. Laeth Nasir for their great work on the editorial team, and of course, thank you to all our readers/users of this book, as I said in the preface of the previous edition: providing good information which helps our readers improve the care of their patients will be our highest marker of success.

Stay well.
For the editors,
Omaha, USA
December 2021

Paul M. Paulman
Lead Editor

Preface to the First Edition

As we celebrate the publication of the 8th edition of Taylor's Family Medicine: Principles and Practice, we are also celebrating the 45th anniversary of the publication of the landmark textbook Taylor's Family Medicine: Principles and Practice, 1st edition.

This book is about people: the patient, the family, and the family physician. It presents health problems of the patient and health care by the physician in the context of mankind's most enduring societal unit – the family.

The objectives in preparation of this book have been:

1. To compile in a single textbook the fundamental principles of family medicine and the methods to implement these principles on a global basis.
2. To describe the approach of the family physician to clinical problems.
3. To help identify the clinical content of family medicine.
4. To provide a data base which can serve as a day-by-day reference source for the resident physician and clinician.
5. To explore the history and philosophy of the family practice movement.

These objectives were pursued by seeking the advice and participation of family medicine educators and practitioners around the world; preparing a book format intended to present data in a logical, cohesive manner; selecting authors based on their interests and contributions in family medicine; considering the priorities family physicians ascribe to achieving competence in various clinical areas; and including chapters telling the evolution of the modern family physician and his focus on the patient in relation to the family.

A new textbook should differ significantly from other literature in the field. The following 94 chapters represent new material prepared specifically for this first edition, including many facts and theories never before in print. There are several chapters giving personal viewpoints on topics pertinent to the specialty. The format employs units of sequential chapters that allow full elucidation of concepts. The broad scope of family medicine is covered, including sections on family medicine education, behavior and counseling, and the full spectrum of clinical medicine. The development of clinical chapters has included the Competence Priority Classification of Behavior, Concepts, and Skills in Family Medicine, a unifying taxonomy that is intended to be academically instructive and clinically relevant.

The editor expresses appreciation to the 128 contributing authors and to the four associate editors: John L. Buckingham, E. P. Donatelle, William E. Jacott, and Melville G. Rosen. Also gratefully acknowledged is the cooperation of the American Academy of Family Physicians, The American Board of Family Practice, the College of Family Physicians of Canada, and the Society of Teachers of Family Medicine. My family – Anita, Diana, and Sharon – shared in the preparation of this book, as did literally hundreds of other persons too numerous to list individually, and to whom the editors, authors, and readers are indebted.

R.B.T

Acknowledgments

We dedicate this book to all the workers who labored to keep us healthy, fed, and safe during the COVID-19 pandemic. There will never be adequate recognition or rewards for these incredible men and women; nevertheless, we'd like to add our thanks.

We have many more people to thank: Dr. Robert Taylor has continued to inspire us in his role as founder of this series of reference books; his advice and counsel have been invaluable.

Saskia Ellis, our production manager, provided a steady, consistent guiding hand throughout the production process. When it seemed that we had reached insurmountable roadblocks, Saskia was there to let us know how much progress we had made and how we weren't THAT far behind schedule. We appreciate your work, Saskia!

Sylvia Blago has also been inspirational for us and has helped us keep our eye on the prize. Having worked with Sylvia on previous projects, we have had great production experiences and she did not disappoint during this project. Thank you, Sylvia.

Our chapter authors came through with great material, while also caring for their patients and keeping themselves and their families safe from the virus. We are in your debt.

Personal thanks to Dr. Audrey Paulman and Dr. Laeth Nasir, volume editors, for their great efforts to recruit chapter authors and overcome any and all problems in order to bring this book to publication. We look forward to future editions of this reference book from Dr. Laeth Nasir and his team. Future editions of this book will be outstanding.

For the editors,
Paul M. Paulman
Editor

Contents

Contributors

Asma Abu-Zanat Department of Family and Community Medicine, University of Jordan, Aamman, Jordan

Alan M. Adelman Family and Community Medicine, Penn State University College of Medicine, Hershey, PA, USA

Temitope I. Afon Department of Family Medicine, Medical College of Georgia, Augusta University, Augusta, GA, USA

Jumana Al-Deek AdventHealth Family Medicine Residency, Winter Park, FL, USA

Lana Alhalaseh The University of Jordan, Aamman, Jordan

Jason B. Alisangco Fort Belvoir Family Medicine Department, Fort Belvoir Community Hospital, Fort Belvoir, VA, USA

Heidi Allespach Department of Family Medicine and Community Health, University of Miami Miller School of Medicine, Miami, FL, USA

Basmah M. Alnshash School of Medicine, University of Jordan, Jordan University Hospital, Amman, Jordan

Maram Alsmairat Department of Family and Community Medicine, University of Jordan, Aamman, Jordan

Patrick Anderl Family Medicine, Univeristy of Nebraska Medical Center, Omaha, NE, USA

Garland Anderson II Department of Family Medicine, Louisiana State University School of Medicine, New Orleans, LA, USA

Tanya Anim College of Medicine, Family Medicine Residency Program at Lee Health, Florida State University, Tallahassee, FL, USA

Tanya E. Anim Department of Family Medicine and Rural Health, Family Medicine Residency Program at Lee Health, Florida State University College of Medicine, Tallahassee, FL, USA

Baha M. Arafah Division of Clinical and Molecular Endocrinology, University Hospitals-Cleveland Medical Center, Case Western Reserve University School of Medicine, Cleveland, OH, USA

Carlos A. Arango Department of Pediatrics, University of Florida College of Medicine, Jacksonville, FL, USA

Corin Archuleta UNMC Family Medicine Residency Program, Omaha, NE, USA

Elisabeth L. Backer Department of Family Medicine, University of Nebraska Medical Center, Omaha, NE, USA

Alison K. Bauer Department of Family Medicine, University of Nebraska Medical Center, Omaha, NE, USA

Margaret Baumgarten Family and Community Medicine, Eastern Virginia Medical School, Norfolk, VA, USA

Jennifer Bepko David Grant Family Medicine Residency Program, David Grant Medical Center, Fairfield, CA, USA

Franklin J. Berkey Department of Family and Community Medicine, Penn State College of Medicine, University Park Regional Campus, State College, PA, USA

Karina Isabel Bishop Division of Geriatrics, Gerontology and Palliative Care, University of Nebraska Medical Center, Omaha, NE, USA

Wendy Bocaille West Kendal Baptist Hospital FIU Family Medicine Residency Program, Miami, FL, USA

Seth Bodden Medical College of Wisconsin, Milwaukee, WI, USA

Gabriel Briscoe David Grant Family Medicine Residency Program, David Grant Medical Center, Fairfield, CA, USA

Mallory Mc Clester Brown Department of Family Medicine, University of North Carolina at Chapel Hill, Chapel Hill, NC, USA

Joedrecka S. Brown Speights Department of Family Medicine and Rural Health, Florida State University College of Medicine, Tallahassee, FL, USA

Leslie Bruce AdventHealth Family Medicine Residency, Winter Park, FL, USA

Jingnan Bu Department of Family Medicine, University of Rochester School of Medicine and Dentistry, Rochester, NY, USA

Amy H. Buchanan Stritch School of Medicine, Loyola University Health System, Maywood, IL, USA

Ushimbra Buford Department of Psychiatry, University of Texas Health Science Center at Tyler, Tyler, TX, USA

Stephen D. Cagle Jr Scott Family Medicine Residency Program, Scott Air Force Base, O'Fallon, IL, USA

Thomas L. Campbell Department of Family Medicine, University of Rochester School of Medicine and Dentistry, Rochester, NY, USA

Patrick M. Carey Department of Family Medicine, Uniformed Services University of the Health Sciences, Bethesda, MD, USA

Daniel Carl Salmon Creek Medical Office, Nephrology, Vancouver, WA, USA

Medical College of Virginia Campus, Virginia Commonwealth University, Richmond, VA, USA

Luanne Carlson Department of Family Medicine, Desert Regional Medical Center, Palm Springs, CA, USA

Carlos A. Carmona Pediatrics, AdventHealth, Orlando, FL, USA

Karenn Chan Division of Care of the Elderly, Department of Family Medicine, Faculty of Medicine and Dentistry, University of Alberta, Edmonton, AB, Canada

Man-Kuang Chang Baptist Primary Care, Jacksonville, FL, USA

Sandra Chaparro Florida International University, Miami, FL, USA

Miami Cardiac and Vascular Institute, Baptist Health South Florida, Miami, FL, USA

Lesley Charles Division of Care of the Elderly, Department of Family Medicine, Faculty of Medicine and Dentistry, University of Alberta, Edmonton, AB, Canada

Justin J. Chin Family Medicine Residency Program, Eglin AFB, FL, USA

Molly S. Clark Department of Family Medicine, University of Mississippi Medical Center, Jackson, MS, USA

Lee Coghill Florida State University College of Medicine Family Medicine Residency Program at Lee Health, Fort Myers, FL, USA

Kathy Cole-Kelly Case Western Reserve School of Medicine, Cleveland, OH, USA

Brian Coleman Department of Family and Preventive Medicine, University of Oklahoma Health Sciences Center, Oklahoma, OK, USA

John Colucci David Grant Family Medicine Residency Program, David Grant Medical Center, Fairfield, CA, USA

Aaron Costerisan Family Medicine Residency Program, University of Illinois College of Medicine, Peoria, Peoria, IL, USA

Carlton J. Covey Travis Family Medicine Residency Program, Travis Air Force Base, Fairfield, CA, USA

Paul Crawford Department of Family Medicine, Uniformed Services University of the Health Sciences, Bethesda, MD, USA

Amy Crawford-Faucher Forbes Family Medicine Residency, Allegheny Health Network, Pittsburgh, PA, USA

Wanda Cruz-Knight Family Medicine, University of South Florida Morsani School of Medicine, Clearwater, FL, USA

GME BayCare Medical Group, Tampa, FL, USA

USF-MPM Family Medicine, Clearwater, FL, USA

Teresa Cvengros Department of Family and Community Medicine, Mount Sinai Hospital, Chicago, IL, USA

Jennifer Dalrymple FSU Family Medicine Residency Program at Lee Health, Fort Myers, FL, USA

Daniel Deaton Forbes Family Medicine Residency, Allegheny Health Network, Pittsburgh, PA, USA

Niyomi DeSilva Florida State University College of Medicine Family Medicine Residency at BayCare Health System, Winter Haven, FL, USA

Sara DeSpain UNMC Family Medicine Residency Program, Omaha, NE, USA

Faith Dickerson College of Medicine, University of Arizona, Tucson, AZ, USA

Kristen Dimas Florida State University Family Medicine Residency Program at Lee Health, Fort Myers, FL, USA

Bonnie Dobbs The Medically At-Risk Driver Centre, Department of Family Medicine, Faculty of Medicine and Dentistry, University of Alberta, Edmonton, AB, Canada

Jason Domagalski Medical College of Wisconsin, Menomonee Falls, WI, USA

Philip T. Dooley Family Medicine Residency Program at Via Christi Hospitals, University of Kansas School of Medicine, Wichita, KS, USA

Erik Egeland Department of Family Medicine, Broadlawns Medical Center, Des Moines, IA, USA

W. Suzanne Eidson-Ton Department of Family and Community Medicine and OB/GYN, University of California, Davis, Sacramento, CA, USA

Nadine El Asmar Division of Clinical and Molecular Endocrinology, University Hospitals-Cleveland Medical Center, Case Western Reserve University School of Medicine, Cleveland, OH, USA

Steven Elek IV Navy Medical Center Portsmouth, Portsmouth, VA, USA

Steven Embry Department of Family Medicine, University of Nebraska Medical Center, Omaha, NE, USA

Hannah M. Emerson College of Medicine, University of Arizona, Tucson, AZ, USA

Emily Emmet AdventHealth Family Medicine Residency, Winter Park, FL, USA

Edward Emmett Center of Excellence in Environmental Toxicology, Perelman School of Medicine, Philadelphia, PA, USA

Susan Evans Department of Family Medicine, University of Nebraska College of Medicine, Omaha, NE, USA

Ashley Falk Florida State University College of Medicine Family Medicine Residency at BayCare Health System, Winter Haven, FL, USA

Nathan P. Falk Florida State University College of Medicine Family Medicine Residency at BayCare Health System, Winter Haven, FL, USA

Omofolarin B. Fasuyi Department of Family Medicine, Morehouse School of Medicine, Atlanta, GA, USA

Kelly Bossenbroek Fedoriw Department of Family Medicine, UNC – Chapel Hill, Chapel Hill, NC, USA

Charles Fleischer College of Medicine, Florida State University, Tallahassee, FL, USA

Angelique S. Forrester Family Medicine Residency Program, Eglin AFB, FL, USA

Louisa Foster The Center for Mindful Living, Omaha, NE, USA

Brian Frank Department of Family Medicine, Oregon Health and Science University, Portland, OR, USA

Daniel J. Frayne MAHEC Family Health Center at Biltmore, Mountain Area Health Education Center, Asheville, NC, USA

Nicholas Galioto Department of Family Medicine, Broadlawns Medical Center, Des Moines, IA, USA

D. Garcia 96th Medical Group, Eglin Air Force Base, FL, USA

Scott G. Garland Florida State University College of Medicine Family Medicine Residency at BayCare Health System, Winter Haven, FL, USA

Todd W. B. Gehr Division of Nephrology/Department of Internal Medicine, Virginia Commonwealth University Medical College of Virginia Campus, Richmond, VA, USA

Faraz Ghoddusi 9th Medical Group, Beale Air Force Base, Beale AFB, CA, USA

Lawrence Gibbs Methodist Health System Family Medicine Residency, Dallas, TX, USA

Alfred C. Gitu Florida State University College of Medicine Family Medicine Residency Program at Lee Health, Fort Myers, FL, USA

Sandra J. Gonzalez Department of Family and Community Medicine, Baylor College of Medicine, Houston, TX, USA

Mark Duane Goodman Department of Family Medicine, Creighton University, Omaha, NE, USA

Paul Gordon Family and Community Medicine, University of Arizona, College of Medicine, Tucson, AZ, USA

Jennifer L. Grana Family and Community Medicine, Penn State University College of Medicine, Hershey, PA, USA

Michael Greene Department of Family Medicine, Alegent Creighton Clinic John Galt, Omaha, NE, USA

Judith Green-McKenzie Division of Occupational Medicine, Department of Emergency Medicine, Perelman School of Medicine, University of Pennsylvania, Philadelphia, PA, USA

Craig Griebel Family Medicine Residency at Methodist Medical Center, Peoria, IL, USA

Marjorie Guthrie Department of Family and Community Medicine, St. Louis University, St. Louis, Belleville, IL, USA

Cecilia Gutierrez Department of Family Medicine and Public Health, UCSD School of Medicine, University of California, San Diego, San Diego, CA, USA

Michael D. Hagen Department of Family and Community Medicine, University of Kentucky College of Medicine, Lexington, KY, USA

Matthew Halfar Department of Family Medicine, Creighton University, Omaha, NE, USA

Suzanne Leonard Harrison Florida State University College of Medicine, Tallahassee, FL, USA

Esmat Hatamy Department of Family Medicine and Public Health, UCSD School of Medicine, University of California, San Diego, San Diego, CA, USA

William Hay Department of Family Medicine, University of Nebraska Medical Center, Omaha, NE, USA

Christopher R. Heron Family and Community Medicine, Penn State University College of Medicine, Hershey, PA, USA

Timothy Herrick Department of Family Medicine, Oregon Health and Science University, Portland, OR, USA

Jacqueline Hidalgo Florida State University Family Medicine Residency Program at Lee Health, Fort Myers, FL, USA

Keeley Hobart Department of Family and Community Medicine, TTUHSC School of Medicine, Lubbock, TX, USA

Sabrina Hofmeister Family and Community Medicine, Medical College of Wisconsin, Milwaukee, WI, USA

Jason J. Hofstede Family Medicine Residency Program, Eglin AFB, FL, USA

Shermeeka Hogans-Mathews College of Medicine, Florida State University, Tallahassee, FL, USA

Diane Holden Nellis Family Medicine Residency, Las Vegas, NV, USA

Hannah Hornsby Department of Family Medicine, University of Nebraska Medical Center, Omaha, NE, USA

Stephen Horras David Grant Family Medicine Residency Program, David Grant Medical Center, Travis AFB, CA, USA

Chad Hulsopple Department of Family Medicine, Uniformed Services University of the Health Sciences, Bethesda, MD, USA

Ryan Hunter Department of Family Medicine, University of Nebraska Medical Center, Omaha, NE, USA

Daniel Hunter-Smith Adventist La Grange Family Medicine Residency, Adventist La Grange Memorial Hospital, LaGrange, IL, USA

Mark K. Huntington Center for Family Medicine, Sioux Falls, SD, USA
Department of Family Medicine, University of South Dakota Sanford School of Medicine, Vermillion, SD, USA

Norman Hurst Family Medicine Residency, David Grant Medical Center, Travis AFB, CA, USA

Rose Anne Illes Florida State University Family Medicine Residency Program at Lee Health, Fort Myers, FL, USA

Douglas J. Inciarte West Kendall Baptist Health/Florida International University, Herbert Wertheim College of Medicine, Family Medicine Residency Program, Florida, SW, USA

Gretchen Irwin University of Kansas School of Medicine-Wichita, Wichita, KS, USA

Cristina S. Ivan Indiana University School of Medicine, Indianapolis, IN, USA

Ruba M. Jaber School of Medicine, University of Jordan, Amman, Jordan

Alexandrea Jacob Broadlawns Medical Center, Des Moines, IA, USA

Anusha Jagadish AdventHealth Family Medicine Residency, Winter Park, FL, USA

Samantha Jakuboski Stritch School of Medicine, Loyola University Health System, Maywood, IL, USA

M. Jawad Hashim Department of Family Medicine, United Arab Emirates University, Al-Ain, United Arab Emirates

Christopher Jensen Department of Family Medicine, University of Nebraska Medical Center, Omaha, NE, USA

Brian Jobe Department of Family Medicine, LSU Health Sciences Center Shreveport, Alexandria, LA, USA

Lisa M. Johnson Department of Family Medicine and Rural Health, Florida State University College of Medicine, Tallahassee, FL, USA

Brett C. Johnson Travis Family Medicine Residency Program, Travis Air Force Base, Fairfield, CA, USA

Anne Marie Kennedy UNMC Family Medicine Residency Program, Omaha, NE, USA

Aruna Khan Florida State University Fort Myers Family Medicine Residency Program at Lee Health, Fort Myers, FL, USA

Birgit Khandalavala Department of Family Medicine, University of Nebraska Medical Center, Omaha, NE, USA

J. Khandalavala Department of Obstetrics and Gynecology, Dignity Health, Omaha, NE, USA

Lainey Kieffer Department of Family Medicine and Community Health, University of Miami Miller School of Medicine, Miami, FL, USA

Gemma Kim Department of Family Medicine, Desert Regional Medical Center, Palm Springs, CA, USA

Tae K. Kim Department of Family Medicine, Desert Regional Medical Center, Palm Springs, CA, USA

Trista Kleppin Mount Sinai Hospital, Chicago, IL, USA

Jade Koide Resident Education, Kaiser Permanente, Portland, OR, USA

Niraj R. Kothari Division of Nephrology/Department of Internal Medicine, Virginia Commonwealth University Medical College of Virginia Campus, Richmond, VA, USA

Alicia Kowalchuk Department of Family and Community Medicine, Baylor College of Medicine, Houston, TX, USA

Jamie L. Krassow Family Medicine Residency Program, Eglin AFB, FL, USA

Department of Family Medicine, Uniformed Services University, Bethesda, MD, USA

Clarissa Kripke Office of Developmental Primary Care, Department of Family and Community Medicine, University of California, San Francisco, CA, USA

Archana M. Kudrimoti Department of Family and Community Medicine, University of Kentucky, KY Clinic, Lexington, KY, USA

Mindy J. Lacey College of Medicine, University of Nebraska, Omaha, NE, USA

Amy E. Lacroix Division of General Pediatrics, University of Nebraska Medical Center, Omaha, NE, USA

Deborah L. Lam Department of Ophthalmology, UW Medicine, University of Washington, Seattle, WA, USA

Francesco Leanza Department of Family and Community Medicine, Faculty of Medicine, University Health Network, University of Toronto, Toronto, ON, Canada

Daniel T. Lee Department of Family Medicine, David Geffen School of Medicine at UCLA Health System, Santa Monica, CA, USA

Jeff Leggit Department of Family Medicine, Uniformed Services University of the Health Sciences, Bethesda, MD, USA

KelliAnn Leli David Grant Family Medicine Residency Program, David Grant Medical Center, Travis AFB, CA, USA

Robert S. Levine Department of Family and Community Medicine, Baylor College of Medicine, Houston, TX, USA

Gerald Liu Atrius Health, Weymouth, MA, USA

Nicholas Longstreet David Grant Family Medicine Residency Program, David Grant Medical Center, Travis AFB, CA, USA

Mila Lopez HonorHealth Medical Group, Scottsdale, AZ, USA

Sarah Louie Community Physicians Group, UC Davis, University of California, Davis, CA, USA

Kanishk Makhija Neurology, Jefferson Hospital Group, Philadelphia, PA, USA

Sophia Malary Carter West Kendal Baptist Hospital FIU Family Medicine Residency Program, Miami, FL, USA

FIU-Herbert Wertheim College of Medicine, Miami, FL, USA

Baptist Health Group, Family Medicine Center, Miami, FL, USA

Rajat Malik AdventHealth Family Medicine Residency, Winter Park, FL, USA

Emma M. Mancini Pediatrics, AdventHealth, Orlando, FL, USA

Emily M. Manlove Indiana University School of Medicine, Bloomington, IN, USA

Andrea Maritato Department of Family Medicine and Community Health, Icahn School of Medicine at Mount Sinai, New York, NY, USA

Institute for Family Health, New York, NY, USA

Ryan Mark Department of Family Medicine, Uniformed Services University of the Health Sciences, Bethesda, MD, USA

Katharine Marshall Department of Internal Medicine, Providence Health and Systems, Portland, OR, USA

Peter Mitchell Martin Department of Family Medicine, University of Nebraska Medical Center, Omaha, NE, USA

Mylynda Beryl Massart Department of Family Medicine, University of Pittsburg, UPMC-Primary Care Precision Medicine, Pittsburgh, PA, USA

Douglas M. Maurer Office of the Surgeon General Defense Health Headquarters, Falls Church, VA, USA

Susan H. McDaniel Department of Family Medicine, University of Rochester School of Medicine, Rochester, NY, USA

Joan Younger Meek Department of Clinical Sciences, Florida State University College of Medicine, Orlando, FL, USA

Raj Mehta AdventHealth Family Medicine Residency, Winter Park, FL, USA

Maria C. Mejia Department of Family and Community Medicine, Baylor College of Medicine, Houston, TX, USA

Michael Dale Mendoza Department of Family Medicine, University of Rochester School of Medicine and Dentistry, Rochester, NY, USA

Monroe County Department of Public Health, Monroe County, NY, USA

Melanie Menning Department of Family Medicine, University of Nebraska Medical Center, Omaha, NE, USA

Anna Meola Eastern Connecticut Health Network Family Medicine Residency, Manchester, CT, USA

T. Jason Meredith Department of Family Medicine, University of Nebraska Medical Center, Omaha, NE, USA

Ashley Morrison Penn State College of Medicine, Hershey, PA, USA

Josiah Moulton Family Medicine Clinic, Hill AFB, UT, USA

Sahil Mullick Hospitalist, CHI Health Creighton University Medical Center – Bergan Mercy Campus, Omaha, NE, USA

Creighton University Department of Family Medicine Residency Program, Omaha, NE, USA

Herbert L. Muncie Department of Family Medicine, Louisiana State University School of Medicine, New Orleans, LA, USA

Rahmat Na'Allah Department of Family and Community Medicine, University of Illinois College of Medicine, Peoria, Family Medicine Residency Program, Peoria, IL, USA

Arwa Nasir Department of Pediatrics, University of Nebraska Medical Center, Omaha, NE, USA

Laeth S. Nasir Department of Family Medicine, Creighton University School of Medicine, Omaha, NE, USA

Seif L. Nasir University of Nebraska Medical Center, Omaha, NE, USA

Warren P. Newton Department of Family Medicine, University of North Carolina, Chapel Hill, NC, USA

American Board of Family Medicine, Lexington, KY, USA

Christine Q. Nguyen Department of Family Medicine, Mayo Clinic, Jacksonville, FL, USA

Benjamin Noble Department of Family Medicine, University of Nebraska Medical Center, Omaha, NE, USA

Bonnie G. Nolan Family Medicine Residency Program, Eglin AFB, FL, USA

David R. Norris Department of Family Medicine, University of Mississippi Medical Center, Jackson, MS, USA

Mary Pfost Norton Florida State University College of Medicine, Tallahassee, FL, USA

David T. O'Gurek Department of Family and Community Medicine, Lewis Katz School of Medicine at Temple University, Philadelphia, PA, USA

Linda Oge Department of Family Medicine, Louisiana State University School of Medicine, New Orleans, LA, USA

Folashade S. Omole Department of Family Medicine, Morehouse School of Medicine, Atlanta, GA, USA

Trevor Owens Florida State University College of Medicine Family Medicine Residency at BayCare Health System, Winter Haven, FL, USA

J. F. Pagel Rocky Mt. Sleep, Pueblo, CO, USA

University of Colorado School of Medicine – Pueblo Family Medicine Residency Program, Pueblo, CO, USA

Carolina S. Paredes-Molina Department of Family Medicine, Mayo Clinic, Jacksonville, FL, USA

Bumsoo Park Departments of Family Medicine and Urology, University of Michigan Medical School, Ann Arbor, MI, USA

Surbhi B. Patel College of Medicine, University of Arizona, Tucson, AZ, USA

Paul M. Paulman Department of Family Medicine, University of Nebraska Medical Center, Omaha, NE, USA

Allen Perkins Department of Family Medicine, University of South Alabama, Mobile, AL, USA

Dianna Pham Florida State University College of Medicine Family Medicine Residency at BayCare Health System, Winter Haven, FL, USA

Micah Pippin Family Medicine, LSUHS-Shreveport Family Medicine Residency, Alexandria, LA, USA

Monica L. Plesa Department of Family Medicine, David Geffen School of Medicine at UCLA Health System, Santa Monica, CA, USA

Sara M. Pope Kaiser Permanente Washington Family Medicine Residency, Seattle, WA, USA

Fiona R. Prabhu Department of Family and Community Medicine, TTUHSC School of Medicine, Lubbock, TX, USA

Emily Prazak Kaiser Permanente Washington Family Medicine Residency, Seattle, WA, USA

George G. A. Pujalte Department of Family Medicine, Mayo Clinic, Jacksonville, FL, USA

Natasha J. Pyzocha 98point6, Seattle, WA, USA

Nuha W. Qasem School of Medicine, Hashemite University, Zarqa, Jordan

Jeffrey D. Quinlan Department of Family Medicine, Uniformed Services University of the Health Sciences, Bethesda, MD, USA

Naureen B. Rafiq Department of Family Medicine, Creighton University, Omaha, NE, USA

Kenyon Railey Department of Family Medicine and Community Health, Duke University School of Medicine, Durham, NC, USA

Kalyanakrishnan Ramakrishnan Department of Family and Preventive Medicine, University of Oklahoma Health Sciences Center, Oklahoma, OK, USA

Daniel Ramon West Kendall Baptist Health/Florida International University, Herbert Wertheim College of Medicine, Family Medicine Residency Program, Florida, SW, USA

Carl Rasmussen Department of Family Medicine, St. Luke's Health System, Duluth, MN, USA

Stephen D. Ratcliffe Lancaster Health Center, Lancaster, PA, USA

Lauren Redlinger Department of Family and Community Medicine, St. Louis University, St. Louis, Belleville, IL, USA

Katherine Reeve Yale New Haven Health Northeast Medical Group, Uncasville, CT, USA

Jordan Rennicke Department of Family Medicine, University of Nebraska Medical Center, Omaha, NE, USA

Karl T. Rew Departments of Family Medicine and Urology, University of Michigan Medical School, Ann Arbor, MI, USA

Santos Reyes-Alonso West Kendal Baptist Hospital FIU Family Medicine Residency Program, Miami, FL, USA

Genevieve Riebe Family and Community Medicine, University of Arizona, College of Medicine, Tucson, AZ, USA

Ashley M. Rietz Department of Family Medicine, University of North Carolina at Chapel Hill School of Medicine, Chapel Hill, NC, USA

Janelle K. Riley Naval Branch Health Clinic, Fallon, NV, USA

Timothy D. Riley Penn State College of Medicine, Hershey, PA, USA

Michael Rivera-Rodríguez West Kendall Baptist Hospital, Miami, FL, USA

Stephanie E. Rosener United Family Medicine Residency Program, Allina Health, Saint Paul, MN, USA

George Rust Department of Behavioral Sciences and Social Medicine, Center for Medicine and Public Health, Florida State University College of Medicine, Tallahassee, FL, USA

Mark Ryan Department of Family Medicine and Population Health, Virginia Commonwealth University School of Medicine, Richmond, VA, USA

Samir Sabbag Department of Psychiatry, Natividad Medical Center, Salinas, CA, USA

Devdutta G. Sangvai Department of Family Medicine and Community Health, Duke University School of Medicine, Durham, NC, USA

Ram Sankaraneni Department of Neurology, Creighton University School of Medicine, Omaha, NE, USA

John W. Saultz Department of Family Medicine, Oregon Health and Science University, Portland, OR, USA

Shailendra Saxena Department of Neurology, Creighton University School of Medicine, Omaha, NE, USA

Peter Schindler Department of Family Medicine, University of Nebraska Medical Center, Omaha, NE, USA

E. Robert Schwartz Department of Family Medicine and Community Health, University of Miami Miller School of Medicine, Miami, FL, USA

Dean A. Seehusen Department of Family Medicine, Medical College of Georgia, Augusta University, Augusta, GA, USA

William Seigfreid Department of Family Medicine, University of Nebraska Medical Center, Omaha, NE, USA

Alap Shah Department of Family and Community Medicine, Adventist La Grange Memorial Hospital Family Medicine Residency, La Grange, IL, USA

Deepa Sharma Family Medicine, Baptist Health Medical Group, Miami, FL, USA

Nina Sharma Cardiac Critical Care/Transplant, University of Washington Medical Center, Seattle, WA, USA

University of Washington School of Pharmacy, Seattle, WA, USA

Sonya R. Shipley Department of Family Medicine, University of Mississippi Medical Center, Jackson, MS, USA

Amy Sikes Department of Family Medicine, Texas Tech University Health Sciences Center, Lubbock, TX, USA

Sanjay Singh Department of Neurology, Creighton University School of Medicine, Omaha, NE, USA

Amy Skiff Florida State University College of Medicine Family Medicine Residency Program at Lee Health, Fort Myers, FL, USA

Charles Kent Smith University Hospitals-Cleveland Medical Center, Case Western Reserve University School of Medicine, Cleveland, OH, USA

Craig W. Smith Department of Family and Community Medicine, St. Louis University, St. Louis, MO, USA

Jillian Soto Department of Family Medicine, Medical College of Georgia, Augusta University, Augusta, GA, USA

Tyler Spradling FSU Family Medicine Residency Program at Lee Health, Fort Myers, FL, USA

Dan Stein Department of Family Medicine, Oregon Health and Science University, Portland, OR, USA

Laurey Steinke Department of Biochemistry and Molecular Biology, University of Nebraska Medical Center, Omaha, NE, USA

Bianca Stewart AdventHealth Family Medicine Residency, Winter Park, FL, USA

Cyneetha Strong Department of Family Medicine and Rural Health, Florida State University College of Medicine, Tallahassee, FL, USA

Courtney Kimi Suh Department of Family Medicine, Loyola University Stritch School of Medicine, Maywood, IL, USA

Irvin Sulapas Department of Family and Community Medicine, Baylor College of Medicine, Houston, TX, USA

Robert B. Taylor Department of Family and Community Medicine, Eastern Virginia Medical School, Norfolk, VA, USA

Oregon Health Science University, Portland, OR, USA

Vincent Tichenor Family Medicine Clinic, Barksdale AFB, LA, USA

Diego R. Torres-Russotto Department of Neurology, Movement Disorders Division, University of Nebraska College of Medicine, Omaha, NE, USA

Marirose Trimmier Department of Family Medicine, University of South Alabama, Mobile, AL, USA

Jean Triscott Division of Care of the Elderly, Department of Family Medicine, Faculty of Medicine and Dentistry, University of Alberta, Edmonton, AB, Canada

Alexander Tu College of Medicine, University of Nebraska, Omaha, NE, USA

Greg Vanichkachorn Division of Preventive, Occupational, and Aerospace Medicine, Rochester, Minnesota, USA

Anthony J. Viera Department of Family Medicine and Community Health, Duke University School of Medicine, Durham, NC, USA

Chelsey Villanueva David Grant Family Medicine Residency Program, David Grant Medical Center, Fairfield, CA, USA

Nicki Vithalani Palliative Medicine, Geisinger Health System, Lewistown, PA, USA

Kirsten Vitrikas Family Medicine Residency, David Grant Medical Center, Travis AFB, CA, USA

Linda J. Vorvick Department of Family Medicine, UW Medicine, University of Washington, Seattle, WA, USA

Cezary Wójcik Oregon Health Sciences University, Portland, OR, USA

Kamal C. Wagle Indiana University School of Medicine, Indianapolis, IN, USA

Gwendolyn Warren David Grant Family Medicine Residency Program, David Grant Medical Center, Travis AFB, CA, USA

L. Michael Waters Department of Community Health and Family Medicine, University of Florida College of Medicine, Jacksonville, FL, USA

James Watson Department of Family Medicine, University of Nebraska Medical Center, Omaha, NE, USA

Kari Beth Watts Family Medicine Residency Program, University of Illinois College of Medicine, Peoria, Peoria, IL, USA

Erin Wendt David Grant Family Medicine Residency Program, David Grant Medical Center, Fairfield, CA, USA

Ryan West Nellis Family Medicine Residency, Nellis AFB, Las Vegas, NV, USA

Richard M. Whalen Department of Family Medicine, Eastern Virginia Medical School, Norfolk, VA, USA

Timothy D. Wilcox U.S. Naval Hospital Guam, Tutuhan, Guam

Ashley Wilk Florida State University College of Medicine Family Medicine Residency at BayCare Health System, Winter Haven, FL, USA

Thad Wilkins Department of Family Medicine, Medical College of Georgia, Augusta University, Augusta, GA, USA

James Hunter Winegarner San Antonio Military Medical Center, Fort Sam Houston, TX, USA

James Winger Department of Family Medicine, Loyola University Chicago Stritch School of Medicine, Maywood, IL, USA

Hailon Wong Florida State University Fort Myers Family Medicine Residency Program at Lee Health, Fort Myers, FL, USA

Amanda S. Wright Marian University College of Osteopathic Medicine, Indianapolis, IN, USA

Matthew Wright UNMC Family Medicine Residency Program, Omaha, NE, USA

Roger J. Zoorob Department of Family and Community Medicine, Baylor College of Medicine, Houston, TX, USA

Max Zubatsky Department of Family and Community Medicine, St. Louis University, St. Louis, MO, USA

Abbreviations

ACE	Angiotensin-converting enzyme
ACTH	Adrenocorticotropic hormone
AIDS	Acquired immunodeficiency syndrome
ALT	Alanine aminotransferase (SGPT)
ANA	Antinuclear antibody
AST	Aspartate aminotransferase (SGOT)
bid	Twice a day
BP	Blood pressure
bpm	Beats per minute
BS	Blood sugar
BUN	Blood urea nitrogen
CBC	Complete blood count
CHF	Congestive heart failure
Cl⁻	Chloride
CO_2	Carbon dioxide
COPD	Chronic obstructive pulmonary disease
CPR	Cardiopulmonary resuscitation
CSF	Cerebrospinal fluid
CT	Computed tomography
cu mm	Cubic millimeter
CXR	Chest X-ray
d	Day, daily
dL	Deciliter
DM	Diabetes mellitus
ECG	Electrocardiogram
ESR	Erythrocyte sedimentation rate
FDA	United States Food and Drug Administration
FM	Family medicine
FP	Family physician
g	Gram
GI	Gastrointestinal
Hb	Hemoglobin
Hg	Mercury
HIV	Human immunodeficiency virus
HMO	Health maintenance organization
hr	Hour

hs	Hour of sleep, at bedtime
HTN	Hypertension
IM	Intramuscular
INR	International normalized ratio
IU	International unit
IV	Intravenous
K^+	Potassium
kg	Kilogram
L	Liter
LD or LDH	Lactate dehydrogenase
mEq	Milliequivalent
μg	Microgram
mg	Milligram
min	Minute
mL	Milliliter
mm	Millimeter
mm^3	Cubic millimeter
MRI	Magnetic resonance imaging
Na^+	Sodium
NSAID	Nonsteroidal anti-inflammatory drug
po	By mouth (per os)
PT	Prothrombin time
PTT	Partial thromboplastin time
q	Every
qd	Every day, daily
qid	Four times a day
qod	Every other day
RBC	Red blood cell
SC	Subcutaneous
sec	Second
SGOT	See AST
SGPT	See ALT
STD	Sexually transmitted disease
TB	Tuberculosis
tid	Three times a day
TSH	Thyroid stimulating hormone
U	Unit
UA	Urine analysis
WBC	White blood cell, white blood count
WHO	World Health Organization

Part XV

The Eye

The Red Eye

73

Gemma Kim, Tae K. Kim, and Luanne Carlson

Contents

General Principles

Definition/Background

Red eye is one of the most common ocular conditions that presents in the primary care setting. Most cases are benign; however, some may cause permanent vision loss. Many conditions can be treated by primary care physicians. Therefore, it is important for the provider to be able to determine those cases that require urgent ophthalmic consultation. Most causes of red eye can be diagnosed by

G. Kim (✉) · T. K. Kim · L. Carlson
Department of Family Medicine, Desert Regional Medical Center, Palm Springs, CA, USA
e-mail: Luanne.Carlson@tenethealth.com

© Springer Nature Switzerland AG 2022
P. M. Paulman et al. (eds.), *Family Medicine*,
https://doi.org/10.1007/978-3-030-54441-6_76

taking a detailed patient history and careful eye examination. Obtaining certain elements in the history can aid in determining whether an ophthalmic consultation is required. Key elements in the history include pain, decreased vision, foreign body sensation, photophobia, trauma, use of contact lens, and discharge. The assessment of clinical signs should include the location of the redness (eyelids, conjunctiva, cornea, sclera and episclera, or intraocular), unilateral or bilateral involvement, associated symptoms (pain, itching, visual decrease or loss), and other ocular (mucopurulent discharge, watering, blepharospasm, lagophthalmus) or systemic (fever, nausea) findings [1]. Equally important is to perform a thorough ophthalmologic examination, including visual acuity, penlight examination, and fundus examination.

Almost half of the eye problems presenting in the primary care setting include conjunctivitis, keratoconjunctivitis sicca, and corneal abrasions [2]. Other less common causes include episcleritis, scleritis, iritis, herpes keratitis, trichiasis, and acute angle-closure glaucoma (see Table 1).

Conjunctivitis

Acute conjunctivitis affects approximately six million people annually and consists of approximately 1% of all primary care visits in the United States [3, 4]. It is estimated that 70% of all patients with acute conjunctivitis present to primary care and urgent care centers [5]. Conjunctivitis, commonly referred to as pinkeye, is the inflammation of the mucous membrane that lines the inside surface of the eyelids and the outer surface of the eye. The causes of acute conjunctivitis can be divided into infectious (e.g., bacterial, viral, chlamydial) or noninfectious (e.g., allergic, nonallergic/irritants). The most prominent signs consist of generalized conjunctival injection with gritty discomfort, mild photophobia, and variable amounts of discharge with no loss of visual acuity [1]. Generally, viral conjunctivitis and bacterial conjunctivitis are self-limiting conditions, and serious complications are rare. Since there is

no specific diagnostic test to differentiate viral from bacterial conjunctivitis, most cases are treated using broad-spectrum antibiotics [2].

Bacterial Conjunctivitis

Bacterial conjunctivitis is caused by a wide range of gram-positive and gram-negative organisms; however, gram-positive organisms are more common [6]. *Staphylococcus aureus* is more common in adults, while *Staphylococcus epidermidis*, *Streptococcus pneumoniae*, *Haemophilus influenzae*, and *Moraxella catarrhalis* are more common in children. The incidence of *Haemophilus influenzae* has decreased as more children are immunized. Gram-negative organisms include *Escherichia coli* and *Pseudomonas* species. Hyperacute bacterial conjunctivitis is usually caused by *Neisseria gonorrhoeae* and is considered a sight-threatening infection that requires immediate ophthalmologic evaluation with hospitalization for systemic and topical therapy. It is usually transmitted from the genitalia to the hands and then to the eyes. It is characterized by a profuse purulent discharge present within 12 h of infection [7]. Additional symptoms include redness, lid swelling, and tender preauricular adenopathy. Gram staining of the purulent discharge reveals gram-negative diplococci.

History
Acute bacterial conjunctivitis initially presents with tearing and irritation in one eye but usually spreads to the opposite eye within 2–5 days. It is highly contagious and causes a rapid onset of generalized conjunctival redness, purulent discharge (yellow, white, or green), gritty discomfort, swelling of the eyelid, early morning crusting of the eyelids, and usually no loss of vision. However, one should suspect a gonococcal infection if the patient presents with profuse amounts of purulent discharge associated with a rapid progression of redness, irritation, and pain. *Neisseria gonorrhoeae* confirmed in a child should raise concern for sexual abuse. For *Neisseria meningitides*, one should consider meningitis.

Table 1 Differential diagnosis of the red eye

	Etiology	Eye pain	Discharge	Visual acuity	Pupillary changes	Corneal involvement	Intraocular pressure	Immediate referral
Bacterial conjunctivitis	Gram + and gram - organisms	Pain with gritty sensation	Mild to moderate purulent discharge	Unchanged	None	Possible	Normal	No
Viral conjunctivitis	Adenovirus (most common)	Pain with gritty sensation	Watery	Unchanged	None	None	Normal	No
Chlamydial conjunctivitis	*Chlamydia trachomatis*	Irritated	Watery to mucopurulent	Unchanged	None	Corneal scarring with trachoma	Normal	No, unless trachoma is suspected
Allergic conjunctivitis	Environmental allergens	Gritty sensation	Watery	Unchanged	None	None	Normal	No
Keratoconjunctivitis sicca	Tear evaporation or deficiency	Irritated, gritty sensation	Watery	Fluctuating or blurry	None	Corneal ulcers and scarring in severe cases	Normal	No
Corneal abrasion/foreign body	Trauma, chemical exposure, foreign body	Moderate to severe	Watery	Usually unchanged	None	Can cause corneal erosions, ulceration and scarring	Normal	Yes, most foreign bodies or globe involvement
Episcleritis	Idiopathic, possible association with systemic disease	Mild	Watery	Unchanged	None	None	Normal	No
Scleritis	Associated with systemic disease	Severe, constant piercing pain	Watery	Unchanged	None	None	Normal	Yes
Iritis	Infection or immune-mediated disease	Gradual onset of aching pain	Minimal and watery	Blurred	Constricted and sluggishly reactive to light	Normal	Normal	Yes

(continued)

Table 1 (continued)

	Etiology	Eye pain	Discharge	Visual acuity	Pupillary changes	Corneal involvement	Intraocular pressure	Immediate referral
Herpes keratitis	Predominantly HSV-1	Pain with foreign body sensation	Watery	Blurred	None	Recurrent infections cause reduced corneal sensation	Normal	Yes
Trichiasis	Abnormal positioning of the eyelids	Irritation	Watery	Untreated can cause vision loss	None	Can cause corneal scarring	Normal	Yes
Acute glaucoma	Narrowing of the ant. chamber	Severe throbbing	Watery	Decreased	Partially dilated, nonreactive	Swelling	Elevated	Yes

Physical Examination

For acute bacterial conjunctivitis, visual acuity is preserved with normal pupillary reaction and absence of corneal involvement. Additional findings include conjunctival injection and swelling of the eyelid, with mild to moderate purulent discharge. Patients will often describe that their eyelids are stuck together upon wakening due to the mucopurulent discharge. For hyperacute bacterial conjunctivitis, there is chemosis (swelling of the conjunctiva) with possible corneal involvement, pseudomembrane formation, and preauricular lymphadenopathy. Patients will complain of severe pain with copious amounts of purulent discharge and diminished vision.

Laboratory Findings

In most cases of bacterial conjunctivitis, the diagnosis and the identification of the presumed organism are based on history and clinical presentation. Further studies to identify the organism and determine its sensitivity to antibiotics are reserved for more severe cases or those that are unresponsive to initial treatment [8]. If a gonococcal infection is suspected, gram staining will reveal gram-negative diplococci.

Treatment

Most cases of bacterial conjunctivitis if uncomplicated are self-limited regardless of antibiotic therapy [9]. However, antibiotics are indicated for conjunctivitis caused by gonorrhea or chlamydia and in those patients that wear contact lenses [10]. It has also been shown that antibiotics cause earlier reduction of symptoms and therefore can be prescribed. Initial preferred treatment options include erythromycin ophthalmic ointment or trimethoprim-polymyxin B drops (see Table 2). For children or for those whom it is difficult to administer eye medications, ointment is preferred as it still maintains a therapeutic effect although none may have been directly applied to the conjunctiva. Because ointment can blur the vision and cause the eyes to feel sticky, drops are recommended for adults who require clear vision for driving or work. Sulfacetamide ophthalmic drops are not considered first line due to potential allergic reactions. Fluoroquinolones are effective and well tolerated but are usually reserved for more severe infections or contact lens wearers. For those who wear contact lenses, contact lens use should be discontinued, lens case discarded, and lenses disinfected or replaced. Once antibiotics have been completed and the eye has cleared and remains free of discharge for 24 h, contact lens wear may be resumed. Bacterial conjunctivitis that is chronic, resistant to initial antibiotic treatment, or caused by gonorrhea or chlamydia requires immediate referral to an ophthalmologist.

Viral Conjunctivitis

Viral conjunctivitis is a common, self-limiting condition that is most commonly caused by adenovirus, which consists of 65–90% of viral conjunctivitis cases [11]. Other viruses which are less likely to spread include herpes simplex virus, varicella zoster virus, picornavirus (enterovirus 70, Coxsackie A24), poxvirus (molluscum contagiosum, vaccinia), and human immunodeficiency virus (HIV). Adenoviruses 8, 19, and 37 are associated with epidemic keratoconjunctivitis, which is highly contagious, while adenoviruses 3 and 7 cause pharyngoconjunctival fever which is characterized by high fevers, sore throat, and preauricular lymphadenopathy [9]. Enterovirus 70 and Coxsackie A24 cause acute hemorrhagic conjunctivitis, which is characterized by the rapid onset of painful conjunctivitis and subconjunctival hemorrhage. Although benign and resolving within 5–7 days, it can cause a polio-like paralysis developing in approximately one in 10,000 patients infected with enterovirus 70 [12]. Conjunctivitis caused by herpes simplex virus is usually unilateral with watery discharge and ipsilateral vesicular facial rash [9]. Herpes zoster virus, commonly known as shingles, can involve the eye when the first and second branches of the trigeminal nerve are involved. Ocular involvement most commonly affects the eyelids (45.8%) followed by the conjunctiva (41.1%) [13]. Herpes zoster ophthalmicus represents approximately 10–25% of all cases of herpes zoster [14].

Table 2 Acute bacterial conjunctivitis treatment options

Medication	Dosage form	Adult dosage	Pediatric dosage	Comments
Erythromycin (Ilotycin)	0.5% ointment	Apply 1 cm ribbon up to 6×/ day × 7–10 days	Apply 1 cm ribbon up to 6×/ day × 7–10 days	Ointment recommended for children
Trimethoprim-polymyxin B (Polytrim)	10,000 units/ 1 mg/ml sol	One drop every 3 h × 7–10 days	>2 months: 1 drop every 3 h × 7–10 days	Drops better for adults
Bacitracin-polymyxin B (AK-Poly-Bac, Polycin)	500 units/ 10,000 units/ g ointment	Apply 0.25–0.5 in. ribbon every 3–4 h × 7–10 days	Apply 0.25–0.5 in. ribbon every 3–4 h × 7–10 days	Ointment recommended for children
Sulfacetamide (Bleph-10)	10% ointment 10% solution	0.5 in. ribbon every 3–4 h and qhs × 7–10 days one to two drops every 2–3 h × 7–10 days	>2 months: 0.5 in. ribbon every 3–4 h and qhs × 7–10 days one to two drops every 2–3 h × 7–10 days	Not first line due to potential sulfa allergy
Gentamycin (Garamycin)	0.3% ointment 0.3% solution	0.5 in. ribbon bid-tid one to two drops every 4 h	>1 month: 0.5 in. ribbon bid-tid one to two drops every 4 h	May cause ocular burning
Tobramycin (Tobrex)	0.3% solution	One to two drops every 4 h	>2 months: one to two drops every 4 h	May cause ocular burning
Azithromycin (AzaSite)	1% solution	One drop bid × 2 days, then qd × 5 days	>1 year: one drop bid × 2 days, then qd × 5 days	May cause ocular burning
Ciprofloxacin (Cifloxan)	0.3% solution	One to two drops every 2 h while awake and then every 4 h while awake × 5 days	>1 year: one to two drops every 2 h while awake and then every 4 h while awake × 5 days	Reserved for severe infections or contact lens wearers
Levofloxacin (Iquix, Quixin)	0.5% solution	One to two drops every 2 h while awake and then every 4 h while awake × 5 days	>1 year: one to two drops every 2 h while awake and then every 4 h while awake × 5 days	Reserved for severe infections or contact lens wearers
Ofloxacin (Ocuflox)	0.3% solution	One to two drops every 2–4 h × 2 days and then one to two drops qid × 5 days	>1 year: one to two drops every 2–4 h × 2 days and then 1–2 drops qid × 5 days	Reserved for severe infections or contact lens wearers
Gatifloxacin (Zymar, Zymaxid)	0.5% solution	One drop every 2 h up to 8×/day × 1 day and then one drop bid-qid × 6 days	>1 year: one drop every 2 h up to 8×/day × 1 day and then 1 drop bid-qid × 6 days	Reserved for severe infections or contact lens wearers
Moxifloxacin (Vigamox, Moxeza)	0.5% solution	One drop tid × 7 days	>1 year: one drop tid × 7 days	Reserved for severe infections or contact lens wearers

History

The patient with acute viral conjunctivitis initially presents with a unilateral red eye with watery discharge and itching. Many times, the other eye becomes affected a few days later. Typically, there is absence of visual involvement or photophobia. Symptoms are typically mild with spontaneous remission in 1–2 weeks [1]. Pain, photophobia, and subconjunctival hemorrhages may be associated with keratoconjunctivitis or acute hemorrhagic conjunctivitis. Commonly, cases of acute viral conjunctivitis occur during or after an upper respiratory infection or with exposure to a person with an upper respiratory infection as it is highly contagious and spreads through direct contact via contaminated fingers, medical instruments, swimming pool water, or other personal items [2].

Physical Examination

For acute viral conjunctivitis, visual acuity is unaffected with normal pupillary reaction and absence of corneal involvement. Additional findings include follicular injection/erythema and swelling of the eyelid, with watery clear discharge. Keratoconjunctivitis is associated with preauricular lymphadenopathy and possible corneal infiltrates. Pharyngoconjunctivitis can be associated with subconjunctival hemorrhage. Herpes simplex virus causes a unilateral follicular conjunctivitis with an ipsilateral vesicular rash [9]. When involving the eye, herpes zoster can cause vesicular lesions in the distribution of the ophthalmic division of the trigeminal nerve with possible blepharitis, keratitis, uveitis, ophthalmoplegia, or optic neuritis [1]. Molluscum contagiosum usually presents as a unilateral follicular conjunctivitis with umbilicated lesions at the eyelid margin.

Laboratory Findings

Generally, viral conjunctivitis is diagnosed on clinical features alone. Laboratory testing is typically not necessary unless symptoms are severe, chronic, or recurrent infections or in patients who fail to respond with treatment. There are rapid immunochromatographic tests available to diagnose adenoviral infections in the office. In addition, Giemsa staining of conjunctival scrapings can aid in characterizing an inflammatory response. Fluorescein staining may reveal dendrites on the cornea for herpes simplex infections.

Treatment

As most cases of viral conjunctivitis are self-limiting and there is no effective treatment available, treatment is mostly supportive and can include cold compresses, saline rinse, ocular antihistamines, and artificial tears. These agents treat only the symptoms and not the disease itself. Antiviral medications and topical antibiotics are not indicated. Use of antibiotic eye drops can increase the risk of spreading the infection to the other eye due to contaminated droppers [11]. Treatment for ocular herpetic infections usually consists of a combination of oral antivirals and topical steroids and warrants immediate ophthalmology referral to monitor for sight-threatening corneal involvement. Molluscum treatment options include excision or cryotherapy of the lesions. Patients with molluscum do not need to be isolated from others while symptomatic [9]. If symptoms do not resolve after 7–10 days or if corneal involvement is suspected, referral to ophthalmologist is indicated.

Family and Community Issues

Patients should be counseled that since viral conjunctivitis although self-limiting is highly contagious, it is important to prevent spread by practicing strict handwashing and avoid sharing personal items with those infected. In cases of adenoviral conjunctivitis, the replicating virus is present 10 days after the appearance of symptoms in 95% of the patients but only in 5% by day 16 [8]. Due to the high risk of spread, children should be refrained from attending daycare and school for up to 1 week [9].

Chlamydial Conjunctivitis

Chlamydial conjunctivitis is a bacterial infection of the eye caused by *Chlamydia trachomatis*.. Chlamydial conjunctivitis can be divided into two types: trachoma and inclusion conjunctivitis. *Chlamydia trachomatis* serotypes A through C cause trachoma and are characterized by a severe follicular reaction which can develop into scarring of the eyelid, conjunctiva, and cornea leading to vision loss. It is the leading infectious cause of blindness worldwide [15]. It is endemic in developing countries with limited resources and is seen only sporadically in the United States. Chlamydial serotypes D through K cause inclusion conjunctivitis, which causes a unilateral chronic follicular conjunctivitis that usually occurs in young adults or neonates (ophthalmia neonatorum) via the birth canal from infected mothers. Chlamydial inclusion conjunctivitis is sexually transmitted from the hand to eye or from the genitalia to eye.

History

Chlamydial conjunctivitis should be suspected in sexually active patients with chronic follicular conjunctivitis that is not responsive to standard antibacterial treatment [16]. There is usually an absence of symptoms from the genital tract; however, males may have symptomatic urethritis and females may have salpingitis or chronic vaginal discharge. Ophthalmia neonatorum, also called neonatal conjunctivitis, usually occurs in the first 4 weeks of life. The incubation period is typically 7 days after delivery but can vary from 5 to 14 days if there was a premature rupture of membranes [17]. Among those neonates with known exposure to chlamydia, 30–50% will develop conjunctivitis [18].

Physical Examination

The patient usually presents with a red, mildly irritated eye with scant watery discharge to severe mucopurulent discharge with eyelid and conjunctival swelling [18]. A palpable preauricular lymph node may be present on the affected side. Vision is usually not affected, and there is usually no history of recent upper respiratory infection. Trachoma causes chronic follicular conjunctivitis that leads to entropion, trichiasis, conjunctival, and corneal scarring causing permanent vision loss.

Laboratory Findings

Diagnosis is usually made based on history and clinical presentation. However, conjunctival scrapings revealing elementary bodies via direct fluorescent antibody stain or polymerase chain reaction testing on scrapings are diagnostic. Culture of conjunctival scrapings can be performed but may take weeks to grow.

Treatment

For newborns, topical therapy is not indicated as more than 50% of affected neonates have concurrent lung, nasopharynx, and genital tract infections [10]. Recommended treatment is a systemic course of erythromycin ethylsuccinate (EryPed) 50 mg/kg/day in four divided doses per day for 14 days [19]. In order to treat inclusion conjunctivitis in adults, a systemic course of oral tetracycline (Sumycin) 250 mg four times per day for 3 weeks, erythromycin stearate (Erythrocin) 250 mg four times per day for 3 weeks, doxycycline 100 mg twice per day for 10 days, or azithromycin 1 g single dose is administered to treat the infection. Topical antibiotics may suppress the ocular symptoms but do not treat the genital disease. Pregnant patients should be treated with erythromycin since tetracyclines can cross the placenta. Sexual partners should also be treated to prevent reinfection and possible coinfection with gonorrhea should be tested.

Allergic Conjunctivitis

Allergic conjunctivitis is a type 1, IgE-mediated hypersensitivity to allergens such as pollen, animal dander, and other environmental allergens [8] and affects up to 40% of the population in the United States [20]. Seasonal allergic conjunctivitis is the most common form consisting of 90% of all allergic conjunctivitis in the United States, usually worse in the spring and summer [21]. It is often encountered in patients with atopic diseases, such as allergic rhinitis (hay fever), eczema, and asthma [22]. Perennial allergic conjunctivitis is similar to seasonal allergic conjunctivitis but occurs throughout the year, and the symptoms tend to be less severe. Other types of ocular allergies include vernal keratoconjunctivitis, atopic keratoconjunctivitis, contact allergy (contact dermatitis), and giant papillary conjunctivitis [23].

History

The hallmark for allergic conjunctivitis is itching along with watery eyes, redness, gritty discomfort, eyelid swelling, and nasal congestion. Vernal keratoconjunctivitis is more common in warmer climates and affects young patients and resolves by age 20. Atopic keratoconjunctivitis is the ocular version of atopic eczema or dermatitis. Contact ocular allergy is caused by contact with an allergen. Giant papillary conjunctivitis is commonly associated with contact lens use or ocular implants.

Physical Examination

Allergic conjunctivitis commonly presents with bilateral dilatation of the conjunctival blood vessels, large cobblestone papillae under the upper lid, conjunctival swelling (chemosis), and watery to mucoid discharge [1]. Redness or conjunctival injection is mild to moderate. Visual acuity is unaffected with normal pupillary reaction and absence of corneal involvement. Vernal keratoconjunctivitis is characterized by the giant papillae found under the upper eyelid. In atopic keratoconjunctivitis, the eyelid skin may have a fine sandpaper-like texture with mild to severe conjunctival injection and chemosis [23]. Giant papillary conjunctivitis may cause giant, medium, or small papillae under the upper lid similar to vernal conjunctivitis [23].

Laboratory Findings

Allergic conjunctivitis is diagnosed based primarily on history and clinical presentation. Giemsa staining of conjunctival scrapings can help characterize the inflammatory response and may reveal eosinophils. Allergy testing via direct skin testing or radioallergosorbent test (RAST) is indicated mostly for patients with systemic allergy or may be indicated for some with ocular allergy.

Treatment

Patients with allergic conjunctivitis should be advised to refrain from rubbing their eyes as this causes mast cell degranulation and worsening of their symptoms. Cool compresses may reduce eyelid swelling, and use of artificial tears throughout the day may help to clear out potential allergens. Patients should also refrain from wearing contact lenses as allergens have the ability to adhere to the contact lens surface. In addition, avoidance of known allergens may reduce exacerbations. Medical therapies that are topical include antihistamine/vasoconstrictor combination products, antihistamines with mast cell stabilizers, and glucocorticoids, which are reserved for resistant cases and should be used under the supervision of an ophthalmologist. Systemic oral antihistamines, such as loratadine (Claritin), fexofenadine (Allegra), and cetirizine (Zyrtec), are often used for the management of allergies in general; however, topical ocular medications are found to be more effective when ocular symptoms primarily predominate.

Keratoconjunctivitis Sicca

Keratoconjunctivitis sicca or dry eye is a condition caused by decreased tear production or poor tear quality causing inadequate moisture to the eye surface. More common in adults over age 50 (women greater than men) and may be associated with underlying autoimmune disease such as rheumatoid arthritis, Sjogren's syndrome and lupus, as well as use of certain medications such as anticholinergics, antihistamines, beta-blockers and hormone replacement therapy (especially estrogen-only pills). Chronic untreated symptoms can result in corneal ulcers and permanent scarring [1, 24].

History

Common complaints of keratoconjunctivitis sicca are soreness, burning, redness, gritty discomfort, and photophobia. Sometimes excessive tearing presents (secondary to reflex secretion), and other times unable to produce tears upon crying. Dry eyes can follow trachoma, in which the lacrimal gland ducts and conjunctival goblet cells are damaged.

Physical Examination

Keratoconjunctivitis sicca often presents with mild to moderate redness or conjunctival injection with or without watery discharge. Blurred vision or partial loss may be present. Poor tear film and corneal desiccation lead to punctate lesions that are evident with fluorescein staining and blue light examination.

Laboratory Findings

Keratoconjunctivitis sicca is diagnosed based primarily on history and clinical presentation. However, use of one or more tests may be utilized to further objectify the diagnosis including the Schirmer test, tear breakup time measurement, and tear meniscometry [2, 25]. If autoimmune disease is suspected as the underlying cause of keratoconjunctivitis sicca, serum antibody testing can be performed (e.g., rheumatoid factor [RF], antinuclear antibody [ANA], antinuclear cytoplasmic antibodies [ANCA], cyclic citrullinated peptides [anti-CCP], anti-Ro [SS-A], and anti-La [SS-B] antibodies) [24].

Treatment

Treatment is initially managed by frequent and liberal application of artificial tears such as hypromellose eye drops and ocular lubricants several times daily and at bedtime. Use of a humidifier can help to decrease tear loss in dry environments. If incomplete relief, cyclosporine eye drops (0.05%, one drop in each eye every 12 h) or lifitegrast ophthalmic solution (5%, one drop in each eye every 12 h) may be used to increase tear production in adults and adolescents greater than 16 years of age [1, 26]. Severe cases not responsive to topical therapies require referral for consideration of temporary (using plugs) or permanent (using cautery) occlusion of lacrimal canaliculi [27, 28].

Other Causes of Red Eyes

Corneal Abrasion/Corneal Foreign Body

Corneal abrasions and foreign bodies interrupt the epithelial layer of the cornea resulting in the exposure of the basement membrane. Usually due to mechanical or chemical trauma, corneal or epithelial disease (e.g., dry eye), contact lens use, or foreign body superficially adherent or embedded within the cornea. Corneal foreign bodies need to be identified and removed as soon as possible to prevent infection and ocular necrosis [2, 29]. Corneal abrasion can be a complication of trachoma secondary to constant corneal trauma of affected lashes and inadequate tears. This is the leading cause of blindness in trachoma as it often progresses to corneal erosions, ulceration, and scarring [15].

History

Patients present with usually unilateral acute onset marked tearing, redness, blepharospasm, moderate to severe pain, foreign body sensation, photophobia, and possible decreased visual acuity dependent on location of the defect along the cornea. Symptoms can be present without known trauma other than aggressive eye rubbing. Bilateral symptoms may be present when associated with chemical exposure, burns, or contact lens use. Suspicion for foreign body should be high if patient engaged in landscape, construction, or manufacturing job without the use of eye protection.

Physical Examination

Corneal disruption can be confirmed by fluorescein examination under blue light and preferably utilizing a slit lamp. Instillation of topical anesthetic (e.g., proparacaine or tetracaine) may be needed for pain control during exam. A check for foreign bodies should include under the eyelids and in the conjunctival fornices [29]. A Seidel's test should be performed if there is concern for corneal laceration or globe rupture that may not be grossly obvious. A Seidel's test is performed by placing fluorescein dye gently against the bulbar conjunctiva. In the case of a positive sign, the oozing aqueous humor at the site of penetration through the cornea appears under ultraviolet light as a "dark waterfall," clearing away excess fluorescein on the cornea. It should be noted that an in intraocular foreign body does not necessarily change visual acuity [30].

Laboratory Findings

There are no specific laboratory tests for the diagnosis of corneal abrasion or foreign body. They are primarily based on clinical history and physical examination.

Treatment

Corneal foreign bodies require immediate removal or urgent transfer to ophthalmology. If removal performed in office, documentation of a negative Seidel's test is good practice to confirm that there was no iatrogenic penetration of the cornea during the procedure. Treatment of corneal abrasions consists of prophylactic antibiotic eye drops and/or ointment (ciprofloxacin 0.3% solution, ofloxacin 0.3% solution, erythromycin 0.5% ointment, gentamycin 0.3% ointment or solution; see Table 2) and topical pain control drops (diclofenac, 0.1% solution, one drop four times daily or ketorolac, 0.5% solution, one drop four times daily). Oral opioid analgesics (e.g., hydrocodone/acetaminophen [Vicodin], oxycodone/acetaminophen [Percocet]) can be used to relieve moderate to severe pain and have been found to allow patients to sleep more comfortably at night. All contact lens wearers, and those whose symptoms do not improve within 24 h, require immediate referral to an ophthalmology specialist [29, 30].

Episcleritis

Episcleritis is a benign inflammatory disease that affects the episclera, which is the thin layer of tissue that is beneath the conjunctiva but is superficial to the sclera. It is usually self-limiting and resolves within 3 weeks. Most cases occur mostly in young to middle-aged females but can affect any age group. The etiology is mainly idiopathic with a minority of cases associated with an underlying systemic disease, such as rheumatoid arthritis, inflammatory bowel disease, vasculitis, and systemic lupus erythematosus [31]. Episcleritis is classified into two types. In the diffuse type, the redness involves the whole episclera, whereas, in the nodular type, the redness involves a smaller contained area.

History

Patients usually present with an abrupt onset of mild eye pain, redness, watery eyes, and mild photophobia. The pain associated with episcleritis is typically mild when compared to the pain experienced with scleritis. The diffuse type of episcleritis may be less painful than the nodular type. Eye involvement may be either localized or diffuse. There is no associated discharge and vision is not affected.

Physical Examination

There is unilateral or bilateral localized or diffuse redness of the episclera. There may be mild pain with palpation. Vision is not affected and there is no edema or thinning of the sclera. A slit-lamp biomicroscope can help visualize any changes in the sclera to differentiate between episcleritis which is benign and scleritis which causes more destructive inflammation. In addition, phenylephrine eye drops can cause transient clearing of the episcleral redness so that a more careful examination of the sclera can be made.

Laboratory Findings

There are no specific laboratory tests for the diagnosis unless a systemic disease is suspected as the cause of the episcleritis. In this case, blood tests, such as rheumatoid factor, antibodies to cyclic citrullinated peptides (anti-CCP), antineutrophil cytoplasmic antibodies (ANCA), and antinuclear antibody testing (ANA), can be drawn targeted to specific inflammatory diseases.

Treatment

Since episcleritis is self-limiting and does not cause vision loss, the treatment is based on symptom relief. Treatment options include topical lubricants/artificial tears and topical glucocorticoids for severe cases [2]. Topical nonsteroidal anti-inflammatory drugs (NSAIDs) are not indicated and have been shown to have no significant benefit versus placebo [32]. Referral to ophthalmology is recommended to definitively confirm episcleritis versus scleritis and for recurrent or worsening of symptoms.

Scleritis

Scleritis is a painful and destructive inflammatory disease that affects the sclera, which comprises 90% of the outer coat of the eye. It is associated with an underlying systemic disorder, such as rheumatoid arthritis, Wegener's granulomatosis, and systemic lupus erythematosus, in up to 50% of patients [33]. The sclera is divided into an anterior and posterior compartment. Inflammation can occur in either compartment but rarely does it affect both. Approximately 90% of scleritis involves the anterior compartment which can be further subdivided into diffuse, nodular, and necrotizing. Diffuse anterior scleritis is the most common, least severe, and usually does not recur. Nodular anterior scleritis is the second most common and tends to be recurrent. Necrotizing anterior scleritis is the least common, most severe, and more likely to cause ocular complications. Posterior scleritis can also be subdivided into diffuse, nodular, and necrotizing but is more rare and difficult to assess clinically.

History

Patients present with a gradual onset of severe, constant, piercing pain that involves the eye and radiates to the face and periorbital region. Tenderness and redness may affect the entire eye or a more localized area. Because the extraocular muscles insert into the sclera, movement of the eye tends to exacerbate the pain. The pain is usually worse at night or in the early morning hours, causing awakening from sleep. Patients also experience headache, watery eyes, and photophobia.

Physical Examination

Examination reveals a characteristic violet-bluish hue of the globe with scleral edema and vasodilatation of the episcleral plexus and superficial vessels. The globe is usually tender to the touch. Using slit-lamp biomicroscopy, one can visualize inflamed scleral vessels which are adherent to the sclera and cannot be moved with a cotton-tipped applicator, whereas the more superficial vessels of the episclera are movable. Although phenylephrine eye drops cause blanching of the superficial episcleral vessels, the deep vessels are not affected which can aid in the differentiation between scleritis and episcleritis.

Laboratory Findings

Like episcleritis, there are no specific laboratory tests for the diagnosis of scleritis. If history and physical examination indicate a systemic inflammatory condition, specialized serologic tests can be drawn. There are some imaging studies that are useful in the evaluation of scleritis, such as ultrasonography of the orbit which can confirm scleral thickening and CT and magnetic resonance imaging of the orbit which can visualize orbital lesions associated with systemic disease processes.

Treatment

If suspected, immediate referral to ophthalmology is warranted. Two-thirds of patients with scleritis require high-dose corticosteroids or the combination of corticosteroids with an immunosuppressive agent [31]. If an underlying systemic disease is suspected or known, referral to rheumatology may be indicated.

Iritis

Iritis is the inflammation of the anterior uveal tract, also referred to as anterior uveitis. It can be caused by infection such as from a wound or corneal ulcer, or it can be caused by a systemic immune-mediated disease. Spondyloarthritides, such as ankylosing spondylitis and reactive arthritis (Reiter syndrome), are the most common systemic immune diseases associated with anterior uveitis. Uveitis can occur in up to 37% of spondyloarthropathy patients, of which most are positive for the human leukocyte antigen (HLA)-B27 allele [34, 35]. Ten to 30% of patients with juvenile idiopathic arthritis develop chronic anterior uveitis, and it remains a cause of blindness in childhood [36]. Other associated systemic diseases include sarcoidosis, inflammatory bowel disease, and Behçet's disease.

History

Patients present with a gradual onset of pain (often described as an ache) developing over hours to days with the exception of trauma. Ocular erythema and excessive tearing are commonly present. In addition, photophobia with blurred vision is commonly noted. Iritis can be unilateral, bilateral, or recurrent affecting either eye, dependent on the etiology or associated disease process.

Physical Examination

The eyelids, lashes, and lacrimal ducts are not involved. Conjunctival examination reveals hyperemic injection surrounding the cornea. If discharge is present, it is minimal and watery. The pupil is constricted in the affected eye and is sluggishly reactive to light. Visual acuity may be decreased in the affected eye, but extraocular movement is not affected. Both direct and consensual photophobia may be present. With slit-lamp biomicroscopy examination, keratic precipitates (white blood cells) can be visualized in the anterior chamber which is a hallmark of iritis. With severe inflammation, the leukocytes in the anterior chamber can settle and form a hypopyon, which is an accumulation of purulent material that can be visualized without magnification.

Laboratory Findings

Iritis (anterior uveitis) is diagnosed based primarily on history and clinical presentation. Slit-lamp biomicroscopy is required to properly assess the presence of leukocytes or protein accumulation in the aqueous humor within the anterior chamber of the eye. If a systemic immune-mediated disease is suspected from the patient's history and examination, diagnostic testing to confirm the specific diagnosis is warranted.

Treatment

If iritis is suspected, immediate referral to ophthalmology is warranted. Although leukocytes may be present on examination, antibiotics are not indicated. Iritis is a diagnosis of exclusion and can be associated with serious complications, such as band keratopathy, posterior synechiae, intraocular hypertension, glaucoma, cataract formation, and increased risk of herpes keratitis. If an underlying systemic disease is suspected or known, referral to rheumatology may be indicated.

Herpes Keratitis

Herpes keratitis is caused by a recurrent herpes simplex virus (IISV) infection in the cornea. It is very common in humans as both subtypes, HSV-1 and HSV-2, have humans as their only natural host. HSV-1 accounts for most oral, labial, and ocular infections and HSV-2 accounts for most genital infections. However, there is quite a bit of overlap of their distributions. HSV-1 causes over 95% of ocular HSV infections, excluding neonatal infections [37]. HSV infection is the leading cause of corneal blindness in the United States despite the fact that only a very low percentage of infected individuals develop ocular disease. Ocular HSV-1 infections are predominately unilateral; however, up to 12% of cases involve both eyes in which the infection tends to be more severe and occurs in younger individuals [38].

History

Primary HSV infection typically presents as an acute oropharyngitis type of illness. Following the initial infection, the virus may go into a latent period within any of the divisions of the trigeminal nerve. It is the reactivation of the latent HSV that causes the primary ocular infection. Patients will present with a unilateral blepharoconjunctivitis with a vesicular rash on the eyelids and follicular conjunctivitis. Patients may present with pain, photophobia, foreign body sensation, blurred vision, tearing, and conjunctival redness.

Physical Examination

Examination may reveal mild conjunctival injection with hyperemic injection surrounding the limbus (ciliary flush). After staining of the eye with fluorescein dye, the typical branching corneal ulcer (dendritic ulcer) with terminal bulbs associated with HSV infection may be seen [39]. With resolution of the infection, patients can develop subepithelial scarring and recurrent infections can lead to focal or diffuse reduction in corneal sensation.

Laboratory Findings

The diagnosis of herpes keratitis is mostly based on clinical history and examination. The dendritic lesions are usually pathognomonic for HSV infection. Laboratory confirmation is rarely indicated, and serologic testing is not recommended due to the prevalence of latent disease and the frequency of recurrences. In severe cases or when clinical findings are atypical, ocular scrapings of epithelial lesions can be sent for viral culture, detection of viral antigen, or detection of viral DNA.

Treatment

Treatment of herpes keratitis is dependent on whether the infection is caused by active viral replication or due to an immune response from a prior infection. Regardless, HSV keratitis warrants immediate referral to an ophthalmologist. For most cases, topical corticosteroids are not indicated as it may worsen the infection.

Trichiasis

Trichiasis is an eyelid abnormality in which the eyelashes are misdirected and grow back toward the eye causing irritation of the cornea and conjunctiva. It can be caused from congenital defects, infection, autoimmune conditions, and trauma. If left untreated, permanent scarring of the cornea can occur, leading to vision loss.

History

The history is essential in directing the clinical examination and formulation of the correct diagnosis. Important questions to ask include recent history of a severe eye infection or travel to a developing country where trachoma is commonly seen, history of herpes zoster ophthalmicus, ocular cicatricial pemphigoid (autoimmune disorder), Stevens-Johnson syndrome, eyelid surgery, or trauma.

Physical Examination

The irritation from the eyelashes causes constant eye irritation, pain, redness, excessive tearing, and sensitivity to light.

Laboratory Findings

There are no specific laboratory tests for the diagnosis of trichiasis. It is primarily based on clinical history and physical examination.

Treatment

For immediate relief, the eyelashes can be plucked out; however, regrowth usually occurs. For more severe cases or for recurrent disease, permanent removal of the affected eyelashes using a radio-frequency device, electrolysis, or cryosurgery can be performed to prevent scarring of the cornea and permanent vision loss. In some cases, corrective eyelid surgery may be indicated.

Acute Closed-Angle Glaucoma

Acute glaucoma is associated with a narrowing of the anterior chamber with obstruction of the aqueous humor from the posterior chamber to the anterior chamber of the eye. This obstruction leads to a rapid increase in intraocular pressure. Acute glaucoma is an ocular emergency and can lead to permanent blindness if left untreated. Primary angle-closure glaucoma is more common in females and those with family history. It is also more prevalent in Eskimos and Southeast Asian populations with a higher risk in individuals over 40 years of age [40]. As people age, the lens of the eye enlarges and pushes the iris forward decreasing the area where the aqueous humor drains thereby increasing the risk for angle-closure glaucoma.

History

Patients present with severe throbbing eye pain, redness, blurred vision, profuse tearing, haloes around lights (due to corneal swelling), nausea, vomiting, and headaches. In acute attacks, it is common for unilateral eye involvement and more severe symptoms. Some may experience intermittent episodes of angle closure and elevated intraocular pressure without a full-blown attack, which is referred to as subacute angle-closure glaucoma. These patients typically are asymptomatic and may experience mildly blurred vision or haloes around lights. These symptoms usually self-resolve once the angle reopens. It is important to review current medications as certain medications can cause drug-induced secondary angle-closure glaucoma.

Physical Examination

Examination requires slit-lamp biomicroscopy which can confirm corneal edema due to the sudden elevation in intraocular pressure. There may also be dilatation of episcleral and conjunctival vessels, shallow anterior chambers, erythema surrounding the iris, and inflammatory cells within the anterior chamber. Tonometry will reveal eye pressures above 21 mmHg and may be as high as 40–80 mmHg. Gonioscopy can be performed to assess the drainage angle of the eye, and ophthalmoscopy can be used to assess the optic nerves for any damage or abnormalities.

Laboratory Findings

There are no specific laboratory tests to confirm the diagnosis of acute glaucoma. It is diagnosed based on clinical history and examination via slit-lamp biomicroscopy.

Treatment

If acute angle-closure glaucoma is suspected, immediate referral to an ophthalmologist is indicated to initiate treatment and prevent permanent vision loss. Initially medications are used to decrease intraocular pressure in preparation for laser iridotomy (treatment of choice), which creates holes in the iris so that the aqueous humor may drain freely from the posterior chamber to the anterior chamber, thereby reducing intraocular pressures.

Conclusion

There are various causes of red eye, and many may be diagnosed based on clinical history and focused examination. In the primary care setting, it is of great importance to be able to determine those cases that require immediate referral to an ophthalmologist. Indications for immediate or emergent referral include unilateral painful red eye that is associated with nausea and vomiting, severe ocular pain or visual loss in association with a red eye, corneal infiltrates or ulcers seen with fluorescein staining, and hypopyon (purulent exudate contained in the anterior chamber of the eye).

References

1. Wirbelauer C. Management of the red eye for the primary care physician. Am J Med. 2006;119:302–6.
2. Cronau H, Kankanala RR, Mauger T. Diagnosis and management of red eye in primary care. Am Fam Physician. 2010;82(2):137–44.
3. Udeh BL, Schneider JE, Ohsfeldt RL. Cost effectiveness of a point-of-care test for adenoviral conjunctivitis. Am J Med Sci. 2008;336(3):254–64.
4. Shields T, Sloane PD. A comparison of eye problems in primary care and ophthalmologic practices. Fam Med. 1991;23(7):544–6.
5. Kaufman HE. Adenovirus advances: new diagnostic and therapeutic options. Curr Opin Ophthalmol. 2011;22(4):290–3.
6. Leibowitz HM. Antibacterial effectiveness of ciprofloxacin 0.3% ophthalmic solution in the treatment of bacterial conjunctivitis. Am J Ophthalmol. 1991;112 (Suppl):29S–33.
7. Wan WL, Farkas GC, May WN, Robin JB. The clinical characteristics and course of adult gonococcal conjunctivitis. Am J Ophthalmol. 1986;102:575.
8. Leibowitz HM. The red eye. N Engl J Med. 2000;343:345–51.
9. LaMattina K, Thompson L. Pediatric conjunctivitis. Dis Mon. 2014;60:231–8.
10. Azari AA, Barney NP. Conjunctivitis a systemic review of diagnosis and treatment. JAMA. 2013;310(16):1721–30.
11. O'Brien TP, Jeng BH, McDonald M, Raizman MB. Acute conjunctivitis: truth and misconceptions. Curr Med Res Opin. 2009;25(8):1953–61.
12. Wright PW, Strauss GH, Langford MP. Acute hemorrhagic conjunctivitis. Am Fam Physician. 1992;45:173–8.
13. Puri LR, Shrestha GB, Shah DN, Chaudhary M, Thakur A. Ocular manifestations in herpes zoster ophthalmicus. Nepal J Ophthalmol. 2011;3(2):165–71.
14. Ragozzino MW, Melton LJ 3rd, Kurland LT, Chu CP, Perry HO. Population-based study of herpes zoster and its sequelae. Medicine. 1982;61:310–6.
15. Resnikoff S, Pascolini D, Etya'ale D. Global data on visual impairment in the year 2002. Bull World Health Organ. 2004;82:844–51.
16. Høvding G. Acute bacterial conjunctivitis. Acta Ophthalmol. 2008;86(1):5–17.
17. Darville T. Chlamydia trachomatis infections in neonates and young children. Semin Pediatr Infect Dis. 2005;16(4):235–44.
18. Hammerschlag MR. Chlamydial and gonococcal infections in infants and children. Clin Infect Dis. 2011;53(Suppl 3):S99–102.
19. American Academy of Pediatrics. Chlamydia trachomatis. In: Pickering LK, editor. Red book: 2012. Report of the committee on infectious diseases. Elk Grove Village: American Academy of Pediatrics; 2012. p. 276–81.
20. Bielory BP, O'Brien TP, Bielory L. Management of seasonal allergic conjunctivitis: guide to therapy. Acta Ophthalmol. 2012;90(5):399–407.

21. Bielory L. Allergic conjunctivitis: the evolution of therapeutic options. Allergy Asthma Proc. 2012;33(2):129–39.

22. Bielory L, Friedlaender MH. Allergic conjunctivitis. Immunol Allergy Clin N Am. 2008;28(1):43–58.

23. Friedlaender MH. Ocular allergy. Curr Opin Allergy Clin Immunol. 2011;11(5):477–82.

24. Messmer EM. The pathophysiology, diagnosis, and treatment of dry eye disease. Dtsch Arztebl Int. 2015;112:71–81.

25. Lemp MA, Bron AJ, Baudouin C, Benitez Del Castillo JM, Geffen D, Tauber J, et al. Tear osmolarity in the diagnosis and management of dry eye disease. Am J Ophthlamol. 2011;151(5):792–798.e1.

26. Stonecipher K, Perry HD, Gross RH, Kerney DL. The impact of topical cyclosporine A emulsion 0.5% on the outcomes of patients with keratoconjunctivitis sicca. Curr Med Res Opin. 2005;21(7):1057–63.

27. Mataftsi A, Subbu RG, Jones S, Nischal KK. The use of punctal plugs in children. Br J Ophthalmol. 2012;96(1):90–2.

28. Ohba E, Dogru M, Hosaka E, et al. Surgical punctal occlusion with a high heat-energy releasing cautery device for severe dry eye with recurrent punctal plug extrusion. Am J Ophthalmol. 2011;151(3):483.e1–7.e1.

29. Wipperman JL, Dorsch JN. Evaluation and management of corneal abrasions. Am Fam Physician. 2013;87(2):114–20.

30. Srinivasan S, Murphy CC, Fisher AC, Freeman LB, Kaye SB. Terrien marginal degeneration presenting with spontaneous corneal perforation. Cornea. 2006;25(8):977–80.

31. Jabs DA, Mudun A, Dunn JP, Marsh MJ. Episcleritis and scleritis: clinical features and treatment results. Am J Ophthalmol. 2000;130:469–76.

32. Williams CP, Browning AC, Sleep TJ, et al. A randomized, double-blind trial of topical ketorolac vs artificial tears for the treatment of episcleritis. Eye. 2005;19(7):739–42.

33. Okhravi N, Odufuwa B, McCluskey P, Lightman S. Scleritis. Surv Ophthalmol. 2005;50:351–63.

34. Suhler EB, Martin TM, Rosenbaum JT. HLA-B27-associated uveitis: overview and current perspectives. Curr Opin Ophthalmol. 2003;14(6):378–83.

35. Chang JH, McCluskey PJ, Wakefield D. Acute anterior uveitis and HLA-B27. Surv Ophthalmol. 2005;50(4):364–88.

36. Bou R, Iglesias E, Anton J. Treatment of uveitis associated with juvenile idiopathic arthritis. Curr Rheumatol Rep. 2014;16(8):437.

37. Pavan-Langston D. In RA Swartz (ed): Herpes Simplex of the Ocular Anterior Segment. Malden, MA, Blackwell Science, Inc. 2000.

38. Kaye S, Choudhary A. Herpes simplex keratitis. Prog Retin Eye Res. 2006;25(4):355–80.

39. Hill GM, Ku ES, Dwarakanathan S. Herpes simplex keratitis. Dis Mon. 2014;60:239–46.

40. Patel K, Patel S. Angle-closure glaucoma. Dis Mon. 2014;60:254–62.

Ocular Trauma

74

T. Jason Meredith, Steven Embry, Ryan Hunter, and
Benjamin Noble

Contents

Introduction

Fifty percent of ocular trauma cases will initially present to an outpatient primary care provider's office [1]. It is imperative that family medicine physicians be able to recognize common ocular injuries, perform a thorough ophthalmologic exam, and most importantly, promptly triage these patients to improve the likelihood of vision preservation. The most frequent etiologies for eye injuries include athletic and workplace-related

T. J. Meredith (✉) · S. Embry · R. Hunter · B. Noble
Department of Family Medicine, University of Nebraska
Medical Center, Omaha, NE, USA
e-mail: jason.meredith@unmc.edu;
steven.embry@unmc.edu; ryan.hunter@unmc.edu;
ben.noble@unmc.edu

© This is a U.S. Government work and not under copyright protection in the U.S.; foreign copyright protection
may apply 2022
P. M. Paulman et al. (eds.), *Family Medicine*,
https://doi.org/10.1007/978-3-030-54441-6_176

injuries, and these injuries disproportionally affect younger men [1–5]. Basketball is commonly cited as the sport with the greatest occurrence of eye injuries, and employees of manufacturing/construction companies lead the way among occupational injuries [3, 5]. Ocular trauma can lead to significant morbidity and disability, including permanent blindness, and therefore necessitates prompt evaluation and management.

This chapter aims to discuss the common yet varied forms of blunt, penetrating, and caustic eye-related traumatic injuries (Table 1). Each

Table 1 Categorization of ocular trauma

Blunt trauma	Caused by forceful impact, non-penetrating
Penetrating trauma	Injury with an entrance wound
Closed globe	Eyewall remains intact
Open globe	Full-thickness injury of ocular surface
Anterior segment	Involving the cornea, ant. chamber, iris or lens
Posterior segment	Involving the vitreous, retina or ocular nerve
Anterior chamber	The space between the cornea and iris

Modified from Refs. [6, 8]

section will cover the pathophysiology, important history and physical exam findings, and management of these injuries.

Ocular Examination

A focused, systematic eye examination is essential to appropriate diagnosis of ocular trauma. The examination begins immediately upon patient contact by assessing the level of patient distress and noting any gross abnormalities with the ocular and periocular anatomy. A primary evaluation, including an abbreviated history and focused physical exam, should be completed to assess for injuries that require emergent intervention to preserve the globe and its function prior to a more generalized examination [6, 7]. This abbreviated history should focus on mechanism of injury, gross visual acuity, and whether the patient wears corrective lenses/contacts. The goal of this primary evaluation is to assess for immediate ocular emergencies such as globe rupture, large foreign body, orbital compartment syndrome, or caustic/chemical injury (Fig. 1). Once these immediate threats to the eye and its function are reasonably excluded, a more thorough history and physical exam should ensue.

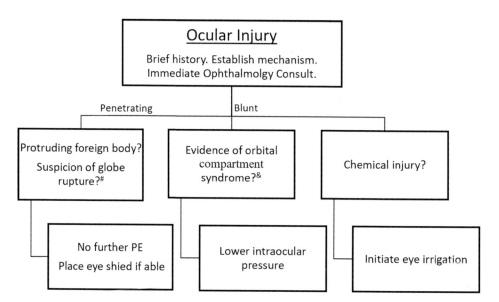

Fig. 1 True ocular emergencies. #Vitreous extrusion, a peaked or eccentric pupil, and severe subconjunctive hemorrhage. &Painful proptosis, pain with eye movements, tense orbits to palpation

A complete ocular examination should begin with assessment of visual acuity. This simple check provides a wealth of knowledge and is the best predictor for potentially blinding conditions [4, 8]. A Snellen eye chart is the test of choice for assessing visual acuity. If the patient is unable to see the largest Snellen letters, even at close distance, then the provider may proceed by determining the ability to count fingers, detect purposeful movement, or simply whether light perception is possible [8]. Barring significant intracranial injury, reduced visual acuity should be assumed to have come from damage to the structures of the anterior or posterior segment of the eye (Table 1). Additional testing will assist in determining the location of the insult. Physicians should start with pupillary response to light and then proceed with direct evaluation with an ophthalmoscope or slit lamp.

Normal pupil reactivity is demonstrated through bilateral pupillary constriction to unilateral light exposure. Pupil reactivity is best appreciated by the "swinging flashlight test," in which the examiner alternates shining light directly into each eye and observing bilateral pupillary response. If the affected eye constricts with contralateral light exposure but is nonreactive and/or appears to actually dilate with direct light exposure as the light is shifted from the contralateral side, a relative afferent pupillary defect (RAPD) is diagnosed [8]. The presence of a RAPD is highly suggestive of an injury to the optic nerve or retina.

Following pupillary response, the gross anatomy of the anterior and posterior segments is evaluated using an ophthalmoscope or slit lamp. During this portion of the examination, mydriatics may be given to improve examination quality (Table 2).

The remainder of the examination involves assessing the periocular and superficial orbital structures including sclera, conjunctiva, eyelids, extraocular muscles, and surrounding bony orbit. While examining the six cardinal eye movements, patients should also be questioned on diplopia symptoms as this may be an indication of extraocular muscle entrapment or nerve paresis [6].

If the patient reports a foreign body sensation and the object is not immediately obvious, the eyelids should be everted for inspection. This should also prompt evaluation for a potential corneal abrasion through the use of fluorescein staining. To apply this stain, moisten the strip with saline or topical anesthetic (Table 2) and place the strip on the palpebral conjunctiva. Ask the patient to blink which will distribute the stain. Cobalt blue light, which is available on most ophthalmoscopes, can then be shone on the eye to highlight corneal irregularities.

In certain settings, radiographic procedures may be desired for further confirmation of the suspected diagnosis. Both computed tomography (CT) and ultrasound have a high degree of sensitivity and specificity for detecting many ocular abnormalities [9]. In clinical practice, the availability of CT scanners and the skill required to complete ocular ultrasound makes CT the imaging modality of choice. CT imaging is preferred

Table 2 Commonly used medications

Topical anesthetics[a]
Tetracaine 0.5%
Proparacaine hydrochloride 0.5%
Mydriatics + cycloplegics
MOA: paralyze iris sphincter (mm)
Tropicamide 0.5% or 1%
Cyclopentolate hydrochloride 0.5% or 1%
Pure mydriatics
MOA: stimulate pupillary dilator (mm)
Phenylephrine hydrochloride 2.5%[b]
Anti-inflammatories
Topical NSAIDs
(a) Diclofenac 0.1%
(b) Ketorolac 0.4%
Topical steroids should not be prescribed by family physicians
Antibiotics
Non-contact wearers:
Erythromycin 0.5%
Contact wearers[c]:
Ciprofloxacin 0.3%
Tobramycin 0.3%
Gentamicin 0.3%

Modified from Refs. [8, 10]
[a]Never prescribe! Corneal toxicity with repeated use
[b]Can be safely combined with low dose tropicamide in adults for additive effect
[c]Pseudomonas coverage

over magnetic resonance imaging (MRI) due to cost, speed of image obtainment, and concern of metal ocular foreign body movement with MRI.

Periocular Injuries

Eyelid Lacerations

Eyelid lacerations are commonly associated with blunt or penetrating trauma, particularly in those who wear corrective lenses [4, 7]. Proper management is essential for preservation of cosmesis as well as structural function. Many eyelid lacerations will require management by an ophthalmologist. If definitive management is not immediately available, delayed closure of 24–36 h in isolated eyelid lacerations has not been shown to lead to significant complications [4, 10, 11].

When confronted with an eyelid laceration, ruling out concurrent injuries which threaten the preservation of the globe and its function must be ensured prior to addressing the laceration. History should focus on the mechanism of injury, ocular function, sensation of foreign body, and tetanus immunization status [7]. Once emergent injuries are successfully ruled out, the laceration should be carefully examined to determine its location and depth. Small superficial cutaneous wounds that do not involve the eyelid margin can be managed by primary or secondary intention and do not require referral [10]. Of note, skin adhesives are not recommended for use around the eye. Ophthalmology or plastic surgery should be involved if any of the following characteristics are present: full thickness lesions, involvement of the lid margin, proximity to the medical canthus, lacrimal duct or sac affected, or presence of ptosis signifying levator palpebrae involvement [7, 10].

Orbital Fractures

The bony orbit is comprised of the frontal, sphenoid, zygomatic, maxillary, and ethmoid bones. Fractures of these bones are common blunt trauma from motor vehicle accidents, falls, and sports-related injuries [12]. The most common type of orbital fracture is the orbital zygomatic fracture, which follows trauma to the inferolateral orbital rim. Other common fractures involve the nasoethmoid bone, orbital floor, and orbital roof, each of which are exceedingly thin. Clinical presentation will vary, and it is not uncommon for simultaneous fractures to occur [13].

Orbital rim fractures present with pain, particularly to palpation, as well as periorbital ecchymosis. Nasoethmoid fractures may also lead to subcutaneous emphysema due to sinus involvement and are a risk for medial rectus muscle entrapment [14]. Orbital floor fractures, also known as orbital "blowout fractures," commonly occur secondary to the increased intraocular pressure associated with blunt trauma. This type of fracture may classically lead to inferior rectus muscle entrapment which causes impaired upward gaze, enopthalmos (posterior globe displacement in the orbit), diplopia with ocular movements, and numbness in the infraorbital nerve distribution [15]. Since this type of fracture has sinus involvement, antibiotic prophylaxis is indicated. Oral cephalexin (250–500 mg QID for 10 days) is an appropriate choice [10].

An orbital CT scan is the test of choice for confirmation of a suspected fracture, and the physical exam should also rule out any co-occurring ocular injuries such as abrasions, hyphema, and lens or retinal injuries, as these often co-occur in many orbital fracture cases [16].

Once a fracture is diagnosed, ophthalmology should be notified. Consider involving ENT or plastic surgery based upon the location of the fracture and noted comorbid injuries. Surgical intervention is not always necessary and is decided on a case-by-case basis [16].

Subconjunctival Hemorrhage

Subconjunctival hemorrhage (SCH) is generally a self-limited condition which may be seen in patients as a consequence of repeated/prolonged Valsalva (i.e., straining in constipation, repeated emesis, childbirth), or direct trauma [17]. Although typically mild, patients who are on blood thinners or those that occur with significant ocular trauma may be quite striking in presentation. A protuberant conjunctiva or circumferential hemorrhage should immediately raise suspicion for occult globe rupture and be managed accordingly. SCH in infants may also be suggestive of non-accidental trauma when its onset occurs outside the peripartum period [18]. Treatment of most subconjunctival hemorrhages is supportive, as they are typically benign and resolve in a few weeks.

Open Globe Injury

An open globe injury is a full-thickness insult to the ocular surface (i.e., cornea or sclera) and is a true ocular emergency (Fig. 1). Direct penetrating injuries are the most common causes, but blunt trauma may also cause globe rupture as forces are transmitted to anatomic weak points in the eye wall (such as the limbus or the coronal equator of the globe) [19].

Open globe injuries are not always immediately apparent, and suspicion must always be maintained in the setting of trauma. Findings that suggest globe rupture include vitreous extrusion, a peaked or eccentric pupil, and severe (i.e., bullous or circumferential) subconjunctival hemorrhage. Orbital CT is the gold standard imaging modality when further evaluation is warranted, but ultrasound may also be beneficial in the hands of an experienced practitioner [20].

Patients with open globe injuries are at high risk for permanent ocular damage, extrusion/prolapse of ocular contents, and development of a post-traumatic infection of the vitreous. As such, initial management consists of minimizing increases to intraocular pressure, administering infection prophylaxis, and avoiding use of eye drops of any kind, including fluorescein and topical anesthetics. Management strategies include [21, 22]:

1. No further physical manipulation of the eye or periocular structures
2. Emergent referral to ophthalmology
3. Application of an eye shield, not an eye patch
4. Avoidance of IOP elevation:

(a) Make the patient strict NPO status (including medications)
(b) Elevate the head of bed >30°
(c) Consider prophylactic intravenous antiemetics
5. Administration of empiric intravenous antibiotics. Do not use topical formulations
(a) Vancomycin (15 mg/kg) AND ceftazidime (50 mg/kg)
6. Administration of appropriate tetanus prophylaxis

Anterior Segment Injuries

Corneal Abrasions and Non-Penetrating Foreign Bodies

Non-penetrating foreign bodies are a common presenting complaint in the primary care setting. Patient presentation likely will involve eye pain, tearing, light sensitivity and a reported foreign body sensation. If concern for penetrating injury is low, removal of a visible foreign body may be attempted. Fluorescein dye should be used to evaluate for possible corneal abrasions caused by movement of the body across the ocular surface.

Removal of non-penetrating foreign bodies should be attempted in a stepwise manner after instillation of a topical anesthetic (Table 2):

1. By irrigation with water or isotonic crystalloid
2. By retrieval with cotton-tipped applicator or similar soft contact
3. By instrumentation by an ophthalmologist

If a corneal abrasion is present, antibiotic prophylaxis should be administered to reduce the risk of infectious keratitis, whether or not foreign body removal is successful [23]. Ointment formulations, such as azithromycin, are preferred due to their additional lubricating effect. If the patient is a contact lens wearer, antibiotic selection should cover *Pseudomonas* species (Table 2).

Abrasions and other corneal injuries, when present, should be reassessed regularly with fluorescein to ensure proper healing [23]. Most defects heal gradually over 3–5 days and are accompanied by steady decreases to symptoms. Lesions that do not follow this pattern, the development of corneal opacities, or change in visual acuity should prompt urgent ophthalmology referral. Ocular steroids, while often used to relieve eye irritation, inhibit epithelial healing and should not be used in these patients [23]. Topical anesthetics may be used acutely during the initial evaluation; however, it is critical to never prescribe these medicines to any patient as prolonged/recurrent use is associated with permanent corneal toxicity. Systemic analgesics may be used for as needed pain relief.

Ultraviolet Light Injury

Ultraviolet (UV) light at a high enough intensity can also lead to diffuse corneal injury known as UV keratitis. Common scenarios include improper eye protection during such activities as welding (Arc Welder's Keratitis) and tanning bed use, or snow blindness secondary to prolonged UV reflection off of snowy surfaces [10, 23]. Patients typically have a delayed presentation of several hours, and the pain can be quite severe. Fluorescein staining will demonstrate diffuse superficial punctate lesions across the cornea [23]. Corneal injury secondary to UV light is treated similarly to corneal abrasions with topical antibiotics and systemic analgesics. Referral guidelines are also the same.

Traumatic Iritis and Hyphema

The force of blunt ocular trauma can lead to traumatic iritis, an acute inflammatory state in the anterior segment involving the iris and ciliary body. Patients typically present with eye pain, tearing, significant photophobia, and visual disturbances. Inspection of the eye classically demonstrates an erythematous dilation of the vessels immediately surrounding the limbus of the eye (known as ciliary flush) [8]. During pupillary assessment, the patient may report increased pain in the affected eye when light is shone in the contralateral eye. If present, this is pathognomonic for iritis [8, 10]. In the setting of trauma, if signs and symptoms of iritis are present, the clinician should also closely evaluate for a commonly co-occurring hemorrhage in the anterior chamber of the eye known as a traumatic hyphema [6].

Hyphema refers to frankly visible blood in the anterior chamber of the eye between the cornea and pupil. The etiology of traumatic hyphema formation is likely due to a sudden increase in intraocular pressure, which creates a shearing force on the vessels of the ciliary body or iris [24]. The diagnosis is made clinically by visualizing the pooling blood behind the cornea. Sitting a patient upright will facilitate blood pooling inferiorly, making hyphemas easier to detect [24].

Initial symptomatic management includes dim lighting, placing an eye shield, and elevating the head. Most hyphemas spontaneously resolve, but there is a risk of rebleed, intraocular hypertension, and corneal injury; which can lead to permanent visual impairment [25]. Therefore, once the diagnosis is made, an ophthalmology consult should ensue.

Lens Injuries

The crystalline lens is the focusing apparatus of the eye and due to its unique structure and anterior position is at high risk of injury from blunt or penetrating insult. The lens itself is encased in a transparent capsule and is suspended in place by thin zonules just posterior to the iris and anterior to the vitreous [8]. With sufficient force, the transmission of energy from blunt trauma can disrupt the protein composition of the crystalline lens and/or damage its associated structures including the lens capsule [26]. This disruption of lens proteins, or the infiltration of foreign substances secondary to capsule rupture, can lead to rapid cataract formation [26, 27]. Direct ophthalmoscopic findings, particularly with dilated eye exam, may include opacification of the lens leading to an abnormal red reflex and obscuration of fundus visualization [6, 27]. A careful dilated eye examination is also crucial to evaluate for lens subluxation/dislocation, indicative of damage to the filamentous zonules which suspend the lens [26, 27]. Any evidence of cataract formation or lens subluxation should prompt consultation with ophthalmology.

Posterior Segment Injuries

Retinal Detachment and Vitreous Hemorrhage

The retina is a thin neurovascular structure which lines the inside surface of the posterior globe and is responsible for transmitting visual signals to the optic nerve [8]. In blunt trauma injuries, energy transmission through the vitreous can cause a traction injury, separating the retina from its underlying structures leading to compromise of sensory input. Retinal detachment should be suspected if the patient reports new monocular flashes of light (known as photopsias) or floaters in their visual field. Patients with extensive detachment may also experience decreased visual acuity and/or demonstrate a RAPD in the affected eye [8, 28]. Definitive diagnosis is achieved through visualization of abnormal surface architecture of the retina with ophthalmoscopic examination. Ocular ultrasound is also sensitive and specific for making the diagnosis [9].

Bleeding into the vitreous of the eye may also occur following a post-traumatic retinal detachment if vascular structures are compromised. If the hemorrhage is significant, these patients will have decreased visual acuity, a RAPD, as well as a diminished or absent red reflex [8]. Regardless of the etiology, when faced with a suspected retinal detachments and/or vitreous hemorrhage, urgent referral to an ophthalmologist is indicated for definitive management. Table 3 summarizes the signs and symptoms which should prompt ophthalmology consultation discussed in this chapter.

Retrobulbar Hemorrhage and Ocular Compartment Syndrome

The bony orbit is relatively incapable of accommodating increases in intracavitary pressure.

Table 3 Signs and symptoms that warrant ophthalmology referral

Loss of vision, diplopia, or abnormal visual field	Embedded foreign body
Suspected globe rupture	Complex eyelid laceration
Painful proptosis	Hyphema
Reported flashes or floaters	Pain with ocular movements
Irregular pupil	Photophobia

Modified from Refs. [4, 27, 33]

Retrobulbar hemorrhage is a rare, but potentially catastrophic complication of orbital/midface trauma. Bleeding into the retrobulbar space causes a rise in intracavitary pressure. If the pressure is great enough, it can precipitate a compartment syndrome of the orbit, which is a true ophthalmic emergency (Fig. 1). Irreversible ischemic injury can occur to the retina and optic nerve leading to monocular blindness in as little as 60 min [29].

Retrobulbar hemorrhage is a clinical diagnosis and should be suspected in all cases of facial trauma, especially if the patient has a known bleeding diathesis or is on anticoagulation. If compartment syndrome is developing, the patient will typically present with painful proptosis, pain with extraocular eye movements, decreased visual acuity, and tense orbits to palpation [29, 30]. Presence of a RAPD is an ominous sign, indicating that ischemic retinal/optic nerve damage is already developing [30]. Tonometry will confirm increased intraocular pressure (IOP >22 mmHg). If diagnosis remains uncertain, advanced imaging with CT can assist [9]. Immediate ophthalmologic surgical consultation is warranted. Until definitive surgical evaluation, management strategies to reduce swelling and IOP may improve outcomes [10, 30]:

1. Elevate head of bed to >30°
2. Make the patient NPO and consider prophylactic antiemetics
3. Methylprednisolone 125 mg IV
4. Acetazolamide 500 mg IV (avoid in sulfa allergic patients)
5. Timolol 0.5%, one drop in affected eye

Chemical Injuries

Chemical injuries are another ocular emergency as rapid and permanent damage may ensue (Fig. 1) [31, 32]. The mainstay of treatment for all suspected chemical injuries is copious irrigation, ophthalmology consultation, and prophylactic topical antibiotic administration. Normalization of pH should only be performed with water or isotonic crystalloid. Instillation of topical analgesia should be performed if blepharospasm occurs in response to pain, in order to promote eye lid opening and enhance ease of irrigation [31]. Contact lenses should be removed if present. After irrigation for least 30 min, pH neutrality (7.0–7.3) may be assessed with a pH strip. After irritative symptoms have resolved and pH neutrality has been sustained, empiric topical antibiotics (Table 2) should be prescribed [31, 32].

Of note, alkaline exposures generally pose a greater risk to the eye, in part due to the lack of physiologic base buffering in the body [32]. Greater irrigation time may be required before pH neutrality is sustained in patients with base exposures (e.g., wet concrete, ammonia, oven cleaner, drain cleaner).

References

1. McGwin GJ, Xie A, Owsley C. Rate of eye injury in the United States. Arch Ophthalmol. 2005;123(7):970–6.
2. Matsa E, Shi J, Wheeler KK, McCarthy T, McGregor ML, Leonard JC. Trends in US emergency department visits for pediatric acute ocular injury. JAMA Ophthalmol. 2018;136:895.
3. Haring RS, Sheffield ID, Canner JK, Schneider EB. Epidemiology of sports-related eye injuries in the United States. JAMA Ophthalmol. 2016;134 (12):1382–90.
4. Toldi JP, Thomas JL. Evaluation and management of sports-related eye injuries. Curr Sports Med Rep. 2020;19:29–34.
5. Peate WF. Work-related eye injuries and illnesses. Am Fam Physician. 2007;75:1017–24.
6. Levine LM. Pediatric ocular trauma and shaken infant syndrome. Pediatr Clin N Am. 2003;50:137–48.
7. Chang EL, Rubin PA. Management of complex eyelid lacerations. Int Ophthalmol Clin. 2002;42(3):187–201.
8. Harper R, Basic Ophthalmology AR. Essentials for medical students. 10th ed. San Francisco: American Academy of Ophthalmology; 2016.
9. Ojaghihaghighi S, Lombardi KM, Davis S, Vahdati SS, Sorkhabi R, Pourmand A. Diagnosis of traumatic eye injuries with point-of-care ocular ultrasonography in the emergency department. Ann Emerg Med. 2019;74 (3):365–71.
10. Cydulka RK, Fitch MT, Joing S, Wang VJ, Cline D, Ma OJ, et al. Tintinalli's emergency medicine manual. 8th ed. New York: McGraw-Hill Medical; 2018.
11. Chiang E, Bee C, Harris GJ, Wells TS. Does delayed repair of eyelid lacerations compromise outcome? Am J Emerg Med. 2017;35(11):1766–7.
12. Cruz AAV, Eichenberger GCD. Epidemiology and management of orbital fractures. Curr Opin Ophthalmol. 2004;15:416–21.
13. Manolidis S, Weeks BH, Kirby M. Classification and surgical management of orbital fractures: experience with 111 orbital reconstructions. J Craniofac Surg. 2002;13:726.
14. Segrest DR, Dortzbach RK. Medial orbital wall fractures: complications and management. Ophthalmic Plast Reconstr Surg. 1989;5:75.
15. Converse JM, Smith B. Enophthalmos and diplopia in fractures of the orbital floor. Br J Plast Surg. 1957;9:265–74.
16. Burnstine MA. Clinical recommendations for repair of orbital facial fractures. Curr Opin Ophthalmol. 2003;14:236.
17. Mimura T, Usui T, Yamagami S, Funatsu H, Noma H, Honda N, Amano S. Recent causes of subconjunctival hemorrhage. Ophthalmologica. 2010;224(3):133.
18. DeRidder CA, Berkowitz CD, Hicks RA, Laskey AL. Subconjunctival hemorrhages in infants and children: a sign of nonaccidental trauma. Pediatr Emerg Care. 2013;29(2):222.
19. Kuhn F, Morris R, Witherspoon CD, Heimann K, Jeffers JB, Treister G. A standardized classification of ocular trauma. Ophthalmology. 1996;103(2):240.
20. Crowell EL, Koduri VA, Supsupin EP, Klinglesmith RE, Chuang AZ, Kim G, Baker LA, Feldman RM, Blieden LS. Accuracy of computed tomography imaging criteria in the diagnosis of adult open globe injuries by neuroradiology and ophthalmology. Acad Emerg Med. 2017;24(9):1072.
21. Colby K. Management of open globe injuries. Int Ophthalmol Clin. 1999;39(1):59.
22. Al-omran A, Abboud E, El-asrar A. Microbiologic spectrum and visual outcome of posttraumatic endophthalmitis. Retina. 2007;27:236–42.
23. Whipperman J, Dorsch J. Evaluation and management of corneal abrasions. Am Fam Physician. 2013;87 (2):114–20.
24. Brandt MT, Haug RH. Traumatic hyphema: a comprehensive review. J Oral Maxillofac Surg. 2001;59:1462.
25. Walton W, Von Hagen S, Grigorian R, Zarbin M. Management of traumatic hyphema. Surv Ophthalmol. 2002;47:297.
26. Salehi-Had H, Turalba A. Management of traumatic crystalline lens subluxation and dislocation. Int Ophthalmol Clin. 2010;50(1):167–79.

27. Micieli JA, Easterbrook M. Eye and orbital injuries in sports. Clin Sports Med. 2017;36(2):299–314.

28. Hollands H, Johnson D, Brox AC, Almeida D, Simel DL, Sharma S. Acute-onset floaters and flashes: is this patient at risk for retinal detachment? JAMA. 2009;302 (20):2243–9.

29. Lima V, Burt B, Leibovitch I, Prabhakaran V, Goldberg RA, Selva D. Orbital compartment syndrome: the ophthalmic surgical emergency. Surv Ophthalmol. 2009;54(4):441–9.

30. Chen YA, Singhal D, Chen YR, Chen CT. Management of acute traumatic retrobulbar haematomas: a 10-year retrospective review. J Plast Reconstr Aesthet Surg. 2012;65(10):1325–30.

31. Spector J, Fernandez W. Chemical, thermal, and biological ocular exposures. Emerg Med Clin North Am. 2008;26:125–36.

32. Fish R, Davidson R. Management of ocular thermal and chemical injuries, including amniotic membrane therapy. Curr Opin Ophthalmol. 2010;21:317–21.

33. Rodriguez JO, Lavina AM, Agarwal A. Prevention and treatment of common eye injuries in sports. Am Fam Physician. 2003;67(7):1481–8.

Linda J. Vorvick and Deborah L. Lam

Contents

John E. Sutherland and Richard C. Mauer are
acknowledged for authoring prior edition.

L. J. Vorvick (✉)
Department of Family Medicine, UW Medicine,
University of Washington, Seattle, WA, USA
e-mail: lvorvick@u.washington.edu; lvorvick@uw.edu

D. L. Lam
Department of Ophthalmology, UW Medicine, University
of Washington, Seattle, WA, USA
e-mail: deblam@u.washington.edu

Presenting complaints of eye disorders need to be quickly divided into complaints that are serious and require an emergent or urgent examination and treatment and complaints that are less serious. Urgent symptoms include recent visual loss, double vision, pain, floaters, flashes, and photophobia. Less serious symptoms, which can be evaluated less urgently, include vague ocular discomfort, tearing, mucous discharge, burning, or eyelid symptoms.

The basic eye examination includes testing for visual acuity with the Snellen chart or starting at 3 years old with a picture chart or matching chart [1]. Along with visual acuity, confrontation visual fields, ocular motility testing, pupillary examination, intraocular pressure measurement, corneal staining, and ophthalmoscopy are essential elements of a complete urgent exam [2].

The Pupil

The pupil regulates the amount of light that enters the eye. Normal pupils are round, regular in shape, and nearly equal in size. The pupillary examination is designed primarily to detect neurologic abnormalities that disturb the size of the pupils. Pupillary reflexes include the direct light reflex and the indirect, or consensual, reflex, a response to light falling on the opposite eye. The measurement of pupil size in dim light assesses the motor (efferent) limb of the pupillary reflex arc; the evaluation of pupil response to direct light assesses both the motor and the sensory (afferent) limbs; the swinging light test (testing for the consensual reflex) assesses only the sensory limbs.

Constriction of the pupil to less than 2 mm is called miosis, if it does not dilate in the dark. Topical cholinergic-stimulating drops and systemic narcotics are the most frequent causes.

Dilatation of the pupil to more than 6 mm is called mydriasis, with failure to constrict to light stimulation. Topical atropine-like drops, trauma, and oculomotor nerve abnormalities are the most common causes.

Anatomic variation in the diameter of the pupil is less than 1 mm. It is best to determine this parameter in the dimmest light possible, measuring with the pupil gauge found on the near vision card. True inequality of pupil size (anisocoria) is caused by drugs, injury, inflammation, angle-closure glaucoma, ischemia, paralysis of the sphincter pupillae muscle (dilated) and dilator pupillae muscles (constricted), Horner syndrome, neuronal lesions (Argyll Robertson pupil), or, most commonly, physiologic variations [3]

The Eyelids

The eyelids protect the cornea, aid in the distribution and the elimination of tears, and limit light entering the eye. Abnormalities can occur in the skin, mucous membranes, glands, and muscles [3].

Congenital Abnormalities

The most common congenital variation is an epicanthus, which is a vertical skinfold in the medial canthal region. This may simulate an esotropia (pseudostrabismus) [1].

Positional Abnormalities

Entropion

Entropion is the inversion of the lid margin. Etiologies are age-related (involutional), cicatricial, spastic, and congenital. Involutional entropion of aging is common, causing misdirected eyelashes (trichiasis) that irritate the eye. Secondary conditions include conjunctivitis, corneal ulcers, keratitis, and tearing. Treatment includes lubricating agents, and topical antibiotic ointment. Everting the eyelid margin away from the globe and taping can be temporary while awaiting definitive surgical procedures for symptomatic patients [4].

Ectropion

Eversion of the lid margin, or ectropion, can be age-related, cicatricial, mechanical, allergic, and congenital. Severe cases may follow Bell's palsy. Ocular manifestations include chronic conjunctivitis, keratitis, epiphora, and keratinization of the lid. Treatment options are similar to those for entropion [5].

Blepharoptosis

The etiology of blepharoptosis lies either in the innervation or the structure of the levator palpebrae superioris muscle, leading to a drooping upper eyelid and a narrow palpebral fissure. The congenital type can be unilateral or bilateral. Acquired forms include dehiscence of the levator aponeurosis, neuropathy, intracranial disorders, Horner syndrome, myotonic dystrophy, and myasthenia gravis. Surgical therapy is the only successful management strategy [6].

Inflammation

Blepharitis

Blepharitis is an inflammatory condition of the lid margin oil glands. It may be infectious, usually due to *Staphylococcus aureus*, involving the eyelash roots, glands, or both. It has been described as "acne" of the eyelids. Individuals who have acne rosacea or seborrheic dermatitis of the scalp and face are particularly vulnerable. Symptoms include swelling, redness, debris of the lid and lashes, itching, tearing, foreign body sensation, and crusting around the eyes on awakening. Management of blepharitis is primarily lid hygiene using warm compresses with baby shampoo or an eyelid cleansing agent applied with a finger, washcloth, or cotton-tipped applicators. Nightly application of bacitracin or erythromycin ointment to the lid margins is helpful when there are signs of secondary infection. For severe or recurrent cases, systemic therapy with tetracycline or doxycycline can be used for several months [7].

Hordeolum

Also known as a stye, an external hordeolum is an inflammation of the ciliary follicles or accessory glands of the anterior lid margin. It is a painful, tender, red mass near the lid margin, often with pustule formation and mild conjunctivitis. An internal hordeolum, which presents in a similar manner, involves an infection of the meibomian gland away from the lid margins. Treatment is usually simple for this self-limited condition: intermittent hot, moist compresses plus topical ophthalmic antibiotics such as tobramycin, bacitracin, erythromycin, gentamicin, or sulfacetamide to prevent infection of the surrounding lash follicles. One method to hasten drainage of the external hordeolum is to epilate (remove a hair and its root) the lash, which effectively creates a drainage channel. Occasionally an incision or puncture for drainage and administration of systemic antistaphylococcal antibiotics are necessary [8].

Chalazion

A chalazion (lipogranuloma) is a chronic granuloma that may follow and be secondary to inflammation of a meibomian gland. During its chronic phase, it is a firm, painless nodule up to 8 mm in diameter that lies within the tarsus and over which the skin lid moves freely. It usually begins as an internal hordeolum. Asymptomatic chalazia usually resolve spontaneously within a month. Treatment options for persistent chalazia include an intralesional long-acting corticosteroid injection, which may cause hypopigmentation, or a surgical incision and curettage with a clamp [8].

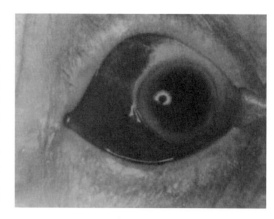

Fig. 1 Subconjunctival hemorrhage

Dermatitis

Dermatitis may be either infectious or of contact etiology. Contact dermatitis is common because of exposure to sensitizing irritants such as neomycin, atropine, cosmetics, lotions, soaps, nickel, thimerosal (often in artificial tears), chloramphenicol, poison ivy, and others. Manifestations include erythema, vesiculation, scaling, edema, and itching. Therapy, most importantly, is the removal of the offending agent. During the acute stages, cool compresses, antihistamines, and topical corticosteroids provide relief. Occasionally, systemic steroids are necessary such as for severe poison ivy dermatitis. The most common infectious causes are impetigo, erysipelas, and herpes zoster, with treatment the same as indicated for other locations [8].

Conjunctiva

Subconjunctival Hemorrhage

Subconjunctival hemorrhage not caused by direct ocular trauma is usually the result of a sudden increase in intrathoracic pressure, as when sneezing, coughing, or straining to evacuate. Rupture of a conjunctival blood vessel causes a bright red, sharply delineated area surrounded by normal-appearing conjunctiva (Fig. 1). The blood is located underneath the bulbar conjunctiva and gradually fades in 2 weeks. Usually no cause is found, but it is seen with hypertension, with anticoagulation, and

in neonates or their mothers as a result of labor and delivery. No treatment is indicated [9].

Pingueculum and Pterygium

A pingueculum is an area of the nasal or temporal bulbar conjunctiva that contains epithelial hyperplasia, a harmless yellow-white, plaque-like thickening.

A pterygium is a triangular elevated mass consisting of vascular growth of the conjunctiva, usually nasal, that migrates onto the corneal surface. Environmental factors such as prolonged sunlight exposure and exposure to heat, wind, and dust contribute to its formation. It may be unsightly and uncomfortable, and it may interfere with vision.

Occasionally inflammatory discomfort of either a pingueculum or pterygium may require a mild topical steroid or nonsteroidal anti-inflammatory drop [3].

Surgical removal may be necessary if vision is impaired or for excessive irritation.

Recurrence may occur, but using a conjunctival autograft or amniotic membrane graft may decrease the recurrence [3, 10].

Lacrimal System

Epiphora

Epiphora is a condition in which tearing occurs because of either hypersecretion or impaired drainage of tears through the lacrimal passages. Causes include muscle weakness, allergy, ectropion, occlusive scarring, glaucoma, dacryocystitis, canaliculitis, and inflammation [3]. In infancy, it is usually due to congenital nasolacrimal duct obstruction, which has a high rate of spontaneous resolution during the first year. Nasolacrimal duct massage may help [1].

Dry Eye

The tear film is a complex, delicately balanced fluid composed of contributions from a series of glands. Alacrima, decreased or absent tears, occurs with keratoconjunctivitis sicca, associated with the autoimmune systemic complex of Sjogren syndrome, most frequently from rheumatoid arthritis or thyroid diseases. Other causes of dry eye can be blepharospasm, blepharitis, allergies, systemic medications, and toxins [10]. Tear film deficiency also causes nonspecific symptoms of burning, foreign body sensation, photophobia, itching, and a "gritty" sensation. Physical findings include hyperemia, loss of the usual glossy appearance of the cornea, and a convex tear meniscus less than 0.3 mm in height. Treatment is difficult and lifelong with artificial tears containing methylcellulose, polyvinyl alcohol, or 2% sodium hyaluronate four times a day to hourly. Punctal occlusion with a silicone plug or permanent punctal closure via thermal cautery can produce dramatic symptomatic improvement. Severe cases occasionally require mucolytic agents or autologous serum tears. Topical cyclosporine treatment is used in the treatment of dry eye and has shown to have clinical benefits [7, 11, 12].

Dacryocystitis

Dacryocystitis is a painful inflammation of the lacrimal sac resulting from congenital or acquired obstruction of the nasolacrimal duct. Even though congenital nasolacrimal duct obstruction occurs commonly in infants, dacryocystitis is rare and is commonly associated with nasolacrimal duct cysts. In adults, it is idiopathic or the result of an obstruction from infection, a facial trauma, or a dacryolith, rarely neoplasm. The medial lower lid location has a domed mass that is tender and painful, with discharge and tearing. Treatment includes hot packs with topical and systemic antibiotics for penicillinase-producing staphylococcal organisms. Incision and drainage may be performed for select cases; if the acute episode has resolved and is now chronic, surgical correction may be considered (dacryocystorhinostomy with silicone intubation) [8].

Dacryoadenitis

Dacryoadenitis, an enlargement of the lacrimal gland, may be granulomatous, lymphoid, or infectious in origin. If acute, this lesion is painful, tender, suppurative, and inflamed; if chronic, it may manifest simply as a swollen, hard mass. Treatment of dacryoadenitis is determined by its etiology and ranges from supportive heat therapy and massage to incision and drainage, followed by the use of systemic antibiotics and, if not responsive, by steroids [8].

Orbit

Preseptal (periorbital) and postseptal (orbital) cellulitis are bacterial infections of the periocular tissue that are serious and potentially vision threatening and lethal. Preseptal cellulitis involves only the lid structures and periorbital tissues anterior to the orbital septum. Postseptal cellulitis involves tissue behind the septum, which children and adolescents have it more commonly than adults. Routes of infection include trauma, bacteremia, upper respiratory infection, and sinusitis. Cellulitis should be considered in every patient with swelling of the eye. Critical signs include pain, fever, erythema, tenderness, swelling, and conjunctival injection. With postseptal infection, impaired ocular motility, afferent pupillary defect, proptosis, and visual loss also occur. Cavernous sinus thrombosis may develop. Leukocytosis is usually present, and a peripheral white blood cell count of more than 15,000/mm^3 suggests bacteremia. Computed tomography (CT) of the orbit is indicated to identify the extent of infection [8].

A bacterial pathogen is identified as the cause of periorbital cellulitis in only 30% of cases. Treatment must cover gram-positive and gram-negative anaerobes and potential methicillin-resistant *Staphylococcus aureus*. Antimicrobial therapy should be intravenous, and guidelines suggest amoxicillin/clavulanic or ceftriaxone with metronidazole as empiric treatment. Emergency consultation with hospitalization should be obtained from both an ophthalmologist and an otolaryngologist [8, 13].

Retina

Disorders of the retina often present with complaints of decreased vision. Assessing visual acuity, examining the eye, and looking for underlying medical problems are important to direct appropriate referral and care.

Arterial Occlusive Retinal Disease

Central artery occlusion (CRAO) is a severe sudden loss of vision due to an embolic or thrombotic occlusion, or obstruction, of the central retinal artery. It is usually painless and is usually monocular. Occasionally it is preceded by symptoms of amaurosis fugax, lasting 5–20 min. A cherry-red spot is often seen in the central macula. Treatment consists of immediate decompression of the eye by pharmacologic or anterior chamber paracentesis. It is important to evaluate for giant cell arteritis as this can cause a CRAO [14].

Branch retinal artery occlusion (BRAO) is a painless, less severe, more peripheral embolic phenomenon in the retinal arterial circulation, where an immediate blank or dark area is noted in the patient's visual field. It is almost always monocular. Treatment is based on finding the systemic source of the problem. Common causes include carotid plaques and cardiac valvular disease [14].

Venous Occlusive Retinal Disease

Central and branch retinal vein occlusions (CRVOs, BRVOs) must be suspected with unilateral loss of vision. A CRVO presents as a sudden loss of vision secondary to compression of the venous return by a retinal artery, causing thrombosis at that location. If an occlusion occurs at the optic nerve head, it is a CRVO; if it is seen more peripherally, it is a BRVO. The CRVO is diagnosed by the presence of flame-shaped and blot hemorrhages throughout the entire retinal field, often obscuring the view of the underlying retina (Fig. 2) [14].

A BRVO causes less severe visual loss, often not noticed by the patient. It leads to stasis of the venous flow more peripherally, which if it involves the macula causes central loss of vision. Here again, flame-shaped hemorrhages are present upon examination [14]. Treatment involves intravitreal injections of anti-vascular endothelial growth factor (anti-VEGF) therapies or laser [15].

Retinal Detachment

The annual incidence of retinal detachment is 12.9:100,000. People with high myopia and lattice degeneration of the retina have about 1% chance of a retinal detachment. Retinal detachment can occur in about 10% of patients with

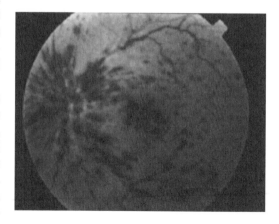

Fig. 2 Central retinal vein occlusion

vitreous detachment which commonly occurs between the ages of 60 and 80 years. A frequent symptom of retinal detachment is a gray curtain or cloud covering a portion of the visual field. These symptoms may be preceded by a quick flash of light and a new onset of many small black floaters. On physical examination with a dilated pupil, one sees a corrugated bulbous elevation of the retina. If a detachment can be surgically repaired immediately, prior to a macular detachment, the resulting visual acuity is much better [16].

Diabetic Retinopathy

Early detection of diabetic retinopathy is important. Diabetics should have regular ophthalmologic examinations.

Nonproliferative Diabetic Retinopathy

Nonproliferative diabetic retinopathy is graded as mild, moderate, or severe. With the more severe retinopathy, cotton wool spots are present, and dot and blot hemorrhages and lipid accumulation are seen throughout the retina (Fig. 3). If there is thickening of the retina in the central macular zone, diabetic macular edema is present and can cause profound visual loss. Laser and intravitreal injections are used to stabilize and improve visual function [14, 17, 18].

Proliferative Diabetic Retinopathy

Proliferative diabetic retinopathy is diagnosed when neovascularization is detected at the optic nerve or elsewhere in the retina. It poses a risk of retinal and vitreous hemorrhage, tractional retinal detachment, fibroglial proliferation, and retinal fibrosis. With a dilated pupil, a lacy network of fine vessels is seen, indicating retinal ischemia (Figs. 4 and 5). Panretinal photocoagulation (PRP) eliminates the mid-peripheral retina. PRP may cause some night and central vision loss but prevents progressive severe visual loss [14, 18, 19].

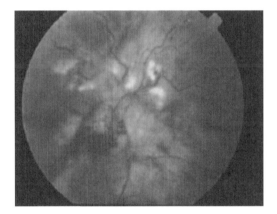

Fig. 4 Proliferative diabetic retinopathy

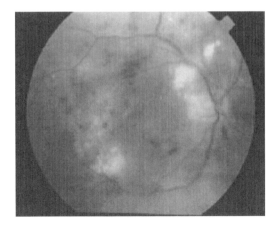

Fig. 3 Nonproliferative diabetic retinopathy

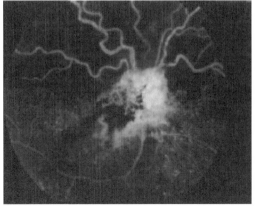

Fig. 5 Angiogram of proliferative diabetic retinopathy

Amaurosis Fugax

Amaurosis fugax is the sudden, painless, monocular loss of vision, described as a curtain or a shade being pulled down or up, blanketing the field of vision. It totally resolves in 5–30 min. A cholesterol plaque in the carotid artery, or rarely, a calcific cardiac valvular condition, is the etiology. Treatment is directed toward anticoagulation or antiplatelet therapy. Based on the patient's risk threshold, surgical intervention, such as carotid endarterectomy or stenting, is undertaken [2].

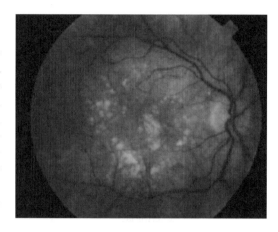

Fig. 6 Dry age-related macular degeneration

Ocular Migraine

Ocular migraine is a common condition in individuals over age 40. It presents often as a migraine aura, a fortification scotoma of jagged, multicolored lights that expand in a gradual fashion across the entire field of vision, leaving in its wake a darker or blank scotoma. Often associated with the migraine symptoms is a queasy feeling. If the episode lasts longer than 1 h, the diagnosis is in question. The eye examination at the time is entirely normal. Treatment is directed to the underlying migraine. Neuroimaging may also be considered if the symptoms are not classic or the duration exceeds 1 h [2, 14].

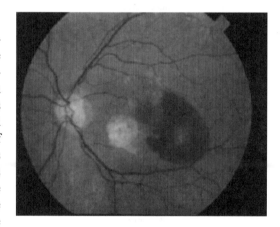

Fig. 7 Wet age-related macular degeneration

Macular Degeneration

Macular degeneration is an aging phenomenon of the inner retina that results in visual loss due to deterioration of the retinal photoreceptors. There are two types of macular degeneration: dry and wet.

Dry Age-Related Macular Degeneration

Dry age-related macular degeneration presents with slow visual loss in the central field of vision. Often the first signs are reduced reading vision and later scotoma in the central field of vision as the severity increases. There is a loss of photoreceptor function in the central macular zone (Fig. 6) [14].

Neovascular Age-Related Macular Degeneration

Neovascular age-related macular degeneration presents with sudden visual loss and hemorrhage in the central macular zone. The underlying retina develops a defect, allowing the choroidal vessels to grow through the retinal pigment epithelium (Fig. 7). The patient presents with a dark or distorted spot in the central field of vision. As the hemorrhage progresses, the vision deteriorates further. Any sudden change in vision of a patient with macular degeneration should result in immediate referral to an ophthalmologist, as neovascular age-related macular degeneration can be treated by intravitreal injection of anti-vascular endothelial growth factors or in some instances laser therapy [14, 20].

Optic Nerve

Optic Disc Edema

Optic nerve disc edema is a common end point for several ocular disorders that result in swelling of the optic nerve head and hemorrhage in the surrounding peripapillary retina. Blood vessel margins are often blurred as they cross over the optic nerve, and splinter hemorrhages are present, distinguishing this disorder from pseudopapilledema (Fig. 8). The ocular causes of disc edema include the following: optic neuritis, anterior ischemic optic neuropathy (arteritic and nonarteritic), ischemic papillitis as in diabetes, and increased intracranial pressure. When optic disc head edema is secondary to increased intracranial pressure, it is termed papilledema. Papilledema occurs in both eyes but may be asymmetric [21, 22].

Pseudopapilledema

Pseudopapilledema is a benign, anomalous appearance of the optic nerve head due to optic disc drusen, often seen during a normal eye examination. The optic nerve head has an elevated, lumpy appearance. No nerve fiber layer edema or splinter retinal hemorrhages are seen, as would be seen with disc edema [22].

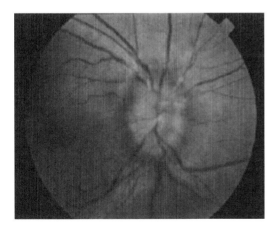

Fig. 8   Optic nerve head edema (papilledema)

Lens

Cataracts, or a clouding of the lens of the eye, are increasingly common among our aged population in the United States. The three of the more common types of cataract can be described based on the location of the lenticular opacity.

A nuclear sclerotic cataract is the hardening of the central nucleus of the lens and leads to gradual yellowing of the nucleus. With further progression, it may turn brown. Frequently this type of cataract is not appreciated at an early stage because of the gradual progression and bilateral aspect of presentation.

Cortical cataract is the whitening of the peripheral lens cortex. As the opacity progresses more centrally, more visual deprivation results. Frequently people complain of glare from lights with this type of cataract. Occasionally, double vision is noted, as cortical opacity splits light into different focal points.

Posterior subcapsular cataracts are the most visually disabling, and the progression can be rapid. Near vision is more impaired than distance vision. The disorder is often seen in patients on chronic steroids (topical or systemic) or diabetes.

The diagnosis can be easily made by dilating the pupil and using the red reflex test. Examination indicators are a hazing over with a nuclear sclerotic cataract, a spoke-like defect with a cortical cataract, and a central dark opacity with a posterior subcapsular cataract. Treatment normally is surgical, but if the patient is not a surgical candidate, chronic dilation of the pupil improves the vision in some patients. Visual recovery from surgery is frequently rapid [23].

Glaucomas

Primary Open-Angle Glaucoma

Primary open-angle glaucoma (POAG) is a relatively common disorder whose incidence increases with advancing age. There is an obstruction of aqueous outflow at the level of the trabecular meshwork. Predisposing factors include a family history of glaucoma, severe blunt trauma to the eye, and possibly high myopia. In 2018, the prevalence of POAG for adults 40 and older in the globally is estimated to be 3.5% [24].

Glaucoma can occur without elevated intraocular pressure. Computer-based visual field testing can be used to screen for glaucoma, but the US Preventive Services Task Force does not recommend for or is not against screening. Physical exam findings of glaucoma show damage to the optic nerve. Elevated intraocular pressure does tend to raise the risk threshold of developing glaucoma. The diagnosis is based on a triad of findings: increased intraocular pressure, optic nerve head cupping, and visual field defect. A cup/disc ratio of more than 0.60 is often a diagnostic clue, as is asymmetry between the two eyes. When a family history of glaucoma is present, or an enlarged cup-to-disc is seen, referral to an ophthalmologist is indicated (Figs. 9 and 10).

The treatment options are pharmacologic lowering of intraocular pressure, laser trabeculoplasty to attempt to increase the aqueous outflow, or surgical decompression of the eye by trabeculectomy or aqueous shunts [14, 24–27].

Angle-Closure Glaucoma

An acute angle-closure glaucoma attack is precipitated by abrupt closure in the aqueous outflow. The iris, with slight dilation, occludes the trabecular meshwork, resulting in progressively increasing pressure within the eye. The acute symptoms include pain, decreased vision, halos around lights, nausea, and vomiting. Examination reveals a cloudy or "steamy" appearance of the cornea, a nonreactive mid-dilated pupil, an area of injection around the limbus, and elevated intraocular pressure. Immediate referral to an ophthalmologist is mandatory. A laser iridotomy is often necessary, and close monitoring is needed in the uninvolved eye [27].

Oculomotor Motility

Strabismus

Strabismus is commonly defined as a deviation of the visual axis. This ocular misalignment can be found at almost any age. The malalignment of the eyes prevents binocular vision. Esotropia (in-turning of one eye) or exotropia (out-turning of one eye) are identified by examining the eyes of the newborn and children for symmetric corneal light reflex and using the cover/uncover test. At birth most infants have a small degree of exotropia that resolves during the first few months of life. Infants can reliably fix with both eyes by 4 months old. An abnormal cover/uncover test or caregiver report of deviation after 4 months old needs evaluation for potential amblyopia [1].

The treatment of strabismus is based on first correcting any refractive disorder, patching for amblyopia if present, and, lastly, surgically

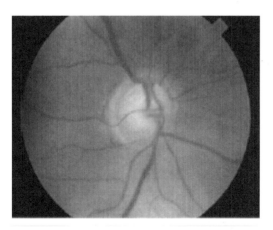

Fig. 9 Chronic open-angle glaucoma with loss of axons; note the centrally excavated optic cup

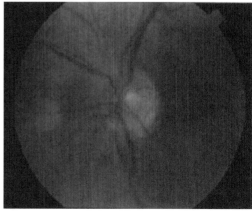

Fig. 10 Normal optic nerve with a healthy, nonexcavated optic cup

realigning the eyes. Visual outcome is best when the problem is diagnosed early [1, 28].

Amblyopia

Amblyopia is defined as a poorly sighted eye secondary to some form of visual deprivation at an early age. Treatment is best when started at a younger age. The US Preventive Services Task Force recommends assessing visual acuity at least once between 3 and 5 years of age to detect amblyopia. Amblyopia is seen in association with strabismus and with refraction disorders [28].

Strabismus produces amblyopia by preventing image stimulation in the fovea of the deviated eye. Occasionally, the diagnosis is made using a red reflex test with a direct ophthalmic scope held about 3 feet from the child's eyes. A difference in the red reflex may indicate a refractive error, amblyopia, or an opacity in the ocular media [28].

Anisometropia is a difference in the refractive status between the eyes leading to amblyopia. Treatment of amblyopia is aimed at restoring the suppressed visual input by occluding the more favored eye with a patch, colored lenses, or pharmacologic intervention. Treatment is more successful when started under 7 years old, but older children may benefit from treatment [1, 28].

Optical Defects

Refractive Disorders

A refractive disorder occurs because the focal point of light does not fall on the retina. In addition to glasses, excimer laser surgery has produced safe and accurate correction of refractive disorders. Laser-assisted in situ keratomileusis (LASIK) is the most common refractive procedure performed today. In LASIK, the corneal stroma is remodeled with computer-controlled assistance to focus images on the retina of the eye. Recovery is usually within days to weeks. Complications, although rare, include under- and overcorrections, diffuse keratitis, and infection. Phakic intraocular lenses are an emerging option for surgical correction with very high myopia [29].

Accommodation Loss or Presbyopia

Accommodation, the ability to adjust the optic power of the eye, decreases from childhood to about age 75. In the normal human eye, as accommodation occurs, the ciliary body contracts, relaxing the zonules (or fibers) to the lens of the eye, and an active increase in lens curvature occurs, increasing the optical power of the eye. As the eye ages, hardening (sclerosis) of the lens reduces the elasticity of the lens capsule and plasticity of the lens core, resulting in a loss of accommodative amplitude. To correct this loss, reading glasses and monocular vision using contacts are prescribed. Options for surgical treatment include LASIK to achieve monovision and multifocal or accommodating intraocular lenses if cataract surgery is indicated [30].

References

1. Bell AL, Rodes ME, Kellar LC. Childhood eye examination. Am Fam Physician. 2013;88(4):241–9.
2. Vorvick L, Reinhardt R. A differential guide to 5 common eye complaints. J Fam Pract. 2013;62(7):345–55.
3. Dupré AA, Wightman JM. Chapter 19. Red and painful eye. In: Walls RM, Hockberger RS, Gausche-Hill M, editors. Rosen's emergency medicine: concepts and clinical practice. 9th ed. Philadelphia: Elsevier; 2018.
4. Boboridis KG, Bunce C. Interventions for involutional lower lid entropion (review). Cochrane Database Syst Rev. 2011;(12):CD002221. https://doi.org/10.1002/14651858.CD002221.pub2.
5. Michels KS, Czyz CN, Cahill KV, Foster JA, Burns JA, Everman KR. Age-matched, case-controlled comparison of clinical indicators for development of entropion and ectropion. J Ophthalmol. 2014;2014:231487. https://doi.org/10.1155/2014/231487. PMID: 24734167 PMCID: PMC3964688.
6. Chang S, Lehrman C, Itani K, Rohrich RJ. A systematic review of comparison of upper eyelid involutional ptosis repair techniques: efficacy and complication rates. Plast Reconstr Surg. 2012;129(1):149–57.
7. Dunlop AL, Wells JR. Approach to red eye for primary care practitioners. Prim Care. 2015;42(3):267–84. PMID: 26319338.
8. Deibel JP, Cowling K. Ocular inflammation and infection. Emerg Med Clin North Am. 2013;31:387–97.

9. Meltzer DI. Painless red eye. Am Fam Physician. 2013;88(8):533–4.

10. Rezvan F, Khabazkhoob M, Hooshmand E, Yekta A, Saatchi M, Hashemi H. Prevalence and risk factors of pterygium: a systematic review and meta-analysis. Surv Ophthalmol. 2018;63(5):719–35. https://doi.org/10.1016/j.survophthal.2018.03.001. PMID: 29551597.

11. Thulasi P, Djalilian AR. Update in current diagnostics and therapeutics of dry eye disease. Ophthalmology. 2017;124(11):S27–33. https://doi.org/10.1016/j.ophtha.2017.07.022. PMID: 29055359.

12. American Academy of Ophthalmology Cornea/External Disease Panel, Hoskins Center for Quality Eye Care. Preferred practice pattern® guidelines. Dry eye syndrome. San Francisco: American Academy of Ophthalmology; 2018. https://doi.org/10.1016/j.ophtha.2018.10.023.

13. Atfeh MS, Khalil HS. Orbital infections: five-year case series, literature review and guideline development. J Laryngol Otol. 2015;7:670–6. https://doi.org/10.1017/S0022215115001371.

14. Pelletier AL, Rojas-Roldan L, Coffin J. Vision loss in older persons. Am Fam Physician. 2016;94(3):219–26. PMID: 27479624.

15. Braithwaite T, Nanji AA, Lindsley K, Greenberg PB. Anti-vascular endothelial growth factor for macular oedema secondary to central retinal vein occlusion. Cochrane Database Syst Rev. 2014;(5):CD007325. https://doi.org/10.1002/14651858.CD007325.pub3.

16. D'Amico DJ. Primary retinal detachment. N Engl J Med. 2008;359:2346–54.

17. Virgili G, Parravano M, Evans JR, Gordon I, Lucenteforte E. Anti-vascular endothelial growth factor for diabetic macular oedema: a network meta-analysis. Cochrane Database Syst Rev. 2018;(10):CD007419. https://doi.org/10.1002/14651858.CD007419.pub6.

18. Cheung N, Mitchell P, Wong TY. Diabetic retinopathy. Lancet. 2010;376(9735):124–36. https://doi.org/10.1016/S0140-6736(09)62124-3. PMID: 20580421.

19. Evans JR, Michelessi M, Virgili G. Laser photocoagulation for proliferative diabetic retinopathy. Cochrane Database Syst Rev. 2014;(11):CD011234. https://doi.org/10.1002/14651858.CD011234.pub2.

20. Solomon SD, Lindsley K, Vedula SS, Krzystolik MG, Hawkins BS. Anti-vascular endothelial growth factor for neovascular age-related macular degeneration. Cochrane Database Syst Rev. 2019;(3):CD005139. https://doi.org/10.1002/14651858.CD005139.pub4.

21. Micieli JA, Margolin E. A 55-year-old man with severe papilledema. JAMA. 2015;313(9):963–4.

22. Chiang J, Wong E, Whatham A, Hennessy M, Kalloniatis M, Zangerl B. The usefulness of multimodal imaging for differentiating pseudopapilloedema and true swelling of the optic nerve head: a review and case series. Clin Exp Optom. 2015;98:12–24.

23. Thompson J, Lakhani N. Cataracts. Prim Care. 2015;42(3):409–23. https://doi.org/10.1016/j.pop.2015.05.012. PMID: 26319346.

24. Jonas JB, Aung T, Bourne RR, Bron AM, Ritch R, Panda-Jonas S. Glaucoma. Lancet. 2017;390 (10108):2183–93. https://doi.org/10.1016/S0140-6736(17)31469-1. Epub 2017 May 31. PMID: 28577860.

25. Vass C, Hirn C, Sycha T, Findl O, Sacu S, Bauer P, Schmetterer L. Medical interventions for primary open angle glaucoma and ocular hypertension. Cochrane Database Syst Rev. 2007;(4):CD003167. https://doi.org/10.1002/14651858.CD003167.pub3.

26. Burr J, Azuara-Blanco A, Avenell A, Tuulonen A. Medical versus surgical interventions for open angle glaucoma. Cochrane Database Syst Rev. 2012;(9):CD004399. https://doi.org/10.1002/14651858.CD004399.pub3.

27. Prum BE Jr, Rosenberg LF, Gedde SJ, Mansberger SL, Stein JD, Moroi SE, Herndon LW Jr, Lim MC, Williams RD. Primary open-angle glaucoma preferred practice pattern® guidelines. Ophthalmology. 2016;123(1):P41–P111. https://doi.org/10.1016/j.ophtha.2015.10.053. Epub 2015 Nov 12. PMID: 26581556.

28. Bradfield YS. Identification and treatment of amblyopia. Am Fam Physician. 2013;87(5):348–52.

29. Barsam A, Allan BDS. Excimer laser refractive surgery versus phakic intraocular lenses for the correction of moderate to high myopia. Cochrane Database Syst Rev. 2014;(6):CD007679. https://doi.org/10.1002/14651858.CD007679.pub4.

30. Wolffsohn JS, Davies LN. Presbyopia: effectiveness of correction strategies. Prog Retin Eye Res. 2019;68:124–43. https://doi.org/10.1016/j.preteyeres.2018.09.004. Epub 2018 Sep 19. PMID: 30244049.

Part XVI

The Ear, Nose, and Throat

Gretchen Irwin

Contents

Acute Otitis Media

Acute otitis media (AOM), an infection most often caused by *Streptococcus pneumoniae*, *Haemophilus influenzae*, or *Moraxella catarrhalis*, will affect one in four children by age 10 [1]. Differentiating the infectious AOM from the noninfectious otitis media with effusion (OME) is a critical skill for accurate diagnosis as both conditions demonstrate fluid trapped in the middle ear on physical exam.

G. Irwin (✉)
University of Kansas School of Medicine-Wichita,
Wichita, KS, USA
e-mail: girwin2@kumc.edu

© Springer Nature Switzerland AG 2022
P. M. Paulman et al. (eds.), *Family Medicine*,
https://doi.org/10.1007/978-3-030-54441-6_79

Epidemiology

Acute otitis media is a common diagnosis in young children. Each year in the United States, more than 2.2 million episodes of acute otitis media occur [2]. Risk factors for acute otitis media include male gender, Native American ethnicity, having multiple siblings in the home, premature birth, bottle-fed status, tobacco smoke exposure, family history of recurrent AOM, and attendance at an out-of-home day care [3, 4]. Typically, incidence peaks in the first year of life and declines after age 5 years with more than 80% of children having an acute otitis media infection before starting school [5]. Additionally, children with earlier onset of first episode of AOM may be more likely to have recurrent disease and complications leading to morbidity and mortality [4].

Diagnosis

Acute otitis media is a clinical diagnosis that should be based on history and physical exam findings. The American Academy of Pediatrics published guidelines in 2013 to help clinicians to limit over diagnosis and subsequent overtreatment of AOM. Bulging of a tympanic membrane with either associated intense erythema or recent onset of ear pain or new onset of otorrhea not explained by otitis externa are common presentations of AOM [6]. Middle ear effusion alone is not sufficient to diagnose acute otitis media, as otitis media with effusion (OME) may also present in this manner [6]. The major factor that distinguishes acute otitis media and otitis media with effusion is that OME is not an infectious process and as such there should not be signs of infection such as an erythematous tympanic membrane or otalgia.

Treatment

Treatment for AOM has been controversial in recent years as guidelines designed to promote watchful waiting in lieu of immediate antibiotic therapy often had poor adoption by physicians [7].

Current guidelines published by the American Academy of Pediatrics in 2013 emphasize the need for adequate analgesia for children during an AOM episode and offer clear definitions of children who would be most likely to benefit from observation rather than immediate antibiotic therapy. A Cochrane review of 13 randomized controlled trials that included 3401 children and 3938 episodes of acute otitis media concluded that antibiotics did not significantly reduce pain in the immediate infection phase or abnormal tympanometry findings in the long term [8]. Severe complications were rare regardless of treatment with antibiotics or watchful waiting; however, adverse effects such as vomiting, diarrhea, or rash were common with 1 child affected for every 14 children treated [8].

Analgesia

Acute otitis media is associated with significant pain that may persist for up to 7 days, despite antibiotic therapy [9]. Both oral and topical medication choices exist to alleviate pain associated with AOM. Oral ibuprofen or acetaminophen as well as topical procaine, phenazone, or benzocaine has all been shown to be effective for AOM-related pain [10, 11]. Narcotic pain medications, antihistamines, and decongestants are associated with significant side effects that outweigh any potential analgesic benefit for AOM [10, 12]. Other pain relief options may include naturopathic remedies or osteopathic manipulation though randomized controlled trials that demonstrate effectiveness of these options are limited [13, 14].

Antibiotic Therapy

All children older than 6 months with evidence of acute otitis media with otorrhea or who have severe symptoms should receive immediate antibiotic therapy [6]. Severe symptoms include toxic appearance, persistent otalgia for more than 48 h, temperature greater than 39 °C in the last 48 h, or uncertain ability to follow-up [6]. Severe bulging of the tympanic membrane may also be a sign that antibiotic treatment is warranted. Additionally, children less than 2 years of age with bilateral acute otitis media should receive immediate antibiotic therapy [6].

First-line antibiotic treatment for acute otitis media remains amoxicillin 80–90 mg/kg/day [3]. Currently, amoxicillin (90 mg/kg/day)-clavulanate (6.4 mg/kg/day) remains the second-line choice for antibiotic treatment of otitis media. However, new studies suggest that lower doses of clavulanate (2.85 vs. 6.4 mg/kg/day) may provide similar effectiveness with less diarrhea or diaper rash [15].

Special circumstances that may necessitate the use of an alternative antibiotic are described in Table 1.

Children less than 2 years of age should be treated for 10 days with antibiotics, while older children may be offered a 5–7-day course of therapy [6]. Any child who fails to improve after appropriate antibiotic therapy should be considered a candidate for tympanocentesis and culture of middle ear fluid to guide therapy [6].

Observation

Children who are older than 6 months with unilateral AOM without otorrhea or severe symptoms or children older than 2 years with bilateral AOM without otorrhea or severe symptoms are candidates for observation rather than immediate antibiotic therapy [6]. Severe complications are rare regardless of whether or not a child receives antibiotics [8]. No child should be offered observation as a treatment option if there is concern that the child will not be able to return for evaluation or obtain antibiotics if they fail to improve in 48–72 h of onset of symptoms [6]. As 78% of AOM episodes will resolve spontaneously and antibiotic side effects such as rash and diarrhea are common, observation in well-chosen patients is a reasonable option [17].

Surgical Options

Children who have more than three episodes of AOM within a 6-month period or more than four episodes of AOM within a year should be referred for evaluation for tympanostomy tubes [18]. Tympanostomy tubes may result in improved hearing initially though continued superiority to watchful waiting with respect to improved hearing is not sustained at 12–24 months [19]. Referral should focus on a careful weighing of risks and benefits of tympanostomy placement individualized for each child.

Complications

Acute otitis media can be associated with significant complications. Hearing loss may be a temporary result of fluid within the middle ear. Unfortunately, fluid may remain for weeks or months following an episode of AOM. Though hearing loss may be frustrating for both child and parents during this time, little evidence exists that speech and language delays result from this hearing loss alone [20–22]. Of note, however, rarely permanent sensorineural hearing loss may occur as a result of AOM.

Balance problems, tympanic membrane perforation, and cholesteatoma may also result from acute otitis media with recurrent episodes increasing risk [23]. Chronic suppurative otitis media, mastoiditis, petrositis, labyrinthitis, meningitis,

Table 1 When to use antibiotics other than amoxicillin for AOM [6, 16]

Special circumstance	Antibiotic choice instead of amoxicillin
Child had amoxicillin in prior 30 days	Amoxicillin-clavulanate (90 mg/kg/day amoxicillin and 6.4 mg/kg/day clavulanate)
Child has concurrent bacterial conjunctivitis	Amoxicillin-clavulanate (90 mg/kg/day amoxicillin and 6.4 mg/kg/day clavulanate)
Child has penicillin allergy	Cefdinir, cefuroxime, cefpodoxime, or ceftriaxone
Child has tympanostomy tubes in place	Topical ciprofloxacin/dexamethasone
Child on amoxicillin not improving in 48–72 h	Amoxicillin-clavulanate (90 mg/kg/day amoxicillin and 6.4 mg/kg/day clavulanate), ceftriaxone, or clindamycin

abscess in the brain or epidural space or thrombosis of the lateral sinus, cavernous sinus, or carotid artery may also result from acute otitis media. Thankfully, these complications are rare. Of note, no studies have demonstrated an increase in meningitis or mastoiditis since implementation of observation guidelines in children [4].

Prevention

Effective prevention strategies would yield large benefits given the prevalence of AOM. While no targeted acute otitis media vaccine exists, introduction of higher-valent pneumococcal vaccines as well as increased influenza vaccination rates have resulted in risk reduction for AOM [24–26]. Supplementation with vitamin D and zinc has been shown to be beneficial only in children with documented nutritional deficiencies [27–29]. Xylitol, a polyol sugar alcohol found in raspberries, has been demonstrated to be effective at preventing acute otitis media though current dosing requirements of administration five times daily make its use limited [30]. Formula-fed infants may benefit from probiotics such as *Lactobacillus rhamnosus* GG, and *Bifidobacterium lactis* Bb-12 [31]. However, exclusive breastfeeding may be more beneficial as a risk reduction strategy than probiotic-supplemented formula [3]. Overall, more research into the role of probiotics is needed as early studies are promising, but limited evidence exists to identify the optimal strain, duration, dose frequency or timing of probiotic administration [32]. In infants, eliminating exposure to passive tobacco smoke and reducing pacifier use after 7 months of life may also lead to reduced incidence of AOM [3].

Otitis Externa

Otitis externa may result from infectious or allergic causes that lead to inflammation of the external auditory canal. Usually inflammation is diffuse throughout the ear canal. Three forms of otitis externa have been described, namely, acute otitis externa (AOE) which lasts for less than 6 weeks, chronic otitis externa (COE) which lasts for more than 3 months and malignant otitis externa. AOE is likely to be the result of a bacterial infection whereas COE most often results from allergy or underlying dermatologic condition [33].

Epidemiology

While the exact incidence of otitis externa is unknown, estimates suggest 10% of people will be affected at some time throughout their lives [34]. Acute otitis externa tends to occur in warm, humid climates and in individuals with narrow ear canals [33]. While children aged 7–12 may be affected, acute otitis externa is seen more commonly in adults [33]. Risk factors for disease include ear trauma such as from cotton swab use, hearing aids, and dermatologic conditions such as eczema or psoriasis. Water exposure is also a risk factor leading to the common name for AOE of swimmer's ear.

Pathophysiology

Acute otitis externa is most often caused by bacterial infection with *Pseudomonas aueriginosa* accounting for 22–62% of infections and *Staphlyococcus aureus* accounting for 11–34% of cases [35]. Polymicrobial infection is common. While only accounting for 10% of cases of acute otitis externa, infection with *Aspergillus niger* and *Candida* species has been reported after prolonged antibiotic use [33]. Polymicrobial infections have also been reported.

Cerumen provides a critical protective function in the ear by limiting exposure of skin to moisture and creating an acidic pH that is inhospitable to bacterial growth. Removal of cerumen with cotton swabs eliminates this protective barrier and creates a trauma to the ear canal that can result in infection. Similarly, water exposure can cause epithelial breakdown also leading to infection [36].

Diagnosis

Most often, patients with acute otitis externa present with symptoms of ear inflammation such as pain, itching or fullness with sudden onset

[37]. Pain is often worsened with manipulation of the pinna or tragus. Additionally, patients may experience otorrhea, hearing loss or jaw pain [37].

Diagnosis of acute otitis externa should be made clinically with history and otoscopic examination of the affected ear. Visualization, or inability to do so, of an intact tympanic membrane is an important physical examination element to guide treatment. Findings of ear canal edema or erythema are also common. Secretions may be present and can be collected for culture, though it is not necessary to do so. Individuals who are immunocompromised or experience frequent infections may benefit from culture.

A differential diagnosis should include consideration for other infections such as perichondritis, erysipelas, otitis media with perforation and herpes zoster oticus as well as eczema, cholesteatoma and carcinoma of the external auditory canal [36].

Treatment

Acute otitis externa is best treated with pain control and topical therapies. Oral antibiotics should only be offered if the patient has poorly controlled diabetes mellitus, immunosuppression, or if the infection has spread beyond the ear canal [38]. Both antiseptic and antibiotic medications can be utilized for treatment with similar effectiveness [38].

Because there are many effective regimens, consideration of side effects, cost and dosing schedule are important when choosing a treatment strategy. For example, neomycin is effective, but ototoxic and cannot be used with a perforated eardrum. Too, neomycin may cause contact dermatitis, worsening itching, and irritation, in up to 30% of patients [39–42]. Fluoroquinolones are often preferred due to twice daily dosing and safety even if the eardrum is ruptured. However, these tend to be more expensive than other options. Some clinicians will offer ophthalmological antibiotic preparations as off label treatment for otitis externa due to cost considerations [38, 43]. Many of the combination regimens will include corticosteroids to lessen edema and hasten resolution of pain and itching [44].

Up to 20–40% of patients receive systemic antibiotics for treatment of acute otitis externa despite efficacy of topical options [20, 21]. Such treatment can increase risk of side effects and antibiotic resistance without offering improved treatment rates. Table 2 describes commonly prescribed regimens.

Regardless of medication chosen, any topical therapy will not be effective if significant cerumen is occluding the canal or if significant edema is present. Also, debris may contain exotoxins such as *Pseudomonas* exotoxin A that can promote inflammation. Gentle suction or direct visualization may be used to remove any cerumen or debris, though irrigation should be avoided in those patients who do not have an intact tympanic membrane, who are immunocompromised, or who have diabetes mellitus as an increased risk of malignant otitis externa has been reported

Table 2 Common topical preparations for acute otitis externa [45]

Component	Cost	Frequency of dosing	Comments	Ok if eardrum perforation
Acetic acid 2% solution	$	Four to six times daily	May increase pain and irritation	No
Acetic acid 2%/hydrocortisone 1% solution	$$$	Four to six times daily	May cause local irritation	No
Neomycin/polymyxin B/hydrocortisone solution	$$	Three to four times daily	Risk of contact hypersensitivity	No
Ciprofloxacin 0.2% solution	$$	BID	Single-use containers	Yes
Ciprofloxacin 0.2%/hydrocortisone 1% suspension	$$$$	BID		Yes
Ciprofloxacin 0.3%/dexamethasone 0.1% suspension	$$$$	BID		Yes
Ofloxacin 0.3% solution	$$$	Daily-BID		Yes

[46]. An ear wick may be used with canal edema to improve drug delivery.

Topical medications should be placed into the ear with the patient lying with the affected ear up. Further, patients should be cautioned that once drops are instilled, a 3–5-min waiting period is necessary before sitting up to allow the medication to be effective [37].

Typical treatment courses are 7 days, though this may be extended to 10 days if patient is not improving. Improvement can be expected within 72 h and significant symptoms beyond 72 h should prompt reevaluation of the patient. Referral to an otolaryngologist is indicated if there is lack of expected improvement, inability to remove debris, or suspected malignant otitis externa.

Over the counter medications such as acetaminophen and ibuprofen are also helpful for pain control. Of note, benzocaine should be avoided as it can lead to contact dermatitis and worsening of symptoms. Patient should be cautioned to avoid water immersion of an affected ear until treatment is concluded. Too, hearing aids should be avoided until pain is improved.

Complications

Infection may extend to surrounding structures, causing chondritis, perichondritis, or facial cellulitis. Over time, patients with chronic infection may develop canal stenosis and conductive hearing loss.

Prevention

Episodes of acute otitis externa may be prevented by avoiding water exposure by either using well-fitting earplugs or using a hair dryer on the lowest setting to dry ears after swimming. Acetic acid 2% drops may also be helpful in acidifying the pH of the ear canal.

Chronic Otitis Externa

Chronic otitis externa is defined as acute otitis externa lasting more than 3 months or with more than four episodes per year [45]. Rather than resulting from bacterial infection, chronic otitis externa is often the result of an underlying skin condition such as atopic dermatitis or psoriasis [45]. Symptoms typically include itching and conductive hearing loss. Unlike acute otitis externa, pain is a rare finding [47]. The physical examination may show erythematous skin with either dry, scaling, or moist debris noted [47]. More than half of individuals have both ears affected [47]. Of most concern with chronic otitis externa is conductive hearing loss as well as chronic fibrosis of the canal which can make it difficult to fit hearing aids [45].

Treatment for chronic otitis externa includes removal of all irritants such as shampoo and soap as well as careful attention to keeping the ear canal dry as much as possible. Too, any underlying skin or autoimmune disease should be treated to improve the overall condition as well as the chronic otitis externa [45].

Malignant (Necrotizing) Otitis Externa

Malignant otitis externa occurs most often in elderly men with diabetes mellitus or immunosuppression [48]. Malignant otitis externa causes destruction of the external auditory canal, perichondritis, and osteomyelitis of the lateral skull base, thus early diagnosis is essential.

Symptoms of malignant otitis externa include intense, nonspecific ear pain, conductive hearing loss, and otorrhea with exam findings of granulations, polyps, or exposed bone [24]. Any individual not responding as predicted to therapy for otitis externa or with severe symptoms should be closely evaluated for malignant otitis externa. Imaging should include both fluorodeoxyglucose positron emission tomography/magnetic resonance imaging as well as high resolution computed tomography to detect osteitis before bone erosions can be appreciated [49]. Additionally, biopsy of the external auditory canal, to rule out tumor or cholesteatoma, and cultures, to guide antibiotic treatment, should be obtained.

Treatment of malignant otitis externa should include at least 4–6 weeks of antibiotics tailored to culture findings [48]. While awaiting sensitivities from culture specimens, empiric therapy directed against *Pseudomonas aeruginosa* is appropriate. Surgery may be needed to remove necrotic tissue.

References

1. Majeed A, Harris T. Acute otitis media in children. BMJ. 1997;315:321–2.
2. Ahmed S, Shapiro NL, Bhattacharyya N. Incremental health care utilization and costs for acute otitis media in children. Laryngoscope. 2014;124(1):301–5.
3. Teele DW, Klein JO, Rosner B, et al. Epidemiology of otitis media during the first seven years of life in children in greater Boston: a prospective cohort study. J Infect Dis. 1989;160(1):83–94.
4. Ladomenou F, et al. Predisposing factors for acute otitis media in infancy. J Infect. 2010;61(1):49–53.
5. Schilder AG, Chonmaitree T, Cripps AW, Rosenfeld RM, Casselbrant ML, Haggard MP, Venekamp RP. Otitis media. Nat Rev Dis Primers. 2016;2:16063.
6. Liberthal AS, Carroll AE, Chonmaitree T, Ganiats TG, et al. The diagnosis and management of acute otitis media. Pediatrics. 2013;131:e964–99.
7. Coco A, Vernacchio L, Horst M, Anderson A. Management of acute otitis media after publication of the 2004 AAP and AAFP clinical practice guideline. Pediatrics. 2010;125(1):214–20.
8. Venekamp RP, Sanders SL, Glasziou PP, et al. Antibiotics for acute otitis media in children. Cochrane Database Syst Rev. 2015;2015(6):CD000219.
9. Rovers MM, Glasziou P, Appelman CL, et al. Antibiotics for acute otitis media: an individual patient data meta-analysis. Lancet. 2006;368(9545):1429–35.
10. Bertin L, Pons G, d'Arthis P. A randomized, double blind, multicentre controlled trial of ibuprofen versus acetaminophen and placebo for symptoms of acute otitis media in children. Fundam Clin Pharmacol. 1996;10:387–92.
11. Adam D, Federspil P, Lukes M. Therapeutic properties and tolerance of procaine and phenazone containing ear drops in infants and very young children. Arzneimittelforschung. 2009;59(10):504–12.
12. Coleman C, Moore M. Decongestants and antihistamines for acute otitis media in children. Cochrane Database Syst Rev. 2008;2008(3):CD001727.
13. Posadzki P, Lee MS, Ernst E. Osteopathic manipulative treatment for pediatric conditions: a systematic review pediatrics. Pediatrics. 2013;132:140–52. https://doi.org/10.1542/peds.2012-3959.
14. Sarrell EM, Mandelberg A, Cohen HA. Efficacy of naturopathic extracts in the management of ear pain associated with acute otitis media. Arch Pediatr Adolesc Med. 2001;155:796–9.
15. Hoberman A, Paradise JL, Rockette HE, et al. Reduced-concentration clavulanate for young children with acute otitis media. Antimicrob Agents Chemother. 2017;61(7):e00238–17.
16. Wright D, Safranek S. Treatment of otitis media with perforated tympanic membrane. Am Fam Physician. 2009;79(8):650–4.
17. Sanders S, Glasziou PP, Del Mar C, Rovers MM. Antibiotics for acute otitis media in children. Cochrane Database Syst Rev. 2004;2004(1): CD000219. https://doi.org/10.1002/14651858. CD000219.pub2.
18. Higgins T, et al. Medical decision analysis: indications for tympanostomy tubes in RAOM by age at first episode. Otolaryngol Head Neck Surg. 2008;138 (1):50–6.
19. Steele DW, Adam GP, Di M, et al. Effectiveness of tympanostomy tubes for otitis media: a meta-analysis. Pediatrics. 2017;139(6):e20170125.
20. Roberts JE, Rosenfeld RM, Zeisel SA. Otitis media and speech and language: a meta-analysis of prospective studies. Pediatrics. 2004;113:e238.
21. Casby MW. Otitis media and language development: a meta-analysis. Am J Speech Lang Pathol. 2001;10:65.
22. Shekelle P, Takata G, Chan L, et al. Diagnosis, natural history, and late effects of otitis media with effusion. Evidence report/technology assessment no. 55. Agency for Healthcare Research and Quality, Rockville. 2003. http://archive.ahrq.gov/downloads/pub/evidence/pdf/otdiag/otdiag.pdf. Accessed 19 Mar 2020.
23. Bluestone CD. Clinical course, complications and sequelae of acute otitis media. Pediatr Infect Dis J. 2000;19:S37.
24. Casey J, Adlowitz D, Pichichero M. New patterns in the otopathogens causing acute otitis media six to eight years after introduction of the pneumococcal conjugate vaccine. Pediatr Infect Dis J. 2010;29(4):304–9.
25. Pichichero M, Kaur R, Scott D, et al. Effectiveness of 13-valent pneumococcal conjugate vaccination for protection against acute otitis media caused by *Streptococcus pneumoniae* in healthy young children: a prospective observational study. Lancet Child Adolesc Health. 2018;2(8):561–8.
26. Mohd N, Ho J, Mohd A. Influenza vaccines for preventing acute otitis media in infants and children. Cochrane Database Syst Rev. 2017;10(10):CD010089.
27. Marchisio P, Consonni D, Baggi E, Zampiero A, et al. Vitamin D supplementation reduces the risk of acute otitis media in otitis-prone children. Pediatr Infect Dis J. 2013;32(10):1055–60.
28. Abba K, Gulani A, Sachdev H. Zinc supplements for preventing otitis media. Cochrane Database Syst Rev. 2010;2010(2):CD006639.
29. Marchisio P, et al. Effectiveness of a propolis and zinc solution in preventing acute otitis media in children with a history of recurrent acute otitis media. Int J Immunopathol Pharmacol. 2010;23(2):567–75.
30. Azarpazhooh A, Lawrence H, Shah P. Xylitol for preventing acute otitis media in children up to 12 years of age. Cochrane Database Syst Rev. 2016;2016(8): CD007095.
31. Rautava S, Salminen S, Isolauri E. Specific probiotics in reducing the risk of acute infections in infancy – a randomised double blind, placebo-controlled study. Br J Nutr. 2009;101(11):1722–6.

32. Scott A, Clark H, Julien B, et al. Probiotics for preventing acute otitis media in children. Cochrane Database Syst Rev. 2019;6(6):CD012941.
33. Hajioff D, MacKeith S. Otitis externa. BMJ Clin Evid. 2015;2015:0510.
34. Raza SA, Denholm SW, Wong JC. An audit of the management of otitis externa in an ENT casualty clinic. J Laryngol Otol. 1995;109:130–3.
35. Roland PS, Stroman DW. Microbiology of acute otitis externa. Laryngoscope. 2002;112(7 Pt 1):1166–77.
36. Neher A, Nagl M, Scholtz AW. Otitis externa. HNO. 2008;56:1067–80.
37. Rosenfeld RM, Schwartz SR, Cannon CR, et al. Clinical practice guideline: acute otitis externa. Otolaryngol Head Neck Surg. 2014;150(Suppl 1):S1–24.
38. Kaushik V, Malik T, Saeed SR. Interventions for acute otitis externa. Cochrane Database Syst Rev. 2010;2010(1):CD004740.
39. Sander R. Otitis externa: a practical guide to treatment and prevention. Am Fam Physician. 2001;63:927–37.
40. Sood S, Strachan DR, Tsikoudas A, Stables GI. Allergic otitis externa. Clin Otolaryngol Allied Sci. 2002;27:233–6.
41. Rutka J. Acute otitis externa: treatment perspectives. Ear Nose Throat J. 2004;83(9 Suppl 4):20–1.
42. Devos SA, Mulder JJ, van der Valk PG. The relevance of positive patch test reactions in chronic otitis externa. Contact Dermatitis. 2000;42:354–5.
43. Rosenfeld RM, Singer M, Wasserman JM, Stinnett SS. Systematic review of topical antimicrobial therapy for acute otitis externa. Otolaryngol Head Neck Surg. 2006;134(4):24–48.
44. Mosges R, Schroder T, Baues CM, Sahin K. Dexamethasone phosphate in antibiotic ear drops for the treatment of acute bacterial otitis externa. Curr Med Res Opin. 2008;24(8): 2339–47.
45. Wiegand S, Berner R, Schneider A, Lundershausen E, Dietz A. Otitis externa. Dtsch Arztebl Int. 2019;116 (13):224–34.
46. Rubin J, Yu VL, Kamerer DB, Wagener M. Aural irrigation with water: a potential pathogenic mechanism for inducing malignant external otitis? Ann Otol Rhinol Laryngol. 1990;99 (2 Pt 1):117–9.
47. Kesser BW. Assessment and management of chronic otitis externa. Curr Opin Otolaryngol Head Neck Surg. 2011;19:341–7.
48. Mahdyoun P, Pulcini C, Gahide I, et al. Necrotizing otitis externa: a systematic review. Otol Neurotol. 2013;34:620–9.
49. van Kroonenburgh AMJL, van der Meer WL, Bothof RJP, van Tilburg M, van Tongeren J, Postma AA. Advanced imaging techniques in skull base osteomyelitis due to malignant otitis externa. Curr Radiol Rep. 2018;6(1):3.

Disorders of the Oral Cavity

Nicholas Galioto and Erik Egeland

Contents

The mouth has been described as a window to general health. Oral health can directly affect overall health and can have a significant impact on the overall quality of life of the individual patient [1]. Disease in the mouth can cause systemic disease such as endocarditis, make chronic disease management such as diabetes more difficult, or lead to adverse pregnancy outcomes [2, 3]. In addition, a thorough oral exam may provide clues to the timely diagnosis of systemic infections, immunologic diseases, hematologic conditions, and nutritional disorders [2, 3].

N. Galioto (✉) · E. Egeland
Department of Family Medicine, Broadlawns Medical Center, Des Moines, IA, USA
e-mail: ngalioto@broadlawns.org

© Springer Nature Switzerland AG 2022
P. M. Paulman et al. (eds.), *Family Medicine*,
https://doi.org/10.1007/978-3-030-54441-6_80

Caries

Dental caries or tooth decay is the most common chronic disease worldwide [1]. Fifty percent of children between the ages of 6 and 8 years old have dental caries, and nearly 24% of adults age 24–64 have untreated dental caries [3–5]. Dental caries develops through the complex interaction of oral microorganisms (*Streptococcus mutans* and lactobacilli), metabolizing dietary sugars into lactic acid creating an acidic environment [3, 5–6]. This acidic environment leads to demineralization of the tooth's protective enamel coating and subsequent tooth decay. When the subsequent caries or decay penetrates through the full thickness of the enamel to reach the underlying dentin layer, patients will begin to typically experience mild intermittent tooth pain or sensitivity to thermal changes or sugary foods. This process is also known as reversible pulpitis and is treated through the mechanical removal of the decayed area and restoration through the placement of a dental filling [1, 4, 6]. As the demineralization process progresses, areas of dental caries may become brown or black stained making them more visible to the naked eye. If the caries goes untreated, irreversible pulpitis may ensue resulting in severe persistent dental pain despite removal of any inciting stimulus. The patient with irreversible pulpitis will often present with poorly localized pain or even pain referred to the opposite jaw [4, 6]. Once again definitive treatment involves mechanical removal of the decay through restoration, root canal or extraction by a dentist. Insufficient evidence exists in the literature to recommend antibiotic therapy, unless infection has spread to the surrounding soft tissue [4–6].

Dental exams should begin by the time patients are 1 year of age. However, the most cost-effective intervention for prevention is the public health policy of adding 0.7–1.0 parts per million of fluoride to the municipal water supply [4]. Fluoride's mechanism of action helps to strengthen tooth enamel and also has a bacteriostatic effect. Whether or not local water has been fluoridated, the effectiveness of topical fluoride has been well established. When compared with mouth rinses or gels, fluoridated toothpastes have a similar degree of effectiveness for the prevention of dental caries in children [4]. Parents should introduce tooth brushing with a smear of low-fluoride toothpaste to children as the first teeth erupt and younger than 2 years of age. Children 2–5 years of age should use a pea-sized amount of fluoride toothpaste [1]. The use of mouth rinses and gels at home is not recommended for children younger than 6 years. Tooth brushing with fluoridated toothpaste twice a day after meals is recommended as an effective way to prevent tooth decay on exposed surfaces, and flossing daily helps prevent plaque build-up on interdental surfaces. Children and adolescents should also be considered for dental sealants when they are most likely not to be compliant with daily dental hygiene regimes [1, 6]. Sealants are resinous materials that are professionally applied to the biting surfaces of teeth most susceptible to decay (molars and premolars). These sealants create a barrier against acid environments and bacterial penetration. Within the adult population, medications that decrease saliva production can be an added risk factor for carries formation [1, 3]. Additionally, dietary changes such as reducing the amount and frequency of foods with caffeine or high sugar content may further decrease dental caries rates [1, 3].

Periodontal Diseases

Periodontal disease is an inflammatory response caused mainly by bacterial colonization within the subgingival dental plaque. Though bacterial colonization is an essential component to the development of periodontal disease, certain conditions such as Down syndrome, Papillion–Lefevre syndrome, diabetes, xerostomia, medications, and smoking may further dispose a patient to periodontal disease [3, 4]. Some evidence also suggests that the presence of chronic periodontal disease may exacerbate the progression of certain diseases such as diabetes and cardiovascular disease and maybe associated with an increased incidence of preterm labor [4, 5, 7]. Periodontal disease can be divided into gingivitis and periodontitis.

Gingivitis

Gingivitis is characterized by reversible inflammation of the gums. Patients present with erythematous swollen tender gums that bleed with routine brushing or flossing. Halitosis may also be present. Pregnancy or other hormonal changes may increase the prevalence of gingivitis in female patients [7]. Medications such as phenytoin, calcium channel blockers, and cyclosporine can also lead to increased inflammatory or non-inflammatory gingival hyperplasia [5]. Care should include removing any offending agents such as medications and tobacco and improved daily oral hygiene. General measures for treating and future prevention include improved oral hygiene with frequent tooth brushing, daily flossing, and use of warm saline or chlorhexidine gluconate 0.12% rinses [1, 4, 5]. Mouth rinses containing essential oils such as Listerine has been shown to be as effective as chlorhexidine but with less tooth staining [4, 5]. Antibiotics are not necessary unless patient presents with acute necrotizing ulcerative gingivitis also known as Vincent's disease or trench mouth [6]. Trench mouth is caused by anaerobic bacteria (*Treponema*, *Selenomonas*, *Fusobacterium*, and *Prevotella intermedia*) and typically presents in patients whose host defenses are compromised by poor oral hygiene, poor nutrition, or systemic illness. Clinically the gingival tissue is denuded with punched-out crater-like areas of necrosis and is accompanied by pain, fetid breath odor, fever, malaise, and cervical lymphadenopathy. In addition to the general measures for treating gingivitis, patients should be prescribed penicillin VK 500 mg orally every 6 h or metronidazole 500 mg orally twice daily [6]. Patients should be given a 7-day course of either regime depending on patient allergy history and/or prescriber preference.

Periodontitis

If left untreated, chronic gingivitis over a period of months to years progresses to periodontitis. Persistent exposure of the mouth to plaque-associated bacteria leads to a local and systemic inflammatory response. This inflammatory response leads to the destruction of the tooth's underlying supporting tissue and alveolar bone. Clinical presentation may demonstrate deep inflamed painful gums with deep gum pockets that bleed easily, heavy tooth plaque, receding gums with exposed root, and loose teeth. Proliferation of bacteria within the deep gum pockets can lead to periodontal abscess formation, which in addition to pain and swelling is further characterized by suppurative drainage. The most common organisms implicated in periodontitis are gram-negative bacteria such as *Actinobacillus actinomycetemcomitans*, *Porphyromonas gingivalis*, and spirochetes [6]. General measures for treating periodontitis should be aggressive plaque descaling by a dentist, incision and drainage of local abscess, and good oral hygiene practices as outlined in the gingivitis section. Antibiotics are indicated when an abscess spreads to the deeper tissues of the oral cavity causing facial swelling and lymphadenopathy or if generalized periodontitis exists where the patient has multiple loose teeth [4–5]. Antibiotic regimes include doxycycline 100 mg daily, metronidazole 500 mg orally twice daily, or topical application of metronidazole, doxycycline, or minocycline [4–5]. Periodontitis is a common and serious condition affecting approximately 20% of all adults and is the leading cause of tooth loss [5]. Besides causing focal oral disease, multiple studies demonstrate an association between periodontitis and cardiovascular disease, worsening diabetes, and increased risk for preterm labor [5, 7]. However, no study has demonstrated whether treating or preventing periodontal disease leads to improved systemic disease outcomes [5].

Candidiasis

Candida species are normal inhabitants of the gastrointestinal tract and present as part of the normal oral flora in 60% of healthy adults [3, 5, 8]. Certain local and systemic factors may make certain individuals more susceptible to oral candidal infections. These include infection with human immunodeficiency virus (HIV), diabetes or glucose intolerance, xerostomia, malnutrition, presence of dentures, patients with cancer, medications (broad spectrum antibiotics, inhaled or systemic steroids, chemotherapy), and reduced immunity related to age [3, 5, 8]. Oral candidiasis is common in infants, affecting 1–37% of newborns [8]. Diagnosis is usually made through a history of risk factors and symptoms. The most common presentation is of painless adherent curd-like white patches along the oral mucosa and/or tongue. These white patches can be partially wiped off using a tongue blade or gauze and diagnosis confirmed either by culture or by preparing a potassium hydroxide slide looking for hyphae. Oral candidiasis may also present as erythema of the oral mucosa especially in denture wearers and/or as angular cheilitis/perleche (painful, erythematous fissures at the corners of the mouth). Common treatments include nystatin suspension 100,000 U/ml four to six times daily, Mycelex (clotrimazole) troches 10 mg five times a day, or fluconazole (Diflucan) 200 mg orally on day one then 100–200 mg daily [3, 5, 8]. Infants should be treated with nystatin suspension 0.5 ml in each cheek, massaging the cheeks to spread throughout the oral cavity. Fluconazole 6 mg/kg orally on day one and 3 mg/kg thereafter may be used as an alternative for resistant cases. All regimes are used for an average of 7–14 days [5, 8]. All pacifiers and bottle nipples should be boiled. In breastfed infants, mother's nipples may be treated if needed, with topical antifungal creams or ointment. The use of probiotics for either prophylaxis or adjunctive treatment of recurrent or primary candidiasis has shown some favorable benefit; however, further studies are needed to confirm effectives, dosages, and side effects [9].

Stomatitis

Characterized by inflammation of the mucosal lining of the mouth, lesions are erythematous, painful, and can be ulcerated. Most common conditions include hand–foot–mouth disease, herpetic stomatitis, and recurrent aphthous

stomatitis/ulcers. Additional causes include herpangina, nicotinic stomatitis, and denture-related stomatitis. Any remaining causes are considered rare and uncommon. The most common forms of stomatitis present with shallow ulcerations less than 1 cm in diameter and resolve spontaneously over 10–14 days [5, 8]. Patients usually present with complaints of burning sensation, localized pain, irritation with certain foods, and intolerance to temperature changes. Recurrent aphthous ulcers or "canker sores" affects 5–21% of the population and etiology remains unclear [8]. Treatment focus is on providing topical relief. Topical agents that can be used include 2% viscous lidocaine or topical steroid such as Kenalog in Orabase applied in small amounts with a cotton swab three to four times daily. Additionally various combinations of "Magic Mouthwash" can be compounded for a swish and spit rinse three to four times daily. Suggested compounds mixed in equal parts have consisted of a thick base coating liquid such as Maalox, Mylanta, Carafate, or Nystatin mixed with, diphenhydramine, plus 2% viscous lidocaine or hydrocortisone. Caution should be noted that overuse of products containing lidocaine may cause cardiac arrhythmias. Since disease course is generally self-limited, when an ulcer persists beyond 3 weeks, other causes should be considered. Nutritional deficiencies, such as folate, B_{12}, B_6, or iron, drug reactions, Behcet's disease, Reiter's syndrome, inflammatory bowel disease, celiac sprue, lichen planus, and HIV infection have all been associated with recurrent aphthous ulcers [5, 8, 10]. Additionally, squamous cell cancer may present as a non-healing or non-resolving ulcer, and biopsy of the ulcer should be considered [5].

Lichen Planus

Lichen planus is a chronic inflammatory condition that is most likely a T cell-mediated autoimmune disease [11]. Lichen planus affects approximately 1–2% of the population, more often in those over age 40 and a slight predilection in perimenopausal women [5, 8, 12]. In women with oral lichen planus, 20% of them will also have concomitant involvement of the vulva and vagina [11, 12]. Patients with lichen planus have also showed a greater prevalence for exposure to hepatitis C (HCV), making it appropriate to screen patients with lichen planus for HCV infection [12]. There are four forms of oral lichen planus: reticular, atrophic, bullous, and erosive. The reticular form is the most common and manifests as asymptomatic bilateral white lace striations on the oral mucosa. The atrophic form presents as erythematous atrophic-appearing lesions within the oral mucosa and may be more painful than the reticular form. The bullous form manifests as fluid-filled vesicles, while the erosive form leads to ulcerated erythematous, painful lesions. Patients can often have a burning sensation within their mouth. Management options should start with good oral hygiene, avoiding irritating foods and tobacco products. Medium- to high-potency topical steroids are first-line therapy to treat symptomatic lichen planus [5, 12]. Clobetasol 0.05% or fluocinonide 0.05% is applied twice daily to lesions [11, 12]. Patients with widespread oral disease or diffuse ulcerations may not adequately respond to corticosteroids alone. Topical calcineurin inhibitors such as pimecrolimus 1% (Elidel) or tacrolimus 0.1% (Protopic) or topical retinoids can be effective second line or adjunctive forms of therapy for these patients [11, 12]. Patients refractory to standard topical therapies may have using oral retinoids such as alitretinoin [13].

Glossitis

Geographic tongue also known as known as benign migratory glossitis affects 1–14% of the population and is of unknown etiology [14, 15]. Geographic tongue is characterized by areas of papillary atrophy that appear smooth and are surrounded by raised wavy borders. The regions of atrophy spontaneously resolve and migrate giving the tongue a topographic map appearance. The condition is benign, but some patients may have sensitivity to hot or spicy foods. Treatment for symptomatic patients may include bland foods, use of topical steroids triamcinolone 0.1%

(Oralone) or antihistamine mouth rinses which can also be used to help reduce tongue sensitivity [14, 15].

In fissured tongue, deep groves develop within the tongue usually due to the physiologic deepening of normal tongue fissures secondary to aging. The deeper fissures can lead to food trapping causing inflammation of the tongue and halitosis. Gentle brushing of the tongue is useful in symptomatic patients. Down's syndrome, Sjogren syndrome, Melkersson–Rosenthal syndrome, psoriasis, and geographic tongue have all been associated with fissured tongue [14].

Hairy tongue results from the accumulation of keratin on the filiform papillae of the dorsal tongue leading to hypertrophy of the papillae. The hypertrophied papillae tend to resemble elongated hairs. Bacteria and debris get trapped in the elongated hairs causing discoloration of the tongue. Color of the tongue can range from white to tan to black. This condition is most often associated with smoking, poor oral hygiene, and antibiotic use [4, 14, 16]. Most patients are asymptomatic but some may experience halitosis or abnormal taste. Daily debridement with a soft toothbrush or tongue scrapper can remove the keratinized tissue.

Oral hairy leukoplakia is characterized by white hairy-appearing lesions on the lateral borders of the tongue either in a unilateral or bilateral fashion. This condition is associated with Epstein–Barr super infection or immunocompromised condition [14, 16]. In the absence of a known immunocompromised condition, testing for human immunodeficiency virus (HIV) should be considered. Treatment consists of the use of antiviral medications though recurrences are common. Acyclovir (Zovirax) 800 mg orally five times daily or ganciclovir 100 mg orally three times a day for 1–3 weeks may be used [14].

Atrophic glossitis results from the atrophy of the filiform papillae and is also referred to as smooth tongue. The tongue has a smooth glossy appearance with a red or pink background, and the patient will often complain of a painful sensation within the tongue. Atrophic glossitis is most commonly caused by nutritional deficiencies [14]. Nutritional deficiencies of iron, folic acid, riboflavin, niacin, and B_{12} are most often implicated [14]. Other possible etiologies include syphilis, candidal infection, amyloidosis, celiac disease, Sjogren syndrome, protein malnutrition, and xerostomia [14].

Halitosis

Halitosis is an unpleasant or offensive odor emanating from the oral cavity. In approximately 80% of the cases, halitosis is caused by conditions of the oral cavity [17]. The most likely cause of oral malodor is the accumulation of food debris and bacterial plaque along the teeth and tongue. The oral malodor arises from the microbial degradation of these organic substrates into volatile sulfur-containing gas compounds. Though the majority of cases of halitosis originate in the oral cavity, non-oral etiologies may include infections of the upper or lower respiratory tract, metabolic disturbances, carcinomas, systemic diseases, and medications [17]. Therefore, before halitosis can be managed effectively, an accurate diagnosis must be made. Achieving an accurate diagnosis starts with first determining whether the source of the odor is of an oral or non-oral etiology. One of the simplest ways to distinguish oral from non-oral etiologies is to compare the smell coming from the patient's mouth with that exiting the nose. To perform this sniff test, have the patient tightly hold their lips together and forcibly blow air through the nostrils. Repeat the test with the patient holding their nostrils closed and passively breathing through their mouth. One can then compare the odors emanating from each cavity and further characterize the intensity and quality of the odor. A systemic origin may be suspected in the case where the odor from the mouth and nose are of the same intensity and quality [18].

As noted, the majority of cases of halitosis originate from the oral cavity. The oral cavity should be inspected for evidence of gingivitis, periodontal disease, and oral cancers. All of which can produce foul putrid-smelling breath. In patients where a rigorous oral hygiene regime of twice daily brushing, flossing, and professional cleaning does not improve the problem, the tongue especially the posterior region should be suspected [17, 18]. The posterior tongue can be assessed by obtaining a gentle scrapping of the area using a plastic spoon. The spoon can be smelled to compare the odor with the overall mouth odor [17]. Gentle but thorough tongue cleaning using either a tongue scrapper or toothbrush should be added to the daily oral hygiene routine. Faulty dental restorations or dentures can be another etiology of bad breath. The odor from dentures may have a somewhat sweet though unpleasant nature and can be more easily identified when the dentures are placed in a sealed plastic bag and smelled after a few minutes [17]. Saliva also affects bad breath. Xerostomia or dry mouth may be a contributor to halitosis secondary to decreased salivary flow and the resultant increased risk for dental infections. A transient odor associated with acute tonsillitis is common especially in children. Tonsillectomy, however, is rarely indicated for chronic halitosis [17, 18].

Nasal sources are second in frequency to oral etiologies as causes of halitosis [17, 18]. Nasal odor is often indicative of sinus infection, but may also signal an obstruction to normal air flow that could occur with nasal polyps, craniofacial anomalies, or foreign body (especially in small children). Nasal discharge can have a fetid cheesy odor [17]. The lungs are also a source of some odors secondary to infection and/or metabolic disorders. A pulmonary source is suggested when the odor intensity increases during expiration. Lung abscess, necrotic tumors, tuberculosis, and bronchiectasis are all possible infections causing bad breath. Because of the associated pus production and tissue necrosis with these diseases, a putrid foul odor similar to rotting meat is produced [17]. Hepatic failure, renal failure, and diabetes are all systemic diseases that may contribute to or present as halitosis. Hepatic failure or cirrhosis may have a mousy, musty, or rotten egg smell, while the uremia from kidney failure can impart a fishy ammonia-type smell to the breath [17]. Trimethylaminuria is a rare genetic metabolic condition that can also produce a foul fishy odor [17, 18]. Diabetes is best known for its distinct sweet fruity odor [17]. GI causes are rarely implicated, though some sources have reported halitosis can be intensified or aggravated by the presence of a *Helicobacter pylori* (*H. pylori*) infection

[17, 19]. *H. pylori* is thought to contribute to the development of halitosis by increasing the production of volatile sulfur compounds (VSC). Reduction or elimination of *H. pylori* in patients with antibacterial therapy therefore may have in the indirect consequence of improving halitosis symptoms by decreasing overall VSC production [19]. Probiotic studies using Lactobacillus strains have not shown clear and definitive benefits in the management of halitosis [20].

Temporomandibular Disorders

Temporomandibular joint (TMJ) disorders are a constellation of conditions characterized by pain and/or dysfunction of the TMJ and surrounding tissues. Incidence is approximately 15% in the general population, although a much smaller percentage seeks medical care for their symptoms [21] TMJ disorders are thought to be three to four times more common in women, with onset of symptoms usually in the first half of life [21]. In most cases, these disorders lack organic pathology, are self-limited, and resolve spontaneously [21–22]. Underlying causes of TMJ disorders and treatment options are poorly understood. Behavioral, psychological, and structural factors all appear to contribute to the formation of TMJ disorders. The diagnosis of TMJ disorders is based largely on history and physical examination [21]. Patients complain of pain, clicking or popping of the jaw, and occasionally limited range of motion. Pain severity is often poorly correlated with the degree or presence of organic pathology. Examination may reveal tenderness of the TMJ and/or muscles of mastication. Occasionally there is palpable crepitus or audible clicks; however, these findings are also commonly found in asymptomatic individuals as well. Based on clinical findings, TMJ disorders are divided into intra-articular or extra-articular (involving muscles of mastication) categories [21]. The differential diagnosis of TMJ disorders should include, but not limited to, dental caries/abscess, oral lesions/ulcerations, osteoarthritis, rheumatoid arthritis, temporal arteritis, and claudication of the masticatory muscles [21, 22]. Oral habits such as frequent gum chewing or bruxism may aggravate symptoms or cause inflammation within the joint. Imaging is rarely useful in the diagnosis of TMJ disorders, since most symptoms are self-limited and should be reserved for patients with persistent symptoms where conservative therapy has failed or internal joint derangement is suspected from degenerative articular disease, fracture, or dislocation. To screen for organic pathology, the panoramic radiograph is the preferred initial study [21, 22]. More advanced imaging such as ultrasound, CT or MRI should be ordered based on the findings of the panoramic film. Patient education should be at the forefront of treating nonorganic and chronic TMJ disorders [21, 22]. It is important for patients to understand that TMJ is generally not related to oral pathology and these disorders are self-limiting and nonprogressive in the absence of any systemic disease. The mainstay and most common dental treatment for TMJ has been dental splinting or interocclusal orthosis. Dental splints work to primarily open the mouth, release muscle tension, and prevent teeth clenching or grinding [21, 22]. Generally most patients perceive the splint to be effective in providing symptomatic improvement. Cognitive behavioral therapy, muscle relaxation techniques, biofeedback, physical therapy, and acupuncture have all shown to be helpful in at least temporarily reducing the pain associated with TMJ [21, 22]. Nonsteroidal anti-inflammatory agents are frequently utilized as first-line pain medications. Other medications to be considered include corticosteroids, muscle relaxants, antiepileptics, anxiolytics, and tricyclic antidepressants. Caution should be used in utilizing selective serotonin or serotonin-norepinephrine reuptake inhibitors, as these medications can induce bruxism [21, 22]. Botox may be effective in treating TMJ disorders, but current evidence is inconclusive [21]. Referral for surgical evaluation is rarely indicated in the absence of organic pathology [21, 22].

Oral Cancer

Cancers of the oral cavity and oropharynx are the ninth most common cancer in the United States [23]. African-Americans have a higher incidence than Caucasians, and males have a slight predominance over their female counterparts [23]. Patients are typically over age 40 at time of presentation. Squamous cell carcinomas account for approximately 90% of all oral cancers [5, 23, 24]. Oral cancers most commonly occur on the anterior two-thirds of the tongue, floor of the mouth, hard palate, buccal mucosa, and vermillion border of the lower lip [24]. The major risk factors for developing oral cancer are tobacco use of any kind and heavy alcohol consumption [5, 23]. Over 75% of all head and neck cancers are linked to one or both of these risk factors, and there does appear to be a synergistic effect when the two are used concomitantly [5]. Despite decreased smoking rates over recent years, the incidence of oropharyngeal cancers have continued to rise while those of oral cancers have decreased [24]. Oropharyngeal cancers include those found on the posterior one-third of the tongue, soft palate, or tonsils [24]. The increased incidence of oropharyngeal cancers is largely explained by the rise in human papillomavirus (HPV)-positive cancers [24–25]. The vast majority of HPV-related oropharyngeal cancers is caused by HPV-16 [25]. These cancers tend to occur more frequently in middle-aged Caucasian males with sexual behavior as the main risk factor [25]. Other potential risk factors for oral and oropharyngeal cancers include ultraviolet light exposure, history of previous head and neck radiation, HIV, and chronic mechanical irritation from poor fitting dentures or restorations. Overall 5-year survival rate for oral cancer is 50–55%, but if detected at an early stage, survival rates can approach 90% [5]. HPV-related oral cancers tend to have better survival rates and lower rates of recurrence [5, 25]. Oral cancers can be subtle and asymptomatic in the early stages and may present as a solitary chronic ulceration, red or white lesion, indurated lump, fissure, or enlarged cervical lymph node. Other concerning symptoms include bleeding, unexplained mouth or ear pain, odynophagia, chronic sore throat, or hoarseness. Oral leukoplakia is the most commonly known premalignant lesion and is defined as a white patch or plaque that cannot be explained by another clinical cause [5, 23]. Similar red lesions are called erythroplakia, and combined red and white lesions are known as speckled leukoplakia or erythroleukoplakia. Erythroplakia and erythroleukoplakia are more likely than leukoplakia to microscopically demonstrate dysplastic or cancerous changes [23]. Any abnormality, ulcer, white, red, or mixed lesion that is not resolving in 3–4 weeks, especially after removing any irritating precipitant such as tobacco, alcohol, and ill-fitting dental restorations, should be considered for biopsy to exclude malignancy [5, 23]. Treatment generally involves surgery and/or radiation therapy. Radiation therapy and/or chemotherapy can be used for patients not amenable to surgery or palliation for unresectable tumors. Counseling of patients regarding risk factors (tobacco, alcohol, sun exposure, and sexual habits) and providing HPV vaccination to adolescent patients can help reduce the future incidence of oral cancers [25]. The American Cancer Society recommends that adults 20 years or older have thorough oral cavity exams as part of any cancer-related check-up [24]. The United States Preventive Services Task Force has found inadequate evidence to make any similar recommendation [24].

Other Oral Lesions

Bony Tori

Tori are benign, non-neoplastic bony protuberances that arise from the cortical plate. They are more common along the hard palate of the mouth but can also arise from the floor of the mouth. Those that form along the hard palate are known as palatal torus or torus palatines, while those located along the lingual aspect of the mandible are known as mandibular torus or torus mandibularis. The overall prevalence in the general population is 3%; palatal tori are three to four times more common than mandible tori [5, 23]. These lesions are thought to be congenital anomalies though they usually do not develop until adulthood. They can be confused for cancerous growths. Bony tori are usually painless and do not cause any symptoms. No management is necessary; unless the tori are interfering with oral function, denture fabrication, or subject to recurrent traumatic ulceration, then surgical removal by an oral surgeon is recommended [5, 23].

Mucocele

Mucoceles are benign fluid-filled sacs which result from disruption of a salivary gland duct with extravasation of mucus into the surrounding tissue, usually secondary to mild local trauma such as biting [26]. Most frequently they occur on the lower lip and are more prevalent in children and young adults [23, 26]. Patients typically present with a pinkish/blue dome-shaped fluctuant papule or nodule. The underlying gelatinous sac can often be felt with palpation. Patients are seldom symptomatic, but often find the lesions irritating because of the recurrent trauma that occurs while eating. Lesions will often resolve on their own due to spontaneous rupture. If the lesion becomes symptomatic, it can be excised, which should include the entire cyst to prevent recurrence. Once excised, the specimen should be sent for pathologic examination to rule out neoplastic changes [5, 23]. As with any lesion in the mouth that does not resolve on its own within 3–4 weeks, consideration should be given for further assessment and pathologic examination either by biopsy or excision [5].

Pyogenic Granuloma

A pyogenic granuloma or lobular capillary hemangioma is an acquired benign vascular growth on the skin and mucous membranes, occurring more often in children and young adults [27]. Pyogenic granulomas appear as erythematous rapidly growing lesions which develop in response to local irritation, trauma, immunosuppression, or increased hormone levels related to pregnancy [7, 23]. These lesions may be smooth or lobulated, easily bleed when touched, and are non-painful. Oral pyogenic granulomas vary in size and most often develop along the gingival border, but can be found anywhere within the oral mucosa. Treatment is generally necessitated by the risk for recurrent bleeding, ulceration, cosmetic concerns, and the low likelihood of spontaneous regression. Options for treatment include surgical excision, laser therapy, systemic or topical therapies, especially beta-blockers [27–29]. Recurrence is uncommon but can be as high as 15% [29]. Pyogenic granulomas induced by pregnancy, however, are more likely to reoccur due to the associated hormonal changes, but are also more likely to spontaneously resolve following childbirth. Therefore observation alone may be an adequate treatment in this patient population [7, 23].

References

1. Stephens MB, Wiedemer JP, Kushner GM. Dental problems in primary care. Am Fam Physician. 2018;98(11):654–60.
2. Chi AC, Neville BW, Krayer JW, Gonsalves WC. Oral manifestations of systemic disease. Am Fam Physician. 2010;82(11):1381–8.
3. Gonslaves WC, Wrightson WC, Henry RG. Common oral conditions in older persons. Am Fam Physician. 2008;78(7):845–52.
4. Nguyen DH, Martin JT. Common dental infections in the primary care setting. Am Fam Physician. 2008; 77(5):797–802, 806. PubMed
5. Silk H. Diseases of the mouth. Prim Care Clin Off Pract Mar. 2014;41(1):75–90. CrossRef
6. Edwards PC, Kanjirath P. Recognition and management of common acute conditions of the oral cavity resulting from tooth decay, periodontal disease, and trauma: an update for the family physician. J Am Board Fam Med. 2010;23:285–94. CrossRef PubMed
7. Silk H, Douglass AB, Douglass JM, Silk L, Martin JT. Oral health during pregnancy. Am Fam Physician. 2008;77(8):1139–44.
8. Gonsalves WC, Chi AC, Neville BW. Common oral lesions: part I. Superficial mucosal lesions. Am Fam Physician. 2007;75:501–7. PubMed
9. Hu L, Zhou M, Young A, Zhao W, Yan Z. In vivo effectiveness and safety of probiotics on prophylaxis and treatment of oral candidiasis: a systematic review and meta-analysis. BMC Oral Health. 2019;19:140.
10. Ilia V, et al. Effectiveness of vitamin B12 in treating recurrent aphthous stomatitis: a randomized, double-blind, placebo controlled trial. J Am Board Fam Med. 2009;22:9–16. CrossRef
11. Eisen D, Carrozzo M, Bagan Sebastian J-V, Thongprason K. Oral lichen Planus: clinical features and management, mucosal disease series number V. Oral Dis. 2005;11:338–49.
12. Usatine RP, Tinitigan M. Diagnosis and treatment of lichen planus. Am Fam Physician. 2011;84(1):53–60. PubMed
13. Kunz M, Uroseivic-Maiwald M, Goldinger SM, Frauchiger AL, Dreier J, Belloni B, Mangana J, Jenni D, Dippel M, Cozzio A, Guenova E, Kamarachev j FLE, Drummer R. Efficacy and safety of oral alitretinoin in severe oral lichen planus-results of prospective pilot study. J Eur Acad Dermatol Venereol. 2016;30:293–8.

14. Reamy BV, Derby R, Bunt CW. Common tongue conditions in primary care. Am Fam Physician. 2010; 81(5):627–34.

15. Gushiken de Campos W, Esteves CV, Fernandes LG, Doimaneschi C, Lemos Junior CA. Treatment of symptomatic benign migratory glossitis: a systematic review. Clin Oral Investig. 2018;22:2487–249.

16. Perrin E, Ota KS. Tongue lesion with sensation of fullness in the mouth. Am Fam Physician. 2011; 83(7):839–40.

17. Rosenberg M. Clinical assessment of bad breath: current concepts. J Am Dent Assoc. 1996;127(4):475–82.

18. Porter SR, Scully C. Oral malodour (halitosis). Br Med J. 2006;333:632–5.

19. Dou W, Juan L, Liming X, Jianhong Z, Hu Z, Sui Z, Wang J, Xu L, Wang S, Yin G. Halitosis and helicobacter pylori infection ameta-analysis. Medicine. 2016;95:36.

20. Yoo J-II, In-Soo S, Jae-Gyu J, Yeon-Mi Y, Jae-Gon K, Dae-Woo L. The effect of probiotics on halitosis: a systematic review and meta-analysis. Probiotics Antimicrob Protein. 2019;11:150–7.

21. Gauer RL, Semidey MJ. Diagnosis and treatment of temporomandibular joint disorders. Am Fam Physician. 2015;91(6):378–86.

22. Buescher JJ. Temporomandibular joint disorders. Am Fam Physician. 2007;76:1477–82. PubMed

23. Gonsalves WC, Chi AC. Neville, common oral lesions: part II. Masses and neoplasia. Am Fam Physician. 2007;75:509–12. PubMed

24. Moyer VA. Screening for oral cancer: US preventive service task force recommendation statement. Ann Intern Med. 2014;160:55–60.

25. Chaturvedi AK, et al. Human papillomavirus and rising oropharyngeal cancer incidence in the United States. J Clin Oncol. 2011;29(32):4294–301. CrossRef PubMed PubMedCentral

26. Chi AC, Lambert PR III, Richardson MS, Neville BW. Oral mucoceles: a clinicopathologic review of 1,824 cases, including unusual variants. J Oral Maxillofac Surg. 2011;69:1086–93.

27. Dany M. Beta-blockers for pyogenic granuloma: a systematic review of case reports, case series, and clinical trials. J Drugs Dermatol. 2019;18(10): 1006–10.

28. Plachouri KM, Georgiou S. Therapeutic approaches to pyogenic granuloma: an updated review. Int J Dermatol. 2019;58:642–8.

29. Lee LW, Goff KL, Lam JM, Low DW, Yan AC, Castelo-Soccio L. Treatment of pediatric pyogenic granulomas using B-adrenergic receptor antagonists. Pediatr Dermatol. 2014;31(2):203–7.

Selected Disorders of the Ear, Nose, and Throat

78

Jamie L. Krassow, Justin J. Chin, Angelique S. Forrester, Jason J. Hofstede, and Bonnie G. Nolan

Contents

The information in this book chapter is written by the authors only and is not of the opinion nor does it represent any of views of the United States Department of Defense nor the United States Air Force.

J. L. Krassow (✉)
Family Medicine Residency Program, Eglin AFB, FL, USA

Department of Family Medicine, Uniformed Services University, Bethesda, MD, USA

J. J. Chin · A. S. Forrester · J. J. Hofstede · B. G. Nolan
Family Medicine Residency Program, Eglin AFB, FL, USA
e-mail: Jason.J.Hofstede.mil@mail.mil

Adult Hearing Loss

General Principles

Hearing impairment affects over 30 million people in the United States and is the fourth leading cause of disability worldwide [1, 2]. As hearing loss is primarily associated with increasing age, its prevalence is expected to rise with an aging population [2]. Hearing loss can significantly degrade quality of life and physical function and has been associated with cognitive decline, dementia, and depression [3, 4].

Pathophysiology

There are three different types of hearing loss: adult – (1) conductive hearing loss, (2) sensorineural hearing loss, and (3) mixed conductive and sensorineural hearing loss.

Conductive hearing loss is secondary to anomalies of the outer or middle ear, which may be due to obstruction of the external auditory canal, impairment of the tympanic membrane function, or middle ear pathology [1, 2]. Examples of conditions that cause conductive hearing loss include (but are not limited to) cerumen impaction, foreign body in the auditory canal, otitis externa or media, exostoses or osteomas of the external auditory canal, tympanic membrane perforation, tympanosclerosis, cholesteatoma, and otosclerosis [1].

Sensorineural hearing loss is due to dysfunction of the inner ear or neural pathways to the auditory cortex. Age-related hearing loss, or presbycusis, is the most common type of sensorineural hearing loss and usually affects high frequencies before progressing to lower frequencies [1, 2]. Noise exposure due to occupational, recreational, or accidental noise also results in sensorineural hearing loss. Prolonged and chronic noise exposure to levels of greater than 85 dB or sudden noise exposure of greater than 130 dB can lead to permanent and irreversible hearing loss [1]. Exposure to ototoxic medications (diuretics, salicylates, aminoglycosides, chemotherapeutics, etc.) can lead to sensorineural hearing loss, which may be temporary and reversible if identified early. Autoimmune hearing loss is characterized by a rapidly progressive or fluctuating bilateral sensorineural hearing loss with poor speech discrimination as well as vertigo and disequilibrium [1, 2]. Infections such as meningitis or labyrinthitis may also lead to hearing loss [1]. Sudden hearing loss occurring within 72 h window and unilateral hearing loss are additional categories of hearing loss that may occur due to a variety of reasons which include but are not limited to fracture to the temporal bone or other trauma to the inner ear, acoustic neuromas, or other cerebellopontine angle tumors, autoimmune, infectious, or may be considered idiopathic [2, 4].

Evaluation and Diagnosis

Hearing loss may simply be identified by asking, "Do you have trouble hearing?" Other hearing loss questionnaires exist, such as the "Hearing Handicap Inventory for the Elderly – Screening Version." Positive answers should further be questioned as to duration of hearing loss, if it has been sudden or gradual hearing loss, and whether it is unilateral or bilateral. It is important to ask occupational history as well as history of noise exposure. Further information may be elicited regarding family history of hearing loss, chronic medical problems, medication use, and any associated tinnitus, dizziness, or other ear problems [4].

The physical exam should consist of examining the auricle and periauricular tissues. An otoscope may be used to evaluate the external auditory canal for any cerumen or foreign objects. The tympanic membrane should be evaluated for surface anatomy, color, and mobility. The pneumatic bulb will aid in evaluating the tympanic membrane movement and aeration of the middle ear. Tuning fork tests can help differentiate between conductive and sensorineural hearing loss [1, 4]. Finally, evaluate the head, neck, and cranial nerves if clinically indicated [1].

Objective evaluation of hearing is commonly performed by pure tone audiometry. This is a diagnostic test that gives information on hearing loss to include the type and degree of hearing loss at a specific frequency threshold [1, 4]. A speech discrimination test can assess a patient's ability to understand speech and identify good candidates for hearing amplification with hearing aids [4]. Tympanometry is another simple test performed in the office, which evaluates the mobility of the tympanic membrane and function of the middle ear and Eustachian tube. Imaging may be indicated to further evaluate certain cases such as those with asymmetric or sudden hearing loss [1].

Treatment

A three-tiered approach is recommended for treatment of hearing loss: adult – assessment, education/counseling, and technology [4]. If a concern of hearing loss is identified and proper equipment is not available in the primary care office for appropriate evaluation, further assessment by audiology and/or otolaryngology is indicated [1, 5]. Counsel on and eliminate environmental noise and ototoxic agents if possible. Technological intervention is important, not only for hearing improvement but also for social and emotional function as well as for communication and cognition [3, 5].

In some cases, the only treatment option is hearing amplification. Hearing aids have several models to include those which fit behind the ear or in the canal. Assisted listening devices may be used for those unable to utilize hearing aids. Recent legislation in the United States has required the FDA to create a new class of over-the-counter hearing devices, which should increase access and decrease costs for hearing-impaired patients in the near future [2, 4]. Cochlear implant surgery is an option for those with severe sensorineural hearing loss [1, 4, 5]. Many etiologies of conductive hearing loss may also be corrected with surgery [1].

Referral to rehabilitation services may help teach patients to use nonverbal clues and vocational modification to ensure safe functioning despite his or her hearing impairment [1, 4].

Prevention

Prevention of some types of hearing loss may be impossible; however, prevention of exposure to ototoxic agents is possible by carefully choosing medications and discontinuing offending agents. Additionally, noise-induced sensorineural hearing loss may be prevented by screening for noise exposure, counseling about proper hearing protection, and avoidance of overexposure [1, 4].

Pediatric Hearing Loss

General Principles

Pediatric hearing loss is one of the most common sensory birth condition abnormalities in the United States affecting 1 to 3 per 1000 newborns [6–8]. Early detection of hearing loss before the age of 6 months is essential to prevent delays in language and other developmental milestones [7]. Although children with hearing loss often have complex needs, the consequences are treatable if hearing loss is detected and treated early in life [6].

Pathophysiology

Hearing loss in the neonate or child can be classified as congenital, acquired, or idiopathic. Of the congenital etiologies, it can be further classified as either syndromic or non-syndromic (non-syndromic can be autosomal recessive, autosomal dominant, or X-linked). Of the acquired cases of hearing loss, the great majority is considered environmental. Environmental risk factors to the neonate include cytomegalovirus, rubella, measles, syphilis, and exposure to alcohol. Other risk

factors for neonates and children may include exposure to ototoxic drugs such as aminoglycosides or antineoplastic agents, hypoxic ischemic injury, or hyperbilirubinemia [7, 8].

Hearing loss may also develop later in childhood. Additional risk factors of childhood hearing loss include family history of childhood hearing loss, history of admission to the neonatal intensive care unit for greater than 5 days, history of mechanical ventilation/oxygenation requirement, craniofacial anomalies, infections associated with late onset hearing loss, head trauma, chemotherapy, recurrent otitis media, and caregiver concern [6, 7].

Hearing loss can be defined by degree, configuration, and type of loss. There are two major types of Hearing loss: adult – conductive hearing loss and sensorineural hearing loss. Conductive hearing loss is caused by problems with the outer or middle hear, whereas sensorineural hearing loss is caused by problems with the inner ear, auditory nerve, or central auditory pathway. Some children have mixed conductive and sensorineural hearing loss [2, 3].

Evaluation and Diagnosis

Newborn hearing screening is mandated in nearly every state in the United States. There are two main screening methods in the United States: the otoacoustic emission (OAE) test and the automated auditory brainstem response (AABR) test. The OAE allows for individual ear testing at any age and assesses for middle ear pathology. The AABR test evaluates the function of the auditory pathway to include the auditory nerve. The AABR is also often used as a follow up test if the OAE is failed during the initial newborn hearing exam. The Joint Committee on Infant Hearing (JCIH) recommends that infants who are admitted to the neonatal intensive care unit (NICU) for greater than 5 days be screened with the AABR [7].

If an infant does not pass initial screening tests, additional evaluation and referral should be completed before 3 months of age with intervention by 6 months of age. Other diagnostic tests exist but are primarily completed by an audiologist. These tests include diagnostic auditory brainstem response, tympanometry, diagnostic otoacoustic emissions, and behavioral hearing assessment [7].

The physical exam should consist of particular attention to head size and symmetry, jaw size and symmetry, facial movement and symmetry, as well as external and middle ear morphology. Signs of the head and neck exam which may be related to hearing loss include malformation of the auricle or ear canal, dimpling or skin tags around the auricle, cleft lip or cleft palate, asymmetric facial structures, microcephaly, or tympanic membrane abnormalities. Many times, the physical exam will be normal. CT, MRI, and lab tests may further be ordered if clinically indicated [9].

Treatment

Any abnormal hearing test requires intervention. Appropriate referrals include those to otolaryngology, audiology, speech and language pathology, and a genetics specialist. Referrals to early intervention programs are essential. Early intervention services should be provided by professionals with expertise in hearing loss, speech and language pathology, and audiology. An ophthalmologic evaluation may also be appropriate if syndromic associations are identified [7].

Hearing aids are devices that amplify sound and transmit to the ear with the desired frequencies depending on the patient's diminished areas. These benefit patients with sensorineural hearing loss and some with conductive hearing loss. Assistive listening devices can be used in public places to help override poor acoustics [7].

Surgical implants are also an option in care for patients with severe hearing loss: adult – bone-anchored hearing aids are beneficial in children older than 5 who suffer from permanent conductive hearing loss. Cochlear implants amplify sound for children that are at least 1 year old and have profound bilateral sensorineural hearing loss [7].

Tinnitus

General Principles

Tinnitus is the perception of continuous or intermittent sound within the ears or head without an objective external stimulus. The noise has been described as ringing, buzzing, clicking, pulsations, roaring, hissing, sizzling, music, or voices. Although much of what we understand about tinnitus remains an enigma, it is considered a symptom, not a disease in and of itself. Tinnitus is often associated with sensorineural hearing loss, making inner ear or auditory tract dysfunction a viable source of tinnitus; however, the precise mechanisms and possible sites of involvement remain unclear [10]. Even when tinnitus is not severe, the perception can be extremely bothersome and often interferes with the daily activities of symptomatic individuals [10–12].

Pathophysiology

While there is no clear etiology of tinnitus, investigators suspect possible lesions or cochlear alterations within the limbic and nervous systems as the source of irregular neuronal activity in the lower auditory pathway. It is theorized that this stimulation of the auditory tract is the perceived sensations we collectively characterized as tinnitus [13]. There are some known risk factors for tinnitus [11, 13]:

- Exposure to high levels of recreational and occupational noise
- Ototoxic drugs: salicylates, quinine, aminoglycosides, antibiotics, antineoplastic agents
- Otologic diseases: otosclerosis, Meniere's disease, vestibular schwannoma (acoustic neuroma)
- Obesity
- Alcohol use
- Smoking
- Arthritis
- Hypertension
- Anxiety
- Depression
- Dysfunction of the temporal mandibular joint
- Hyperacusis

Tinnitus is most notable in patients who have been exposed to hazardous levels of industrial, recreational, or military-related noise [11]. Other underlying associations to tinnitus include nerve damage from brain trauma or lesions, inner ear damage, acute ear infections, foreign objects in the ear, allergies, ototoxic medications (aminoglycosides, aspirin, chemotherapeutics), stress, or low serotonin activity [11, 13].

Tinnitus can be characterized in several different ways, but most commonly, it is characterized as either "objective" or "subjective" tinnitus. Objective tinnitus can be heard by the examiner, usually with a stethoscope, and it is generally referred to as "pulsatile" tinnitus. If it synchronized with the heartbeat, it may be considered vascular in origin. If it is not, it may be originating from the middle ear or palatal muscles. Subjective tinnitus, on the other hand, is only heard by the patient. The tinnitus may be chronic or intermittent. It may be heard in one ear, both ears, or centrally within the head. The onset may be abrupt or insidious, and the severity may change with time as well [12, 13].

Evaluation and Diagnosis

The severity and sensation of tinnitus significantly vary among affected individuals. There is no current standardized guideline for the evaluation of tinnitus. Although serious pathology leading to tinnitus is rare, it is important to get a complete medical history to understand of any possible underlying causes [11, 12]. Assess the character of the tinnitus: (1) subjective versus objective, (2) location and quality, and (3) distinguished chronicity (chronic is considered at least 6 months duration). Subjective idiopathic tinnitus is the most commonly diagnosed type of tinnitus. There are several questionnaires to evaluate tinnitus to include the "Tinnitus Handicap Inventory" (THI) and the "Tinnitus Functional Index" [11]. Evaluate for any associated hearing loss and tympanic membrane dysfunction [12].

If asymmetric tinnitus is associated with asymmetric hearing loss or any other neurological deficits, further investigation and imaging is indicated. Likewise, for any heartbeat-synchronous pulsatile tinnitus, further evaluation with advanced imaging is indicated: this may include but is not limited to CT, MRI, CT

angiography, MRI angiography, or ultrasound. If the tinnitus is unilateral and pulsatile or the tinnitus is associated with vertigo, it is recommended that the patient be referred to a specialty clinician [11].

Treatment

There have been multiple medications, to include complementary and alternative, studied to evaluate treatment of tinnitus, but none so far have demonstrated statistically significant improvements [11, 12]. There have been medical interventions studied such as transcranial magnetic stimulation, electromagnetic stimulation, low-level laser therapy, and acupuncture; however, none of these has shown consistent improvement of tinnitus either [11].

Sound therapy or sound maskers, which produce sound to cover the tinnitus, have not shown statistically significant improvement. Sound technologies, such as hearing aids (if the patient has associated hearing loss), may help mask tinnitus by increasing the overall level of ambient sound delivered to the patient. Cochlear implants may also help to mask tinnitus and improve perception of external noise; however, these are only for patients with profound sensorineural hearing loss [11].

Much of the treatment involved for treating tinnitus is truly aimed at treating the comorbid conditions associated with tinnitus such as anxiety, depression, hearing loss, and sleep disorders. Psychological and behavioral interventions are recommended to improve associated distress [11, 12].

Mindfulness-based cognitive therapy (MBCT) uses mediation techniques to address the burdens of tinnitus [14]. The goal of MBCT is to reframe an individual's outlook on the unpleasant experience of living with a chronic condition. This technical approach focuses on helping individuals adapt to distressing experiences by validating their personal thoughts, emotions, and sensations. Once acceptance is achieved, theorists believe the patient can focus on improving adaptive behaviors to combat the distressing experience such as tinnitus [14].

A recent study by Takahashi et al. expands on reports investigating the impact of psychological background on patients with tinnitus. Investigators argue that in order to improve the treatment of tinnitus, grading systems and protocols should take into consideration both psychological state and severity of tinnitus perception by affected individuals. Currently, THI does not incorporate the psychological background of patients with tinnitus into its severity grading system. Limited reports have found depression to be a significant factor on how the severity and sensation of tinnitus was perceived. Studies have found that patients with moderate to severe tinnitus have better therapeutic response to interventions when their psychiatric conditions were treated concurrently. This discovery has led some healthcare professionals to advocate for developing new protocols and parameters that utilize the Hospital Anxiety and Depression Scale (HADS) and the Diagnostic and Statistical Manual of Mental Disorders (DSM-V)'s criteria for major depression and catastrophic events in addition to the THI when grading tinnitus severity and assessing for therapeutic intervention [10].

Unfortunately, there is no single effective treatment regimen to cure or significantly alleviate tinnitus. It is important to treat or eliminate comorbid conditions. Any surgical otologic disorders should be evaluated by otolaryngology [11].

Prevention

Because there is no effective treatment for most cases of tinnitus, the focus should be on prevention of known causes: reduce exposure to ototoxic drugs as well as avoid occupational and recreational loud noises [12].

Salivary Gland Inflammation and Salivary Stones

General Principles

Saliva plays an important role in the oral and digestive health. Composed of enzymes, electrolytes, and other molecules, saliva is an enrichened fluid that provides lubrication for the function of swallowing as well as aids in the digestion of starches through with salivary amylase [15]. Saliva also acts as a layer of protection against dental caries and oral pathogens. Major salivary glands include the parotid, submandibular, and sublingual glands. Additionally, there are minor salivary glands lining the oral cavity, pharynx, lips, and tongue [15]. Inflammatory conditions of the glands, also known as sialadenitis, are most common in the major salivary glands, with obstructive sialadenitis accounting for approximately one-half of benign salivary disorders treated in a primary care setting [15]. Other causes of inflammation of the salivary glands include infections (viral and bacterial), autoimmune disorders, and neoplasm of the salivary gland. While neoplasm of the salivary glands is relatively rare, they make up about 6% of all head and neck tumors [15]. Inflammation may be acute or chronic and can lead to salivary stone formation which will further enhance the inflammation in some cases [16].

Pathophysiology

Salivary gland stones, also known as sialoliths, develop when calcified mass forms within the salivary duct or gland [17]. The accumulation of salivary calculi can lead to mechanical obstruction within the duct, thus predisposing the gland to inflammation. The precise mechanisms leading to the developing of salivary stone are unclear. The "retrograde theory" of sialolith development postulates the migration of bacteria or food debris into the salivary gland ducts which later serves as a nidus for stone formation [17]. Another popular theory suggests that a localized inflammatory process causing the calcification of a mucus plug leads to the formation of sialoliths [18]. Other potential risk factors include use of tobacco products such as cigarettes. Very few studies have shown significant correlation between poor hygiene and salivary gland inflammation and stone development [17].

Acute bacterial sialadenitis is most often seen in the parotid gland in medically debilitated patients. Debilitation and dehydration may lead to the stasis of salivary flow which can generate stone precipitation and strictures of the salivary ducts. This environment favors bacterial infection, most commonly from *Staphylococcus aureus*, streptococcal species, and *Haemophilus influenzae* [15, 16]. Other infectious etiologies include *Mycobacterium*, *Toxoplasma*, and *Actinomyces* species [16].

Acute viral sialadenitis is most commonly found in the setting of mumps in children aged 4 through 6. Other viral causes include *Cytomegalovirus*, lymphocytic choriomeningitis virus, Coxsackie virus A, echo virus, and parainfluenza virus type C [16]. Predisposing factors for noninfectious acute sialadenitis include autoimmune disorders such as Sjogren's syndrome as well as chronic metabolic conditions such as diabetes mellitus and hypothyroidism [15].

Chronic sialadenitis is characterized by repeated episodes of pain and edema. Affected patients will often complain of intermittent pain and swelling of the gland, which is exacerbated during prandial salivary stimulation [14]. Furthermore, commonly prescribed medications such as diuretics, antihypertensive, antihistamines, antipsychotics, and antidepressants are known to decrease the salivary flow rate, which may play a limited role in facilitating stone formation and sialolithiasis [18, 19].

Neoplasms may be benign or malignant. Malignancies of the salivary gland are rare, encompassing only 16% of all salivary gland neoplasm cases [15].

Evaluation and Diagnosis

Acute bacterial sialadenitis has characteristic clinical findings of salivary gland pain and edema. Mucopurulent material can sometimes be expressed at the orifice of the nearby salivary duct [15, 16]. Acute viral sialadenitis is most commonly due to mumps offending the parotid gland, which is characterized by parotid edema with symptoms of fever, malaise, myalgias, and headaches in the weeks preceding the incubation period. Some children can experience recurrent viral sialadenitis. This can last weeks and recur every few months. Viral serology may help to confirm the diagnosis.

Chronic sialadenitis has characteristic findings of repeated episodes of pain and edema of the salivary glands. Generally, this occurs from little to no salivary flow and due to stones, strictures, or stenosis. It is sometimes possible to palpate the stone along the nearby duct [15].

Neoplasms typically present as painless, asymptomatic, slow-growing masses. Malignant neoplasms may present with findings such as facial paresis, fixation of the mass, and lymphadenopathy. Specialty referral to an otolaryngologist for further evaluation and possible biopsy is essential for an accurate diagnosis. A CT scan with contrast or MR with MR sialography may also be used to identify the mass's characteristics [15].

CT is the preferred modality for acute sialadenitis due to its sensitivity to calcification and spatial resolution. Extensive dental artifacts on CT imaging are a common limitation of this modality [19]. Ultrasound and MRI are also options; the clinical scenario will ultimately dictate the appropriate diagnostic imaging necessary for further evaluation. When imaging is inconclusive, further referral for US-guided fine needle aspiration and cytology may be indicated [19].

Treatment

Acute bacterial sialadenitis is treated by empiric antimicrobial therapy (i.e., Augmentin, etc.). Increasing salivary volume and flow by increasing hydration and utilizing sialagogues is also recommended. Salivary gland massage may also be useful.

Recurrent parotitis of childhood and chronic sialadenitis in adults are treated similarly as in acute cases as outlined above. It generally resolves spontaneously over time. Anti-inflammatory medications may also be considered.

Viral parotitis or mump treatment is primarily supportive and focuses on hydration and pain control. Mumps usually resolves spontaneously within weeks. Any stones contributing to acute or chronic sialadenitis may need surgical removal if conservative management fails [15].

Prevention

Vaccination has reduced the incidence of mumps by 99%. It is important to promote hydration and use sialagogues for enhancement of saliva production and prevention of stone formation [16].

Xerostomia

General Principles

Xerostomia is the subjective sensation of dry mouth. Its prevalence increases with age and tends to be higher in women than in men [20]. Major and minor salivary glands produce the saliva, which is composed of electrolytes, organic compounds, and water. Normal salivary function is to aid in digestion through oral processing and swallowing of food. Saliva protects the oral cavity by cleansing it, sustaining a neutral pH, preventing tooth demineralization, and adding an antimicrobial effect [21].

Pathophysiology

Xerostomia can occur with the reduction in the quantity, flow rate, or composition of the saliva produced. Hyposalivation is a pathological condition in which there is insufficient or decreased production of saliva [21]. Some cases of xerostomia may correlate with hyposalivation while others do not. Symptoms of xerostomia may range from oral discomfort to significant oral disease such as dental caries, periodontitis, dental erosion, and intraoral candidiasis that can negatively impact a patient's health, dietary habits, and quality of life [20, 21].

There are several causes of xerostomia such as dehydration, poor nutritional status, head or neck radiation, chemotherapy, salivary gland aplasia, Sjögren's syndrome, depression, smoking, and a variety of medications [21]:

- Antihypertensives
- Anticholinergics
- Antidepressants
- Antipsychotics
- Anxiolytics
- Diuretics
- Muscle relaxants
- Diuretics
- Muscle relaxants
- Sedatives
- Antiepileptics
- Antiparkinsonisms
- Antihistamines
- Cytotoxics
- Analgesics

Evaluation and Diagnosis

As with all ailments, a thorough medical history and exam are the chief means of attaining a diagnosis. It is important to identify any diseases that may put the patient at risk for the development of xerostomia or if the patient is on a medication regimen that may be inducing xerostomia, which is more common [20]. Patients may complain of dry mouth or other symptoms from dry mouth like a burning sensation or difficulty with speech and swallowing. He or she may also note a change in taste. On exam, the mucosal surfaces may be dry and the tongue swollen and dry, erythematous and atrophic oral mucosa, angular cheilitis or peeling lips [21].

Treatment

Treatment is aimed at identifying the underlying cause. Underlying systemic medical conditions such as Sjogren's disease, lymphoma, sarcoidosis, or amyloidosis may lead to xerostomia; treatment of these conditions may help the symptoms of dry mouth. If a medication is identified as causation, then it should be changed or eliminated if possible. It is important to encourage hydration, especially in the elderly and those with poor nutrition. Avoidance of food and drinks such as alcohol, sugar, and caffeine, which may lead to dry mouth or dental caries, is an essential dietary modification. Furthermore, if the patient is a current tobacco user, tobacco cessation should be encouraged [21].

There are a number of over-the-counter treatments available – toothpastes, rinses, lozenges, sprays, gels, oral patches, and chewing gums. Research suggests that when used in conjunction with prescription medication, the benefits can be additive, but when used alone, their efficacy is undetermined.

Two systemic medications available in the United States which may help stimulate saliva production (sialagogues): pilocarpine or cevimeline drops [21].

Hoarseness

General Principles

Hoarseness (or dysphonia) is a term used to describe a symptom or sign of altered voice quality [22]. The change in voice may be an alteration in quality, pitch, and loudness or may be described as breathy, strained, rough, or raspy [22, 23]. It is a common problem in the United States adult population affecting up to one-third of all adults at some point in time and leads to 2.5 million dollars in lost work cost [22].

Pathophysiology

The larynx houses the vocal folds, which are responsible for the production of sound as airflows pass these structures. The larynx extends from the base of the tongue to the trachea and is innervated by the superior and recurrent laryngeal nerves. There is a multitude of etiologies which may cause hoarseness. In general, these etiologies may be from irritants, inflammation, neuromuscular, psychiatric, systemic, or neoplastic disorders [23]. Table 1 outlines details of each of these categories.

Evaluation and Diagnosis

A careful history and physical exam are important to understand the etiology of the patient's

Table 1 Etiologies of hoarseness (or dysphonia) in the adult population [23]

Irritants and inflammation	Acute laryngitis: viral, vocal abuse, allergies Chronic laryngitis: smoking, voice abuse, laryngopharyngeal reflux, allergies, inhaled corticosteroids
Neuromuscular	Vocal cord paralysis: Injury to recurrent laryngeal nerve, head and neck surgery (especially thyroid surgery), endotracheal intubation, mediastinal or apical immersion of lung cancer Muscle tension dystonia Spasmodic dysphonia (laryngeal dystonia)
Psychiatric	Stress and other psychiatric disorders
Systemic	Parkinson's disease Myasthenia gravis Multiple sclerosis Hypothyroidism Acromegaly Inflammatory arthritis
Neoplasms	Laryngeal papillomatosis Laryngeal leukoplakia Dysplasia or squamous cell carcinoma (risk factors: Smoking, alcohol use, chronic reflux)

hoarseness. Evaluate the onset and duration of voice changes. In the medical history, it is prudent to ask about any recent upper respiratory infections, allergies, or chronic medical problems. Assess for any associated symptoms of gastroesophageal reflux. In the social history, it is important to discuss any environmental exposures, tobacco use, or alcohol use. In addition, vocations in singing, teaching, and of the clergy are more at risk for this condition. Learning of any recent surgeries is also key. Associated symptoms such as cough, dysphagia, and odynophagia are important and may lead to more serious underlying causes of hoarseness [22, 23].

During the physical exam, it is important to assess for rhinorrhea, sneezing, or watery eyes which may suggest a more benign cause such as allergies or viral irritation; however, findings such as lymphadenopathy, stridor, and weight loss may be more concerning for serious etiologies such as malignancies. Stridor may indicate airway obstruction due to mass [23].

Laryngoscopy may be performed at any point in time. Different recommendations exist as to when direct visualization is required. More recent guidelines suggest direct visualization is indicated if hoarseness persists for greater than 4 weeks [22]. The procedure should be done in the primary care office or referred to a specialist who has this capability. Direct visualization of the larynx should be done sooner if there is any suspicion of serious underlying condition. In case of tobacco or alcohol use, a neck mass, hemoptysis, dysphagia, odynophagia, neurological symptoms, unexplained weight loss, aspiration of a foreign body, and persistent symptoms after surgery or if the hoarseness significantly impairs the quality of life of the patient, then visualization is more urgent [22, 23].

Imaging, such as a CT or MRI, may be used to assess specific pathology; however, it is recommended that direct visualization be performed prior to any imaging [22].

In cases of pediatric hoarseness, it is generally indicated for the patient to be referred to otolaryngology and speech and language pathology early [24].

Treatment

If hoarseness duration is less than 2 weeks (acute), it is more likely to be benign. Reassurance is appropriate but also address and treat any underlying etiologies such as viral infections, allergies, and reflux. If reflux is suspected through history or visualization of chronic laryngitis, then a trial of a high-dose proton pump inhibitor (PPI) is warranted; however, isolated dysphonia should not be treated with PPI therapy without visualization first. Likewise, antibiotics are usually not indicated in treating hoarseness [22, 23]. If corticosteroids are on the patient's medication list, the clinician may recommend a decrease or alteration in the dose or type of corticosteroid used for 4 weeks. Inhaled fluticasone (Flovent) is the most common offending agent [23]. Oral corticosteroids to treat hoarseness are not recommended without visualization of the larynx [22]. If there is a systemic condition which has a known symptom of hoarseness (such as hypothyroidism), optimize treatment for the condition, and reassess after 4 weeks.

If laryngoscopy is completed and no serious pathology is found, it is recommended the patient be referred for vocal hygiene training and voice therapy by a speech and language pathologist.

Surgery may be indicated for any findings of benign or malignant masses, glottic insufficiency, or if airway obstruction is a risk [22, 23].

Prevention

Educate of the patient on measures to reduce voice disorders: adequately hydrate with water, use amplification devices to reduce voice strain, rest the voice briefly, and provide indoor air humidification. Additionally, educate the patient on avoidance of triggers such as tobacco smoke, certain medications, environmental irritants or allergens, and vocational abuse of the voice [22, 23].

Epistaxis

General Principles

Epistaxis is a common condition that can affect up to 60% of the general population [25]. Up to 9% of the pediatric population experiences recurrent epistaxis. Epistaxis is generally categorized as anterior (90%) or posterior (10% of cases but more severe). Epistaxis has a bimodal distribution 2–10 and 50–80 years of age [25, 26]. Anterior epistaxis generates from either Kiesselbach's plexus or the anterior inferior turbinate [26]. Posterior epistaxis results from bleeding of the posterior edge of the nasal septum or the posterior lateral nasal wall mucosa [29].

Pathophysiology

The etiology of epistaxis can be divided into two general causes: local and systemic. Local causes refer to specific complications to the nasal mucosa. Systemic causes refer to more systemic etiologies causing epistaxis to be more likely [25, 29]. See Table 2 for a list of local and systemic causes of epistaxis.

In children, the most common etiology of anterior epistaxis is trauma (usually nose picking) [29]. Idiopathic nose bleeding occurring at night is also common in children but is eventually outgrown. Posterior epistaxis in children is most often due to juvenile nasopharyngeal angiofibroma, which is most commonly seen in teenage boys. Similar to adults, systemic disease of childhood may also lead to epistaxis such as (1) vascular anomalies: hereditary hemorrhagic telangiectasia (Rendu-Osler-Weber syndrome); (2) hematologic problems (genetic or acquired) such as primary idiopathic thrombocytopenic purpura, leukemia, or aspirin use; or (3) coagulopathies (genetic or acquired) such as von Willebrand disease, hemophilia, warfarin use, liver diseases leading to coagulopathy, or drug-related thrombocytopenic purpura [28].

Evaluation and Diagnosis

Anterior epistaxis is generally obvious to the examiner, and blood loss is usually not significant.

Table 2 Local and systemic causes of epistaxis [25, 29]

Local causes	Systemic causes
Trauma	Hypertension
Nose picking	Antiplatelet medications
Foreign objects stuck in nose	Hereditary hemorrhagic telangiectasia
Neoplasms or polyps (nasopharyngeal angiofibroma)	Hemophilia
Rhinitis or sinusitis (chronic, acute, allergic)	Leukemia
Medications (inhaled corticosteroids)	Liver disease
Irritants (occupational exposures, cigarettes, etc.)	Medications (aspirin, anticoagulants, NSAIDS)
Septal perforation	Platelet dysfunction
Vascular malformations or telangiectasia	Thrombocytopenia
Environmental: Dry and low humidity	

Posterior epistaxis may be associated with a large volume of blood loss but may present insidiously with symptoms such as nausea, hematemesis, hemoptysis, or melena [25, 27]. It is important to identify the likely source of bleeding (anterior or posterior) as well as inquire about the history leading up to the epistaxis episode in order to understand if further workup is necessary. Estimate the volume of blood loss, time of onset, frequency of any prior episodes, any medical comorbidities, acute respiratory infections, use of medications, recreational drug use, and any recent surgery or trauma. In more severe cases, airway protection and hemodynamic stability must be considered. Any concern of clinical instability should be managed in the emergency department [26, 27, 29].

In stable scenarios, the physical exam may be performed with the aid of a vasoconstrictor spray or gauze soaked in a vasoconstrictor. Physical exam ideally should be done with nasal speculum and light source. This in combination with an anesthetic may be helpful during the physical exam to successfully identify the source of bleeding [25, 26].

Treatment

Because 90% of epistaxis cases are anterior, most cases of epistaxis are treated successfully with conservative therapies [26]. Initial treatment consists of pinching the lower portion of the nose against the anterior nasal septum placing pressure along the ala for several minutes. Cotton-tipped applicators or cotton balls can be used to place pressure against the source of bleeding. These items may be soaked in topical vasoconstrictors or decongestants if needed [25–27]. It is important to tilt the head forward, not backward, in order to avoid pooling of the blood, which can lead to airway obstruction [26]. If direct pressure is not helpful, silver nitrate sticks or electrocautery may be applied to the area of bleeding. Apply the cauterization instrument directly to the source of bleeding to avoid any excessive soft tissue damage; do not cauterize blindly [25, 27]. Avoid cauterizing bilaterally due to risk of septal necrosis and perforation. If bilateral cauterization is needed, it is optimal to perform cauterization 4–6 weeks apart [26, 27].

If this initial management is unsuccessful, nasal packing may be an effective next step. There is data showing that using tranexamic acid (TXA) soaked pledgets before nasal packing may stop bleeding within 10 min of application in up to 71% of subjects [27]. There are many commercial products or commercial nasal tampons available for nasal packing. The principle is to localize the source and apply packing to stop the site of bleeding. The packing may be left in for several days [26, 27]. If anterior packing is unsuccessful, then one can move to posterior packing, which is a more complex procedure. If this is necessary, specialty consultation and admission to the hospital are recommended due to complexity and risks involved in the procedure. Toxic shock syndrome is a risk in the setting of any type of packing techniques. Anti-staphylococcal antibiotic (oral or topical) may be considered as prophylactic therapy, with special attention for patients who are immunocompromised, have heart valve disease or receiving posterior nasal packing [27]. Similar to posterior packing for persistent anterior bleeding, posterior bleeding should be treated in the hospital setting and with specialty consultation. Additional intervention may be indicated such as arterial embolization or arterial ligation [25–27].

In summary, epistaxis, in particular anterior epistaxis, is a common condition that can be treated in the outpatient setting with conservative measures; however, in cases of persistent bleeding or posterior epistaxis, more invasive measures performed with specialty consultation in the hospital may be necessary.

Prevention

If recurrent anterior epistaxis persists, consider underlying etiologies. If underlying pathology is ruled out, various treatments may be helpful in prevention such as humidification of air, application of petroleum jelly to the local area to maintain humidity, or application of antiseptic creams.

Abstain from alcohol and avoid hot drinks that cause vasodilation [27, 29].

Foreign Bodies in the Ear and Nose

General Principles

Foreign bodies lodged in the ear and nose are a problem commonly seen in children and patients with mental handicaps. At times, it can be difficult to diagnose as the object placement may not have been observed by the parent or caregiver. Common foreign bodies found in the ear or nose include beads, rubber erasers, toy parts, pebbles, food, marbles, and button batteries [30–32].

Pathophysiology

Although a nasal foreign body can be found in any portion of the nasal cavity, it is most commonly found in one of two places: below the inferior turbinate and anterior to the middle turbinate.

A foreign body within the ear is usually lodged at the point where the external auditory canal narrows into a bony cartilaginous junction. If lodged too far, the tympanic membrane can be damaged [30, 32].

Evaluation and Diagnosis

A nasal cavity foreign body may be asymptomatic; however, it may also present as unilateral, malodorous, mucopurulent nasal discharge or intermittent epistaxis. Other complications include posterior dislodgement with risk of aspiration, trauma due to initial placement or self-removal attempts, and infection [31].

When evaluating a patient for a nasal foreign body, it is useful to apply a topical vasoconstriction agent to reduce mucosal edema, such as 0.5% phenylephrine or oxymetazoline [30, 32]. Anesthesia may also be accomplished with a topical spray such as 4% lidocaine. If no foreign body is visualized on physical exam, a plain film of the sinus or CT scan may be considered [30].

A foreign object in the ear may also be asymptomatic or an incidental finding on exam. Symptoms can include otitis, hearing loss, or purulent drainage. It is important to appropriately visualize the object in order to decrease trauma. If it is not easily visualized or if there is evidence of a perforated tympanic membrane, it may be necessary to refer to a specialty physician. Topical anesthesia of the ear is generally not required for foreign body removal [30].

Treatment

In most cases, a foreign object in the nose or ear is not an emergency, so removal may be delayed if it is not easily achieved in the family physician's office. It is appropriate, then, to refer to an otolaryngologist. In the event a caustic object is present (batteries, etc.) irrigation should not be used, and a referral is urgent [30].

Removal of a nasal cavity foreign object may be completed by several different techniques. Most commonly, if the object is in the anterior passage, it may be graspable with a forceps, curved hooks, cerumen loops, or suction catheter [32]. A balloon tip catheter may be used by lubricating the balloon tip, passing the tip past the foreign body, inflating, and then pulling forward [31]. The "parental kiss" is a less invasive option in children in which the parent provides a puff of air through the child's mouth with the unaffected nostril occluded, providing positive pressure to expel the foreign body [30–32]. Once the object is removed, it is important to reinspect the nasal cavity for any additional objects or localized trauma. If the object is not successfully removed, it may be necessary to refer to an otolaryngologist.

Removal of a foreign object within the external auditory canal may be performed using similar techniques as mentioned above. Irrigation is another option, which may be helpful to flush out small objects closer to the tympanic membrane [30, 32]. If a live insect is present, it is important that it be killed prior to removal. Alcohol, 2% lidocaine, or mineral oil may be instilled in the canal [32]. This should be done only if the tympanic membrane is intact. If the object is not

easily graspable, however, there are higher rates of complications such as canal lacerations and tympanic membrane damage. In the event of unsuccessful removal, high risk of trauma, or if there is need for anesthesia, specialty referral is recommended [30].

References

1. Michels TC, et al. Hearing loss in adults: differential diagnosis and treatment. Am Fam Physician. 2019;100(2):98–108.
2. Cunningham LL, Tucci DL. Hearing loss in adults. N Engl J Med. 2017;377:2465–73.
3. Rutherford BR, et al. Sensation and psychiatry: linking age-related hearing loss to late-life depression and cognitive decline. Am J Psychiatry. 2018;175:215–24.
4. Contrera KJ, et al. Hearing loss health care for older adults. J Am Board Fam Med. 2016;29:394–403.
5. Phan NT, et al. Diagnosis and management of hearing loss in elderly patients. Aust Fam Physician. 2016 Jun;45(6):366–9.
6. Judge PD, et al. Medical referral patterns and etiologies for children with mild-to-severe hearing loss. Ear Hear. 2019;40(4):1001–8.
7. Stewart JE, Bentley JE. Hearing loss in pediatrics: what the medical home needs to know. Pediatr Clin N Am. 2019;66(2):425–36.
8. Wroblewska-Seniuk K, et al. Sensorineural and conductive hearing loss in infants diagnosed in the problem of universal newborn hearing screening. Int J Pediatr Otorhinolaryngol. 2018;105:181–6.
9. Lin J, Oghalai JS. Towards an etiologic diagnosis: assessing the patient with hearing loss. Adv Otorhinolaryngol. 2011;70:28–36.
10. Takahashi M, et al. An improved system for grading and treating tinnitus. Auris Nasus Larynx. 2018;45 (4):711–7. https://doi.org/10.1016/j.anl.2017.11.012.
11. Pichora-Fuller MK, Santaguida P, Hammill A, et al. Evaluation and treatment of tinnitus: comparative effectiveness. Comparative effectiveness review no. 122 (Prepared by the McMaster University evidence-based practice center under contract no. 290-2007-10060-I). AHRQ publication no. 13-EHC110-EF. Rockville: Agency for Healthcare Research and Quality; 2013 [cited 29 Aug 2014]. Available from: www.effective healthcare.ahrq.gov/reports/final.cfm
12. Baguley D, McFerran D, Hall D. Tinnitus Lancet. 2013;382(9904):1600–7.
13. Donnelly K. Tinnitus. In: Caplan B, DeLuca J, Kreutzer J, editors. Encyclopedia of clinical neuropsychology: Springer reference www.springerreference.com. Berlin/Heidelberg: Springer; 2011 [cited 29 Aug 2014]. Available from: http://www.springerreference.com/index/chapterdbid/183592

14. McKenna L, Marks EM, Vogt F. Mindfulness-based cognitive therapy for chronic tinnitus: evaluation of benefits in a large sample of patients attending a tinnitus clinic. Ear Hear. 2018;39(2):359–66.

15. Wilson KF, Meier JD, Ward PD. Salivary gland disorders. Am Fam Physician. 2014;89:882–8.

16. Mazziotti S. Salivary glands, inflammation, acute, chronic. In: Baert A, editor. Encyclopedia of diagnostic imaging: Springer reference www.springerreference.com. Berlin/Heidelberg: Springer; 2008 [cited 25 Oct 2014]. Available from: http://www.springerreference.com/index/chapterdbid/137299

17. Hung SH, Huang HM, Lee HC, Ching Lin H, Kao LT, Wu CS. A population-based study on the association between chronic periodontitis and sialolithiasis. Laryngoscope. 2016;126(4):847–50.

18. Kraaij S, Karagozoglu KH, Kenter YA, Pijpe J, Gilijamse M, Brand HS. Systemic diseases and the risk of developing salivary stones: a case control study. Oral Surg Oral Med Oral Pathol Oral Radiol. 2015;119:539–43.

19. Ugga L, Ravanelli M, Pallottino AA, Farina D, Maroldi R. Diagnostic work-up in obstructive and inflammatory salivary gland disorders. Work-up diagnostico nella patologia ostruttiva e infiammatoria delle ghiandole salivari. Acta Otorhinolaryngol Ital. 2017;37(2):83–93.

20. Astrom AN, Lie SSA, Ekback G, Gulcan F, Ordell S. Self-reported dry mouth among ageing people: a longitudinal cross-national study. Eur J Oral Sci. 2019;127:130–8.

21. Donaldson M, Goodchild JH. A Systematic Approach to Xerostomia Diagnosis and Management. Compend Contin Educ Dent. 2018;39(suppl 5):1–9.

22. Francis DO, Smith LJ. Hoarseness guidelines redux toward improved treatment of patients with dysphonia. Otolaryngol Clin N Am. 2019;52:597–605.

23. House SA, Fisher EL. Hoarseness in Adults. Am Fam Physician. 2017;96(11):720–8.

24. Zur K. Hoarseness and pediatric voice disorders. In: Kountakis S, editors. Encyclopedia of otolaryngology, head and neck surgery: Springer reference www.springerreference.com. Berlin/Heidelberg: Springer; 2013. [cited 26 Oct 2014]. Available from: http://www.springerreference.com/index/chapterdbid/370684

25. Womack JP, Kropa J, Jimenez SM. Epistaxis: Outpatient Management. Am Fam Physician. 2018;98 (4):240–5.

26. Becker A. Epistaxis. In: Kountakis S, editor. Encyclopedia of otolaryngology, head and neck surgery: Springer reference www.springerreference.com. Berlin/Heidelberg: Springer; 2013 [cited 27 Sept 2014]. Available from: http://www.springerreference.com/index/chapterdbid/370724

27. Krulewitz NA, Fix ML. Epistaxis. Emerg Med Clin North Am. 2019;37(1):29–39.

28. Abuzeid M. Pediatric epistaxis. In: Elzouki A, editor. Textbook of clinical pediatrics: Springer reference www.springerreference.com. Berlin/Heidelberg: Springer; 2012 [cited 27 Sept 2014]. Available from: http://www.springerreference.com/index/chapterdbid/324084

29. Wong AS, Anat DS. Epistaxis: a guide to assessment and management. J Fam Pract. 2018 Dec;67(12): E13–20.

30. Oyama LC. Foreign bodies of the ear, nose and throat. Emerg Med Clin N Am. 2019;37:121–30.

31. Dann L, et al. Nasal foreign bodies in the paediatric emergency department. Ir J Med Sci. 2019;188: 1401–5.

32. Grigg S, Grigg C. Removal of ear, nose and throat foreign bodies: a review. AJGP. 2018;47(10):682–5.

Part XVII

The Cardiovascular System

Hypertension

Kenyon Railey, Mallory Mc Clester Brown, and
Anthony J. Viera

Contents

K. Railey · A. J. Viera (✉)
Department of Family Medicine and Community Health,
Duke University School of Medicine, Durham, NC, USA
e-mail: kenyon.railey@duke.edu;
anthony.viera@duke.edu

M. M. C. Brown
Department of Family Medicine, University of North
Carolina at Chapel Hill, Chapel Hill, NC, USA
e-mail: mallory_mcclester@med.unc.edu

© Springer Nature Switzerland AG 2022
P. M. Paulman et al. (eds.), *Family Medicine*,
https://doi.org/10.1007/978-3-030-54441-6_82

General Principles

Hypertension, also referred to as high blood pressure (BP), is one of the most common conditions seen in adult primary care practices. In 2016, there were nearly 33 million visits to provider offices with essential hypertension as the principle diagnosis [1]. In 2017, age-adjusted prevalence data in the United States reveals that 46% of adults aged ≥ 20 years have hypertension, which equates to an estimated 116.4 million men and women [2]. Worldwide, at least 1.39 billion adults have high blood pressure [3].

Hypertension remains a major risk factor for cardiovascular and cerebrovascular disease. From a population health perspective, the elimination of hypertension could reduce cardiovascular mortality by 30% in men and 38% in women, which translates to a larger impact on mortality for all risk factors among females and all but smoking cessation among males [4]. In addition to a reduction of mortality, management of uncontrolled hypertension substantially reduces the risk of heart failure, stroke, myocardial infarction, and chronic kidney disease.

As knowledge and analysis of population trends deepen, it has become apparent that certain populations bear a greater burden of illness from hypertension and its consequences both in the United States and globally. There is a widening disparity of prevalence and control among individuals from low- and middle-income countries compared to those from high-income countries [5]. In addition, regarding race/ethnicity, non-Hispanic blacks in the United States have higher age-adjusted prevalence and unmet treatment goals for hypertension than other racial groups. When compared to non-Hispanic white patients, there is a larger proportion of Mexican-Americans and people of other races/ethnicities not receiving treatment for hypertension despite the indication [5].

The diagnosis and management of hypertension has been complicated by the release of multiple guidelines in the last decade which are supported by varying degrees of evidence. In addition to age, race/ethnicity, and comorbid condition-specific management recommendations, these guidelines contain potentially conflicting recommendations for diagnostic and treatment thresholds. Thankfully, they are consistent regarding the first-line pharmacological treatments recommended which include diuretics, angiotensin-converting enzyme (ACE) inhibitors, angiotensin receptor blockers (ARBs), and calcium channel blockers. In addition, among all guidelines, recommendations are consistent regarding renewed emphasis on and reaffirmation of the importance of accurate diagnosis, lifestyle modifications, and individualized management approaches.

Overall, management of hypertension remains a challenge in primary care. Providers are tasked with accurately detecting high blood pressure, managing comorbidities, minimizing side effects, maintaining quality of life, and promoting healthy lifestyle choices, all with the goal of reducing cardiovascular risk.

Detection and Diagnosis

There is ample evidence to support the benefits of screening for high blood pressure in adults. In the landmark report made by the seventh Joint National Committee (JNC 7) in 2003, recommendations were made to screen adults every 2 years if blood pressure was recorded as less than 120/80 mm Hg and every 1 year for systolic blood pressures 120–139 mm Hg or diastolic pressures 80–90 mm Hg [6]. The report from the eighth Joint National Committee (JNC 8) did not address nor define the diagnosis of hypertension in its 2014 guideline [7]. Rather, the 2014 guideline focused on management principles based upon age (greater than or younger than 60) as well as comorbid conditions like diabetes and chronic kidney disease.

The American Academy of Family Physicians (AAFP) supports the US Preventive Services Task Force (USPSTF) clinical preventive service recommendations on this topic which suggests screening all adults over 18 for hypertension. The USPSTF recommends annual screening for adults aged 40 years or older and for those at increased risk for high blood pressure. Persons deemed at increased risk include those who have high-normal blood pressure (130 to 139/85 to 89 mm Hg), those who are overweight or obese, and African Americans. Adults aged 18–39 years with normal blood pressure (<130/85 mm Hg) who do not have other risk factors should be rescreened every 3–5 years. It is important to note that previous recommendation statements from the USPSTF did not differentiate blood pressure measurement protocols nor create a reference standard for measurement confirmation. The most current USPSTF recommendation, however, added to the yearly screening guidance by including language regarding method of measurement, specifically assessing the diagnostic accuracies of office blood pressure measurement, ambulatory blood pressure monitoring (ABPM), and home blood pressure monitoring (HBPM). The USPSTF concluded that obtaining measurements outside of the clinical setting is necessary for diagnostic confirmation before starting treatment [8].

Guidelines and typical practice patterns suggest that the diagnosis should be based on at least two separately recorded elevated blood pressure readings. In a patient with a single greatly elevated blood pressure reading in the office setting who already has hypertensive-related target organ damage, the diagnosis can generally be made without follow-up readings. Table 1 gives an overview of office-based blood pressure and hypertension classifications based on current guidelines. This table includes information from the 2018 European Society of Cardiology (ESC) and the European Society of Hypertension (ESH) definition of high blood pressure, which is defined as office systolic blood pressure value of >140 mm Hg and/or diastolic blood pressure value of >90 mm Hg [9].

Traditionally, blood pressure is recorded in the office with an auscultatory or oscillometric method manually or via an automated device. Patients should be seated quietly for at least 5 min in a chair with feet on the floor and arm supported. Transient elevations in blood pressure can occur as a result of certain substances like nicotine, alcohol, cocaine, or caffeine in addition to commonly utilized medications like nonsteroidal anti-inflammatory medications, antidepressants, oral contraceptives, and decongestants [10]. Table 2 outlines some more of these common substances. As mentioned, the JNC 8 report does not address screening intervals, nor does the American College of Cardiology (ACC)/

American Heart Association (AHA) guideline, which was released as an update to the JNC 7. It does, however, conclude that the diagnosis of hypertension should be based on accurate measurement and confirmation, which ultimately aligns with other US and international guidelines [9, 10, 11].

The USPSTF found convincing evidence that ABPM is the best method for diagnosing hypertension. However, ABPM is not widely available. The USPSTF found good quality evidence that HBPM may be an acceptable alternative [8]. Both ABPM and HBPM permit recognition of white coat hypertension (i.e., elevated blood pressure level that occurs only in clinical settings), thus helpful in confirmation of a hypertension diagnosis. HBPM also facilitates self-monitoring of blood pressure, which likely has benefits in awareness, adherence, and ultimately blood pressure reduction. Home blood pressure measurement technique is also important, and providers should instruct patients on proper monitoring protocols. The 2017 ACC/AHA guidelines provided a reference regarding the relationship between HBPM blood pressure readings, ABPM readings, and corresponding office-based measurements, which is summarized in Table 3 [10]. Note that the threshold for stage 1 and stage 2 hypertension based on these guidelines is achieved with lower HBPM and ABPM measurements.

Approach to the Patient

Cornerstones in the evaluation of patients with newly diagnosed hypertension include (1) assessing overall cardiovascular mortality

Table 1 Classification of blood pressure level for adults

Guideline (year released)	Normal blood pressure	Elevated blood pressure or prehypertension[a]	Stage 1 hypertension[b]	Stage 2 hypertension[b]
JNC 7 (2003)	<120/80	120–139/80–89	140–159/90–99	>160/100
JNC 8 (2014)	Not defined	Not defined	Not defined	Not defined
ACC/AHA (2017)	<120/80	120–129/80	130–139/80–89	>140/90
ESC/ESH (2018)	120–129/80–84	130–139/85–89	140–159/90–99	160–179/100–109

[a]Prehypertension category was removed from JNC 8 and AHA/ACC guidelines.
[b]ESC/ESH guidelines use "Grade" language instead of "Stage" and defines Grade 3 HTN as >180/110.

Table 2 Drugs that may cause blood pressure (BP) elevation

Drug	Common examples
Estrogen	Oral contraceptives, hormone replacement therapy
Herbals	Ephedra, ginseng
Illicit drugs	Amphetamines, cocaine
Nonsteroidal anti-inflammatories	Ibuprofen, naproxen
Psychiatric agents	Fluoxetine, lithium, tricyclic agents (TCAs)
Steroids	Prednisone
Sympathomimetics	Over-the-counter nasal decongestants

Table 3 ACC/AHA corresponding values of SBP/DBP for clinic, HBPM, daytime, nighttime, and 24-h ABPM measurements

Office measurement	HBPM	Daytime ABPM	Nighttime ABPM	24-hour ABPM
120/80	120/80	120/80	100/65	115/75
130/80	130/80	130/80	110/65	125/75
140/90	135/85	135/85	120/70	130/80
160/100	145/90	145/90	140/85	145/90

ABPM indicates ambulatory blood pressure monitoring, *BP* blood pressure, *DBP* diastolic blood pressure, *HBPM* home blood pressure monitoring, *SBP* systolic blood pressure.
Source. [10].

Table 4 Cardiovascular disease risk factors common in patients with hypertension

Age (>55 men or >65 women)
Chronic kidney disease
Cigarette smoking
Diabetes obesity (body mass index >30)
Dyslipidemia/hypercholesterolemia
Family history of hypertension
Family history of premature cardiovascular disease (first-degree male relative <55 years, female <65 years)
Microalbuminuria or GFR <60 mL/min
Obstructive sleep apnea
Overweight/obesity
Physical inactivity/low fitness level
Poor/unhealthy diet
Psychosocial stress

should inquire about a patient's history of previously elevated blood pressures and specific conditions like diabetes, hyperlipidemia, and obstructive sleep apnea as well as specific risk factors. Table 4 outlines some of the well-documented modifiable and fixed risk factors common in patients with high blood pressure. Given evidence of disparities of disease prevalence and burden previously mentioned, stress and even discrimination have been linked to hypertension [12], so providers should strongly consider asking patients and their families about social determinants of health that may influence decision-making, adherence, and overall wellness.

Physical Examination

Each patient newly diagnosed with hypertension should have a physical exam including more than one blood pressure measurement with adherence to proper technique. At least at the initial diagnosis, blood pressure should be measured in both arms in addition to assessments in both the standing and sitting positions. In subsequent visits, the arm with the higher reading should be used. The exam should also include (1) calculation of the body mass index (BMI), (2) evaluation of the optic fundi, (3) exam of the neck including palpation of the thyroid gland and auscultation for

risk and presence of comorbid cardiovascular disease risk factors, (2) investigating for secondary causes of high blood pressure, and (3) determining if the patient has evidence of end-organ damage. A thorough history and physical examination with targeted laboratory and diagnostic studies will assist the clinician in a comprehensive evaluation toward these goals.

History

Hypertension is the result of a complex interaction between genetic predisposition and various environmental exposures including diet, physical activity, and medication/substance use. Physical inactivity, being overweight or obese, and excess intake of alcohol or nicotine contribute to a large proportion of underlying hypertension. Providers

carotid bruits, (4) cardiac exam, (5) lung exam, (6) abdominal examination with special attention for enlarged kidneys, masses, abdominal aortic pulsation, and abdominal or renal bruits, (7) examination of the lower extremities for pulses and edema, and (7) a neurological evaluation.

Laboratory Tests and Diagnostic Procedures

Laboratory and diagnostic testing are valuable tools not only in determining the presence of end-organ damage at the time of diagnosis but also in identifying secondary causes of hypertension. In addition, baseline laboratory tests are also important in cardiovascular risk factor profiling which facilitates effective treatment planning. Recommended tests include serum potassium and sodium levels, blood urea nitrogen, and creatinine level. An electrocardiogram (ECG), blood glucose, hematocrit, and fasting lipid panel are also recommended, if not done previously, to help assess overall cardiovascular risk. The ECG also may reveal target organ damage in the form of left ventricular hypertrophy or prior myocardial infarction (Q waves). Optional tests include a TSH level and calcium. A decision to perform other tests such as a chest radiograph, uric acid level, or echocardiogram are appropriate if indicated based on findings from history, physical exam, or ECG or in instances of historical clues suggesting a secondary cause of hypertension.

Secondary Causes

Though most cases of hypertension are considered idiopathic or primary, it is important to consider secondary causes of hypertension at the time of diagnosis. Secondary causes of hypertension are identifiable and potentially reversible causes of elevated blood pressures. It is estimated that one of these specific and remediable causes is identified in approximately 10% of patients (9). The most common secondary causes are obstructive sleep apnea, renal artery stenosis, and hyperaldosteronism. Secondary hypertension should be suspected in younger patients (less than 30 years of age) as well as in patients with treatment-resistant high blood pressure. As noted in Table 2, there are multiple substances and medications that cause elevations in blood pressure. A trial off potentially offending medications (if possible), or a change in diet, may be warranted before embarking on pharmacologic treatment. Specialty colleague consultation is often necessary in the evaluation of secondary hypertension due to the complex measurements and data interpretation necessary to properly diagnose these conditions.

Management

Benefits of Treatment

In clinical trials, antihypertensive therapy has been associated with reductions in stroke incidence averaging 35–40%; myocardial infarction, 20–25%; and heart failure, more than 50% [13]. These data support the importance of treating patients to not only reduce BP but to also, more importantly, prevent the morbidity and mortality associated with hypertension.

The panel members appointed to the eighth Joint National Committee (JNC 8) provided an evidence-based update to BP treatment goals. Per their report, in the general population aged ≥ 60 years, pharmacologic treatment should be initiated to lower BP at systolic BP ≥ 150 mm Hg or diastolic BP ≥ 90 mm Hg and treat to a goal systolic BP <150 mm Hg and goal diastolic BP <90 mm Hg. This recommendation is made with Grade A (i.e., highest level) evidence. For patients <60 years of age, expert opinion recommendation is to initiate treatment with a systolic BP of ≥ 140 mm Hg and treat to a goal of <140 mm Hg, and grade A recommendation is to initiate pharmacologic treatment to lower BP at diastolic BP ≥ 90 mm Hg and treat to a goal <90 mm Hg. In the population aged ≥ 18 years with chronic kidney disease (CKD) or diabetes, the recommendation is to initiate pharmacologic treatment at systolic BP ≥ 140 mm Hg or diastolic BP ≥ 90 mm Hg and treat to goal $<140/90$ mm Hg [7].

The 2017 ACC/AHA guidelines recommend incorporating cardiovascular risk estimates with BP levels to determine when to initiate antihypertensives. The guidelines suggest initiating medication in those at high cardiovascular risk when systolic BP is 130 mm Hg or greater or diastolic BP is 80 mm Hg or greater. In those at lower risk, they suggest initiating antihypertensives when systolic BP is 140 mm Hg or greater or diastolic BP is 90 mm Hg or greater (10). High risk is defined as a history of clinical cardiovascular disease or an estimated 10-year atherosclerotic cardiovascular disease (ASCVD) risk of 10% or higher according to the pooled cohort equations. Clinical disease is defined as coronary artery disease, heart failure, or stroke [10]. A target close to 120/80 mmHg is generally better than a higher BP target.

Nonpharmacologic Interventions

All patients with blood pressures above normal should be treated with nonpharmacologic interventions: heart-healthy diet, reducing sodium intake, potassium supplementation, increasing physical activity, limiting alcohol consumption, and losing body weight for those who are overweight [10]. Table 5 is a summary of some key recommendations for lifestyle changes that lower blood pressure. For overall cardiovascular disease risk reduction, all patients who smoke should be counseled about smoking cessation and provided with assistance modalities.

The DASH eating plan emphasizes intake of vegetables, fruits, and whole grains. Additionally, low-fat dairy products, poultry, fish, legumes, and nuts should be included. Diet should be rich in calcium and potassium. Intake of sweets, sugar-sweetened beverages, and red meats should be limited. Sodium intake should be no more than 2400 mg each day. Research has shown that a DASH eating plan with no more than 1600-mg sodium has effects similar to single drug therapy [14].

Adults with elevated BP should be encouraged to engage in aerobic physical activity to lower BP. The recommendation is to include three to four sessions per week lasting an average of 40 min per session and involving moderate- to vigorous-intensity physical activity [15].

Some research has shown increased blood pressure to be positively correlated to more than 2 ounces/day of alcohol. Therefore, it is important to limit alcohol intake [16]. Alcohol should be limited to no more than one ounce (30 mL) of ethanol per day for women and no more than two ounces (60 mL) per day for men.

Pharmacologic Treatment

When deciding on pharmacologic therapy, the individual patient characteristics, including age, race, sex, family history, cardiovascular risk factors, and concomitant disease states, should be considered. Additionally, the patient's ability to afford the prescribed therapy as well as their compliance must be considered.

In the general population, including those with diabetes, initial antihypertensive treatment should include a thiazide-type diuretic, calcium channel blocker (CCB), ACE inhibitor, or ARB. In the

Table 5 Lifestyle recommendations for hypertension

Recommendation	Description	Approximate systolic BP reduction
DASH eating plan	Diet rich in fruits, vegetables, and low-fat dairy with reduced fat intake	8–14 mm Hg
Exercise	Regular aerobic activity at least 30 min per day	4–9 mm Hg
Reduced dietary sodium intake	Maximum 2400 mg (ideally 1600 mg) of sodium daily	2–8 mm Hg
Moderate alcohol drinking	Maximum 2 ounces ethanol per day for men; maximum 1 ounce per day for women	2–4 mm Hg
Weight loss	Achieve/maintain BMI of 18.5–24.9 kg/m²	5–20 mm Hg

population aged ≥ 18 years with chronic kidney disease (CKD), initial (or add-on) antihypertensive treatment should include an ACE inhibitor or ARB to improve kidney outcomes. This recommendation applies to all CKD patients with hypertension regardless of race or diabetes status. Note that an ACE inhibitor and ARB should not be used together [17].

The main objective of hypertension treatment is to attain and maintain goal blood pressure. If goal BP is not reached within a month of treatment, the initial drug dose should be increased or a second drug such as a thiazide-type diuretic, CCB, ACE inhibitor, or ARB should be added. If the goal BP cannot be reached with two agents, a third drug should be added [7]. It has been suggested that a 6-month period of undertreated hypertension increases cardiovascular morbidity [18] (Fig. 1).

Not at goal BP as defined by 2014 JNC-8, 2017 ACC/AHA, or 2018 ESC/ESH guidelines

Choose from thiazide-type diuretic, ACE-inhibitor or ARB, or CCB. Consider combination if BP more than 20/10 mm Hg above goal.

If not at goal after reasonable time, either increase dose of current medication (if it is not already at moderate to maximum dose) or add another agent from a different class

---

Fig. 1 Evidence-based simplified algorithm for hypertension treatment

Diuretics

Thiazide-type diuretics (chlorthalidone, hydrochlorothiazide) increase renal excretion of sodium and chloride at the distal segment of the renal tubule which results in decreased plasma volume, cardiac output, and renal blood flow and increased renin activity. With these agents, potassium excretion is increased, while calcium and uric acid elimination is decreased. Because of its greater potency and longer duration, chlorthalidone should be preferred over hydrochlorothiazide, especially when used alone. Potential side effects of all thiazide-type diuretics include hyponatremia, hypokalemia, dizziness, fatigue, muscle cramps, gout attacks, and impotence. Special attention should be paid when starting these agents in patients with diabetes, elevated cholesterol, or gout as thiazides can worsen each of these conditions. None of these conditions is a contraindication, however.

Loop diuretics and potassium-sparing diuretics can be used as adjunct therapy when thiazide-type diuretics are not sufficient (e.g., in patients with decreased glomerular filtration rate). Loop diuretics (furosemide, torsemide, and bumetanide) inhibit sodium and chloride reabsorption in the proximal and distal tubules and the loop of Henle. Side effects include diarrhea, headache, blurred vision, tinnitus, muscle cramps, fatigue, or weakness. When used in high doses in patients with significant renal disease, ototoxicity may occur.

Potassium-sparing diuretics (spironolactone, triamterene, amiloride) are useful for preventing potassium wastage that occurs with thiazide and loop diuretics. Spironolactone competitively inhibits the uptake of aldosterone at the receptor site in the distal tubule, in turn reducing the effect of aldosterone. This drug is an evidence-based fourth-line medication for resistant hypertension (described below). Main adverse effects to be aware of include gynecomastia and hyperkalemia. Triamterene and amiloride are typically used more specifically to stop potassium loss, and both have side effect profiles similar to the thiazide diuretics [19].

ACE Inhibitors

ACE inhibitors block the conversion of angiotensin I to angiotensin II, resulting in decreased aldosterone production with subsequent increased sodium and water excretion. As a result, renal blood flow is increased and peripheral resistance decreases. Renin and potassium levels typically increase. Major side effects include cough, angioedema, and the possibility of acute renal failure (in patients with renal artery stenosis). Importantly, this class of medication can cause syncope in patients who are salt, or volume, depleted. This drug class is teratogenic in the human fetus and should therefore be avoided in pregnancy and in women who may become pregnant.

ACE inhibitors have little effect on insulin and glucose levels or lipid levels, making them a good choice for most diabetics and patients with hyperlipidemia. ACE inhibitors are a particularly good choice for patients with congestive heart failure, peripheral vascular disease, and renal insufficiency as well.

Angiotensin Receptor Antagonists

ARBs bind to angiotensin II receptors, blocking the vasoconstrictor and aldosterone-secreting effects of angiotensin II. Aldosterone production decreases, while plasma renin and angiotensin II levels rise. There is no notable change in the serum potassium level, renal plasma flow, glomerular filtration rate, heart rate, cholesterol level, or serum glucose.

ARBs are generally well-tolerated but can cause hyperkalemia. ARBs are also teratogenic and should be avoided in patients of childbearing age. The major use of ARBs is for patients who cannot tolerate an ACE inhibitor due to cough.

Calcium Channel Blockers

CCBs reduce the influx of calcium across cell membranes in myocardial and smooth muscles. This in turn dilates coronary arteries, as well as peripheral arteries. This dilation reduces total peripheral resistance leading to decreased BP. Structural differences exist between agents in this class, which lead to different adverse effect profiles as well as differences in their effect on cardiac conduction. Verapamil and diltiazem (non-dihydropyridines) work to slow the conduction through the AV node and prolong the effective refractory period in the AV node.

Dihydropyridines (e.g., amlodipine, nifedipine) increase cardiac output and have a more profound vasodilatory effect, making them the preferred CCBs for hypertension.

The main noteworthy side effect of dihydropyridine CCBs is peripheral edema, but they can also cause constipation, flushing, and tachycardia. CCBs are contraindicated in patients with heart block, acute myocardial infarction, and cardiogenic shock. CCBs have no effect on glucose metabolism or lipid levels. CCBs are a particularly good choice for patients with migraine headaches, angina, chronic obstructive pulmonary disease or asthma, peripheral vascular disease, renal insufficiency, supraventricular arrhythmias, and diabetes.

Beta-Blockers

Beta-blockers are not indicated for first-line treatment of uncomplicated hypertension but are recommended for patients following a myocardial infarction and for patients with congestive heart failure. Beta-blockers antagonize the effects of sympathetic nerve stimulation or circulating catecholamines at beta-adrenergic receptors, which are widely distributed throughout the body. Beta-1 receptors are predominant in the heart (and the kidney), while beta-2 receptors are predominant in other organs such as the lung, peripheral blood vessels, and skeletal muscle. In the kidney, the blockade of B1 receptors inhibits the release of renin from the juxtaglomerular cells and thereby reduces the activity of the renin-angiotensin-aldosterone system. In the heart, blockade of B1 receptors in the sinoatrial (SA) node reduces heart rate, and blockade of the B1 receptors in the myocardium decreases contractility. It is likely a combination of these effects that leads to BP reduction. The overall clinical response to beta-blockers is a decreased heart rate, decreased cardiac output, lower blood pressure, decreased renin production, and bronchiolar constriction.

The side effect profile of beta-blockers depends on their receptor selectivity. In those without intrinsic sympathomimetic activity, the heart rate is slowed, a decrease is seen in cardiac output, and an increase is noted in peripheral vascular resistance. Bronchospasm may also be the cause. Typical side effects seen with these agents include fatigue, erectile dysfunction, dyspnea, cold extremities, cough, drowsiness, and dizziness. These agents tend to increase the triglyceride level and decrease the HDL level but have little effect on blood glucose levels. Beta-blockers should not be used in patients with sinus bradycardia, second- or third-degree heart block, cardiogenic shock, cardiac failure, and/or severe COPD/asthma.

Central Acting Drugs

Methyldopa, clonidine, guanfacine, and guanabenz are central alpha-2 agonists. These agents act to decrease dopamine and norepinephrine production in the brain, resulting in decreased sympathetic nervous activity throughout the body. BP declines with the decrease in peripheral resistance. Methyldopa is unique in its adverse effect profile as it can induce autoimmune disorders such as those with positive Coombs' and antinuclear antibody (ANA) tests, hemolytic anemia, and hepatic necrosis. The other agents can lead to sedation, dry mouth, and dizziness. Importantly, abrupt clonidine withdrawal can lead to rebound hypertension.

Alpha-Blockers

Alpha-1 receptor blockers, such as prazosin, terazosin, and doxazosin, block the uptake of catecholamines by smooth muscle cells. In the peripheral vasculature, this results in vasodilation. A marked reduction in BP may be noted with the first dose of these drugs; therefore, it is recommended they be started at low doses and slowly titrated upward. Side effects of these agents include dizziness, sedation, nasal congestion, headaches, and postural effects. They have no effect on lipid levels, glucose, exercise tolerance, or electrolytes. These agents are probably best reserved for men with hypertension and comorbid BPH symptoms.

Vasodilators

Hydralazine and minoxidil dilate peripheral arterioles, resulting in a fall in BP. Several other responses simultaneously occur including a sympathetic reflex which leads to increased heart rate, renin and catecholamine release, and venous constriction. The kidneys retain sodium and water. Side effects include tachycardia, flushing, and headache. A beta-blocker and a loop diuretic are usually used with these drugs to minimize side effects. These agents are used mainly for resistant hypertension.

Special Considerations

Hypertensive Emergency

A hypertensive emergency is described as a severe elevation in BP accompanied by evidence of impending or progressive target organ dysfunction. Note that the actual BP measurement is not likely as important as the rate of the rise in blood pressure since patients with chronic hypertension often tolerate higher BP levels than normotensive individuals.

The most common origin of hypertensive emergency is an abrupt increase in BP in patients with chronic hypertension, which may be related to medication noncompliance. Hypertensive emergency can also be caused by certain medications or substances. Examples include withdrawal syndrome from antihypertensives including clonidine and beta-blockers as well as stimulant intoxication with cocaine, methamphetamine, and phencyclidine (PCP).

Clinical manifestations of target organ damage usually involve derangements in the neurologic, cardiac, or renal systems. The patient with hypertensive emergency may present with encephalopathy, pulmonary edema, myocardial infarction, or unstable angina.

Upon presentation, a focused physical exam should include repeated BP recording in both arms. Direct ophthalmoscope exam should be completed with special attention to look for papilledema. A brief neurologic examination should be done to assess for focal deficits and to assess for altered mental status. The cardiac and pulmonary examination should be complete with attention to possible arrhythmias and pulmonary edema. Abdominal exam should focus on palpating for abdominal masses and tenderness as well as auscultation for abdominal bruits. Peripheral pulses should be palpated.

The immediate goal when treating hypertensive emergency is to reduce the systolic by no more than 25%, within the first hour, and if the patient is then stable, to 160/100–110 mm Hg over the ensuing 2–6 h [10]. Treatment should be more aggressive for certain patients, however. For adults with a compelling condition like severe preeclampsia/eclampsia or pheochromocytoma crisis, blood pressure should be reduced to less than 140 mm Hg during the first hour. For patients with aortic dissection, blood pressure should be reduced to less than 120 mm Hg in that same time [10]. The selection of an antihypertensive agent is an individualized one. Beta-blockers, vasodilators, dopamine agonists, and calcium channel blockers are all potential agents. The selection of which medication should be based on the drug's pharmacology, the underlying pathophysiology of the patient's hypertension, the degree of target organ damage, the rate of desired blood pressure decline, and the presence of comorbidities [10].

Hypertension Treatment in Older Adults

While current JNC 8 guidelines and the USPSTF recommend treating patients over age 60 to a blood pressure of <150/90, several studies are in support of tighter blood pressure control in order to reduce cardiovascular events. The Hypertension in the Very Elderly Trial (HYVET) was one of the first large-scale clinical trials to establish the benefit of lowering blood pressure in patients 80 years and older [20]. The Systolic Blood Pressure Intervention Trial (SPRINT) was a sentinel clinical trial that compared cardiovascular outcomes in patients with increased cardiovascular risk who were randomized to an intensive blood pressure goal of less than 120 mm Hg or a standard blood pressure goal of less than 140 mm Hg [21]. A subanalysis of the SPRINT trial was completed on patients over the age of 75 which also supported more intensive blood pressure control as a way of preventing cardiovascular events, even in frail older adults. On the other hand, several cohort studies of adults 80 years of age and over have shown that participants with low

blood pressure at baseline had higher all-cause mortality rates [22–25]. These findings suggest that lowering BP among the oldest-old might be harmful. While these findings could be related to patient selection, frailty or other poor health indicators, or confounding causality, the current recommendations for adults over the age of 75 remain to control blood pressure to <150/90 mm Hg.

"Race"-Based Treatment

JNC 7 was one of the first hypertension guidelines to mention race-specific recommendations for treatment of high blood pressure. In the JNC 7, thiazide diuretics were considered as the first-line therapy for black patients [6]. The JNC 8 guidelines were similar in the recommendation of thiazide-type diuretics being considered first line, but also added that calcium channel blockers should be used as the antihypertensive treatment of choice in the general black population, including those with diabetes [7]. The authors of this chapter chose to deemphasize these race-specific recommendations since a large body of anthropological and contemporary genetic evidence suggests that "race" is a social construct, not a biological one. Insights into genetic variation support the notion that humans are essentially the same, and there is greater variation within identified racial groups than across groups [26]. In addition, while there is ample evidence from clinical trials that demonstrate differences in cardiovascular outcomes among populations in the United States, the participation of various racial/ethnic groups other than white populations in multiple trials has been inconsistent, inadequate, or not measured [27]. Since there are multiple complex factors that affect blood pressure control in patients of all racial/ethnic backgrounds (i.e., socioeconomic standing, lifestyle, clinical inertia, and even discrimination or bias), the interpretation of medical literature and guidelines utilizing "race" is challenging. Until future studies analyze concepts of ancestry, which incorporates ethnicity, geography, and genetics, clinicians should take care with "race"-based recommendations, and instead approach patients in an individualized manner, prioritizing care that is simultaneously culturally aware and evidence based.

References

1. Rui P, Okeyode T. National ambulatory medical care survey: 2016 national summary tables. 2016. Available from: https://www.cdc.gov/nchs/data/ahcd/namcs_summary/2016_namcs_web_tables.pdf
2. Virani SS, Alonso A, Benjamin EJ, Bittencourt MS, Callaway CW, Carson AP, American Heart Association Council on Epidemiology and Prevention Statistics Committee and Stroke Statistics Subcommittee, et al. Heart disease and stroke statistics-2020 update: a report from the American Heart Association. Circulation. 2020;141(9):e139–596.
3. Mills KT, Bundy JD, Kelly TN, Reed JE, Kearney PM, Reynolds K, et al. Global disparities of hypertension prevalence and control: a systematic analysis of population-based studies from 90 countries. Circulation. 2016;134(6):441–50.
4. Patel SA, Winkel M, Ali MK, Narayan KMV, Mehta NK. Cardiovascular mortality associated with 5 leading risk factors: national and state preventable fractions estimated from survey data. Ann Intern Med. 2015;163(4):245–53.
5. Al Kibria GM. Racial/ethnic disparities in prevalence, treatment, and control of hypertension among US adults following application of the 2017 American College of Cardiology/American Heart Association guideline. Prev Med Rep. 2019;14 https://doi.org/10.1016/j.pmedr.2019.100850.
6. Chobanian AV, Barkis GL, Black HR, et al. The seventh report of the joint national committee on prevention, detection, evaluation, and treatment of high blood pressure: the JNC 7 report. JAMA. 2003;289(19):2560–72.
7. James PA, Oparil S, Carter BL, Cushman WC, Dennison-Himmelfarb C, Handler J, et al. 2014 evidence-based guideline for the management of high blood pressure in adults: report from the panel members appointed to the eighth Joint National Committee (JNC 8). JAMA. 2014;311(5):507–20.
8. US Preventative Services Task Force. Final recommendation statement: High blood pressure in adults: screening. 2016. Available at: https://www.uspreventiveservicestaskforce.org/Page/Document/RecommendationStatementFinal/high-blood-pressure-in-adults-screening
9. Williams B, Mancia G, Speiring W, Rosei EA, Azizi M, Burnier M, et al. 2018 ESC/ESH Guidelines for the management of arterial hypertension: the task force for the management of arterial hypertension of the European Society of Cardiology (ESC) and the European Society of Hypertension (ESH). J Hypertens. 2018;36(12):2284–309.
10. Welton PK, Carey RM, Aronow WS, Casey DE, Collins KJ, Himmerlfarb CD, et al. ACC/AHA/AAPA/ABC/ACPM/AGS/APhA/ASH/ASPC/NMA/PCNA Guideline for the Prevention, Detection, Evaluation, and Management of High Blood Pressure in Adults. Am Coll Cardiol. 2018;71(19):e127–248.
11. Woolsey S, Brown B, Ralls B, Friedrichs M, Stults B. Diagnosing hypertension in primary care clinics according to current guidelines. J Am Board Fam Med. 2017;30(2):170–7.
12. Dolezsar CM, McGrath JJ, Herzig AJM, Miller SB. Perceived racial discrimination and hypertension: a comprehensive systematic review. Health Psychol. 2014;33(1):20–34.
13. Neal B, MacMahon S, Chapman N. Effects of ACE inhibitors, calcium antagonists, and other blood-pressure-lowering drugs: results of prospectively designed overviews of randomised trials. Blood pressure lowering treatment trialists' collaboration. Lancet. 2000;356(9246):1955–64.
14. Sacks FM, Svetkey LP, Vollmer WM, et al. Effects on blood pressure of reduced dietary sodium and the dietary approaches to stop hypertension (DASH) diet. DASH-Sodium Collaborative Research Group. N Engl J Med. 2001;344(1):3–10.
15. Eckel RH, Jakicic JM, Ard JD, et al. AHA/ACC guideline on lifestyle management to reduce cardiovascular risk: a report of the American College of Cardiology/American Heart Association task force on practice guidelines. J Am Coll Cardiol. 2014;63(25) Pt B:2960–84.
16. Gordon T, Doyle JT. Alcohol consumption and its relationship to smoking, weight, blood pressure and blood lipids. Arch Intern Med. 1986;146(2):262–5.
17. Mann JF, et al. Renal outcomes with telmisartan, ramipril, or both, in people at high vascular risk (the ONTARGET study): a multicentre, randomised, double-blind, controlled trial. Lancet. 2008;372(9638):547–53.
18. Julius S, et al. Outcomes in hypertensive patients at high cardiovascular risk treated with regimens based on valsartan or amlodipine: the VALUE randomised trial. Lancet. 2004;363(9426):2022–31.
19. Calhoun DA, Jones D, Textor S, et al. Resistant hypertension: diagnosis, evaluation, and treatment. A scientific statement from the American Heart Association professional education committee of the council for high blood pressure research. Circulation. 2008;117:e510–26.
20. Beckett NS, Peters R, Fletcher AE, Staessen JA, Liu L, Dumitrascu D, et al. Treatment of hypertension in patients 80 years of age or older. N Engl J Med. 2008;358(18):1887–98.
21. Wright JT Jr, Fine LJ, Lackland DT, et al. Evidence supporting a systolic blood pressure goal of less than 150 mm Hg in patients aged 60 years or older: the minority view. Ann Intern Med. 2014;160(7):499–503.
22. Molander L, Lovheim H, Norman T, Nordstrom P, Gustafson Y. Lower systolic blood pressure is associated with greater mortality in people aged 85 and older. J Am Geriatr Soc. 2008;56(10):1853–9.

23. Poortvliet RK, Blom JW, de Craen AJ, Mooijaart SP, Westendorp RG, Assendelft WJ, et al. Low blood pressure predicts increased mortality in very old age even without heart failure: the Leiden 85-plus study. Eur J Heart Fail. 2013;15(5):528–33.

24. Ravindrarajah R, Hazra NC, Hamada S, Charlton J, Jackson SHD, Dregan A, et al. Systolic blood pressure trajectory, frailty, and all-cause mortality > 80 years of age: cohort study using electronic health records. Circulation. 2017;135(24):2357–68.

25. Van Bemmel T, Gussekloo J, Westendorp RG, Blauw GJ. In a population-based prospective study, no association between high blood pressure and mortality after age 85 years. J Hypertens. 2006;24(2):287–92.

26. Royal CDM, Dunston GM. Changing the paradigm from 'race' to human genome variation. Nat Genet. 2004;36(S11):S5–7.

27. Ferdinand KC, Ferdinand DP. Race-based therapy for hypertension: possible benefits and potential pitfalls. Expert Rev Cardiovasc Ther. 2008;6(10):1357–66.

Ischemic Heart Disease

Devdutta G. Sangvai, Ashley M. Rietz, and
Anthony J. Viera

Contents

General Principles

Ischemic heart disease (IHD) refers to the condition of inadequate blood supply to the myocardium. It is also commonly referred to as heart disease, coronary heart disease (CHD), or coronary artery disease (CAD). From 2013 to 2016, the total number of people age 20 and older in the United Sates affected by IHD was estimated to be 18.2 million [1]. Each year about 605,000 Americans have their first myocardial infarction (MI), with more than 200,000 experiencing a subsequent event [1]. While deaths from IHD have declined since 2000, it remains the leading killer of both men and women [1, 2]. In addition to the loss of life, IHD has a large financial impact. The National Heart, Lung, and Blood Institute estimates a loss of 218 billion dollars in 2014 including loss of productivity [1].

Angina pectoris, or simply angina, refers to the chest pain that occurs when myocardial oxygen supply cannot keep up with demand. Most patients with IHD experience angina. Thus, the evaluation of angina or chest pain is ultimately what leads to the diagnosis in most instances. Acute coronary syndrome (ACS) is a term used

D. G. Sangvai · A. J. Viera (✉)
Department of Family Medicine and Community Health,
Duke University School of Medicine, Durham, NC, USA
e-mail: devdutta.sangvai@duke.edu;
anthony.viera@duke.edu

A. M. Rietz
Department of Family Medicine, University of North
Carolina at Chapel Hill School of Medicine, Chapel Hill,
NC, USA
e-mail: ashley_rietz@med.unc.edu

© Springer Nature Switzerland AG 2022
P. M. Paulman et al. (eds.), *Family Medicine*,
https://doi.org/10.1007/978-3-030-54441-6_83

to describe a range of conditions associated with sudden, reduced blood flow to the heart [3]. This chapter will review the diagnosis of IHD when patients present with chest pain, distinguish between the acute coronary syndromes, and describe the management of acute coronary syndrome as well as stable IHD.

Diagnosis

History

The first task when evaluating a patient with chest pain is to quickly establish whether it is secondary to a life threatening cause such as an acute MI or other emergent cause such as pulmonary embolism, aortic dissection, or tension pneumothorax, to list a few. It is important to note that few patients with chest pain seen in the primary care setting have emergent or cardiac causes. Most patients presenting with chest pain in the outpatient setting have musculoskeletal (36%), gastrointestinal (19%), or anxiety-related causes (7.5%) [4]. These prevalence estimates reinforce the need for confidence in understanding the presentations of IHD.

The clinical history is one of the most important tools in the evaluation of the patient presenting with chest pain. Typical angina is described as substernal chest pain or discomfort that is provoked by exertion or emotional stress and relieved by rest or nitroglycerin. Its onset is usually not abrupt, and its duration is usually only a few minutes. When the chest pain has two of these criteria, it is classified as atypical angina. Nonanginal chest pain has only one of these clinical features [5]. While certain characteristics of the chest pain history are associated with increased or decreased likelihoods of a diagnosis of ACSs or MI, none of them alone or in combination are sufficient to diagnose a cardiac etiology [6]. Angina can be specified further by the level of exertion needed prior to onset. The tables below outline a general perspective on how to think about chest pain of possible cardiac origin (Tables 1 and 2).

As mentioned above, it is important to note that atypical angina or nonanginal chest pain does not mean that IHD is not the cause, only that the pain

Table 1 Clinical criteria of angina

	Typical	Atypical	Nonanginal
Angina	Substernal chest pain or discomfort; may radiate to arm or jaw. Provoked by exertion or emotional stress. Relieved by rest and/or nitroglycerin.	2 of the three features of typical chest pain. Pain is often located elsewhere, right side or left side of chest, for example.	1 of the three features. Note that "nonanginal" does not necessarily mean not of cardiac origin.

Table 2 Clinical criteria of stable versus unstable angina

	Stable	Unstable [7]
Angina	Symptoms of angina provoked by a consistent level of exertion or emotional stress. Relieved by rest.	Unprovoked chest pain or provoked by less exertion than previously. Generally not relieved by rest or medications. Lasting for longer periods of time.

is much less characteristic. Pretest probability for IHD is assessed by taking into consideration the type of chest pain (typical angina, atypical angina, nonanginal) and a patient's age and sex (Table 3). Additional pretest estimates may take into consideration changing demographics, comorbidities, and improvements in imaging and diagnostics [8]. While pretest probability is helpful, clinicians should not solely rely on this estimate to determine need for further evaluation of a patient with chest pain.

Gender differences make correlating symptoms to anatomic causes challenging. The WISE (Women's Ischemic Syndrome Evaluation) study highlighted that women ultimately diagnosed with IHD did not have typical angina 65% of the time [10]. Women also have a higher likelihood of ACS related to *microvascular etiology* rather than to stenosis of coronary arteries [11]. Finally, some patients lack the chest discomfort and are thus characterized as having silent ischemia.

Table 3 Estimating pretest probability of ischemic heart disease, Diamond Forrester model [9]

Age range	Men			Women		
	Nonanginal	Atypical	Typical	Nonanginal	Atypical	Typical
30–39 years	5.2	21.8	69.7	0.8	4.2	25.8
40–49 years	14.1	46.1	87.3	2.8	13.3	55.2
50–59 years	21.5	58.9	92.0	8.4	32.4	79.4
60–69 years	28.1	67.1	94.3	18.6	54.4	90.6

Other important symptoms to inquire about include pain radiating to arm(s) or jaw, epigastric pain, dyspnea, and any association of the pain with nausea, diaphoresis, or syncope [12]. Such clinical features increase the probability of a myocardial infarction in patients presenting with chest pain. Interestingly, pain radiating to both arms is the clinical feature that has the strongest positive likelihood ratio (approximately 7) for acute MI [13]. Pain that is pleuritic, sharp, or positional tends to lower the likelihood of MI as the etiology [14].

Obtaining a thorough past medical history is extremely valuable when assessing a patient for possible IHD. A history of hypertension, hyperlipidemia, diabetes, and any prior cardiovascular events should be noted.

ACS, in addition to unstable angina (UA), includes ST segment elevation myocardial infarction (STEMI) and non-ST segment elevation myocardial infarction (NSTEMI). In patients with previously stable angina, a change of chest pain from baseline in terms of increase in frequency, new occurrence with lower levels of activity, or increase in length of symptoms also is consistent with UA [3]. UA and MI cannot be differentiated by history alone. The use of electrocardiogram and cardiac biomarkers (discussed below) is essential to distinguishing amongst these clinical entities.

Physical Exam

The physical exam is less helpful in the diagnosis of IHD. The physical exam of the patient presenting with chest pain that may represent underlying IHD begins with an assessment of vital signs. Note the pulse and blood pressure. Significant hypotension may be a manifestation of MI. Diaphoresis may be present, and sweating in association with typical or atypical angina is a much better predictor of STEMI or NSTEMI than UA [13]. A third heart sound or pulmonary crackles on auscultation also would be concerning for possible MI [14]. Tenderness or reproducibility of chest pain on chest wall palpation argues against IHD as a diagnosis but does not necessarily rule it out [15].

Electrocardiogram and Biomarkers

The electrocardiogram (ECG) is a critical component of the evaluation of chest pain suggesting IHD, whether stable or possible ACS. A pathologic Q-wave is indication of prior MI. ECG abnormalities that may indicate myocardial ischemia include changes in the PR segment, the QRS complex, and the ST-segment. In the setting of possible ACS, a careful evaluation of ECG changes can assist in estimating time of the event, amount of myocardium at risk, patient prognosis, and appropriate therapeutic strategies. ST segment elevation found on an ECG is the hallmark sign of an acute STEMI [12]. The ECG alone is often insufficient to make the diagnosis of an acute MI, and the sensitivity and specificity of ECG are increased by serial assessments [16]. ECG changes such as ST deviation may be present in other conditions, such as left ventricular hypertrophy, left bundle branch block, or acute pericarditis. Note that in addition to patients diagnosed at the time of presentation of their chest pain, each year an additional 170,000 Americans experience a "silent" MI [1].

Like the ECG, cardiac biomarkers are an important extension of the history and physical examination in the evaluation of the patient with possible ACS. They are not part of the evaluation of patients with stable IHD. Cardiac troponins, the gold standard, are biochemical markers of active or recent myocardial damage. Increases in cardiac biomarkers, notably conventional cardiac troponins (cTnI or cTnT), or the MB fraction of creatinine kinase (CKMB), signify myocardial injury leading to necrosis of myocardial cells. Patients may present for evaluation before cTn values elevate, and others may have values that do not change on serial measurement [17]. High-sensitive troponin (hsTn) may assist with ruling out MI when not elevated. Elevated hsTn may also signal ischemia without infarction [17].

Troponin levels should be measured on initial assessment, within 6 h after the onset of chest pain, and in the 6–12 h time frame after onset of pain. In addition, it is important to understand that elevations in troponin may be seen for up to 14 days after the onset of myocardial necrosis. The preferred cardiac biomarker is troponin, which has high clinical sensitivity and myocardial tissue specificity [18]. If troponin concentrations are unavailable, then CKMB should be measured. Ideally, both troponin and CKMB should be obtained during evaluation for ACS due to the different concentrations of these biomarkers over time and the added diagnostic value of serial testing.

However, elevated cardiac biomarkers in and of themselves do not indicate the underlying mechanism of injury and do not differentiate between ischemic or nonischemic causes. There are several clinical conditions that have the potential to result in myocardial injury and cause elevations in cardiac biomarkers, including acute pulmonary embolism, heart failure, end stage renal disease, and myocarditis [19]. As a result, cardiac biomarker elevations cannot be utilized in isolation to make a diagnosis of MI.

Stress Testing and Cardiac Imaging

In the evaluation of a patient with possible IHD who is otherwise stable and not experiencing ACS, the first step before ordering or conducting a stress test is to gauge clinical utility. For patients with a low pretest probability, a stress test is unlikely to be helpful. The sensitivity and specificity of a standard exercise tolerance test varies depending on the extent of disease (e.g., >70% stenosis), but in general has a sensitivity of approximately 50–65% and specificity of approximately 75–85% [20, 21]. For example, a 36-year-old woman with atypical chest pain has an estimated pretest probability of 4%. If an exercise tolerance test is positive, her posttest probability of having IHD is only about 9–10%; and if the test is negative, her posttest probability of having IHD is about 2%. The test is most useful for people with a moderate pretest probability, although the testing range spans from 10% to 90%. For people with a high pretest probability, a negative stress test does not reduce the post-test probability sufficiently. In addition to the predicted posttest utility of stress testing, the clinician should take into consideration other factors such as clinical presentation, comorbidities, and other variables in considering stress testing and further diagnostic workup.

Before embarking on standard exercise tolerance testing, it is also important to know that the patient can exercise sufficiently for the test. An ECG should be obtained prior to ordering the stress test to make sure that there are no baseline ECG abnormalities that will make interpretation of the stress test difficult. Patients with a bundle branch block (especially left) or irregularities in the ST segment (e.g., due to digitalis or strain pattern) are not candidates for standard exercise tolerance testing.

There are many alternatives to a standard exercise tolerance stress test, and when considering concomitant imaging, the decision making can seem complicated. Factors to consider are the patient's ability to exercise, previous history of MI, baseline ECG including any rhythm abnormalities. The most common alternative to standard exercise tolerance testing is radionuclide perfusion imaging. It can be accomplished with or without exercise. A radionuclide (e.g., technetium-99 m sestamibi) is injected intravenously and its uptake by the myocardium is compared via imaging during rest and at peak exercise. For patients unable to exercise, adenosine or dipyridamole is used to dilate the coronary arteries and induce a relative difference between stenotic and nonstenotic vessels. Sensitivity and specificity are greater with perfusion testing (approximately 75% and 85%, respectively). Stress echocardiography is another test that can be used to evaluate for possible IHD. Areas of the myocardium that are not perfused will exhibit a wall-motion defect. Like radionuclide imaging, stress echocardiography can be performed with or without exercise, the latter method using dobutamine.

Coronary Angiography

Patients with a positive stress test or those with a high pretest probability or for whom the diagnosis remains equivocal should be referred for possible coronary angiography. Coronary angiography is the gold standard for diagnosing coronary artery disease, and depending on the findings, therapeutic interventions can be accomplished simultaneously.

Management

Acute Coronary Syndrome

Initial management of ACS consists of identifying whether a patient should be managed with an early invasive strategy versus an initial conservative strategy. Early risk stratification should take into account a patient's age and medical history, physical exam, ECG, and cardiac biomarker measurements [3]. A risk assessment tool can be used to predict the patient's risk of recurrent ischemia or death following an ACS event. The Thrombosis and Myocardial Infarction (TIMI) risk score is a scoring system for unstable angina and NSTEMI that incorporates seven variables upon hospital admission and has been validated as a reliable predictor of subsequent ischemic events (Table 4) [3].

For patients presenting with a STEMI with symptom onset within the prior 12 h, reperfusion therapy should be considered [22]. Percutaneous coronary intervention (PCI) is the recommended method of reperfusion when it can be performed with the goal of time from first medical contact to device time of less than or equal to 90 min [22].

Table 4 The thrombosis and myocardial infarction (TIMI) risk score for UA/NSTEMI [3]

Baseline characteristics	TIMI risk score (points)	Rate of composite endpoint (%)[a]
1 point for each of the following: Age ≥ 65 years At least 3 risk factors for IHD[b] Prior coronary stenosis ≥50% ST segment deviation At least 2 anginal events in last 24 h Use of aspirin in last 7 days Elevated serum cardiac biomarkers[c]	0–1	4.7
	2	8.3
	3	13.2
	4	19.9
	5	26.2
	6–7	40.9

[a]All-cause mortality, new or recurrent MI, or severe recurrent ischemia requiring urgent revascularization through 14 days after randomization
[b]Risk factors include family history of IHD, hypertension, hypercholesterolemia, diabetes, or being a current smoker
[c]CKMB fraction and/or cardiac-specific troponin level

If patients are unable to get to a PCI-capable hospital within 120 min of a STEMI, then fibrinolytic therapy should be administered within 30 min of hospital arrival, provided there are no contraindications. The benefits of an early invasive strategy for patients initially presenting with NSTEMI or unstable angina are less certain. A meta-analysis was inconclusive in regard to survival benefit associated with early (typically <24 h) vs. delayed invasive strategy in patients presenting with NSTEMI [23]. However, early invasive coronary angiography is recommended in NSTEMI/unstable angina patients who have refractory angina or hemodynamic or electrical instability [24]. Early invasive strategy is reasonable for higher risk NSTEMI/UA patients previously stabilized who do not have serious comorbidities (e.g., liver or pulmonary failure, cancer) or contraindications to the procedure [old 18 new 25]. There is no clear benefit to PCI for individuals with stable angina, and studies show that medical management is just as effective in preventing mortality [25].

Antiplatelet therapy is a foundational in the management of ACS because it reduces the risk of thrombosis [24]. Well-established antiplatelet therapies in the management of ACS include aspirin, adenosine diphosphate P2Y12 receptor antagonists, and glycoprotein IIb/IIIa inhibitors. Aspirin should be started as soon as possible after an ACS event with an initial loading dose of 162 mg to 325 mg, unless contraindicated. Aspirin should be continued at a dose of 81-mg daily. A P2Y12 antagonist should be added to aspirin for patients with ACS who are medically managed as well as those undergoing PCI [23, 24]. P2Y12 receptor antagonists frequently used in the management of ACS include clopidogrel (Plavix), prasugrel (Effient), and ticagrelor (Brillinta) [26–29]. Triple antiplatelet therapy accomplished by adding GP IIb/IIIa inhibitors has been shown to be efficacious when used during PCI in reducing ischemic complications. However, triple antiplatelet therapy has also been associated with an increased bleeding risk [24].

Parenteral anticoagulants (unfractionated heparin (UFH), low molecular weight heparin (LMWH), fondaparinux, or bivalirudin) are used in combination with antiplatelet agents during the initial management of ACS. The choice of anticoagulant agent is dependent upon the initial management strategy and the recommended duration of therapy varies based on the chosen agent [22, 24].

For patients presenting with unstable angina, NSTEMI, or STEMI, oral beta-blocker therapy should be initiated within 24 h of the onset of the event unless the patient has evidence of low-output state, signs of heart failure, increased risk for cardiogenic shock or other contraindications to therapy [3]. The use of intravenous beta-blockers is reasonable in patients who are hypertensive and do not have contraindications. Beta-blockers decrease cardiac work and reduce myocardial oxygen demand by reducing myocardial contractility, sinus node rate, and AV node conduction velocity. Beta-blocker should be continued in the post MI setting unless contraindicated or not tolerated. The duration of benefit of long-term oral beta blocker therapy is uncertain, but

many clinicians choose to continue beta blockers indefinitely. If patients are experiencing side effects from beta blocker use, it may be reasonable to discontinue therapy at least 1 year after an MI [30]. For patients who are unable to take beta blockers and experience recurrent ischemia, consideration should be given to starting a non-dihydropyridine calcium channel blocker (i.e., verapamil or diltiazem) [3, 22].

As long as no contraindications exist, an angiotensin converting enzyme (ACE) inhibitor or angiotensin receptor blocker (ARB) should be initiated within the first 24 h of patients presenting with ACS who have pulmonary congestion, heart failure, STEMI with anterior location, or left ventricular ejection fraction (LVEF) $\leq$ 40% [3, 22]. ACE inhibitors have been shown to reduce mortality in a broad spectrum of patients following MI, including those with and without LV dysfunction [31–36]. Patients with stable CAD who are not medically optimized (i.e., cannot tolerate a beta blocker or statin), who are not able to be re-vascularized, and/or who have poorly controlled diabetes have shown mortality benefit with continued treatment with ACE inhibitors [37]. When initiating inhibitors of the renin-angiotensin system, it is important to monitor for adverse effects associated with these agents including hyperkalemia, elevations in serum creatinine, and hypotension.

Statin (HmG-CoA reductase inhibitor) therapy is recommended for all patients presenting with ACS who have no contraindications [22, 24]. High-intensity statin therapy following an ACS event was shown to confer an absolute risk reduction of 4% over 2 years compared with a moderate intensity statin for the composite endpoint of death from any cause, recurrent MI, UA requiring rehospitalization, revascularization, and stroke [38]. Statin therapy is beneficial following ACS even in patients with baseline low-density lipoprotein (LDL) cholesterol levels of <70 mg/dL [22, 24]. Recently published American College of Cardiology and American Heart Association Guidelines on treatment of cholesterol recommend high intensity statins (i.e., $\geq$ atorvastatin 40 mg daily or $\geq$ rosuvastatin 20 mg daily) for high-risk patients, which include patients who have an ACS event [39]. Lower dose statins can be considered if patients are >75 years old or if patients cannot tolerate high intensity statins. Ezetimibe and then PCSK9 inhibitors may be utilized in very high risk patients who have LDL levels that remain at 70 or above [39]. Other medications such as colchicine are showing promise to prevent further ischemic events after MI [40].

Stable Ischemic Heart Disease

Stable ischemic heart disease represents an established pattern of angina, a history of myocardial infarction, or the diagnosis of coronary artery disease on catheterization. The goals of managing stable IHD are to prevent progression of disease and reduce the likelihood of cardiovascular disease events (secondary prevention), ultimately reducing premature mortality. The "ABCss" of management are shown in Table 5.

Low-dose aspirin (typically 81-mg) is recommended for all patients for secondary prevention unless it is contraindicated (e.g., allergy) or poorly tolerated. Aspirin inhibits cyclooxygenase, and the resultant reductions in prostaglandin and thromboxane-A prevent platelet aggregation. Numerous studies have demonstrated the benefit of aspirin for secondary prevention.

Control of blood pressure is important in the management of IHD. Recent evidence-based guidelines recommend initiation of treatment for hypertension at blood pressure > 140 mm Hg systolic and/or > 90 mm Hg diastolic in patients with diabetes, CKD, or in patients younger than 60 years old without these comorbidities [33]. These new guidelines support permissive elevation of systolic blood pressure to 150 mm Hg prior to initiation of therapy in patients 60 years and older. See ▶ Chap. 79, "Hypertension" for further discussion of BP-lowering.

Cholesterol Lowering. The ACC/AHA Lipid Guidelines support use of a high-dose statin in all patients less than 75 years old who will tolerate this treatment [39]. The LDL goals seen in previous guidelines are no longer recommended. Consider at least a moderate dose statin in patients older than 75 [39]. Statins are the preferred treatment, but for patients who do not tolerate them or have other risk factors that may classify them as very high risk, ezetimibe, PCSK9 inhibitor, or a bile acid sequestrant can be considered. Niacin and fibrates can be prescribed for patients with elevated triglycerides [39].

Patients with IHD should be counseled to make smoking cessation a priority. See ▶ Chap. 6, "Clinical Prevention" for information on strategies and clinical interventions that may help patients become smoke free.

Options for antianginal therapy include beta-blockers, nitrates and calcium channel blockers. Beta-blockers are the first-line recommendation for control of angina. By reducing myocardial oxygen demand, they reduce the frequency of chest pain episodes and improve exercise tolerance. In addition to their benefit for symptom

Table 5 Management of stable ischemic heart disease

	Recommendation	Comment
Aspirin	81-mg daily unless contraindicated	Clopidogrel can be used for patients allergic to aspirin
Blood pressure lowering medication(s)	Goal BP < 140/90 mm Hg for most patients	Beta-blocker recommended as part of regimen for post-MI patients
Cholesterol lowering medication	Statin therapy	Use at highest tolerated dose
Smoking cessation	Any patient who smokes should be provided recommendation, counseling and resources to quit	
Symptom management	Control angina symptoms with beta-blocker, nitrates, and/or calcium channel blocker	Beta-blocker is first-line; calcium channel blocker should be long-acting nondihydropyridine or dihydropyridine (avoid nifedipine); long-acting nitrate can be added to help manage chronic angina

control, beta-blockers help prevent reinfarction and reduce mortality in patients who have suffered an MI. When beta-blockers are contraindicated or not effective as monotherapy, a nitrate or calcium channel blocker can be used.

Sublingual nitroglycerin or nitroglycerin spray is provided for relief of acute episodes of IHD related chest pain. These preparations can also be used a few minutes before activity to prevent effort-induced angina. A long-acting nitrate (e.g., isosorbide mononitrate) can be provided as a supplement to beta-blocker or calcium channel blocker for controlling chronic angina. Nitrate tolerance is minimized by having a nitrate-free interval of about 12 h.

Anolazine can be considered as an add-on for angina control. It is a sodium channel blocker that reduces oxygen demand by decreasing tension during ventricular relaxation. The medication can be a useful when angina is not controlled with the above strategies or can be prescribed instead of beta-blockers if beta-blockade is contraindicated or poorly tolerated [5]. Ranolazine can be used in patients with bradycardia or low blood pressure.

Lifestyle modifications for all patients include weight loss if overweight, regular physical activity, and an eating plan that is low in saturated fats, trans fats, and cholesterol [5]. Referring a patient to a dietitian may be reasonable.

References

1. Virani SS, Alonso A, Benjamin EJ, Bittencourt MS, Callaway CW, Carson AP, et al. American Heart Association Statistics Committee. Heart disease and stroke statistics – 2020 update: a report from the American Heart Association. Circulation. 2020;141(9):e139–596.
2. Heron M. Deaths: leading causes for 2013. Natl Vital Stat Rep. 2016;65(2):1–95.
3. Amsterdam EA, Wenger NK, Brindis RG, Casey DE, Ganiats TG, et al. AHA/ACC guideline for the management of patients with non–ST-elevation acute coronary syndromes. J Am Coll Cardiol. 2014;64(24):e139–228.
4. Ebell MH. Evaluation of chest pain in primary care patients. Am Fam Physician. 2011;83(5):603–5.
5. Fihn SD, Gardin JM, Abrams J, Berra K, Blakenship JC, Dallas AP, et al. ACCF/AHA/ACP/AATS/PCNA/SCAI/STS guideline for the diagnosis and management of patients with stable ischemic heart disease: a report of the American College of Cardiology Foundation/American Heart Association Task Force on Practice Guidelines, and the American College of Physicians, American Association for Thoracic Surgery, Preventive Cardiovascular Nurses Association, Society for Cardiovascular Angiography and Interventions, and Society of Thoracic Surgeons. Circulation. 2012;126(25):e354–471.
6. Herman LK, Weingart SD, Yong M, Yoon YM, Genes NG, et al. Comparison of frequency of inducible myocardial ischemia in patients presenting to emergency department with typical versus atypical or nonanginal chest pain. Am J Cardiol. 2010;105(11):1561–4.
7. Devon HA, Zerwic JJ. The symptoms of unstable angina: do women and men differ? Nurs Res. 2003;52(2):108–18.
8. Carli MF, Gupta A. Estimating pre-test probability of coronary artery disease. JACC Cardiovasc Imaging. 2019;12(7):1401–4.
9. Diamond GA, Forrester JS. Analysis of probability as an aid in the clinical diagnosis of coronary-artery disease. N Engl J Med. 1979;300(24):1350–8.
10. Pepine CJ, Balaban RS, Bonow RO, Diamond GA, Johnson BD, Johnson PA, et al. National Heart, Lung and Blood Institute; American College of Cardiology Foundation. Women's ischemic syndrome evaluation: current status and future research directions: report of the national heart, lung and blood institute workshop: October 2–4, 2002: section 1: diagnosis of stable ischemia and ischemic heart disease. Circulation. 2004;109(6):e44–6.
11. Reis SE, Holubkov R, Smith AJC, Kelsey SF, Sharaf BL, Reichek N, et al. Coronary microvascular dysfunction is highly prevalent in women with chest pain in the absence of coronary artery disease: Results from the NIILBI WISE study. Am Heart J. 2001;141(5):735–41.
12. Thygesen K, Alpert JS, Jaffe AS, Simoons ML, Chaitman BR, White HD, et al. Third universal definition of myocardial infarction. Circulation. 2012;126(16):2020–35.
13. Gokhroo RK, Ranwa BL, Kishor K, Priti K, Ananthraj A, Gupta S, et al. Sweating: a specific predictor of ST-segment elevation myocardial infarction among the symptoms of acute coronary syndrome: sweating in myocardial infarction (SWIMI) study group. Clin Cardiol. 2015;39(2):90–5.
14. Panju AA, Hemmelgarn BR, Guyatt GH, Simel DL. The rational clinical examination. Is this patient having a myocardial infarction? JAMA. 1998;280(14):1256–63.
15. Chun AA, McGee SR. Bedside diagnosis of coronary artery disease: a systematic review. Am J Med. 2004;117(5):334–43.
16. Fesmire FM, Percy RF, Bardoner JB, Wharton DR, Calhoun FB. Usefulness of automated serial 12-lead ECG monitoring during the initial emergency department evaluation of patients with chest pain. Ann Emerg Med. 1998;31(1):3–11.
17. Januzzi JL. What biomarkers are useful for detection of myocardial ischemia? American College of Cardiology; 2011 [cited 2020 Apr 30]. Available at

https://www.acc.org/latest-in-cardiology/articles/2014/07/18/14/24/what-biomarkers-are-useful-for-detection-of-myocardial-ischemia

18. Reichlin T, Hochholzer W, Bassetti S, Steuer S, Stelzig C, et al. Early diagnosis of myocardial infarction with sensitive cardiac troponin assays. N Engl J Med. 2009;361(9):858–67.

19. Korff S, Katus HA, Giannitsis E. Differential diagnosis of elevated troponins. Heart. 2006;92(7):987–93.

20. Knox MA. Optimize your use of stress tests: a Q&A guide. J Fam Pract. 2010;59(5):262–8.

21. Gianrossi r, Detrano R, Mulvihill D, Lehmann K, Dubach P, Colombo A, et al. Exercise-induced ST depression in the diagnosis of coronary artery disease. a meta-analysis. Circulation. 1989;80(1):87–98.

22. O'Gara PT, Kushner FG, Ascheim DD, et al. ACCF/AHA guideline for the management of ST-elevation myocardial infarction: a report of the American College of Cardiology Foundation/American Heart Association Task Force on Practice Guidelines. J Am Coll Cardiol. 2013;61:e78–140.

23. Navarese EP, Gurbel PA, Andreotti F, Tantry U, Jeong YH, Konzinski M, et al. Optimal timing of coronary invasive strategy in non–ST-segment elevation acute coronary syndromes: a systematic review and meta-analysis. Ann Intern Med. 2013;158:261–70.

24. Jneid H, Anderson JL, Wright RS, Adams CD, Bridges CR, Casey DE, et al. ACCF/AHA focused update of the guideline for the management of unstable angina/non-ST segment myocardial infarction (updating the 2007 guideline and replacing the 2011 focused update): a report of the American College of Cardiology Foundation/American Heart Association Task Force on Practice Guidelines. Circulation. 2012;126(7):1–60.

25. Maron D, Hochman JS, Reynolds HR, Banglore S, O'Brien SM, Boden WE, et al. Initial invasive or conservative strategy for stable coronary disease. NEJM. 2020;382(15):1395–407.

26. CURE Trial Investigators. Effect of clopidogrel in addition to aspirin in patients with acute coronary syndromes without ST-segment elevation. N Engl J Med. 2001;345(7):494–502.

27. Wiviott SD, Braunwald E, McCabe CH, Montalescot G, Ruzyllo W, et al. Prasugrel versus clopidogrel in patients with acute coronary syndromes (TRITON-TIMI 38). N Engl J Med. 2007;357(20):2001–15.

28. Wallentin L, Becker RC, Budaj A, Cannon CP, Emanuelsson H, Held C, et al. Ticagrelor versus clopidogrel in patients with acute coronary syndromes (PLATO). N Engl J Med. 2009;357(11):1045–57.

29. Mehta SR, Tanguay JF, Eikelboom JW, Jolly SS, Joyner CD, Granger CB, et al. Double-dose versus standard-dose clopidogrel and high-dose versus low-dose aspirin in individuals undergoing percutaneous coronary intervention for acute coronary syndromes (CURRENT-OASIS 7): a randomized factorial trial. Lancet. 2010;376(9748):1233–43.

30. Kezerashvili A, Marzo K, De Leon J. Beta blocker use after acute myocardial infarction in the patient with

31. Pfeffer MA, Braunwald E, Moye LA, Basta L, Brown EJ, Cuddy TE, et al. Effects of captopril on mortality and morbidity in patients with left ventricular dysfunction after myocardial infarction: results of the survival and ventricular enlargement trial. N Engl J Med. 1992;327(10):669–77.

32. Kober L, Torp-Pedersen C, Carlsen JE, Bagger H, Eliasen P, Lyngborg K, et al. A clinical trial of the angiotensin-converting enzyme inhibitor trandolapril in patients with left ventricular dysfunction after myocardial infarction. N Engl J Med. 1995;333(25):1670–6.

33. ISIS-4 (Fourth International Study of Infarct Survival) Collaborative Group. ISIS-4: a randomized factorial trial assessing early oral captopril, oral mononitrate, and intravenous magnesium sulphate in 58,050 patients with suspected acute myocardial infarction. Lancet. 1995;345(8951):669–85.

34. Gruppo Italiana per lo Studio della Sopravvivenza nell'infarto Miocardico. GISSI-3: effects of lisinopril and transdermal glyceryl trinitrate singly and together on 6-week mortality and ventricular function after acute myocardial infarction. Lancet. 1994;343(8906):1115–22.

35. The Heart Outcomes Prevention Evaluation (HOPE) Study Investigators. Effects of an angiotensin-converting enzyme inhibitor, ramipril, on cardiovascular events in high-risk patients. N Engl J Med. 2000;342(3):145–53.

36. The EURopean trial On reduction of cardiac events with Perindopril in stable coronary Artery disease (EUROPA) Investigators. Efficacy of perindopril in reduction of cardiovascular events among patients with stable coronary artery disease: randomized, double-blind, placebo-controlled, multicenter trial (the EUROPA study). Lancet. 2003;362(9386):782–8.

37. Braunwald E, Domanski MJ, Fowler SE, Geller NL, Gersh BJ, Hsia J, et al. Angiotensin-converting enzyme inhibition in stable coronary artery disease. N Engl J Med. 2004;351(2):2058–68.

38. Cannon CP, Braunwald E, McCabe CH, Rader DJ, Rouleau JL, Belder R, et al. Intensive versus moderate lipid lowering with statins after acute coronary syndromes. N Engl J Med. 2004;350(15):1495–504.

39. Grundy SM, Stone NJ, Bailey AL, Beam C, Birtcher KK, Blumenthal RS, et al. 2018 AHA/ACC/AACVPR/AAPA/ABC/ACPM/ADA/AGS/APhA/ASPC/NLA/PCNA Guideline on the Management of Blood Chol ACC/AHA guideline on the treatment of blood cholesterol to reduce atherosclerotic cardiovascular risk in adults: a report of the American College of Cardiology/American Heart Association Task Force on Practice Guidelines. J Am Coll Cardiol. 2014;63(25 Pt B):2889–934.

40. Tardif JC, Kouz S, Waters DD, Bertrand OF, Diaz R, Maggioni AP, et al. Effiacay and safety of low-dose colchicine after myocardial infarction. N Engl J Med. 2019;381(26):2497–250.

Cardiac Arrhythmias

Cecilia Gutierrez and Esmat Hatamy

Contents

C. Gutierrez (✉) · E. Hatamy
Department of Family Medicine and Public Health, UCSD
School of Medicine, University of California, San Diego,
San Diego, CA, USA
e-mail: cagutierrez@health.ucsd.edu;
ehatamy@health.ucsd.edu

The electrical activation of heart muscle follows a precise and organized pathway which ensures that contraction and relaxation occur in an efficient way to support effective circulation. Arrhythmias result from an abnormal electrical activation of the heart which may lead to an abnormal rhythm, rate,

© Springer Nature Switzerland AG 2022
P. M. Paulman et al. (eds.), *Family Medicine*,
https://doi.org/10.1007/978-3-030-54441-6_84

or both in the heart cycle. While some arrhythmias are benign and pose no significant cardiovascular compromise, others degrade the mechanical pumping activity and lead to hemodynamic compromise and, in some cases, to collapse and/or death.

Arrhythmias are commonly seen in primary care, and many are diagnosed and managed by primary care physicians, either alone or along with a cardiologist. Although more common among the elderly and those with heart disease, they must be considered in the differential diagnosis of all patients presenting with syncope, lightheadedness, palpitations, fatigue, dyspnea on exertion, and shortness of breath. The main goal in evaluating patients is to first assess cardiopulmonary stability and, in life-threatening situations, activate the emergency response system. In stable patients the work-up focuses on identifying the arrhythmia, its cause(s), its effect on cardiac function, and treating it to improve patients' symptoms and reduce morbidity and mortality.

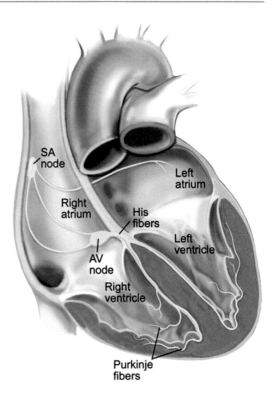

Fig. 1 Diagram of the heart and the electrical conduction system of the heart (From Wang and Estes [1])

Electrophysiology of the Heart

The heart generates its own electrical impulse, an action potential (AP) transmitted through specialized cells and conductive fibers to activate myocardial cells to contract and relax in a highly coordinated fashion. This determines heart rate and rhythm.

In a simplified view, at the molecular level, the generation of the AP is due to unstable transmembrane potential caused by a slow sodium (Na+) leak into the cells, depolarizing the membranes until the threshold that triggers an AP is reached. Cardiac cells have several voltage-gated ion channels, and the in- and outflow of mostly Na, K, and Ca ions through these gated channels (fast and slow) play key roles in generating the AP and repolarizing cell membranes. Through the cycle, cells exhibit absolute and relative refractory periods. Sympathetic and parasympathetic fibers innervate the heart and modulate cardiac function.

Figure 1 [1] shows a schematic and simplified view of the normal electrical conduction system. The AP originates at sinoatrial node (SA), a group of specialized cells in the upper posterior wall of

the right atrium. It is transmitted to the atria and to the atrioventricular node (AV), a group of cells in the posterior region of the atrial septum. In the AV node, the impulse is delayed, allowing atrial contraction to occur before the ventricular activation. The AV node transmits the impulse through the bundle of His, fast-conducting fibers in the upper interventricular septum, which splits into two branches, right and left. Then the impulse continues through the Purkinje fibers, which transmit it to all ventricular cells, resulting in ventricular contraction and ejection of blood into the circulation. Although the AV node, bundle of His, and Purkinje can act as pacemakers, the SA node has the highest intrinsic rate of depolarization, and it serves as the pacemaker. At rest, the SA node triggers APs at a rate of 60 to 100 times per minute. In an ECG this pattern is seen as regular waves known as P, QRS, and T waves, which is normal sinus rhythm (NSR).

Detailed knowledge of the variety of ion channels and their electrophysiology is beyond the scope of this chapter. However, it is essential to point out some highlights which have clinical and pharmacologic significance.

Various types of ion channels exist in myocytes. Some channels are present in all cells, while others only on certain cells, or preferentially on specific areas of the conduction system. Although the major ions involved are Na, K, and Ca, other ions may also play a role and/or serve to modulate their responses. Some channels are fast, while others are slow; some are voltage gated, and some are modulated by local current across gap junctions with adjacent cells, while others are affected by local currents within the cells (e.g., across their sarcoplasmic reticulum), or via special proteins, ion transport mechanisms, and other intracellular signals. Some channels are up- or downregulated, and some have mutations (leading to familial channelopathies). Some channels are transient responding to immediate changes in the cells in ways to achieve homeostasis, while others undergo permanent changes due to long-standing chronic ischemia, scarring, and remodeling.

Three main mechanisms have been identified as the causes of arrhythmias: increased automaticity, triggered activity, and re-entry. Re-entry is the most common cause of arrhythmias. It occurs when the normal electrical impulse does not dissipate and re-excite cardiac cells after the refractory period.

Arrhythmias are described according to where they originate (in the atria or ventricles, along the multiple sites of the electrical conduction system, or on myocardial cells); according to their effect on heart rate (HR) (fast, tachyarrhythmias, > 100 beats per minute, or slow, bradyarrhythmias, < 60 beats per minute); and according to their effect on heart rhythm (regular versus irregular patterns). All these characteristics define a unique pattern in the ECG.

Evaluation of Patients with Arrhythmia

History and Physical Exam (H&P)

Although studies have shown poor correlation between symptoms and actual arrhythmias, the H&P helps to identify potential causes, risk factors, and comorbidities. Elements of the history must consider both cardiac and non-cardiac causes of arrhythmia. As usual, it must include onset, patient's description of symptoms, duration, aggravating and alleviating factors, severity, and course of symptoms. The review of systems must inquire about shortness of breath, palpitations, dizziness, edema, orthopnea, paroxysmal nocturnal dyspnea, fatigue, lightheadedness, chest pain, syncope, orthostatic hypotension, symptoms of sleep apnea, pedal edema, new medications (prescribed or over the counter), herbal and other supplements, symptoms of thyroid disease, and recent illnesses. The social history provides information about the use of recreational drugs, alcohol, and diet pills as possible causes or contributors. Table 1 presents the most common causes of arrhythmias. Rare conditions such as infiltrative heart diseases, pheochromocytoma, and other endocrine conditions must be considered. All patients must have a complete PE, vital signs, and BMI. The cardiovascular exam should include inspection, palpation, percussion and auscultation of the heart, assessment of heart rate and rhythm, presence of murmurs, carotid bruits, patient's JVD, peripheral pulses, and edema.

Table 1 Most common causes of arrhythmias

Cardiac	Non-cardiac
CAD: Myocardial ischemia or infarction	Pulmonary disease
	COPD, PE,
Heart failure	pneumonia
Structural heart disease:	Cor pulmonale
Congenital or acquired	Thyroid disease
Dilated cardiomyopathy	Drug toxicity
Ventricular hypertrophy	Antiarrhythmics
Valvular disease	Beta agonist
Atrial septal defect	inhalers
Ebstein anomaly	Lithium
Epicardial, myocardial, and endocardial diseases:	Drugs that increase QT interval
Infectious, injury, or drug toxicity	Electrolyte abnormalities
Iatrogenic	Recreational drugs
Post-cardiac catheterization	Diet pills
Post-cardiac surgery	Collagen vascular
Post-ablation	disease
Post-ICD placement	Infiltrative disease
	Hypothermia

Evaluation of Cardiac Arrhythmia

Because patient symptoms often do not correlate with actual arrhythmias and the H&P cannot characterize the arrhythmia, the first step is to get an ECG. The ECG provides immediate information of the HR and rhythm and changes in P wave, PR interval, QRS complexes, ST segment, and T waves. Since a normal ECG cannot capture a paroxysmal arrhythmia, a Holter monitor (24-h recording) or an event monitor (7–30 days recording) may be required. In some cases a long-term implantable loop recorder may be necessary [2]. An echocardiogram is also needed to evaluate heart function and assess for possible structural diseases.

Initial blood tests include a complete blood count with differential, a comprehensive metabolic panel, magnesium, lipid panel, and TSH. Additional tests may be necessary depending on the patient's H&P and risk factors. These include stress echocardiogram, nuclear perfusion imaging or cardiac catheterization for ischemia or coronary artery disease, table tilt test for vasovagal syncope, drug screen (if suspected), and urine vanillylmandelic acid and serum metanephrine for evaluation of possible pheochromocytoma.

Treatment Options for Cardiac Arrhythmia

Several options are available to treat arrhythmias. They include cardioversion, drugs with AV nodal suppression, antiarrhythmic drugs acting on different ion channels, radiofrequency ablation, pacemakers, defibrillators, and surgery. Based on best evidence from clinical trials, the most updated knowledge of pharmacology and pathophysiology, the American Heart Association, the American College of Cardiology, the European College of Cardiology, and the Heart Rhythm Society, AHA/ACC/ECC/HRS, have developed guidelines for the evaluation and treatment of arrhythmias [3–8]. These guidelines are frequently revised and updated to include latest knowledge, and they provide a framework for a discussion with patients and their families about treatment options. Therapeutic decisions also must reflect patients' preferences and choices. Prior to initiating a specific therapy, it is essential to identify and treat reversible causes of arrhythmias.

Cardioversion

It is the attempt to return the heart rhythm to NSR and can be achieved by an electrical current shock or by drugs. The goal is to override all abnormal electrical activity and synchronize the heart rhythm again. Unless done in an emergency basis, it requires preparation: IV access, continuous cardiac monitoring, sedation and/or anesthesia, resuscitation equipment, proper anticoagulation, normal electrolytes and short fasting, etc.

Electrical cardioversion is accomplished by delivering a direct current electric shock of 50–360 joules of energy. Shocks are delivered in synchrony with the R or S wave of the QRS complex, to avoid the relative refractory period and minimize triggering of other arrhythmias. One or more shocks may be necessary, starting at the lowest energy. The main indications for cardioversion are unstable or poorly tolerated narrow QRS complex tachycardias (atrial fibrillation (AF) or flutter) and ventricular tachycardia not responsive to drug therapy.

Pharmacological cardioversion and maintenance of NSR has been challenging due to limited long-term efficacy of drugs, the risk of triggering ventricular arrhythmias, and their long-term adverse side effects [3–5]. It is more successful in young patients with healthy hearts who have recently developed an arrhythmia. Most commonly used drugs include ibutilide (Corvert), flecainide (Tambocor), dofetilide, propafenone (Rythmol), and amiodarone (Cordarone, Nexterone, Pacerone). Contraindications for cardioversion include digitalis toxicity, multifocal atrial tachycardia, and suboptimal anticoagulation.

Antiarrhythmic Drug Therapy

Multiple drugs are available to suppress and treat arrhythmias, but their use is complex. Many drugs can trigger arrhythmias, some have serious short- and long-term adverse side effects, some require hospitalization to initiate therapy, some have limited long-term benefit, many have drug interactions, etc. Therefore, the patient should be referred to cardiology.

Antiarrhythmic drugs have various effects on ion channel function; most have more than one action. They may slow down, accelerate, or modify ion movement across cell membranes. They act at various phases of the AP and in unique ways along the specialized conduction system. Advances in electrophysiology and the development of new drugs led to the revision and expansion of the well-established Vaughan-Williams classification of antiarrhythmic drugs [9].

Table 2 presents the new drug classification, mode of action, indications, and contraindications for their use [3, 5, 9–12].

Class 0. This new class identifies drugs that have an effect on the automaticity of the SA node. Ivabradine is a drug that reduces heart rates in inappropriate sinus tachycardia [10].

Class I. These drugs block Na channels and therefore act on the depolarization phase of the cardiac AP. New classification identified a variety of Na^+ channels. Some of these drugs act early or late in the phase of the AP, while others act on voltage gated channels in the atria, Purkinje fibers and ventricles. They are further subdivided into four subclasses according to their effect on the duration of the AP [10]:

- Class Ia agents prolong the initial phase of the AP, thus delaying depolarization. They also increase the effective refractory period. Some examples are quinidine (Qualaquin), procainamide, and disopyramide (Norpace).
- Class Ib. These drugs shorten the duration of the AP by increasing repolarization. Some examples are lidocaine, phenytoin (Phenytek), mexiletine, and tocainide.
- Class Ic. These drugs have no effect on AP duration, but they significantly slow the initial depolarization of the AP and have no effect on refractory period. Some examples are encainide, flecainide (Tambocor), propafenone (Rythmol), and moricizine.

- Class Id. These drugs inhibit late $Na +$ channels after the rapid initial repolarization phase. They shorten AP recovery and increase refractoriness. Examples include ranolazine, GS-458967, and F15845.

Class II. This classification includes drugs that have effect on sympathetic and parasympathetic activity, as well as drugs that act through cell membrane proteins, particularly G-proteins. They have ionotropic, chronotropic, and lusitropic (myocardial relaxation) effects on the heart:

- Class IIa include non-selective (carvedilol and propranolol) and selective (atenolol) $\beta1$ adrenergic blockers. They inhibit Ca^{++} entry and release from the sarcoplasmic reticulum.
- Class IIb. In contrast to class IIa, these drugs stimulate Ca^{++} entry and release from the SR. An example is non-selective isoproterenol.
- Class IIc. These are drugs that act on muscarinic receptors via various G-proteins. An example is atropine.
- Classes IId and IIe. These drugs mediate their effects by inhibiting G-proteins. Examples are carbachol (IId) and adenosine (IIe) [10].

Class III. These drugs block K^+ channels, subtype and auxiliary subunits. They prolong repolarization and refractory period of myocytes:

- Class IIIa. They act on voltage-gated ion channels.
- Class IIIb. They affect specific K^+ channels via specific transmitters.
- Class IIIc. Act on K^+ channels affected by specific transmitters.

Class IV. These drugs are referred as calcium channel modulators. Overall, they delay conduction at the AV node, slowing HR. Subclasses in the surface of cells and within cell membranes (sarcoplasmic reticulum) have been identified. These channels have complex mechanisms affected by local currents, voltage, and Ca homeostasis and intracellular signals. Their activation at different times and sites and their

Table 2 Antiarrhythmic drugs: classification, mode of action, indication, and contraindications

Drug classification		Medication name and MOA	Indications	Contraindications
0 **HCN channel blocker**		Ivabradine: ↓ SAN phase 4 depolarization, ↓ HR, possible ↓ AVN automaticity	Stable angina, chronic HF w HR > 70, potential use in tachyarrhythmia (IST)	Decompensated HF, SSS, BP < 90/50, third degree block (unless there is a pacemaker), severe liver disease
I **Sodium** **Channel** **Blockers**	Ia	Quinidine ↓↓ phase 0 slope	A-fib A-flutter VT, VF	HtoD, digitalis toxicity, complete AV dissociation, myasthenia gravis, Immune thrombocytopenia Thrombocytopenic purpura
		Procainamide ↑ AP duration	A-fib, VT, VF	HtoD, complete HB, second or third degree AVB SLE, torsades de pointes
		Disopyramide ↑ effective refractory period	VT	HtoD, cardiogenic shock, congenital prolonged QT Second or third degree block
		Ajmaline Changes shape and threshold of AP	Use as diagnostic drug to make diagnosis of BS No therapeutic use	Should not be used if BS diagnosis is clear
	Ib	Mexiletine ↓ AP duration	VT	HtoD, cardiogenic shock, second and third degree AVB, if no pacemaker is present
		Phenytoin (rarely used in arrhythmia) ↓ effective refractory period	VT secondary to digoxin	HtoD or other hydantoins Concomitant use with delavirdine or rilpivirine
		Lidocaine ↓ phase 0 slope	VF, VT	HtoD, use of local amide anesthetic
		Tocainide	VF, VT	HtoD, second and third degree AVB, HF, ↓ K, liver and kidney disease
	Ic	Flecainide ↓↓↓ phase 0 slope	PAF, ventricular arrhythmia PSVT, P-atrial flutter	HtoD, RBBB with left hemi-block without pacemaker, second and third degree AVB without pacemaker
		Propafenone ↔ AP duration	PSVT and PAF Without structural heart disease, VT	HtoD, bradycardia, BS, severe bronchospasm, COPD, cardiogenic

(continued)

Table 2 (continued)

Drug classification		Medication name and MOA	Indications	Contraindications
				shock, HF, electrolyte imbalance, marked hypotension. SSS and AVB without pacemaker
	Id	Ranolazine Affects the AP recovery, refractoriness, repolarization reserve, and QT interval	SA, VT, chronic angina in combination with other meds	Prolonged QT syndrome Partial contraindication/ caution: Severe impairment of kidney and liver
LII **Beta blockers** **Most commonly used**	IIa: Non-selective (NS) and selective (S) B1 inhibitors	NS: Carvedilol, nadolol, and propranolol (Inderal) S: Metoprolol, atenolol, bisoprolol, betaxolol, celiprolol, esmolol ↓ SAN and AVN and atrial /vent (ectopic) automaticity ↓ HR and conduction ↓ Chronotropy and ionotropy by inhibition of β1 receptor	VT, PVC, VF ST, A-fib, A-flutter, PAT	HtoD, ↓ BP or shock, severe bradycardia, HB >first degree (unless pacemaker), MI precipitated by cocaine, overt HF with pulmonary edema (start at low dose)
	IIb: Non-selective B adrenergic receptor activators	Isoproterenol ↓ RR and PR interval, stimulates both B1 snd B2 receptors, ↓ VR in SM, renal vascular bed	Cardiac arrest (when electric shock not available HB (not caused by AF, VT)	May have a deteriorating effect in injured or failing heart (↑ ox demand and ↓ effective perfusion) Should be used cautiously with inhaled anesthetic (halothane)
	IIc: Muscarinic receptor inhibitors Only atropine checked	Atropine anisodamine, hyoscine, and scopolamine ACI, which blocks the activity of the AC on M2R, ↑ the AVN conductivity, and ↓ SAN automaticity	Bradycardia, AV block in the setting of acute inferior MI, cardiac arrest/ Brady-asystole Vagal reaction to pain	Acute closed-angle glaucoma
	IId: Muscarinic receptor activators	Carbachol, pilocarpine, methacholine, and digoxin ↓ SAN automaticity, AVN conduction and re-entry	Sinus tachycardia and SV tachyarrhythmias	Asthma, incontinence, peptic ulcer disease, coronary insufficiency Do not use methacholine in

(continued)

Table 2 (continued)

Drug classification		Medication name and MOA	Indications	Contraindications
				hypertension, pregnancy, epilepsy
	IIe: Adenosine A1 receptor activators	Adenosine acts as an ARI MOA: ↓ conduction in AVN, interrupt re-entry pathway	SVT, WPW syndrome	Sinus bradycardia, SSS, Second and third degree heart block in the absence of a functioning pacemaker
LIII K channel Blockers and opener	IIIa: Non-selective K channel blockers	Ambasilide, amiodarone, dronedarone Dofetilide, ibutilide, sotalol Vernakalant Blocks K channels, ↓ repolarization, which leads to ↑ in AP duration and ERP ↓ re-entry Amio: Also ↓ SAN and AVN conduction	VT (w/o structural heart disease or remote MI), VF, AF with AV conduction via accessory pathways VF, PVCs Tachyarrhythmia associated with AF	HtoD, severe bradycardia, syncope without pacemaker, severe sinus node dysfunction, second and third degree AV block (unless with pacemaker) Cardiogenic shock. Prolonged QT Should not be used with class I or lll antiarrhythmics
	IIIb: Metabolically dependent K channel blockers	Nicorandil, penacidil ↓ AP recovery, refractoriness in all cardiac cells but for SAN	Nicorandil used for angina Penacidil: Under investigation for HTN	HtoD, cardiogenic shock, ↓ BP, atient at risk of MI, patients receiving soluble guanylate cyclase stimulators
	IIIc: Transmitter-dependent K channel blocker	Medication under review Prolongs APD and ERP, ↓RR	AF	
IV calcium handling modulators	IVa: Non-selective surface membrane ca channel blockers	Bepridil Verapamil and Diltiazem Blocks ca current, inhibits SAN pacing, AVN conduction, ↑ ERP and AP recovery time and PR interval Block L-type ca channels Most effective at SA and AVN ↓ HR and conduction	B: Angina pectoris and potential management of SVT SVT and VT (w/o structural heat disease), rate control of AF	HtoD. For verapamil: A-fib, A-flutter associated with WPW syndrome SSS, second and third degree AVB without pacemaker, HF with EF < 30%, hypotension HtoD. For diltiazem: All the above, newborns, acute MI with pulmonary congestion, administration within a few hours of IV β-blockers
	IVb: Intracellular ca channel blockers	Flecainide Propafenone Reduced SR ca	Catecholaminergic polymorphic VT	Flecainide: SSS, ↓ or ↑K, MI, second degree HB, RBBB

(continued)

Table 2 (continued)

Drug classification	Medication name and MOA		Indications	Contraindications
		release, reduced cytosolic and SR ca	PAF, A-flutter, PSVT	with left hemi B, chronic HF Propafenone: HF, cardiogenic shock, SSS (w/o pacer), bradycardia, BS
	IVc: Sarcoplasmic reticular ca, ATPase activators	Not clinically approved yet	Not determined yet	Note determined yet
	IVd: Surface membrane ion exchanger	Not clinically approved yet	Not determined yet	Not determined yet
	IVe: Phosphokinase and phosphorylase inhibitors	Not clinically approved yet	Not determined yet	Not determined yet
V: Mechanosensitive channel blockers	Transient receptor potential channel (TRPC3 and TRPC6) blockers	Under investigations: N-(P-amylcinnamoyl) anthranilic acid	Not determined yet	Not determined yet
VI Gap junction channel blockers	Cx (Cx40, Cx43, Cx45) blockers	Under investigations: Carbenoxolone	Not determined yet	Not determined yet
VII upstream target modulators	ACEI Electrophysiological and structural remodeling (fibrotic, hypertrophic, inflammatory)	Captopril, enalapril, delapril, ramipril, quinapril, perindopril, lisinopril, benazepril, imidapril, trandolapril, cilazapril	HTN, heart failure and potential application reducing arrhythmic substrate	H to D, angioedema, bilateral renal artery stenosis, and prior deterioration of kidney function with ACE-I, hyperkalemia, pregnancy May also hold when BP < 90/30
	ARBs Electrophysiological and structural remodeling (fibrotic, hypertrophic or inflammatory)	Losartan, candesartan, eprosartan, telmisartan, irbesartan, olmesartan, valsartan	HTN, heart failure, and potential application reducing arrhythmic substrate	H to D, angioedema, bilateral renal artery stenosis, and prior deterioration of kidney function with ARBs, hyperkalemia, pregnancy
	Omega-3 fatty acids Electrophysiological and structural remodeling (fibrotic, hypertrophic, inflammatory)	Eicosapentaenoic acid, docosahexaenoic acid, docosapentaenoic acid	Post MI reduction of cardiac death, MI, stroke, and abnormal cardiac rhythm	HtoD, hypersensitivity to fish or shellfish, hepatic impairment May increase risk of bleeding
	Statins Electrophysiological and structural (fibrotic, inflammatory) remodeling	Atorvastatin, rosuvastatin, fluvastatin, pravastatin, simvastatin, pitavastatin, others	Post MI reduction of cardiac death, MI, stroke, and abnormal cardiac rhythm	Acute liver disease, pregnancy, lactation, elevation of liver enzymes, and conditions that increase AKI

(continued)

Table 2 (continued)

Drug classification		Medication name and MOA	Indications	Contraindications
II d		Digoxin Inhibits ca-K ATPase, causing ↑ chronotropic and ↓ ionotropic effects	A-fib, A-flutter with RVR, HF	HtoD, VF ↓ dose by 30–50% when using amiodarone and 50% with dronedarone

Data on this table are from references [9–12]

Note: The reader is responsible for checking all drugs and verifying doses according to patient's age, liver/kidney functions, and comorbid conditions

AC, Acetyl choline; ACI, acetyl choline inhibitor; ACEI, angiotensin converting enzyme inhibitor; A-Fib, atrial fibrillation; AP, action potential; AKI, acute kidney injury action potential duration; Amio, amiodarone; ARB, angiotensin receptor blocker; ARI, adenosine receptor inhibitor; AV, atrioventricular; AVB, atrioventricular block; AVN, atrioventricular node; BP, blood pressure; β1S, β1 selective; BS, Brugada syndrome; CAD, coronary artery disease; ERP, effective refractory period; HB, heart block; HCN, hyperpolarization-activated cyclic nucleotide-gated channel; HF, heart failure; HR, heart rate; HTN, hypertension; HtoD, hypersensitivity to drug or its components; IST, inappropriate sinus tachycardia; LV, left ventricular; MI, myocardial infarction, M2R, muscarinic receptor; MOA, mechanism of action; Nβ1S, non-β1 selective; PAF, paroxysmal atrial fibrillation; PAT, paroxysmal atrial tachycardia; PSVT, paroxysmal supraventricular tachycardia; PVC, premature ventricular contraction; RBBB, right bundle branch block; RR, repolarization reserve; SA, stable angina; SAN, sinoatrial node; SLE, systemic lupus erythematous; SR, sarcoplasmic reticulum; SSS, sick sinus syndrome; ST, sinus tachycardia; VA, ventricular arrhythmias; VF, ventricular fibrillation; VT, ventricular tachycardia; w/o, without ; WPW, Wolff-Parkinson-White

modulation by protein kinases are the target of new drug effects:

- Class IVa. They act on surface membranes of cells' Ca channel blockers.
- Class IVb. They act on intracellular Ca channel blockers.
- Class IVc. They act on sarcoplasmic reticulum Ca ATPase activators.
- Class IVd. They act on surface membrane ion exchange inhibitors.
- Class IVe. They act on phosphokinase and phosphorylase inhibitors cellular signals.

Class V. These drugs act on cation mechanosensitive ion channels and transient channels which suppress ectopic activity in hypertrophic cardiomyopathy. These drugs modulate the activity of channels in fibroblasts after cell death.

Class VI. These drugs act on connexins-associated channels. The initiation and propagation of AP is also affected by local currents through gap junctions, hemichannels, and cell-to-cell connections (connexin currents). Blocking gap junction currents can increase or reduce arrhythmias. These channels are important in remodeling process in the heart. Examples are carbenoxolone and peptide analog ZP-123.

Class VII. These drugs act on upstream modulatory targets. Fibrotic changes post-MI and chronic scarring in the heart lead to arrhythmias. This class includes drugs which inhibit remodeling and fibrosis. Examples are those who block the renin-angiotensin-aldosterone inhibitors, omega-3 fatty acids, and statins.

Ablation Therapy

Ablation therapy has gained a prominent role in the treatment of some tachyarrhythmias. Its aim is to deliver radiofrequency energy to destroy abnormal foci and pathways that cause the arrhythmia. The injury to heart tissue is thermal and creates scarring, inflammation, and then necrosis. Electrophysiology studies are used to identify, study, and accurately map the foci of arrhythmia. Indications for ablation therapy include WPW syndrome (usually curable), unifocal atrial tachycardia, AF, and idiopathic VT. Patients with VT may choose this as first-choice therapy. Ablation can be helpful in patients with structural heart disease, when drug therapy is not effective and when patients' ICDs have frequent discharge [4, 6–8, 13–15].

Pacemakers and Defibrillators

Pacemakers and defibrillators are sophisticated computers which can pace, sense, and respond to arrhythmias by inhibiting and/or stimulating electrical activity in the atria, ventricles, or both. Pacemakers can also modulate their responses in a graded fashion. Patients at risk of life-threatening arrhythmias, or when arrhythmias severely compromise their cardiac function, must be referred to a cardiologist for evaluation of pacemaker and/or defibrillator placement. Several studies have demonstrated their effectiveness in preventing sudden death from arrhythmias [5–8].

The ACC/AHA and the North American Society of Pacing and Electrophysiology recommend the implantation of pacemakers in patients with complete third degree AV block; advanced second degree AVB (block of two or more consecutive P waves); symptomatic Mobitz I or Mobitz II AV block; second degree AV block with a widened QRS or chronic bi-fascicular block; and exercise-induced second or third degree AV block (in the absence of myocardial ischemia). They also recommend biventricular pacing for patients with dilated cardiomyopathy (ischemic and non-ischemic); those with an LVEF <35%; those with QRS complexes >0.12 ms; and patients with New York Heart Failure class III or IV, despite optimal medical treatment [4–8].

Patients with implanted pacemakers need to be monitored regularly by cardiologist for proper function and programming, to check the battery life, and to monitor pacemaker activity and patient's clinical symptoms.

Defibrillators deliver unsynchronized electrical shocks to the heart with the aim to stop a lethal arrhythmia and re-establish a viable cardiac rhythm [15, 16]. There are several types of defibrillators: external, transvenous, implantable in the form of a cardioverter-defibrillator (ICD), or as part of a pacemaker. Some have become part of the general public domain, known as automated external defibrillators (AEDs), allowing even the lay public to use them successfully [16]. Today, most defibrillators deliver shocks in a biphasic truncated waveform which is more efficacious while using lower levels of energy to produce defibrillation. Defibrillation is only recommended for ventricular fibrillation and pulseless ventricular tachycardia.

Surgery

Two surgical therapies for atrial fibrillation are available: the obliteration of the left atrial appendage (LAA) and the Cox-Maze procedure, in which surgical disruption of abnormal conduction pathways within the atria is made.

LAA obliteration is a surgical procedure aimed at reducing the risk of thromboembolic events in patients with AF and possibly avoiding long-term anticoagulation. The rationale for obliteration is based on the observation that >90% of the thrombus forms in the LAA and is the main source of thromboembolism [3, 17–20]. Recently, the development of percutaneous procedures to obliterate the left atrial appendage has shown to be equal or superior to warfarin in reducing stroke and adverse cardiovascular events and all-cause mortality [16–20]. This approach should be considered when contraindication for long-term anticoagulation exists [3].

In the Maze procedure, incisions are made in the atria to isolate and interrupt re-entry circuits while maintaining the physiologic activation of the atria. The Maze procedure has undergone multiple revisions since its development, and it is considered for patients who need invasive cardiac surgery for other reasons [21].

Referral to Cardiologist

Cardiology referral is warranted when patients have complex cardiac disease, cannot tolerate the arrhythmia, need rhythm control, require ablation therapy, may benefit from surgical treatment, or need a pacemaker or defibrillator.

Supraventricular Tachyarrhythmias (SVT)

These arrhythmias originate above the ventricles and involve the atria, the AV node, or both for initiation and propagation. These are due to re-entry circuits or accessory pathways, most commonly the AV nodal re-entrant tachycardia, the atrioventricular re-entrant tachycardia, or the atrial tachycardia. In the absence of other conduction defects, the ECG shows a rapid HR with narrow QRS complexes. Wide QRS complexes indicate additional conduction abnormalities distal to AVN, such as bundle branch block and/or accessory pathways. These arrhythmias are treated as ventricular tachycardias.

In an acute setting, IV access and continuous cardiac monitoring are necessary. The first line of therapy is either IV adenosine or IV calcium channel blocker; they are both equally effective in terminating SVT. However, adenosine has quicker action, and it is short lasting. In patients with rare episodes and able to tolerate the episodes, a "pill on the pocket" (flecainide, diltiazem, or propranolol) is a reasonable choice. Patients with persistent or frequent episodes need continuous drug therapy, or they may benefit from radiofrequency ablation therapy which has high success rate in patients with AVN re-entry tachycardia [22].

When evaluating SVT, the following questions should be answered: "What is the ventricular response?", "Does it lead to a narrow or wide QRS?", "Is the arrhythmia regular or irregular?", and "What is the effect on cardiovascular status of the patient?"

Atrial Fibrillation (AF)

AF is the most common SVT seen in primary care. In addition to adverse effects on cardiac function, it increases the risk of stroke. AF has been identified as an independent risk factor for death [4, 22–26]. It worsens heart failure and increases mortality in the setting of myocardial infarct [22–26]. It causes about 10% of strokes, and these are more devastating and a major cause of disability [27–30]. Figure 2 shows the deleterious effect of AF [31].

AF results from uncoordinated atrial activation leading to deterioration of mechanical function. In the ECG, the normal P waves are lost, and irregular impulses reach the AV node and activate the ventricles at an irregular rapid rate, usually between 90 and 170 beats/min. The QRS complex remains narrow unless other conduction abnormalities coexist (Fig. 3). Enhanced automaticity of depolarizing foci and re-entry in one or more circuits are responsible.

AF may result from several disease processes with different prognoses and associated morbidities and mortalities. AF in patients younger than 60 with no underlying heart disease is known as lone AF and has good prognosis. AF due to congenital or acquired valvular disease carries the highest risk for stroke. Valvular vs non-valvular AF is defined by the presence or absence of

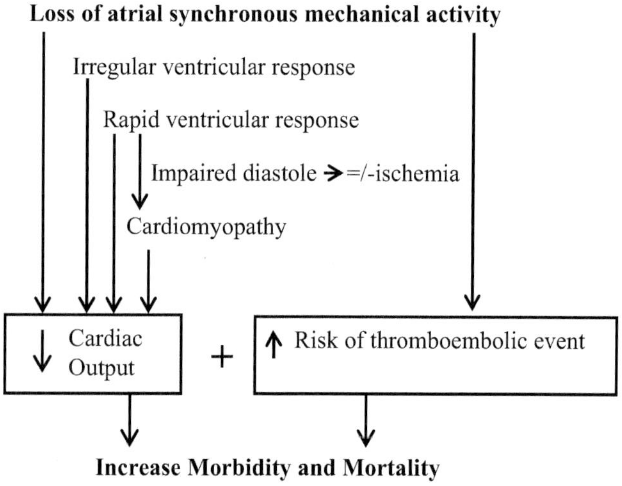

Fig. 2 Clinical implications of atrial fibrillation (Reproduced with permission from Atrial Fibrillation: Diagnosis and Treatment, January 1, 2011, Vol 83, No 1, issue of American Family Physician Copyright © 2011 American Academy of Family Physicians. All Rights Reserved.)

Loss of atrial synchronous mechanical activity

Irregular ventricular response

Rapid ventricular response

Impaired diastole ➔ =/-ischemia

Cardiomyopathy

↓ Cardiac Output + ↑ Risk of thromboembolic event

Increase Morbidity and Mortality

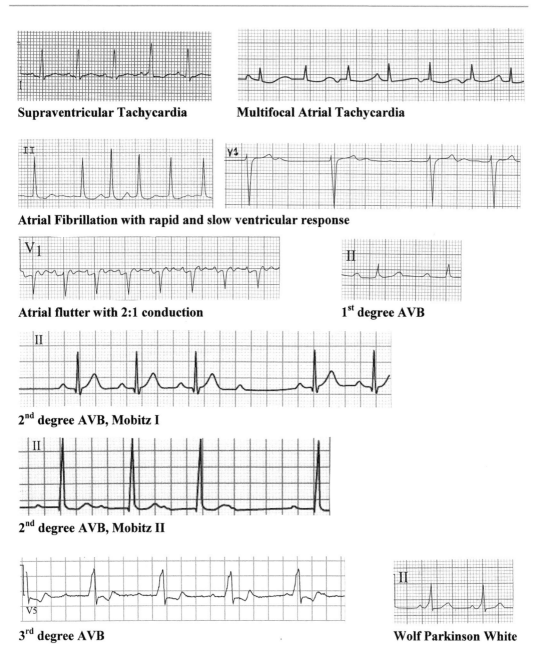

Fig. 3 Supraventricular Arrhythmias

moderate to severe mitral stenosis. Valvular AF that needs valve replacement requires long-term anticoagulation with warfarin [3]. AF due to non-cardiac disease such as hyperthyroidism or pulmonary disease is referred as secondary AF, and treating its cause resolves it. AF treatment and prognosis are affected by its duration and persistence. Paroxysmal AF is defined as episodes of self-resolving AF. Persistent AF lasts for >7 days and can still be terminated by cardioversion. Chronic AF is continuous and unresponsive to cardioversion. Paroxysmal and chronic AF carry the same risk for stroke. Persistent AF causes atrial remodeling (anatomical and physiologic changes) which leads to its perpetuation [3]. Patients with AF may be asymptomatic, have vague symptoms, or present with myocardial infarction, a stroke, or complete hemodynamic collapse. The diagnosis requires the typical ECG pattern: loss of P waves, narrow QRS complexes with a fast and irregular ventricular response. An event or Holter monitor may be needed to capture the arrhythmia.

The management of AF depends on the patient's clinical presentation. In cases of hemodynamic instability, stroke, or myocardial infarction, emergency evaluation and treatment is warranted, including emergency cardioversion.

The long-term treatment of AF poses three main therapeutic challenges: 1. Reverse to NSR by cardioversion or ablation; 2. control the ventricular rate and allow AF to continue; and 3. in either case, start anticoagulation.

Cardioversion can be achieved electrically or pharmacologically. Unless done emergently, or if AF is known to be less than 48 h, cardioversion requires 4 weeks pre- and 4 weeks post-anticoagulation. Pharmacologic cardioversion with antiarrhythmic drugs has limited efficacy. Commonly used drugs include flecainide (Tambocor), propafenone (Rythmol), dofetilide (Tikosyn), amiodarone (Cordarone, Nexterone, Pacerone), dronedarone (Multaq), and sotalol (Betapace, Sorine). Because they can trigger additional arrhythmias and have long-term adverse side effects, it is suggested to refer or co-manage patients with a cardiologist.

Ablation therapy is another way to restore NSR. It is gaining acceptance after the discovery of specific foci that trigger AF. These foci are at or near the pulmonary veins, the crista terminalis, and the coronary sinus [14, 28]. The ACC/AHA/HRS AF guidelines recommend it for patients with recurrent AF who are symptomatic but who have no structural heart disease [3, 4].

Most patients are treated with ventricular rate control vs rhythm control [3, 4, 28–30]. Rate control slows the ventricular response and improves diastolic ventricular filling, reduces myocardial oxygen demand, and improves coronary perfusion and mechanical function. β-blockers, metoprolol, esmolol, and propranolol, and non-dihydropyridine calcium channel blockers (CCB), diltiazem and verapamil, are used to achieve rate control with a goal of <80 during rest and <110 during exercise. More lenient rate control to a resting heart rate of <110 is reasonable in asymptomatic patients with normal left ventricular function. Digoxin is no longer a first or sole choice, but it can be used in addition to β-blockers or CCB [3]. Rhythm control is an option for patients in whom rate control cannot be achieved or who remain symptomatic.

Surgical treatments for AF include left atrial appendage obliteration and the Maze procedure. Both are invasive and are only considered in patients undergoing cardiac surgery for other reasons [17–21].

Anticoagulation

Although anticoagulation increases the risk for bleeding, it significantly reduces the risk of stroke and thromboembolic events, and therefore, it is an essential part of AF treatment. Several stratification tools to assess both the risk of stroke and the risk of bleeding have been developed. In spite of their limitations, they are useful in evaluating patients' risks and benefits for long-term anticoagulation.

The CHAD2DS2-VASc is an acronym that describes the main risk factors for stroke; it has been well established [32]. Table 3 shows the current risk stratification and recommendations for anticoagulation [3]. In general, anticoagulation is recommended for patients whose CHAD2DS2-VASc scores are >2 in males and for female patients >3. Similarly, the ATRIA and HAS-BLED are tools used to assess risk of bleeding [32–35]. Risk factors include anemia, severe renal disease, age, previous bleeding, hypertension, liver disease, labile INR, and drug or alcohol use.

Anticoagulation treatment has changed since the development of non-vitamin K antagonist drugs known as NOACs. Over decades warfarin (Coumadin, Jantoven) had been the cornerstone of anticoagulation therapy.

NOACs include direct thrombin inhibitor dabigatran and the newest factor Xa inhibitors rivaroxaban (Xarelto), apixaban (Eliquis), and edoxaban (Savaysa). All NOACs have been consistently shown to be non-inferior to/or superior to

Table 3 CHAD2DS2-VASc stratification risk for stroke

CHA2DS2-VASc risk factor score	CHA2DS2-VASc total score	Adjusted stroke rate (percent/year)	Anticoagulation recommendation
Congestive heart failure/1 LV dysfunction	0	0	No
Hypertension 1	1	1.3	
Age < 65 0 65–75 1 > 75 2	2	2.2	Unless risk outweighs benefits, recommended options: Warfarin to target INR 2–3
Diabetes 1	3	3.2	Dabigatran 150 mg bid
Stroke/TIA 2 Thromboembolism	4	4.0	Rivaroxaban 20 md qd Apixaban 5 mg bid Edoxaban 60 mg qd
Vascular disease 1	5	6.7	For patients unable/or who refuse
Female gender 1	6	9.8	above choices:
Maximum score 9	7	9.6	Aspirin 81 to 325 mg qd
	8	6.7	Clopidegel 75 md qd
	9	15.2	

Modified from the American Heart Association. http://circ.aha.journals.org/content/early/2014/04/10/CIR.0000000000000040.citation

warfarin in preventing stroke and systemic thromboembolism while having a safer profile, particularly in regard to intracranial bleeding [36–41]. The PROSPER study showed that in patients being treated for acute stroke, NOACs have better long-term outcomes relative to warfarin [40].

Due to warfarin's narrow therapeutic range, multiple drug and food interactions, need for frequent monitoring, and increase risk of bleeding, NOACs are recommended over warfarin in patients who have non-valvular AF, no mechanical valve, and no contraindications.

Warfarin is still the choice for patients who have moderate to severe mitral stenosis and mechanical valve. Many patients still take warfarin due to the higher cost of NOACs. The target goal is measured as the international normalized ratio (INR), and for most patients it is between 2 and 3 with non-valvular AF and an INR of 2.5–3.5 for those with valvular AF.

Warfarin is more effective than aspirin (Bayer Aspirin, Bufferin, Ecotrin) and clopidogrel (Plavix) alone or in combination, but it carries a higher risk for bleeding. It is estimated that warfarin lowers the risk of thromboembolic events by 68% while aspirin by 21% [42–46].

NOACs dosing needs to be adjusted for age, weight, kidney function, and liver disease. Table 4 shows a summary of approved anticoagulants available and their characteristics [36–41].

The main advantages of NOACs over warfarin include fixed dosing, no food interactions, fewer drug interactions, and no need for monitoring. Their major drawback is still high cost. Reversal therapy is now available for dabigatran and factor Xa inhibitors [47, 48]. The FDA has not approved them for valvular AF, pregnant, or lactating patients, and some are contraindicated in patients with advanced kidney disease.

Anticoagulation therapy must consider the patients' preferences. This requires a discussion regarding the risks, benefits, and a shared decision between physicians and patients.

Stopping anticoagulation due to emergencies and/or medical procedures may be necessary. The risk and benefits of doing so must be carefully assessed. Some data has shown worsening outcome when stopping anticoagulation [49]. If interruption is necessary, the recommendation is to bridge using unfractionated heparin or low molecular heparin [3, 4].

Atrial Flutter

Atrial flutter is an organized regular rhythm caused by a re-entry circuit around the tricuspid valve. It is often seen after cardiac surgery or cardiac ablation. AF and atrial flutter can occur

Table 4 Pharmacological properties of approved anticoagulants available for the prevention of thromboembolism in non-valvular atrial fibrillation

Property Mechanism	Warfarin Vitamin K antagonist	Dabigatran Direct thrombin inhibitor	Rivaroxaban Factor Xa inhibitor	Apixaban Factor Xa inhibitor	Edoxaban Factor Xa inhibitor
Dosing	Variable (dose adjusted on basis of the international normalized ratio, INR INR goal is 2–3	150, 110 mg bid 75 bid if CrCl 15–30. Not recommended if CrCl <15	20 mg qd 15 mg if CrCl 15–50 Not recommended if Cr cl < 15	5 mg bid 2.5 mg bid for patients with 2 or more of the following: Cr > 1.5; age > 80y; weight < 60 kg CrCl <15, not defined	30–60 mg qd Avoid if Cr is >95 or < 30 Caution child-Pugh class B or C hepatic impairment
Oral bioavailability	100%	3–7%	60%	58%	64%
Time to effect (hr)	72–96	1–2	2–4	3–4	1–2
Half-life (hr)	40	12–17	5–9	8–15	10–14
Multiple drug and food interactions		Strong P-glycoprotein inducers			Minimal CYP450:3A4 substrate
		Strong P-glycoprotein inhibitors with concomitant kidney dysfunction	Strong P-glycoprotein inhibitors, strong cytochrome P450 inducers and inhibitors		

Cr, creatinine; CrCl, creatinine clearance; hr, hour
Modified from the American Heart Association. http://circ.aha.journals.org/content/early/2014/10/CIR00000000000000040.citation

back and forth and sometimes coexist, but they are different. In atrial flutter waves of depolarization activate the atria to contract regularly at about 280–300 times per minute, and if there are a healthy AVN and no AV node-blocking drugs, there is a 2:1 conduction resulting in a ventricular rate of about 150 beats per minute (Fig. 3). The preferred treatment for atrial flutter is ablation. AV node suppression drugs often change atrial flutter to AF, which may be better tolerated by patients. In the setting of cardiovascular compromise, electrical cardioversion may be necessary using biphasic defibrillator starting at 50 J energy shock.

Atrial or Sinus Tachycardia

Sinus tachycardia (Fig. 3) is in most cases a normal response of the heart to physiologic stressors such hyperthyroidism, dehydration, anemia, hypoxia, etc. A rare type of atrial tachycardia, called inappropriate sinus tachycardia (IST), is diagnosed when all possible causes have been excluded.

Frequent or Premature Atrial Contractions (PACs)

These are not classified as SVT. They generate from a single focus tachycardia but 1:1 P/QRS ratio with a single P wave morphology. When more than one focus triggers the arrhythmia, this is referred as multifocal atrial tachyarrhythmia (MAT). In this case the heart rate is greater than 100 beats/min, and the EKG has at least three different P wave morphologies with variable PP, PR, and RR intervals (Fig. 3). MAT is seen in heart disease, pulmonary disease, hypokalemia, and hypomagnesemia. When patients have different P wave morphologies and heart rate is <100 beats/min, the condition is referred as wandering pacemaker. Therapy is mostly focused at reversing potential causes, and CCB and BB are used to slow heart rate.

Wolff-Parkinson-White (WPW) Syndrome

It occurs when one or more accessory pathways exist bypassing the AVN, allowing the ventricles to activate earlier than normal and resulting in tachy-arrhythmia. The ECG shows a short PR interval with a slurring of the initial part of the QRS, making it wider, which is known as "delta wave" and represents pre-excitation (Fig. 3). Ablation therapy is curative and recommended. Drugs with AV node suppression effect such as BB, CCB, digoxin, and adenosine are contraindicated [5, 7].

Atrioventricular Arrhythmias

Atrioventricular block (AVB) results from an abnormal delay or interruption in the conduction of AP from the atria to the ventricles. This block can occur in the atria and at AVN and the His-Purkinje fibers, and it can be intermittent, complete or incomplete, and uni-fascicular, bi-fascicular, or tri-fascicular depending on the location of the lesion. The severity is described in degrees.

In first degree AVB, the delay conduction is at the AVN, but each AP from the SA reaches the ventricles. The ECC shows a prolonged PR interval, >0.2 s (Fig. 3). Usually this block does not cause significant symptoms, and it does not require treatment. Drugs with nodal suppression effects such as digoxin, verapamil, diltiazem, and beta blockers can be the culprit.

There are two types of second degree AVB, known as Mobitz I and II. Mobitz I occurs when the PR intervals progressively increase in length until a QRS is dropped. This phenomenon is also known as Wenckebach (Fig. 3). In Mobitz II, the PR interval remains constant, but not all APs from the SA are transmitted to the ventricles. Thus, the 1:1 P/QRS ratio is lost, and 2:1 or 3:1 conduction pattern appears. In patients with bi-fascicular block, a pacemaker is recommended.

In third degree AVB, there is complete blockage of conduction between the SA and AV nodes, and the atria and ventricles contract at different rates (Fig. 3). Depending on the ventricular response, the rate may be too slow to sustain appropriate circulation, and in some cases, it can lead to complete heart block. Most patients are symptomatic and require a permanent pacemaker.

Sick Sinus Syndrome (SSS) Also Known as Sinus Node Dysfunction (SND)

SSS describes a bradyarrhythmia caused by a sick SA node unable to be pacemaker, usually as a result of aging or heart disease. The SA node generates AP at a very slow rate leading to severe bradycardia, sinus pauses, and sometimes arrest. As the heart is unable to maintain adequate perfusion, patients experience lightheadedness, pre-syncope, syncope, dyspnea, and angina. Some patients develop brady-tachy syndrome with paroxysmal atrial tachycardia (most commonly AF) in response to the bradycardia. It is crucial to establish a correlation between the arrhythmia and symptoms to make the diagnosis of SSS, and a Holter or an event monitor is required. Treatment is focused at treating reversible causes, such as stopping drugs that suppressed the SA node, correcting electrolyte imbalances and hypoxia. Drug therapy has not been successful, and most patients require the implantation of a pacemaker [5, 7]. Patients with asymptomatic bradycardia do not need treatment but need close follow-up.

Ventricular Arrhythmias (VA)

VA are caused by electrical activation of ventricular cardiac cells without atrial or nodal influences, most commonly triggered by re-entry mechanism. Their characteristic ECG pattern shows wide QRS complexes (>120 ms), bizarre shape, no preceding P wave, and large T wave usually of opposite polarity to the QRS complex. They are serious arrhythmias associated with sudden cardiac death especially among patients with underlying cardiac disease and require cardiology referral. VA are classified according to their frequency, persistence, and effect on ventricular contraction [50].

Premature Ventricular Contractions, PVCs

PVCs show a wide QRS, no preceding P wave, and T wave is large and opposite to the QRS, giving a bizarre appearance (Fig. 4). They may

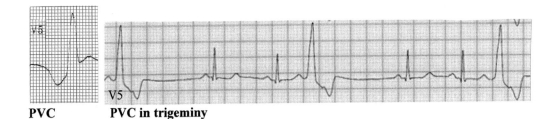

PVC   **PVC in trigeminy**

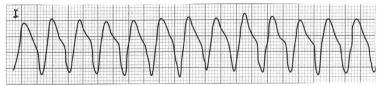

Non-sustained VT

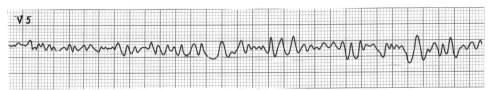

Sustained VT

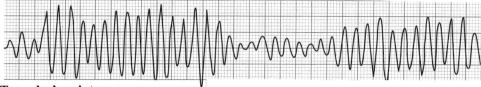

Ventricular Fibrillation

Torsade de pointes

Fig. 4 Ventricular Arrhythmias

be triggered by electrolyte abnormalities (particularly hypokalemia, hypomagnesemia, and hypercalcemia), certain drugs, and stimulants. In addition to check electrolytes, magnesium and calcium, EKG, echocardiogram, a 24 h. Holter monitor is needed to assess their frequency, morphology, and effect on cardiac function.

PVCs are very common in the general population, and isolated events in patients with healthy hearts do not require treatment. However, in the setting of MI, ischemia, HF, and structural heart disease, they warrant immediate cardiology referral. First-line therapy for symptomatic patients is either a β-blocker, or non-dihydropyridine CCB, or antiarrhythmic drugs. Some patients may benefit from electrophysiology study (EPS) and catheter ablation if specific foci are identified. PVCs also can present in bigeminy, trigeminy, or quadrigeminy patterns when followed by one, two, or three normal beats, respectively (Fig. 4). Their clinical significance depends on their frequency, morphology, complexity, and patient's hemodynamic response.

Ventricular Tachycardia (VT)

It is defined as more than 3 PVCs in a row and HR > 100 beats/ min. VT is further characterized by duration and morphology [50]. Non-sustained VT lasts for <30 s. Sustained VT lasts >30 s, is symptomatic, and causes hemodynamic instability. VT may have single morphology (single focus), or may be polymorphic (two or more foci). Polymorphic rhythms are seen in patients with structural and ischemic heart disease, and they are associated with worse prognosis. It is key not to confuse VT with SVT associated with BBB or aberrant conduction since treatment is different.

Sustained VT requires emergent cardioversion and eventual ICD placement. Unstable polymorphic rhythms require defibrillation. Antiarrhythmic drugs (procainamide, amiodarone, and, less commonly, lidocaine) can be given to patients with monomorphic, stable, sustained VT, or when VT is refractory to cardioversion. Transvenous pacing may be necessary until a permanent ICD is placed. Patients with VT and ischemic heart disease benefit from β-blockers, ACEI or ARB, and aggressive treatment of HF. Class I antiarrhythmic agents are contraindicated post-MI and in HF. Patients with syncope should have EPS and ablation therapy if indicated.

Ventricular Fibrillation (VF)

This is life-threatening arrhythmia caused by the activation of multiple foci in the ventricles leading to loss of effective ventricular contraction. The EKG shows chaotic rapid polymorphic QRS complexes (Fig. 4). It requires immediate cardiopulmonary resuscitation and emergent defibrillation. VF is a common cause of cardiac arrest, and the use of automatic external defibrillators in the community is aimed to increase the chances of survival while activating the emergency response system. The most common cause of VF is severe CAD, history of MI, ischemia, and scarring. Patients with dilated cardiomyopathy have high mortality. More rare causes include genetic mutations. Long-term treatment of VF include revascularization, beta blockers, and ICD placement [5, 16, 51, 52].

QT Interval Prolongation

The QT interval in the EKG represents the time from the initial depolarization of the ventricles to their full repolarization. Prolongation of this interval can lead to deadly polymorphic ventricular arrhythmias and sudden death, such as torsades de pointes.

The QT interval varies with heart rate and it is necessary to correct for this. A corrected QT interval (QTc) also varies according to gender, for males 470 ms and for females 480 ms.

Hundreds of genetic mutations in K^+ channels which can cause QT prolongation have been identified. Recent progress in electrophysiology and genetic testing helps to identify and stratify patient's risk for these arrhythmias [53].

In addition to antiarrhythmic drugs, there are commonly used drugs in primary care, which can also prolong QT interval. Some examples include macrolide and fluoroquinolones antibiotics, some antihistamines, methadone, antipsychotic, and others.

Therefore, it is important for physicians to be aware of drugs that can prolong QT interval, their potential additive effects, and magnifying effect in the setting on hypokalemia and hypomagnesemia and any condition that causes hypoxia [54].

Torsades de Pointes

It is a rare form of VT characterized by repeated cycles of QRS complex changing in amplitude and twisting along the isoelectric axis, giving a unique pattern in the ECG (Fig. 4). It is associated with a significant QT prolongation, >600 ms. Although torsades can self-terminate, it can also degenerate into VF. Treatment requires IV magnesium given under continuous cardiac monitoring (even when Mg is normal). Temporary transvenous pacing can be used, with atrial pacing preferred to maintain the atrial filling, except in patients with AVB where ventricular pacing is best. Long-term therapy includes β-blockers (except in congenital torsades) and permanent pacing. In refractory cases an ICD is necessary, and rarely, thoracic sympathectomy is done.

VF and torsades are associated with sudden cardiac death. Since most events occur outside the hospital, recognition by lay persons, activation of the emergency system, immediate CPR, and defibrillation when indicated are key to survival [16, 51]. This has been the reason to install automatic external defibrillators (AEDs) in public places [51].

Summary

Arrhythmias are commonly seen by family physicians in the office. Immediate recognition of arrhythmias causing cardiovascular instability is key to improving patients' survival, sometimes requiring activation of the emergency system. Full evaluation, diagnosis, and treatment are warranted for all patients presenting with an arrhythmia or with suggestive symptoms, despite normal exams and/or EKGs. Reversible causes should be treated as well as comorbidities. Treatment option is tailored to the type of arrhythmia and must reflect a shared decision-making between patients and doctors, based on best available evidence and the patients' preferences.

References

1. Wang PJ, Estes NA. Cardiology patient pages. Supraventricular Tachycardia Circulation. 2002;106(25): e206–8.
2. Giada F, Gulizia M, Francese M, et al. Recurrent unexplained palpitations (RUP) study comparison of implantable loop recorder versus conventional diagnostic strategy. J Am Coll Cardiol. 2007;49:1951–6.
3. January CT, Wann LS, Calkins H, et al. 2019 AHA/ACC/HRS focused update of the 2014 AHA/ACC/HRS guideline for the management of patients with atrial fibrillation. A report of the American College of Cardiology/American Heart Association task force on clinical practice guidelines and the Heart Rhythm Society. Circulation. 2019;140:e125–51. https://doi.org/10.1161/CIR.0000000000000665.
4. Craig TJ, January L, Wann S, et al. 2014 AHA/ACC/HRS guidelines for the Management of Patients with atrial fibrillation: executive summary: a report of the American College of Cardiology/American Heart Association task force on practice guidelines and the Heart Rhythm Society. Circulation Published on line March 28, 2014. http://circ.ahajournals.org/content/suppl/2014/10/CIR.0000000000000040.DC1.html
5. Al-Khatib SM, Stevenson WG, Ackerman MJ, et al. 2017 AHA/ACC/HRS guideline for management of patients with ventricular arrhythmias and the prevention of sudden cardiac death: executive summary: a report of the American College of Cardiology Foundation/American Heart Association task force on clinical practice guidelines and the Heart Rhythm Society. Circulation. 2018;138:e210–71. https://doi.org/10.1161/CIR.0000000000000548.
6. Strickberger SA, Conti J, Daoud EG, et al. Patient selection for cardiac resynchronization therapy: from the council on clinical cardiology subcommittee on electrocardiography and arrhythmias and the quality of care and outcomes research interdisciplinary working group, in collaboration with the Heart Rhythm Society. Circulation. 2005;111(16):2146–50.
7. Page RL, Joglar JA, Caldwell MA, et al. Evidence review committee chair‡. 2015 ACC/AHA/HRS guideline for the management of adult patients with supraventricular tachycardia: a report of the American College of Cardiology/American Heart Association task force on clinical practice guidelines and the Heart Rhythm Society. Circulation. 2016;133: e506–74.
8. Jacobs I, Sunde K, Deakin CD. Et at. Part 6: defibrillation: 2010 international consensus conference on cardiopulmonary resuscitation and emergency cardiovascular care science with treatment recommendations. Circulation. 2010;122(suppl2):S325–37.
9. Lei M, DPhil LW, Terrar D, et al. Modernized classification of cardiac antiarrhythmic drugs. Circulation. 2018;138:1879–96.
10. Mathew ST, Po SS, Thadani U. Inappropriate sinus tachycardia-symptom and heart rate reduction with Ivabradine: a pooled analysis of prospective studies. Heart Rhythm. 2018;15:240–7.
11. Uddin S, Price S. Anti-arrhythmic therapy. In: Hall J, editor. Encyclopedia of intensive care medicine 2012: spring reference. Berlin/Heidelberg: Springer-Verlag; 2012. 2012-08-14 10:55:27 UTC. www.springerreference.com.
12. Micromedex. http://micromedex.com/

13. Holgate A, Foo A. Adenosine versus intravenous calcium channel antagonists for the treatment of supraventricular tachycardia in adults. Cochrane Database Syst Rev 2012, issue 2. Art. No:CD005154. https://doi.org/10.1002/14651858.CD005154.pub3.

14. Calkins H. Catheter ablation to maintain sinus rhythm. Circulation. 2012;125:1439–45.

15. Link MS, Atkins DL, Passman RS, et al. Part 6: electrical therapies: automated external defibrillators, defibrillation, cardioversion, and pacing: 2010 American Heart Association guidelines for cardiopulmonary resuscitation and emergency cardiovascular care. Circulation. 2010;122(18 Suppl 3):S706–19. Erratum in Circulation 2011;123(6):e235

16. Hallstrom AP, Ornato JP, Weisfeldt M, et al. Public-access defibrillation and survival after out-of-hospital cardiac arrest. N Engl J Med. 2004;351:637–46.

17. Reddy VY, Sievert H, Halperin J, et al. Percutaneous left atrial appendage closure vs warfarin for atrial fibrillation. A randomized clinical trial. JAMA. 2014;312:1988–98.

18. Holmes DR, Kar S, Price MJ, et al. Prospective randomized evaluation of the watchman left atrial appendage closure device in patients with atrial fibrillation versus long term warfarin therapy: the prevail trial. J Am Coll Cardiol. 2014;64:1–12.

19. Holmes DR, Doshi SK, Kar S. Left atrial appendage closure as an alternative to warfarin for stroke prevention in atrial fibrillation: a patient-level meta-analysis. J Am Coll Cardiol. 2015;65:2614–23.

20. Vy R, Sievert H, Halperin J, et al. Percutaneous left atrial appendage closure vs warfarin for atrial fibrillation: a randomized clinical trial. JAMA. 2014;312:1988–98.

21. Damiano RJ, Gaynor SL, Bailey M, et al. The long-term outcome of patients with coronary disease and atrial fibrillation undergoing the cox maze procedure. J Thorac Cardiovasc Surg. 2003;126:2016–21.

22. Link MS. Clinical practice. Evaluation and initial treatment of supraventricular tachycardia. N Engl J Med. 2012;376:1438–48.

23. Vidaillet H, Granada JF, Chyou PH, et al. A population-based study of mortality among patients with atrial fibrillation or flutter. Am J Med. 2002;113:365–70.

24. Go AS, Hylek EM, Phillips KA, et al. Prevalence of diagnosed atrial fibrillation in adults: national implications for rhythm management and stroke prevention: the anticoagulation and risk factors in atrial fibrillation (ATRIA) study. JAMA. 2001;285:2370–5.

25. Wang TJ, Larson MG, Levy D, et al. Temporal relations of atrial fibrillation and congestive heart failure and their joint influence on mortality: the Framingham heart study. Circulation. 2003;107(23):2920–5.

26. Pederson OD, Abildstrom SZ, Ottesen MM, et al. Increased risk of sudden and non-sudden cardiovascular death in patients with atrial fibrillation/flutter following acute myocardial infarction. Eur Heart J. 2006;27:290–5.

27. Chen HS, Wen JM, Wu SN, et al. Catheter ablation for paroxysmal and persistent atrial fibrillation. Cochrane Database Syst Rev. 2012;4:CD007101.

28. Sherman DG, Kim SG, Boop BS, et al. Occurrence and characteristics of stroke events in the atrial fibrillation follow-up investigation of sinus rhythm management (AFFIRM) study. Arch Intern Med. 2005;165:1185–91.

29. Hagens VE, Ranchor AV, Van Sonderen E, et al. Effect of rate or rhythm control on quality of life in persistent atrial fibrillation. Results from the rate control versus electrical cardioversion (RACE) study. J. Am Coll Cardiol. 2004;43(2):241–7.

30. Van Gelder IC, Hagens VE, Bosker HA, et al. A comparison of rate control and rhythm control in patients with recurrent persistent atrial fibrillation. N Engl J Med. 2002;347(23):1834–40.

31. Gutierrez C, Blanchard D. Atrial fibrillation: diagnosis and treatment. Am Fam Physician. 2011;83:61–8.

32. Lip GY. Implications of the CHA2DS2-VASc and HAS-BLED scores for thromboprophylaxis in atrial fibrillation. Am J Med. 2011;124:111–4.

33. Pisters R, Lane DA, Nieuwlaat R, et al. A novel user-friendly score (HAS-BLED) to assess 1-year risk of major bleeding in patients with atrial fibrillation: the euro heart survey. Chest. 2010;138:1093–100.

34. Apostolakis S, Lane DA, Guo Y, et al. Performance of the HEMORR(2)HAGES, ATRIA, and HAS-BLED bleeding risk–prediction scores in patients with atrial fibrillation undergoing anticoagulation: the AMADEUS (evaluating the use of SR34006 compared to warfarin or acenocoumarol in patients with atrial fibrillation) study. J Am Coll Cardiol. 2012;60:861–7.

35. Roldan V, Marin F, Fernandez H, et al. Predictive value of the HAS-BLED and ATRIA bleeding scores for the risk of serious bleeding in a "real world" population with atrial fibrillation receiving anticoagulation therapy. Chest. 2013;143:179–84.

36. Connolly SJ, Ezekowitz MD, Yusuf S, et al. Dabigatran versus warfarin in patients with atrial fibrillation. N Engl J Med. 2009;361:1139–51.

37. Patel MR, Mahaffey KW, Garg J, et al. Rivaroxaban versus warfarin in non valvular atrial fibrillation. N Engl J Med. 2011;365:883–91.

38. Granger CB, Alexander JH, McMurray JJ, et al. Apixaban warfarin in patients with atrial fibrillation. N Engl J Med. 2011;365:981–92.

39. Giugliano RP, Ruff CT, Braunwald E, et al. Edoxaban versus warfarin in patients with atrial fibrillation. NEJM. 2013;369:2093–104.

40. Xian Y, Xu H, O'Brien EC, et al. Clinical effectiveness of direct Oral anticoagulants vs warfarin in older patients with atrial fibrillation and ischemic stroke: findings from the patient-centered research into outcomes stroke patients prefer and effectiveness research (PROSPER) study. JAMA Neurol. 2019;76(10):1192–202.

41. Steinberg BA, Piccini JP. Anticoagulation in atrial fibrillation. BMJ. 2014;348:g2116.

42. Ruff CT, Giugliano RP, Braunwald E, et al. Comparison of the efficacy and safety of new oral anticoagulants with warfarin in patients with atrial fibrillation: a meta-analysis of randomized trials. Lancet. 2014;383:955–62.

43. Weitz JI, Connolly SJ, Patel I, et al. Randomized, parallel-group, multicenter, multinational phase 2 study comparing edoxaban, an oral factor Xa inhibitor, with warfarin for stroke prevention in patients with atrial fibrillation. Thromb Haemost. 2010;104:633–41.

44. Aguilar MI, Hart R, Pearce LA. Oral anticoagulants versus antiplatelet therapy for preventing stroke in patients with non-valvular atrial fibrillation and no history of stroke or transient ischemic attacks. Cochrane Database Syst Rev. 2007:CD006186.

45. Perez-Gomez F, Alegria E, Berjon J, et al. Comparative effects of antiplatelet, anticoagulant, or combined therapy in patients with valvular and nonvalvular atrial fibrillation: a randomized multicenter study. J Am Coll Cardiol. 2004; 44(8):1557–66.

46. Connolly S, Pogue J, Hart R, et al. ACTIVE writing group of the ACTIVE investigators. clopidogrel plus aspirin versus oral anticoagulation for atrial fibrillation in the atrial fibrillation clopidogrel trial with Irbesartan for prevention of vascular events (ACTIVE W): a randomized controlled trial. Lancet. 2006;367:1903–12.

47. Pollack CV, Reilly PA, van Ryn J, et al. Idarucizumab for Dabigatran reversal- full cohort analysis. N Engl J Med. 2017;377:431–41.

48. Siegal DM, Curnutte JT, Connolly SJ, et al. Andexanet alpha for the reversal of factor Xa inhibitor activity. N Engl J Med. 2015;373:2413–24.

49. Douketis JD, Spyropoulos AC, Kaatz S, et al. Perioperative bridging anticoagulation in patients with atrial fibrillation. N Engl J Med. 2015;373:823–33.

50. Bacon D, Philips B. Ventricular arrhythmias. In: Hall J., Vincent J. (Ed.) Encyclopedia of intensive medicine spring reference. Springer-Veriag Berlin/Heidelberg 2012. 2012-08-14 10:55:00 UTC. www.springerreference.com.

51. Moss AJ, Zareba W, Hall WJ, et al. Prophylactic implantation of a defibrillator in patients with myocardial infarction and reduced ejection fraction. New Engl J Med. 2002;346:877–33.

52. Huang Y, He Q, Yang LJ, et al. Cardiopulmonary resuscitation (CPR) plus delayed defibrillation versus immediate defibrillation for out-of-hospital cardiac arrest. Cochrane Database Syst Rev 2014, Issue 9. Art. No.: CD 009803. https://doi.org/10.1002/14651858.CD009803.pub2

53. Neira V, Enriquez A, Simpson C, et al. Update on long QT syndrome. J Cardiovasc Electrophysiol. 2019;30:3068–78.

54. Straus SM, Sturkenboom MC, Bleumink GS, et al. Non-cardiac QTc-prolonging drugs and the risk of cardiac sudden death. Eur Heart J. 2005;26:2007–12.

Valvular Heart Disease

Sophia Malary Carter, Wendy Bocaille, and
Santos Reyes-Alonso

Contents

S. Malary Carter (✉)
West Kendal Baptist Hospital FIU Family Medicine
Residency Program, Miami, FL, USA

FIU-Herbert Wertheim College of Medicine, Miami, FL,
USA

Baptist Health Group, Family Medicine Center, Miami,
FL, USA
e-mail: SophiaMal@baptisthealth.net

W. Bocaille · S. Reyes-Alonso
West Kendal Baptist Hospital FIU Family Medicine
Residency Program, Miami, FL, USA
e-mail: WendyBo@baptisthealth.net;
SantosR@baptisthealth.net

© Springer Nature Switzerland AG 2022
P. M. Paulman et al. (eds.), *Family Medicine*,
https://doi.org/10.1007/978-3-030-54441-6_193

Introduction

Valvular heart disease occurs when one or multiple valves of the heart are damaged or diseased. About 2.5% of the US population has valvular heart disease, but it is more common in older adults. About 13% of people born before 1943 have valvular heart disease [1]. In 2017, there were 3046 deaths due to rheumatic valvular heart disease and 24,811 deaths due to non-rheumatic valvular heart disease in the USA. Nearly 25,000 deaths in the USA each year are due to heart valve disease from causes other than rheumatic disease. Valvular heart disease deaths are more commonly due to aortic valve disease [2]. There are several causes of valvular heart disease, including congenital conditions, infections, degenerative conditions (wearing out with age), and conditions linked to other types of heart disease [1]. Valvular heart disease is recognized by finding a heart murmur. Here, even more than elsewhere in cardiology, the physical findings are all important to making a diagnosis and assessing severity. Often, they trump the results of special testing. Murmurs may first be detected in a symptomless patient, perhaps a young would-be athlete at a high school physical examination, or they may be the clue in someone with dyspnea and fluid retention that valvular disease is the reason for their cardiac failure [3]. The family physician is in a particularly challenging position because we will be addressing these potential concerns at every stage of life and often may be dealing with determining the significance of a new heart sound as an incidental finding. Valvular disease may lead to decreased functional status, permanent structural changes, and increased mortality. Timely diagnosis and appropriate testing and consultation are the goals of the family physician, in order to prevent the negative sequelae of inappropriately addressing valvular disease. Learning maneuvers and understanding the sounds present within the heart facilitate appropriate diagnosis [4].

The Third Heart Sound

The third heart sound (S3) is the most difficult heart sound to identify on auscultation. S3 occurs in early diastole (during passive filling) when the ventricle is dilated and noncompliant. It will be heard after

S2, with low frequency. Its significance varies depending on to the age of the patient. It can be interpreted as physiologic in patients under 30 years old with no structural or functional cardiac condition (thyrotoxicosis, pregnancy, and anemia). It is suspicious in patients between 30 and 40 years of age and it is considered pathologic in patients older than 40 years old often correlating with dysfunction or volume overload what is seen in patients suffering from pregnancy, thyrotoxicosis, valvular regurgitations, and excessive fluid overload. Right ventricle S3 is best heard (sometimes only) during inspiration because negative intrathoracic pressure increases RV filling with the patient supine. Left ventricle S3 is then best heard during expiration with patient in left lateral decubitus position [5–7].

The Fourth Heart Sound

The fourth heart sound (S4) is produced by augmented ventricular filling, caused by atrial contraction, near the end of diastole. It is auscultated immediately prior to S1 and it is a result of decreased compliance within the ventricles. S4 is similar to S3 and is best heard with the bell of the stethoscope. During inspiration, RV S4 increases while LV S4 becomes less intense. S4 is typically associated with hypertrophy of the ventricles. The fourth heart sound is best heard at the level of the apex and can be also palpable. In general it is accepted that the presence of S4 is highly associated with pathology although there is some disagreement in regards of the presence of audible S4 in absence of cardiac pathology [7, 8].

Physical Exam and Diagnostic Approach

Auscultating heart murmur can be difficult sometimes. In general physicians must exam the patient in a quiet room minimizing external surrounding noises in order to be able to fully characterize the murmur. First step when examining a murmur is to determine relation with the cardiac cycle since all diastolic murmurs must be considered pathologic until proven otherwise. The second step would be grading the murmur. There are several approaches to determine the grade of the murmur. In general every murmur whose intensity is louder than S1-S2 should be considered Grade III or greater and requires further evaluation with echocardiogram. Grade VI can be heard even without the stethoscope. Grade V can be auscultated with the stethoscope half off the chest wall. Grade IV, V, and VI have associated thrill.

Classification of cardiac murmurs (six):

- **Grade I:** Audible under optimal conditions by an expert.
- **Grade II:** Easy to hear with stethoscope but soft.
- **Grade III:** Moderately loud, no thrill.
- **Grade IV**: Very loud with a palpable thrill, with stethoscope on chest.
- **Grade V:** Audible with stethoscope partly off chest with a thrill.
- **Grade VI:** Audible without a stethoscope with a thrill.

Most of the murmurs foundin children and adults are benign innocent murmurs in adults [8]. In general and for practice purposes further workup is warranted in patients with systolic murmurs Grade III or more and in every patient with a diastolic murmur. In such cases an echocardiogram should be ordered as the best initial step.

Physical Maneuvers

Exam room maneuvers may alter the qualities of a murmur and may help to define and diagnose innocent versus pathological murmurs. Maneuvers that increase afterload are better for ruling out murmurs than ruling in. Methods of increased peripheral resistance, such as the patient gripping something hard, decreases outflow from the heart and thus decreases outflow, physiologic, and innocent murmur volumes. Decreased preload maneuvers decrease venous return to the heart, so murmurs affected by filling, including innocent and physiologic murmurs and outflow, mitral valve, and tricuspid valve murmurs, will all have a decrease in audible volume.

Decreasing preload is done best by Valsalva maneuvers. A Valsalva maneuver is executed by asking the patient to take a deep breath, hold it, and bear down like performing a bowel movement.

Increased preload maneuvers increase venous return and filling of the heart. Squatting position is the easiest method to increase preload. Though maybe variable, most outflow murmurs increase in volume when a patient is squatting, and murmurs caused by hypertrophic cardiomyopathy (HCM) or mitral valve prolapse (MVP) decrease in volume [6, 8].

In other words, a larger volume of blood in the heart (increase preload through squatting and lift legs) will increase the audible volume of the murmur except in patients with mitral valve prolapse and hypertrophic cardiomyopathy. Less volume of blood in the heart (decrease preload through Valsalva maneuver) will cause the opposite effect.

Definitions of Severity of Valve Disease

It is important to access the severity of a valvular disease. This allows us to determine if valvular replacement is indicated. Valve replacement are reserved for patient with severe valvular disease. Severity is based on multiple criteria, including symptoms, valve anatomy, valve hemodynamics, and the effects of valve dysfunction on ventricular and vascular function. Indications for intervention and periodic monitoring are dependent on:

1. The presence or absence of symptoms
2. The severity of VHD
3. The response of the LV and/or RV to volume or pressure overload caused by VHD
4. The effects on the pulmonary or systemic circulation [6]

Stages of Valvular Heart Disease

Stage A: Patient with risk factors for developing VHD

Stage B: Patient with a progressive VHD and presence of mild to moderate severity and asymptomatic

Stage C: Patient with asymptomatic severe VHD
- C1: Patient with severe VHD, no symptoms with left/right ventricular function remains compensated
- C2: Patient with severe VHD, no symptoms with decompensated left/right ventricular function

Stage D: Patient with severe VHD who has developed symptoms already [9]

Key Points in Treatment

Treatment and management will be discussed in details under specific topics. In general, valvular diseases are treated either medically or with surgery. Considering that an increase in preload will worsen the severity of the murmur except in mitral valve prolapse and hypertrophic cardiomyopathy, medical management of almost all murmurs must focused on the reduction of the preload and decrease afterload. In MVP and HCM the goal is to improve the filling of the heart. This is achieved by the use of beta blockers (increase filling time/diastole) and avoiding dehydration or any condition that decrease circulating volume.

Aortic Regurgitation (AR)

Aortic regurgitation occurs when the aortic valve does not close tightly due to incompetence of the aortic causing flow from the aorta into the left ventricle during diastole. Causes include idiopathic valvular degeneration, rheumatic fever, endocarditis, myxomatous degeneration, congenital bicuspid aortic valve, syphilis, and connective tissue and rheumatologic disorders. Acute aortic regurgitation is an early diastolic murmur that is the result of the blood flowing retrograde into the left ventricle and has been described as a blowing decrescendo at the left sternal border best heard when patient has held breath after exhalation and is leaning forward [4, 7]. AR can be classified as acute or chronic depending on the onset of presentation. Acute aortic regurgitation derives from a rapid change in the aortic valve causing an acute abnormality, which may arise from etiologies including infective endocarditis or changes in the aorta such as aortic dissection. Acute aortic regurgitation is the result of life-threatening abnormalities, and early diagnosis with echocardiogram or CT imaging is crucial to facilitate rapid surgical intervention [4].

Chronic aortic regurgitation is also a diastolic murmur, and as with all diastolic murmurs, a referral to a cardiologist should be considered for echocardiography and further recommendations [4].

Etiology

Acute aortic regurgitation (AR) may result from abnormalities of the valve, most often endocarditis, or abnormalities of the aorta, primarily aortic dissection. Acute AR may also occur as an iatrogenic complication of a transcatheter procedure or after blunt chest trauma. The acute volume overload on the LV usually results in severe pulmonary congestion, as well as a low forward cardiac output. Urgent diagnosis and rapid intervention are lifesaving [9].

Chronic AR has a wide variety of causes that requires early identification before determining treatment options. Causes can be divided in three groups including conditions that involves the valve itself, the aorta, and diseases affecting both the valve and the aorta [3].

Diseases of the Valve

- Bicuspid aortic valve
- Following endocarditis
- Rheumatic valve disease

Diseases of the Aorta

- Connective tissue disorders
- Marfan syndrome
- Familial aortic ectasia
- Other rare, inherited vascular disorders
- Aortic dissection
- Inflammatory disorders
- Vasculitis (Takayasu disease)

- Giant-cell arteritis
- Syphilis

Diseases Affecting Aorta and Valve

- Spondyloarthropathies
- Ankylosing spondylitis
- Reiter syndrome
- Psoriatic arthropathy

Symptoms and Physical Findings

Acute AR causes symptoms of HF and cardiogenic shock. Patient will present with dyspnea on exertion that can progress to dyspnea at rest, orthopnea, and paroxysmal nocturnal dyspnea (PND), with physical findings typical of left side heart failure such us bilateral symmetric and progressively ascending crackles, associated with tachycardia, hypotension, JVD, and other signs consistent with cardiogenic shock [7].

Chronic AR is typically asymptomatic for years with signs and symptoms of HF developing insidiously. Symptoms associated with chronic aortic regurgitation include syncope, angina, and reduced exercise tolerance. As the disease progresses and left ventricular function begins to decrease, symptoms associated with systolic heart failure may arise including lower extremity edema and increasing dyspnea [4, 7].

The findings on physical examination in patients with chronic AR are primarily related to the increased stroke volume and widened pulse pressure. The peripheral pulses demonstrate an abrupt rise of the upstroke and a quick collapse (water hammer or Corrigan pulse). Apical impulse is hyper-dynamic lateralized to the left and inferiorly. Depending on severity is possible to auscultate a thrill usually over the base of the heart but also can be heard over the carotids and suprasternal notch. The classic murmur of AR is a high-frequency, blowing, and decrescendo diastolic murmur, usually heard in the aortic area but also audible in the left third and fourth intercostal spaces along the sternal border. Initial phases of the disease murmur are mild and present only during early diastole but with progression it starts becoming more like a holodiastolic murmur. AR murmur will increase in intensity with increase preload or afterload maneuvers and will feel less intense with maneuvers that decrease blood pressure, such as standing, amyl nitrate inhalation, or the strain phase of the Valsalva maneuver [10].

Most common signs seen in patients with chronic AR are summarized below [3].

Quincke's sign: Nail bed pulsation
Corrigan's pulse: Visible carotid pulsation
de Musset's sign: Head bobbing to pulse
Müller's sign: Uvula bobbing to pulse
Duroziez's sign: Diastolic bruit with compression of the femoral artery at the groin
Hill's sign: Systolic pressure in the leg >10 mmHg higher than measures at the brachial artery
Traube's sign: Pistol-shot sounds best heard over the femoral artery

Diagnosis of Aortic Regurgitation

The initial diagnosis of any suspected valvular disease is with a transthoracic echocardiogram (TTE) which is the best tool to assess valve anatomy and etiology, concurrent valve disease, and associated abnormalities, such as aortic dilation. Doppler echocardiography provides accurate noninvasive determination of valve hemodynamics. For regurgitant lesions, calculation of regurgitant orifice area, volume, and fraction is performed, when possible in the context of a multiparameter severity grade based on color Doppler imaging, continuous- and pulsed-wave Doppler recordings, and the presence or absence of distal flow reversals. Other more invasive procedures sometimes can be used in order to determine a final diagnosis and stratified severity of AR especially when noninvasive tests like TTE cannot provide accurate information or when there is no correlation between noninvasive imaging and clinical findings. In these cases cardiac catheterization should be considered and will provide valuable information that will help significantly in the decision-making process regarding surgical intervention. Exercise testing can be considered in patients which physician is not sure about the real physical limitations the patient is experiencing. Cardiac magnetic resonance imaging is another option for initial evaluation and further follow-up since it can provide highly accurate assessment of LV volumes, mass, and ejection fraction; it can also provide excellent visualization of the aortic root and ascending aorta.

Cardiac MRI can be used to obtain accurate information regarding regurgitant volumes and flow [9, 10].

Natural History, Complications, and Follow-Up

Aortic regurgitation is a chronic progressive condition which causes significant hemodynamic changes in the heart that leads to compensatory remodeling of the left ventricle over time with a subsequent decreased LV function and can eventually lead to severe HF. Once such remodeling is established the probability of full recovery even with appropriate treatment including valve replacement is minimal. With treatment, the 10 years survival for patients with mild to moderate AR is about 80–95%. With timely valve replacement before HF, long-term prognosis is good, however for those with severe AR and HF is really poor. That is why early diagnosis is important and adequate initial workup and follow-up of these patients in order to intervene in a timely manner [4]. Patients with AR requires appropriate clinical and echocardiographic follow-up. New guidelines have established a regular follow-up with transthoracic echocardiogram (TTE) depending on the severity of the disease. For patient with AR Stage B (Progressive) evaluation is needed with TTE every 3–5 years if mild severity symptoms are present. Patients with AR Stage B (Progressive) will be evaluated with TTE every 1–2 years if moderate severity symptoms are noticed. And for severe asymptomatic (Stage C1) patient will need TTE every 6–12 months with the possibility of more frequent evaluation if LV dilation is present [7, 9].

Medical Therapy and Timing for Surgery

Treatment for acute AR is aortic valve replacement plus treating any underlined medical conditions that led to the AR. Treatment for chronic AR varies depending on symptoms and the degree of LV dysfunction. Patient experiencing symptoms during an exercise testing will require valve replacement before developing signs and symptoms of HF [8]. For asymptomatic patient with chronic AR (Stages B-C), treatment for HTN is recommended when BP is >140/90 (level B recommendation). In patients with severe AR with symptoms and/or LV systolic dysfunction (Stages C2 and D) but prohibited surgical risk guideline–directed medical management (GDMT) for LVEF with ACEI, ARBs and sacubitril-valsartan (Entresto) are recommended (also level B recommendation) [9].

Valve replacement is the goal for treatment of chronic AR. Most recent recommendations are summarized below:

- Surgery is recommended for patients that are symptomatic regardless of LV function
- Asymptomatic patient with LVEF <=55%
- Patients with moderate/severe AR that are undergoing cardiac surgery for other reasons
- Asymptomatic patients with LVEF >55% but left ventricular end systolic diameter >50 mm on echocardiogram, surgery can be considered
- Asymptomatic patients with severe AR and normal LVEF >55%, but with declining EF in at least three serial studies, or if progressive increase LV dilation into the severe range (>65 mm end diastolic dimensions LVEDD) [9]

Aortic Stenosis

Aortic stenosis (AS) is narrowing of the valve orifice obstructing blood flow from the left ventricle to the ascending aorta during systole. Causes include congenital valve disease (unicuspid and bicuspid valve), degenerative sclerosis, and rheumatic disease. Progressive untreated AS will result in a classic triad of syncope, angina, and exertional dyspnea. Eventually heart failure and arrhythmia

may develop. A carotid pulse with small amplitude and crescendo-decrescendo ejection murmur are typical of the disease. Diagnosis is based on physical findings and echocardiography. Asymptomatic patient will not require treatment while symptomatic cases can be treated with balloon valvulotomy (especially in children) and valve replacement more commonly used in adults [7].

Etiology

Aortic stenosis (AS) etiologies are diverse. Causes can be divided for practical purposes in congenital and degenerative calcific disease. Congenital causes are unicuspid aortic valve, usually severe and presents in children, and congenital bicuspid aortic valve with a murmur that can be present since childhood and it is recognized as the most common cause of AS as well as AR. AS secondary to bicuspid aortic valve develops in middle age with associated valve calcification.

Degenerative calcific AS develops usually later in life (late middle age) and it is not associated with any congenital anatomic defect (trileaflet aortic valve). The earliest manifestation is the aortic sclerosis characterized as thickening of the leaflets, with the presence of heart murmur, and a gradient less than 25 mmHg. Progression of this sclerosis is pathologically similar to that of atherosclerosis and it is linked to the same risk factors [11–13].

Another significant cause of AS is rheumatic disease which tends to be much more common in developing countries where rheumatic fever is highly prevalent. Patients who have suffered rheumatic fever can have not only aortic valve disease but also mitral regurgitation/stenosis. Rheumatic valve disease is characterized by fusion of the commissures between the leaflets resulting in stenosis of the orifice which is histologically typical of rheumatic disease [14].

Symptoms and Physical Findings

Congenital AS is usually asymptomatic until around the ages between 10 and 20 years old when symptoms start to develop insidiously. Regardless of the etiology untreated AS ends up a classic triad that includes syncope, angina, and exertional dyspnea. Other clinical manifestations and physical findings are those related to heart failure and arrhythmia, when ventricular fibrillation can be potentially fatal. In general symptoms of AS are absent until AS is severe enough (valve area <1 cm^2, the jet velocity is over 4 m/sec, and/or the transvalvular gradient exceeds 40 mmHg).

Unlike AR there are no visible signs associated with AS. Carotid and other peripheral pulses are diminished and delayed on exam compared to LV contraction (pulsus parvus et tardus). LV impulse is displaced when signs and symptoms start to develop. A palpable fourth heart sound can be felt at the apex with a systolic thrill best felt at the level of the left upper sternal border present in severe cases only. Systolic blood pressure is elevated in mild and moderate cases with a drop when AS becomes severe.

The classic sign on auscultation is a crescendo-decrescendo ejection murmur best heard with the stethoscope placed at the left upper sternal border with the patient sitting and leaning forward. The intensity of the murmur is soft when obstruction is not severe and louder when progresses to a severe form of the disease, when the crescendo phase tends to longer and the decrescendo phase becomes shorter. Murmur is louder with maneuvers that increase left ventricular volume [7, 15].

Diagnosis of Aortic Stenosis

Diagnosis of AS is suspected by symptoms and physical exam and finally confirmed by echocardiography. Medical and interventional treatments rely on an accurate diagnosis and staging of the disease. As any other valvular disease staging is based on the presence of symptoms and hemodynamics identified on echocardiogram. Stage A are patients identified as at risk of having AS and includes patients with congenital aortic disease and aortic sclerosis. Stage B are patients with no symptoms with mild to moderate AS. And Stage D are considered patients with severe AS with the classic clinical manifestations.

Transthoracic echocardiogram (TTE) is the recommended test for an accurate diagnosis of the cause, hemodynamic assessment of the severity, and to determine LV size and systolic function in order to understand prognosis and timing for valve intervention, as well as other associated valvular diseases. Severity of AS can be misinterpreted in the presence of elevated uncontrolled hypertension and thus is recommended to reassess with TTE in such cases when BP is adequately controlled.

Dobutamine stress echocardiography is used to distinguish severe AS with LV systolic dysfunction and primary causes of myocardial dysfunction with less than severe AS.

Aortic valve calcification is a strong predictor of progression and clinical outcome. Calcium deposition can be determined by CT imaging. Agaston score threshold for severe AS in women is 1300 and 2000 in men. CT imaging also is used for procedural planning in patients undergoing TAVI, for measurement of annulus area, leaflet length, and the annular-to-coronary ostial distance.

Cardiac catheterization is used sometimes to determine if the presence of angina is secondary to coronary artery disease or when there is discordance between clinical findings and echocardiographic results. EKG and chest X rays can be useful and may show signs of LVH, axis deviations, electrical blocks, ST-T changes, cardiomegaly, and calcification of the aortic cusps. Exercise stress test can be useful in patients with AS that are asymptomatic and when the functional capacity of the patient is not clear. Exercise-induced angina, early dyspnea on exertion, dizziness, and syncope during test are considered symptoms of AS [7, 9].

Natural History, Complications, and Follow-Up

The natural progression of AS could be either slow or rapid and thus requires regular follow-up and evaluation especially in sedentary elderly patient in which functional status sometimes is unclear. Patients with mild disease are unlikely to develop symptoms due to AS over the course of 5 years. Untreated patient has a mean survival of 5 years after angina starts, 4 years after syncope, and 3 years after signs and symptoms of CHF appear. Progression has significant individual variability. Older patients are more likely to have rapid progression [7, 9, 15, 16]. For asymptomatic patients with severe AS the event-free survival rate is 56–63% at 2 years and 25–33% at 4 to 5 years [17].

Regular follow-up is very important considering that symptoms tend to progress insidiously and patients cannot recognized them clearly. Follow-up visits must include clinical and echocardiographic (TTE) assessments with the main goal of preventing severe irreversible diseases. Stage B patient with mild and moderate disease will require TTE every 3–5 years and 1–2 years, respectively. Stage C1 patient needs to be evaluated with TTE every 6–12 months. Patients classified in higher categories are candidates for interventions and need a different approach [9].

Medical Therapy and Timing for Surgery

Treatment of AS will depend on if the patient is asymptomatic or symptomatic. For asymptomatic patients regular clinical follow-up and TTE are indicated in order to identify early symptoms and signs of AS. Even when there is no medical therapies that have proven to delay the progression it is still recommended a conventional CVD risk assessment and treatment based on guidelines considering that some studies have shown that valve calcification and progression are increased in patients with LDL cholesterol >130 [6, 15, 18]. Patients with associated hypertension must be adequately controlled with close monitoring and careful titration of the medications to avoid hypotension. Hypertensive patients with more severe AS requires a greater degree of caution when treated. There are no studies studying the use of specific antihypertensive medications, although it is known that diuretics decrease the stroke volume and thus should be avoided in AS patients. ACE inhibitors may be beneficial

preventing LV fibrosis, in addition to control of hypertension [6, 17, 19]. Patients requiring medical management must be treated with ACE inhibitors, ARBs, and beta blockers in order to optimize left ventricular systolic dysfunction [4]. Nitrates are contraindicated because of its effects lowering preload. Patients with AS may require antibiotic prophylaxis prior to dental work and other potentially contaminated procedures [3].

Aortic valve replacement (AVR) is the definitive treatment for AS. All symptomatic patients thought to be secondary to AS are candidates for AVR. Asymptomatic patients with severe AS with or without LVEF <50% are also accepted as candidates for AVR. Other clinical scenarios must be evaluated more carefully before recommended surgical intervention [9].

Hypertrophic Obstructive Cardiomyopathy

Etiology

Hypertrophic obstructive cardiomyopathy (HOCM) is a heart condition that arises from genetic mutations in multiple sarcomere genes. These genes are responsible for the proper structural integrity of protein that makes up the contractile apparatus of the heart. There is an incidence of 1 in every 500 individuals worldwide, with an estimated 1% annual mortality rate [20]. It is among the most common causes of sudden cardiac death in young athletes in the USA. Hypertrophic cardiomyopathy is inherited in an autosomal dominant pattern. However, there is varying penetrance depending on the genetic mutation involved [21].

Signs and Symptoms

Individuals tend to have a thickened interventricular septum of the heart leading to left ventricular outflow obstruction. While some patients may be asymptomatic, others present with symptoms due to this outflow obstruction, especially with exertion. This may include chest pain, dyspnea, palpitations, malaise, presyncope, or exertional syncope due to cardiogenic shock. Cardiogenic shock in such patients may not always present with autonomic prodromal symptoms as in the case of other benign syncopal etiologies. Syncope due to cardiogenic shock tends to resolve once cardiac output is restored [22].

Physical Findings

There are no clear specific findings for HOCM, but there are those that would prompt further evaluation leading to this diagnosis. On examination, a systolic ejection murmur can be heard on auscultation. There are different maneuvers that change the intensity of the murmur. Standing and Valsalva strain phase causes decreased venous return to the heart, resulting in decreased left ventricular cardiac output. The left ventricular outflow track is narrowed, and can be exacerbated by anterior motion of the mitral valve leaflets. This then increases the intensity of the murmur. Squatting, handgrip, or supine leg raise, however, causes increased venous return. This volume increases the left ventricular outflow tract and lessens obstruction by systolic anterior motion of the mitral valve. As a result, squatting, handgrip, or supine decreases the intensity of the murmur. Some nonspecific findings for individuals with HOCM include voltage changes as seen on EKG, confirming left ventricular hypertrophy. Echocardiogram and cardiac MRI are specific and diagnostic. Chest X-Ray may reveal left atrial enlargement due to mitral regurgitation [23].

Natural History and Complications

Medical Therapy and Timing of Surgery

Some patients may be hypotensive in response to exercise, or have episodes of ventricular tachycardia resulting in cardiogenic shock and syncope. Complications include sudden cardiac death. There are those that develop heart failure or atrial fibrillation as a sequela of left ventricular dysfunction.

Individuals diagnosed with hypertrophy obstructive cardiomyopathy are to avoid high-intensity physical activity that could further exacerbate cardiac outflow. Patients that are clinically stable can be actively monitored with echocardiogram every one to two years. Those with left ventricular outflow tract obstruction can be managed with nonvasodilating beta blockers as first-line therapy. Non-dihydropyridine calcium channel blockers, including Verapamil and Diltiazem, are second-line agents for those that are unable to tolerate beta blockers. Individuals that develop atrial fibrillation or heart failure as a sequela of poor left ventricular function can be managed by using respective agents for atrial fibrillation and heart failure. In the setting of atrial fibrillation, anticoagulation therapy is indicated irrespective of CHA2DS2-VASc score. Other more invasive measures such as implantable defibrillators may be indicated for those with increased risk of sudden cardiac death. Those increased risks include prior history of cardiac arrest, a family history of sudden cardiac death, ventricular tachycardia, or recurrent exertional syncope [24].

Mitral Stenosis

Etiology

The most common cause of mitral stenosis is rheumatic heart disease. Rheumatic mitral stenosis is commonly seen in developing countries more so than developed countries. If seen in developed countries such as the USA, the outbreak tends to arise from increased virulence of streptococcal strain or from someone that is from an area with high prevalence of the disease. Rheumatic mitral stenosis is caused by cross-reactivity of the streptococcal antigen and the valvular tissue, and not due to an infectious process on the valve. This cross-reactivity causes an inflammatory process to occur that damages the mitral valve. Calcifications of the mitral valve leaflets, fusion of the leaflet commissures, and fibrotic changes to the chordae tendinae can occur. The severity of this inflammatory process in addition to recurrence determines the extent of the structural damage. Other causes of mitral stenosis, although less common, include congenital, systemic rheumatic disease (as seen in patients with systemic lupus erythematosus, rheumatoid arthritis) as well as radiation therapy as seen in patients with a history of Hodgkin's lymphoma [25].

Signs and Symptoms

Individuals tend to present with shortness of breath and exertional dyspnea. Due to increased left atrial pressure and resultant pulmonary edema, some patients may present with hemoptysis. Hoarseness and cough due to compression of the recurrent laryngeal nerve by increased left atrial pressure can also be seen. Hoarseness would be part of a constellation of other symptoms as seen in cardiovocal syndrome (Ortner's Syndrome) [26].

Physical Examination

On auscultation, a loud first heart sound can be heard, accompanied by an opening snap and mid-diastolic rumble. This can be best heard at the cardiac apex. Mitral stenosis, when severe, can cause pulmonary hypertension from increased left atrial pressure. Patients with pulmonary hypertension can develop mitral facies, with pink-purplish patches noted on examination due to capillary vasodilation. Patients that develop right heart failure can present with edema. Chest X-ray imaging may show dilated pulmonary vessels, and flattening of left heart border due to left atrial enlargement [27].

Natural History and Complications
Medical Therapy and Timing of Surgery

Mitral stenosis is generally slow to progress from asymptomatic to severe. Thus asymptomatic patients can be monitored by echocardiograms. The frequency of echocardiograms is every 3–5 years when the mitral valve area is >1.5 cm squared; then, in severe mitral stenosis, it is every 1–2 years when the mitral valve area is 1.0–1.5 cm squared; then it is once a year when the mitral valve area is <1.0 cm squared [28].

Patients with rheumatic mitral stenosis associated with atrial fibrillation, left atrial thrombus, or prior history of an embolic events should be placed on anticoagulation. Patients with tachycardia at rest or with exertion are considered symptomatic and may benefit from a beta blocker to manage symptoms. Surgical/operative management may be indicated in some instances.

Mitral Regurgitation

Etiology

Mitral regurgitation can be classified as acute versus chronic, and divided into primary versus secondary depending on the etiology.

In primary mitral regurgitation, there is organically or structurally a component of the mitral valve (leaflets, chordae tendinae, annulus, or papillary muscles) that is defective, incompetent, or damaged resulting in backflow during systole. The leading cause of primary mitral regurgitation, and mitral regurgitation in general, is mitral valve prolapse among other degenerative mitral valve diseases. Although uncommon in the USA, rheumatic heart disease often results in mitral regurgitation in the first two decades of life. Other causes of primary mitral regurgitation include infective endocarditis, trauma, mitral annular calcifications, or drug induction [29].

Mitral regurgitation due to secondary causes arise from functional incompetence of the valve, and not due to structural defect. This is typically seen in patients with coronary artery disease or cardiomyopathy. Patients with coronary artery disease, including those with a history of myocardial infarction, can have resultant regional wall motion abnormalities. This leads to improper closure of mitral valve leaflets. In patients with hypertrophic cardiomyopathy, mitral regurgitation can occur due to anterior motion of the mitral leaflets. In dilated cardiomyopathy, findings are a result of dilation of the annulus and displacement of the papillary muscles.

Signs and Symptoms

In acute mitral regurgitation, patients can present with symptoms of hypotension, pulmonary edema, and cardiogenic shock. Such a scenario would be considered a cardiac emergency and can be seen in patients with infectious endocarditis and inferior myocardial infarction due to rupture of papillary muscles. In chronic mitral regurgitation, there is a compensatory left atrial enlargement and left ventricular dilation that allows for adequate support of cardiac backflow and increased preload. In this setting, patients may not always be symptomatic. In severe cases of chronic mitral regurgitation, patient can present with exertional dyspnea and fatigue. Patients with mitral valve prolapse may complain of palpitations. Although less common than in mitral stenosis, patient may present with hemoptysis, thromboembolism, and symptoms of right heart failure.

Physical Examination

On auscultation, a holosystolic murmur can be heard best at the cardiac apex, with radiation to the axilla. The murmur can be blowing with a high-pitched S3. The murmur is louder with leg raise, squatting, and hand grip, as this increases venous return and arterial pressures. Standing tends to decrease the murmur, as this reduces venous return. Some patients have paroxysmal or persistent atrial fibrillation as a consequence of mitral regurgitation. A midsystolic click followed by systolic murmur can sometimes be heard in patients with mitral valve prolapse [30].

Natural History and Medical Therapy

Some studies show that vasodilators improve hemodynamic compensation in acute mitral regurgitation. They tend to reduce aortic pressure, decrease afterload as well as the regurgitant flow. Timely surgical intervention may still be indicated. Surveillance with echocardiogram is key in closely following for any progressive changes with mitral regurgitation. Echo every 3–5 years for mild mitral regurgitation, every 1–2 years for moderate, and 6–12 months in severe mitral regurgitation [31].

Cardiovascular Evaluation of the Young Athlete

Pre-participation screening of young athletes is used to identify any relevant history, physical findings, or symptoms that would raise concern for sudden cardiac death. Young athletes, defined as those under the age of 35, who suffer from sudden cardiac death (SCD) likely had an underlying structural or nonstructural cardiac condition [32]. Structural causes can arise from congenital coronary anomalies or hypertrophic obstructive cardiomyopathy (HOCM). Nonstructural causes such as in Wolf Parkinson White, Long QT Syndrome, and Brugada Syndrome are other possibilities. Even though SCD is rare, it is important to identify any young athletes at risk and further investigate.

Screening should include a focused history and physical examination. Young athletes should be asked if they have experienced symptoms of chest pain, heart palpitations, exertional dyspnea, presyncopal episodes, or syncope especially in the absence of autonomic prodromal symptoms [33]. Any history of myocarditis, endocarditis, elevated cholesterol, elevated blood pressure, or murmurs should be noted. A thorough family history should be taken to determine if any family members younger than 50 years of age died unexpectedly, or passed away from SCD [34, 35]. On physical examination, murmurs should prompt further workup. Although some connective tissue disorders such as Marfan syndrome have a genetic predisposition, there are some mutations that can arise de novo. As such, general inspection is an important component of any examination. Physical features suspicious for Marfan syndrome such as abnormal arm length to height ratio should prompt further cardiac evaluation.

Obtaining an EKG as part of the pre-participation evaluation is still an ongoing debate. When seen, EKG findings help to solidify a diagnosis. In HOCM, EKG findings of left ventricular hypertrophy can be seen. In Wolf Parkinson White, EKG would show shortened PR interval, delta wave, and widened QRS. However, the absence of EKG findings does not rule out the possibility of a cardiac condition, especially in the setting of red flags on history. In some instances, patients with cardiac conditions can have a normal EKG, making history taking a reliable tool in screening young athletes [36].

Even with a thorough history and physical examination, there is the chance of overlooking a patient at risk. Having an automated defibrillator in sight and being CPR certified helps to reduce an adverse outcome in symptomatic patients [37].

References

1. Otto CM, Bonow RO. Valvular heart disease: a companion to Braunwald's heart disease. 4th ed. Philadelphia: Elsevier Saunders; 2014.
2. Centers for Disease Control and Prevention, National Center for Health Statistics. Underlying Cause of Death 1999–2017 on CDC WONDER Online Database, released December, 2018. Data are from the Multiple Cause of Death Files, 1999–2017, as compiled from data provided by the 57 vital statistics jurisdictions through the Vital Statistics Cooperative Program. Accessed at http://wonder.cdc.gov/ucd-icd10.html on Oct 24, 2019.
3. Ashar BH, Miller RG, Sisson SD. The Johns Hopkins internal medicine board review. 4th ed.
4. Paulman P, Taylor RB, Paulman AA, Nasir LS. Family medicine, principles and practice. 7th ed; 2017.
5. Nishimura RA, Otto CM, Bonow RO, Carabello BA, Erwin 3rd JP, Guyton RA, et al. AHA/ACC guideline for the management of patients with valvular heart disease: executive summary: a report of the American College of Cardiology/American Heart Association Task Force on Practice Guidelines. Circulation. 2014;129(23):2440–922020. ACC/AHA guideline for the management of patients with valvular heart disease: a report of the American College of Cardiology/American Heart Association Joint Committee on Clinical Practice Guidelines. J Am Coll Cardiol. 2020. Epublished https://doi.org/10.1016/j.jacc.2020.11.018.
6. Ashley EA, Niebauer J. Cardiology explained. London: Remedica; 2004.
7. The Manual Merck of diagnosis and therapy. 18th ed; 2006.
8. Maganti K, Rigolin VH, Sarano ME, Bonow RO. Valvular heart disease: diagnosis and management. Mayo Clin Proc. 2010;85(5):483–500.
9. 2020 ACC/AHA guideline for the management of patients with valvular heart disease: a report of the American College of Cardiology/American Heart Association Joint Committee on Clinical Practice Guidelines. J Am Coll Cardiol. 2020. Epublished https://doi.org/10.1016/j.jacc.2020.11.018.
10. Maganti K, Rigolin VH, Sarano ME, Bonow RO. Valvular heart disease: diagnosis and management. Mayo Clinic Proc. 2010; https://doi.org/10.4065/mcp.2009.0706.
11. Bonow RO, Carabello BA, Chatterjee K, et al. ACC/AHA 2006 guidelines for the management of patients with valvular heart disease. J Am Coll Cardiol. 2006;48:1–148.
12. Lung B, Gohlke-Barwolf C, Tornos P, et al. For the working group on valvular heart disease: recommendations on the management of the asymptomatic patient with valvular heart disease. Eur Heart. 2002; J23:1252–66.
13. Otto CM. Evaluation and management of chronic mitral regurgitation. N Engl J Med. 2001;345:740–6. Otto CM: Valvular aortic stenosis: disease severity and timing of intervention, J Am Coll Cardiol 47:2141–51, 2006.
14. Eveborn GW, Schirmer H, Heggelund G, et al. The evolving epidemiology of valvular aortic stenosis the Tromsø study. Heart. 2013;99:396.
15. Otto CM, Burwash IG, Legget ME, et al. Prospective study of asymptomatic valvular aortic stenosis. Clinical, echocardiographic, and exercise predictors of outcome. Circulation. 1997;95:2262.
16. Rosenhek R, Zilberszac R, Schemper M, et al. Natural history of very severe aortic stenosis. Circulation. 2010;121:151.
17. Rosenhek R, Binder T, Porenta G, et al. Predictors of outcome in severe, asymptomatic aortic stenosis. N Engl J Med. 2000;343:611.
18. Pohle K, Mäffert R, Ropers D, et al. Progression of aortic valve calcification: association with coronary atherosclerosis and cardiovascular risk factors. Circulation. 2001;104:1927.
19. Gosavi S, Channa R, Mukherjee D. Systemic hypertension in patients with aortic stenosis: clinical implications and principles of pharmacological therapy. Cardiovasc Hematol Agents Med Chem. 2015;13:50.
20. Semsarian C, Ingles J, Maron MS, Maron BJ. New perspectives on the prevalence of hypertrophic cardiomyopathy. J Am Coll Cardiol. 2015;65:1249.
21. Richard P, Charron P, Carrier L, et al. Hypertrophic cardiomyopathy: distribution of disease genes, spectrum of mutations, and implications for a molecular diagnosis strategy. Circulation. 2003;107:2227.
22. Ommen SR, Mital S, Burke MA, Day SM, Deswal A, Elliott P, Evanovich LL, Hung J, Joglar JA, Kantor P, Kimmelstiel C, Kittleson M, Link MS, Maron MS, Martinez MW, Miyake CY, Schaff HV, Semsarian C, Sorajja P. 2020 AHA/ACC guideline for the diagnosis and treatment of patients with hypertrophic cardiomyopathy: a report of the American College of

Cardiology/American Heart Association Joint Committee on Clinical Practice Guidelines. J Am Coll Cardiol. 76(25):e159–240.

23. Maron BJ. Clinical course and management of hypertrophic cardiomyopathy. N Engl J Med. 2018;379:655.

24. Silbiger JJ. Abnormalities of the mitral apparatus in hypertrophic cardiomyopathy: echocardiographic, pathophysiologic, and surgical insights. J Am Soc Echocardiogr. 2016;29:622.

25. Zühlke L, Engel ME, Karthikeyan G, et al. Characteristics, complications, and gaps in evidence-based interventions in rheumatic heart disease: the global rheumatic heart disease registry (the REMEDY study). Eur Heart J. 2015;36:1115.

26. Chandrashekhar Y, Westaby S, Narula J. Mitral stenosis. Lancet. 2009;374:1271.

27. Marcus RH, Sareli P, Pocock WA, Barlow JB. The spectrum of severe rheumatic mitral valve disease in a developing country. Correlations among clinical presentation, surgical pathologic findings, and hemodynamic sequelae. Ann Intern Med. 1994;120:177.

28. Topilsky Y, Michelena H, Bichara V, et al. Mitral valve prolapse with mid-late systolic mitral regurgitation: pitfalls of evaluation and clinical outcome compared with holosystolic regurgitation. Circulation. 2012;125:1643.

29. Baumgartner H, Falk V, Bax JJ, et al. 2017 ESC/EACTS guidelines for the management of valvular heart disease. Eur Heart J. 2017;38:2739.

30. Enriquez-Sarano M, Akins CW, Vahanian A. Mitral regurgitation. Lancet. 2009;373:1382.

31. Gaasch WH, Meyer TE. Left ventricular response to mitral regurgitation: implications for management. Circulation. 2008;118:2298.

32. Maron BJ, Thompson PD, Ackerman MJ, et al. Recommendations and considerations related to preparticipation screening for cardiovascular abnormalities in competitive athletes: 2007 update. Circulation. 2007;15:1643–55.

33. Sharma S, Estes NA 3rd, Vetter VL, Corrado D. Clinical decisions. Cardiac screening before participation in sports. N Engl J Med. 2013;369:2049.

34. American Academy of Pediatrics, American Academy of Family Physicians, Am College of Sports Med. Preparticipation Physical Evaluation, 5th ed. American Academy of Pediatrics, Elk Grove Village, IL 2019.

35. Harmon KG, Asif IM, Maleszewski JJ, et al. Incidence, cause, and comparative frequency of sudden cardiac death in National Collegiate Athletic Association athletes: a decade in review. Circulation. 2015;132:10–9.

36. Corrado D, Pelliccia A, Heidlbuchel H, et al. Recommendations for interpresteations of 12lead electrocardiogram in the athlete. Eur Heart J. 2010;31:243.

37. Holst AG, Winkel BG, Theilade J, et al. Incidence and etiology of sports-related sudden cardiac death in Denmark – implications for preparticipation screening. Heart Rhythm. 2010;7:1365–71.

38. Otto CM, Nishimura RA, Bonow RO, Carabello BA, Erwin JP 3rd, Gentile F, Jneid H, Krieger EV, Mack M, McLeod C, O'Gara PT, Rigolin VH, Sundt TM 3rd, Thompson A, Toly C. ACC/AHA guideline for the management of patients with valvular heart disease: a report of the American College of Cardiology/American Heart Association joint committee on clinical practice guidelines. Circulation. 2021;2020:143. https://doi.org/10.1161/CIR.0000000000000923.

Heart Failure

Sandra Chaparro and Michael Rivera-Rodríguez

Contents

S. Chaparro (✉)
Florida International University, Miami, FL, USA

Miami Cardiac and Vascular Institute, Baptist Health South
Florida, Miami, FL, USA
e-mail: sandrach@baptisthealth.net

M. Rivera-Rodríguez
West Kendall Baptist Hospital, Miami, FL, USA
e-mail: michaelrive@baptisthealth.net

© Springer Nature Switzerland AG 2022
P. M. Paulman et al. (eds.), *Family Medicine*,
https://doi.org/10.1007/978-3-030-54441-6_192

Definition

Heart failure (HF) is a syndrome in which the heart is unable to pump blood at a sufficient output to meet tissue requirements, or in which the heart can do so only with an elevated filling pressure. The heart's failure to pump is caused by impairment of cardiac contractility (systolic dysfunction) or cardiac filling (diastolic dysfunction). HF is associated with a variety of interrelated structural, functional, and neurohumoral changes. Structurally, this could result from left ventricle dilation, hypertrophy, or both. Functionally, systolic or diastolic dysfunction can cause reduced ventricular filling or ejection of blood, and to compensate, activation of the sympathetic nervous system and renin-angiotensin-aldosterone systems occurs. These neurohormonal changes increase blood pressure and blood volume, further enhancing venous return (preload), stoke volume, and cardiac output to compensate for the cardiac dysfunction. Despite these compensatory mechanisms, the ability of the heart to contract and relax declines with time. These changes also cause HF symptoms of dyspnea on exertion, fluid retention, and fatigue. Because some patients present without signs or symptoms of volume overload, the term "heart failure" is preferred over "congestive heart failure." Early recognition is important because without appropriate therapies and interventions, HF can progressively worsen [1].

Epidemiology

Heart failure is an ongoing public health challenge in the USA. Americans over 40 years old have a 20% lifetime risk of developing HF [1]. With aging of the population, the prevalence of HF continues to rise over time. An estimated 6.2 million American adults $\geq$20 years of age had HF between 2013 and 2016, compared with an estimated 5.7 million between 2009 and 2012.

The prevalence of HF will increase 46% from 2012 to 2030, resulting in >eight million people ≥18 years of age with HF [2]. Worldwide, there are an estimated 23 million people with HF [3]. The prevalence of HF is highly variable across the world. Prevalence of HF risk factors also varies worldwide, with hypertension being most common in Latin America, the Caribbean, Eastern Europe, and sub-Saharan Africa. Ischemic heart disease is most prevalent in Europe and North America. Valvular heart disease is more common in East Asia and Asia-Pacific countries [3]. The overall prognosis of HF is poor with a 50% mortality rate within 5 years of symptom onset. Appropriate management of HF can significantly stabilize the disease with improvement in symptoms, cardiac function, and survival [1].

Hypertensive men and women have a substantially greater risk for developing HF than normotensive men and women [4]. The incidence of HF is greater with higher levels of blood pressure, older age, and longer duration of hypertension. Long-term treatment of both systolic and diastolic hypertension reduces the risk of HF by approximately 50% [4]. Obesity and insulin resistance are also important risk factors for the development of HF. The presence of clinical diabetes markedly increases the likelihood of developing HF in patients without structural heart disease and adversely affects the outcomes of patients with established HF [1]. Fortunately, the appropriate treatment of hypertension, diabetes mellitus, and dyslipidemia can significantly reduce the development of HF.

Classification

HF is classified based on the left ventricular ejection fraction (EF). The echocardiogram will define HF preserved EF (HFpEF) as greater than 50%, mid-range EF (HFmrEF) between 49 and 41%, and reduced EF (HFrEF) as lower than 40% [5]. Symptom severity is graded according to the New York Heart Association (NYHA) functional class designations (class I, no limitation in normal physical activity; class II, mild symptoms only during normal activity; class III, marked symptoms during daily activity, comfortable only at rest; and class IV, severe limitations and symptoms even at rest). While the NYHA classification is a simple way to classify HF symptoms, it is nevertheless a subjective measure affected by the patient and physician expectations. The American College of Cardiology (ACC) and the American Heart Association (AHA) created HF stages that emphasize the progressive nature of HF and defines the appropriate therapeutic approach for each stage. Table 1 demonstrates the overlap and progression of the ACC/AHA stages and NYHA classes [1]. HFrEF has effective evidence-based therapies that improve morbidity and mortality, while HFpEF still lacks the same amount of therapies.

Table 1 Classification of HF: ACC/AHA HF stage and NYHA functional class

ACC/AHA HF Stage[1]		NYHA Functional Class[2]	
High risk, no structural heart disease	A	Not applicable	—
Asymptomatic but with structural heart disease (MI, reduced LVEF, valvular disease)	B	Asymptomatic	I
Current or history of symptomatic HF with cardiac structural abnormalities	C	Symptoms with significant exertion	II
		Symptoms on minor exertion	III
Refractory end-stage heart failure	D	Symptomatic at rest	IV

ACC/AHA American College of Cardiology/American Heart Association, NYHA New York Heart Association, MI Myocardial Infarction, LVEF Left Ventricular Ejection Fraction
*Arrows indicate potential directions of stage progression

Approach to the Patient

The approach to determining the cause and severity of heart failure (HF) includes the history, physical examination, and diagnostic tests. Initial tests include an electrocardiogram, initial blood tests, echocardiogram, and assessment for coronary artery disease. Demonstration of an underlying cardiac cause is key to the diagnosis of HF. This is usually a myocardial abnormality causing systolic and/or diastolic ventricular dysfunction. However, abnormalities of the valves, pericardium, endocardium, heart rhythm, and conduction can also cause HF (and more than one abnormality is often present). It is crucial to identify the underlying cardiac problem for therapeutic reasons, as the precise pathology determines the specific treatment used.

Diagnosis

History

A detailed history and physical examination should be obtained in patients presenting with HF to identify cardiac and noncardiac disorders or behaviors that might cause or accelerate the development or progression of HF. Typical symptoms include dyspnea, orthopnea, paroxysmal nocturnal dyspnea, fatigue, and ankle swelling. Other symptoms of right-sided heart failure that may be present but are more nonspecific include abdominal bloating, right upper-quadrant discomfort, and early satiety. In patients with idiopathic dilated cardiomyopathy, a three-generational family history should be obtained to aid in establishing the diagnosis of familial dilated cardiomyopathy [1].

Physical Examination

Patients should be examined for markers of congestion and reduced peripheral perfusion (Table 2). Patients with more signs of congestion (jugular venous distension, edema, lung rales, and S3 gallop) are at higher risk of cardiovascular death or heart failure hospitalization independent of symptoms, natriuretic peptides, and validated risk scores. As a

Table 2 Initial evaluation for diagnosing symptoms and signs in heart failure with reduced ejection fraction

Typical symptoms
Dyspnea
Orthopnea
Paroxysmal nocturnal dyspnea
Fatigue
Reduced exercise tolerance
Ankle swelling
Cough
Abdominal distension
Wheeze
Abdominal bloating
Early satiety
Bendopnea
More specific signs
Elevated jugular venous pressure
Positive abdominojugular reflux
S3 (gallop rhythm)
Laterally displaced apical impulse
Less specific signs
Lung rales
Peripheral edema
Ascites
Cool and/or mottled extremities
Narrow proportional pulse pressure (pulse pressure: Systolic blood pressure ratio 0.25)
Murmur of valvular regurgitation or stenosis
Weight loss and cachexia (advanced HF)

Modified from Murphy et al. [6]

result of compensatory upregulation in lymphatic drainage, patients with chronic HF may lack lung rales or peripheral edema, even when pulmonary capillary wedge pressure is elevated [6]. The clinical assessment of left-sided filling pressures relies heavily on the presence of symptoms (e.g., dyspnea, paroxysmal nocturnal dyspnea, orthopnea, and S3 gallop) and evidence of elevation in right-sided filling pressures (e.g., jugular venous distension, hepatojugular reflux, and edema). Markers of low cardiac output state include diminished peripheral pulses, cool extremities, pallor, peripheral cyanosis, sluggish capillary refill, presence of pulsus alternans, and a low pulse pressure.

Laboratory and Imaging

A number of laboratory tests can aid in the diagnosis of HF and can help risk stratify patients with known HF. At the time of diagnosis, laboratory work should focus on evidence of end-organ involvement, including assessment of renal function and liver abnormalities. Initial testing involves the measurement of natriuretic peptides, electrocardiography, chest X-ray, and echocardiogram. Further laboratory assessment should be considered based on suspicion of other causes or if findings suggest further investigation (Table 3).

B-Type Natriuretic Peptide

B-Type natriuretic peptide (BNP) is a cardiac neurohormone secreted from the ventricles in response to stretching and increased wall tension from volume and pressure overload. Cleavage of the prohormone proBNP produces biologically active BNP as well as biologically inert NT-proBNP. Changes in natriuretic peptide levels in response to HF therapy have been shown to correlate with changes in pulmonary wedge pressure. The measurement of natriuretic peptide levels in patients presenting with dyspnea in the emergency department outperforms clinical judgment for the diagnosis of HF (Table 4). It is important to realize that natriuretic peptides can be elevated in disease processes other than HF (e.g., acute pulmonary embolism, COPD, cor pulmonale, anemia, renal failure, sepsis, atrial fibrillation, and myocardial infarction).

Electrocardiogram

An electrocardiogram (ECG) is a useful initial test to evaluate the heart for structural or physiological abnormalities. An abnormal ECG increases the likelihood of the diagnosis of HF, but has low specificity. It is most useful in evaluating other possible causes of HF or reasons for a worsened clinical status. HF is unlikely in patients presenting with a completely normal ECG (sensitivity 89%) [7]. Therefore, the routine use of an ECG is mainly recommended to rule out HF. Signs of previous MI or ischemia, left ventricle hypertrophy, left bundle branch block (LBBB), or atrial fibrillation can all be present and assist in guiding further treatment options. A LBBB in the presence of HF is a very poor prognostic sign with

Table 3 Laboratory evaluation for heart failure and selected alternate causes

Initial tests
BNP or NTproBNP level (Heart failure)
Complete blood count (Anemia, infection)
Serum electrolytes (Diuretics, cause of arrhythmia)
Liver profile (Hepatic congestion, alcoholism)
Renal function (Renal disease, volume overload)
Thyroid stimulating hormone (Thyroid disorders)
Urinalysis (Renal disease)
Other tests for alternative causes
Arterial blood gases (Hypoxia, pulmonary disease)
Blood cultures (Endocarditis, systemic infection)
Human immunodeficiency virus (Cardiomyopathy)
Lyme serology (Bradycardia/heart block)
Thiamine level (Deficiency, beriberi, alcoholism)
Troponins, creatinine kinase-MB (Myocardial infarction)
Ferritin, iron levels (Hemochromatosis)
Urine or serum drug screen (Cocaine use)
Tests for comorbid conditions, risk management
A1C level (Diabetes mellitus)
Lipid panel (Hyperlipidemia, cardiovascular risk)

Sources: King et al. [21]
BNP B-type natriuretic peptide; *NTproBNP* N-terminal pro-B-type natriuretic peptide

Table 4 Uses of natriuretic peptides as part of the initial evaluation for diagnosing HFrEF

To rule in acute heart failure
NT-proBNP >450 pg/mL BNP >100 pg/mL
To rule out acute heart failure
NT-proBNP <300 pg/mL10 BNP <50 pg/mL
To rule out chronic heart failure
NT-proBNP <125 pg/mL BNP <35 pg/mL
Factors that increase natriuretic peptides
Advancing age Atrial fibrillation or other arrhythmia Kidney failure Weight loss and cachexia (advanced HF)
Factors that decrease natriuretic peptides
Obesity Pericardial constriction

Modified from Murphy et al. [6]
BNP B-type natriuretic peptide; *HFrEF* heart failure with reduced ejection fraction; *NT-proBNP* N-terminal pro–B-type natriuretic peptide

increased one-year mortality overall and from sudden cardiac death [8]. A QRS interval of >0.12 and a LBBB pattern in a HF patient would be a consideration to refer to a cardiologist or electrophysiologist to evaluate for an implantable device after medical optimization.

Chest Radiograph

A chest radiograph in HF can reveal cephalization, interstitial or alveolar edema, the presence of effusions, or Kerley B lines. The absence of these findings does not rule out HF. Of note, the chest radiograph can help identify other etiologies of dyspnea such as pneumonia, COPD, thoracic mass, or pneumothorax.

Cardiac Imaging

Echocardiography is the most important imaging tool to diagnose HF. It provides assessment of chamber dimensions, biventricular function, valvular stenosis/regurgitation, wall thickness, wall motion, and filling pressures/patterns (diastolic function), including hemodynamics.

Cardiac magnetic resonance imaging, although not readily available, provides high anatomical resolution of all aspects of the heart and surrounding structure, leading to its recommended use in known or suspected congenital heart diseases [1]. It can also evaluate ischemia and identify inflammatory or infiltrative causes of HF without radiation exposure. Cardiac magnetic resonance imaging allows accurate assessment of biventricular function, quantitation of valvular regurgitation and/or stenosis, tissue characterization, and assessment of both microvascular and epicardial perfusion. It can assist in the diagnosis of the underlying etiology of cardiomyopathy, such as infiltrative cardiomyopathies, myocarditis, prior infarction, suggesting an ischemic etiology. Also, a cardiac magnetic resonance is an excellent method to assess myocardial viability in patients with impaired LV function and significant coronary disease when deciding on the utility of revascularization.

Given that 50% of HFrEF cases are of ischemic etiology, patients with a new diagnosis of HFrEF

usually require an evaluation for coronary artery disease, although other patient-specific factors (e.g., advanced age, multiple severe comorbidities, noncandidates for revascularization, or choosing not to undergo coronary revascularization procedures) should be considered prior to referral. Coronary angiography is the criterion standard test for identification of obstructive epicardial coronary artery disease, although noninvasive testing with coronary-computed tomography angiography may be considered in patients with low pretest probability for coronary atherosclerosis. Stress testing is less useful because of lower sensitivity and specificity [6].

Special Testing

Hemodynamic monitoring is indicated in patients with clinically indeterminate volume status, those refractory to initial therapy, patients with hypotension, and/or worsening renal function particularly if intracardiac filling pressures and cardiac output are unclear.

To allow physicians to discuss prognostic information with patients and aid in decision-making, a commonly utilized model is the Seattle Heart Failure Model (SHFM). The model also allows the clinician to add or subtract an assortment of treatment regimens, including medical therapies and devices, to assess how these changes affect mortality. There is a simple, free, online score calculator that is readily accessible.

Differential Diagnosis

Patients with HF may present with complaints of decreased exercise tolerance, fluid retention, or both. Many of the symptoms and signs of HF are nonspecific, so other potential causes should be considered such as cardiac and noncardiac causes. Cardiac causes include arrhythmias, structural heart disease, valvular disease, and myocardial infarction. Noncardiac causes include processes that increase the preload (volume overload and renal failure), increase the afterload (hypertension), reduce the oxygen-carrying capacity of the blood (anemia, pulmonary diseases), or increase demand (sepsis).

Treatment

In heart failure management, the goals are to reduce mortality and morbidity by improving functional status and health-related quality of life, reducing symptoms, and decreasing the risk of hospitalization [9]. Based on the severity of the illness, nonpharmacologic therapies include dietary sodium and fluid restriction and physical activity as appropriate. Figure 1 shows a treatment

strategy for the use of drugs (and devices) in patients with HFrEF. The recommendations for each treatment will be summarized ahead.

Heart Failure with Reduced Ejection Fraction

The standard therapy for HFrEF includes loop diuretics for fluid and symptom control as well as angiotensin-converting enzyme inhibitor (ACEI), an angiotensin receptor blocker (ARB), or an angiotensin receptor neprilysin inhibitor (ARNI), and beta-blocker therapy,

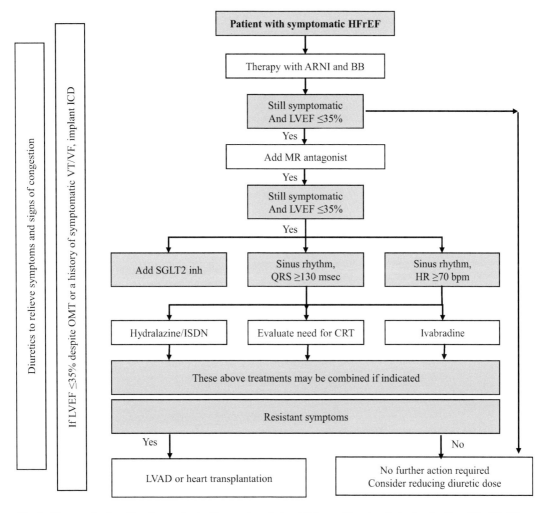

Fig. 1 Therapeutic algorithm for a patient with symptomatic heart failure with reduced ejection fraction. (Modified from Ponikowski P, et al. [22])

mineralocorticoid receptor antagonist (MRA), and more recently SGLT-2 inhibitors to improve morbidity and mortality. Appropriate starting doses of drug therapies and evidence-based targets are listed in Table 5.

Diuretics

Diuretics are an important treatment for patients with HF and evidence of volume overload. They also have not been proven to have a long-term mortality benefit [1]. The goal of loop diuretic therapy is to manage fluid retention and achieve and maintain a euvolemic state. The majority of HF patients are treated with loop diuretics, such as furosemide, bumetanide, or torsemide. Torsemide has the advantage of greater, and more consistent, bioavailability following oral dosing, Diuretic resistance can be due to inadequate diuretic dose, excess sodium intake, reduced diuretic absorption, impaired diuretic urinary excretion (due to chronic kidney disease, advanced age, or poor cardiac output), and concomitant medications (e.g., nonsteroidal anti-inflammatory agents). Treatment approaches to refractoriness to loop diuretics include increased dose, dividing into multiple daily doses, switching from furosemide to torsemide, and adding a thiazide diuretic, such as chlorothiazide or metolazone. It is important to monitor electrolytes as well as the renal function during titration of diuretics. Initial,

Table 5 Medications in heart failure with reduced ejection fraction

Drugs for mortality and morbidity benefit	Initial doses	Target doses
Angiotensin-converting enzyme inhibitors		
Captopril (Capoten)	6.25 mg TID	50 mg TID
Enalapril (Vasotec)	2.5 mg BID	10–20 mg BID
Fosinopril (Monopril)	5–10 mg daily	40 mg daily
Lisinopril (Zestril, Prinivil)	2.5–5 mg daily	20–40 mg daily
Perindopril (Aceon)	2 mg daily	8–16 mg daily
Quinapril (Accupril)	5 mg BID	20 mg BID
Ramipril (Altace)	1.25–2.5 mg daily	10 mg daily
Trandolapril (Mavik)	1 mg daily	4 mg daily
Angiotensin receptor blockers		
Candesartan (Atacand) Losartan (Cozaar) Valsartan (Diovan)	4–8 mg daily 25–50 mg daily 20–40 mg BID	32 mg daily 50–100 mg daily 160 mg BID
β-Blockers		
Bisoprolol (Zebeta)	1.25 mg daily	10 mg daily
Carvedilol (Coreg)	3.125 mg BID	50 mg BID
Carvedilol CR (Coreg CR)	10 mg daily	80 mg daily
Metoprolol succinate CR/XL (Toprol XL)	12.5–25 mg daily	200 mg daily
Aldosterone antagonists		
Eplerenone (Inspra) Spironolactone (Aldactone)	25 mg 2.5–25 mg daily	50 mg daily 25 mg daily or BID
Vasodilators: Hydralazine and isosorbide dinitrate		
Fixed dose hydralazine and isosorbide dinitrate (BiDil)	37.5 mg/20 mg TID	75 mg/40 mg TID
Hydralazine and isosorbide dinitrate (Apresoline and Isordil)	25–50 mg and 20–30 mg TID or QID	300 mg and 120 mg daily in TID doses
Angiotensin receptor neprilysin inhibitor		
Sabubitril/Valsartan (Entresto)	49 mg/51 mg BID	97 mg/103 mg BID
SGLT-2 inhibitors		
Dapagliflozin (Farxiga)	10 mg daily	10 mg daily
Empagliflozin (Jardiance)	10 mg daily	10 mg daily

Modified from: Maddox et al. [14]
BID twice daily; *TID* three times daily; *QID* four times daily

Table 6 Diuretic dose therapies

Drugs for symptom control		Initial doses	Maximum doses
Loop diuretics	Drug/Dose equivalents		
Bumetanide (Bumex) Furosemide (Lasix) Torsemide (Demadex)	1 mg PO/1 mg IV 40 mg PO/80 mg IV 20 mg PO/20 mg IV	0.5–1.0 mg/dose 20–40 mg/dose 5–10 mg/dose	10 mg/day 600 mg/day 200 mg/day
Thiazide diuretics (Combination with loops)			
Hydrochlorothiazide (HydroDiuril) Metolazone (Zaroxolyn)		25 mg daily 2.5 mg daily	100 mg daily 10 mg daily

Modified from: Yancy et al. [1]

maximum, and equipotent oral and intravenous (IV) dose equivalents are listed in Table 6.

Renin-Angiotensin System Inhibition

Renin-angiotensin system inhibition with ACE Inhibitor, ARB, or ARNI angiotensin-converting enzyme inhibitors (ACEI) reduce morbidity and mortality in HFrEF. Clinical trials clearly establish the benefits of ACEI in patients with mild, moderate, or severe symptoms of HF. ACEI can produce angioedema and should be given with caution to patients with low systemic blood pressures, renal insufficiency, or elevated serum potassium. They also inhibit kininase and increase levels of bradykinin, which can induce cough but also may contribute to their beneficial effect through vasodilation [10].

Angiotensin receptor blockers (ARBs) do not inhibit kininase and are associated with a much lower incidence of cough and angioedema than ACE inhibitors. Long-term therapy with ARBs produces hemodynamic, neurohormonal, and clinical effects consistent with those expected after interference with the renin-angiotensin system and have been shown to reduce morbidity and mortality, especially in ACE inhibitor–intolerant patients.

In ARNI, an ARB (valsartan) is combined with an inhibitor of neprilysin (sacubitril), an enzyme that degrades natriuretic peptides, bradykinin, adrenomedullin, and other vasoactive peptides. In a landmark trial that compared the first approved ARNI, valsartan/sacubitril, with enalapril in symptomatic patients with HFrEF tolerating an adequate dose of either ACE inhibitor or ARB, the ARNI reduced the composite endpoint of cardiovascular death or HF hospitalization significantly, by 20% [11]. The benefit was seen to a similar extent for both death and HF hospitalization and was consistent across subgroups. The use of ARNI is associated with the risk of hypotension and renal insufficiency and may lead to angioedema as well.

Beta-Blockers

Use of beta-blockers is recommended for all patients with current or prior symptoms of HFrEF, unless contraindicated, to reduce morbidity and mortality [1]. Carvedilol (Coreg), metoprolol succinate (Toprol XL), and bisoprolol (Zebeta) are recommended and have proven mortality benefits over other beta-blockers likely due to how they inhibit the sympathetic nervous system which is activated in HF. Even among these three proven beta-blockers, there are some differences. Beta-blockers benefit mortality and disease progression in addition to ACEI therapy and are recommended early after the diagnosis of HFrHF with initiation at low doses along with low-dose ACEI and appropriate titration (Table 5). Beta-blockers should be hemodynamically stable with minimal to no fluid retention before initiation and are contraindicated with bradycardia, hypotension, hypoperfusion, second- or third-degree atrioventricular block, or severe asthma or COPD [1].

Mineralocorticoid Receptor Antagonists

Mineralocorticoid receptor antagonists (MRA) are recommended in patients with NYHA class

II–IV HF and who have LVEF of 35% or less, unless contraindicated, to reduce morbidity, mortality, and HF hospitalization. MRA block receptors bind aldosterone and, with different degrees of affinity, other steroid hormone (e.g., corticosteroids and androgens) receptors. Caution should be exercised when MRAs are used in patients with impaired renal function and in those with serum potassium levels >5.0 mmol/L. Regular checks of serum potassium levels and renal function should be performed according to clinical status.

Hydralazine and Isosorbide

The combination of hydralazine and isosorbide dinitrate is recommended to reduce morbidity and mortality for patients self-described as African Americans with NYHA class III–IV HFrEF receiving optimal therapy with ACE inhibitors and beta-blockers, unless contraindicated [1]. It can be useful to reduce morbidity or mortality in patients with current or prior symptomatic HFrEF who cannot be given an ACE inhibitor or ARB or ARNI because of drug intolerance, hypotension, or renal insufficiency, unless contraindicated.

Ivabradine

Ivabradine is an agent that selectively inhibits current in the sinoatrial node, providing heart rate reduction without affecting blood pressure, myocardial contractility, or intracardiac conduction. Ivabradine can be beneficial to reduce HF hospitalization for patients with symptomatic (NYHA class II-III) stable chronic HFrEF who are receiving guideline medical therapy, including a beta-blocker at maximum tolerated dose, and who are in sinus rhythm with a heart rate of 70 bpm or greater at rest [10].

Digoxin

Digoxin may be considered in patients in sinus rhythm with symptomatic HFrEF to reduce the risk of hospitalization (both all-cause and HF

hospitalizations) [5]. Digoxin level should be monitored a week after initiation for a goal level less than 1 ng/mL, also toxicity risk is higher in the elderly, causing hypomagnesemia, hypokalemia, and renal dysfunction.

New Therapies Awaiting Guideline Recommendation

SGLT-2 Inhibitors

The US Food and Drug Administration recently approved the use of dapagliflozin for treatment of HFrEF, irrespective of diabetes status, and it is anticipated that dapagliflozin will be added to guideline-directed medical therapy for all patients with HFrEF in the 2021 American College of Cardiology/American Heart Association heart failure guideline [6]. The DAPA-HF (Dapagliflozin and Prevention of Adverse Outcomes in Heart Failure) trial evaluated the effect of dapagliflozin in patients with HFrEF with and without type 2 diabetes [12]. Dapagliflozin reduced the primary end point of worsening heart failure or cardiovascular death, cardiovascular mortality, and all-cause mortality compared with placebo. SGLT2 inhibitors are contraindicated in patients with type 1 DM, type 2 DM with risk factors for ketoacidosis, or severely impaired or rapidly declining kidney function. In the DAPA-HF trial, dapagliflozin demonstrated a reduction in CV death and HF hospitalization in patients with and without type 2 diabetes (T2D) [12]. In addition, the EMPEROR-reduced (Empagliflozin Outcome Trial in Patients with Chronic HFrEF) trial demonstrated a reduction in HF hospitalization/CV death from empagliflozin treatment in patients with HFrEF with and without diabetes [13]. As such, it is clear that SLGT2 inhibitors exhibit a beneficial class effect in patients with HFrEF.

Vericiguat

Vericiguat is an oral soluble guanylate cyclase stimulator that increases activity of the second messenger cyclic guanosine monophosphate (cGMP), which is involved in regulation of protective cardiovascular, kidney, and metabolic actions. The VICTORIA (Vericiguat Global Study in Subjects with Heart Failure with Reduced Ejection Fraction) trial enrolled patients with higher-risk HFrEF than those included in other contemporary clinical trials, and found that vericiguat reduced the composite primary outcome of cardiovascular death or first heart failure hospitalization over median follow-up of 10.8 months, although this was driven by the reduction in heart failure hospitalization [15]. Given its vasodilation properties, vericiguat resulted in symptomatic hypotension in 9.1% of patients, although these were not significantly higher than placebo.

Omecantiv Mecarbil

This is a novel cardiac myosin activator, or myotrope – significantly reduces the combined risk of first heart failure events or cardiovascular death in patients with chronic HFrEF, as shown in the GALACTIC-HF trial [16]. The benefit was modest, with an absolute reduction of 2.1% and a relative reduction of 8% over a median follow-up of about 22 months. One of the benefits is that it is well tolerated and does not affect the blood pressure nor the heart rate.

How to Initiate Therapies

The ACC Expert Consensus recommends titration of therapies as follows: In a patient with new-onset stage C HFrEF, the writing committee recommends that either an ARNI/ACEI/ARB or beta-blocker should be started. In some cases, an ARNI/ACEI/ARB and a beta-blocker can be started at the same time. Regardless of the initiation sequence, both classes of agent should be up-titrated to the maximum tolerated or target doses in a timely fashion (every 2 weeks). Initiation of an ARNI/ACEI/ARB is often better tolerated when the patient is still congested, whereas beta-blockers are better tolerated when the patient is less congested with an adequate resting heart rate; beta-blockers should not be initiated in patients with decompensated signs or symptoms. Only evidence-based beta-blockers (bisoprolol, carvedilol, and metoprolol succinate) should be used in patients with HFrEF. With recent clinical trial data supporting the use of SGLT2 inhibitors in a reasonably broad spectrum of HFrEF severity, the addition of this class of therapy to the regimens of patients with HFrEF provides improvements in clinical outcomes and in patient-reported outcome measures [14].

Adverse Therapies

Non-dihydropyridine calcium channel blockers (CCBs) are not indicated for the treatment of patients with HFrEF. Diltiazem and verapamil have been shown to be unsafe in patients with HFrEF. There is a variety of dihydropyridine CCBs; some are known to increase sympathetic tone and they may have a negative safety profile in HFrEF. There is only evidence on safety for amlodipine [5].

Implantable Devices

Implantable cardioverter defibrillators (ICDs) are effective in preventing bradycardia and correcting potentially lethal ventricular arrhythmias. Sudden cardiac death (SCD) from cardiac arrest and ventricular arrhythmias is estimated to occur in a third to half of all HF deaths, thus automatic ICDs are indicated. ICD implantation is recommended only after a sufficient trial (minimum 3 months) of optimal medical therapy (OMT) has failed to increase the LVEF to 35% [1]. In primary prevention, ICDs are recommended for HF patients with a reasonable life expectancy (>1 year), no history of recent MI (within 40 days), NYHA Class II–III and a LVEF ≤35%, or NYHA Class I and a LVEF <30% [1]. In secondary prevention, ICDs are recommended for patients with history of cardiac arrest, ventricular fibrillation, or sustained ventricular tachycardia regardless of the EF [1]. Multiple studies have proven the benefit in NYHA Class II–III reducing mortality by 23–31%. Subcutaneous defibrillators may be as effective as conventional ICDs with a lower risk from the implantation procedure. They may be the preferred option for patients with difficult access or who require ICD explantation due to infection. A wearable ICD (an external defibrillator with leads and electrode pads attached to a wearable vest) that is able to recognize and interrupt VT/ventricular fibrillation may be considered for a limited period of time in selected patients with HF who are at high risk for sudden death but otherwise are not suitable for ICD implantation. However, no prospective randomized clinical trials evaluating this device have been reported [5].

Cardiac Resynchronization Therapy

Cardiac resynchronization therapy (CRT) involves implantation of pacing leads to the right and left ventricles via the coronary sinus, which are timed to pace at an interval maximizing synchrony. CRT is indicated for patients with NYHA Class III or IV symptoms, a LVEF $\leq 35\%$, a QRS interval ≥ 0.15 ms, a left bundle branch block (LBBB) pattern, and sinus rhythm to improve mortality and hospitalizations. Studies of CRT include dNYHA Class II, a QRS ≥ 0.12 ms, or a non-LBBB pattern, resulting in varying mortality and hospitalization decreases from 19% to 37%. CRT also improves symptoms and quality of life in these studies. Patients who meet criteria for CRT and an ICD should receive a combined device, unless contraindicated [1].

Transcatheter Mitral Valve Repair

Transcatheter mitral valve repair (tMVR) may be considered for patients with HFrEF and severe secondary mitral regurgitation (MR) after the use of maximally tolerated guideline-directed medical therapy [17]. In the COAPT (Cardiovascular Outcomes Assessment of the MitraClip Percutaneous Therapy for Heart Failure Patients with Functional Mitral Regurgitation) trial, there was a significant reduction in the primary end point of heart failure hospitalization and the secondary end point of all-cause mortality in patients treated with tMVR compared with placebo.

Wireless Pulmonary Artery Pressure

Patients with persistent NYHA class III symptoms may be considered for implantation of a wireless pulmonary artery pressure monitor. In the CHAMPION trial, the device reduced heart failure hospitalizations, and there was a statistically nonsignificant reduction in mortality over a mean follow-up period of 18 months [6].

Cardiac Rehabilitation

A prescribed exercise training program modestly reduced clinical events when added to optimal medical therapy. After adjustment for prognostic variables, the risk of all-cause mortality and hospitalization was 11% lower in cardiac rehabilitation participants, and cardiovascular mortality and heart failure hospitalization was reduced by 15%. Cardiac rehabilitation was safe, with no excess risk of cardiovascular adverse events or hospitalization after exercise [6].

Heart Failure with Preserved Ejection Fraction

HFpEF has been defined by the European Society of Cardiology (ESC) as preserved left ventricular EF (LVEF $\geq 50\%$), with evidence of diastolic dysfunction or structural heart disease, in the context of classic signs and symptoms of heart failure and elevated natriuretic peptides [5]. HFpEF represent about a third to one-half of the total number of HF patients [18].

The H2FPEF score and the HFpEF nomogram are recently validated highly sensitive tools employed for risk assessment of subclinical heart failure. These tools are based on clinical and echocardiographic parameters, including body mass index (BMI) > 30 kg/m2 (H); use of two or more antihypertensive medications (H); the presence of atrial fibrillation (F); pulmonary hypertension (pulmonary artery systolic pressure > 35 mmHg) (P); elderly with an age > 60 years (E); and elevated filling pressures (E/e' > 9) [18]. With a score of 0–1 consider a noncardiac cause, a score of 2–5 with abnormal natriuretic peptides and abnormal wedge pressure, or a score of 6–9 is diagnostic of HFpEF.

Clinical trials in HFpEF have produced largely neutral results to date and most management is directed toward associated conditions (e.g., hypertension) and symptoms (e.g., edema). Overall with HFpEF, no treatment has been well validated to show a reduction in morbidity and mortality. The treatment of HFpEF is directed by management of associated conditions (e.g., hypertension, atrial fibrillation, sleep apnea, obesity, and diabetes) and symptoms [1]. Amyloidosis is also an increasingly common cause of HFpEF and must be excluded in patients suspected of HF [18]. In the near future, SGLT2 inhibitors trials will be showing results in this patient population.

Acute Heart Failure

Acute heart failure (AHF) refers to rapid onset or worsening of symptoms and/or signs of HF. It is a life-threatening medical condition requiring urgent evaluation and treatment [5]. AHF may present as a first occurrence, or, more frequently, as a consequence of acute decompensation of chronic HF, and may be caused by primary cardiac dysfunction or precipitated by extrinsic factors, often in patients with chronic HF. Acute myocardial dysfunction (ischemic, inflammatory, or toxic), acute valve insufficiency, or pericardial tamponade are among the most frequent acute primary cardiac causes of AHF. Clinical classification is based on bedside physical examination in order to detect the presence of clinical symptoms/signs of congestion (wet versus dry) and/or peripheral hypoperfusion (cold versus warm). Initial diagnosis of AHF should be based on a thorough history assessing symptoms, prior cardiovascular history and potential cardiac and noncardiac precipitants, as well as on the assessment of signs/symptoms of congestion and/or hypoperfusion by physical examination and further confirmed by appropriate additional investigations such as ECG, chest X-ray, laboratory assessment (with natriuretic peptides biomarkers), and echocardiography. An arterial blood gas and lactic acid are warranted to accurately assess acid-base abnormalities and hypoxia. Invasive hemodynamic monitoring can be considered when there is evidence of impaired perfusion, uncertainty of fluid status, uncertainty of systemic or pulmonary vascular resistance, worsening renal function, or a need for vasoactive agents [1].

The initial goal of treatment should be stabilization to control hypoxemia or hypotension that can cause under perfusion of vital organs, the heart, kidneys, and brain [5]. Intravenous loop diuretics are the first-line therapy to treat pulmonary edema and volume overload by lowering central venous capillary wedge pressures and improving hemodynamic status. Loop diuretic dosing should be equal or 2.5 times higher than the patient's normal oral dose (for dosing and equivalents, see Table 6). A continuous infusion of loop diuretics is not more effective than IV bolus therapy. If necessary, adding a second diuretic to potentiate a diuresis is an option, either with oral hydrochlorothiazide, metolazone, or spironolactone. Careful monitoring of congestive symptoms, volume status, blood pressure, oxygenation, daily intake and out-take, and daily weights should be utilized. To reduce adverse effects of treatment, daily monitoring of renal function, for overdiuresis or azotemia, and electrolyte disturbances to appropriately replace depleted potassium and magnesium is considered [1]. Intravenous vasodilators, nitroglycerin or nitroprusside, are recommended for persistent congestive symptoms and rapid symptom relief in acute pulmonary edema or severe hypertension not responding to diuretics alone [19]. Inotropic agents such as dobutamine or milrinone are indicated in AHF when LVEF is reduced and hypotension causes diminished perfusion and end-organ dysfunction (low-output syndrome). When initiating a vasodilator or inotropic therapy, consideration should be given for cardiology or pulmonary consultation. In patients with HFrEF experiencing a symptomatic exacerbation of HF requiring hospitalization during chronic maintenance treatment with guideline-directed medical therapy (GDMT), it is recommended that GDMT be continued in the absence of hemodynamic instability or contraindications [1].

Referrals

Early identification and timely referral of select patients to a heart failure specialist is critical so that those with advanced disease can be considered for heart transplantation or LVAD placement. This window of opportunity is missed if referral is delayed until multiorgan failure develops, as such patients may no longer candidates for these therapies. A useful acronym "I-NEED-HELP" was developed to assist clinicians recognize such appropriate patients [20] (Table 7).

Counseling and Patient Education

HF management and self-care behavior are complicated by ageing, comorbid conditions, cognitive impairment, frailty, and limited social support. HF is also a leading cause of hospital admission in the older adult, where it is associated with increased hospital length of stay and risk of mortality [9]. Counseling patients with HF education and strategies for self-care are critically important to enhance treatment compliance, improve transitions of care and manage worsening signs and symptoms of fluid retention. Although frequently utilized, there is limited evidence to support the daily 2–3 gram sodium restriction or the 1.5–2 L fluid restriction recommended by current guidelines. Daily weights are important to detect early fluid retention, and a weight gain of 2 lb. in a day or ≥ 5 lb. in a week should prompt contacting or seeing a

Table 7 When to refer to advanced heart failure

I	IV inotropes
N	NYHA III/IV or persistently elevated natriuretic peptides
E	End organ dysfunction
E	Ejection fraction $\leq 35\%$
D	Defibrillator shocks
H	Hospitalizations >1
E	Edema despite escalating diuretics
L	Low BP, high heart rate
P	Prognostic medication – Progressive intolerance or down-titration of GDMT

Modified from Yancy et al. [20]

health care provider. Exercise training or regular physical activity is highly recommended as safe and effective to improve symptoms and functional status. Formal cardiac rehabilitation can be useful and effective when clinically stable to improve functional capacity, exercise duration, quality of life, and mortality [9].

Prevention

Effective systems of care coordination with special attention to care transitions should be deployed for every patient with chronic HF that facilitate and ensure effective care that is designed to achieve GDMT and prevent hospitalization [1]. Every patient with HF should have a clear, detailed, and evidence-based plan of care that ensures the achievement of GDMT goals, effective management of comorbid conditions, timely follow-up with the health care team, appropriate dietary and physical activities, and compliance with secondary prevention guidelines for cardiovascular disease. Palliative and supportive care is effective for patients with symptomatic advanced HF to improve quality of life [1].

Management of HF often entails adherence to a complex medication regimen in conjunction with dietary sodium restriction and limitation of fluid intake. In addition, HF usually occurs in the context of one or more comorbid conditions, such as hypertension, diabetes mellitus, and coronary artery disease, which further increase the complexity of care. A significant proportion of early HF readmissions are due to nonadherence to medications or diet, inadequate patient education, or lack of timely follow-up. Heart failure disease management (HFDM) is an opportunity to provide a patient-centered, multidisciplinary, coordinated approach to care that incorporates optimization of the medication regimen, effective patient education, and close follow-up designed to improve clinical outcomes, including quality of life, readmission rates, and survival. Performance measures based on professionally developed clinical practice guidelines should be used with the goal of improving quality of care for HF [1].

References

1. Yancy CW, Jessup M, Bozkurt B, Butler J, Casey DE Jr, Drazner MH, et al. 2013 ACCF/AHA guideline for the management of heart failure: executive summary: a report of the American College of Cardiology Foundation/American Heart Association Task Force on practice guidelines. Circulation. 2013;128(16):1810–52.

2. Virani SS, Alonso A, Aparicio HJ, Benjamin EJ, Bittencourt MS, Callaway CW, Carson AP, et al. Heart disease and stroke statistics-2021 update: a report from the American Heart Association. Circulation. 2021;143:e00.

3. Gaziano TA, Bitton A, Anand S, Abrahams-Gessel S, Murphy A. Growing epidemic of coronary heart disease in low- and middle-income countries. Curr Probl Cardiol. 2010;35(2):72–115.

4. Kannel WB. Incidence and epidemiology of heart failure. Heart Fail Rev. 2000;5(2):167–73.

5. Ponikowski P, Voors AA, Anker SD, Bueno H, Cleland JG, Coats AJ, et al. 2016 ESC Guidelines for the diagnosis and treatment of acute and chronic heart failure: The Task Force for the diagnosis and treatment of acute and chronic heart failure of the European Society of Cardiology (ESC). Developed with the special contribution of the Heart Failure Association (HFA) of the ESC. Eur J Heart Fail. 2016;18(8):891–975.

6. Murphy SP, Ibrahim NE, Januzzi JL Jr. Heart failure with reduced ejection fraction: a review. JAMA. 2020;324(5):488–504.

7. Madhok V, Falk G, Rogers A, Struthers AD, Sullivan FM, Fahey T. The accuracy of symptoms, signs and diagnostic tests in the diagnosis of left ventricular dysfunction in primary care: a diagnostic accuracy systematic review. BMC FamPract. 2008;9:56.

8. Baldasseroni S, Opasich C, Gorini M, Lucci D, Marchionni N, Marini M, et al. Left bundle-branch block is associated with increased 1-year sudden and total mortality rate in 5517 outpatients with congestive heart failure: a report from the Italian network on congestive heart failure. Am Heart J. 2002;143(3):398–405.

9. Heart Failure Society of America, Lindenfeld J, Albert NM, Boehmer JP, Collins SP, Ezekowitz JA, et al. HFSA 2010 comprehensive heart failure practice guideline. J Card Fail. 2010;16(6):e1194.

10. Yancy CW, Jessup M, Bozkurt B, Butler J, Casey DE Jr, Colvin MM, et al. 2017 ACC/AHA/HFSA Focused Update of the 2013 ACCF/AHA Guideline for the Management of Heart Failure: A Report of the American College of Cardiology/American Heart Association Task Force on Clinical Practice Guidelines and the Heart Failure Society of America. Circulation. 2017;136(6):e137–e61.

11. McMurray JJ, Packer M, Desai AS, Gong J, Lefkowitz MP, Rizkala AR, et al. Angiotensin-neprilysin inhibition versus enalapril in heart failure. N Engl J Med. 2014;371(11):993–1004.

12. McMurray JJV, Solomon SD, Inzucchi SE, Kober L, Kosiborod MN, Martinez FA, et al. Dapagliflozin in patients with heart failure and reduced ejection fraction. N Engl J Med. 2019;381(21):1995–2008.

13. Packer M, Anker SD, Butler J, Filippatos G, Pocock SJ, Carson P, et al. Cardiovascular and renal outcomes with empagliflozin in heart failure. N Engl J Med. 2020;383(15):1413–24.

14. Writing C, Maddox TM, Januzzi JL Jr, Allen LA, Breathett K, Butler J, et al. 2021 Update to the 2017 ACC Expert Consensus Decision Pathway for Optimization of Heart Failure Treatment: Answers to 10 Pivotal Issues About Heart Failure With Reduced Ejection Fraction: A Report of the American College of Cardiology Solution Set Oversight Committee. J Am Coll Cardiol. 2021; Feb 16;77(6):772–810.

15. Teerlink JR, Diaz R, Felker GM, JJV MM, Metra M, Solomon SD, et al. Cardiac Myosin Activation with Omecamtiv Mecarbil in Systolic Heart Failure. N Engl J Med. 2020; Jan 14;384(2):105–116.

16. Butler J, Anstrom KJ, Armstrong PW. Comparing the Benefit of Novel Therapies Across Clinical Trials: Insights From the VICTORIA Trial. Circulation. 2020;142(8):717–9.

17. Bonow RO, O'Gara PT, Adams DH, Badhwar V, Bavaria JE, Elmariah S, et al. 2020 Focused Update of the 2017 ACC Expert Consensus Decision Pathway on the Management of Mitral Regurgitation: A Report of the American College of Cardiology Solution Set Oversight Committee. J Am Coll Cardiol. 2020;75(17):2236–70.

18. Adamczak DM, Oduah MT, Kiebalo T, Nartowicz S, Beben M, Pochylski M, et al. Heart failure with preserved ejection fraction: a concise review. Curr Cardiol Rep. 2020;22(9):82.

19. Heart Failure Society of America, Lindenfeld J, Albert NM, Boehmer JP, Collins SP, Ezekowitz JA, et al. HFSA 2010 comprehensive heart failure practice guideline. J Card Fail. 2010;16(6):e1–194.

20. Yancy CW, Januzzi JL Jr, Allen LA, Butler J, Davis LL, Fonarow GC, et al. 2017 ACC Expert Consensus Decision Pathway for Optimization of Heart Failure Treatment: Answers to 10 Pivotal Issues About Heart Failure With Reduced Ejection Fraction: A Report of the American College of Cardiology Task Force on Expert Consensus Decision Pathways. J Am Coll Cardiol. 2018;71(2):201–30.

21. King M, Kingery J, Casey B. Diagnosis and evaluation of heart failure. Am Fam Physician. 2012;85(12):1161–8.

22. Ponikowski P, Voors AA, Anker SD, Bueno H, Cleland JGF, Coats AJS, Falk V, González-Juanatey JR, Harjola V-P, Jankowska EA, Jessup M, Linde C, Nihoyannopoulos P, Parissis JT, Pieske B, Riley JP, Rosano GMC, Ruilope LM, Ruschitzka F, Rutten FH, van der Meer P. 2016 ESC Guidelines for the diagnosis and treatment of acute and chronic heart failure. Eur J Heart Fail. 2016;18:891–975.

Cardiovascular Emergencies

84

Andrea Maritato and Francesco Leanza

Contents

A. Maritato (✉)
Department of Family Medicine and Community Health,
Icahn School of Medicine at Mount Sinai, New York, NY,
USA

Institute for Family Health, New York, NY, USA
e-mail: amaritato@institute.org

F. Leanza
Department of Family and Community Medicine, Faculty
of Medicine, University Health Network, University of
Toronto, Toronto, ON, Canada

© Springer Nature Switzerland AG 2022
P. M. Paulman et al. (eds.), *Family Medicine*,
https://doi.org/10.1007/978-3-030-54441-6_87

General Principles

Cardiovascular death remains the number one cause of death in the United States. It causes more deaths than lung cancer, breast cancer, prostate cancer, colon cancer, stroke, and chronic lower respiratory diseases combined [1, 2]. While most of these conditions require specialist care, often in a hospital setting, patients will present with these complaints to their family physician, and one must be able to recognize and assess them. Furthermore, family physicians will continue to care for these patients as they live with these conditions. These patients will turn to their family physician for information, second opinions, and advice. This chapter will look at some of these conditions.

Cardiogenic Shock

Shock is caused when oxygen demand exceeds available supply. This can be caused by increased demand of tissue due to infection, metabolic or endocrine disease, decreased supply due to hypovolemia, or a combination of the two. Sometimes, inability of tissue to use oxygen can contribute as well.

There are five categories of shock: cardiogenic, obstructive, hypovolemic, distributive, and endocrine (see Table 1).

When oxygen supply to tissues is decreased, cells can extract more oxygen from red blood cells to meet demands. However, this can only compensate so much, and once supply drops below a critical level, this mechanism can no longer meet the demands of the tissues (compensated vs decompensated shock).

Cardiogenic shock is due to primary cardiac dysfunction. While there may be adequate volume, the heart is unable to circulate it, and tissues suffer from hypoperfusion and hypoxia.

Myocardial infarction (MI) is the most common cause of cardiogenic shock. Arrhythmias, valve rupture, myocarditis, endocarditis, cardiomyopathy, and contusion after chest wall trauma can cause cardiogenic shock as well [3].

Pathophysiology

Ischemia reduces both contractility and relaxation of the heart. This leads to reduced cardiac compliance and reduced filling. As a result, stroke volume is reduced. This in turn reduces cardiac output (cardiac output = stroke volume X heart rate), which then reduces blood pressure. Compensatory mechanisms such as the sympathetic nervous system and the renin-angiotensin system increase heart rate, afterload, and fluid retention. These in turn cause increased oxygen demand on the heart which already has an inadequate supply [4]. This further widens the gap between oxygen need and available oxygen, exacerbating shock and end-organ dysfunction.

Definition

Cardiogenic shock is defined as a systolic BP < 80–90 mmHg in the absence of hypovolemia and must be associated with end-organ damage such as cold extremities, oliguria, or mental status changes. This can also be measured as reduced cardiac index (CI) < 2.2 l/min/m^2 (cardiac output to body surface area)

Table 1 Shock classification

Name	Causes	Examples
Cardiogenic	Myocardial disease	MI Myocarditis
Obstructive	Mechanical blockage of blood flow beyond the heart	Pulmonary embolus Cardiac tamponade
Hypovolemic	Loss of circulating volume	Blood loss Third spacing
Distributive	Vasodilation and relative inadequate circulating volume	Sepsis Neurogenic shock Anaphylaxis
Endocrine	Thyroid disease Adrenal insufficiency	Thyroid storm Stopping steroid use abruptly

or elevated pulmonary capillary wedge pressure > 15 mmHg [4].

Despite numerous advances in revascularization, medications, and mechanical support, cardiogenic shock is still the number one cause of mortality due to acute myocardial infarction (AMI). Overall, however, the rate of cardiogenic shock has decreased from around 7.5% (range 5–15%) in the 1970s to around 4% in 2003 [5].

Patients who develop cardiogenic shock during a hospitalization for AMI are more than ten times more likely to die than patients hospitalized for AMI who do not develop cardiogenic shock.

Patients who develop cardiogenic shock after an AMI tend to be older, be female, and have a do-not-resuscitate (DNR) order, a history of diabetes mellitus (DM), a history of heart failure (HF), or prior MI.

Management

If a patient develops cardiogenic shock from any cause, the keys to management are improving perfusion and oxygenation. Ideally, PaO$_2$ (partial pressure of arterial oxygen) levels should be maintained at more than 60 mmHg using bilevel

positive airway pressure (BPAP) or intubation as needed. Maintain hemoglobin >8 to allow for adequate oxygen delivery. Fluid resuscitation needs to be monitored carefully as improving filling pressures is important but must be balanced against fluid overload.

Vasopressors such as norepinephrine (Levophed), dopamine, and dobutamine and intraaortic balloon pump counterpulsation (IABP) are used to give BP support while stabilizing and preparing the patient for revascularization procedures. While dopamine was originally considered the first-line vasopressor in cardiogenic shock, recent evidence suggests better outcomes with norepinephrine. Dobutamine doesn't help hypotension and should only be used in patients who have less hypotension, i.e., SBP > 80 mm Hg, in conjunction with vasodilators [6].

Results from the GUSTO-I and SHOCK trials suggest improved survival with emergent revascularization in patients with cardiogenic shock. Percutaneous coronary interventions (PCI) have a class 1A indication in AMI with cardiogenic shock as do coronary artery bypass grafts (CABG) if the patient has suitable coronary anatomy [5]. A class 1A indication means that there are multiple randomized controlled trials showing that the procedure is both effective and useful.

Cardiopulmonary Resuscitation (CPR)

CPR was developed in the 1960s and has been saving lives ever since.

Every 5 years, the International Consensus of CPR and Emergency Cardiovascular Care (ECC) Conference convenes and evaluates the guidelines. The most recent conference took place in 2015, and the American Heart Association (AHA) guidelines for CPR and ECC were updated.

In a major shift, the usual "A-B-C" (airway-breathing-circulation) protocol was changed to "C-A-B" (circulation-airway-breathing). This change was made to stress that reduced time to first compressions and early use of a defibrillator are the priorities for survival. The AHA has found that oxygen demand is lessened during cardiac arrest, and therefore pumping blood to a victim's brain is more important than oxygen [7]. In fact, bystander hands-only CPR, where compressions are done without breaths, shows similar outcomes to conventional CPR in adults [8].

The compression rate has been changed from "at least 100 compressions a minute" to "no slower than 100 compressions per minute and no faster than 120 compressions per minute" [9].

Compression depth is now 2 in. for adults as opposed to 1½–2 in. for adults. The depth has changed for children as well [10]. The latest recommendations also suggest not compressing further than 2.4 in. for adults [9].

Minimizing interruptions to compressions is also emphasized by changes in pulse checks. These should not last for more than 10 s, and if an obvious pulse isn't noted, compressions should continue. Again, trying to confirm a faint pulse may delay in needed compressions, and there are rarely significant injuries caused by chest compressions to patients who were not in cardiac arrest.

Additional changes include the removal of atropine (AtroPen) from the pulseless electrical activity (PEA) and asystole protocol.

Waveform capnography has been added to confirm endotracheal tube placement and quality of compressions. Cricoid pressure is no longer recommended during airway management.

Therapeutic hypothermia has been shown to improve outcomes for comatose patients after out-of-hospital arrests with a presenting rhythm of ventricular fibrillation (VF). New evidence shows a wider range of temperatures are acceptable. Providers should select a temperature between 32 and 36 degrees Celsius and maintain it for at least 24 h [9].

Aortic Dissection

Classification

There are two classification systems used: DeBakey and Standford (see Tables 2 and 3).

Table 2 DeBakey classifications

Type I	Originates in the ascending aorta and propagates to at least the arch
Type II	Originates in and is confined to the ascending aorta
Type IIIA	Dissection tear only in the descending thoracic aorta
Type IIIB	Tear extending below the diaphragm [12]

Table 3 Stanford classifications

| Type A | All dissections that involve the ascending aorta |
| Type B | All dissections that do not involve the ascending aorta |

Additionally, there are newer classifications based on other characteristics that pertain to suitability for endovascular repair, in particular, the DISSECT mnemonic: duration of dissection (D) less than 2 weeks, 2 weeks to 3 months, and more than 3 months from initial symptoms; intimal tear location (I) in the ascending aorta, arch, descending, abdominal, or unknown; size of the aorta (S); segmental extent (SE); clinical complications (C) such as aortic valve compromise, tamponade, rupture, and branch malperfusion; and thrombosis (T) of the false lumen and the extent [12].

There are three syndromes included in acute aortic disease: aortic dissection, aortic intramural hematoma (IMH), and penetrating atherosclerotic ulcer (PAU). Aortic dissections comprise 90% of acute aortic disease. Classic aortic dissection occurs when there is an intimal flap between the true lumen and the false lumen. An IMH occurs when there is bleeding into the aortic wall without a tear. This occurs by rupture of the vasa vasorum into the media of the aortic wall. This can happen either spontaneously or by a penetrating atherosclerotic ulcer [11].

Aortic dissection is often seen later in life, occurring after age 50. In cases that occur in younger patients, physicians should consider underlying connective tissue disorders such as Marfan's syndrome, Ehler-Danlos syndrome, or familial forms of dissection.

Chronic hypertension is the number one cause of aortic dissection and occurs in 75% of cases. Smoking, dyslipidemia, direct blunt trauma, and cocaine and methamphetamine use can all contribute to aortic dissection [12].

Aortic dissection is twice as prevalent in men as women. The incidence is hard to determine as patients may die before reaching care but is estimated to be between 2 and 3.5 cases per 100,000 patient-years [13].

Symptoms

More than 90% of patients with aortic dissection present with pain. Of the patients that present with pain, 90% describe it as severe. The pain is abrupt and maximal at outset and is described as sharp, tearing, or stabbing. Some patients may have uncommon presentations which can confound the diagnosis. They may present with acute heart failure, stroke, or syncope and either not have pain or not mention pain due to other distracting symptoms.

Type A dissections occur in 65% of cases and are more commonly seen in patients between 50 and 60 years of age. Type A dissections are lethal with a 1–2% mortality rate per hour after onset of dissection. Patients usually have symptoms of immediate, severe chest pain and/or back pain. Patients can also have abdominal pain, syncope, and/or stroke. Acute heart failure is also possible if the dissection involves the aortic valve. Type A dissections are surgical emergencies. Medical treatment alone results in approximately 20% mortality in the first 24 h. Mortality increases as time passes, with 50% mortality by day 30. Surgery improves chance of survival, but the 24-h mortality is still high at 10%.

Type B dissections occur more commonly over age 60. Type B dissections have similar presentations with chest and back pain as the common symptoms. Type B dissections are treated medically, and uncomplicated type B dissections have 10% mortality at day 30 [14].

Diagnosis

A routine chest x-ray (CXR) will be abnormal in 60–90% of patients, but 12–15% of patients can have normal CXR, and this cannot be used to exclude the diagnosis.

Electrocardiography (ECG) may be completely normal or extremely abnormal if the dissection involves the coronary circulation. This too cannot be used to exclude the diagnosis.

According to the International Registry of Acute aortic Dissection (IRAD) which is a clearinghouse of information on aortic dissections, transthoracic echocardiography (TTE), or transesophageal echocardiography (TEE), was used as the initial imaging test in 33% of patients, computed tomography (CT) in 61%, magnetic resonance imaging (MRI) in 2%, and angiography in 4%. For confirmation or further evaluation, TTE/TEE was used in 56% of patients, CT in 18%, MRI in 9%, and angiography in 17% [14].

CT is useful for allowing clinicians to evaluate involvement of surrounding organs, local anatomy, and possible ruptures or leaks. However, CT must be done with contrast in order to detect a false lumen and is contraindicated in patients with nephropathy. Contrast-induced nephropathy is a complication even for patients without underlying renal disease. CT imaging is limited by cardiac motion artifact as well as streak artifact from any implanted devices.

MRI is better than CT at seeing the aortic valve and coronary arteries. It does not require radiation or iodinated contrast material. However, MRI is not readily available in all sites and requires the patient to undergo imaging for a longer period of time. Also certain medical devices make it impossible to use MRI [13].

TTE has excellent specificity in the range of 93–96%, but the sensitivity is lower at only 77–80%. As such, a normal TTE does not rule out an aortic dissection. TEE, on the other hand, has both excellent sensitivity at around 98% and specificity at around 95%. Like all ultrasonography, both modalities are operator dependent [13]. This may be a concern in smaller centers where aortic dissection isn't diagnosed frequently.

Additionally, biomarkers are now being looked at for information regarding aortic dissection as it is a disease of the medial layer of the aorta. Currently, only D-dimer has any clinical value though other biomarkers are being studied. D-dimer has a sensitivity of 97% and a specificity of 47%. Therefore, a negative D-dimer may exclude the disease [12].

Management

Initial management for any type of dissection should include stabilizing the patient, controlling pain, lowering blood pressure, and reducing left ventricular contraction with beta-blockers. Initial blood pressure management is aimed at getting systolic blood pressure < 130 mmHg. IV beta-blockers are the first-line therapy. These should be used to control heart rate as well, aiming for a pulse <60 BPM. Nitroprusside (Nipride, Nitropress) can be used but only in conjunction with beta-blockers as nitroprusside can increase LV contractility. If a patient has a contraindication to a beta-blocker, verapamil (Calan, Isoptin SR, Veralan) or diltiazem (Cardizem, Cartia XT, Dilacor XR, Dilt-CD, Taztia XT, Tiazac) can be used. While stabilizing the patient, additional management depends on whether the patient has a type A or type B dissection.

Type A Dissections

Type A dissections should be managed as surgical emergencies. Medical management of type A dissections has a 20% mortality rate in the first 24 h and 30% in the first 48 h. Surgical management leads to improved outcomes for these patients. The aim of surgical management is to prevent aortic rupture, pericardial effusions which can lead to cardiac tamponade and death, and aortic regurgitation which can impair coronary artery blood flow leading to myocardial infarction and death. At 30 days, the mortality rate for type A dissections managed surgically is between 17% and 26%. If managed medically, the 30-day mortality is between 55% and 60% [13, 15]. The patient's hemodynamic stability immediately prior to surgery is a key predictor of how well the patient will do during and after surgery. Therefore, it is critical that surgery not be delayed for type A dissections.

Type B Dissections

Type B dissections have traditionally been managed medically. Uncomplicated type B dissections should be managed medically, and those that only require medical management have a low mortality rate around 6%. Additionally, the 5-year survival rate for these patients with optimal medical management is 89% [15]. The overall mortality rate for type B dissections treated medically was 10.7% in the International Registry of Acute aortic Dissection (IRAD), while those requiring surgery had a 31% mortality rate. Surgical management is required for complications such as limb ischemia, impending or actual rupture, increasing aortic diameter, intractable pain, or retrograde dissection (type A). Looking at 571 patients in the IRAD with type B dissection, 32% were complicated. The type of surgery required affected the mortality rate for type B dissections requiring surgery. Open surgical repairs had 33% mortality, whereas those who had an endovascular repair had only an 11% mortality rate [13]. As a result, endovascular procedures have a 1A recommendation for surgical repair of complicated type B dissections [14A]. About 25% of type B dissections are complicated at presentation [15].

Almost all patients with a type B dissection require intravenous antihypertensives with most requiring more than one antihypertensive medication during hospitalization. Beta-blockers, calcium channel blockers, nitroglycerin (Nitrolingual, NitroMist, Nitrostat), and nitroprusside were the most common initial antihypertensives used in one study of 129 patients. Mean hospital stay is more than 2 weeks with most patients spending a week in the intensive care unit as well [16]. All patients went home on an oral antihypertensive medication. These patients should be closely followed for at least the first 6 months after discharge as most complications that require intervention occur within this time frame. These patients are at risk for future dissections, aneurysms, and rupture. Systemic hypertension, advanced age, aortic size, and a patent false lumen are characteristics that put patients at higher risk for complications. Estimates are that 1/3 of all patients with original medical management will have an aneurysm, further dissection, or surgical requirement within 5 years [17].

Beta-blockers are the cornerstone of therapy as they affect both BP and contractility and are recommended even for patients with well-controlled BP. Ideal BP control should be <120/80 mmHg. Smoking cessation and risk factor modification for atherosclerotic disease are also key components for chronic management of aortic dissection. Surveillance with CT or MRA should occur at 1, 3, 6, and 12 months. After the first 12 months, imaging can be continued annually. Primary care doctors can oversee this surveillance along with cardiologists or cardiothoracic surgeons as appropriate.

Cardiac Syncope

Syncope is defined as sudden temporary loss of consciousness (LOC) with complete spontaneous recovery. It is very important to obtain a good history and physical exam in order to determine if the patient experienced syncope or if another diagnosis is more likely. If the patient did indeed have a syncopal event, the history and physical exam will help the clinician distinguish between the five types of syncope: cardiac, reflex mediated, neurologic, orthostatic, and psychogenic (see Table 4) [18].

The differential for syncope includes seizures, dizziness, presyncope, drop attacks, vertigo, and near sudden cardiac death events [19]. The history can usually elicit which of these the patient experienced. The input of any witnesses is vital as the patient often does not remember the event or does not remember the entirety of the event. Studies have shown that the elements that distinguish seizure from syncope include disorientation after the event (postictal phase), tongue-biting, frothing at the mouth, and loss of consciousness for more than 5 min. An aura preceding and a headache after the event also suggest seizure [20]. Urinary or fecal incontinence can be seen with either condition but is more common in seizures.

Cardiac syncope is important to distinguish from other causes as it is associated with an increased risk of death from all causes, such as stroke, and from cardiac causes, such as myocardial infarction or arrhythmia. Cardiac syncope is the second most common type of syncope and is seen in about 10–20% of cases. Patients tend to be older, have a cardiac history, and/or have risk factors for cardiac disease such as diabetes and HTN. They may also have palpitations, syncope related to exercise, and/or a family history of sudden cardiac death. They may complain of chest pain or shortness of breath in addition to the syncopal episode. Ventricular tachycardia (VT) is the most common tachyarrhythmia that leads to syncope. Supraventricular tachycardia (SVT) can lead to syncope but this is less common. More often, patients with SVT have less severe symptoms such as lightheadedness, palpitations, and shortness of breath. Bradyarrhythmias such as sick sinus syndrome can also lead to syncope. A massive pulmonary embolism and aortic stenosis are obstructive causes of cardiac syncope. Increased age and male sex, both risk factors for cardiac disease, also suggest a cardiac etiology for syncope.

Risk Factors for Serious Adverse Events After a Syncopal Episode

The San Francisco Syncope Rule (SFSR) is a tool used to determine if a patient has an increased risk of death after a syncopal episode. Systolic blood pressure <90 mmHg, shortness of breath, congestive heart failure, ECG abnormalities, and hematocrit <30 were all predictors of serious outcomes [3S]. Another tool is the Risk stratification Of Syncope in the Emergency department (ROSE) rule. This states that if any of the following seven risks are present, the patient should be considered high risk: BNP > 300 pg/ml, HR <50, hemoglobin <9, positive fecal occult blood, chest pain, ECG with Q waves, or oxygen saturation <94% [21].

Another study looked at death or significant cardiac arrhythmias in the year after a syncopal episode and found that the four most important risk factors were age > = 45, a history of heart failure, a history of ventricular arrhythmia, and an abnormal ECG. Patients with none of these risks had a 4–7% chance of death or a significant

Table 4 Types of syncope

Name	Situation	Prevalence (%)	Risk of death
Cardiac	Exertional, arrhythmias, palpitations, unprovoked	18	2X increased risk of death from any cause
Reflex mediated	Vasovagal, situational, micturition, defecation, sight of blood	24	None
Neurologic	Steal syndrome, TIAs, neurologic symptoms	10	Increased risk of death
Orthostatic	Dehydration, medication, alcohol, occurs with standing	8	None
Psychogenic	Depression, anxiety, normal exam findings, panic attacks	2	None

All other episodes of syncope are of unknown etiology, 38%

cardiac arrhythmia as opposed to those with three or four of these risks who had a 58–80% chance [21].

History and Physical Exam

Diagnosing and distinguishing between types of syncope, history, and physical exam allow for more accurate diagnosis than any other modality, establishing the cause up to 65% of the time [18]. ECG was next at only 10%.

It is important when taking the history to ask about the patient's position prior to and at the time of the event, last PO intake including fluids, recent exertion, any situational stressors, any new or recently taken medications or drugs, the presence of palpitations or dyspnea, and any family history of cardiac disease and sudden cardiac death. Also ask if the patient has experienced prior episodes of syncope. It is also important to know if the patient has a personal cardiac history including a pacemaker or defibrillator.

The physical exam should include vitals particularly any orthostatic changes and oxygen saturation, cardiac murmurs, arrhythmias, any neurologic changes, or any gastrointestinal blood loss.

Testing

Routine lab testing has little diagnostic value in assessing syncope with <3% of cases having any significant lab abnormalities [21]. It may be reasonable to check glucose, CBC, and BNP in certain patients.

Carotid massage can be used to check for neurally mediated carotid sinus hypersensitivity in patients over age 40 only after ruling out the presence of bruits. This test should not be performed in patients with a history of transient ischemic attack (TIA), recent stroke, or neurologic findings on exam. The test is positive if the patient experiences a pause in heart rate for >3 s or whose systolic BP drops by more than 50 mmHg. The test should be done in the supine and upright positions [20]. While this is mentioned in most texts, it is not often done in practice.

ECG should be ordered for patients where cardiac syncope is suspected. The ECG can establish the diagnosis in 5–10% of cases of syncope. One should look for QT prolongation, delta waves, and short PR interval which suggest Wolff-Parkinson-White (WPW) syndrome, bundle branch block (BBB), and particularly right BBB with ST elevation which is seen in Brugada syndrome. One should also look for ST elevations suggestive of myocardial infarction, bradycardia, second- or third-degree atrioventricular (AV) node block, SVT, or VT. Any abnormality in the ECG should raise the concern for a cardiac cause of syncope and increased mortality [20].

Telemetry is often ordered for patients who present with syncope but does not frequently help identify the cause. Holter monitoring and more recently loop monitoring may be useful in cases of suspected arrhythmia. These allow for longer periods of monitoring with implantable loop recorders being able to monitor patients for more than 12 months. Symptoms attributable to arrhythmias can be found with loop recorders in 50–85% of cases [21].

Stress testing and cardiac catheterization should only be used in cases where myocardial ischemia is highly suspected.

Echocardiography is useful to evaluate for structural cardiac abnormalities. It is also useful for determining left ventricular ejection fraction (EF) as an EF <35% is an indication for an implantable cardioverter-defibrillator (ICD). These patients are at high risk for arrhythmias and sudden cardiac death. In these patients, syncope is an ominous sign. Echocardiography is also useful in establishing aortic stenosis as the cause of syncope. This should be suspected in older adults presenting with syncope during exertion.

Electrophysiologic (EP) testing can be useful in establishing the diagnosis for patients suspected of having sick sinus syndrome, heart block, ventricular tachycardia (VT), or supraventricular tachycardia (SVT). Those patients with structural heart abnormalities, ECG abnormalities, a clinical history that suggests arrhythmia, or a family history of sudden death should undergo EP testing.

Management

Management of cardiac syncope depends on the underlying cause. If the cause is ischemic, patients should receive optimal medical management along with surgical interventions as needed. Most arrhythmias will require ICD implantation. Patients with sick sinus syndrome and AV node block can be treated with pacemakers. WPW can be treated with catheter ablation therapy.

Sudden Cardiac Death

Sudden cardiac death (SCD) affects between 300,000 and 500,000 people in the United States annually. SCD is usually caused by VT decompensating to ventricular fibrillation (VF) though it may also result from heart failure, bradyarrhythmias, heart block, or pulmonary emboli. SCD is responsible for more deaths annually in the United States than stroke, lung cancer, and breast cancer combined. Worldwide, it is responsible for 50% of overall cardiac deaths [22]. It is the most common presenting sign of coronary artery disease. Risks for SCD include decreased left ventricular EF, acute MI, prior MI, prior ventricular arrhythmia, and congestive heart failure.

Seventy-five percent of cases occur in men with a fourfold to sevenfold higher risk of SCD in men than women <65 years of age. After age 65, the ratio of SCD in men to women is 2:1 or less [22]. Pre-menopausal women have some cardioprotection that decreases their risk of SCD and cardiac disease. However, in women over age 40, coronary artery disease is the most common cause of SCD. Further, women with SCD are less likely to have severely reduced left ventricular ejection fraction or known heart disease which makes it that much harder to establish a risk profile for women.

Studies show that more than 50% of people with SCA had warning symptoms before the event; however, they often went unrecognized or minimized. The most common symptoms were chest pain and dyspnea. Women experienced dyspnea more than chest pain.

Risk factors for SCD (or SCA) are the same as for coronary heart disease (CHD): smoking, obesity, inactivity, dyslipidemia, diabetes, hypertension, and family history of CHD [23].

Primary Prevention

Given that the first arrhythmic event is usually fatal in SCD (or perhaps more appropriately, sudden cardiac arrest (SCA)), it is critical to try to identify people who are at high risk for these events and intervene early. People with known cardiac disease and ejection fraction (EF) < 30–40% are known to be at very high risk for SCD. An EF < 30% is the biggest independent predictor for SCD, and reduced EF predicts SCD in both ischemic and nonischemic dilated cardiomyopathies. The American College of Cardiology (ACC), American Heart Association (AHA), and Heart Rhythm Society (HRS) published guidelines recommending ICD implantation in people with EF less than 30–35% with heart failure [24]. Therefore, it is critical that any patient with known cardiac disease have an evaluation for ejection fraction. Patients with low functional capacity who don't have a reasonable expectation to live more than 1 year are not candidates for ICDs.

Secondary Prevention

Three studies have shown that ICDs decrease mortality in patients with aborted SCD, VT, or VF. Therefore, any patient with a history of VT, VF, SCA, or aborted SCD should be evaluated for possible ICD implantation. VT or VF that occur within 48 h of an MI do not need to be evaluated for ICD placement.

Hypertrophic Cardiomyopathy

Definition

Hypertrophic cardiomyopathy (HCM) is defined as LV hypertrophy associated with nondilated ventricles that is not caused by cardiac or other systemic illness. HCM affects approximately 600,000 people in the United States. Most of those have no symptoms and most have a normal life expectancy. Those that do die from SCD suffer from ventricular tachyarrhythmias. This occurs most often in asymptomatic patients younger than 35. The other two serious complications of HCM are atrial fibrillation (AF) and heart failure with dyspnea.

The complications of HCM are caused by left ventricular outflow tract (LVOT) obstruction, arrhythmias, myocardial ischemia, diastolic dysfunction, and mitral regurgitation [25]. It is critical to establish whether LVOT obstruction is present as management strategies are based largely on this complication.

Diagnosis

The diagnosis of HCM is made by transthoracic echocardiography (TTE) and more recently, cardiac MRI. Once HCM is diagnosed, first-degree relatives should be screened with TTE. Patients with HCM can undergo genetic testing. If a patient screens positive for one of the genetic markers of HCM, first-degree relatives can be screened with genetic testing as well.

If a patient is diagnosed with HCM, ECG, and Holter monitoring should be done to look for any tachyarrhythmias. This should be repeated annually or whenever the patient has worsening symptoms of HCM [25].

Children of patients with HCM should be screened annually with TTE starting at age 12 or earlier if puberty or growth spurt begins before age 12. Children in intense competitive sports should also be screened earlier. Adult relatives can be surveyed every 5 years with TTE.

Management

Providers should aggressively manage patients with asymptomatic HCM by evaluating them for other risk factors for cardiovascular disease as these may contribute to complications of HCM. These patients should not participate in strenuous activities or competitive sports. Patients with resting or provoked LVOT obstruction should not be given high-dose diuretics or pure vasodilators as these are harmful. Beta-blockers should be used as first-line medications for symptoms of dyspnea and angina. If patients cannot tolerate these, verapamil can be used. Disopyramide (Norpace) can be added to a beta-blocker or verapamil if symptoms cannot be controlled; however, it should not be used alone. Dihydropyridine calcium channel blockers such as amlodipine (Norvasc) should not be used in patients with HCM who have LVOT obstruction. ACE inhibitors have not been shown to be useful or harmful in the treatment of symptoms of HCM. Beta-blockers can be used in children but watch for side effects such as depression or difficulty in school.

Surgical interventions such as septal reduction or alcohol septal ablation should only be considered in cases of refractory LVOT obstruction and symptoms that interfere with daily living despite optimal medical management. These should only be performed at experienced centers.

Implantable cardiac defibrillators (ICDs) have been shown to decrease mortality in patients with HCM and tachyarrhythmias. Patients with HCM should receive risk stratification for SCD to determine if an ICD if appropriate. These include prior personal cardiac arrest, history of VF, sustained VT, sudden cardiac arrest (SCA) (recurrence is 10% per year), family history of SCD, unexplained syncope, documented nonsustained VT, or LV thickness $> = 30$ mm [25]. An ICD can be implanted in children as well who have any of these high-risk factors.

Patients with HCM, regardless of symptoms, should not participate in intense or competitive sports. One third of all SCD in young athletes are due to HCM. Low-intensity aerobic exercise is recommended.

References

1. Heron MD. Leading causes for 2012. Natl Vital Stat Rep, CDC. 2015;64(10):1–93.
2. Cancer Facts and Figures 2013, American Cancer Society.
3. Gaieski, D, Mikkelsen, M. Evaluation of and initial approach to the adult patient with undifferentiated hypotension and shock. Uptodate. 2020.
4. Terblanche M, Assmann N. Shock. In: Petrou M, editor. Cardiovascular critical care. Chichester: Wiley. 2010. p. 1–15.
5. Goldberg RJ, Spencer F, Gore J, Lessard D, Yarzebski J. Thirty-year trends (1975–2005) in the magnitude of, management of, and hospital death rates associated with cardiogenic shock in patients with acute myocardial infarction: a population-based perspective. Circulation. 2009;119(9):1211–9.
6. Hochman JS, Reyentovich A. Prognosis and treatment of cardiogenic shock complicating acute myocardial infarction. Suggests dobutamine for LESS ill patients not the very sickest. 2015.
7. Field JM, Hazinski MF. 2010 American heart association guidelines for cardiopulmonary resuscitation and emergency cardiovascular care science. Circulation. 2010;122:640–56.
8. Pozner CN. Basic life support in adults. UpToDate, 2015.
9. American Heart Association. 2015 Guidelines update for CPR and ECC, Oct 15, 2015.
10. American Heart Association. Advanced cardiovascular life Support provider manual. 2015.
11. Manning WJ. Aortic intramural hematoma. UpToDate, 2013.
12. Nienaber CA, Clough RE. Management of acute aortic dissection. Lancet. 2015;385:800–11.
13. Mann DL. Aortic disease. In: Braunwald's heart disease-textbook of cardiovascular medicine. 10th ed. Philadelphia: Elsevier; 2015. p. 1277–311.
14. Nienaber CA, Eagle KA. Aortic dissection: new frontiers in diagnosis and management, part I: from etiology to diagnostic strategies. Circulation. 2003;108:628–35.
15. Sidloff D, Choke E, Stather P, Bown M, Thompson J, Sayers R. Mortality from thoracic aortic diseases and associations with cardiovascular risk factors. Circulation. 2014;130:2287–94.
16. Estrera AL, Miller CC, Safi HJ, Goodrick JS, Keyhanii A, Porat EE, Achouh PE, Meada R, Azizzadeh A, Dhareshwar J, Allaham A. Outcomes of medical management of acute type B aortic dissection. Circulation. 2006;114(suppl I):I-381–9.
17. Nienaber CA, Eagle KA. Aortic dissection: new frontiers in diagnosis and management, part II: therapeutic management and follow-up. Circulation. 2003;108:772–8.
18. Benditt D. Syncope in adults: clinical manifestations and initial diagnostic evaluation. Uptodate. 2020.
19. Kapoor WN. Current evaluation and management of syncope. Circulation. 2002;106:1606–9.
20. Calkins HG, Zipes DP. Hypotension and syncope. In: Braunwald's heart disease-textbook of cardiovascular medicine. 10th ed. Philadelphia: Elsevier; 2015. p. 861–71.
21. Gauer RL. Evaluation of syncope. Am Fam Physician. 2011;84(6):640–50.
22. Myerburg RJ, Castellanos A. Cardiac arrest and sudden cardiac death. In: Braunwald's heart disease-textbook of cardiovascular medicine. 10th ed. Philadelphia: Elsevier; 2015. p. 821–60.
23. Podrid PJ. Overview of sudden cardiac arrest and sudden cardiac death. Uptodate. 2019.
24. Turakhia MP. Sudden cardiac death and implantable cardioverter-defibrillators. Am Fam Physician. 2010;82(11):1357–66.
25. Gersh BJ, Barry MJ. 2011 ACCF/AHA guideline for the diagnosis and treatment of hypertrophic cardiomyopathy: a report of the American College of Cardiology Foundation/American Heart Association task force on practice guidelines. Circulation. 2011;124(24):e783–831.

Venous Thromboembolism

85

Lawrence Gibbs, Josiah Moulton, and Vincent Tichenor

Contents

Introduction

DVT and PE have shared pathophysiology and together, along with superficial venous thrombosis, comprise the spectrum of venous thromboembolism (VTE). PE is the most serious of these, causing up to 10% of deaths in the hospital setting, and represents the most common preventable cause of death in patients with misdiagnosed

L. Gibbs (✉)
Methodist Health System Family Medicine Residency,
Dallas, TX, USA
e-mail: lawrencegibbs@mhd.com

J. Moulton
Family Medicine Clinic, Hill AFB, UT, USA

V. Tichenor
Family Medicine Clinic, Barksdale AFB, LA, USA

© This is a U.S. Government work and not under copyright protection in the U.S.; foreign copyright protection may apply 2022
P. M. Paulman et al. (eds.), *Family Medicine*,
https://doi.org/10.1007/978-3-030-54441-6_88

or improperly treated PE or DVT [1]. Even though the number of in-hospital deaths due to PE has decreased in the US, up to 30% of patients still die within the first year of diagnosis [2]. It is critical to maintain a high clinical suspicion in patients at risk of VTE and apply current diagnostic tools appropriately in order to initiate prompt therapy.

Pathophysiology

The major theory describing the pathogenesis of VTE is a triad derived from the extensive research of Virchow almost 100 years after his passing. This theory states that thrombosis occurs due to a combination of endothelial injury, hemodynamic changes (such as stasis or turbulence), and changes in the balance or properties of blood components involved in the coagulation cascade (i.e., inherited or acquired states of hypercoagulability) [3]. The role of inflammation is apparent by the increased frequency of DVT and PE formation in chronic inflammatory conditions such as inflammatory bowel diseases and systemic vasculitis [4]. C-reactive protein elevation has been linked to increased VTE risk. In the Atherosclerosis Risk in Communities (ARIC) study, an elevated C-reactive protein above the 90th percentile was associated with a 76% increased risk of VTE formation compared to lower percentiles [4]. Endothelial injury and stasis also increase VTE risk via increasing coagulation factors and preventing adequate mixing of anti-clotting factors, respectively [4, 5]. Local injury from indwelling devices, such as pacemaker leads or long-term indwelling central venous catheters, also increases upper extremity DVT formation [5].

Inherited and acquired thrombophilias affecting anticoagulant or pro-coagulant pathways lead to hypercoagulopathy [6]. Common inherited disorders include factor V Leiden mutation, which causes resistance to degradation by activated protein C, G2021A mutation, and deficiencies in proteins C and S, and antithrombin III. Hyperhomocysteinemia spans both categories, as it involves inheriting a defective enzyme, but is acquired through dietary folate, B6 and B12

deficiency [7]. Antiphospholipid antibody syndrome is an acquired autoimmune disorder characterized by abnormal levels of lupus anticoagulant, anti-β-2 glycoprotein-1, and anti-cardiolipin antibodies that increase the risk of recurrent VTE [8].

Inherited coagulopathies are among the rare, but significant risk factors for development of VTE, particularly in younger populations. However, thrombophilia testing remains controversial as absolute VTE risk is only mildly affected by these disorders, and currently available thrombophilia tests are insufficient to identify inherited risks of VTE [8]. The majority of patients with VTE should not be tested for thrombophilia, and most patients with inherited thrombophilia can accurately be identified based on the patient's personal and family history of VTE and not require testing [8]. Of those risks mentioned, family history of an unprovoked VTE in a first-degree relative, especially under age 50, may be more important in terms of counseling patients on their inherent risk (i.e., during pregnancy) than specific testing results [8, 9].

Epidemiology

Only myocardial infarction and stroke are more common in terms of cardiovascular disease than VTE [1]. The annual frequency of first-time VTE in adults is 1–2:1000 (rising to 1:200 in those over age 70), and if left untreated, the 30-day mortality rate for a first-time DVT is 5% and as high as 33% for those with a PE [9, 10]. The incidence of VTE increased significantly from 2001 to 2009 and may in part reflect improvement in imaging quality and increased use of diagnostic studies [9].

Approximately 33% of patients with VTE have recurrence within the following 10 years [10]. Predictors of recurrence include prior VTE, increased age, increased BMI, male gender, active cancer, and leg paresis among others. VTE accounts for approximately 1% of hospital admissions in the USA annually, and two-thirds of VTE cases occur in patients who have been hospitalized within the past 90 days [7]. Hospitalization, illness with resulting inflammation, recent surgery, and chemotherapy can all increase the risk of VTE by up to 100-fold [6, 7].

Men over age 45 are typically higher risk than similarly aged women, but women are 2–4 times higher risk during pregnancy, and the risk to postpartum women is as much as 5 times that during pregnancy [9]. In terms of race, the age-adjusted VTE incidence for those of European descent appears to be 104–183 per 100,000. Most data indicate the risk for African-Americans is slightly higher than this, but the risk may differ based on the region in the USA. The risks in Asian and Native Americans are estimated to be much lower [5, 9]. Among the highest incidence of VTE in the community include patients with a central venous catheter or transvenous pacemaker (9%) nursing home patients (10%) and active cancer (20%) [9]. Cancer may increase the risk of VTE in various ways such as through the elaboration of pro-inflammatory products which activate the coagulation cascade or through a tumor compressing vessels which causes stasis. The incidence of VTE during the first 6 months after a cancer diagnosis is 12.4 per 1,000 [11].

Modifiable risk factors for VTE include obesity, hypertension, tobacco use, dyslipidemia, diabetes, diet, stress, hormone replacement therapy, and contraceptive use. Patients with a BMI >30 have a two- to threefold higher risk for VTE, and may be related to impaired venous return or increased coagulation and inflammation [7]. Regarding contraceptive use, while the levonorgestrel intrauterine device imparts no additional risk, first- and third-generation oral contraceptives are at higher risk than second-generation contraceptives, and the depomedroxyprogesterone injection carries a threefold increased risk for VTE from baseline [9]. Table 1 includes further risk factors for VTE.

The most significant sequelae of VTE are venous stasis syndrome, venous ulcers, and chronic thromboembolic pulmonary hypertension. The 20-year incidence of venous stasis syndrome after VTE and proximal DVT is close to 25% and 40%, respectively, while that of venous ulceration is 3.7% [6].

Table 1 Risk factors for venous thromboembolism

Strong risk factors (odds ratio ≥ 10)
Fracture (hip or leg)
Hip or knee replacement
Major general surgery
Major trauma
Spinal cord injury
Moderate risk factors (odds ratio 2–9)
Arthroscopic knee surgery
Central venous lines
Chemotherapy
Congestive heart or respiratory failure
Hormone replacement therapy
Malignancy
Oral contraceptive therapy
Paralytic stroke
Pregnancy/Postpartum
Previous venous thromboembolism
Thrombophilia
Weak risk factors (odds ratio ≤ 2)
Bed rest >3 days
Immobility due to sitting (e.g. prolonged car or air travel)
Increasing age
Laparoscopic surgery (e.g. cholecystectomy)
Obesity
Pregnancy/Antepartum
Varicose veins

Used with permission from Anderson FA, Spencer FA. Risk factors for venous thromboembolism. Circulation. 2003;107(23):I9–I16

Diagnosis

Evaluating the history, signs, symptoms, and the individual's risk factors for VTE is essential for the diagnosis of DVT and PE (see Table 1). Patients with symptomatic DVT classically present with unilateral calf or thigh swelling, warmth, and tenderness. However, peripheral arterial disease (PAD), trauma, infection, and compartment syndrome may share these features. Likewise, patients suspicious for PE commonly present with one or more symptoms of chest pain, tachypnea, tachycardia, dyspnea, cough, and syncope. Concurrent DVT symptoms may also be present in those with suspected PE. Congestive heart failure (CHF), acute coronary syndrome (ACS), and chronic obstructive pulmonary disease (COPD) share similar signs and symptoms as PE and may confound the diagnosis [12].

Clinical Approach

Because none of the signs and symptoms of DVT or PE are specific, clinical probability assessment is an essential component in the diagnosis. Clinical prediction rules that incorporate signs, symptoms, and patient risk factors are frequently utilized to categorize patients as low, moderate, or high probability of having VTE [13]. Numerous guidelines recommend the use of validated clinical prediction rules to assess pretest probability of VTE to guide diagnostic decision-making [12, 14, 15].

A variety of formal scoring systems have been developed and validated to assist in stratifying patients with suspected DVT or PE [12]. Wells' DVT criteria is frequently used for DVT assessment and assigns a pretest probability category based on risk factor scoring. Patients are determined to be low (≤0), moderate (1–2), or high risk (≥3) for DVT based on their scores [15]. Wells' DVT criteria are shown in Table 2. Meanwhile, Wells' PE criteria [16] and the modified Geneva criteria [17] have similar predictive value and assist providers in determining pretest probability for PE [14]. Similar to the Wells' DVT criteria, the physician assigns points for different clinical criteria to obtain a pretest probability score. For the Wells' PE criteria, a patient's pretest probability is considered low for scores less than 2, moderate for scores between 2 and 6, and high for scores greater than 6. Wells' and the modified Geneva criteria are shown in Table 3. Simpler, two-tier/dichotomous versions of the Wells' and Geneva scores do exist (e.g., low risk vs high risk), but caution is advised since prospective validation of these models is still needed [14]. Also, though some suggest a simple gestalt approach to pretest probability, determination based on experience is often inaccurate and should be used cautiously [12]. Pretest probability for DVT or PE, along with test availability and risk, should guide subsequent D dimer and diagnostic imaging (see algorithm) [18]. For those patients at low risk for PE determined by Wells'

Table 2 Wells' DVT Criteria

Variable	Points
Active cancer (treatment ongoing or within previous 6 months of palliative treatment)	1
Paralysis, paresis, or recent plaster immobilization of the lower extremities	1
Recently bedridden for >3 days or major surgery within 4 weeks	1
Localized tenderness alone the distribution of the deep venous system	1
Entire lee swollen	1
Calf swelling by >3 cm when compared with the asymptomatic leg	1
Pitting edema (greater in the symptomatic leg)	1
Collateral superficial veins (not varicose)	1
Alternative diagnosis as likely or more likely than that of deep-vein thrombosis	-2
Analysis	
Probability of DVT is low	≤0
Probability of DVT is moderate	1 or 2
Probability of DVT is high	≥3

Reprinted from Wells PS, Anderson DR, Bormanis J, et al. Value of assessment of pretest probability of deep-vein thrombosis in clinical management. The Lancet 1997;350:1795–1798, with permission from Elsevier

criteria, the Pulmonary Embolism Rule Out Criteria (PERC rule) can be used to effectively rule out PE (<1% of low-risk patients who are PERC negative will develop PE within 30 days) [18, 19].

D-Dimer Testing

D-dimers are a byproduct of fibrinolysis formed by the degradation of fibrin within a clot and are acutely elevated in VTE [12]. The use of D-dimer testing with diagnostic algorithms that include pretest probability assessments can effectively exclude VTE in roughly 30% of patients suspected of having DVT or PE [2, 20]. Current assays are fast, readily available, and highly sensitive for DVT (over 93%) and PE (over 95%), but not nearly as specific [14]. False positives can be seen in patients with malignancy, infection, recent surgery or trauma, and pregnancy [13]. It is worth noting that since D-dimer levels increase naturally with age, for patients 50 years or older, using an

Table 3 PE clinical decision rules

Wells rule variable [16]	Points	Revised Geneva score variable [17]	Points
Clinical signs and symptoms of DVT (minimum of leg swelling and pain with palpation of deep veins)	3	Age > 65	1
An alternative diagnosis is less likely than PE	3	Previous DVT or PE	3
Heart rate > 100	1.5	Surgery (under general anesthesia) or fracture (of the lower limbs) within 1 month	2
Immobilization or surgery in the previous 4 weeks	1.5	Active malignant condition (solid or hematologic, currently active or considered cured <1 year)	2
Previous DVT/PE	1.5	Unilateral lower-limb pain	3
Hemoptysis	1	Hemoptysis	2
Malignancy (on treatment, treated in the last 6 months or palliative)	1	Heart rate 75–94 beats min^{-1}	3
		Heart rate > 94 beats min^{-1}	5
		Pain on lower – limb deep venous palpation and unilateral edema	4
Clinical probability		*Clinical probability*	
Low	<2 total	Low	0–3 total
Intermediate	2–6 total	Intermediate	4–10 total
High	>6 total	High	>10 total

Reprinted from Klok FA, Kruisman E, et al. Comparison of the revised Geneva score with the Wells rule for assessing clinical probability of pulmonary embolism. J Thromb Haemost. 2008;6(1): 40–44

age-adjusted D-dimer, defined as a patient's age multiplied by 10, may be more accurate at ruling out VTE than using the typical fixed D-dimer cutoff of 500 ug/L [20, 21]. This approach appears very useful in ruling out PE, but prospective validation of its use to rule out DVT is currently ongoing [2].

exclude the diagnosis of DVT [14]. Repeat CUS 1 week later is recommended for this group [13]. Some limitations include decreased reliability in detecting calf and upper extremity thrombi or poorer detection of thrombi isolated to the pelvis and difficulty distinguishing between old and new clots [12].

Compression Ultrasound (CUS)

Widely available and noninvasive, CUS is the imaging procedure of choice for the diagnosis of DVT, with a sensitivity and specificity of 95% and 98%, respectively, when performed by a well-trained operator [14]. Inability to compress a vein with the transducer is diagnostic for DVT, while signs of distention, decreased flow, and abnormal Doppler signal support the diagnosis [13]. In patients with moderate to high pretest probability of DVT, negative CUS alone, especially if just proximal vessels were tested, cannot

Venography

Once considered the gold standard for DVT detection, venography involves injecting contrast into the venous system to assess for filling defects or collateral flow. The PIOPED II trial demonstrated CT venography to be diagnostically equivalent at identifying DVT compared to CUS at the risk of higher contrast and radiation exposure [22]. Currently, venography is reserved for times when noninvasive tests cannot be performed or when noninvasive tests yield results counter to clinical suspicion [12].

Computed Tomographic Pulmonary Angiography (CTPA)

Multi-detector CT angiography has replaced conventional pulmonary angiography as the reference standard for diagnosing PE with high sensitivity and specificity of up to 100% and 97%, respectively [23]. Not only does it meet or exceed pulmonary angiography in ability to rule out PE, but it also generates diagnostic information that may suggest alternative or additional diagnoses [23]. Additionally, the PIOPED II trial showed that for those with high or intermediate pretest probability and positive CTPA results or those with low pretest probability and normal CTPA results, predictive values in the mid-90s were achieved [22]. Due to increased ionizing radiation and contrast exposure, consider ventilation-perfusion (V/Q) scanning for pregnant women, obese patients, or those with compromised renal function [12, 18].

Ventilation-Perfusion (V/Q) Scanning and V/Q SPECT

Ventilation-perfusion (V/Q) lung scans are reported as low, intermediate, or high likelihood for the presence of PE. A normal scan effectively excludes PE (negative predictive value of 100%) [23], while high pretest probability and a high-probability V/Q scan have a positive predictive value of 96% [18]. Unfortunately, approximately two-thirds of scans are not definitive and fall in the intermediate/non-diagnostic range [18]. As with CTPA, results discordant with pretest probability require further workup. Advances in V/Q single-photon emission CT (SPECT) have increased its sensitivity and specificity while limiting non-diagnostic results, which plague typical planar V/Q scans [18]. Though not available in all centers, its interobserver variability and diagnostic accuracy (both sensitivity and specificity of 96–97%) are superior to planar V/Q scans [24]. A single systematic review and meta-analysis also showed V/Q SPECT to be equivalent to CTPA

in terms of diagnostic accuracy while allowing less radiation exposure but at a cost approximately twice that of CTPA [25].

Other Diagnostic Testing

Pulmonary angiography may still be considered in select cases where clinical suspicion for PE remains high despite negative prior testing, but it is more invasive and requires higher contrast exposure than CTPA [12]. Those with normal angiography results have a 3-month VTE incidence less than 2% with 0.3% incidence of fatal PE [26]. Meanwhile, the PIOPED III trial did show magnetic resonance angiography and venography (MRA and MRV) to have good sensitivity and specificity at detecting PE, but their high percentage of technically inadequate results currently do not support routine use [18, 27]. Additionally, tests like a chest x-ray showing pleural infiltrates, or engorged central pulmonary artery vasculature with a paucity of peripheral vessels, or an electrocardiogram showing right bundle branch block with the a S1Q3T3 pattern may increase suspicion for PE but are not specific [12] (Fig. 1).

Management

Management of VTE centers on initial stabilization of the patient, selection of anticoagulation therapy, and determining treatment duration. Providers may start empiric pharmacological treatment in high-risk patients (based on pretest probability) while undergoing testing, and delay treatment until testing is finished for low-risk patients, but there is insufficient data to support that administering anticoagulation prior to imaging improves morbidity or mortality [18]. A distal DVT is less likely to embolize than a proximal DVT, and a DVT that does not extend within a period of 2 weeks is unlikely to extend into the proximal veins. Therefore, for acute isolated distal DVT in a patient without severe symptoms or risk factors (i.e., positive D-Dimer, extensive thrombosis, thrombus near proximal veins,

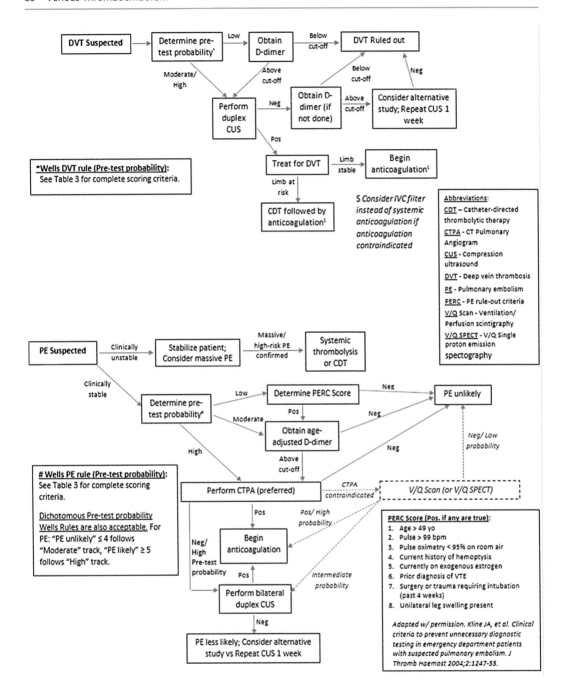

Fig. 1 Diagnostic algorithms for DVT (top) and PE (bottom) [14, 15, 18]

absence of reversible provoking factor, prior VTE, or inpatient status), the physician may delay anticoagulation and repeat imaging of the deep veins in 2 weeks [28]. Similarly, for asymptomatic patients with small, sub-segmental PEs and no DVT, recent guidelines suggest clinical surveillance over anticoagulation [28].

Initial Management

Given the variation of severity in patients who present with PE, the provider must ensure hemodynamic stability. For patients who are stable (such as with an isolated single DVT of the leg or segmental PE with hemodynamic stability), initial therapy can be initiated with a goal to move to long-term anticoagulation. However, in more critical situations, such as acute massive PE, PE in a patient who is hypotensive, PE with significant right ventricular strain (i.e., cardiac biomarker elevations or right ventricular strain shown on echocardiogram or CTPA), or extensive acute proximal DVT, early thrombolysis may be needed in addition to respiratory and hemodynamic support [28]. Early lysis of the thrombus and reducing post-thrombotic morbidity [28, 29] may be achieved through venous infusion of a thrombolytic agent (systemic thrombolysis) or delivery into the thrombus via catheter-direct thrombolysis (CDT). Current guidelines still prefer systemic thrombolysis over CDT [28] as most data show that systemic thrombolysis and CDT have similar effectiveness [30], but the resources required for systemic thrombolysis are more widely available. However, in certain circumstances (such as severe PE or failure of systemic thrombolysis), CDT may be more appropriate assuming the resources and expertise to perform the procedure are available [2]. Emerging techniques, such as pharmacomechanical thrombectomy (PMT), are still being developed, and no specific guidelines yet exist regarding them. Once the patient is stable, the treatment focus may be shifted toward anticoagulation, which is broadly the same in patients with PE or DVT [13, 28].

Anticoagulation has traditionally been accomplished with initial treatment with unfractionated heparin (UH) or low-molecular-weight heparin (LMWH) to achieve immediate anticoagulation, along with a vitamin K antagonist (VKA, typically warfarin) to achieve long-term anticoagulation [31]. Initial treatment with subcutaneous UH, LMWH, or fondaparinux is required to allow time for the VKA to begin to work [32], after which frequent testing via PT/INR is required to ensure the VKA is dosed within an effective range [28, 33].

UH has long been utilized in the initial treatment of VTE and when given intravenously (IV), is dosed via a nomogram based on periodic monitoring of the patient's activated partial thromboplastin time (aPTT) [34]. IV UH is preferred in patients with PE who will likely undergo thrombolysis (due to its shorter action and easier reversibility), those with impaired subcutaneous absorption, or those with increased bleeding risk [31]. UH carries the risk of heparin-induced thrombocytopenia (HIT), hemorrhage, and anaphylaxis. The risk of hemorrhage increases with age, comorbidities, and previous bleeding. Due to the risk of HIT, patients on heparin should have their platelet count monitored daily. Despite UH's long history of use, LMWH and fondaparinux have become the favored initial treatment for uncomplicated VTE as both have equal efficacy, increased bioavailability, and less frequent dosing when compared to heparin [32].

While the traditional regimen of bridging initial subcutaneous anticoagulation with long-term oral anticoagulation is still a viable method of treatment, evidence has shown that immediate therapy with either rivaroxaban or apixaban can safely replace the traditional regimen, eliminating the need for the use of heparin injections or frequent monitoring required by VKAs [28, 35, 36]. Direct oral anticoagulants (DOACs) are now preferred as first-line anticoagulant therapy in most patients [28, 33, 37] due to their rapid onset of action, predictable pharmacokinetic profile, and comparative effectiveness for treating VTE compared to LMWH and warfarin [2]. An exception to this management strategy is VTE associated with malignancy where most guidelines recommend that the patient be anticoagulated with LMWH for the duration of their treatment [28, 31, 37]. However, evidence from recent randomized control trials (Hokusai-VTE Cancer [38], SELECT-D [39], and CARAVAGGIO [40]) shows that DOACs (edoxaban, rivaroxaban, and apixaban) are non-inferior to LMWH for treatment of VTE in patients with cancer without significant increased bleeding risk (highest risk found in those with gastrointestinal malignancies) and could be an option for this group of patients.

Outpatient initial management may be appropriate in low-risk patients. Criteria for outpatient therapy include patients with good cardiorespiratory reserve, no excessive bleeding risks, a creatinine clearance greater than 30 mL/min, and ability to safely self-administer the medication [28, 33]. Well-validated clinical scores, like the Pulmonary Embolism Severity Index (PESI) and simplified-PESI (sPESI), can also be used to provide objective measures of a patient's appropriateness for initial outpatient management and hospital discharge [33]. Each provides reliable identification of patients at low 30-day mortality risk using baseline indicators of PE severity and the individual's comorbidities and potentially aggravating conditions. For the sPESI, a high-risk patient meets at least one of the following requirements: age over 80 years old, history of cancer, chronic cardiopulmonary disease (i.e., chronic obstructive pulmonary disease or congestive heart failure), pulse over 100 beats per minute, systolic blood pressure under 100 mmHg, or oxygen saturation less than 90% [33]. See Table 4 for a summary of treatment options.

Long-Term Anticoagulation

Goals of long-term anticoagulation therapy include preventing clot propagation, preventing possible PE (primary or subsequent), and minimizing complications. Resolution of an existing clot is not a direct goal of anticoagulation therapy [13, 28]. Recommended duration of therapy varies based on clinical circumstances, with a minimum treatment length of 3 months [28, 31]. Generally (with the exception of UH), the initial form of anticoagulation can be continued as the patient's long-term anticoagulation agent. However, given that LMWH and fondaparinux are both administered subcutaneously, it is typically favored to transition to an oral anticoagulant.

VKAs, LMWH, fondaparinux, and direct oral anticoagulants (DOACs) may be used to provide long-term anticoagulation [31]. The longest used

agent is warfarin, a VKA. Warfarin was previously preferred due to time-proven efficacy, oral administration, reversibility, and low cost. However, periodic lab testing, narrow therapeutic window, need for dosage adjustments, and its interactions with many drugs and foods may limit its use [31]. When using warfarin for long-term anticoagulation, initial therapy should be continued for a minimum of 5 days and at least 24 h after the patient's international normalized ratio (INR) is above 2.0. The initial subcutaneous or IV therapy provides adequate anticoagulation, while the vitamin K-dependent clotting factors are depleted. The goal INR value for treatment is 2.5, with an acceptable range of 2.0–3.0 [28, 31]. Various tables and algorithms are available to guide warfarin dosing based on INR testing. One such validated protocol suggests monthly INR testing for patients within their therapeutic window, and weekly testing for those outside of this range, which is supported by groups like the American Society of Hematology [37].

LMWH is also a viable option with similar efficacy and risk profile when compared to warfarin for long-term anticoagulation [41]. LMWH is advantageous due to its ease of dosing, wide therapeutic window, no need to monitor, and fewer drug/food interactions compared to warfarin. However, it is also more expensive than warfarin, more difficult to reverse, requires subcutaneous dosing, and carries a risk of drug-induced osteoporosis. LMWH is preferred in patients with malignancy for long-term treatment by most guidelines [28, 37]. Fondaparinux is a subcutaneous agent that is similar to LMWH in use and may also be used in long-term treatment [31, 37].

DOACs are quickly becoming the treatment of choice for long-term anticoagulation as evidence supports their effectiveness compared to warfarin for long-term therapy [35, 36, 42]. Also, most current guidelines recommend these as first-line treatment for VTE that is not associated with malignancy due to continued evidence demonstrating their safety and efficacy [28]. Compared with LMWH treatment followed by long-term VKA treatment, DOACs are non-inferior for recurrent VTE and have a lower risk of major bleeding [43]. Meta-analyses have also

Table 4 VTE treatment options [2, 28, 31, 33, 43]

Parenteral anticoagulants

Agent	Mechanism	Dosing	Half-life	Metabolism	Antidote	Monitoring	Miscellaneous
Heparin	Binds antithrombin	IV: 80 U/kg bolus, then 18 u/kg/h (adjust w/ aPTT) SC: 333 U/kg, then 250 u/kg q12 h	90 min	Depolymerization	Protamine	aPTT (1.5–2.0 × Normal)	
LMWH (enoxaparin)	Binds antithrombin	SC: 1 mg/kg BID (daily if CrCl<30); 1.5 mg/kg daily (BMI < 30)	3–4 h	Depolymerization, desulphation	Protamine	None required	Max dose 180 mg/day
LMWH (Dalteparin)	Binds antithrombin	SC: 100 U/kg q12h or 200 U/kg once daily	3–4 h	Depolymerization, desulphation	Protamine	Anti-Xa levels if CrCl <30 mL/mm	Max dose 18,000 U/day
Fondaparinux	Indirect factor Xa inhibitor	SC: 5.0 mg daily (<50 kg); 7.5 mg daily (50–100 kg); 10 mg daily (>100 kg)	17–21 h	Insignificant	None	None required	CrCl 30–50 mL/min, use with caution; if CrCl<30 mL/min: use alternative agent.

Oral anticoagulants

Agent	Mechanism	Dosing	Half-life	Drug interactions	Antidote	Monitoring	Parenteral anticoagulation	Miscellaneous
Vitamin K antagonist (warfarin)	Indirect thrombin inhibition	Initial dose 5–10 mg daily, changes based on INR	36 h	CYP2C9, CYP1A2, CYP3A4	Vitamin K	INR (2.0–3.0)	Initially required, 5–10 days	Ok in patients with CrCl<30 mL/min and those on potent P-glycoprotein inhibitors or CYP450 3A4 inhibitors or inducers.

Drug	Class	Dosing	Half-life	Metabolism/interactions	Reversal agent	Monitoring	Parenteral bridging	Renal considerations
Dabigatran[a]	Direct thrombin inhibitor	150 mg BID; CrCl 30–50 or age > 75 yo: 110 mg BID; CrCl 15–30: 75 mg BID	14–17 h	P-glycoprotein inducers/inhibitors	Idarucizumab	None required	Initially required, 5–10 days	CrCl <15, not defined
Apixaban[a,b]	Factor Xa inhibitor	10 mg BID for 7 days, then 5 mg BID. 2.5 mg BID if treating beyond 6 mos	8–12 h	CYP3A4/5. P-glycoprotein inducers/inhibitors	Andexanet alfa	None required	None required	2.5 mg BID if at least 1 criterion is met: Serum Cr ≥ 1.5 mgdL, age 80 yo, weight 60 kg or less
Rivaroxaban[a,b]	Factor Xa inhibitor	15 mg BID for 21 days, then 20 mg daily (15 mg daily if CrCl 15–50). 10 mg daily if treating beyond	7–11 h	CYP3A4, CYP2J2, P-glycoprotein inducers/inhibitors	Andexanet alfa	None required	None required	If CrCl <30, consider alternative agent.
Edoxaban[a,b]	Factor Xa inhibitor	30 mg (if ≤60 kg, or CrCl 15–50) or 60 mg daily (if >60 kg & CrCl >50)	6–11 h	P-glycoprotein inducers/inhibitors	None	None required	Initially required, 5–10 days	CrCl <15, consider alternative agent

aPTT activated partial thromboplastin time, *BID* twice daily, *BMI* body mass index, *CrCl* Creatinine clearance (mL/min), *INR* international normalized ratio, *IV* intravenous, *SC* subcutaneous

[a]Limited data in those with creatinine clearance (CrCl) less than 30, antiphospholipid syndrome, heparin-induced thrombocytopenia, BMI >40 kg/m^2, or VTE at unusual sites

[b]Generally avoided if concurrent use of azole antimycotics (e.g., ketoconazole), certain protease inhibitors (e.g., ritonavir), and antiepileptic drugs (e.g., carbamazepine & phenytoin). Note: information on conversion to and from DOACs and warfarin can be found in reference [31] (eTable A). https://www.aafp.org/afp/2017/0301/hi-res/afp20170301p295-ta.gif (Accessed March 1, 2020)

shown good tolerability in elderly patients [44]. In addition, as mentioned above, evidence for DOACs effectiveness and safety for treatment of VTE in patients with cancer is growing [38–40].

Length of Therapy and Extended Anticoagulation

The length of therapy for anticoagulation depends upon the clinical picture surrounding the VTE with the standard length of anticoagulation therapy being at least 3 months. Anticoagulation that lasts for 3–6 months is considered "long-term anticoagulation," whereas anticoagulation extending beyond 3–6 months without a scheduled stop date is considered "extended anticoagulation" [2]. The decision to extend therapy beyond 3 months is based on balancing the benefits of treatment (i.e., reduction in VTE recurrence based on patient risk factors) and the risks of treatment (i.e., increased bleeding) [2, 31]. For provoked VTE (i.e., a VTE with a known cause such as surgery or non-surgical risk factors), whether a DVT of the leg or PE, anticoagulation can be stopped after 3 months as long as there is no recurrence. For those with unprovoked VTE, the decision to extend anticoagulation beyond 3 months should be based on their bleeding risk. If they have a low or moderate bleeding risk, extended therapy (no scheduled stop date) is preferred. If they have a high bleeding risk, 3 months of therapy is preferred [28, 33]. Reasons to treat for longer than 6 months include those with a first or second unprovoked PE or proximal DVT of the leg, patients with active cancer and VTE, or those with genetic thrombophilias, so long as they are at low or moderate risk of bleeding [28, 31]. Prediction models for quantifying bleeding risk like the HAS-BLED or VTE-BLEED scores can be used to help the clinician stratify bleeding risk [33]. For extended therapy with DOACs beyond 6 months, current guidelines recommend the use of the prophylactic doses of apixaban and rivaroxaban (2.5 mg twice per day and 10 mg daily, respectively) [2, 33].

Additional Therapy

Daily low-dose aspirin (~100 mg) after the initial anticoagulation treatment period may be considered, particularly in patients on extended anticoagulation who elect to stop anticoagulation [28, 33]. Pooled results of the randomized, multicenter WARFASA and ASPIRE trials showed a 32% reduction in the rate of recurrence of VTE in patients receiving aspirin following anticoagulation therapy [45]. The use of compression stockings can be justified to lessen symptoms of existing acute or chronic post-thrombotic syndrome (PTS), but are not recommended for the use of prevention of PTS [28]. Inferior vena cava (IVC) filters are reserved for those with PE or proximal DVT and a contraindication to or a complication from anticoagulant treatment [28]. They have not been shown to reduce recurrent PE in previously anticoagulated patients who have additional risk factors for recurrence [33].

Prevention

Recognizing those factors that increase one's risk for VTE is essential for prevention. Extended or life-long anticoagulation may be appropriate for those with multiple risk factors. ▶ Chap. 55, "Athletic Injuries," discusses VTE prophylaxis for hospitalized and surgical patients in more detail.

Superficial Vein Thrombosis and Superficial Thrombophlebitis

Traditionally considered to be a more benign and self-limiting condition, thrombosis of the superficial venous system is often considered distinct from deep vein thrombosis and, as a result, studied less [46]. Superficial vein thrombosis (SVT) is currently the preferred term for a thrombus in the superficial vein system (especially the axial veins like the great and small saphenous veins), while the term superficial thrombophlebitis can more appropriately be used to describe confirmed thrombus accompanying phlebitis (inflammation within a vein) of the tributary veins. Phlebitis can develop for a variety of reasons including injury, infection, or thrombus [47]. The distinction between SVT and superficial thrombophlebitis is important because thrombosis of axial veins can lead to thromboembolism, especially if the proximal aspect of the larger axial veins is affected [46]. Patients with superficial venous thrombosis are at higher risk of developing DVT [31].

The risks for developing SVT and superficial thrombophlebitis are similar to those previously described for VTE (Table 1) and include advanced age, obesity, active cancer, previous thromboembolic episodes, pregnancy, oral contraceptive use, hormone replacement therapy, recent surgery, autoimmune diseases, and varicose veins (this last one being unique to SVT) [46]. Phlebitis and thrombosis of the lower extremities are more likely to occur in varicose veins, which account for over 60% of SVT cases, while lack of physical activity and trauma are among the risk factors for the development of a clot in varicosities [48]. The most consistent risk factor for developing phlebitis or thrombosis of the upper extremities involves the use of venous cannulation, and while this discussion focuses more on lower extremity conditions, the same principles may be applied to the upper extremities with regard to SVT [49]. Saphenous vein thrombosis is thought to be more common than DVT, and the great saphenous vein is more commonly involved than the small saphenous vein [48, 49].

On exam, one can expect to find pain, redness, and swelling along the path of a superficial vein [48]. If a thrombus is present, it may appear as a thickened cord, especially if it persists when the extremity is raised, and may be accompanied by low-grade fever. High fever or redness extending significantly past the margin of the vein should prompt evaluation for suppurative infection, and is usually associated with invasive procedures [46]. Superficial thrombus is usually identified with the use of duplex ultrasound, which will also help to identify whether DVT is present; however, some favor a period of observation in isolated findings of thrombophlebitis remote from the great and small saphenous veins [46].

Patients with isolated uncomplicated phlebitis not involving the saphenous veins, with no other risk factors for DVT, can be treated symptomatically with repeat evaluation in 7–10 days. Treatment depends on several variables, including size, location, and severity of symptoms [46]. For the management of uncomplicated thrombi at low risk for VTE (>5 cm from the saphenofemoral or saphenopopliteal junction, <5 cm in length, and no other risk factors), supportive therapy with elevation of the affected extremity, cool/warm compresses, non-steroidal anti-inflammatory drugs (NSAIDS), encouraging patient mobility, and possibly compression stockings in appropriate candidates are preferred initial therapies [46]. Most uncomplicated cases respond to supportive care within a few days and pain usually resolves in a week. Ultrasound should be performed if extension does occur, and the thrombosed vessel may still be palpable for months after resolution of pain [46, 50].

For higher-risk thrombi (i.e., SVT ≤5 cm from the saphenofemoral or saphenopopliteal junction, a thrombosed segment ≥5 cm in length, or other medical risk factors for VTE), anticoagulation should be considered [46]. Suggested therapies include subcutaneous fondaparinux (2.5 mg daily), subcutaneous low-molecular-weight heparin (enoxaparin 40 mg daily), or oral rivaroxaban (10 mg daily) for 45 days [46, 50]. If anticoagulation is not possible, or if thrombus recurs, ligation or excision may be needed to prevent extension. Antibiotics should be used only if signs of infection are present [46].

References

1. Stein PD, Matta F. Epidemiology and incidence: the scope of the problem and risk factors for development of venous thromboembolism. Clin Chest Med. 2010;31:611–28.
2. Tritschler T, Kraaijpoel N, Le Gal G, Wells PS. Venous thromboembolism: advances in diagnosis and treatment. JAMA. 2018;320(15):1583–94.
3. Bagot CN, Arya R. Virchow and his triad: a question of attribution. Br J Haematol. 2008;143(2):180.
4. Folsom AR, Lutsey PL, Astor BC, et al. C-reactive protein and venous thromboembolism: a prospective

investigation in the ARIC cohort. Thromb Haemost. 2009;102:615–9.

5. Joffe HV, Kucher N, Tapson VF, et al. Upper-extremity deep vein thrombosis: a prospective registry of 592 patients. Circulation. 2004;110:1605–11.

6. Heit JA. The epidemiology of venous thromboembolism in the community. Arterioscler Thromb Vasc Biol. 2008;28:370–2.

7. Cushman M. Epidemiology and risk factors for venous thrombosis. Semin Hematol. 2007;44(2):62–9.

8. Connors JM. Thrombophilia testing and venous thrombosis. N Engl J Med. 2017;377:1177–87.

9. Heit JA, Spencer FA, White RH. The epidemiology of venous thromboembolism. J Thromb Thrombolysis. 2016;41:3–14.

10. Centers for Disease Control and Prevention. Venous thromboembolism (blood clots). Data and statistics. February 7, 2020. http://www.cdc.gov/ncbddd/dvt/data.html. Accessed 20 Mar 2020.

11. Piccioli A, Falanga A, Baccaglini U, et al. Cancer and venous thromboembolism. Semin Thromb Hemost. 2006;32:694–9.

12. Wilbur J, Shian B. Diagnosis of deep venous thrombosis and pulmonary embolism. Am Fam Physician. 2012;86:913–9.

13. Wells P, Anderson D. The diagnosis and treatment of venous thromboembolism. Hematol Am Soc Hematol Educ Program. 2013;2013:457–63.

14. Wells PS, Ihaddadene R, Reilly A, Forgie MA. Diagnosis of venous thromboembolism: 20 years of progress. Ann Intern Med. 2018;168:131–40.

15. Lim W, LeGal G, Bates SM, et al. American Society of Hematology 2018 guidelines for management of venous thromboembolism: diagnosis of venous thromboembolism. Blood Adv. 2018;2(22):3226–56.

16. Wells PS, Anderson DR, Rodgers M, et al. Derivation of a simple clinical model to categorize patients' probability of pulmonary embolism: increasing the model's utility with simpliRED D-dimer. Thromb Haemost. 2000;83:416–20.

17. Ten Cate-Hoek AJ, Prins MH. Management studies using a combination of D-dimer test result and clinical probability to rule out venous thromboembolism: a systematic review. J Thromb Haemost. 2005;3:2465–70.

18. Kline JA. Diagnosis and exclusion of pulmonary embolism. Thromb Res. 2018;163:207–20.

19. Singh B, Mommer SK, Erwin PJ, et al. Pulmonary embolism rule-out criteria (PERC) in pulmonary embolism–revisited: a systematic review and meta-analysis. Emerg Med J. 2013;30(9):701–6.

20. van Es N, Kraaijpoel N, Klok FA, et al. The original and simplified Wells rules and age-adjusted D-dimer testing to rule out pulmonary embolism: an individual patient data meta-analysis. J Thromb Haemost. 2017;15:678–84.

21. Righini M, Van Es J, Den Exter PL, et al. Age-adjusted d-dimer cutoff levels to rule out pulmonary embolism: the ADJUST-PE study. JAMA. 2014;311(11):1117–24.

22. Stein PD, Fowler SE, Goodman LR, PIOPED II Investigators, et al. Multidetector computed tomography for acute pulmonary embolism. N Engl J Med. 2006;354:2317–27.

23. Remy-Jardin M, Pistolesi M, Goodman LR, et al. Management of suspected acute pulmonary embolism in the era of CT angiography: a statement from the Fleischner society. Radiology. 2007;245:315–29.

24. Bajc M, Schümichen C, Grüning T, et al. EANM guideline for ventilation/perfusion single photon emission computed tomography (SPECT) for diagnosis of pulmonary embolism and beyond. Eur J Nucl Med Mol Imaging. 2019;46(12):2429–2451.

25. Phillips JJ, Straiton J, Staff RT. Planar and SPECT ventilation/perfusion imaging and computed tomography for the diagnosis of pulmonary embolism: a systematic review and meta-analysis of the literature, and cost and dose comparison. Eur J Radiol. 2015;84 (7):1392–400.

26. van Beek EJ, Brouwerst EM, Song B, et al. Clinical validity of a normal pulmonary angiogram in patients with suspected pulmonary embolism – a critical review. Clin Radiol. 2001;56(10):838–42.

27. Stein PD, Chenevert TL, Fowler SE, et al. Gadolinium-enhanced magnetic resonance angiography for pulmonary embolism: a multicenter prospective study (PIOPED III). Ann Intern Med. 2010;152(7):434. W143.

28. Kearon C, Akl EA, Ornelas J, et al. Antithrombotic therapy for VTE disease: CHEST guideline. Chest. 2016;149:315–52.

29. Jeff MR, McMurtry MS, Archer SL, et al. Management of massive and submassive pulmonary embolism, Iliofemoral deep vein thrombosis, chronic thromboembolic pulmonary hypertension: a scientific statement from the American Heart Association. Circulation. 2011;123:1788–830.

30. Watson L, Broderick C, Armon MP. Thrombolysis for acute deep vein thrombosis. Cochrane Database Syst Rev 2016;11:CD002783.

31. Wilbur J, Shian B. Deep venous thrombosis and pulmonary embolism: current therapy. Am Fam Physician. 2017;95(5):295–302.

32. Büller HR, Davidson BL, Decousus H, Matisse Investigators, et al. Fondaparinux or enoxaparin for the initial treatment of symptomatic deep venous thrombosis: a randomized trial. Ann Intern Med. 2004;140 (11):867–73.

33. Konstantinides SV, Meyer G, Becattini C, et al. 2019 ESC guidelines for the diagnosis and management of acute pulmonary embolism developed in collaboration with the European Respiratory Society (ERS). Eur Heart J. 2020;41:543–603.

34. Raschke RA, Reilly BM, Guidry JR, et al. The weight-based heparin dosing nomogram compared with a "standard care" nomogram. A randomized controlled trial. Ann Intern Med. 1993;119(9):874.

35. Bauersachs R, Berkowitz SD, Brenner B, EINSTEIN Investigators, et al. Oral rivaroxaban for symptomatic venous thromboembolism. N Engl J Med. 2010;363 (26):2499–510.

36. Agnelli G, Buller HR, Cohen A, AMPLIFY Investigators, et al. Oral apixaban for the treatment of acute venous thromboembolism. N Engl J Med. 2013;369(9):799.

37. Witt DM, Nieuwlaat R, Clark NP, et al. American Society of Hematology 2018 guidelines for management of venous thromboembolism: optimal management of anticoagulation therapy. Blood Adv. 2018;2(22):3257–91.

38. Raskob GE, van Es N, Verhamme P, Hokusai VTE Cancer Investigators, et al. Edoxaban for the treatment of cancer-associated venous thromboembolism. N Engl J Med. 2018;378(7):615–24.

39. Young AM, Marshall A, Thirlwall J, et al. Comparison of an oral factor Xa inhibitor with low molecular weight heparin in patients with cancer with venous thromboembolism: results of a randomized trial (SELECT-D). J Clin Oncol. 2018;36:2017–23.

40. Agnelli G, Becattini C, Meyer G, et al. Apixaban for the treatment of venous thromboembolism associated with Cancer. N Engl J Med. 2020; https://doi.org/10.1056/NEJMoa1915103.

41. Andras A, Sala Tenna A, Crawford F. Vitamin K antagonists or low-molecular-weight heparin for the long term treatment of symptomatic venous thromboembolism. Cochrane Database Syst Rev. 2012;10: CD002001.

42. Schulman S, Kearon C, Kakkar AK, RE-COVER Study Group, et al. Dabigatran versus warfarin in the treatment of acute venous thromboembolism. N Engl J Med. 2009;361(24):2342–52.

43. Kakkos SK, Kirkilesis GI, Tsolakis IA. Efficacy & safety of the new oral anticoagulants dabigatran, rivaroxaban, apixaban, & edoxaban in the treatment and secondary prevention of venous thromboembolism: systemic review & meta-analysis. Eur J Vasc Endovasc Surg. 2014;48(5):565–75.

44. Geldhof V, Vandenbriele C, Verhamme P, et al. Venous thromboembolism in the elderly: efficacy and safety of non-VKA oral anticoagulants. Thromb J. 2014;12:21.

45. Prandoni P, Noventa F, Milan M. Aspirin & recurrent venous thromboembolism. Phlebology. 2013;28(1):99–104.

46. Cosmi B. Management of superficial vein thrombosis. J Thromb Haemost. 2015;13(7):1175–83.

47. Di Nisio M, Wichers IM, Middeldorp S. Treatment for superficial thrombophlebitis of the leg. Cochrane Database Syst Rev. 2018;(2):CD004982. https://doi.org/10.1002/14651858.CD004982.pub6.

48. Litzendorf ME, Satiani B. Superficial venous thrombosis: disease progression and evolving treatment approaches. Vasc Health Risk Manag. 2011;7:569.

49. Decousus H, Quéré I, Presles E, POST Study Group, et al. Superficial venous thrombosis and venous thromboembolism: a large, prospective epidemiologic study. Ann Intern Med. 2010;152(4):218.

50. Decousus H, Prandoni P, Mismetti P, et al. Fondaparinux for the treatment of superficial-vein thrombosis in the legs. N Engl J Med. 2010;363(13):1222.

Selected Disorders of the Cardiovascular System

Philip T. Dooley and Emily M. Manlove

Contents

P. T. Dooley (✉)
Family Medicine Residency Program at Via Christi
Hospitals, University of Kansas School of Medicine,
Wichita, KS, USA
e-mail: philip.dooley@ascension.org;
pdooley@umich.edu

E. M. Manlove
Indiana University School of Medicine, Bloomington, IN,
USA
e-mail: emanlove@iu.edu

© Springer Nature Switzerland AG 2022
P. M. Paulman et al. (eds.), *Family Medicine*,
https://doi.org/10.1007/978-3-030-54441-6_89

Peripheral Artery Disease

The prevalence of peripheral artery disease (PAD) increases with age from <5% before age 60 to over 20% after age 74 with over 80% of PAD patients identified as current or former smokers [1]. Coronary artery disease (CAD) and cerebrovascular disease occur two to four times more often in patients with lower extremity PAD compared to those without PAD. The amputation rate in the general PAD population is 1% or less per year but is significantly more common in current smokers and diabetics (7–15-fold increase). Recent trials have reported a combined rate of myocardial infarction (MI), stroke, and vascular death of 4–6%, while epidemiological studies report annual mortality of 4–6%. Unfortunately, too few patients with PAD receive guideline-directed management and therapy (GDMT) to reduce morbidity and mortality from CAD and other cardiovascular diseases [2].

Presentation and Diagnosis

Intermittent claudication, defined as fatigue, discomfort, cramping, or pain that occurs in lower extremity muscle groups during exercise which is relieved by rest (in 10 min or less), is the presenting symptom in 10–35% of patients. Atypical lower extremity pain (including numbness, tingling, or paresthesia) is the presenting symptom in 40–50% of cases, although in many of these patients, PAD is an incidental finding and not the cause of their leg pain. When combined with cases found through screening, 20–50% of patients are asymptomatic from their PAD at the time of diagnosis. Acute limb ischemia (ALI), where symptoms are present for less than 2 weeks, is characterized by the 6 "Ps": pain, paralysis, paresthesias, pulselessness,

pallor, and poikilothermia. ALI represents a medical emergency which is subdivided into three severities: viable (no immediate threat), threatened, and irreversible (major tissue loss or permanent nerve damage is inevitable). Critical limb ischemia (CLI) includes chronic rest pain ($\geq$2 weeks), nonhealing ulcers/wounds, or gangrene due to occlusive arterial disease. CLI is the presentation in 1–2% of cases, and after 1 year only 50% will be alive with both legs (25% will die and 25% will have at least one amputation). Additional signs on physical exam include diminished pulses and vascular bruits, while dependent rubor, early pallor when elevating the limb, reduced capillary refill, hair loss, and muscle wasting are signs of chronic ischemia. Arterial ulcerations are typically quite painful unless neuropathy is also present as can occur in patients with concomitant diabetes mellitus.

A resting ankle-brachial index (ABI) in both legs is recommended for diagnosis of lower extremity PAD and should be reported as follows: noncompressible >1.40, normal 1.00 to 1.40, borderline 0.91 to 0.99, or abnormal $\leq$0.90 [2]. A toe-brachial index should be used in patients with noncompressible vessels ($\leq$0.70 diagnoses PAD). Patients with typical exertional claudication and a normal or borderline resting ABI should complete an exercise treadmill ABI. Further imaging is reserved for patients in whom revascularization is considered or who continue to experience lifestyle-limiting claudication despite GDMT. Anatomic assessment may be completed with duplex ultrasound (which localizes diseased segments and grades lesion severity), MR angiography (especially good for evaluation of arterial dissection and wall morphology), or CT angiography (when MR is contraindicated). Invasive angiography is often the first-line choice for patients with CLI but remains a second-line choice for patients without CLI if they are candidates for revascularization.

Differential Diagnosis

Atherosclerosis is the most common cause of PAD, just as it is for CAD and stroke. Lower extremity PAD may also be caused by thromboembolism, trauma, vasculitis, physiological entrapment syndromes, fibromuscular dysplasia, or congenital abnormalities [2]. The differential considerations for claudication include neurogenic claudication (due to lumbar disk disease, spinal stenosis, or osteophytic changes), osteoarthritis (hip, foot, or ankle), severe venous obstructive disease, chronic compartment syndrome, symptomatic Baker's cyst, or shin splints (in younger persons). The differential considerations for nonhealing wounds include trauma, infection, malignancy, autoimmune injury, drug reactions, neuropathic, microangiopathy, or venous ulceration.

Intervention

Atherosclerotic cardiovascular disease (ASCVD) risk factors, including hypertension and diabetes, should be managed according to current evidence-based guidelines [2]. Statins are recommended for all patients with PAD. Tobacco cessation is essential, and pharmacologic therapies should be combined with behavioral treatment if there are no contraindications. Antiplatelet therapy (aspirin 75–325 mg or clopidogrel 75 mg daily) is recommended for all patients with PAD to decrease the risk of myocardial infarction, ischemic stroke, and vascular death. Vorapaxar (2.5 mg daily with aspirin or clopidogrel), a novel antiplatelet agent which is contraindicated in patients with a history of transient-ischemic attack or stroke, and rivaroxaban (2.5 mg BID with low dose aspirin) are also FDA approved for patients with both PAD and CAD; however, their use is limited by an increased risk of bleeding complications [3]. Supervised exercise training for a minimum of 30–45 minutes, three times per week for at least 12 weeks, improves intermittent claudication [2]. Cilostazol (100 mg twice per day) is the first-line pharmacologic treatment for claudication in the absence of heart failure (HF). Pentoxifylline is no longer recommended as a second-line therapy since the evidence now shows that it has no benefit. Oral vasodilator prostaglandins, vitamin E, chelation therapy, and homocysteine lowering with B-complex vitamins should also not be used to treat PAD. While warfarin anticoagulation should not be used to decrease the risk of cardiovascular ischemic events, it may have a role in improving graft patency. Consultation for surgical or endovascular revascularization is indicated for occupation or lifestyle-limiting symptoms where nonsurgical therapy has failed or for signs or symptoms of ischemia at rest.

Pericarditis

Acute pericarditis is an inflammation of the pericardium, the avascular fibrous sac that surrounds the heart. Constrictive pericarditis is a term reserved for post-inflammatory changes affecting the pericardium, resulting in impaired diastolic filling of the heart. Acute pericarditis is relatively common and accounts for 5% of emergency room admissions for chest pain [4]. Some cases are mild and patients may not present for medical care; others can be life-threatening. There are numerous etiologies of pericardial inflammation (Table 1). In developed countries, 80–90% of cases are idiopathic, as no specific cause is found after routine evaluation. These cases are typically thought to be viral in origin. The remaining cases are most often found to be related to post-cardiac injury syndromes, autoimmune disease, and malignancy. Tuberculosis remains the leading cause of pericardial disease in the developing world.

Presentation and Diagnosis

Patients typically present with chest pain. The pain is often sharp, severe, retrosternal, exacerbated with breathing, and relieved with sitting

Table 1 Etiologies of pericarditis

Infectious
Viral: Coxsackievirus, echovirus, Epstein-Barr virus, cytomegalovirus, adenovirus, parvovirus B19, human herpesvirus 6
Bacterial: Tuberculosis, *Coxiella burnetii*, rare other bacteria (pneumococcus, meningococcus, gonococcus, haemophilus, streptococcus, staphylococcus, chlamydia, mycoplasma, legionella, leptospira, listeria)
Fungal: Histoplasma (more likely in immunocompetent patients), aspergillus, *Blastomyces*, candida (more likely in immunosuppressed patients)
Parasitic: *Echinococcus*, toxoplasma (overall very rare)
Autoimmune
Pericardial injury syndromes: Post-myocardial infarction syndrome, post-pericardiotomy syndrome
Connective tissue diseases: Systemic lupus erythematosus, Sjögren syndrome, rheumatoid arthritis, systemic sclerosis, systemic vasculitides, Behçet's syndrome, sarcoidosis, amyloidosis
Autoimmune diseases: Familial Mediterranean fever, tumor necrosis factor receptor-associated periodic syndrome (TRAPS)
Neoplastic
Primary tumors: Pericardial mesothelioma (overall rare)
Secondary metastatic tumors: Lung cancer, breast cancer, lymphoma
Other
Trauma: Blunt chest trauma, penetrating thoracic injury, esophageal perforation, radiation
Metabolic: Uremia, myxedema (rare)
Drugs: Lupus-like syndrome (procainamide, hydralazine, isoniazid, phenytoin), hypersensitivity pericarditis with eosinophilia (penicillins), direct toxic effects (doxorubicin and daunorubicin; often associated with cardiomyopathy)

Source: Little and Freeman [5]

forward. This pain may mimic other diagnoses. Acute pericarditis is diagnosed if at least two of four key findings are present: chest pain consistent with pericarditis, pericardial friction rub ("Velcro-like" sounds heard best at the apex), typical electrocardiogram (ECG) changes (diffuse upsloping ST elevation with PR depression), or significant pericardial effusion (seen on echocardiogram) [4]. The auscultative and electrographic signs may be transient, and repeated examination may be warranted.

Patients with pericarditis may report a viral prodrome. Many have sinus tachycardia and low-grade fever. Signs of systemic inflammation commonly arise, such as elevated white blood cell count, erythrocyte sedimentation rate (ESR), and C-reactive protein (CRP). Troponin may be elevated. Rarely, patients will present with cardiac tamponade and likely will have chest pain and dyspnea. Exam shows jugular venous distention, muffled heart sounds, hypotension, and a paradoxical pulse.

Once the diagnosis of pericarditis is confirmed, the next step is to search for the cause of inflammation. This can be tailored to the patient's presentation and history, to identify possible treatable or life-threatening etiologies outlined in Table 1. Diagnostic pericardiocentesis is typically done only for large effusions. If the diagnosis is not confirmed, but clinical suspicion remains for pericarditis, routine lab evaluation can be done with frequent reexamination and repeat ECG. At times, CT or MRI is used to show pericardial thickening.

Differential Diagnosis

Differential considerations for acute pericarditis include most cardiac syndromes. This includes acute myocardial infarction (AMI), pulmonary embolus, aortic dissection, cardiac contusion, and myocarditis. Consideration must also be given to the other structures in the thorax, to include mediastinitis, esophageal spasm, esophagitis, gastroesophageal reflux, costochondritis, and pneumonia. The ECG changes of pericarditis may be confused with early repolarization [4]. Often the most difficult distinction to make is between acute pericarditis and AMI. Cardiac catheterization may be performed. There will be a lack of angiographic evidence of CAD in cases of acute pericarditis.

Intervention

Initial management of acute pericarditis focuses on treating the underlying cause, if possible. Otherwise, most idiopathic or viral pericarditis resolves spontaneously or with simple, first-line treatment. Nonsteroidal anti-inflammatory drugs (NSAIDs) and colchicine are the basis of the treatment regimen. Often aspirin is used, especially in post-MI patients, but at higher anti-inflammatory doses (650 mg every 6 h) [5]. Indomethacin (50 mg every 8 h) and ibuprofen (600 mg every 8 h) can also be used. NSAIDs can be discontinued or tapered after 7–10 days if the patient's pain is resolved. Some clinicians use the CRP level to guide discontinuation. A proton-pump inhibitor is often used in conjunction for gastric protection. Colchicine (0.5 mg twice daily if weight >70 kg, once daily if weight <70 kg) is used in addition to NSAIDs to decrease the likelihood of persistent symptoms and the risk of recurrent pericarditis [4]. Colchicine is typically continued for 3 months. Corticosteroids do have strong anti-inflammatory properties, but their use is associated with an increased chance of recurrence. They may be required in refractory cases. Patient's lacking high-risk indicators can be managed in the outpatient setting (Table 2). Bacterial pericarditis, while rare, can be life-threatening. In addition to antibiotics, intrapericardial fibrinolysis can be effective to prevent evolution to constrictive pericarditis.

Adequate treatment of acute pericarditis is key to prevent recurrent pericarditis or constrictive pericarditis. If symptoms recur, NSAID therapy should be reinstated. Colchicine should be added if it was not used in the initial case. The most significant complication of acute pericarditis is constrictive pericarditis. Since diastolic filling of the heart is impaired by a fibrotic pericardium, patients develop symptoms of HF and fluid overload. If the initial case of acute pericarditis was not recognized, the diagnosis may not be initially clear. At times the constriction is transient, but

Table 2 Predictors of poor outcome in pericarditis

Fever >38 °C
Symptoms developing over several weeks in association with an immunosuppressed state
Traumatic pericarditis
Pericarditis in a patient receiving oral anticoagulants
Large pericardial effusion (>20 mm echo-free space or evidence of tamponade)
Failure to respond to nonsteroidal anti-inflammatory drugs

Source: Little and Freeman [5]

patients often require pericardiectomy for treatment.

Bacterial Endocarditis

Infectious endocarditis (IE) is an infection of the endocardial surface mainly due to bacteria but rarely may be caused by fungi and protozoa [6]. Bacterial endocarditis (BE) may give rise to the classic though not universally found lesion of IE: the valvular vegetation. These vegetations may interfere with valvular function leading to HF and may embolize to produce a wide variety of focal and systemic signs and symptoms. The overall incidence of IE in the United States has risen to 13 cases per 100,000 patient-years, with a slight male predominance (58%) and a median age of 61 years [7, 8]. While valvular disease is still a major risk factor, it is now uncommonly due to rheumatic heart disease, having dropped from 50% of cases to less than 5% over the last 40 years. Untreated BE is almost uniformly fatal; therefore, if BE is suspected, aggressive evaluation and treatment, to include early surgery in some cases, are essential. In-hospital mortality rates have been stable over the past 25 years at 15–20% with 1-year mortality of almost 40%.

Effective management of BE relies on targeting treatment to specific organisms. Gram-positive bacteria (predominantly *streptococci*, *staphylococci*, and *enterococci*) are the most common cause of IE and now account for over 90% of the cases with a known organism, in part due to an increasing incidence of *Staphylococcus aureus* [7]. Fungal, protozoal, and gram-negative causes increase with prosthetic valve endocarditis (PVE) and other invasive cardiovascular devices [6]. The HACEK group (*Haemophilus* species, *Actinobacillus actinomycetemcomitans*, *Cardiobacterium hominis*, *Eikenella corrodens*, and *Kingella kingae*) occurs in 2% of cases worldwide. Intravenous drug users (IVDUs) have a very high incidence of right-sided valvular involvement, especially the tricuspid valve which is uncommon in non-IVDUs. Nosocomial BE is most commonly related to indwelling catheters or invasive procedures. BE caused by HACEK most commonly occurs in native valve, non-IVDUs.

Presentation and Diagnosis

Though the primary lesion in BE is in the heart itself, many of its presenting signs and symptoms reflect the systemic nature of the disease [6]. Fever, myalgias, fatigue, headache, and abdominal pain are common in all types of BE. Heart failure is the most common complication and develops in approximately 30% of cases. Vegetations can embolize to almost any location, causing distant infection or infarction. Right-sided embolic events may lead to specific complaints of chest pain, cough, and hemoptysis. Left-sided embolic events can present as mental status changes, stroke, myocardial infarction, splenic infarction, and renal abscess. Stroke occurs in approximately 9–13% of patients, while myocardial infarction occurs in 3–7% of cases [7]. Other complications of BE include osteomyelitis, septic arthritis, and mycotic aneurysms.

With the exception of Janeway lesions, which occur in only 5% of cases, few physical findings are highly specific for BE. Likewise, Roth's spots (2%), Osler's nodes (3%), splinter hemorrhages (8%), and splenomegaly (11%) are relatively uncommon since the diagnosis of IE is now occurring earlier in the clinical course [7, 8]. Cardiac murmurs are most often regurgitant with a new murmur occurring 48% of the time and worsening of an old murmur is present in an additional 20% of cases. With the exception of blood cultures, laboratory evaluation is frequently of less value

in making the early diagnosis of BE compared to the history and examination. Antibiotic therapy should not be given prior to blood culture collection, particularly in patients with known valvular heart disease and an unexplained fever [8, 9]. Antimicrobial therapy can be delayed in patients with a chronic or subacute presentation to allow for the collection of three sets of blood cultures from peripheral sites with the first and third drawn at least 1 h apart from each other [6]. At least two, but preferably three, sets of blood cultures separated by 30 min should be obtained from patients who present in severe sepsis or septic shock. Other laboratory findings and imaging may reflect other complications as mentioned above. Blood culture negative IE (as high as 31% of IE) may require serologic testing or PCR of surgical specimens to identify the causative organism [9]. ECG may reveal conduction abnormalities, indicating the extension of an aortic valve infection to a valve ring abscess, which carries a worse prognosis.

The 1994 Duke criteria were modified in 2000 to redefine "possible IE" (reducing the number of patients in this category) and modify the major and minor criteria (increasing the sensitivity) [10]. The diagnosis of "definite IE" is arrived at either through one of two pathologic criteria or through one of several combinations of major and minor clinical criteria (Table 3). The clinical criteria emphasize two main areas: positive blood cultures and evidence of endocardial involvement (Table 4). The second major criterion takes advantage of both transthoracic echocardiography (TTE) and transesophageal echocardiography (TEE) as a safe yet highly sensitive means for identifying endocardial lesions. Guidance as to when TEE is preferred over TTE was added to the major criteria definitions as part of the modifications in 2000.

The Duke criteria have been extensively studied and found to have a sensitivity around 80% while maintaining a specificity of 92–99% [6, 8, 9]. These criteria have also been validated for both the adult and pediatric populations, as well as special groups such as those with PVE. However, since an adequate amount of clinical data must be collected before the Duke criteria can be applied, early empiric therapy should not

Table 3 Definition of infective endocarditis according to the modified Duke criteria, with modifications shown in boldface

Definite infective endocarditis
Pathologic criteria
Microorganisms demonstrated by culture or histologic examination of a vegetation, a vegetation that has embolized, or an intracardiac abscess specimen
Pathologic lesions; vegetation or intracardiac abscess confirmed by histologic examination showing active endocarditis
Clinical criteria[a]
2 major criteria
1 major criterion and 3 minor criteria
5 minor criteria
Possible infective endocarditis
1 major criterion and 1 minor criterion
3 minor criteria
Rejected
Firm alternate diagnosis explaining evidence of infective endocarditis
Resolution of infective endocarditis syndrome with antibiotic therapy for ≤4 days
No pathologic evidence of infective endocarditis at surgery or autopsy, with antibiotic therapy for ≤4 days
Does not meet criteria for possible infective endocarditis, as above

Source: Li et al. [10], "Proposed Modifications to the Duke Criteria for the Diagnosis of Infective Endocarditis," *Clinical Infectious Diseases*, 2000; 30:633–8, by permission of the Infectious Diseases Society of America
[a]See Table 4 for definitions of major and minor criteria

be delayed if IE is suspected. In this regard, the criteria are best used to assist in sculpting medical therapy and determining a need for surgical intervention.

Differential Diagnosis

Virtually any systemic infection should be considered in the differential diagnosis of IE. These include, but are not limited to, pneumonia, meningitis, pericarditis, abscess, osteomyelitis, tuberculosis, and pyelonephritis. Noninfectious etiologies to be considered include stroke, myocardial infarction, rheumatic fever, vasculitis, malignancy, and fever of unknown origin.

Intervention

Once the diagnosis of IE is suspected, antibiotic therapy should be instituted without delay after blood cultures are obtained [6, 9]. Because bacteria in valvular vegetations are relatively protected from host immune defenses, antibiotics chosen to treat IE must be bactericidal, and regimens for their administration must be aggressive and of adequate duration to completely eradicate the organism and prevent relapse. Empiric therapy should be guided by local resistance patterns, but as a general rule for all native valves and prosthetic valves greater than 12 months after surgery, treatment may begin with ampicillin-sulbactam (3.0 g IV q6h) and gentamicin (1.5 mg/kg IV/IM q12h or 1.0 mg/kg IV/IM q8h). In patients with a β-lactam allergy, vancomycin (15/mg IV q12h) and ciprofloxacin (400 mg IV q12h or 500 mg PO q12h) may replace ampicillin-sulbactam. Empiric therapy for prosthetic valves less than 12 months after surgery may begin with vancomycin (15 mg/kg IV q12h), gentamicin (1.5 mg/kg IV/IM q12h or 1.0 mg/kg IV/IM q8h), and rifampin (600 mg PO q12h). The full course of antibiotics is tailored to culture results with some native valve regimens as short as 2 weeks, while all PVE regimens last a minimum of 6 weeks (Tables 5 and 6).

At least two sets of blood cultures should be collected every 24–48 h until a negative culture is

Table 4 Definition of terms used in the modified Duke criteria for the diagnosis of infective endocarditis (IE) with modifications shown in boldface

Major criteria
Positive blood culture for IE
Typical microorganisms consistent with IE from 2 separate blood cultures:
Viridans streptococci, *Streptococcus bovis*, HACEK group, *Staphylococcus aureus*
Community-acquired enterococci, in the absence of a primary focus
Microorganism consistent with IE from persistently positive blood cultures, defined as follows:
At least 2 positive cultures of blood samples drawn >12 h apart
All of 3 or a majority of ≥4 separate cultures of blood (with first and last drawn at least 1 h apart)
Single positive blood culture for *Coxiella burnetii* or antiphase I IgG titer ≥1:800
Evidence of endocardial involvement
Echocardiogram positive for IE (TEE recommended in patients with prosthetic valves, rated at least "possible IE" by clinical criteria, or complicated IE [paravalvular abscess]; TTE as first test in other patients), defined as follows:
Oscillating intracardiac mass on valve or supporting structures, in the path of regurgitant jets, or on implanted material in the absence of an alternative anatomic explanation
Abscess
New partial dehiscence of prosthetic valve
New valvular regurgitation (worsening or change in preexisting murmur not sufficient)
Minor criteria
Predisposition: Predisposing heart condition or injection drug use
Fever: Temperature >38 °C
Vascular phenomena: Major arterial emboli, septic pulmonary infarcts, mycotic aneurysm, intracranial hemorrhages, conjunctival hemorrhages, and Janeway lesions
Immunologic phenomena: Glomerulonephritis, Osler's nodes, Roth's spots, and rheumatoid factor
Microbiologic evidence: Positive blood culture but does not meet a major criterion as noted above[a] *or* serological evidence of active infection with organism consistent with IE
Echocardiographic minor criteria eliminated

Note: *TEE* transesophageal echocardiography, *TTE* transthoracic echocardiography
Source: Li et al. [10], "Proposed Modifications to the Duke Criteria for the Diagnosis of Infective Endocarditis," *Clinical Infectious Diseases*, 2000; 30:633–8, by permission of the Infectious Diseases Society of America
[a]Excludes single-positive cultures for coagulase-negative staphylococci and organisms that do not cause endocarditis

obtained. The first day of therapy for determining the duration of antibiotics is the day when blood cultures were initially negative (if initial cultures were positive). If a native valve is replaced or repaired with prosthetic material during the initial course of antibiotics, European guidelines recommend continuation of native valve treatment, while US guidelines now state that there is no consensus regarding regimen selection in this situation. If the resected tissue is culture positive, then the first day of a complete course for PVE should be the day of surgery (if blood cultures were negative before the operation). If the resected tissue is culture negative, the previously completed days of treatment can be subtracted from the total required duration of treatment. When multiple antibiotics are recommended, they should be given simultaneously or in short succession to maximize pharmacologic synergy.

Careful attention should be given to identifying and treating complications. HF in particular must be treated aggressively, since there is a dramatic worsening of prognosis as HF becomes more severe. Therapy of HF should be initiated with GDMT, but the timing of surgical intervention should be given particular emphasis as the mortality without surgery when HF is present may exceed 50%. To that end, early consultation with cardiovascular surgery, infectious disease, and cardiology is warranted for all patients with

Table 5 Antibiotic regimens for native valve endocarditis

Viridans group streptococci and *Streptococcus gallolyticus (bovis)* (highly penicillin susceptible: MIC ≤0.12 µg/mL)
Penicillin G IV or ceftriaxone IV/IM for 4 weeks[a]
[Penicillin G IV or ceftriaxone IV/IM] and gentamicin IV/IM for first 2 weeks[a,b]
Vancomycin IV for 4 weeks (with trough of 10–15 µg/mL)
Viridans group streptococci and *Streptococcus gallolyticus (bovis)* (relatively penicillin resistant: MIC >0.12 to ≤0.5 µg/mL)
Penicillin G IV for 4 weeks and gentamicin IV/IM for first 2 weeks[a]
Ceftriaxone IV/IM for 4 weeks if the isolate is susceptible
Vancomycin IV for 4 weeks (with trough of 10–15 µg/mL)
Viridans group streptococci (fully penicillin resistant: MIC >0.5 µg/mL), *Abiotrophia defectiva*, and *Granulicatella* species
Infectious disease consultation required to determine duration:
[Ampicillin IV or penicillin G IV] and gentamicin as done for *Enterococcus* species
Ceftriaxone IV/IM if the isolate is susceptible and gentamicin
Vancomycin IV (with trough of 10–15 µg/mL)
Streptococcus pneumoniae, *Streptococcus pyogenes*, groups B, C, F, and G β-hemolytic streptococci
Consult infectious disease as there is little published evidence to guide therapy
Staphylococci
Oxacillin-susceptible
Nafcillin IV (preferred if brain abscess also present) or oxacillin IV for 6 weeks
For 2 weeks for uncomplicated right-sided IE
Cefazolin IV for 6 weeks (in patients with non-anaphylactic penicillin reactions)
Vancomycin IV for 6 weeks (with trough of 10–20 µg/mL, in patients with immediate-type hypersensitive reactions to β-lactams)
Daptomycin IV for 6 weeks (in patients with immediate-type hypersensitive reactions to β-lactams; or for 2 weeks for uncomplicated right-sided IE)
Oxacillin-resistant
Vancomycin IV for 6 weeks (with trough of 10–20 µg/mL)
Daptomycin IV for 6 weeks (or for 2 weeks for uncomplicated right-sided IE)
Enterococcus susceptible to penicillin, vancomycin, and gentamicin or streptomycin
Gentamicin should be given in three divided doses, with peak of 3–4 µg/mL and trough of <1 µg/mL
[Ampicillin IV or penicillin G IV] and gentamicin IV/IM for 4 weeks (symptom duration <3 months)
[Ampicillin IV or penicillin G IV] and gentamicin IV/IM for 6 weeks (symptom duration ≥3 months)
Vancomycin IV (if unable to tolerate β-lactam; with trough of 10–20 µg/mL) and gentamicin IV/IM for 6 weeks
Ampicillin IV and ceftriaxone IV for 6 weeks (for patients with CrCl <50 mL/min, or if gentamicin resistant and rapid streptomycin serum concentrations not available)
Streptomycin may replace gentamicin, if isolate is sensitive to the former and resistant to the latter, with a peak of 20–35 µg/mL and a trough of <10 µg/mL
Enterococcus resistant to penicillin but susceptible to aminoglycoside and vancomycin
Gentamicin should be given in three divided doses, with peak of 3–4 µg/mL and trough of <1 µg/mL
β-lactamase-producing strain
Ampicillin-sulbactam IV and gentamicin IV/IM for 6 weeks
Vancomycin IV and gentamicin IV/IM for 6 weeks
Intrinsic penicillin resistance
Vancomycin IV and gentamicin IV/IM for 6 weeks
Enterococcus resistant to penicillin, aminoglycoside, and vancomycin
Linezolid IV/PO for >6 weeks
Daptomycin IV for >6 weeks
HACEK microorganisms
Ceftriaxone IV/IM for 4 weeks (cefotaxime or another 3rd-/4th-generation cephalosporin may be used)

(continued)

Table 5 (continued)

Ampicillin-sulbactam IV for 4 weeks
Ciprofloxacin IV/PO for 4 weeks (third-line treatment due to limited published in vivo evidence for IE; levofloxacin or moxifloxacin may be used)
Culture-negative endocarditis
Cefepime IV and vancomycin IV for acute presentations (days of symptoms)
Ampicillin-sulbactam IV and vancomycin IV for subacute presentations (weeks of symptoms)
Duration to be determined with infectious disease consultant

Source: Baddour et al. [6]

[a]Ampicillin is a reasonable alternative to penicillin if a penicillin shortage exists

[b]The 2-week regimen is not appropriate for patients with known abscesses, impaired 8th cranial nerve function, creatinine clearance <20 mL/min, or infection with *Abiotrophia, Granulicatella,* or *Gemella* species

suspected IE. Nearly 50% of patients will undergo surgical intervention, and in general, surgery should not be delayed because of active IE [6, 8]. Reinfection of newly implanted valves occurs in 2–3% of cases; however, surgery is associated with a marked reduction of in-hospital mortality. Indications for surgical intervention are listed in Table 7.

Patients who survive an episode of IE remain at increased risk for recurrent infection for the rest of their life. All patients should undergo a complete dental evaluation for the eradication of sources and education on the need for lifelong follow-up care with a dental professional. IVDUs should be referred to a drug treatment program. At the completion of therapy, all patients should have an echocardiogram repeated in order to establish a new baseline for valvular function and morphology. They should be educated on the signs and symptoms of IE and HF as well as any procedural antibiotic prophylaxis that may be needed in the future. Patients who were exposed to aminoglycosides are at risk for ototoxicity, and *Clostridium difficile* diarrhea may present up to 4 weeks after the last dose of antibiotics. All survivors of IE should have ≥3 sets of blood cultures drawn prior to starting antibiotics for a subsequent febrile illness.

Prevention

Prevention of IE in those with abnormal valvular architecture is covered in detail in ► Chap. 60, "Medical Care of the Surgical Patient." In those with normal native valves, prevention is mainly an issue of education on the avoidance of IV drug use.

Cardiomyopathy

The American Heart Association (AHA) published a scientific statement in 2006 which updated the definition and classification of the cardiomyopathies (CMs) [11]. The primary CMs mainly, or only, involve the heart muscle, while the myocardial dysfunction of the secondary CMs represents just one of the many organs damaged by a systemic disorder. This chapter focuses on the primary CMs which are further subdivided into three categories: genetic, mixed (genetic and nongenetic), and acquired. The AHA definition of the CMs specifically excludes myocardial dysfunction directly caused by other cardiovascular abnormalities such as systemic hypertension, valvular heart disease, congenital heart disease, and ischemia from ASCVD.

Most CMs present with the typical manifestations of either heart failure with reduced ejection fraction (HFrEF) or heart failure with preserved ejection fraction (HFpEF) [12]. Management of the CMs typically includes early consultation with a cardiologist well versed in the pertinent and complex issues surrounding diagnosis and treatment. Possible treatments include lifestyle changes, pharmacologic modification of the neurohormonal axes which contribute to HF progression (angiotensin-converting enzyme inhibitors [ACE-Is], angiotensin receptor blockers [ARBs], aldosterone

Table 6 Antibiotic regimens for endocarditis of prosthetic valve or valvular prosthetic material

Viridans group streptococci and *S. gallolyticus (bovis)* (penicillin susceptible: MIC ≤0.12 µg/mL)
[Penicillin G IV or ceftriaxone IV/IM] for 6 weeks ± gentamicin IV/IM for 2 weeks[a]
Vancomycin IV for 6 weeks (with trough of 10–15 µg/mL)
Viridans group streptococci and *S. gallolyticus (bovis)* (penicillin resistant: MIC >0.12 µg/mL)
[Penicillin G IV or ceftriaxone IV/IM] for 6 weeks and gentamicin IV/IM for 6 weeks[a]
Vancomycin IV for 6 weeks (with trough of 10–15 µg/mL)
Streptococcus pneumoniae, Streptococcus pyogenes, groups B, C, F, and G β-hemolytic streptococci
Consult infectious disease as there is little published evidence to guide therapy
Staphylococci
Oxacillin-susceptible
[Nafcillin IV or oxacillin IV] plus rifampin IV/PO for ≥6 weeks and gentamicin IV/IM for first 2 weeks
Cefazolin IV replaces nafcillin/oxacillin in patients with non-anaphylactic penicillin reactions
Oxacillin-resistant (or in patients with immediate-type hypersensitive reactions to β-lactams)
Vancomycin IV for ≥6 weeks plus rifampin IV/PO for ≥6 weeks and gentamicin IV/IM for first 2 weeks
Enterococcus susceptible to penicillin, vancomycin, and gentamicin or streptomycin
Gentamicin should be given in three divided doses, with peak of 3–4 µg/mL and trough of <1 µg/mL
[Ampicillin IV or penicillin G IV] and gentamicin IV/IM for 6 weeks (symptom duration ≥3 months)
Vancomycin IV (if unable to tolerate β-lactam; with trough of 10–20 µg/mL) and gentamicin IV/IM for ≥6 weeks
Ampicillin IV and ceftriaxone IV for 6 weeks (for patients with CrCl <50 mL/min, or if gentamicin resistant and rapid streptomycin serum concentrations not available)
Streptomycin may replace gentamicin, if isolate is sensitive to the former and resistant to the latter, with a peak of 20–35 µg/mL and a trough of <10 µg/mL
Enterococcus resistant to penicillin but susceptible to aminoglycoside and vancomycin
Gentamicin should be given in three divided doses, with peak of 3–4 µg/mL and trough of <1 µg/mL
β-lactamase-producing strain
Ampicillin-sulbactam IV and gentamicin IV/IM for 6 weeks
Vancomycin IV and gentamicin IV/IM for 6 weeks
Intrinsic penicillin resistance
Vancomycin IV and gentamicin IV/IM for 6 weeks
Enterococcus resistant to penicillin, aminoglycoside, and vancomycin
Linezolid IV/PO for >6 weeks
Daptomycin IV for >6 weeks
HACEK Microorganisms
Ceftriaxone IV/IM for 6 weeks (cefotaxime or another 3rd-/4th-generation cephalosporin may be used)
Ampicillin-sulbactam IV for 6 weeks
Ciprofloxacin IV/PO for 6 weeks (third-line treatment due to limited published in vivo evidence for IE; levofloxacin or moxifloxacin may be used)
Culture-negative endocarditis
Early (≤1 year after surgery)
Vancomycin, cefepime, rifampin, and gentamicin
Late (>1 year after surgery)
Vancomycin and ceftriaxone
Duration to be determined with infectious disease consultant

Source: Baddour et al. [6]

[a]Ampicillin is a reasonable alternative to penicillin if a penicillin shortage exists

antagonists, beta-blockers, ARB-neprilysin inhibitor), invasive electrophysiology (cardiac resynchronization, implanted cardioverter defibrillator [ICD]), arrhythmia suppression (pharmacologic and nonpharmacologic), surgery (septal myomectomy, heart transplantation), and therapies targeted

Table 7 Indications for surgery in infectious endocarditis (IE)

Early surgery (before completion of antibiotics, during initial hospitalization)[a]
Valve dysfunction causing signs or symptoms of heart failure
Left-sided IE caused by *S. aureus*, fungi, or other highly resistant organisms
New heart block
Annular or aortic abscess
Destructive (valve dehiscence, rupture) or penetrating lesions/fistulas
Persistent bacteremia or fevers for more than 5–7 days after starting appropriate antibiotics
Recurrent emboli and persistent or enlarging vegetations despite appropriate antibiotic therapy
Native valve endocarditis with severe regurgitation and mobile vegetations >10 mm
Relapse of prosthetic valve endocarditis
Complete removal of pacemaker or defibrillator with proven infection of pocket or leads
Surgery (variable timing)
Repair rather than replacement of right-sided IE when possible, especially in intravenous drug users
Prosthetic valve endocarditis with recurrence of bacteremia after complete course of antibiotics and negative blood cultures with no other source of infection
Complete removal of pacemaker or defibrillator when valvular IE is caused by S. aureus or fungi
Complete removal of pacemaker or defibrillator when undergoing valve surgery for IE

Source: Baddour et al. [6] and Nishimura, et al. [8]

[a]Early surgery is still appropriate in patients with a stroke provided there is no evidence or extensive neurological damage and no intracranial hemorrhage. If either of those findings is present, surgery should be delayed at least 4 weeks in a hemodynamically stable patient

at specific underlying causes (chelation, phlebotomy, bone marrow transplant, etc.).

Hypertrophic Cardiomyopathy (Genetic)

Hypertrophic cardiomyopathy (HCM) is defined as "a disease state characterized by unexplained left ventricular (LV) hypertrophy associated with non-dilated ventricular chambers in the absence of another cardiac or systemic disease that itself would be capable of producing the magnitude of hypertrophy evident in a given patient" [13]. Over 1500 autosomal dominant mutations have been identified in at least 8 genes that encode sarcomere proteins (3 other genes are still considered potentially causative). HCM is seen throughout the world with a global prevalence of approximately 0.2% which in the United States represents at least 600,000 individuals.

Presentation and Diagnosis

Most affected individuals likely have a normal life expectancy; however, in those who develop symptoms, HCM manifests in three different patterns which are not mutually exclusive: sudden cardiac death (SCD), atrial fibrillation/stroke, and HF that may progress to end-stage disease. SCD due to ventricular tachyarrhythmia may be the initial presentation of HCM with the highest risk in patients <35 years of age.

Dynamic left ventricular outflow tract (LVOT) obstruction, defined as an outflow gradient ≥30 mmHg, is typically caused by a narrowing between the hypertrophied ventricular septum and anterior displacement of the mitral valve during systole. Basal obstruction is present at rest, while labile obstruction is only present when physiologically provoked. LVOT obstruction is increased by activities that increase myocardial contractility (e.g., strenuous exercise) or by maneuvers or agents that decrease afterload (e.g., Valsalva, diuretics). Conversely, obstruction is decreased by agents that decrease myocardial contractility (e.g., beta-blockers) or by maneuvers that increase afterload (e.g., squatting).

In addition to common HF symptoms such as fatigue, dyspnea, and orthopnea, patients with

HCM often complain of palpitations (due to atrial fibrillation caused by left atrial enlargement), pre-syncope, and syncope. Since most HCM is nonobstructive (outflow gradient <30 mmHg at rest and with provocation), auscultation generally reveals no murmur. Patients with LVOT often demonstrate a 3–4/6 systolic murmur heard over both the left sternal border (due to outflow obstruction) and apex with radiation to the axilla (due to mitral regurgitation). An S_4 is often heard due to increased filling from the enlarged atria. Pulmonary congestion is rare except with severe outflow obstruction or end-stage HCM (when systolic and diastolic dysfunction become manifest) or with atrial fibrillation. The ECG usually reveals a wide array of nonspecific changes including LV hypertrophy, ST changes, T wave inversion, left atrial enlargement, and Q waves. 24-hour electrocardiographic monitoring is recommended to identify patients who may be a candidate for an ICD, due to ventricular tachycardia, and may also identify atrial fibrillation or flutter. The chest radiograph is often normal or suggestive of atrial enlargement. TTE with Doppler imaging is essential and may be combined with exercise testing to identify labile obstruction. The transesophageal approach may help define subtle mitral valve abnormalities or guide surgical intervention. Cardiovascular magnetic resonance imaging (CMR) can diagnose HCM in patients where echocardiography is inconclusive, or hypertrophy is limited to areas that are poorly visualized on echocardiography, such as the anterolateral wall or apex.

Family history, morphology on imaging, response to a short period of deconditioning, and genetic testing can be used to differentiate between HCM and other conditions with LV hypertrophy including physiologic remodeling ("athlete's heart"), hypertensive heart disease, and metabolic or infiltrative storage diseases. In patients with a confirmed mutation, genetic counseling and testing of first-degree relatives is critical as mutation-positive family members may benefit from early identification and treatment, while mutation-negative family members need no further evaluation.

Intervention

All patients with HCM should be counseled to avoid particularly strenuous activity, avoid certain competitive athletics, undergo risk stratification for SCD, and have comorbid ASCVD risk factors managed according to current guidelines since comorbid coronary disease significantly reduces survival in HCM patients. All asymptomatic patients should receive an annual clinical evaluation. Asymptomatic patients with obstructive physiology should maintain proper hydration while avoiding vasodilators, high-dose diuretics, and environmental situations which may cause vasodilation.

Non-vasodilating beta-blockade is the first-line treatment for symptomatic patients since the negative inotropic and chronotropic effects decrease outflow obstruction through increased diastolic filling time and decreased filling pressures. Patients without obstructive physiology who also have a reduced ejection fraction (EF <50%) should be managed according to the current HF guidelines. End-stage HCM may present as a dilated cardiomyopathy. Patients without obstruction who have a preserved EF and remain symptomatic after, or do not tolerate, beta-blockade may be managed with verapamil, diltiazem, diuretics, ACE-I, or ARB.

For symptomatic patients with obstruction, negative inotropic agents other than beta-blockers may be used with caution since the vasodilating properties of verapamil and diltiazem may lead to decreased filling, increased obstruction, and sudden death in patients with severe obstruction. Oral disopyramide may be added to a beta-blocker or verapamil if symptoms persist, but it should not be used as monotherapy. If medical management fails, surgical myectomy by experienced operators achieves technical success in 90–95% of appropriately selected patients. Alcohol septal ablation can be used in patients who are not candidates for open-heart surgery.

In HCM patients with atrial fibrillation, anticoagulation with a vitamin K antagonist to an international normalized ratio (INR) of 2.0–3.0 or a direct oral anticoagulant (dabigatran, rivaroxaban, apixaban, edoxaban) is strongly recommended regardless of the patient's

CHA$_2$DS$_2$-VASc score. Rate control may be achieved with beta-blockers, verapamil, or diltiazem with AV node ablation and pacemaker placement reserved for failures of medical management. First-line agents for rhythm control include disopyramide (with a rate control agent) or amiodarone. Catheter ablation and AV nodal ablation with pacemaker implantation remain rhythm control options in refractory cases.

Arrhythmogenic Right Ventricular Cardiomyopathy (Genetic)

Arrhythmogenic right ventricular cardiomyopathy (ARVC) is caused by a progressive replacement of the myocardium by fibrofatty tissue [14]. The disease is more common in men with a prevalence estimated as 1 in 2000–5000, and it usually demonstrates autosomal dominant transmission with variable penetrance. Mutations identified to date implicate a degenerative process of the cardiomyocyte involving the intercellular mechanical junction (desmosome). Symptoms may include palpitations (due to ventricular tachycardia [VT] of a left bundle branch block morphology), syncope, or aborted sudden death with initial presentation most likely after puberty but before 60 years of age. Sudden cardiac death occurs with an annual incidence of 0.1–3.0% in adults, and ventricular fibrillation (VF) can occur at any age.

The diagnosis is challenging and requires a high index of suspicion since there is no single gold standard test. The current highly specific criteria from an expert task force combine the results of multiple tests (echocardiography, CMR, endomyocardial biopsy, ECG, Holter, exercise stress) using major and minor criteria. Modifications to the original criteria for first-degree relatives of affected patients increased the overall sensitivity.

Treatment focuses on the prevention of sudden cardiac death. As with HCM, all affected individuals should limit strenuous activity and competitive athletic participation since this has been shown to increase the risk of life-threatening arrhythmias. Universal pre-participation screening in a region of Italy with a high prevalence of ARVC has reduced the annual incidence of SCD in young competitive athletes from 3.8 to 0.4 per 100,000. While an ICD is reasonable in patients with hemodynamically stable VT, medical therapy with beta-blockers or amiodarone can be used. An ICD is strongly recommended in patients with a history of cardiac arrest, syncope, VF, or hemodynamically unstable VT. As with HCM, oral anticoagulation is recommended for patients with ARVC and AF.

Other Genetic Cardiomyopathies

Other less common genetic cardiomyopathies include left ventricular non-compaction, conduction system disease, and the ion channelopathies (long QT syndrome, Brugada syndrome, catecholaminergic polymorphic ventricular tachycardia, short QT syndrome, and idiopathic ventricular fibrillation) [11].

Dilated Cardiomyopathy (Mixed)

Dilated cardiomyopathy (DCM) is characterized by an increase in LV volume with an associated reduction in LVEF that is not caused by another cardiovascular condition [15]. The previously estimated prevalence of 1 in 2700 may have underestimated the true disease burden by an order of magnitude, and DCM could be twice as common as HCM. Up to 48% of patients currently diagnosed with idiopathic DCM likely have a familial cardiomyopathy. The DCM phenotype is seen in other primary and secondary cardiomyopathies, particularly in their end stage, but these etiologies are no longer considered primary DCM. Some of the causes previously classified as DCM include myocarditis, infiltrative disease (amyloidosis, sarcoidosis, hemochromatosis), peripartum cardiomyopathy, HIV, connective tissue disease, substance abuse (alcohol, cocaine), and doxorubicin administration. HF caused by ASCVD, valvular heart disease, systemic hypertension, and congenital heart disease may also share the

DCM phenotype. While the DCM phenotype as a whole has a poor prognosis, with 25% mortality at 1 year and 50% mortality at 5 years, truly idiopathic DCM appears to have a better prognosis than many of the secondary cardiomyopathies with less than 50% mortality at 10 years.

Patients with DCM often present with generalized symptoms of fatigue and dyspnea worsening over months to years. The classic HF symptoms of orthopnea and paroxysmal nocturnal dyspnea are also common. Physical examination reveals pulmonary and, less often, systemic venous congestion. Laboratory tests are recommended to identify other cardiovascular conditions or systemic diseases which may result in the DCM phenotype. The ECG may be normal but often shows T wave changes, septal Q waves, atrioventricular conduction abnormalities, and bundle branch blocks. Sinus tachycardia and supraventricular dysrhythmias are common, especially atrial fibrillation, while non-sustained ventricular tachycardia occurs in 20–30%. Echocardiogram with Doppler imaging is still the first-line test for diagnosis. As in HCM, CMR provides imaging of the entire myocardium while still assessing valvular regurgitation, dyssynchrony, and even ischemia when combined with late gadolinium contrast. Treatment for DCM should adhere to the current evidence-based guidelines for the management of HF as discussed in ▶ Chap. 83, "Heart Failure."

Primary Restrictive Nonhypertrophied Cardiomyopathy (Mixed)

Severe diastolic dysfunction is the hallmark of the restrictive cardiomyopathy (RCM) phenotype; LV size, shape, and systolic function are either normal or nearly so [16]. This phenotype may be seen in both HCM and hypertensive HF as well as many secondary cardiomyopathies. These include infiltrative diseases such as hemochromatosis and amyloidosis (the most common systemic cause of RCM), scleroderma, carcinoid, sarcoidosis, radiation therapy, and anthracycline use. Primary restrictive nonhypertrophied cardiomyopathy, or idiopathic RCM, is the least common etiology and

occurs both sporadically and in familial forms [11].

The pathophysiology is characterized by decreased cardiac output, increased jugular venous pressure, and pulmonary congestion [16]. Biatrial enlargement accounts for an increased incidence of atrial fibrillation and frequent thromboembolic events. Both right- and left-sided HF symptoms are common presenting scenarios. Examination reveals increased jugular venous pulse and decreased pulse pressure. An S_3 gallop due to abrupt cessation of early rapid filling is common. Echocardiography is essential to rule out other causes of the patient's symptoms and to assess filling rates and pressures. The myocardium may also demonstrate patterns on echocardiography that are suggestive of a specific secondary etiology. CMR or even biopsy may be necessary in some cases to distinguish RCM from constrictive pericarditis.

Treatment with diuretics is indicated for congestive symptoms, and beta-blockers may also help with symptom control as described in HFrEF management guidelines. Transplantation is considered in refractory cases, and there may be less chance of recurrence with idiopathic RCM compared to the secondary cardiomyopathies.

Myocarditis (Acquired)

Myocarditis is an inflammatory disease of the heart muscle [17]. The gold standard diagnosis is by histologic and immunologic criteria from endomyocardial biopsy (EMB); however, the diagnosis is often made clinically. Due to the discrepancies in diagnosis, the true incidence of myocarditis is difficult to estimate. It affects children and adults, but it is more common in younger patients. Myocarditis may be caused by infections (most commonly viral), autoimmune disease, medications, and toxins (Table 8). There is significant geographical variation with parvovirus B19 and human herpes virus-6 extremely common in some areas, while coxsackievirus type B remains common in other regions [18].

The inflammation of myocarditis is first caused by either direct microbial damage or toxic damage

Table 8 Etiologies of myocarditis

Infection		
Bacteria	Staphylococcus, streptococcus, pneumococcus, meningococcus, gonococcus, salmonella, *Corynebacterium diphtheriae, Haemophilus influenzae*, mycobacterium, *Mycoplasma pneumonia*, brucella	Diphtheria is a common cause in areas without adequate vaccination
Spirochetes and rickettsia	Borrelia (Lyme disease), leptospira, *Coxiella burnetii* (Q fever), *Rickettsia rickettsii* (Rocky Mountain spotted fever), *Orientia tsutsugamushi* (scrub typhus)	Patients with Lyme myocarditis can be co-infected with *Ehrlichia* or babesia
Fungi	Aspergillus, actinomyces, *Blastomyces*, candida, *Coccidioides*, cryptococcus, histoplasma, mucormycoses, nocardia, sporothrix	
Protozoans and parasites	*Trypanosoma cruzi, Toxoplasma gondii, Entamoeba*, leishmania, *Trichinella spiralis, Echinococcus granulosus, Taenia solium*	*Trypanosoma cruzi* (Chagas disease) is a common cause in Central and South America, may also have bundle branch block
Viruses	RNA viruses: Coxsackieviruses A and B, echoviruses, polioviruses, influenza A and B viruses, respiratory syncytial virus, mumps virus, measles virus, rubella virus, hepatitis B virus, dengue virus, yellow fever virus, chikungunya virus, Junin virus, Lassa fever virus, rabies virus, human immunodeficiency virus-1 (HIV)	Viral myocarditis is the most common cause in the developed world Myocarditis is found in autopsies of more than 50% of patients with HIV (may also be due to antiviral medications)
	DNA viruses: Adenovirus, parvovirus B19, cytomegalovirus, human herpesvirus 6, Epstein-Barr virus, varicella zoster virus, herpes simplex virus, variola virus, vaccinia virus	
Autoimmune/immune-mediated disease		
Allergens	Tetanus toxoid, vaccines, serum sickness	
	Drugs: Penicillin, cefaclor, colchicine, furosemide, isoniazid, lidocaine, tetracycline, sulfonamides, phenytoin, phenylbutazone, methyldopa, thiazides, amitriptyline	Drug-induced hypersensitivity can improve after withdrawal of the drug; steroid treatment may be required
Alloantigens	Heart transplant rejection	
Autoantigens	Infection-negative lymphocytic myocarditis, infection-negative giant cell myocarditis	Considered idiopathic if no viruses are found on EMB
	Associated with autoimmune or immune-oriented disorders: systemic lupus erythematosus, rheumatoid arthritis, Churg-Strauss syndrome, Kawasaki disease, inflammatory bowel disease, scleroderma, polymyositis, myasthenia gravis, insulin-dependent diabetes mellitus, thyrotoxicosis, sarcoidosis, Wegener's granulomatosis, rheumatic heart disease (rheumatic fever)	Cardiac sarcoidosis (idiopathic granulomatous myocarditis) must have negative stains for infectious causes for diagnosis
Toxins		
Drugs	Amphetamines, anthracyclines, cocaine, cyclophosphamide, ethanol, fluorouracil, lithium, catecholamines, hemetine, interleukin 2, trastuzumab, clozapine	
Heavy metals	Copper, iron, lead	

(continued)

Table 8 (continued)

Physical agents	Radiation, electric shock	
Misc.	Scorpion sting, snake and spider bites, bee and wasp stings, carbon monoxide, inhalants, phosphorus, arsenic, sodium azide, pheochromocytoma, beriberi	

Note: *RNA* ribonucleic acid, *DNA* deoxyribonucleic acid
Source: Caforio et al. [19], Fung [18]

[19]. Myocyte death causes the release of cytokines and activation of the immune system. This exposes antigens that are normally hidden from the immune system which induces both a cellular and humoral immune response. This immune response may resolve, as in acute myocarditis, or persist and result in chronic myocarditis. Ongoing destruction and remodeling of the myocardial tissue will eventually lead to the DCM phenotype.

Presentation and Diagnosis

Some patients have minimal symptoms and may never present to a clinician, while others have a severe course of illness and develop severe, life-threatening symptoms. The European Society of Cardiology has described four main presentations of significant acute myocarditis (Table 9). The most common presenting symptom is dyspnea, but patients will frequently report chest pain or palpitations. Because myocarditis is often caused by viral infection, the patient may report respiratory or gastrointestinal illness 1–4 weeks before symptom onset. Myocarditis should be considered as a possible diagnosis for patients presenting with any cardiac syndrome [18]. These include AMI, HF, pericarditis, arrhythmias, heart block, and SCD. Myocarditis must be excluded in a suspected case of sudden infant death syndrome. The evaluation is complicated by the fact that all of these conditions may coexist with myocarditis.

All patients suspected to have myocarditis should first be evaluated with ECG and echocardiogram. The findings of these studies in myocarditis are variable as described in Table 9. Troponin, ESR, and CRP are often elevated and

should be measured. Routine viral serology is not recommended. If the initial evaluation of the patient still indicates myocarditis is likely, the patient should be managed in a center capable of hemodynamic monitoring, cardiac catheterization, and EMB. Patients will frequently require cardiac catheterization to rule out acute coronary syndrome (ACS) as the cause for their symptoms, as there is significant overlap in presentation. CMR is being used more frequently in the evaluation of myocarditis, but current evidence does not justify using it for definitive diagnosis. EMB is safe when done by an experienced clinician and can guide specific therapies.

Intervention

If the patient is hemodynamically unstable, they must be stabilized for transfer to the appropriate care team and intensive care initiated. Ventricular assist devices or extracorporeal membrane oxygenation may be used, often as a bridge to transplant. Stable patients may decompensate quickly, so at a minimum, they should be hospitalized for initial evaluation and observation [19]. All patients with HF should be treated according to current guidelines which include diuretics, beta-blockers, and ACE-I or ARB. Arrhythmias should also be managed according to current guidelines. Digoxin is not recommended as animal studies have shown that it may increase myocardial injury [17]. Temporary pacing may be required if complete heart block is present. ICDs are often not indicated until the acute phase of myocarditis has subsided, as the arrhythmia may also subside. All patients with myocarditis should avoid NSAIDs, as they may increase mortality [19]. Exercise should be avoided

Table 9 Clinical presentation of patients with myocarditis

Clinical presentation	Diagnostic and clinical findings	Length of illness
Chest pain similar to acute MI	ST/T wave changes (ST segment elevation or depression, T wave inversion), elevated troponin (may have time course similar to acute MI or may be elevated for a prolonged period of time), no angiographic evidence of coronary artery disease	Several hours or days
New onset or worsening heart failure	Absence of CAD, no known cause of heart failure, impaired systolic function (LV or RV) seen on echocardiogram, nonspecific ECG signs, bundle branch block, AV block, and/or ventricular arrhythmias	2 weeks to 3 months
Chronic heart failure with symptoms and recurrent exacerbations	Absence of CAD, no known cause of heart failure, impaired systolic function (LV or RV) seen on echocardiogram suggestive of dilated cardiomyopathy or nonischemic cardiomyopathy, nonspecific ECG signs (see point 2 above)	More than 3 months
"Life-threatening condition" in the absence of CAD and known heart failure	Life-threatening arrhythmias and aborted sudden death, cardiogenic shock, *or* severely impaired LV function	Any duration

Note: *CAD* coronary artery disease, *LV* left ventricle, *RV* right ventricle, *ECG* electrocardiogram
Source: Caforio et al. [19], Fung [18]

until complete resolution and for at least 6 months in competitive athletes. There are no specific preventive measures for myocarditis.

Specific therapies may be indicated in certain cases, especially if an etiology is found on EMB. Antiviral treatment with ribavirin and interferon alfa has shown some benefit; however, it is most helpful early in the course of the viral illness, and myocarditis is often diagnosed too late. Interferon beta has been shown to be effective in some chronic cases. Intravenous immunoglobulin is often used, particularly in pediatric cases; however, the overall data supporting its use is inconclusive, especially for adults. Immunosuppressive therapy can play a role in some cases, especially giant cell myocarditis and chronic myocarditis with DCM unresponsive to traditional treatment. Immunosuppressive agents include cyclosporine, azathioprine, and prednisone.

Stress-Induced ("Takotsubo") Cardiomyopathy (Acquired)

Stress-induced cardiomyopathy, or apical ballooning syndrome, first described in Japan, is characterized by a ventricle which resembles an octopus trap (a takotsubo) which is triggered by acute physical or psychological stress [15]. It is more common in postmenopausal women with a presentation that mimics ACS, often with ST elevation and elevated cardiac enzymes, and is seen in 1–2% of patients undergoing angiography for ACS. Subsequent studies demonstrate no evidence of ischemia, no pheochromocytoma, and no myocarditis. The LV dysfunction often resolves within days to weeks after initial presentation.

Peripartum Cardiomyopathy (Acquired)

Peripartum cardiomyopathy (PPCM) shares the DCM phenotype and develops within the last trimester of pregnancy or first 5 months postpartum with an incidence of 1 in 300–4350 live births [15]. Risk factors include multiparity, advanced maternal age, long-term tocolysis, and African descent. It is a diagnosis of exclusion that requires no identifiable cause of HF and no history of heart disease prior to diagnosis. Many patients experience spontaneous recovery in the first 6 months after diagnosis and have an excellent prognosis; however, if cardiomegaly persists past 4–6 months, mortality increases to 50% at 6 years. PPCM can recur in subsequent pregnancies with the highest risk in patients whose LVEF has not normalized. GDMT for HFrEF must be adjusted if the patient is still pregnant or breastfeeding. Anticoagulation is particularly important due to a high rate of venous thromboembolism. European guidelines suggest that bromocriptine may improve outcomes in patient with severe PPCM, but this is controversial, and bromocriptine will inhibit lactation [20].

Tachycardia-Induced Cardiomyopathy (Acquired)

The severity of tachycardia-induced cardiomyopathy is correlated with the duration and rate of the inciting tachycardia [15]. Any ventricular tachycardia, frequent premature ventricular complexes, or supraventricular tachycardia with rapid ventricular response may induce this largely reversible cardiomyopathy. Treatment is directed at correcting the causative tachycardia, and subsequent improvement of the cardiomyopathy, while not guaranteed, is expected.

Pulmonary Hypertension and Cor Pulmonale

Pulmonary hypertension (PH) is a complex disease with multiple etiologies. Regardless of the underlying cause, it is defined by a mean pulmonary artery pressure >25 mmHg at rest measured by right heart catheterization (RHC) [21]. The World Health Organization (WHO) classifies PH into five groups based on etiology and pathophysiology (Table 10). All etiologies of PH are felt to

Table 10 Classification and epidemiology of pulmonary hypertension (PH)

WHO classification		Associated diseases	% of all PH cases	Others
Group 1	Pulmonary arterial hypertension (PAH)	Idiopathic (IPAH), familial, "associated with" (connective tissue disorder, congenital systemic-to-pulmonary shunts, portal hypertension, HIV infections, drugs, and toxins), persistent pulmonary hypertension of the newborn, others	4.2%	PAH 15 cases/million adult population IPAH 5.9 cases/million adult population
Group 2	Pulmonary hypertension with left heart disease	Left-sided atrial or ventricular heart disease, left-sided valvular heart disease	78.7%	Up to 60% of with severe LV systolic dysfunction have PH Almost all patients with symptomatic mitral valve disease have PH
Group 3	Pulmonary hypertension associated with lung diseases and/or hypoxemia	Chronic obstructive pulmonary disease (COPD), interstitial lung disease, sleep-disordered breathing, alveolar hypoventilation disorders, chronic exposure to high altitude, developmental abnormalities	9.7%	More than 50% of patients with advanced COPD have PH
Group 4	Pulmonary hypertension due to chronic thrombotic and/or embolic disease	Proximal pulmonary arteries, distal pulmonary arteries, non-thrombotic pulmonary embolism (tumor, parasites, foreign material)	0.6%	Incidence is 0.5–2% of survivors of acute pulmonary embolism
Group 5	Miscellaneous	Sarcoid, histiocytosis X, lymphangiomatosis, compression of pulmonary vessels (adenopathy, tumor, fibrosing mediastinitis)	6.8%	These cases cannot otherwise be classified

Note: *LV* left ventricle, *HIV* human immunodeficiency virus
Source: Galiè et al. [22] and McLaughlin et al. [24]

have one or more underlying pathophysiologic mechanisms: vascular injury, an alteration in the balance of vasodilatation and vasoconstriction, and thrombotic changes in the pulmonary vasculature. Rarely, PH can be familial, and 70% of these cases have been associated with mutations of the BMPR2 gene [22]. The right ventricle (RV) is a low-pressure chamber with thin walls, as it normally pumps against the low resistance of the pulmonary vascular bed [23]. With the increased resistance of PH, the RV can hypertrophy and/or dilate, causing right ventricular failure (RVF). While RVF can result from any type of PH, the term "cor pulmonale" has historically been used to describe RVF secondary to diseases affecting the function or structure of the lungs, which would imply WHO group 3 disease.

Presentation and Diagnosis

The presentation of PH is very nonspecific, so the physician's challenge is to be aware of the risk factors for PH and to have an appropriate index of suspicion. The goal of the evaluation and early consultation is to identify an underlying cause, prognosis, and treatment options. The most common presenting symptoms include dyspnea (initially only with exertion), fatigue, chest pain, pre-syncope/syncope, lower extremity edema, and palpitations. Physical exam may be benign at first. With more severe PH, one may appreciate an S_3 heart sound, the holosystolic murmur of tricuspid regurgitation, or the early diastolic murmur of pulmonic regurgitation. As PH progresses, signs of RVF may develop with increased jugular venous distention, RV heave, and a prominent P2. Significant RVF may be evidenced by an S_4 heart sound, peripheral edema, hepatomegaly, and ascites.

If a patient has signs, symptoms, or history suggestive of PH, echocardiography is the next diagnostic step [21]. If there is evidence of PH, the most common causes of PH should be considered first (left heart disease, lung disease, and hypoxia; group 2 and 3 disease). A focused evaluation can include further history taking, ECG, X-ray, pulmonary function tests, blood gas analysis,

polysomnography, and high-resolution computed tomography. Chest radiograph may show increased hilar structures and enlarged RV and right atrium. ECG usually reveals normal sinus rhythm with right chamber enlargement and a strain pattern. If the diagnosis of heart or lung disease is confirmed, and there are no signs of severe PH or RVF, the physician can continue with appropriate care for the underlying disease. If severe PH or RVF is present, the patient should be referred to a PH expert center for further investigation, including RHC. If heart or lung disease is not evident, the next step is to search for chronic thromboembolic pulmonary hypertension (CTEPH, group 4) with V/Q scintigraphy. This should be done even if the patient does not have a known history of pulmonary embolism, as CT pulmonary angiography may not be sensitive enough to confidently rule out group 4 disease [25]. Patients with CTEPH will also require referral and RHC. If this evaluation does not elucidate a cause of PH, broad work-up for pulmonary arterial hypertension (PAH, group 1) and miscellaneous other causes (group 5) is needed at a PH referral center.

Differential Diagnosis

CAD and cardiomyopathies leading to RVF may present with the same symptoms and signs as PH. The nonspecific presentation of the disease often results in significant diagnostic delays.

Intervention

Treatment of PH primarily focuses on supportive care and management of the underlying disease process [25]. All patients should use supplemental oxygen as needed to keep oxygen saturation ≥90% during rest, exercise, and sleep. If patients have RVF, it should be treated appropriately, typically with diuretics and salt restriction. Patients with CTEPH require long-term anticoagulation. These patients may also require pulmonary thromboendarterectomy, which can be curative. Pulmonary rehabilitation may be valuable for some patients to counter deconditioning. Patients should remain active and exercise but avoid isometric exercises which can increase risk of syncope. Female patients should be counseled to avoid pregnancy, a high-flow state that can worsen symptoms.

Several specific therapies exist for patients with PAH (WHO group 1). Vasodilator response testing should be completed during RHC to identify appropriate candidates since an empiric trial of therapy in a nonresponder can have negative hemodynamic outcomes. Pharmacologic options include calcium channel blockers, prostacyclin derivatives, endothelin receptor antagonists, and drugs that target nitric oxide pathways [26]. These group 1-specific drugs are typically not used for group 2–5 disease and may worsen outcomes in those patients. The choice of agent is based on severity of disease; oral medicines are used in lower-risk patients, while parenteral therapies are reserved for higher-risk patients. The 6-minute walk test or graded treadmill test can be used for risk stratification. The presence of RVF is a poor prognostic factor [23]. Patients with group 1 disease may also benefit from anticoagulation, typically with warfarin to an INR of 1.5–2.5. Lung transplantation may be considered in patients with group 1 disease who fail medical therapy and in group 3 patients who progress to end-stage lung disease.

References

1. Hirsch AT, Haskal ZJ, Hertzer NR, Bakal CW, Creager MA, Halperin JL, et al. ACC/AHA 2005 practice guidelines for the management of patients with peripheral arterial disease (lower extremity, renal, mesenteric, and abdominal aortic): a collaborative report from the American Association for Vascular Surgery/Society for Vascular Surgery, Society for Cardiovascular Angiography and Interventions, Society for Vascular Medicine and Biology, Society of Interventional Radiology, and the ACC/AHA Task Force on Practice Guidelines (Writing Committee to Develop Guidelines for the Management of Patients With Peripheral Arterial Disease). Circulation. 2006;113:e463–654. CrossRef PubMed

2. Gerhard-Herman MD, Gornik HL, Barrett C, Barshes NR, Corriere MA, Drachman DE, et al. AHA/ACC guideline on the management of patients with lower extremity peripheral artery disease: a report of the American College of Cardiology/American Heart Association Task Force on Clinical Practice Guidelines. Circulation. 2016;135:e726–79. CrossRef PubMed

3. Kaplovitch E, Rannelli L, Anand SS. Antithrombotics in stable peripheral artery disease. Vasc Med. 2019;24(2):132–40. CrossRef PubMed

4. LeWinter MM. Acute pericarditis. N Engl J Med. 2014;371(25):2410–6. CrossRef PubMed

5. Little WC, Freeman GL. Pericardial disease. Circulation. 2006;113(12):1622–32. CrossRef PubMed

6. Baddour LM, Wilson WR, Bayer AS, Fowler VG Jr, Tleyjeh IM, Rybak MJ, et al. Infective endocarditis in adults: diagnosis, antimicrobial therapy, and management of complications: a statement for healthcare professionals from the American Heart Association: endorsed by the Infectious Diseases Society of America. Circulation. 2015;132(15):1435–86. CrossRef PubMed

7. Bor DH, Woolhandler S, Nardin R, Brusch J, Himmelstein DU. Infective endocarditis in the U.S., 1998–2009: a nationwide study. PLoS One. 2013;8(3): e60033. CrossRef PubMed

8. Nishimura RA, Otto CM, Bonow RO, Carabello BA, Erwin JP III, Fleisher LA, et al. AHA/ACC Focused Update of the 2014 AHA/ACC guideline for the management of patients with valvular heart disease: a report of the American College of Cardiology/American Heart Association Task Force on Practice Guidelines. J Am Coll Cardiol. 2017;70(2):252–89. CrossRef PubMed

9. Habib G, Hoen B, Tornos P, Thuny F, Prendergast B, Vilacosta I, et al. ESC guidelines for the management of infective endocarditis: the Task Force for the Management of Infective Endocarditis of the European Society of Cardiology (ESC). Endorsed by: European Association for Cardio-Thoracic Surgery (EACTS), the European Association of Nuclear Medicine (EANM). Eur Heart J. 2015;36(44):3075–128. CrossRef PubMed

10. Li JS, Sexton DJ, Mick N, Nettles R, Fowler VG Jr, Ryan T, et al. Proposed modifications to the Duke criteria for the diagnosis of infective endocarditis. Clin Infect Dis. 2000;30(4):633–8. CrossRef PubMed

11. Maron BJ, Towbin JA, Thiene G, Antzelevitch C, Corrado D, Arnett D, et al. Contemporary definitions and classification of the cardiomyopathies: an American Heart Association Scientific Statement from the Council on Clinical Cardiology, Heart Failure and Transplantation Committee; Quality of Care and Outcomes Research and Functional Genomics and Translational Biology Interdisciplinary Working Groups; and Council on Epidemiology and Prevention. Circulation. 2006;113(14):1807–16. CrossRef PubMed

12. Brieler J, Breeden MA, Tucker J. Cardiomyopathy: an overview. Am Fam Physician. 2017;96(10):640–6. PubMed PubMedCentral

13. Elliott PM, Anastasakis A, Borger MA, Borggrefe M, Cecchi F, Charron P, et al. ESC guidelines on diagnosis

and management of hypertrophic cardiomyopathy: the Task Force for the Diagnosis and Management of Hypertrophic Cardiomyopathy of the European Society of Cardiology (ESC). Eur Heart J. 2014;35(39):2733–79. CrossRef PubMed

14. Towbin JA, McKenna WJ, Abrams DJ, Ackerman MJ, Calkins H, Darrieux FCC, et al. HRS expert consensus statement on evaluation, risk stratification, and management of arrhythmogenic cardiomyopathy. Heart Rhythm. 2019;16(11):e301–72. CrossRef PubMed

15. Bozkurt B, Colvin M, Cook J, Cooper LT, Deswal A, Fonarow GC, et al. Current diagnostic and treatment strategies for specific dilated cardiomyopathies: a scientific statement from the American Heart Association. Circulation. 2016;134(23):e579–646. CrossRef PubMed

16. Muchtar E, Blauwet LA, Gertz MA. Restrictive cardiomyopathy: genetics, pathogenesis, clinical manifestations, diagnosis, and therapy. Circ Res. 2017;121(7):819–37. CrossRef PubMed

17. Canter CE, Simpson KP. Diagnosis and treatment of myocarditis in children in the current era. Circulation. 2014;129(1):115–28. CrossRef PubMed

18. Fung G, Luo H, Qiu Y, Yang D, McManus B. Myocarditis. Circ Res. 2016;118(3):496–514. CrossRef PubMed

19. Caforio AL, Pankuweit S, Arbustini E, Basso C, Gimeno-Blanes J, Felix SB, et al. Current state of knowledge on aetiology, diagnosis, management, and therapy of myocarditis: a position statement of the European Society of Cardiology Working Group on Myocardial and Pericardial Diseases. Eur Heart J. 2013;34(33):2636–48. 2648a–2648d. CrossRef PubMed

20. Regitz-Zagrosek V, Roos-Hesselink JW, Bauersachs J, Blomström-Lundqvist C, Cífková R, De Bonis M, et al. ESC Guidelines for the management of cardiovascular diseases during pregnancy. Eur Heart J. 2018;39(34):3165–241. CrossRef PubMed

21. Hoeper MM, Bogaard HJ, Condliffe R, Frantz R, Khanna D, Kurzyna M, et al. Definitions and diagnosis of pulmonary hypertension. J Am Coll Cardiol. 2013;62(25):D42–50. CrossRef PubMed

22. Galiè N, Hoeper MM, Humbert M, Torbicki A, Vachiery JL, Barbera JA, et al. Guidelines for the diagnosis and treatment of pulmonary hypertension: the Task Force for the Diagnosis and Treatment of Pulmonary Hypertension of the European Society of Cardiology (ESC) and the European Respiratory Society (ERS), endorsed by the International Society of Heart and Lung Transplantation (ISHLT). Eur Heart J. 2009;30(20):2493–537. CrossRef PubMed

23. Han MK, McLaughlin VV, Criner GJ, Martinez FJ. Pulmonary diseases and the heart. Circulation. 2007;116:2992–3005. CrossRef PubMed

24. McLaughlin VV, Archer SL, Badesch DB, Barst RJ, Farber HW, Lindner JR, et al. ACCF/AHA 2009 expert consensus document on pulmonary hypertension a report of the American College of Cardiology Foundation Task Force on Expert Consensus Documents and the American Heart Association developed in collaboration with the American College of Chest Physicians; American Thoracic Society, Inc.; and the Pulmonary Hypertension Association. J Am Coll Cardiol. 2009;53(17):1573–619. CrossRef PubMed

25. Mandel J, Poch D. In the clinic. Pulmonary hypertension. Ann Intern Med. 2013;158(9):ITC5-1-16. CrossRef PubMed

26. Thenappan T, Ormiston ML, Ryan JJ, Archer SL. Pulmonary arterial hypertension: pathogenesis and clinical management. BMJ. 2018;360:j5492. CrossRef PubMed

Part XVIII

The Respiratory System

Obstructive Airway Disease

87

Timothy D. Riley and Ashley Morrison

Contents

Asthma

General Principles

Definition/Background

Asthma is a respiratory disease characterized by chronic airway inflammation and is defined by symptoms including shortness of breath, wheeze, chest tightness and cough along with variable limitation in expiratory airflow [1]. Advances in medical therapy have greatly increased the options for treatment for patients with asthma; however it remains one of the most common major non-communicable diseases and has a substantial impact on quality of life. Adequate care of patients suffering from asthma involves the triad of systematic chronic care plans, support for self-management, and appropriate medical therapy [2].

Epidemiology

Asthma afflicts around 300 million people worldwide, ranking 16th among the leading causes of years lived with disability and 28th among the leading causes of burden of disease. While high-income countries have a higher asthma prevalence, low- to middle-income countries account for most asthma-related mortality [3]. In 2018, 7.5% of children and 7.7% of adults in the USA had been diagnosed with asthma, including 9.1% of females and 6.2% of males. Impoverished persons or those less

T. D. Riley (✉) · A. Morrison
Penn State College of Medicine, Hershey, PA, USA
e-mail: triley1@pennstatehealth.psu.edu;
amorrison2@pennstatehealth.psu.edu

© Springer Nature Switzerland AG 2022
P. M. Paulman et al. (eds.), *Family Medicine*,
https://doi.org/10.1007/978-3-030-54441-6_172

than 100% of the poverty threshold are more likely to suffer from asthma (10.8%) compared to those at 450% of the poverty threshold (6.5%) [4].

Classification

Asthma may be classified as intermittent, mild persistent, moderate persistent, or severe persistent as detailed in Table 1.

There are several different clinical phenotypes of asthma that have been identified including allergic asthma, non-allergic asthma, adult-onset asthma, asthma with persistent airflow limitation, and asthma with obesity [1].

Diagnosis

The diagnosis of asthma should be based on detailed history and physical examination in combination with spirometry and/or peak expiratory flow.

History

Patients with respiratory symptoms should be asked about a history of allergies, atopic dermatitis, and symptoms starting in childhood, all of which increase the likelihood that symptoms are secondary to asthma. Family history of allergy

and asthma also increase the likelihood of asthma [1].

Respiratory symptoms including wheeze, shortness of breath, cough and/or chest tightness are suggestive of asthma. Table 2 lists features that increase and decrease likelihood of asthma as a diagnosis [1].

Physical Examination

The most common abnormality on physical is expiratory wheezing; however, there are often no abnormalities detected on exam, especially if the patient is not in an acute exacerbation. Wheezing may also be caused by inhaled foreign body, tracheomalacia, or respiratory infections. Other signs on physical exam such as nasal polyps or atopic dermatitis would not be specific for asthma but suggest associated conditions such as allergy and atopy [1].

Laboratory and Imaging

Laboratory testing for specific immunoglobulin E may suggest the presence of atopy which increases the likelihood a patient that has respiratory symptoms is suffering from allergic-type asthma; however this test is not specific for asthma itself. Similarly, skin prick testing suggests the presence of atopy but is not a specific diagnostic test for asthma [1].

Table 1 Classification of asthma severity in adults and adolescents age $\geq$ 12 years [1]

	Intermittent	Mild persistent	Moderate persistent	Severe persistent
Symptoms	$\leq$2 days/week	>2 days/week but not daily	Daily	Throughout the day
Nighttime awakenings	$\leq$2x/month	3–4x/month	>1x/week but not nightly	7x/week
SABA[a] use for symptom control	$\leq$2 days/week	>2 days/week but not daily and not more than once on any day	Daily	Several times/day
Interference with normal activity	None	Minor limitation	Some limitation	Extremely limited
FEV$_1$[a] (% predicted)	>80%	>80%	60–80%	<60%
FEV1/FVC[a]	Normal	Normal	Reduced 5%	Reduced >5%
Asthma exacerbations requiring oral systemic corticosteroids	0–1/year	$\geq$2/year	Generally, more frequent and intense events indicate greater severity	Generally, more frequent and intense events indicate greater severity

[a]SABA, short-acting beta agonist; FEV$_1$, forced expiratory volume in 1 s; FVC, forced vital capacity [5]

Table 2   Characteristic symptom features of asthma [1]

Features that increase probability of asthma	Features that decrease probability of asthma
Often worse at night or early morning	Isolated cough with no other respiratory symptoms
Vary over time and in intensity	Chronic production of sputum
Symptoms are triggered by viral infections, exercise, allergen exposure, or environmental irritants	Shortness of breath associated with dizziness, light-headedness, or peripheral tingling
Having more than one symptom of wheeze, cough, shortness of breath, chest tightness	Exercise-induced dyspnea with noise on inspiration
	Chest pain

Imaging does not play a role in diagnosis of asthma but may evaluate for other causes of respiratory symptoms such as pneumonia, congestive heart failure, lung cancer, etc.

Special Testing

Spirometry is the preferred initial test to measure presence and severity of airflow obstruction in adults [6]. Improvement of the forced expiratory volume in 1 s (FEV1) of $\geq 12\%$ and 200 mL is suggestive of asthma.

Once a diagnosis of asthma has been made, peak expiratory flow (PEF) monitoring may be used in the short term to establish a baseline and initial response to treatment [1].

Nitrous oxide is a biological mediator that has been implicated in pathophysiology of lung diseases including asthma. Measurement of fractional nitrous oxide concentration (FE_{NO}) in exhaled breath is a quantitative method of measuring airway inflammation and can also predict corticosteroid responsiveness [7].

Bronchial provocation tests are another way to test for airflow limitation. Challenge agents include methacholine, histamine, exercise, and inhaled mannitol. These tests are moderately sensitive but not very specific for the diagnosis of asthma, as multiple chronic lung conditions can also cause abnormal results [1].

Differential Diagnosis

The differential diagnosis of asthma in adults is listed in Table 3 [6]. In children aged 6–11 who present with recurrent infections and productive cough, bronchiectasis and primary ciliary dyskinesia must be considered. A heart murmur may suggest congenital heart disease as a possible cause of symptoms. If a child presents with excessive cough and mucous production as well as gastrointestinal symptoms, cystic fibrosis should be considered [1].

Treatment

Medications/Immunizations and Chemoprophylaxis

Choice of initial treatment is based on the patient's presenting symptom severity and frequency. For those age 12 and above with infrequent asthma symptoms (less than twice a month) and with no risk factors for exacerbations, the preferred initial treatment is with as-needed low-dose inhaled corticosteroid (ICS)-formoterol, or with an ICS whenever a short-acting beta agonist (SABA) is taken. Sole prescription of SABAs is no longer recommended. If a patient presents with symptoms twice a month or more but less than daily, a daily low-dose ICS with as-needed SABA or as-needed low-dose ICS-formoterol is recommended. For patients with asthma symptoms most days or nighttime awakenings due to asthma once a week or more, it is recommended to initiate treatment with a low-dose ICS-long-acting beta agonist (LABA) as maintenance and reliever therapy, known as the single maintenance and reliever therapy (SMART) approach [8]. Maintenance-only ICS-LABA with as-needed SABA or medium-dose ICS with as-needed SABA may also be used for these patients. If a patient presents initially with severe uncontrolled asthma or in an acute exacerbation, start regular controller treatment with a high-dose ICS or medium-dose ICS-LABA and consider a short course of oral corticosteroids [1].

Table 3 Differential diagnosis – cough and/or dyspnea [1, 12]

Chronic cough and/or dyspnea		Acute cough and/or dyspnea	
Source	Differential	Source	Differential
Pulmonary	Asthma	Pulmonary	Asthma exacerbation
	Lung cancer		Pulmonary embolism
	Interstitial lung disease		Pneumothorax
	Bronchiectasis		Pleural effusion
	Obliterative bronchiolitis	Infectious	Pneumonia
	Diffuse pan-bronchiolitis		Bronchitis/bronchiolitis
	Sarcoidosis	Cardiovascular	Congestive heart failure exacerbation
Infectious	Tuberculosis		Ischemic heart disease
	Atypical mycobacterial infections		Arrhythmia (e.g., atrial fibrillation)
Cardiovascular	Congestive heart failure	Irritants	Smoke, dust, or chemical exposure
	Ischemic heart disease		
Upper airway	Chronic allergic rhinitis		
	Upper airway cough syndrome		
Gastrointestinal	Gastroesophageal reflux		
Medications	ACE inhibitors		
Irritants	Smoke, dust, or chemical exposure		
Genetic	Cystic fibrosis		

After starting initial treatment, in most circumstances obtaining a measure of lung function with PFTs is beneficial. Review patient's response to initial therapy and consider step-down treatment after good control has been maintained for 3 months [1] (Fig. 1).

Treatment of asthma exacerbations in adults is dependent on exacerbation severity. For mild (peak expiratory flow rate [PEFR] > 75%) to moderate (PEFR 50–75%) exacerbations, outpatient management is appropriate with increased frequency of SABA or short-acting muscarinic antagonist (SAMA) use, temporarily quadrupling ICS, and systemic corticosteroids if no response to initial therapy. The recommended steroid dose is 1 mg/kg/day of prednisolone (or equivalent) per day up to 50 mg for 5–7 days. For severe exacerbations (PEFR 33–50%), management in an emergency room or urgent care facility is warranted with increased frequency of SABA or SAMA use along with systemic corticosteroids and consideration of a single dose of IV magnesium sulfate. Inpatient hospitalization is indicated if improvement is not obtained with these measures or the patient is pregnant or has one or more of the following: respiratory rate greater than 25/min, heart rate greater than 110/min, inability to speak in full sentences in one breath, or adherence concerns. For patients with life-threatening exacerbations (PEFR<33%) who may present with worsening hypoxia, hypercapnia, altered level of consciousness, hypotension, or cyanosis, treatment in an intensive care unit is required with possible noninvasive ventilation or intubation [9].

For children aged 5–11, SABA therapy is recommended to treat symptoms of intermittent asthma. Moderate or severe exacerbations due to viral respiratory infections which are common in children should be treated with a short course of oral corticosteroids, 1–2 mg/kg/day up to a maximum of 40 mg/day for 3–5 days. Daily low-dose ICS is the preferred step 2 treatment, while alternative treatment options include cromolyn, leukotriene antagonists (LTRA), nedocromil, and theophylline. For step 3 care, a low-dose ICS plus LABA, LTRA, or theophylline and medium-dose ICS are equivalent options. The preferred step 4 treatment is medium-dose ICS and LABA, and the preferred step 5 treatment is high-dose ICS and LABA. For step 6 care, oral systemic corticosteroids long term added on to high-dose ICS and LABA is preferred [1].

Box 3-5A. Personalized management for adults and adolescents to control symptoms and minimize future risk

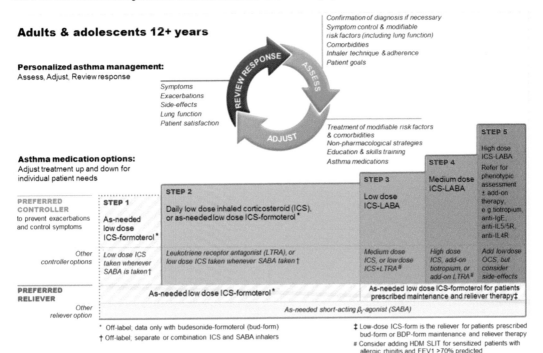

Fig. 1 Asthma management. (Reprinted with permission [1])

Referrals

In general, asthma is managed by primary care physicians, but in certain instances referral to a pulmonologist is indicated (Table 4) [6].

Counseling

Patient Education and Activation

Patient education is key in effectively managing asthma and preventing complications. A comprehensive strategy includes skills training to ensure effective use of inhalers and guided self-management with self-monitoring of symptoms or peak flow with a written action plan. For children and adolescents with asthma, a written asthma management plan should be provided for the student's school, and prompt, reliable access to medication should be ensured. Review of inhaler technique is important for all patients.

Prevention

Exposure to tobacco smoke should be eliminated if possible and those who smoke should be given cessation resources. Patients with obesity should be counseled on weight reduction strategies and distinguishing asthma symptoms from symptoms that may be due to deconditioning, mechanical restriction, or sleep apnea. Low socioeconomic status and inability to afford medications are associated with increased emergency department visits for asthma exacerbations and should be addressed [10]. Those with confirmed food allergies should be counseled on avoidance strategies and prescribed with injectable epinephrine. Allergen-specific immunotherapy may help reduce exacerbations in patients where allergy plays a significant role. Adults with asthma should be screened for occupational triggers and removed from them as soon as possible. Avoidance of indoor allergens such as mold, dust mites, and pets can be helpful in

Table 4 Criteria for referral for asthma [6]

	Prominent systemic features (myalgia, fever, weight loss)
Unclear diagnosis	
Unexpected clinical findings (crackles, cyanosis, clubbing, cardiac disease)	Chronic sputum production
Unexplained restrictive spirometry	CXR shadowing
Suspected occupational asthma	Marked blood eosinophilia
Monophonic wheeze or stridor	Poor response to asthma treatment
Persistent non-variable breathlessness	Severe asthma attack

some, but these strategies can be complicated and expensive [1].

Family and Community Issues

According to epidemiological studies, approximately 21.5% of adults with asthma suffer from work-exacerbated asthma (WEA), defined as pre-existing asthma which is exacerbated by workplace conditions. WEA is associated with more symptomatic days and utilization of healthcare resources and is similar to occupational asthma in that both are associated with unemployment and loss of income. The possibility of WEA or occupational asthma should be ascertained by asking about relatedness of a patient's symptoms to the workplace [11].

Chronic Obstructive Pulmonary Disease

General Principles

Definition and Background

Chronic obstructive pulmonary disease (COPD) is a syndrome of abnormal lung physiology characterized by irreversible obstructive limitation in airflow (Fig. 2) [12]. The disease is defined by measurement through spirometry [12, 13]. Emphysema and chronic bronchitis often accompany and may be confused with COPD. Emphysema is an anatomic diagnosis, referring to destruction of alveoli. Chronic bronchitis refers to chronic cough with sputum production for at least 3 months in 2 consecutive years. Either or both of these diagnoses can occur together with or separate from COPD [12]. COPD patients may experience

exacerbations, characterized by increased dyspnea, cough, and sputum production and purulence [13]. Triggers for exacerbations include viral infections, bacterial infections, and environmental causes such as pollution. Exacerbations typically last 7–10 days, but symptoms may persist for more than 8 weeks [12].

Epidemiology

COPD is common and deadly. 11.7% of the population worldwide suffered from the disease in 2010, resulting in three million deaths [12], making it the most common cause of death from chronic lung disease worldwide [14]. Cigarette smoking is the most common cause of COPD. Other tobacco smoke and secondhand smoke and smoking marijuana also increase risk [12]. Other potential causes of COPD include occupational exposure, including dust and fumes, and smoke from indoor cooking [12, 13]. Patients with asthma and chronic bronchitis are more likely to develop COPD. Alpha-1 antitrypsin deficiency is a rare genetic cause of the disease [12]. Associated conditions are listed in Table 5 [12, 13].

Classification

The 2020 Global Initiative for Chronic Lung Disease (GOLD) COPD classification system recommends a "grade (number) group (letter)" classification for each patient with COPD (Fig. 3) [12]. Symptom assessment tools include the Modified British Medical Research Council (mMRC), a brief questionnaire which assesses breathlessness and predicts future mortality risk (Table 6) [15]. The COPD Assessment Test (CAT) is more comprehensive but longer [16]. The mMRC is reproduced here for its simplicity.

Fig. 2 Pathophysiology of COPD [12]

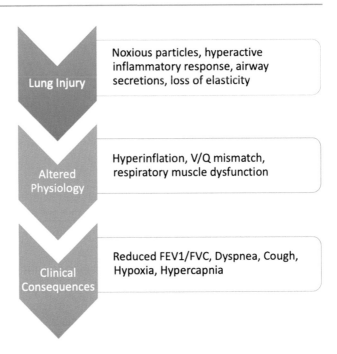

Table 5 Comorbid conditions with COPD [12, 13]

Condition	Examples and comments
Cardiac	Ischemic heart disease, heart failure, cardiac arrhythmias, peripheral vascular disease and hypertension
Lung cancer	Only among patients whose COPD is caused by smoking
Osteoporosis	Associated with smoking and frequent use of systemic steroids
Diabetes	Worsened by systemic steroid use
Gastroesophageal reflux disease	Associate with increased risk of exacerbations and progression
Anxiety and depression	Often underdiagnosed, associated with poor prognosis and suicidality

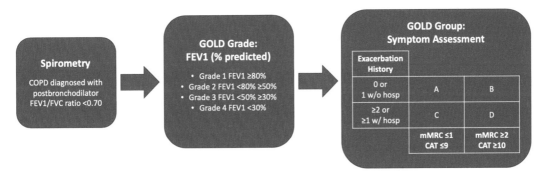

Fig. 3   GOLD 2020 classification system [1]

Exacerbations are classified as mild (requiring only short-acting bronchodilators [SABDs]), moderate (requiring SABDs with antibiotics and/or oral corticosteroids), or severe (requiring hospitalization with or without acute respiratory failure). Multiple instruments assess prognosis in COPD patients. The BODE index (body mass index, obstruction, dyspnea, and exercise

Table 6 Modified British Medical Research Council (mMRC) Score [11]

Statement	mMRC grade
I only get breathless with strenuous exercise.	0
I get short of breath when hurrying on the level or walking up a slight hill.	1
I walk slower than people of the same age on the level because of breathlessness, or I have to stop for breath when walking on my own pace on the level.	2
I stop for breath after walking about 100 meters or after a few minutes on the level.	3
I am too breathless to leave the house or I am breathless when dressing or undressing.	4

Table 7 Risk factors for COPD [1]

Modifiable	Non-modifiable
Tobacco exposure	Family history
Occupational smoke, chemical, or dust exposure	Low birth weight
Cooking or heating smoke exposure	Anatomic lung abnormalities
	Severe childhood lung infections

assessed by 6-min walk test) predicts 4-year survival [17]. The ADO index (age, dyspnea, airflow obstruction) incorporates age, mMRC, and FEV1 and predicts 3-year mortality without the 6-min walk test [13].

Diagnosis

History

The most common presentation for patient with COPD is chronic cough and dyspnea. Cough is not necessarily productive. Dyspnea is typically worse with exertion. Risk factors should be assessed (Table 7). Weight loss, fatigue, and anorexia occur later in the course of the disease [12].

Symptom severity should be assessed through the mMRC or CAT questionnaires. Patients with known COPD should be evaluated for triggers, the presence or absence of sputum as well as its volume, and healthcare utilization, particularly hospitalizations (duration, need for critical care or mechanical ventilation) [12].

Physical Examination

Physical examination has low specificity and sensitivity for diagnosis. Physical signs can include decreased breath sounds, lung hyperinflation with chest expansion, and prolonged forced expiration. With severe disease, pulmonary hypertension can result in cor pulmonale leading to leg swelling. In the context of an acute exacerbation, wheezing and rhonchi are common. The presence of rales suggests heart failure or pulmonary fibrosis [12].

Laboratory and Imaging

Complete blood count with peripheral eosinophil absolute count and percentage can help direct therapy [13]. Vitamin D levels should be checked. CRP may be useful in directing antibiotic use during exacerbations [12]. Alpha-one antitrypsin deficiency screening is recommended for all patients diagnosed with COPD [12, 13]. Chest X-ray is indicated for all nonsmokers with chronic cough who do not take ACE inhibitors [18] and may be useful in identifying comorbidities among patients with COPD [12]. Chest X-ray should also be obtained in the context of severe COPD exacerbations [12]. Chest CT is necessary prior to consideration of lung volume reduction surgery or lung transplant but is otherwise not routinely indicated [12, 13].

Special Testing

Spirometry demonstrating post-bronchodilator FEV1/FVC ratio of less than 0.70 determines the diagnosis of COPD [12]. This cutoff results in over-diagnosis in the elderly and under-diagnosis in younger patients [13]. The American Thoracic Society/European Respiratory Society guidelines recommend FEV1/FVC less than the lower limit of normal (LLN) as a diagnostic cutoff [19]. However, patients with FEV1/FVC greater than the LLN but less than 0.70 have worse outcomes [13]. Patients with post-bronchodilator spirometry demonstrating FEV1/FVC ratio of 0.6 to 0.8 should be repeated due to variability in test results. Spirometry should be repeated annually [12].

Oximetry is indicated with symptoms concerning for respiratory failure [12, 13]. Arterial or capillary blood gas should be considered in the setting of hypoxia to evaluate for hypercapnia. The 6-min walk test and paced shuttle walk test are standardized measures of exercise capacity [12].

Differential Diagnosis

Multiple conditions can mimic COPD. The differential diagnoses are summarized in Table 3.

Treatment

Treatment of Chronic COPD

The goals of chronic COPD treatment are to reduce symptoms, risk of exacerbations, disease progression, and death. Treatment includes behavioral techniques, medications, oxygen and ventilatory support, and surgery.

Behavioral counseling is recommended to foster understanding of disease process and progression, management of breathlessness and stress, energy conservation, and the role of the patient and provider. Counseling should include a written action plan for exacerbations. Smoking cessation can reduce progression of disease and risk of exacerbations, and other triggers should be avoided as well. Nutrition should be assessed and addressed through supplements where appropriate. Regular exercise has been shown to be beneficial. Pulmonary rehabilitation, a combination of exercise and counseling, has been shown to be highly effective at improving quality of life and exercise tolerance in patients with moderate to severe COPD (GOLD Groups B, C, and D) [12].

Multiple classes of medications are used to treat chronic COPD (Table 8); however medication treatment does not appear to change the trajectory of decreased lung function over time

[12]. Medications are typically delivered through inhalers, which come in multiple formats and are frequently used inappropriately [12, 13]. Teaching and assessment of proper inhaler technique and adherence is essential. Nebulized delivery is only more effective for patients who are unable to adequately tolerate inhaler administration [12].

SABAs and SAMAs are effective for mild disease. More persistent symptoms should be treated with a long-acting muscarinic antagonist (LAMA) or LABA. If either of these classes alone are ineffective, they can be combined. Side effects of beta agonists include tremor, arrhythmia, and hypokalemia. Muscarinic antagonist side effects include dry mouth. Ipratropium has been associated with increased risk of cardiovascular events, an effect not seen to date with tiotropium. Nebulized LAMAs delivered by facemask can precipitate acute glaucoma [12].

Inhaled corticosteroids alone do not improve outcomes in patients with COPD. Combination ICS + LABA treatment has been shown to reduce the risk of exacerbations and hospitalizations in patients with moderate disease who have frequent exacerbations, particularly those with serum eosinophil counts of $\geq$300 cells/μL [12]. Eosinophil counts of $\leq$100 cells/μL are associated with poor response to inhaled corticosteroids [12, 13]. For appropriately selected patients (persistent symptoms on LAMA + LABA, with asthma or high eosinophil count), the combination of LABA, LAMA, and ICS is more effective than LABA + LAMA [20, 21]. ICS treatment is associated with hoarseness, oral thrush, bruising, and in severe COPD increased risk of pneumonia [12, 13]. Figure 4 demonstrates use of GOLD Group assignment as a guide for medication selection.

Phosphodiesterase-4 (PDE4) inhibitors work by reducing inflammation. They decrease moderate and severe exacerbations for patients with chronic bronchitis or severe COPD with an FEV1 of <50%. Side effects include diarrhea, reduced appetite, weight loss, and abdominal pain but diminish with time [12].

In patients with frequent exacerbations, azithromycin 250 milligrams per day or 500 milligrams three times a week reduce exacerbation frequency. It is less effective in smokers.

Table 8 COPD medications[a,b]

Generic (trade)	Delivery methods	Typical adult dosing [22]
Short-acting beta agonists (SABA)		
Albuterol (Proventil, Ventolin, ProAir)	Inhaler	2 inh every 4–6 h as needed with spacer
	Nebulizer	2.5 mg every 4–6 h as needed
Levalbuterol (Xopenex)	Inhaler	2 inh every 4 h as needed with spacer
	Nebulizer	0.63 mg three times daily
Short-acting muscarinic antagonists (SAMA)		
Ipratropium (Atrovent)	Inhaler	2 inh four times daily
	Nebulizer	0.5 mg every 4–6 h
Short-acting beta agonist/short-acting muscarinic antagonist combinations		
Albuterol/ipratropium (Combivent)	Inhaler	1 inh four times daily
	Nebulizer	1 vial (3 ml) (ipratropium 0.5 mg/albuterol 2.5 mg) every 6 h
Long-acting beta agonists (LABAs)		
Arformoterol (Brovana)	Nebulizer	15 mcg twice daily
Formoterol	Inhaler (Foradil)	12 mcg every 12 h
	Nebulizer (Perforomist)	20 mcg twice daily
Indacaterol (Arcapta)	Inhaler	75 mcg (1 inh) once daily
Olodaterol (Striverdi)	Inhaler	2 inh once daily
Salmeterol (Serevent)	Inhaler	1 inh twice daily
Long-acting muscarinic antagonists (LAMAs)		
Aclidinium bromide (Tudorza Pressair)	Inhaler	400 mcg (1 inh) twice daily
Glycopyrrolate (Lonhala Magnair, Seebri Neohaler)	Inhaler	15.6 mcg (1 capsule) inhaled twice daily
	Nebulizer	25 mcg (1 vial) inhaled twice daily
Revefenacin (Yupelri)	Nebulizer	175 mcg (1 vial) once daily
Tiotropium (Spiriva)	Spiriva Respimat 2.5 mcg/actuation	5 mcg (2 inh) once daily
	Spiriva Handihaler	18 mcg (1 capsule) once daily
Umeclidinium (Incruse Ellipta)	Inhaler	62.5 mcg (1 inh) once daily
LABA/LAMA combinations		
Formoterol/aclidinium (Duaklir Pressair)	Inhaler 12 mcg/400 mcg per actuation	1 inh twice daily
Formoterol/glycopyrrolate (Bevespi Aerosphere)	Inhaler 4.8 mcg/9 mcg per actuation	2 inh twice daily
Indacaterol/glycopyrrolate (Utibron Neohaler)	Inhaler 27.5 mcg/ 15.6 mcg per capsule	1 capsule inh twice daily
Vilanterol/umeclidinium (Anoro Ellipta)	Inhaler 25 mcg/62.5 mcg per actuation	1 inh once daily
Olodaterol/tiotropium (Inspiolto Respimat)	Inhaler 2.5 mcg/2.5 mcg per actuation	2 inh once daily

(continued)

Table 8 (continued)

Generic (trade)	Delivery methods	Typical adult dosing [22]
LABA/inhaled corticosteroid combinations		
Formoterol/budesonide (Symbicort)	Inhaler 4.5 mcg/160 mcg	2 inh twice daily
Formoterol/mometasone (Dulera)	Inhaler 5 mcg/100 mcg	2 inh twice daily
Salmeterol/fluticasone (Advair Diskus)	Inhaler 50 mcg/250 mcg	1 inh twice daily
Vilanterol/fluticasone furoate (Breo Ellipta)	Inhaler 25 mcg/100 mcg	1 inh once daily
LABA/LAMA/inhaled corticosteroid combinations		
Vilanterol/umeclidinium/fluticasone furoate (Trelegy Ellipta)	Inhaler 25 mcg/62.5 mcg/ 100 mcg	1 inh once daily
Methylxanthines		
Aminophylline	Intravenous	Loading dose: 5.7 mg/kg Maintenance dose: variable
Theophylline	Immediate release: solution Sustained release: oral pill	Immediate release: 300 mg/24 h divided q6–8h, increasing q3d to max 600 mg/24 h Sustained release (12 or 24 h formulations): 300 mg/24 h, increasing q3d to max 600 mg/24 h
Phosphodiesterase-4 Inhibitors		
Roflumilast (Daliresp)	Oral pill	250 mcg daily for 4 weeks, then 500 mcg daily
Mucolytic agents		
N-acetylcysteine (Acetadote)	Nebulized	See dosing instructions

Inh = oral inhalation
[a]Only formulations available in the USA are listed
[b]Information from Ref. [1] unless otherwise stated

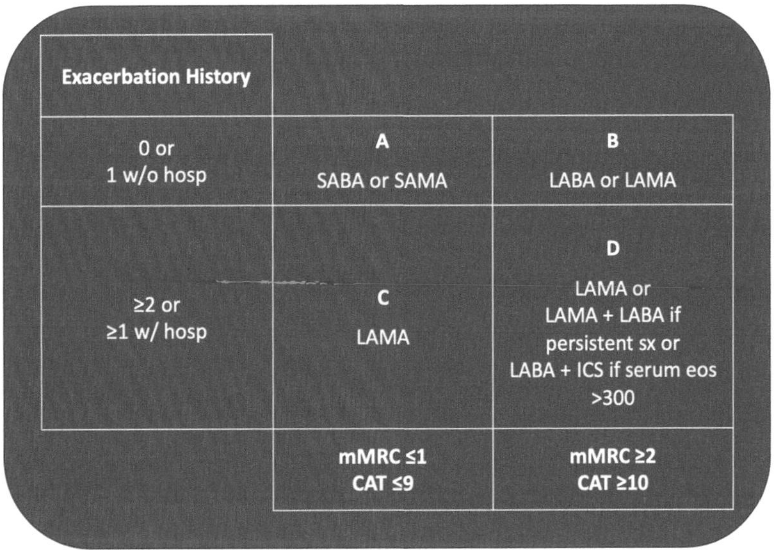

Fig. 4 GOLD Group and associated medications [1]

Azithromycin is known to prolong the QTc interval, and frequent use can lead to antibiotic resistance as well as reversible hearing loss [12, 13].

Medications of poor or uncertain efficacy for chronic use include mucolytics, oral glucocorticoids, methylxanthines, biologics, and statins. Mucolytic N-acetylcysteine may reduce exacerbations, though which patients will benefit is uncertain, and it has not been studied in patients taking modern inhaled medications. Chronic daily oral corticosteroids are not recommended for COPD as they result in significant side effects including steroid myopathy, which reduces functional capacity and increases risk of respiratory failure [12, 13]. Methylxanthines (e.g., theophylline) act as bronchodilators and improve FEV1, but given their narrow therapeutic window and risk of life-threatening arrhythmias and seizures, they are not recommended unless other long-acting bronchodilators are unavailable [12].

Oxygen (O2) and ventilatory support can be helpful for patients with severe disease. Those with resting O2 saturation < 89% who use oxygen > 15 h per day demonstrate improved survival. O2 supplementation does not improve mortality or hospitalization for patients with stable COPD and exertional hypoxemia, but it can mitigate exertional dyspnea. Hypercapnic patients discharged from the hospital may benefit from positive pressure ventilation [12].

Procedures for COPD include surgery and bronchoscopic interventions. Lung volume reduction surgery removes part of the lung to optimize ventilatory mechanics and has been shown to improve mortality for patients with severe emphysema, upper lobe emphysema, and poor post-rehab exercise capacity. It is less effective for patients with homogeneous emphysema, high exercise capacity, and decreased diffusion capacity. Bullectomy can improve dyspnea and exercise tolerance when large bullae are present. Lung transplant is indicated for patients who are not candidates for other surgeries and who have severe progressive COPD. Transplant improves health status and functional capacity but not necessarily mortality and is associated with complications including rejection, bronchiolitis obliterans, and infection. Bronchoscopic

interventions include endobronchial valves, thermal ablation, and nitinol coils and have been shown to improve exercise capacity and quality of life [12].

Referral to pulmonology is appropriate for patients with persistently impaired quality of life or recurrent hospitalization despite optimized medical therapy and pulmonary rehab. Indications for hospice include disabling dyspnea and recurrent hospitalization. End of life discussion should start early due to difficulty accurately predicting prognosis. Palliative care for end-stage COPD focuses on treatment of symptoms such as dyspnea, for which effective interventions include opiates, neuromuscular electrical stimulation, chest wall vibration, oxygen, pulmonary rehabilitation, fans blowing air onto the face, and noninvasive ventilation. Benzodiazepines have not been shown to be effective. Depression, panic, anxiety, and fatigue can be improved by pulmonary rehab, cognitive behavioral therapy, and mind-body interventions [12].

Treatment of Acute COPD Exacerbations

The goals of treating COPD exacerbations include reducing severity and preventing recurrences. Indications for hospitalization are listed in Table 9. Written action plans reduce risk of hospitalization during exacerbations [12].

COPD exacerbations are treated with a combination of bronchodilators, oral corticosteroids, antibiotics, and/or oxygen and ventilatory support. Bronchodilators can be given via any available delivery method. Continuous nebulizers should be avoided. Inhalers dosed hourly for 2–3 h then every 2–4 h are recommended for acute symptoms. Combinations of SABA + SAMA are more effective than either alone. Oral corticosteroids (prednisolone [Prednisone] 40 mg daily for ≤5–7 days) improve rates of treatment success, reduce relapse, and improve symptoms but are associated with increased risk of pneumonia, sepsis, and death. Antibiotics for 5–7 days are indicated in COPD exacerbations featuring increased sputum purulence, but not when sputum is white or clear. Normal C-reactive protein may indicate that antibiotics are not needed [12]. First-line antibiotics include trimethoprim-sulfamethoxazole

Table 9 Indications for hospitalization during COPD exacerbation [12, 13]

Category	Examples
Acute respiratory signs and symptoms	Resting dyspnea
	Tachypnea
	Hypoxia
	Respiratory failure
Acute central nervous system symptoms	Confusion
Failure of outpatient treatment	Persistent symptoms despite oral steroids, antibiotics, and bronchodilators
Life-threatening comorbidities	Heart failure
	New-onset arrhythmia
Inadequate social support	Lack of monitoring or transportation

(Bactrim), amoxicillin-clavulanic acid (Augmentin), macrolide such as azithromycin (Zithromax), or a tetracycline such as doxycycline (Vibramycin) [12, 13]. Patients with hypoxia should receive supplemental O2 with a goal O2 saturation between 88% and 92%. Arterial blood gases may be beneficial to monitor for CO2 retention. Noninvasive positive pressure ventilation is preferred over intubation for patients with acute respiratory failure. Intubation should be reserved for patients that are unable to tolerate noninvasive ventilation. Hospitalized patients should be monitored for fluid balance and nutrition and offered DVT prophylaxis and assistance with smoking cessation. After discharge, they should be contacted within 48 h and seen within 7 days to ensure stability. Pulmonary rehab and follow up within 3 months are recommended [12].

Prevention

Routine screening for COPD is not recommended. Smoking cessation is the most important preventative intervention and can be facilitated by counseling, pharmacotherapy, and nicotine replacement [12]. Excessive work or home exposure to dust, smoke, or pollution should be avoided. Influenza vaccination is recommended annually [12, 13]. Pneumococcal polysaccharide vaccine (PPSV23 [Pneumovax]) is recommended for all patients with COPD and all patients who smoke. Pneumococcal conjugate vaccine (PCV 13 [Prevnar]) is recommended for COPD patients age 65 or older or those who are frail or require frequent systemic steroids [13]. Vitamin D supplementation can reduce exacerbation frequency. Legislative bans can reduce smoking rates [12].

References

1. Global strategy for asthma management and prevention. 2019. Global initiative for asthma website. https://ginasthma.org/gina-reports. Accessed 24 Apr 2020.
2. Elward KS, Pollart SM. Medical therapy for asthma: updates from the NAEPP guidelines. Am Fam Physician. 2010;1:1241–51.
3. Dharmage SC, Perret JL, Custovic A. Epidemiology of asthma in children and adults. Front Pediatr. 2019;7:246.
4. Most recent asthma national data. 2018. Centers for disease control and prevention website. https://www.cdc.gov/asthma/most_recent_national_asthma_data.htm. Accessed 30 Apr 30 2020.
5. Guidelines for the Diagnosis and Management of Asthma (EPR-3) Guidelines. 2012. National Heart, lung and blood institute website. https://www.nhlbi.nih.gov/health-topics/guidelines-for-diagnosis-management-of-asthma. Accessed 3 Apr 2020.
6. BTS/SIGN British Guideline on the Management of Asthma. 2019. British Thoracic Society website. https://brit-thoracic.org.uk/quality-improvement/guidelines/asthma/. Accessed 14 May 2020.
7. Dweik RA, Boggs PB, Erzurum SC, Irvin CG, Leigh MW, Lundberg JO, Olin A, Plummer AL, Taylor DR. An official ATS clinical practice guideline: interpretation of exhaled nitric oxide levels (FENO) for clinical applications. Am J Respir Crit Care Med. 2011;184:602–15.
8. Tripple JW, Ameredes MS, Calhoun WJ. Outpatient management of chronic asthma in 2020. JAMA. 2020;323:561–2.
9. Zaidan MF, Ameredes BT, Calhoun WJ. Management of acute asthma in adults in 2020. JAMA. 2020;323(6):563–4.
10. Brite J, Alper HE, Friedman S. Association between socioeconomic status and asthma-related emergency

department visits among world trade center rescue and recovery works and survivors. JAMA Netw Open. 2020;(3):e201600.

11. Henneberger PK, Redlich CA, Callahan DV, Harber P, Lemiere C, Martin J, Tarlo SM, Vandenplas O, Toren K. An official American thoracic society statement: work-exacerbated asthma. Am J Respir Crit Care Med. 2011;184:368–78.

12. GOLD 2020 citation: © 2020, Global Initiative for Chronic Obstructive Lung Disease, available from www.goldcopd.org, published in Fontana.

13. Riley CM, Sciurba FC. Diagnosis and outpatient management of chronic obstructive pulmonary disease: a review. JAMA. 2019;321(8):786–97. https://doi.org/10.1001/jama.2019.0131. Review.

14. GBD 2016 Causes of Death Collaborators. Global, regional, and national age-sex specific mortality for 264 causes of death, 1980–2016: a systematic analysis for the Global Burden of Disease Study 2016. Lancet. 2017;390(10100):1151–210. https://doi.org/10.1016/S0140-6736(17)32152-9. Erratum in: Lancet. 2017;390(10106):e38. PubMed PMID: 28919116; PubMed Central PMCID:PMC5605883.

15. Fletcher CM. Standardised questionnaire on respiratory symptoms: a statement prepared and approved by the MRC Committee on the Aetiology of chronic bronchitis (MRC breathlessness score). BMJ. 1960;2:1662.

16. Jones PW, Harding G, Berry P, Wiklund I, Chen WH, Kline Leidy N. Development and first validation of the COPD assessment test. Eur Respir J. 2009;34(3):648–54.

17. Celli BR, Cote CG, Marin JM, Casanova C, Montes de Oca M, Mendez RA, Pinto Plata V, Cabral HJ. The body-mass index, airflow obstruction, dyspnea, and exercise capacity index in chronic obstructive pulmonary disease. N Engl J Med. 2004;350(10):1005–12.

18. Benich JJ, Carek PJ. Evaluation of the patient with chronic cough. Am Fam Physician. 2011;84(8):887–92.

19. Langan RC, Goodbred AJ. Office spirometry: indications and interpretation. Am Fam Physician. 2020;101(6):362–8.

20. Lipson DA, Barnhart F, Brealey N, Brooks J, Criner GJ, Day NC, Dransfield MT, Halpin DMG, Han MK, Jones CE, Kilbride S, Lange P, Lomas DA, Martinez FJ, Singh D, Tabberer M, Wise RA, Pascoe SJ, IMPACT Investigators. Once-daily single-inhaler triple versus dual therapy in patients with COPD. N Engl J Med. 2018;378(18):1671–80. https://doi.org/10.1056/NEJMoa1713901. Epub 2018 Apr 18.

21. Papi A, Vestbo J, Fabbri L, Corradi M, Prunier H, Cohuet G, Guasconi A, Montagna I, Vezzoli S, Petruzzelli S, Scuri M, Roche N, Singh D. Extrafine inhaled triple therapy versus dual bronchodilator therapy in chronic obstructive pulmonary disease (TRIBUTE): a double-blind, parallel group, randomized controlled trial. Lancet. 2018;391(10125):1076–84. https://doi.org/10.1016/S0140-6736(18)30206-X. Epub 2018 Feb 9. Erratum in: Lancet. 2018 Feb 26. PubMed PMID: 29429593.

22. Lexi-Comp. https://online.lexi.com/lco/action/login. Accessed 2/12/2020.

Pulmonary Infections

Fiona R. Prabhu, Keeley Hobart, Irvin Sulapas, and
Amy Sikes

Contents

F. R. Prabhu (✉) · K. Hobart
Department of Family and Community Medicine,
TTUHSC School of Medicine, Lubbock, TX, USA
e-mail: fiona.prabhu@ttuhsc.ed;
keeley.hobart@ttuhsc.edu

I. Sulapas
Department of Family and Community Medicine, Baylor
College of Medicine, Houston, TX, USA
e-mail: irvin.sulapas@bcm.edu

A. Sikes
Department of Family Medicine, Texas Tech University
Health Sciences Center, Lubbock, TX, USA
e-mail: amy.sikes@umchealthsystem.com

© Springer Nature Switzerland AG 2022
P. M. Paulman et al. (eds.), *Family Medicine*,
https://doi.org/10.1007/978-3-030-54441-6_91

Introduction

Pneumonia is a lung infection involving the alveoli and can be caused by a variety of microbes including bacteria, viruses, and fungi. It is the leading infectious cause of hospitalization and death in the United States [1].

Most instances of pneumonia are attributable to self-infection with one or more types of microbes that originate in the nose and mouth. In healthy individuals, typical upper airway bacterial residents such as *Streptococcus pneumoniae* and *Haemophilus influenzae* are the most common bacteria causing community-acquired pneumonia. Other causes of pneumonia include *Staphylococcus aureus*, *Klebsiella pneumonia*, *Pseudomonas aeruginosa*, and *Escherichia coli* that are generally seen in patients at higher risk for resistant bacteria.

In those with a serious impairment of their immune system, opportunistic microbes are more readily apparent such as fungi, viruses, and mycobacteria [1].

There are many mechanisms used by the lungs to resist infection. Physical mechanisms are structure of the upper airway, branching of the bronchial tree, sticky mucous layer lining the airways, cilia that propel mucous upward, and the cough reflex. If microbes do reach the alveoli, the immune system is usually able to destroy them [1].

A variety of strategies have been used to reduce the incidence of pneumonia. Elements of a healthy lifestyle that reduce the incidence are adequate nutrition, dental hygiene, and not smoking. For those with lung disease or impaired clearance of mucous, aerobic exercise, deep breathing maneuvers, and cough assist devices can facilitate expectoration and lung hygiene. Immunity to certain microbes can be enhanced by immunization [1].

Bacterial Pneumonia

General Principles

Definition/Background/Epidemiology

Pneumonia is a common infection in the parenchyma of the lower respiratory tract that can affect all age populations. There is significant morbidity and mortality associated with pneumonia, especially in the very young and elderly populations. Pneumonia is the leading cause of death in children younger than 5 years of age worldwide [2]. The average yearly incidence of pneumonia, specifically community-acquired pneumonia, is 5–11 per 1000, with most incident cases occurring in the winter months [3]. It is passed from person to person by viral particles on respiratory droplets.

Decisions on how to treat, whether to admit to the hospital or treat outpatient and potential prognosis, depend upon the most likely pathogen and the current clinical picture. In most cases, the pathogen is never isolated – only suspected – prior to initiation of treatment.

Classification

Pneumonia classification is based upon a variety of factors – age, clinical presentation, and comorbidities. Additionally, patients are further classified according to their risk factors for multidrug-resistant bacteria.

The best approach is a good history and physical exam in combination with knowledge of the most common causes of pneumonia for the presenting age patient being seen.

In 2019, the American Thoracic Society (ATS) and the Infectious Diseases Society of America (IDSA) updated the community-acquired pneumonia (CAP) guidelines [4]. Previous guidelines classified pneumonia based on the site of care (outpatient, inpatient, or ICU) and utilized terms such as healthcare-associated pneumonia, hospital-acquired pneumonia, and ventilator-associated pneumonia. These terms have been eliminated in the new guidelines and instead base classifications solely on the severity of illness and risk factors for multidrug-resistant bacteria. The IDSA/ATS CAP severity criteria have been validated and can be used to define severe community-acquired pneumonia. Validated definition includes either one major criterion or three or more minor criteria.

2007 Infectious Diseases Society of America/American Thoracic Society Criteria for Defining Severe Community-Acquired Pneumonia
Minor Criteria

Respiratory rate $\geq$ 30 breaths/min.
PaO_2/F_1O_2 ratio $\leq$ 250
Multilobar infiltrates
Confusion/disorientation
Uremia (blood urea nitrogen level $\geq$ 20 mg/dL)
Leukopenia (white blood cell count <4000 cells/mL)
Thrombocytopenia (platelet count <100,000 mL)
Hypothermia (core temperature < 36 °C)
Hypotension requiring aggressive fluid resuscitation
Major Criteria
Septic shock with need for vasopressors Respiratory failure
If a patient does not meet severe criteria, in general, it is safe to attempt treatment as an outpatient. The inpatient categories are then further classified by patient specific factors such as prior respiratory isolation of either MRSA or *Pseudomonas*, recent hospitalization and parenteral antibiotics (within 90 days), and locally validated risk factors for MRSA and/or *P. aeruginosa*.

In children, the suspected organism that has caused the pneumonia is based upon the age of the child: [3].

- *Birth to 3 weeks*: Group B streptococcus, *Haemophilus influenzae* type b (Hib), *Listeria monocytogenes*, and cytomegalovirus
- *3 Weeks to 3 months*: *Streptococcus pneumoniae*, *Chlamydia trachomatis*, respiratory syncytial virus (RSV) or other respiratory viruses, and *Bordetella pertussis*
- *4 Months to 4 years*: RSV and other respiratory viruses, *S. pneumoniae*, and group A streptococci
- *5–18 Years*: *S. pneumoniae*, *Mycoplasma pneumoniae*, and *Chlamydia pneumoniae*

Approach to the Patient

The most important point to consider when evaluating for pneumonia is the patient's age, the time of year, social habits, existing disease processes, travel history, or other exposure history – animals, geography, and other people. This information is best obtained from a thorough history and physical exam.

Diagnosis

History
The most common presenting symptoms in an immunologically competent patient include sudden or recent onset of:

- Cough with purulent sputum
- Dyspnea
- Fever $\pm$ chills
- Pleuritic chest pain

Other important information to obtain from the patient is with regard to recent hospitalizations, current resident location (in elderly patients), medical history, and recent medication (antibiotic) use.

Physical Exam

Physical exam findings can vary from one patient to another, let alone one age population to another. The following exam findings are the most consistent findings in patients with pneumonia:

Vital signs:

- Temperature > 100 °F (37.8 °C)
- Tachypnea (>20 breaths/min)
- Tachycardia (>100 beats/min)
- Decreased pulse oximetry readings on room air (<92%)

General:

- Septic appearance

Respiratory exam:

- Increased tactile fremitus
- Crackles, rhonchi
- ± Egophony
- Dullness to percussion
- Decreased breath sounds/air movement

Make sure to look for red flags in patients presenting with pneumonia-type symptoms. Red flag symptoms:

- Accessory muscle use (sternal retractions)
- Grunting
- Nasal flaring
- Altered mental status
- Apnea

The presence any of these symptoms may indicate a more severe infection requiring admission to an intensive care unit.

Laboratory and Imaging

Chest radiography is the test of choice in patients with clinically suspected CAP. The presence of an infiltrate or consolidation on X-ray is required for the diagnosis of CAP (Fig. 1).

Chest radiography should be performed in:

Any patient with at least one of the following abnormal vital signs:

- Temperature > 37.8 °C (100 °F)
- Heart Rate > 100 beats/min
- Respiratory rate > 20 breaths/min

Or

Any patient with at least two of the clinical findings:

- Decreased breath sounds
- Crackles (rales)
- Absence of asthma

Routine laboratory testing is not required to establish diagnosis in an outpatient setting. Laboratory testing recommendations differ, though, for patients who are requiring admission to hospital or the intensive care unit for treatment. These include:

- Complete blood count (CBC)
- Basic metabolic panel (BMP)
- Sputum gram stain and culture
- Blood cultures drawn from two separate sites
- Arterial blood gas (ABG) if patient is experiencing respiratory distress

For patients who are being treated empirically for MRSA or *Pseudomonas*, lower respiratory tract specimens should be cultured. These specimens can come from expectorated sputum or from a bronchoalveolar lavage (BAL) [4].

Special Testing

In patients presenting with severe CAP, special testing for urinary antigens of *Streptococcus pneumoniae* and *Legionella pneumoniae* serogroup 1 has been approved [6]. Recent guidelines, however, recommend against urinary antigen testing for *Streptococcus pneumoniae* and *Legionella* [4].

Differential Diagnosis

The following might be considered in the differential based upon the patient's signs, symptoms, and comorbidities:

- Influenza
- Viral pneumonia

Fig. 1 X-ray of infiltrates in pneumonia [7]

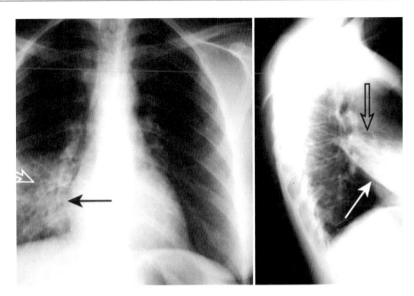

- Atypical pneumonia
- Acute bronchitis
- COPD exacerbation
- Congestive heart failure (CHF)
- Pleural effusion
- Pulmonary embolism

Treatment

Medications

Severity of illness is the most important first determination to make in treatment for a patient with pneumonia; this should direct the "site-of-care" decision (hospital vs. outpatient, ICU vs. medical ward). Two scoring systems for assisting with the decision on hospitalization are the pneumonia severity index (PSI) and the CURB-65 (confusion, uremia, respiratory rate, low blood pressure, age 65 years or greater). Using one of these criteria, in addition to the clinical picture of the patient, will help guide the appropriate medication and site of treatment [4]. In the 2019 guidelines, the PSI is recommended over the CURB-65. The PSI has been shown to more consistently serve as a decision aid to increase outpatient treatment of patients with CAP and has potential to decrease unnecessary variability in admission rates, the high cost of inpatient pneumonia treatment, and the risk of hospital-acquired complications.

After deciding to admit a patient to the hospital for treatment, the next decision to be made is whether or not the patient needs ICU treatment. As mentioned, previously, according to the Infectious Diseases Society of America/American Thoracic Society, there are several clinical criteria that should be considered for ICU admission – meeting three or more of the following:

- Tachypnea, RR >25–30 breaths/min
- PaO_2 or FiO_2 ratio <250
- Multilobar infiltrates
- Altered mental status/confusion
- BUN >20 (uremia)
- White blood cell count <4000
- Thrombocytopenia, platelet count <150 k
- Temperature <36 °C
- Hypotension/septic shock requiring aggressive fluid hydration [4]

Severity of illness, presence of comorbidities and/or risk factors for MRSA or *P. aeruginosa* guides antibiotic choice for treatment. In most cases, it can be difficult to establish exact organism(s) affecting a patient; therefore, empiric antibiotic therapy guidelines have been established.

For patients who do not meet severity criteria requiring inpatient or intensive care unit admission, with or without comorbidities, treatment can be attempted outpatient. *S pneumoniae* is still the most common cause of community-acquired pneumonia and is the main target of antibiotic therapy. The 2019 ATS/IDSA guidelines highlight using amoxicillin as a first-line agent for outpatient CAP treatment. Previously, macrolides were recommended as first-line outpatient CAP antibiotic treatment, but increasing macrolide resistance in the United States has emerged, causing a shift away from this practice.

If attempting outpatient community-acquired pneumonia treatment in a patient with comorbidities (i.e., diabetes mellitus, alcoholism, malignancy, asplenia or chronic heart, liver, lung or renal disease), combination therapy with amoxicillin/clavulanate or cephalosporin *and* a macrolide or doxycycline *or* monotherapy with a respiratory fluoroquinolone is recommended (Table 1).

For inpatient treatment of pneumonia, the same severity criteria are applied to determine patient treatment. For nonsevere inpatient pneumonia, recommended empiric treatment is a beta-lactam + macrolide OR respiratory fluoroquinolone. For severe inpatient pneumonia, the recommended treatment would be a beta-lactam + macrolide or beta-lactam + fluoroquinolone. As the new guidelines eliminate the term healthcare-associated pneumonia, it is recommended that patients in nursing homes or with recent hospitalization only be treated for methicillin-resistant *Staphylococcus aureus* (MRSA) and *Pseudomonas aeruginosa* if they meet criteria for locally validated risk factors or antibiotic-resistant bacteria. Risk factors would include previous respiratory isolation of MRSA or *P. aeruginosa* or recent hospitalization AND receipt of parenteral antibiotics within the last 90 days. It is also recommended that sputum and blood cultures should be ordered for any patients started empirically on anti-MRSA or antipseudomonal antibiotics to allow for more rapid de-escalation when culture findings are negative for these bacteria.

Bacterial pneumonia is typically treated for a minimum of 5–14 days, with length of treatment being dependent upon degree of illness at presentation, age, comorbidities, initial response, and whether patient was hospitalized/ICU or not. Attention should be directed at monitoring length of intravenous therapy and recognizing when to switch to oral therapy. Once a patient is clinically improving and requiring no intervention to maintain hemodynamic stability, he/she can safely be switched to oral therapy to complete the course of treatment [4].

In addition to following the most updated guidelines, it is also important to be aware of local epidemiological data, as well as potential antibiotic-resistant changes with typical bacterial pneumonia treatment [5].

Table 1 Initial treatment strategies for outpatients with community-acquired pneumonia

	Standard regimen
No comorbidities or risk factors for MRSA or *Pseudomonas aeruginosa* (risk factors for MRSA/*P. aeruginosa* include prior respiratory isolation of MRSA or *P. aeruginosa* or recent hospitalization AND receipt of parenteral antibiotics in the last 90 days)	Amoxicillin or Doxycycline or Macrolide (if local pneumococcal resistance is <25%)
With comorbidities (such as chronic heart, lung, liver, or renal disease; diabetes mellitus, alcoholism, malignancy, or asplenia)	Combination therapy with amoxicillin/clavulanate or cephalosporin AND Macrolide or doxycycline OR Monotherapy with respiratory fluoroquinolone

Patient Education

Decreasing a patient's chance of becoming ill with pneumonia is an important part of a primary care physician's job [6]:

- Counsel patients who smoke on the importance of smoking cessation.
- Encourage scheduled vaccinations.
- Educate patients on accepted hand hygiene standards: wash hands regularly with soap and warm water for at least 20 s.
- Disinfect frequently touched surfaces.
- Teach them about cough etiquette: cover the mouth and nose with a tissue when they cough or sneeze, and put used tissues in the waste basket.
- If they do not have a tissue, teach them to cough or sneeze into their upper sleeve or elbow, not their hands.

Prevention

Immunizations

Vaccinations against preventable illnesses have long been proven effective in overall patient and population morbidity and mortality. Risk for infection with the most common bacterial pneumonia – *Streptococcus pneumoniae* – can be decreased with immunization. According to the Centers for Disease Control, the following vaccinations are important for prevention of pneumonia:

- Pneumococcal
- *Haemophilus influenzae* type b
- Pertussis (whooping cough)
- Influenza (flu) – yearly
- Measles [2, 7]

Atypical Pneumonias

Mycoplasma Pneumoniae

General Principles

M. pneumoniae is considered the most common "atypical" pathogen for community-acquired pneumonia (CAP). The prevalence of *M. pneumoniae* in adults with pneumonia can range between 1.9% and 32.5%. Outbreaks can occur in institutional settings such as schools and military bases [8]. It is usually transmitted from close person to person contact via respiratory droplets. The average incubation period is around 2–3 weeks [9], and infections tend to occur during the summer and early fall. *M. pneumoniae* pneumonia is most frequently seen among children around 5–15 years of age [10].

Approach to the Patient

Diagnosis

History and Physical
The onset of symptoms is typically gradual over the course of several days. Common symptoms include sore throat, muscle pain, headache, malaise, and chills. Patients also complain of a cough that is initially dry but becomes productive over the course of the infection. The cough is typically worse at night. Sinus pressure and otalgia can also occur. The lung exam can be normal on initial examination but can develop into scattered rales or wheezes during its progression. Extra-pulmonary complications can include maculopapular rashes, arthralgia, aseptic meningitis, transverse myelopathy, and Guillain-Barré syndrome. Since the progression is gradual, a patient may not seek medical attention until a few days to a week.

Laboratory and Imaging: Special Testing
Obtaining a chest radiograph may reveal diffuse, interstitial infiltrates [10] and may be more prominent if the illness has been present for at least 2 weeks [9]. Traditionally a throat culture was obtained; however, the incubation period in a culture can take up to 3 weeks. Nuclear acid amplification testing (NAATs) is now considered the "gold standard" and has a high sensitivity and shorter turnaround time [10, 11]. A cold agglutinin test can be used as well and usually appears by the end of the first week of illness. Around 72–92% of patients with pneumonia and positive cold agglutinins ($>$1:32) will develop a serologic response to *M. pneumoniae*. Serology can be obtained by complement fixation (CF) or enzyme immunoassay (EIA) [8, 11].

Treatment
With the absence of a cell wall, *Mycoplasma pneumoniae* is typically resistant to glycopeptides, fosfomycin, and beta-lactam antimicrobials. Macrolides (erythromycin, azithromycin), tetracyclines (doxycycline), and fluoroquinolones (levofloxacin, moxifloxacin) are the typical therapies used to treat *M. pneumoniae*. If central nervous system involvement is suspected, consider the use of tetracyclines. In a patient with an impaired immune system and a suspicion of a systemic infection outside the respiratory system, consider the use of a fluoroquinolone [11]. Macrolides, particularly azithromycin, tend to be the most active against *M. pneumoniae* in in vitro studies [8]. The duration of antibiotic treatment is typically 5 days of azithromycin or 7–14 days with a tetracycline or fluoroquinolone.

Prevention
Use of appropriate hand hygiene and cough etiquette.

Chlamydial Infection

General Principles
Chlamydia is a set of gram-negative obligate intracellular organisms. It includes *Chlamydia trachomatis*, *Chlamydophila* (formerly *Chlamydia*) *pneumoniae*, and *Chlamydophila psittaci*. *C. trachomatis* generally presents as a genital tract or ocular infection, but the latter two can present itself as an atypical pneumonia. Around 10% of cases of community-acquired pneumonia (CAP) are related to *C. pneumoniae* [12].

Approach to the Patient

Diagnosis

History and Physical
Along with other atypical pneumonias, patients can present with productive cough, sore throat [13], sinus congestion, and malaise.

Patients who have psittacosis, caused by *C. psittaci*, tend to have a history with exposure to infected birds, which is also known as parrot fever, ornithosis or avian chlamydiosis [14]. *C. psittaci* comprises around 1% of all community-acquired pneumonia cases, and less than 50 cases a year of psittacosis are reports in the United States [14, 15]. It often presents in young to middle-aged adults. Symptoms include abrupt fever, headache, dry cough, myalgia, and malaise.

Laboratory and Imaging: Special Testing
Chest radiographs may show infiltrates. For diagnosis, oropharyngeal swabs can be used to culture *Chlamydophila* species. Serology tests, EIA, and polymerase chain reaction (PCR) can be used as well [13]. Laboratory testing may show abnormal liver enzymes, hyponatremia, elevated BUN/creatinine levels, and elevated erythrocyte sedimentation rate (ESR) and C-reactive protein (CRP). The patient may also have a normal white blood cell count with a "left shift" [14]. A chest

radiograph can reveal interstitial or lobar infiltrates [16]. As with *C. pneumoniae*, *C. psittaci* can be diagnosed with serologic testing.

Treatment
Tetracyclines such as doxycycline (100 mg orally twice daily) or tetracycline (500 mg orally four times per day) for 7–10 days are the treatment of choice for both *C. pneumoniae* and *C. psittaci* [14]. Macrolides (azithromycin) can be used as well and are usually the choice for empiric treatment for atypical pneumonia [13, 16]. For children, macrolides are the treatment of choice.

Prevention
Counsel patients about the importance of hand hygiene and cough etiquette [17].

Viral Pneumonia

General Principles

Worldwide, 900,000 children aged less than 5 years die from pneumonia every year. Despite advances, a cause is not always ascertained in a patient with pneumonia. Recent prospective pneumonia etiology studies have failed to detect a pathogen in greater than 50% of adults and approximately 20% of children hospitalized with pneumonia. In these same studies, viruses were more commonly detected than bacteria in both adults and children, accounting for greater than 25% of detections in adults and greater than 70% in children [18].

Epidemiology
More studies are showing that viral pathogens are an important cause of community-acquired pneumonia (CAP), including viruses other than influenza. In a large epidemiological study conducted by the Centers for Disease Control and Prevention despite an extensive diagnostic workup performed, no pathogen was detected in 62% of cases, vital pathogen was detected as the single pathogen in 22% of cases, bacterial pathogens were detected in 11% of cases, and co-infection virus-bacteria were detected in 3% of cases.

Among the viral pathogens, human rhinovirus was the most commonly detected followed by influenza virus [19].

In the EPIC (Etiology of Pneumonia in the Community) study among the 2222 children with pneumonia, the most commonly detected viruses were respiratory syncytial virus (28%), human rhinoviruses (27%), human metapneumovirus (13%), adenoviruses (11%), parainfluenza 1 to 3 viruses (7%), influenza A and B viruses (7%), and coronaviruses (CoV, 5%) [18].

As of the time of writing this chapter, there has been a declaration of a pandemic with COVID-19 which is part of the group of coronaviruses responsible for severe acute respiratory syndrome (SARS) and Middle East Respiratory Syndrome (MERS). Coronaviruses are single-stranded RNA viruses, and there are six that have been identified in humans. In SARS, nosocomial transmission was an important factor in epidemic spread. In MERS, direct contact with dromedaries in the 2 weeks before illness onset was a strong association [20].

Transmission

For influenza and RSV, droplet and fomite transmission are the most common methods of transmission.

Influenza has an incubation period of 1–3 days, and viral shedding begins before the appearance of symptoms and within the first 24 h of inoculation. Viral shedding peaks on the second day and in healthy adults is no longer detectable 6–10 days later. In children and immunocompromised adults, prolonged viral shedding occurs up to 21 days [21]. RSV viral shedding has a mean of 6.7 days with a range of up to 21 days [22].

Approach to Patient

Diagnosis

History

Infants with RSV initially present with rhinorrhea and decreased appetite followed by a cough

within 1–3 days. Soon after the cough, sneezing, fever, and wheezing occur. In very young infants, the only symptoms may be irritability, decreased activity, and apnea [22].

In adults the presentation is similar to that of community-acquired pneumonia, but they may have symptoms of an upper respiratory infection for less than 5 days prior. The symptoms of an upper respiratory infection are rhinorrhea, sore throat, cough, headache, fatigue, and fever [6].

Physical Examination

The physical examination should target the following areas: general appearance and vital signs, head, eyes, ears, nose, and throat, cardiac, and pulmonary and thorax.

General appearance and vital signs are important in discerning the severity of illness. Is the patient lethargic or confused? Is the patient tachycardic or hypotensive? These are signs of more severe illness and most likely will require hospitalization.

Examination of the head, eyes, ears, nose, and throat can provide evidence for a preceding upper respiratory infection which would indicate a more viral etiology.

On cardiac examination, if there is a new gallop or murmur, then that can indicate increased severity of illness.

Pulmonary and thorax examinations are done to look for abnormal breath sounds and evidence of a consolidation or effusion which again can indicate a higher level of severity (Table 2) [6].

Treatment

Medications are given based on etiology of viral pneumonia. Influenza is treated with oseltamivir (although peramivir can also be used) [19].

Herpes simplex and varicella zoster are treated with acyclovir. No antiviral treatment of proven value is available for other viral pneumonias, and a high clinical suspicion for bacterial superinfection should be maintained. For RSV infection, high-risk infants and young children likely to benefit from immunoprophylaxis based on gestational age, certain underlying medical

Table 2 Laboratory and imaging recommendations for viral pneumonia [23]

Office-based	
RSV	Antigen detection test supplemented by cell culture
Sensitivity of antigen detection tests range from 80% to 90% and is reliable in young children
Real-time polymerase chain reaction (RT-PCR) assays are more sensitive in older children and adults who may have a lower viral load
Influenza	Rapid influenza diagnostic tests
Sensitivity tests range from 50% to 70% and specificity tests range from 90% to 95%
Hospital-based	
Serology	Complete blood count with differential – To assess severity of infection
Electrolytes – To assess hydration, kidney function, and glucose
Blood culture for bacterial pathogens
Sputum	Culture and sensitivity for bacterial pathogens
Nasopharyngeal	For RSV and influenza
Chest X-ray	Initially, to assess for presence of consolidation or effusion
CT of chest	For those not responding to initial therapy
Specialized testing	
Serology	Titers for acute and convalescent phase – More important for seroprevalence and epidemiological studies

conditions, and RSV seasonality, palivizumab is available. This is a monoclonal antibody given in monthly intramuscular injections during RSV season [23]. In immunocompromised patients, ribavirin has been used anecdotally for severe parainfluenza and human metapneumovirus infections; cidofovir for severe adenovirus infection in both immunocompromised and immunocompetent patients; and ganciclovir in CMV pneumonitis [19].

For coronoviruses, symptomatic and supportive care are, again, the mainstay of therapy. The most commonly prescribed antiviral regimens in the clinical settings are ribavirin, interferons, and lopinavir/ritonavir [20].

Family and Community Issues

Prevention using standard precautions and droplet precautions for at least 5 days is recommended. Wash hands frequently and correctly with soap and water for at least 20 s, or use alcohol-based hand gels. Use respiratory hygiene measures such as masks or tissues to cover the mouth for patients with respiratory illness. Avoid sharing cups and utensils. Clean contaminated surfaces.

Yearly influenza vaccination is recommended, and for those whom vaccination is contraindicated, antiviral chemoprophylaxis is recommended. Encourage patients to alert providers when they present for a visit and have symptoms of respiratory infection [22, 21].

Tuberculosis

General Principles

Definition

Tuberculosis is caused by *Mycobacterium tuberculosis* (MTB). This is a large nonmotile rod-shaped obligate aerobic bacterium requiring oxygen for survival. It is commonly introduced to the body through inhalation of droplet nuclei. MTB is usually found in well-aerated upper lobes of the lungs. MTB is a facultative intracellular parasite that is engulfed by macrophages. MTB is released into the alveoli upon death of the macrophage, and the health of the host's immune system is the key factor in expression of TB disease [24].

Epidemiology

One-third of the world's populations is infected with tuberculosis (TB). In 2012, nearly nine million people around the world became sick with TB disease, and there were approximately 1.3 million TB-related deaths worldwide. TB is a leading killer of people who are HIV-infected. A total of 8920 TB cases (or 2.8 per 100,000 persons) were reported in the United States in 2019 [25]. Up to 13 million people in the United States are living with latent TB infection [25].

Classification

MTB may be cleared by the host immune system or may progress to latent TB infection or to primary TB. Latent tuberculosis infection (LTBI) means that the host immune system has used the cellular immune system mediated by T-helper cells to contain MTB in a granuloma. 5–10% of persons with LTBI are at risk of progressing to active TB disease. Immunocompromised persons (HIV, cancer, on immunosuppressing medications) are at greater risk for progression to active TB disease [24].

Approach to the Patient

Diagnosis

Screening

The Centers for Disease Control (CDC) recommends that high-risk populations be screened for latent infection. This includes HIV patients, IV drug users, healthcare workers who serve high-risk populations, and contacts of individuals with pulmonary tuberculosis. A validated risk assessment questionnaire may be used to identify children who are likely to benefit from screening.

History/Physical Examination

Classic clinical features of pulmonary tuberculosis include chronic cough, sputum production, appetite loss, weight loss, fever, night sweats, and hemoptysis. Extrapulmonary tuberculosis occurs in 10–42% of patients. In HIV-infected persons, the risk of active tuberculosis increases soon after infection with HIV. Those with a CD4 count of less than 200 cells/mm^3 may have an atypical presentation of tuberculosis with subtle infiltrates, pleural effusion, hilar lymphadenopathy, and other forms of extrapulmonary tuberculosis. At CD4 counts of less than 75 cells/mm^3, pulmonary findings may be absent, and disseminated tuberculosis is more frequent. Disseminated tuberculosis presents as a nonspecific chronic febrile illness with widespread organ involvement [24].

Laboratory/Imaging

Latent infection is diagnosed using the tuberculin skin test (TST) or interferon-gamma release assay (IGRA).

In the TST a small amount of tuberculin is injected into the dermis of the skin creating a small, pale bump. In 2–3 days the TST must be read by a trained healthcare worker. A positive reaction is induration measured in millimeters. Those people who have previously been vaccinated with bacillus Calmette-Guérin (BCG) may have a false-positive TST [26]. IGRA measures a person's immune reactivity to MTB. White blood cells from most persons infected with MTB will release interferon-gamma when mixed with antigens derived from MTB. IGRA requires a single patient visit and results can be available within 24 h. Vaccination with BCG does not cause a false-positive IGRA test. However, IGRA is more expensive than TST [26].

Active tuberculosis infection is diagnosed using sputum microscopy and culture along with chest radiography. Three sputum samples are obtained for acid-fast bacilli (AFB). In addition a nucleic acid amplification test (NAAT), a complete blood count, and electrolytes are also ordered. Sputum culture is more sensitive than smear staining, facilitates identification of the mycobacterium species by nucleic acid amplification, and evaluates drug sensitivity. Cultures may take 4–8 weeks [26]. 40–50% of TB cases are AFB smear negative and 15–20% have negative cultures [26]. Chest X-ray is often normal but hilar adenopathy is the most common abnormality found in as much as 65% of cases. Hilar changes can occur 1–8 weeks after skin test conversion. The findings often resolve within the first year of detecting a positive skin test for primary TB [24]. Pleural effusions are also common in active TB infection.

Treatment

Treatment depends on whether latent or active infection is diagnosed.

Latent infection is treated with isoniazid 300 mg daily for at least 6 months and preferably for 9 months. Alternative treatment regimens are listed on the Centers for Disease Control and

Prevention website. All treatment regimens require directly observed therapy – a person employed by the state health department administers and ensures that the patient diagnosed with latent infection takes their medication [27].

Active drug-susceptible TB is treated with a four-drug regimen: isoniazid (INH), rifampin (RIF), ethambutol (EMB), and pyrazinamide (PZA). There is an intensive phase of treatment for 2 months followed by a continuation phase of either 4 or 7 months for a total of 6 to 9 months of treatment. There are four different regimens recommended by the Centers for Disease Control. The 4-month continuation phase is used in most patients. The 7-month continuation phase is recommended for the following groups: those with cavitary pulmonary TB and the sputum culture obtained at 2 months of treatment which is positive; those whose intensive phase of treatment did not include PZA; patients with HIV who are not receiving antiretroviral treatment during TB treatment; and patients being treated with once weekly INH and rifapentine and whose sputum culture obtained at the completion of the intensive phase is positive.

Pyridoxine supplementation is recommended to prevent isoniazid-induced neuropathy [27]. If there is multidrug-resistant disease, then initial treatment is based on local disease patterns and pending drug-susceptibility results; later-generation fluoroquinolones are preferred (e.g., moxifloxacin or levofloxacin) [27].

For those with active TB, sputum analysis should be done weekly until sputum conversion is documented. Patients who receive pyrazinamide should undergo baseline and periodic serum uric acid assessments. Those who receive long-term ethambutol therapy should undergo baseline and periodic visual acuity and red-green color perception testing. Also patients should be monitored for toxicity with baseline and periodic liver enzymes, complete blood cell count, and serum creatinine [27].

Drug-resistant TB is caused by TB bacteria that are resistant to at least one first-line anti-TB drug. Multidrug-resistant TB is resistant to more than one anti-TB drug and at least INH and RIF. Extensively drug-resistant TB is a rare type of multidrug-resistant TB that is resistant to isoniazid and rifampin, plus any fluoroquinolone, and at least one of three injectable second-line drugs (i.e., amikacin, kanamycin, or capreomycin). Extensively drug-resistant TB is of special concern for people with HIV infection or other conditions that can weaken the immune system [27].

Causes of multidrug-resistant TB include drugs used to treat TB that are misused or mismanaged (e.g., people do not complete a full course of TB treatment); healthcare providers prescribe the wrong treatment (wrong dose or length of time); drugs for proper treatment are not available; drugs are of poor quality [27].

Family and Community Issues

Tuberculosis is required to be reported to local public health authorities. For control of pulmonary tuberculosis, control of infectivity is most efficiently achieved through prompt specific drug treatment. It takes 2–4 weeks for vital organisms to disappear in the sputum and 4–8 weeks to be cleared in the sputum.

Patients with sputum smear-positive TB who live in congregate settings should be placed in an airborne infection isolation room with negative pressure ventilation. Patients should cover their nose and mouth while sneezing. Persons entering rooms where TB patients reside should wear personal respiratory protective devices capable of filtering particles less than 1 micromillimeter in diameter. Patients whose sputum is negative for bacteria and who do not cough and who are known to be on adequate drug treatment do not require isolation. Handwashing and good housekeeping practices must be maintained according to policy [17].

Histoplasmosis

General Principles

Definition/Background and Epidemiology

Histoplasmosis is a pulmonary infection caused by *Histoplasma* – a fungus found in soil with large amounts of bird and bat guano [28]. People acquire histoplasmosis after breathing in the microconidia (microspores) from the air, often after participating in activities that disturb the soil. Although most people who breathe in the spores become mildly ill, moderate infection may present with a fever, cough, and/or fatigue. Not every person infected with this spore becomes ill; but in patients with weakened immune systems, the infection can become severe, especially if it becomes a systemic infection [28].

Anyone is susceptible to histoplasmosis if they live or have traveled to an area where *Histoplasma* lives in the soil. In the United States, *Histoplasma* mainly lives in soil in the central and eastern states, especially in the Ohio and Mississippi River valleys. *Histoplasma* has been reported worldwide, with localized foci located in Central America, Europe, Africa, and Asia [29]. Outdoor activities often associated with this fungus include cave spelunking, mining, construction/demolition, excavation, chimney cleaning, and farming/gardening.

There are specific populations who are at higher risk for developing the severe forms of histoplasmosis. This population includes patients who have weakened immune response (HIV/AIDS, previous organ transplant, or who are on chronic immune-suppressing medications), infants, and older adults (55 and older).

Approach to the Patient

Diagnosis

History
A majority of patients either will have no symptoms or will present with subacute influenza-like symptoms – dry cough, fever, myalgias, and fatigue – possibly weeks to months after exposure. In patients with acute illness, presenting symptoms can include high fever, headache, nonproductive cough, chills, weakness, pleuritic chest pain, and fatigue. Patients who are immunocompromised are at increased risk for systemic dissemination.

For patients not living in the areas of highest incidence, travel and activity history are important factors in diagnosing this illness.

Physical Examination
In general, the physical exam findings for any acute pulmonary infection will be similar to those for bacterial pneumonia:

- Tachycardia
- Tachypnea, +/− hypoxia
- Decreased or adventitious breath sounds
- Fever >40 °C (102 °F)
- Possible septic appearance

Laboratory and Imaging
Initial presentation resembles community-acquired pneumonia; therefore, the typical lab tests and imaging are completed at that time. These include a CBC and chest X-ray. Based on initial exam and diagnostic findings alone, most patients will likely be treated for a bacterial CAP; not until the patient's condition has worsened or initial antibiotic therapy has failed will additional special testing be completed.

Chest X-ray findings with acute pulmonary histoplasmosis include patchy or diffuse reticulonodular infiltrates; CT scans show +/− mediastinal or hilar lymphadenopathy [30]. At this point, further testing with treatment plan adjustments is recommended.

Special Testing
Definitive testing for histoplasmosis requires cultured growth of the organism, but this can take 4–6 weeks. Several tests are available for diagnosis of histoplasmosis once it is considered the cause of illness. Table 3 provides a list of testing available [29, 30].

For patients who present with diffuse disease or chronic disease with cavitating lesions, HIV testing or differentiation of cause of immunocompromised state should be completed.

Differential Diagnosis
- Pneumonia – bacterial, atypical, viral
- Sarcoidosis

Table 3 Testing methods for histoplasmosis

Diagnostic method	Comments
Antigen detection Urine Serum	Most sensitive if both urine and blood are tested Acute and chronic infection *CON*: Not as useful in immunocompromised patients – Unable to mount antibody response
Culture	Diagnostic *CON*: Takes 4–6 weeks for culture to grow

- Other pulmonary fungal infections – blastomycosis, aspergillosis, coccidioidomycosis
- Lung cancer

Treatment

Medications
Table 4 summarizes the most recent recommendations on treatment of histoplasmosis. There has been a recent change in the treatment recommendations, with increased use of itraconazole. Amphotericin B is still highly recommended for patients with severe pulmonary histoplasmosis and for immunosuppressed patients [38, 29–31].

Prevention and Patient Education
For patients who are immunocompromised, education on high-risk behavior in endemic areas – cave exploration/spelunking, for example – should be provided.

Coccidioidomycosis

General Principles

Definition/Background and Epidemiology
Coccidioides is a dimorphic fungus that is found in the soil of the southwest region of the United States. Coccidioidomycosis is an infection caused by *Coccidioides immitis* or *Coccidioides posadasii*, and it is due to the inhalation of spores [32]. The incidence of reported coccidioidomycosis has increased, from 5.3 per 100,000 population in 1998 to 42.6 per 100,000 in 2011 [33]. The

Table 4 Treatment recommendations for histoplasmosis [29]

Disease acuity	Medications
Mild to moderate	Itraconazole 200 mg orally three times a day for first 3 days and then 200 mg orally once or twice daily for 6–12 weeks
Moderate to severe	Amphotericin B (lipid formulation) 3–5 mg/kg daily IV for 1–2 weeks, followed by itraconazole 200 mg orally three times daily for 3 days and then 200 mg twice daily, for a total of 12 weeks *Plus* Methylprednisolone 0.5–1 mg/kg daily IV for the first 1–2 weeks of therapy, in patients with ARDS[a]

[a]*ARDS* acute respiratory distress syndrome

reports were from the endemic areas of Arizona, California, Nevada, New Mexico, and Utah. Due to population increases in Arizona and California, the number of infections has risen to about 150,000 per year. It is also known as "valley fever" [34], or in California, San Joaquin valley fever.

Approach to the Patient

Diagnosis

History and Physical Examination
Infection is usually acquired by inhalation of the spores and living around the endemic regions of the southwestern United States. Most commonly, coccidioidomycosis usually presents itself as a self-limiting acute or subacute community-acquired pneumonia. This can develop around 7–28 days infection. The patient can present with respiratory complaints, fatigue, or arthralgia. Around 75% of patients with primary pulmonary coccidioidomycosis develop a flu-like syndrome with fever and cough [15]. For some patients, fatigue can last from weeks to months. A few patients (0.5%) infected may develop a progressive pulmonary or disseminated infection (skin, meninges, and bones). Persons of African or Filipino descent and pregnant, diabetic, and

immunosuppressed patients have a higher risk of extrapulmonary complications.

Obtaining an accurate travel history is important. The patient should have been exposed in a region where exposure is possible (southwestern United States). The most common symptom is a respiratory illness, particularly if it involves the lower respiratory tract (i.e., pneumonia). The severity of illness varies from a mild respiratory infection to progressive pulmonary lesions or dissemination. The diagnosis of coccidioidomycosis from other causes is difficult without further testing.

Laboratory and Imaging: Special Testing

A sputum culture growing *Coccidioides* species establishes the diagnosis; however, it could take weeks for the culture to grow. *Coccidioides* species is considered by the Centers for Disease Control (CDC) as a select agent, so there are specific guidelines to oversee its handling [35]. Usually a culture is reserved for patients who require hospitalization. For most patients in an ambulatory setting, serologic testing can be used to diagnose coccidioidomycosis. IgM and IgG anticoccidioidal antibodies are usually the screening test of choice. In 25%–30% of cases, eosinophilia is seen on a white blood cell differential [15].The most common chest radiograph abnormality is airspace opacity (58% of patients), followed by pulmonary nodules (22.8%) and a cavitary lesion (13.2%) [36].

Treatment

If there are no risk factors or no evidence of extensive coccidioidal infection, a majority of patients do not need any antifungal medication. Follow-up visits every 3–6 months for up to 1–2 years are recommended with serial chest radiographs. This is done to document radiographic resolution or to identify extrapulmonary complications. *Coccidioides* nodules generally do not calcify, which is in contrast to histoplasmosis [15]. For patients presenting with a severe illness or have risk factors (i.e., pregnancy), it is recommended to start antifungal therapy. Common antifungals used are ketoconazole 400 mg PO (per os/by mouth) daily, fluconazole 400–800 mg by PO daily, and itraconazole 200 mg PO two to three times per day. For pregnant patients, amphotericin B deoxycholate (0.5–1.5 mg/kg intravenously daily or alternate day) or amphotericin B lipid formulation (2.0–5.0 mg/kg or greater intravenously daily) is used as the antifungal of choice. Depending on the severity, the duration of therapy can range from 3 to 6 months to years.

Prevention

Dust control measures in endemic areas such as face masks, air-conditioned cabs, and wetted soil are recommended. Concurrent disinfection of discharges and soiled surfaces and terminal cleaning must be accomplished [17].

Legionnaire's Disease

General Principles

Definition/Background

Legionnaire's disease is a waterborne, pulmonary infection caused by a gram-negative, nonspore-forming, aerobic bacterium, *Legionella pneumophila*. This pulmonary infection was coined Legionnaire after an outbreak of pneumonia that occurred in people who had attended a convention of the American Legion in Philadelphia in 1976. *Legionella* is the third most common cause of pneumonia in immunocompetent patients [35].

The bacterium, *Legionella pneumophila*, loves warm water and can be found naturally in the environment. This bacterium can live in and be spread to humans from hot tubs, cooling towers, hot water tanks, large plumbing systems, or fountains. The bacteria reside on droplets of water (vapor or mist) and are inhaled from environments containing water features as described above. The incubation period is usually 2–14 days before patients notice any symptoms.

This organism should be suspected in a patient who has had progressive pneumonia-like symptoms and is resistant to standard treatment for CAP.

Epidemiology

Since being discovered, an estimated 8000–18,000 people are hospitalized yearly in the United States with this infection [36]. It is considered the second most common pathogen detected in cases of pneumonia requiring admission to ICUs and is the third most common cause of pneumonia in immunocompetent patients [35, 36]. In the past 10–12 years, there has been a notable increase in the number of cases reported. This infection is most often reported in the fall and summer, peaking in August [36].

Approach to the Patient

Factors to consider in a patient presenting with a pneumonia-type picture and potential diagnosis of *Legionella* are:

- Older age, >65 years of age
- Smoking status
- Male
- COPD or other chronic lung diseases
- Immunosuppressed or immunocompromised
- Lung cancer
- Diabetes mellitus

Diagnosis

Prompt diagnosis and early initiation of therapy are important for adequate treatment of Legionnaire's disease [6].

History and Physical Examination

Many symptoms are associated with Legionnaire's disease, but symptoms that are consistently reported include fever, loss of appetite, dyspnea, cough, headaches, and malaise. Some patients have reported diarrhea, confusion, phlegm, and/or blood-streaked sputum/hemoptysis. In most cases, symptoms have an abrupt start. If not recognized and treated appropriately, a mild infection can rapidly turn fatal.

Additional information to glean from a patient is recent travel history (including hotel or cruise ship stay) within 2 weeks of onset of symptoms [37].

Physical exam findings might include:

- Tachypnea, RR >20
- Temperature > 40 °C (102 °F)
- Mental status changes, confusion
- Rales on auscultation
- Relative bradycardia
- Generalized abdominal tenderness

Use of special scoring systems, like the Modified Winthrop-University Hospital Infectious Disease Division's Weighted Point System for Diagnosing Legionnaire's Disease in Adults, can be crucial in early infection to diagnose correctly for treatment of Legionnaire's disease.

Laboratory and Imaging

Chest X-rays of patients with *Legionella pneumoniae* can appear identical to X-rays from other types of bacterial pneumonia; therefore, additional testing is required. In general, if these patients are admitted to the hospital, standard blood work should be collected (CBC, BMP, blood cultures × 2, sputum culture/g stain). If *Legionella* is being suspected, there are several options in testing for this organism – the choice of test will likely be driven by what is available within the clinic or hospital laboratory.

Special Testing

When Legionnaires' disease is suspected, both a urinary antigen test and *Legionella* culture of a respiratory specimen should be ordered. The culture requires a special medium, buffered charcoal yeast extract agar (BCYE). The "gold standard" and most sensitive test is the isolation of the organisms by culture from sputum or BAL. The disadvantage to culturing *Legionella* is that it can take 5–10 days for results and is a meticulous process. Cultures can yield a sensitivity of 20–80%, with a specificity of 100% [35, 36].

A serum test has been developed utilizing immunofluorescent assay (IFA) and enzyme-linked immunosorbent assay (ELISA). These tests evaluate and aid in diagnosis when the antibody titer increases greater than fourfold [31]. The time required for adequate testing using this method can take up to 3–8 weeks. Sensitivity and specificity of blood serum testing are 70–100% and 100%, respectively [35, 36].

A newer test being used in hospitals is the urinary antigen test. An advantage to this test is a fast turnaround time (<1 h) allowing a shorter time from presentation to diagnosis to targeted treatment. The main disadvantage to using this test for detection of *Legionella* is that it is specific for *L. pneumophila* serogroup 1 only [36]. The urinary antigen test yields a sensitivity and specificity of 80–90% and > 99%, respectively [35, 36].

Differential Diagnosis
- Bronchitis
- Q-fever
- Acute respiratory distress syndrome
- Pneumonia – viral, atypical, bacterial
- Pleural effusion

Treatment

Medications
First-line treatment for *Legionella pneumoniae* follows the guidelines for bacterial CAP – utilizing either a respiratory fluoroquinolone or azithromycin [37, 38, 36] (Table 5).

Immunizations and Chemoprophylaxis
There are no vaccines available for prevention of *Legionella* infections.

Prevention
The most important factor in preventing infection is continued maintenance of water areas, such as hot tubs and heating/cooling water systems.

Table 5 Antimicrobial therapy for *Legionella pneumoniae*

First line	**Levofloxacin** 500 mg IV or orally every 24 h for 7 days or 750 mg IV orally every 24 h for 5 days **Azithromycin** 500 mg IV or 500 mg IV daily for 7–10 days
Second line	**Doxycycline** 100 mg orally twice daily for 5–7 days

Family and Community Issues
Awareness of outbreaks and potential contaminants should be considered when multiple cases within a community are diagnosed with *Legionella*.

Mycobacterium Avium Complex

General Principles

Definition/Background and Epidemiology
Mycobacterium avium complex (MAC) is considered to be nontuberculous mycobacteria. MAC includes several subspecies: *Mycobacterium avium* subsp. *avium*, *M. avium* subsp. *silvaticum*, *M. avium* subsp. *hominissuis*, *M. avium* subsp. *paratuberculosis*, *M. avium* subsp. *intracellulare*, *M. arosiense*, *M. chimaera*, *M. colombiense*, *M. marseillense*, *M. timonense*, *M. bouchedurhonese*, and *M. ituriense* [39].

Nontuberculous mycobacteria (NTM) are normal inhabitants of soil and water. Infections occur because their occupied habitats are shared with humans, animals, fish, and poultry. The habitats include drinking water distribution systems and household plumbing [39].

Patients who receive TNF-α blockers are susceptible to NTM infections, and MAC was the most commonly implicated [40].

Approach to the Patient

Diagnosis

History and Physical Examination
Symptoms are nonspecific. Most patients present with a chronic cough, with or without sputum production or hemoptysis, and slowly progressive fatigue or malaise. Constitutional symptoms such as weight loss, fever, and night sweats are less frequent, occurring in 30–50% of patients, and often indicate advanced disease. Physical examination would be the same as for other types of pneumonia [41].

Laboratory and Imaging
Radiographic abnormalities are more specific and generally follow two distinct patterns. The first is bronchiectasis and nodular lesions mostly

involving the lingual and middle lobe. The second is fibrocavitary lesions that mostly involve the upper lobes and resemble pulmonary tuberculosis [41].

Differential diagnoses for cavitary lesions include pulmonary malignancy, sarcoidosis, and infections by non-mycobacterial pathogens such as fungi and *Nocardia* species [41].

Special Testing
Sputum culture is required to make the diagnosis. This can be from at least two separate expectorated sputum samples or at least one bronchial wash or lavage.

Management
Treatment regimens should consist of a rifamycin (rifampin or rifabutin), ethambutol, and a macrolide (azithromycin or clarithromycin). Therapy can be given daily or intermittently depending on the disease type and severity. Nodular bronchiectasis patterns can usually be treated by three times weekly therapy. Cavitary MAC disease involves daily three-drug therapy in addition to IM streptomycin or IM/IV amikacin usually given three times weekly [40].

Pneumocystis Pneumonia

General Principles

Definition/Background and Epidemiology
Pneumocystis pneumonia (PCP) is an opportunistic infection that occurs in immunocompromised patients, such as persons infected with the human immunodeficiency virus (HIV). Patients who are on chronic immunosuppressive therapy are also at risk [42]. Traditionally the nomenclature of the organism was *Pneumocystis carinii pneumonia* (*P. carinii p*neumonia), but the name has been changed to *Pneumocystis jiroveci* to distinguish the species that affects humans. The acronym "PCP" is still used today (*Pneumocystis p*neumonia) to avoid confusion in medical literature [43]. For patients with acquired immunodeficiency syndrome (AIDS),

PCP is the most common opportunistic infection, but since the introduction of highly active antiretroviral therapy (HAART), the prevalence of PCP has decreased [44]. Most HIV-associated cases of PCP occur in undiagnosed HIV patients [14].

Approach to the Patient

Diagnosis

History and Physical
Patients typically have to be in an immunocompromised state to develop *Pneumocystis* pneumonia. The risk of PCP increases as the T-helper cell count (CD4) decreases in a patient. PCP usually occurs when the CD4 count is less than 200 cells/ mm^3. Symptoms can include a low-grade fever, progressive dyspnea, or a nonproductive cough. Upon physical examination, a patient may have tachycardia and tachypnea. Auscultating the lung can be within normal limits but may reveal nonspecific crackles.

Laboratory and Imaging: Special Testing
With PCP, a chest radiograph can show perihilar interstitial infiltrates, which may become more dispersed as the disease process worsens. The interstitial infiltrates may progress into bilateral consolidations [14]. One may also see lung nodules. If the chest radiograph is normal, a high-resolution computed tomography (CT) scan may show ground-glass opacification or lesions cystic in nature. For diagnosis of PCP, an induced sputum (with hypertonic saline) culture should be the initial test of choice. If the culture is negative and still suspected, bronchoscopy with bronchoalveolar lavage is indicated [43]. In the HIV-infected population, an elevated serum lactate dehydrogenase (LDH) is suggestive of PCP, with levels reaching >500 ml/dL [14].

Treatment
In not acutely ill patients with PCP (PaO2 > 70 mmHg), the treatment of choice is trimethoprim-sulfamethoxazole (TMP-SMX) 20 mg/kg PO daily in two to four divided doses

[14]. For patients who are acutely ill (PaO2 < 70 mmHg, unable to take PO), a 3-week corticosteroid taper should be added in conjunction with TMP-SMX. The patient should take prednisone 40 mg twice daily for 5 days, followed by 40 mg daily on days 6–11, and then 20 mg daily on days 12–21. For those patients who cannot tolerate TMP-SMX, alternative regimens include oral primaquine (30 mg daily) plus clindamycin (600 mg three times daily), atovaquone 750 mg orally twice a day [45], trimethoprim (5 mg/kg orally three times daily) plus dapsone (100 mg orally daily) [46], or pentamidine 4 mg/kg intravenously daily. Glucose-6-phosphate dehydrogenase (G6PD) deficiency must be checked prior to using primaquine or dapsone [44]. The duration of treatment should be 21 days. Following therapy, it is recommended for the patient to start on PCP prophylaxis.

Prevention and Community Issues

For patients with HIV, primary prophylaxis should be started when the CD4 count is less than 200 cells/mm^3. The prophylactic treatment of choice is TMP-SMX at one tablet (single or double strength) by mouth daily. Other options can include dapsone 100 mg PO daily, atovaquone 1500 mg PO daily, or pentamidine 300 mg PO nebulized every 4 weeks. With the introduction of HAART, prophylaxis can be discontinued if the CD4 levels go above 200 cells/mm^3 [42].

References

1. Peters-Golden M. Chapter 15: Pneumonia. In: Schraufnagel DE, editor. Breathing in America: diseases, progress, and hope: American Thoracic Society; 2010. https://www.thoracic.org/patients/patient-resources/breathing-in-america/resources/breathing-in-america.pdf.
2. Is the leading cause of death in children. World Health Organization. https://www.who.int/maternal_child_adolescent/news_events/news/2011/pneumonia/en/. Accessed May 2020. Pneumonia.
3. Sethi S. Merck manual – community-acquired pneumonia. http://www.merckmanuals.com/professional/pulmonary_disorders/pneumonia/community-acquired_pneumonia.html. Accessed May 2020.
4. Metlay JP, Waterer GW, Long AC, et al. Diagnosis and Treatment of adults with community-acquired pneumonia. An official clinical practice guideline of the American Thoracic Society and Infectious Diseases Society of America. Am J Respir Crit Care Med. 2019;200 (7) https://doi.org/10.1164/rccm.201908-1581st.
5. Herring W. Learning radiology. Recognizing the basics. Mosby. 1st ed. Philadelphia: Mosby Elsevier.
6. Watkins R, Lemonovich T. Diagnosis and management of community acquired pneumonia in adults. Am Fam Physician. 2011;83(11):1299–306.
7. Prevention of pneumococcal disease: recommendations of the Advisory Committee on Immunization Practices (ACIP). Centers for Disease Control and Prevention. MMWR Morb Mortal Wkly Rep. 1997;46(RR-08):1–24. http://www.cdc.gov/Features/Pneumonia/
8. Hammerschlag MR. *Mycoplasma pneumoniae* infections. Curr Opin Infect Dis. 2001;14(2):181–6.
9. Clyde WA Jr. Clinical overview of typical *Mycoplasma pneumoniae* infections. Clin Infect Dis. 1993;17(Suppl 1):S32–6.
10. Ojeda Rodriguez JA, et al. Pneumonia, psittacosis. StatPearls [Internet]. Treasure Island: StatPearls Publishing; 2020.
11. Hogerwerf L, et al. Chlamydia psittaci (psittacosis) as a cause of community-acquired pneumonia: a systematic review and meta-analysis. Epidemiol Infect. 2017;145 (15):3096–105.
12. Miyashita N, et al. Prevalence of asymptomatic infection with *Chlamydia pneumoniae* in subjectively healthy adults. Chest. 2001;119(5):1416–9.
13. Grayston JT, et al. Evidence that *Chlamydia pneumoniae* causes pneumonia and bronchitis. J Infect Dis. 1993;168(5):1231–5.
14. White PL, et al. Diagnosis and management of *Pneumocystis jirovecii* infection. Expert Rev Anti Ther. 2017;15(5):435–47.
15. Gabe LM, et al. Diagnosis and management of coccidioidomycosis. Clin Chest Med. 2017;38(3):417–33.
16. Compendium of measures to control *Chlamydia psittaci* infection among humans (psittacosis) and pet birds (avian chlamydiosis). Centers for Disease Control and Prevention (CDC). MMWR Recomm Rep. 2000;49(RR-8):3–17.
17. Heymann DL, editor. Control of communicable diseases manual. 19th ed. Coccidioidomycosis, pp. 139–41. Mycoplasma, pp. 476–78. Pneumocystis carinii, pp. 478–80. Chlamydia, pp. 480–83. Tuberculosis, pp. 625–58.
18. Jain S. Epidemiology of viral pneumonia. Clin Chest Med. 2017;38:1–9.
19. Dandachi D, Rodriguez-Barradas MC. Viral pneumonia: etiologies and treatment. J Investig Med. 2018;66:957–965.
20. Yin Y, Wunderink RG. MERS, SARS, and other coronaviruses as causes of pneumonia. Respirology. 2018;23:130–137.
21. Influenza. Centers for Disease Control and Prevention. http://www.cdc.gov/flu/index.htm. Accessed 2 Oct 2015.

22. Respiratory Syncytial Virus (RSV). Centers for Disease Control and Prevention. http://www.cdc.gov/rsv/. Accessed 31 March 2020.

23. Bradley JS, et al. The management of community-acquired pneumonia in infants and children older than 3 months of age: clinical practice guidelines by the Pediatric Infectious Diseases Society and the Infectious Diseases Society of America. Clin Infect Dis. 2011;53 (7):e25–76.

24. Cruz-Knight W, Blake-Gums L. Tuberculosis: an overview. Prim Care. 2013;40:743–56.

25. Tuberculosis Data and Statistics. www.cdc.gov/tb/statistics/default.htm. Accessed 30 March 2020.

26. Interferon-Gamma Release Assays (IGRAs) – Blood Tests for TB Infection. Cdc.gov/tb/publications/factsheets/testing/igra.htm. Accessed 31 March 2020.

27. Treatment. Cdc.gov/tb/topic/treatment/default.htm. Accessed 31 March 2020.

28. Histoplasmosis. Centers for Disease Control and Prevention. http://www.cdc.gov/fungal/diseases/histoplasmosis/index.html. Accessed 26 February 2020.

29. Smith J, Kauffman C. Pulmonary fungal infections. Respirology. 2012;17:913–26.

30. Hage CA, Knox KS, Wheat LJ. Endemic mycoses: overlooked causes of community acquired pneumonia. Respir Med. 2012;106:770–5.

31. Wheat LJ, Friefeld AG, Kleimman MB, et al. Clinical practice guidelines for the management of patients with histoplasmosis: 2007 update by the Infectious Diseases Society of America. Clin Infect Dis. 2007;45:807–25.

32. Galgiani JN, et al. Coccidioidomycosis. Clin Infect Dis. 2005;41(9):1217–23.

33. Stevens DA, et al. Expert opinion: what to do when there is Coccidioides exposure in a laboratory. Clin Infect Dis. 2009;49(6):919–23.

34. Crum NF, et al. Coccidioidomycosis: a descriptive survey of reemerging disease. Clinical characteristics and current controversies. Medicine. 2004;83(3):149–75.

35. Legionella – About the Disease. Centers for Disease Control and Prevention. http://www.cdc.gov/legionella/about/index.html. Accessed 26 February 2020.

36. Guyard C, Low DE. Legionella infections and travel associated legionellosis. Travel Med. 2011;9: 176–86.

37. Emerging Infectious Centers for Disease Control and Prevention. Pneumonia. www.cdc.gov/pneumonia. Accessed May 2020.

38. Micromedex. http://www.micromedexsolutions.com. Accessed May 2020, used for all current antibiotic reference information.

39. Falkinham JO. Ecology of nontuberculous mycobacteria – where do human infections come from? Semin Respir Crit Care Med. 2013;34: 95–102.

40. Aksamit TR, Philley JV, Griffith DE. Nontuberculous mycobacterial (NTM) lung disease: the top ten essentials. Respir Med. 2014;108:417–25.

41. Van Ingen J. Diagnosis of nontuberculous mycobacterial infections. Semin Respir Crit Care Med. 2013;34:103–9.

42. Thomas CF Jr, et al. *Pneumocystis* pneumonia. N Engl J Med. 2004;350(24):2487–98.

43. Stringer JR, et al. A new name (*Pneumocystis jiroveci*) for Pneumocystis from humans. Emerg Infect Dis. 2002;8(9):891–6.

44. Sepkowitz KA. Opportunistic infections in patients with and patients without acquired immunodeficiency syndrome. Clin Infect Dis. 2002;34(8):1098–107.

45. Cover Cough. www.cdc.gov/flu/protect/covercough.htm. Accessed May 2020.

46. Safrin S, et al. Comparison of three regimens for treatment of mild to moderate *Pneumocystis carinii* pneumonia in patients with AIDS. A double-blind, randomized, trial of oral trimethoprim-sulfamethoxazole, dapsone-trimethoprim, and clindamycin-primaquine. ACTG 108 study group. Ann Intern Med. 1996;124(9):792–802.

Lung Cancer

89

Alap Shah and Daniel Hunter-Smith

Contents

A. Shah
Department of Family and Community Medicine,
Adventist La Grange Memorial Hospital Family Medicine
Residency, La Grange, IL, USA
e-mail: alap.shah@amitahealth.org; alap.shah@ahss.org

D. Hunter-Smith (✉)
Adventist La Grange Family Medicine Residency,
Adventist La Grange Memorial Hospital, LaGrange, IL,
USA
e-mail: daniel.hunter-smith@amitahealth.org

© Springer Nature Switzerland AG 2022
P. M. Paulman et al. (eds.), *Family Medicine*,
https://doi.org/10.1007/978-3-030-54441-6_92

General Principles

In the USA, primary lung cancer is the most common cause of cancer death and, after skin cancer, the second most commonly diagnosed cancer. It is one of the leading causes of morbidity and mortality in the USA. In 2019, there were an estimated 228,150 new cases of, and 142,670 deaths from, primary lung cancer [1]. Lung cancer also imposes a large financial burden on the healthcare system, with 2018 national expenditure for diagnosis and treatment totaling $14.2 billion [2].

However, since 1992, the rates of new cases and deaths from lung cancer in the USA has been steadily decreasing. In 1999, the age-adjusted rate of lung cancer was 71 per 100,000 Americans. By 2016, it had steadily declined to 58 per 100,000 Americans, with a concomitant decrease in death rates as well, across most ethnicities and in both genders [3]. By ethnicity, African-American men, of all subgroups, have consistently had the highest incidence and death rate over the last decade. Although the gap between African-American men and other groups has been closing, this disparity still serves as a reminder of the significance of socioeconomic factors in the incidence and death rates from lung cancer.

Prevention

Efforts at the prevention of lung cancer can be divided into two separate categories: primary prevention through risk factor modification and secondary prevention through early detection of asymptomatic disease.

Primary Prevention

The CDC has declared that reducing tobacco use is a "Winnable Battle." As the vast majority of lung cancers develop in association with cigarette smoking, the primary prevention of most lung cancers can be achieved through increased smoking cessation and decreased smoking initiation. As with other neoplastic disease, there are additional risk factors involved, including environmental and occupational exposure, nutrition, and genetic predisposition.

Cigarette Smoking

It is estimated that tobacco cigarette smoking causes 80% of the lung cancer deaths in women and 90% in men. Men and women who smoke are 23 times and 13 times more likely to develop lung cancer than men and women who do not smoke, respectively. In addition, exposure to secondhand smoke among nonsmokers increases the risk of lung cancer by 20–30% [4]. Promisingly, the overall prevalence of current smokers in the USA has been steadily decreasing: from 1965 to 2017, the percentage of current cigarette smokers decreased from 42.4% to 14.0% [5]. Among high school students, the overall prevalence has also been decreasing: from 1991 to 2015, the percentage of those who smoked a cigarette within the last 30 days decreased from 36.4% to 9.3% [6]. In 1997, the prevalence had peaked at 37.7% in high school boys and 34.7% in high school girls. It has steadily declined to current levels following the 1998 Tobacco Master Settlement Agreement, perhaps demonstrating the importance of public policy in curbing cigarette use among minors. Still, with the decline in combustible cigarette use, there has been a recent increase in the use of electronic nicotine delivery systems among both minors and adults. Their effects on long-term lung cancer risk are as of yet unknown [7].

From the public health perspective, and for the primary physician, encouraging smoking cessation and preventing smoking initiation are among the most important measures that can be taken to prevent lung cancer.

Occupational and Environmental Exposure

It is estimated that occupational carcinogen exposures are responsible for 9% to 15% of cases (approximately 20,000–34,000) of lung cancer in the USA [8]. Lung cancer is known to be associated with a vast number of workplace exposures, most notably tar and soot, heavy metals (including arsenic, chromium, and nickel), asbestos, silica, and radioactive materials. The list of occupations that involve these substances is extensive and includes mining, manufacturing, printing, painting, and ionizing radiation. Cigarette smoking has been shown to potentiate the effects of some of the occupational carcinogens. In the case of asbestos, arsenic, and radiation, the combined carcinogenic effect can be multiplicative.

Air pollution is becoming increasingly recognized as a risk factor for lung cancer. While different geographic areas have varying components of particulate air pollutants, a 2014 meta-analysis by the World Health Organization classified general outdoor air pollution as a Group 1 (highest risk) lung carcinogen. Indoor air pollution from burning biomass is also a well-known risk factor for lung cancer and is an issue more commonly encountered in the developing world.

Ionizing radiation is also classified as a Group 1 lung carcinogen. In the USA, approximately half of an average individual's annual ionizing radiation exposure is iatrogenic, and most of the remainder is from radon-222 exposure. About half of iatrogenic radiation is due to computed tomography (CT), and the rest is from fluoroscopy and nuclear medicine. In the USA, CT scan usage is sharply rising, and it is estimated that in 2007, 1.5–2% of all types of cancers (including lung cancer) were attributable to radiation from CT scans [9]. Non-occupational radon exposure in nonsmokers is estimated to be responsible for approximately 15,000 deaths from lung cancer annually [10]. The EPA has reported that 1 in 15 US homes has radon levels at or above the recommended levels and that lowering levels in these homes could prevent 5,000 lung cancer deaths annually.

Nutrition and Exercise

There is growing evidence that diet and exercise play a role in modifying lung cancer risk. A 2009 review found that the risk for lung cancer was 22% lower in those who ate the highest amount of cruciferous vegetables compared to those who ate a minimal amount [11]. Additionally, a 2018 World Cancer Research Fund report noted that high fruit intake consistently protected against lung cancer (in one analysis, reducing risk by 23% compared to low fruit intake) and that carotenoid-containing foods probably protect against lung cancer [12]. There was also limited evidence suggesting that non-starchy vegetables, selenium, and physical activity were protective against lung cancer, whereas red meat, processed meat, butter, and high overall fat intake were causes of lung cancer. Attempts to isolate the antioxidants thought to be responsible for the protective effects from carotenoid-containing vegetables have not been successful; high-dose vitamin A supplementation in smokers was actually associated with an increased risk of lung cancer.

The interplay of antioxidants contained within foods and the possibility that carotenoids are a marker for a healthier lifestyle rather than protective on their own create uncertainty regarding to the mechanisms of the protective effects of a healthy diet. However, the evidence clearly shows that a diet high in fruits and cruciferous vegetables, combined with physical activity, is a significant part of overall lung cancer prevention.

Genetics

The lifetime risk of being diagnosed with lung cancer in smokers is approximately 17.2% in males and 11.6% in females (compared to 1.3% and 1.4% in nonsmokers, respectively) [13]. That a majority of smokers do not develop lung cancer shows that other factors are involved in the pathogenesis of lung cancer, especially genetic susceptibility. In one study, after adjusting for smoking, age, and gender, a positive family history of lung cancer conferred an odds ratio of developing lung cancer of 1.6, with an increase to 3.6 if two or more family members had been diagnosed [14].

As with other cancers, lung carcinogenesis is a multistep process, involving DNA damage at multiple levels that ultimately causes unchecked cell proliferation. Specifically, mutations within tumor suppressor genes, DNA repair genes, and oncogenes work synergistically to promote tumor growth. Dozens of genes have been noted to have mutations in those with lung cancer, including K-*ras*, *EGFR*, and p53. Recent developments in genomic profiling allow for a million or more genetic variants to be concurrently sequenced, allowing more widespread identification of mutations that may indicate an increased risk of lung cancer. Though genetic testing is not currently used for screening in clinical practice, ongoing research may make it possible that it could one day play a major role in determining susceptibility to lung cancer.

Secondary Prevention

Efforts at secondary prevention have been geared toward early detection through imaging, as other noninvasive tests (serologic, sputum, and breath testing) remain in developmental stages. In 2013, the United States Preventive Services Task Force (USPSTF) recommended annual low-dose computed tomography (CT) screening for high-risk current or former smokers (those with a 30 pack-year history and who have smoked in the last 15 years) aged 55–80 years old, to detect asymptomatic disease.

This recommendation was primarily based on the National Lung Screening Trial (NLST), a landmark trial which enrolled over 53,000 patients in academic medical centers across the USA. The NLST demonstrated a 20% reduction in lung cancer mortality with annual low-dose CT compared to chest X-ray, with a number needed to screen (to prevent one death from lung cancer) of 320 [15]. The subsequent NELSON trial, which enrolled 13,000 men and 2,500 women in the Netherlands and Belgium, showed a reduction in lung cancer-specific mortality of 24% in men and 33% in women over 10 years, with a number needed to screen of 133 in men. The NELSON trial used a protocol based on lung nodule volume (as opposed to nodule diameter, used by previous studies) which significantly reduced false positives and unnecessary harms, a noted concern with the NLST findings. In addition, the NELSON trial used longer intervals between screenings, suggesting that biennial screenings may be as effective as annual screenings in select populations [16, 17].

Since the USPSTF recommendation, analyses have estimated the cost of annual low-dose CT screening to cost between $53,000 and $75,000 per quality-adjusted life-year (QALY) gained which is not dissimilar to the costs of screening mammography and colonoscopy [18].

Classifications

Lung cancer originates from cells in the respiratory epithelium (resulting in small cell lung cancer, adenocarcinoma, squamous cell carcinoma, and large cell carcinoma) and the pleura (resulting in mesothelioma). Much rarer forms of lung cancer include spindle cell carcinoma, giant cell carcinoma, and carcinosarcomas; they are classified

Table 1 Incidence of Lung Cancer type by histology

Lung cancer type by histology	Incidence (%)[a]
Small cell lung cancer (SCLC)	18%
Non-small cell lung cancer (NSCLC)	74%
Adenocarcinoma	46%
Squamous cell carcinoma	25%
Large cell carcinoma	8%
Mesothelioma	<0.02%

[a]Due to a combination of sources, the total may not add up to 100%

as non-small cell lung cancers. The relative incidence of the most common types is shown (*see* Table 1) [19]. In recent decades, adenocarcinoma has become the most prevalent type of lung cancer. This may be due to the widespread use of filtered cigarettes, which allow carcinogens to travel further down the bronchial tree, bypassing protective epithelium. Smoking is associated with nearly all types of lung cancer, but is most closely associated with small cell and squamous cell cancers. In those who have never smoked, adenocarcinoma is the most common type of cancer [20].

The stage of disease is the strongest predictor of survival, though histology also plays an important part in prognosis [21]. Among the major histological types, adenocarcinoma generally has the highest 5-year survival, and small cell has the poorest survival. For localized disease, the 5-year survival is approximately 69% for adenocarcinoma, 46% for squamous cell, 48% for large cell, and 27% for small cell. For regional disease, the survival drops to 42% for adenocarcinoma, 26% for squamous cell, 29% for large cell, and 15% for small cell. With the new implementation of screening CT for lung cancer, cancers may be detected at earlier (more local) stages, which may improve survival and increase the amount of disease amenable to a cure.

Diagnosis

Clinical Presentation

The clinical presentation of a lung cancer is driven by the site of origin and the extent of the disease. It is not uncommon for it to be an asymptomatic finding on a chest X-ray or CT scan of the abdomen or chest obtained while working up another problem. Other common presentations are non-resolving infiltrates after treatment for pneumonia, as a pleural effusion or with persistent chest wall or shoulder pain. Because of the endobronchial origin of many lung cancers, cough, hemoptysis, dyspnea, and unilateral wheezing or stridor may be the original complaint. Patients presenting with advanced disease may have weight loss, anorexia, fatigue, persistent fevers, or clubbing.

Lung cancers are associated with a number of syndromes, which can be divided into general categories: (1) the consequences of tumor invasion of the surrounding tissues, (2) the systematic effects of hormonal substances produced by cancers, and (3) cytokines or antibodies triggered by the immune system's response to the tumor (paraneoplastic syndromes). Local invasion of nerves at the apex of the lung causes Horner's syndrome (cervical sympathetic) or Pancoast syndrome (brachial plexus). Tumor invasion of the mediastinum can block venous return to the heart causing superior vena cava syndrome, invasion of the pericardium causing cardiac tamponade, or erosion into the esophagus causing obstruction or fistulas. Metastatic lesions in the spine can cause spinal cord compression with distal weakness and pain. Tumors can secrete antidiuretic hormone causing hyponatremia, parathyroid hormone causing hypercalcemia, or adrenocorticotrophic hormone leading to Cushing syndrome. These latter hormonal syndromes are more common with SCLC and reflect the neuroendocrine nature of these cancers. The most common paraneoplastic syndrome associated with lung cancer, occurring in 5–15% of patients, is periosteal swelling of the distal phalanges causing clubbing of the fingers. The myasthenia-like Lambert-Eaton syndrome develops from the production of antibodies to the postsynaptic acetylcholine receptor of the motor end plate.

Diagnostic Approach

Typically, patients with lung cancer present with advanced tumors causing a range of symptoms. Diagnostic decisions center on identifying the tumor cell type and accurately staging the extent of the cancer. With increasing frequency, especially in the context of screening for asymptomatic cancers using low-dose CT scans of the chest, diagnostic decisions revolve around the safest way to evaluate small, indeterminate lung nodules. Recent years have seen a rapid expansion in the complexity of diagnostic algorithms for both clinical scenarios. This complexity makes it beyond the scope of this chapter to make any detailed suggestions about workups for particular clinical presentations.

Evaluating a Lung Nodule

Lung nodules may be found incidentally on a chest X-ray or through a screening protocol using a CT scan. Incidental lung nodules should be compared with any prior imaging tests. An indeterminate nodule that can be shown to have been stable for at least 2 years requires no further diagnostic evaluation. Nodules found by chest X-ray that cannot be shown to be stable for 2 years should have a diagnostic, thin-section CT of the chest performed. Further evaluation is determined by the pretest probability of malignancy, the size of the nodule (greater than 8 mm or smaller), and nodule characteristics. Further diagnostic steps may include serial CT studies over 2 years, functional imaging with positron emission tomography (PET), bronchoscopy with biopsy, CT-guided needle biopsy, or surgical wedge resection. Based on the NELSON Trial, measuring nodule volume doubling time improves sensitivity and specificity for nodule characterization [22]. The choice of which technique to use should involve a team approach involving input from radiologists, pulmonologists, thoracic surgeons, and the patient's preferences. The family physician can play a crucial role explaining the risks and benefits of the various options to the patient and helping to make sure the final decision reflects the patient's values.

Staging Non-small Cell Lung Cancer

The diagnostic workup for a patient with a suspected lung cancer is based on the size and location of the suspected tumor, evidence for mediastinal or distant metastatic disease, the efficiency of the proposed workup, the invasiveness and risks of any procedures, the technologies and expertise locally available, and the patient's comorbidities and preferences. Diagnostic technologies are in a period of rapid evolution. It is reasonable to consult a team representing interventional radiology, thoracic surgery, pulmonology, and oncology. Accessing websites from groups such as the National Comprehensive Cancer Network or the American College of Chest Physicians can provide family physicians with current diagnostic guidelines. The family physician should conduct a thorough history and physical examination, including performance status and noting any weight loss. Routine studies should include the following: a CBC with platelets, a comprehensive metabolic profile, a CT scan of the chest and upper abdomen (including the adrenal glands), and a pulmonary function testing. Counseling on smoking cessation should be performed for current smokers. Discuss with the patient and participating consultants a plan for integrating palliative care into the treatment plan. When there is a high clinical suspicion for advanced disease, PET imaging allows for the choice of a diagnostic biopsy site to confirm the highest stage to be assigned to the cancer.

Staging Small Cell Lung Cancer

The diagnostic evaluation for suspected or known small cell lung cancer follows the same outline as for non-small cell lung cancer discussed above. The aim is to categorize the disease as in either a limited or extensive stage. In addition to the general workup reviewed above, a brain MRI is obtained. For equivocal bone lesions on PET imaging, bone imaging with MRI/radiographs as well as bone marrow aspiration/biopsy may be needed [23].

Treatment

Algorithms for treating lung cancer are now evolving rapidly after years of very modest progress. This has come about through an increased understanding of cancer genomics. Tumors harboring specific acquired genetic alterations are being treated with targeted inhibitors of altered enzymes that are driving cancer growth. Monoclonal antibodies targeted at altered epidermal growth factor receptor (EGFR), anaplastic lymphoma kinase (ALK), and receptor tyrosine kinase (ROS1) are producing exciting clinical response rates [24–26]. The list of targeted mutations is growing rapidly [27]. An era of personalized treatment, based on whole tumor genome sequencing, is imminent. The family physician is in the position, working collaboratively with the consulting oncologist, to educate patients about these treatment options and to counsel them about the option of participating in an experimental treatment protocol. In addition, palliative care needs should be addressed throughout the treatment process.

Non-small Cell Carcinoma

Treatment algorithms are driven by stage, pathology, and mutation testing of the tumor. It is now possible to identify genetic mutations in lung cancer cells through circulating tumor DNA (ctDNA). This technology is beginning to replace invasive biopsies in some centers. This genetic focus on the tumor cell is shifting the treatment focus from cytotoxic chemotherapy to personalized choices of targeted monoclonal antibody based therapies [27]. Treatment decisions need to be worked out consensually between the patient and the treatment team of medical oncologists, radiation oncologists, and thoracic surgeons [28]. The family physician can help to facilitate these decisions and advocate for the patient's values and preferences.

Small Cell Carcinoma

The performance status of the patient with limited stage disease drives treatment decisions ranging from concurrent chemotherapy and radiation therapy for high-functioning patients to hospice care for patients with extensive comorbidities. Patients with extensive disease are treated with chemotherapy. Whole brain radiation therapy is used for patients with brain metastases. Palliative external beam radiation therapy can be used for bone metastases, superior vena cava syndrome, lobar obstruction, or spinal cord compression.

Posttreatment Follow-Up

With the earlier detection of lung cancers and more effective treatments, the family physician will be involved with a growing number of patients who have undergone therapy with curative intent who will need surveillance for recurrent disease. Coordinate this care with the treating oncologist. A history and physical examination, along with CT examinations of the lungs, should be done every 4–6 months for the first 2 years and then yearly thereafter. Encourage patients to remain current with influenza and pneumococcal vaccinations [29].

Palliative Care

The family physician can play a key role in ensuring as high a quality of life as possible for patients as they move through the continuum from diagnosis to treatment with intent to cure and finally to end-of-life care. The family physician can educate patients about creating a living will and a durable power of attorney to establish their care preferences. They can explore the patients' interest in the use of complementary and integrative therapies alongside standard cancer therapies. They should question patients about common symptoms such as pain, anorexia, constipation, breathlessness, fatigue, depression, and insomnia and provide care to ameliorate these as much as possible [30–32].

References

1. National Cancer Institute. Lung cancer. 2014. Available from: http://www.cancer.gov/cancertopics/types/lung
2. National Cancer Institute, NIH, DHHS. Cancer trends progress report. Bethesda. 2019. Available from: https://progressreport.cancer.gov
3. U.S. Cancer Statistics Working Group. U.S. cancer statistics data visualizations tool. 2019. Available from: www.cdc.gov/cancer/dataviz
4. U.S. Department of Health and Human Services. The Health Consequences of Involuntary Exposure to Tobacco Smoke: A Report of the Surgeon General. Atlanta, GA: U.S. Department of Health and Human Services, Centers for Disease Control and Prevention, Coordinating Center for Health Promotion, National Center for Chronic Disease Prevention and Health Promotion, Office on Smoking and Health, 2006. https://www.ncbi.nlm.nih.gov/books/NBK44324/
5. Wang TW, Asman K, Gentzke AS, et al. Tobacco product use among adults – United States, 2017. MMWR Morb Mortal Wkly Rep. 2018;67:1225–32.
6. American Lung Association. Key facts about tobacco use among children and teenagers. Updated March 13, 2020.
7. Drope J, Cahn Z, Kennedy R, et al. Key issues surrounding the health impacts of electronic nicotine delivery systems (ENDS) and other sources of nicotine. CA Cancer J Clin 2017;67:449–71.
8. Alberg AJ, Samet JM. Epidemiology of lung Cancer. Chest. 2003;123:21–49.
9. Brenner D, Hall E. Computed tomography – an increasing source of radiation exposure. N Engl J Med. 2007;357:2277–84.
10. Cao X, MacNaughton P, Laurent JC, Allen JG. Radon-induced lung cancer deaths may be overestimated due to failure to account for confounding by exposure to diesel engine exhaust in BEIR VI miner studies. PLoS One. 2017;12(9):e0184298.
11. Lam TK, Gallicchio L, Lindsley K, et al. Cruciferous vegetable consumption and lung cancer risk: a systematic review. Cancer Epidemiol Biomark Prev. 2009;18(1):184–95.
12. World Cancer Research Fund/American Institute for Cancer Research. Diet, Nutrition, Physical Activity and Cancer: A Global Perspective. Continuous Update Project Expert Report, 2018.
13. Villeneuve PJ, Mao Y. Lifetime probability of developing lung cancer, by smoking status, Canada. Can J Public Health. 1994;85(6):385–8.
14. Lissowska J, Foretova L, Dabek J. Family history and lung cancer risk: international multicentre case-control study in eastern and Central Europe and meta-analyses. Cancer Causes Control. 2010;21(7):1091–104.
15. The National Lung Screening Trial Research Team. Reduced lung-cancer mortality with low-dose computed tomographic screening. N Engl J Med. 2011;365:395–409.
16. Koning H, et al. Reduced lung-cancer mortality with volume CT screening in a randomized trial. N Engl J Med. 2020;382:503–13.
17. Duffy S, Field J. Mortality reduction with low-dose CT screening for lung Cancer. N Engl J Med. 2020;382:572–3.
18. Kumar V, Cohen JT, van Klaveren D, et al. Risk-Targeted Lung Cancer Screening: A Cost-Effectiveness Analysis. Ann Intern Med 2018;168:161–9.
19. Herbst RS, Heymach JV, Lippman SM. Lung cancer. N Engl J Med. 2008;359:1367–80.

20. Lortet-Tieulent J, Soerjomataram I, Ferlay J, Rutherford M, Weiderpass E, Bray F. International trends in lung cancer incidence by histological subtype: adenocarcinoma stabilizing in men but still increasing in women. Lung Cancer. 2014;84(1):13–22.

21. Gary GM, Jemal A, McKenna MB, Strauss J, Cummings KM. Lung cancer survival in relation to histologic subtype: an analysis based upon surveillance epidemiology and end results (SEER) data: B4-06. J Thorac Oncol. 2007;2(8):S345–6.

22. Horeweg N, Scholten ET, de Jong PA, et al. Detection of lung cancer through low-dose CT screening (NELSON): a prespecified analysis of screening test performance and interval cancers. Lancet Oncol. 2014;15:1342–50.

23. National Comprehensive Cancer Network Guidelines Version 1. Small cell lung cancer. SCL, 1–6. 2015. Available at http://www.nccn.org/professionals/physician_gls/f_guidelines.asp. Accessed Dec 2014.

24. Solomon DJ, Mok T, Kim DW, et al. First-line crizotinib versus chemotherapy in ALK-positive lung cancer. N Engl J Med. 2014;371:2167–77.

25. Shaw AT, Ou SI, Bang YB, et al. Crizotinib in ROS1-rearranged non-small-cell lung cancer. N Engl J Med. 2014;371:1963–71.

26. Ramalingam SS, Vanstennnkiste J, Planchard D, et al. Overall survival with Osimertinib in untreated, EGFR-mutated advanced NSCLC. N Engl J Med. 2020;382:41–50.

27. Patil PD, Shepherd F, Johnson DH. A career in lung cancer: pushing beyond chemotherapy. Am Soc Clin Oncol Educ Book. 2019;39:583–9.

28. Nagasaka M, Gadgeel SM. Role of chemotherapy and targeted therapy in early-stage non-small cell lung cancer. Expert Rev Anticancer Ther. 18(1):63–70.

29. Colt HG, Murgu SD, Korst RJ, et al. Follow-up and surveillance of the patient with lung cancer after curative-intent therapy, diagnosis and management of lung cancer, 3rd ed: American college of chest physicians evidence-based clinical practice guidelines. Chest. 2013;143(Suppl 5):e437S–54.

30. Ford DW, Koch KA, Ray DE, Selecky PA. Palliative and end-of-life care in lung cancer, diagnosis and management of lung cancer, 3rd ed: American college of chest physicians evidence-based clinical practice guidelines. Chest. 2013;143(Suppl 5):e498S–512.

31. Deng GE, Rausch SM, Jones LW, et al. Complementary therapies and integrative medicine in lung cancer, diagnosis and management of lung cancer, 3rd ed: American college of chest physicians evidence-based clinical practice guidelines. Chest. 2013;143(Suppl 5): e420S–36.

32. Simoff MJ, Lally B, Slade MG. Symptom management in patients with lung cancer, diagnosis and management of lung cancer, 3rd ed: American college of chest physicians evidence-based clinical practice guidelines. Chest. 2013;143(Suppl 5):e455S–97.

Selected Disorders of the Respiratory System

90

T. Jason Meredith, James Watson, and William Seigfreid

Contents

T. J. Meredith (✉) · J. Watson · W. Seigfreid
Department of Family Medicine, University of Nebraska
Medical Center, Omaha, NE, USA
e-mail: jason.meredith@unmc.edu;
james.watson@unmc.edu; william.seigfreid@unmc.edu

P. M. Paulman et al. (eds.), *Family Medicine*,
https://doi.org/10.1007/978-3-030-54441-6_177

There are many respiratory disorders that will commonly be encountered by family physicians that are not addressed in other chapters of this text. This chapter briefly discusses the etiology, epidemiology, presentation, diagnostic criteria, and management of several selected disorders: pulmonary hypertension, pneumothorax, pleural effusion, interstitial lung disease, lung cancer, pulmonary sarcoidosis, and vaping-induced pulmonary injury.

Pulmonary Hypertension

The term pulmonary hypertension (PH) is used to describe a diverse group of disorders causing increased pulmonary arterial pressures; specifically, the mean resting pulmonary arterial pressure is greater than or equal to 25 mmHg. Symptoms may include fatigue and shortness of breath, although many patients are asymptomatic until later in the disease course [1]. The true prevalence of pulmonary hypertension is not clear with estimates ranging from 5 to 52 cases per million people [2]. Pulmonary hypertension can be broadly divided into five groups based on presentation, pathophysiology, and potential treatments [3]. The five groups can then be further subdivided based on the exact etiology of the patient's symptoms. Group 1, or pulmonary arterial hypertension, is associated with drug toxicity, connective tissue disorders, and congenital disease etiologies. Group 2 is due to left heart disease. Group 3 is due to lung disease or hypoxia. Group 4 is due to chronic thromboembolic disease or other pulmonary obstructions. Group 5 is due to unclear or multifactorial mechanisms [Table 1].

Diagnosis

The diagnosis of pulmonary hypertension is difficult as the symptoms tend to be vague and non-specific. Common presenting symptoms include fatigue, dyspnea on exertion, cough, and syncope [4]. Comorbid conditions such as COPD, obstructive sleep apnea, heart failure, and history of chronic thromboembolic disease should raise the index of suspicion, especially if symptoms were previously well controlled and have now worsened. Physical exam findings cannot be used to rule out pulmonary hypertension; however, elevated jugular venous pressure, peripheral edema, and parasternal heave may suggest severe disease [5].

Lab evaluation is not indicated as no specific findings exist. Ancillary testing with electrocardiogram (ECG) and chest X-ray (CXR) may be performed. CXR may reveal right-sided heart enlargement and/or dilation of the pulmonary arteries. ECG may reveal right heart strain, right axis deviation, and right atrial enlargement. Of note, a normal CXR or ECG does not exclude pulmonary hypertension. Pulmonary function testing may aid in the diagnosis of pulmonary hypertension by ruling in underlying conditions including COPD or pulmonary fibrosis. Patients may frequently have decreased diffusion capacity [3].

The most important non-invasive test in diagnosis of pulmonary hypertension is transthoracic echocardiography (TTE). TTE will assess peak tricuspid regurgitation in order to estimate pulmonary artery pressure and assign patients to low-, intermediate-, and high-risk groups. Right heart catheterization remains the gold standard to confirm the diagnosis of pulmonary hypertension [3].

Table 1 Adapted from ECS/ERS guidelines comprehensive clinical classification of pulmonary hypertension [3]

Group 1: pulmonary arterial hypertension	Group 2: left heart disease	Group 3: chronic Lung Disease	Group 4: pulmonary artery obstruction	Group 5: multifactorial/ unclear
Idiopathic Hereditary Schistosomiasis infection Drugs: appetite suppressants, rapeseed oil, benfluorex Connective tissue disorders: systemic sclerosis, Raynaud's disease, SLE, mixed connective tissue disease Congenital heart disease	HFpEF HFrEF Valvular Disease Restrictive cardiomyopathy Constrictive pericarditis Pulmonary vein stenosis	Obstructive sleep apnea COPD Interstitial lung disease Restrictive lung disease Pneumoconiosis	Chronic thromboembolic Malignancy Benign tumors Parasites	Hemolytic anemia Sickle cell disease Thalassemias Gaucher's disease Glycogen storage diseases Sarcoidosis Chronic kidney disease

Based on current recommendations, several populations are at increased risk of developing pulmonary hypertension and therefore should be screened. Individuals with HIV should be screened if they possess an additional risk factor: female sex, hepatitis C positive status, or African American. Additionally, patients with hereditary hemorrhagic telangiectasias, congenital heart disease, and familial pulmonary arterial hypertension be screened as well [4].

Management

The most important aspect of primary care management of PH is early recognition and referral to pulmonary hypertension specialists for definitive management. Family physicians play an important part in the treatment of pulmonary hypertension and should help facilitate treatment once the underlying cause has been identified. There are also disease-specific considerations and monitoring guidance that primary care physicians should keep in mind for patients with pulmonary hypertension. All patients with pulmonary hypertension should receive age- and comorbidity-appropriate vaccinations.

Most published data on treatment of PH is specific to group 1 patients. Every 3–6 months these patients should be seen and undergo ECG to monitor for arrhythmias, dyspnea monitoring, and labs including CBC, BMP, and pro-BNP [3]. Every 6–12 months additional lab evaluation including TSH, troponin, iron studies, and blood gas analysis should

be considered. Iron deficiency frequently exists in these patients and should be treated accordingly. Repeat echocardiogram and right heart catheterization occur every 6–12 months for disease monitoring [3]. Group 1 patients should be encouraged to exercise within the limitations of their symptoms.

Given the increased risk of serious obstetric complications, pregnancy and birth control should be discussed in all female patients with PH. Contraceptive management strategies are controversial as some treatment modalities for PH may interfere with estrogen, and vasovagal reactions during IUD placement may be poorly tolerated [3]. Appropriate preventative health strategies such as vaccinations against influenza and pneumococcal pneumonia should be emphasized.

The goal for patients with group 2 and 3 is optimal management of their underlying medical condition. Patients in group 4 generally benefit from lifelong anticoagulation and oxygen when needed for hypoxemia. There is limited data regarding treatment of group 5 disease. Encouraging social support and end of life planning are important tasks for family physicians in all patients with PH regardless of which group they belong to [3].

Pneumothorax

Pneumothorax is defined as the presence of air in the pleural space. It takes one of the following abnormal circumstances to allow air accumulation in the pleural space: communication between the alveolar spaces and pleura, communication between the atmosphere and pleural space, or gas-producing organisms in the pleural space. From a clinical standpoint, pneumothorax is classified as either spontaneous or nonspontaneous (iatrogenic or traumatic). Spontaneous pneumothorax is further subdivided as primary (without clinically apparent underlying pulmonary disease) and secondary (underlying pulmonary disease) [6].

Primary Spontaneous Pneumothorax

Primary spontaneous pneumothorax (PSP) has long thought to occur due to spontaneous rupture of a subpleural bleb (small thin-walled air pockets); however, recent evidence points to diffuse emphysema-like changes of the lung parenchyma as the more likely cause [7]. The classic patient with PSP is a tall, thin male. The most important risk factor is tobacco smoking, though cannabis smoking also has demonstrated strong association with bullous parenchymal disease [8]. PSP doesn't usually have a known trigger but may be preceded by precipitating factors including atmospheric pressure changes, exposure to loud music, and pollution. These precipitating factors explain why cases of PSP tend to exhibit a clustering effect. PSP has an incidence of 7.4–18 cases/100,000 in males and 1.2–6 cases/100,000 in females per year [6].

Diagnosis

Typically, patients present with an abrupt onset of ipsilateral chest pain with or without dyspnea. Pain may be localized over the site of pneumothorax or radiate to the ipsilateral shoulder. Symptoms can often be minimal and even totally absent (in stark contrast to the presentation of secondary spontaneous pneumothorax). Symptoms also tend to improve following presentation; worsening of symptoms is rare and suggests the development of complications such as hemopneumothorax [8].

Physical exam can be completely normal in small pneumothoraces [6]. Findings that may indicate pneumothorax include decreased or absent breath sounds, percussive hyper-resonance, and reduced ipsilateral chest expansion. Significant hemodynamic compromise (tachycardia, tachypnea, hypoxia, etc.) is usually absent. Radiographic imaging confirms the diagnosis and allows estimation of pneumothorax size, with an upright posteroanterior chest radiograph being the modality of choice. Findings on X-ray include the displacement of the pleural line and absence of lung markings between the pleural edge and chest wall. Inspiratory images alone are sufficient for diagnosis. Occasionally the pneumothorax cannot be detected on simple radiographs, and a CT is required. Ultrasound can also be a very sensitive modality but is not routinely used to evaluate PSP [6, 8].

Management

Therapeutic options for PSP depend on the size of the pneumothorax and the severity of the patient's symptoms. Treatment focuses on evacuation of air, if necessary, and prevention of recurrence. As tension and hemodynamic compromise is rare in PSP, conservative initial management is an option. Assuming mild symptomatology and small size of the pneumothorax (less than 20% or less than 3 cm between the lung and chest wall), outpatient management with observation and close radiographic follow-up is a reasonable option [6]. If air evacuation is necessary, needle aspiration and chest drain insertion are both options; however, no consensus guidelines exist on recommended treatment. Recent evidence suggests that needle aspiration is effective for the initial management of PSP [7]. A large pneumothorax or significant symptoms increase the likelihood that simple aspiration will not be sufficient, thus requiring chest tube placement for definitive management [8].

Recurrence rates for PSP are approximately 33% irrespective of treatment modality. Recurrence prevention with pleurodesis procedure should be offered after a single episode of recurrence to those who are at professional risk (aviation personnel, divers) or if chest tube therapy fails to result in lung expansion [6, 8].

Secondary Spontaneous Pneumothorax

Secondary spontaneous pneumothorax (SSP) results as a complication of underlying lung disease. The most frequent associated underlying disorders are COPD with emphysema, cystic fibrosis, tuberculosis, lung cancer, and lung infections. Because these conditions already represent some level of lung compromise, SSP often presents as a more life-threatening event requiring intervention as opposed to PSP. Incidence is similar to that of PSP with a peak incidence between 60 and 65 years of age [6].

Diagnosis

As opposed to PSP, dyspnea is usually the most prominent clinical feature in SSP; other symptoms including chest pain, cyanosis, hypoxemia, hypercapnia, and acute respiratory failure can also be present and are generally much more severe. As with PSP, imaging with CXR and/or CT scan will confirm the diagnosis. Recurrence is much more common than in PSP; rates up to 80% are seen in conditions such as cystic fibrosis [6].

Management

Management of SSP targets air evacuation, symptomatic control, and prevention of recurrence. As the majority of patients with SSP have significantly decreased pulmonary reserve, most will require pleural drainage. No consensus exists on initial management, but most guidelines recommend immediate chest tube insertion. Given the increase risk of recurrence, prevention by pleurodesis procedure should be performed after the initial event [6].

Tension Pneumothorax

A tension pneumothorax constitutes a life-threatening emergency. It develops as a result of air moving through a pleural defect that acts as a one-way valve, opening during inspiration and closing during expiration, resulting in progressive pneumothorax volumes and further lung collapse. Eventually, shifting of the trachea and mediastinum away from the pneumothorax occurs leading possible cardiopulmonary compromise. Tension pneumothoraxes most often occur secondary to major chest wall trauma. Classically, patients with tension pneumothorax develop jugular venous distension and contralateral tracheal deviation; however, these are very late signs and much less commonly observed in real studies [9]. Acute respiratory distress is often the initial presentation, and cardiovascular collapse can rapidly occur without prompt intervention. Immediate needle decompression by insertion of a large bore needle into the pleural cavity at the midline of the second intercostal space releases the trapped air and results in improved cardiopulmonary status. Following needle decompression, placement of a chest tube and treatment of chest wall injuries are required [6, 9].

Family and Community Issues

Given the strong association between smoking and PSP in addition to its link to underlying respiratory disorders, smoking cessation interventions provide an excellent opportunity for family physicians to intervene at a population level to decrease risk factors for initial PSP, prevent recurrent pneumothoraces, and minimize the risk for underlying respiratory disorders that cause SSP.

Pleural Effusion

Pleural effusions are an accumulation of fluid in the pleural space as a result of disparity in the formation and resorption of pleural fluid. The presence and amount of pleural fluid is typically regulated by capillary oncotic pressure as well as capillary and interstitial hydrostatic pressure. Pleural effusions are very common in clinical practice, with an estimated prevalence of 400 cases/100,000. A plethora of disease processes can cause pleural effusions with the most common being congestive heart failure, hepatic cirrhosis, pulmonary infections, and malignancy [10].

Diagnosis

Patients with pleural effusions can present with a variety of symptoms including dyspnea, pleuritic chest pain, cough, and referred pain to the shoulder or abdomen. Some patients are asymptomatic. Due to the breadth of the differential diagnosis and the presenting complaints, a systematic evaluation must be undertaken to diagnose the underlying cause. Pulmonary exam may reveal decreased breath sounds, percussion dullness, or even a friction rub. Given the prevalence of congestive heart failure as a cause of pleural effusion, a careful cardiac exam can provide valuable insight. A chest radiograph is often the initial diagnostic study, while more sensitive CT is not usually necessary to diagnose a pulmonary effusion [11].

While history and physical examination can provide clues to the causes of pleural effusions, determination of the exact etiology can be very difficult. Thoracentesis and pleural fluid analysis (PFA) are the next steps in the evaluation process; PFA can lead to a definitive or presumptive diagnosis in approximately 95% of cases [10].

The initial step of PFA is determining if the effusion is transudative or exudative. The rationale for differentiating is that a transudative effusion can be effectively treated by addressing the underlying cause such as heart failure or hepatic cirrhosis. If the effusion is exudative, further investigation is required to identify the local pathology causing the effusion. Differentiating transudative from exudative effusions is best achieved by using Light's criteria. Table 2 outlines how pleural and serum protein and LDH are utilized in Light's criteria.

Gross appearance, cell count, and pH studies of the pleural fluid can also be of use. Limitations with Light's criteria do exist. Almost all exudative effusions will be correctly identified; however, in approximately 25% of cases transudates will be misclassified as exudates, usually in the case of diuretic usage in CHF patients. The majority of these errors occur in patients where exudative criteria are barely met and usually in only one of the three elements of Light's criteria [11]. If clinical suspicion exists that the effusion has been misclassified, additional calculations using serum-pleural fluid albumin gradient or serum-pleural fluid protein gradient can be helpful [12].

Transudative Effusions

Transudative effusions occur secondary to processes that increase the hydrostatic pressure or decrease the oncotic pressure in pulmonary capillaries. Additionally, an increase in negative pressure in the pleural space can also lead to these types of effusions. Congestive heart failure and cirrhosis are the two most common causes of transudative effusions [10]. Pleural effusions associated with CHF tend to be bilateral. In contrast, around 80% of effusions from cirrhosis with ascites are right sided. Less common causes of transudative effusions are nephrotic syndrome, urinothorax, peritoneal dialysis, and trapped lung [10].

Exudative Effusions

In contrast to transudates, exudates are caused by local processes that lead to increased capillary permeability causing leakage of serum contents. Malignancy and infections of the pleural space or lung parenchyma commonly produce exudative effusion. A plethora of less common etiologies also cause exudative effusion; these include chylothorax, pulmonary embolism, superior vena cava syndrome, aortic dissection, rheumatoid arthritis, systemic lupus erythematous, liver abscesses, and hepatitis [10].

Table 2 Pleural fluid characteristics

Characteristics	Transudate	Exudate
Pleural fluid protein/serum protein ratio	<0.5	>0.5
Pleural fluid LDH/serum LDH ratio	<0.6	>0.6
Pleural fluid LDH	<2/3 the upper limit of normal serum LDH	>2/3 upper limit of normal serum LDH
pH	>7.40	<7.40
WBC count	<1000/uL	>1000/μL

Adapted from [11]

Management

Ultimately, treatment of pleural effusions targets controlling symptoms and treating the underlying disease process. With appropriate treatment, the majority of the pleural effusions will resolve or cause minimal symptoms. Some effusions may require long-term drainage with placement of a small caliber chest tube and outpatient drainage. In refractory pleural effusions, a pleurodesis procedure can be considered, but this practice is controversial [10].

Family and Community Issues

Given that pleural effusions commonly result from chronic disease processes, family physicians play an important role in their management. Our role ranges from coordinating chronic disease care interventions to formulating long-term goals to end of life discussions. These discussions and management decisions play a large role not only in the physical care and health of patients but also in their and their family's mental and psychological health.

Interstitial Lung Disease

Interstitial lung disease (ILD) is a term used to refer to a wide variety of pulmonary disorders that share similar clinical, radiological, or pathological criteria. Approximately 200 conditions cause interstitial lung disease; these include sarcoidosis, idiopathic pulmonary fibrosis, connective tissue disease manifestations, systemic lupus erythematous, radiation exposure, hypersensitivity pneumonitis, and non-specific fibrosis [13]. Unfortunately, only one in three cases of interstitial lung disease have an identifiable cause [13]. While the diseases that comprise interstitial lung disease are individually rare, together they affect more than 1.9 million people worldwide [14].

Diagnosis

Patients will often present with non-specific cardiopulmonary symptoms including dyspnea and cough. A detailed history will help the physician identify risk factors and previous exposures for one of the many causes of interstitial lung disease. Emphasis should be placed on obtaining smoking history, family history of pulmonary disease, a list of all medications regularly taken at any point in their lifetime, radiation exposure history, and occupational/hobby history. Establishing a patient's exercise tolerance will provide an assessment of the current disease severity [15].

Given the broad spectrum of possible causes and often non-specific initial presenting symptoms, the diagnosis of ILD often occurs through a multidisciplinary team utilizing clinical, radiologic, and pathologic data to establish the definitive diagnosis and severity. Physical examination is not reliable for establishing the diagnosis and may be normal. Crackles may be present on auscultation but may not present in granulomatous causes such as sarcoidosis. Clubbing of the fingers may be present and is a harbinger of severe disease if present [16]. Patients with suspected interstitial lung disease should undergo laboratory testing including urinalysis, complete blood count, complete metabolic panel, ANA, CPK, and aldolase as well as other laboratory testing suggested by the history that may help limit the differential [17]. Patients should receive a chest X-ray and high-resolution chest CT. Pulmonary function testing should also be obtained to help narrow the differential diagnosis [15].

Management

Management principles that apply to all types of interstitial lung disease include smoking cessation and referral to pulmonary rehabilitation. Specific therapy for each type of interstitial lung disease is reliant on an accurate diagnosis and may require referral to multidisciplinary specialist clinics [15].

Lung Cancer

Lung cancer is tied with breast cancer as the most common form of cancer worldwide and carries significant morbidity. In the United States, approximately 230,000 new cases and 142,000 deaths occur from lung cancer every year [18]. The incidence of lung cancer rose sharply in the early 1900s following the rise in cigarette smoking. After the surgeon general's report on the link between tobacco smoking and lung cancer in the 1960s, the incidence of lung cancer has progressively decreased. Besides cigarette smoking, other exposure risk factors including radon, arsenic, asbestos, chromates, chloromethyl ethers, nickel, polycyclic aromatic hydrocarbons, air pollution, second-hand smoke, and even fumes from cooking sources all increase the risk of lung cancer. Men, specifically African American men, are more commonly affected than women [19].

Subtypes

Lung cancer is commonly divided into two major types, small cell and non-small cell. Additionally, four histological subtypes exist: squamous cell, adenocarcinoma, large cell, and small cell. Non-small cell encompasses 80% of lung cancers. Small cell lung cancer (SCLC) possesses the worst prognosis due to its aggressive behavior and rapid doubling time [20]. Classically in SCLC, you will see massive lymphadenopathy and direct mediastinal invasion. SCLC also presents more commonly with paraneoplastic syndromes such as SIADH, ectopic ACTH production, and Lambert-Eaton syndrome [20].

Screening

The high incidence and significant morbidity associated with lung cancer necessitates appropriate screening. Annual low-dose chest CT without contrast is the most appropriate screening modality [21]. When compared to plain radiographs, low-dose CT screening demonstrated a 20% relative risk reduction in mortality. Current guidelines recommend annual low-dose CT in adults age 55–80 who possess a 30-pack year history and currently smoke or have quit within the past 15 years [21].

Diagnosis

Initial presentation of lung cancer can be varied. Most will present with some form of pulmonary complaint such as cough, dyspnea, chest pain, or hemoptysis. Many will also present with the classic symptoms of cancer such as unexplained weight loss and fatigue. Up to 25% of patients will be asymptomatic and only diagnosed because they underwent imaging for another reason. Pulmonary exam may reveal evidence of pleural effusion, wheezing, or pneumonia but most often is largely normal. Because symptoms can be so varied, the clinician must have a high suspicion in the right patient population and undertake appropriate evaluation [22].

The majority of decisions regarding advanced imaging, tissue diagnosis, and treatment options will not be guided by the family physician. Rather, an FP's role is to have an appropriate index of suspicion to initiate the work up in the appropriate patient. The first step in diagnosis is usually plain chest radiographs. Findings can range from a single pulmonary nodule to widespread disease with malignant pleural effusions. The three most important features of a pulmonary nodule that should raise the suspicion for malignancy are size (>20 mm), location in the upper lobes, or edges that are spiculated [20]. Several risk calculators exist that take into account pulmonary nodule characteristics as well as other patient characteristics (age, risk factors, etc.) to calculate malignancy risk of the nodule. Every patient in whom there is a suspicion for lung cancer should undergo a chest CT with IV contrast [20]. Family physician should coordinate further care and evaluation with the appropriate specialists.

Three basic questions need to be answered on patients with diagnosis of lung cancer: what the extent of the disease/metastasis is, what comorbidities exist that may limit treatment options (such as COPD), and are symptoms or evidence of paraneoplastic syndrome present that would require early treatment [20].

Once definitive diagnosis is made by tissue biopsy and treatment begins, the role of the family physician shifts to support and comfort. Assisting with treatment side effect management, addressing depression and other psychiatric comorbidities, and discussing end of life goals all fall within the purview of the patient's family physician.

Family and Community Issues

Given the significant morbidity of this disease as well as its association with smoking, the family physician's primary role needs to be one of primary and secondary prevention. Smoking cessation and appropriate screening are among the most effective things a family physician can do to combat this disease.

Pulmonary Sarcoidosis

Sarcoidosis is a multisystem, granulomatous disease of unclear etiology. Its effects can range from an acute self-limited process to progressive and debilitating multi-organ system dysfunction. Annual incidence is approximately 10 cases/100,000. African Americans are affected at four to ten times the rate of Caucasians; it is quite rare in those of Asian ancestry. Females are also affected at a higher rate than males. Peak age of presentation for men is between 40 and 59 and for women between 50 and 69. Despite extensive research, the etiology and pathogenesis of sarcoidosis is poorly understood. While classically affecting the lungs and intrathoracic lymphatic system, sarcoidosis commonly demonstrates extra-thoracic manifestations [23].

Diagnosis

Given the variety of organ systems that can be affected and lack of definitive diagnostic test for sarcoidosis, clinical suspicion with a thorough evaluation is necessary. As the lung is involved in greater than 90% of cases, patients will often present with pulmonary symptoms such as cough, dyspnea, or chest pain. Additional, non-specific symptoms include fatigue, malaise, fever, and weight loss. Dermatologic, hepatic, and ocular signs and symptoms may also be present [24]. Many cases are asymptomatic and are only incidentally found on radiograph. Physical exam often is normal unless the disease course is aggressive or advanced [24].

The diagnosis of sarcoidosis requires three essential elements: typical clinical and radiographic manifestations, exclusion of other disease processes, and proven histopathologic detection of noncaseating granulomas. Laboratory evaluation consists of complete blood count with differential, complete metabolic panel, urinalysis, HIV testing, and TB testing. Inflammatory markers such as ESR and CRP are non-specific but are often obtained. Classically, serum ACE levels are elevated in 75% of cases of sarcoidosis; however current testing modalities lack both sufficient sensitivity and specificity [25].

Radiographic evaluation plays a very important role in the diagnosis of sarcoidosis. Plain films commonly reveal bilateral hilar adenopathy but can also demonstrate parenchymal infiltrates and/or evidence of fibrosis. High-resolution CT scan of the lungs is often completed as well. PFTs can be useful in assessing respiratory impairment as well as monitoring disease improvement or progression [25].

Definitive diagnosis requires histopathologic findings of noncaseating granulomas. Transbronchial lung biopsy is often the modality of choice to obtain histology specimens. After confirmation of disease presence on pathology, a thorough evaluation for extrapulmonary involvement should be completed including electrocardiogram, echocardiography, and detailed fundoscopic evaluation. Regular visits should occur as almost a quarter of patients develop new system involvement within the first 2 years following initial diagnosis [25].

Management

Management decisions are based on expected prognosis, extent of disease/severity, and the patient's preferences. As many cases of sarcoidosis resolve spontaneously or are asymptomatic, therapy may or may not be necessary [26]. Sarcoidosis progression can be divided into three broad categories: acute disease which resolves within 2–5 years, chronic disease which persists beyond 5 years, and refractory disease which is chronic and progressive. Traditionally, first-line treatment consisted of corticosteroids; in recent years steroid-sparing therapies have gained popularity [26]. Steroids possess the advantages of being available, reliable, effective, and easily titrated; however, the plethora of known side effects and toxicities associated with long-term steroid use makes case by case decision-making imperative. Patients who possess comorbidities such as diabetes, osteoporosis, or psychiatric disorders may benefit from steroid-sparing therapies [27].

In the appropriate patient, treatment guidelines suggest initiating therapy with 10–40 mg of prednisone daily and regular titration until therapeutic response is obtained. This response is usually evident in 3–4 weeks. When adequate response is obtained, the dose can be slowly tapered every 3–4 weeks until the lowest required maintenance dose is determined; a goal of 10 mg of prednisone or less is reasonable [26]. Maintenance therapy usually lasts for at least 6 months. Relapse rates range widely between 14% and 74% with acute disease, usually occurring within the first 6 months of therapy discontinuation [26]. Relapses can occur up to 2 years after discontinuation. Initiation of the previously effective steroid doses usually regains control over symptoms. For patients with predominantly lung symptoms (cough, dyspnea), switching to an inhaled corticosteroid after a 3-month trial with systemic steroids has demonstrated improvement in symptoms [26].

Steroid-sparing treatment options such as methotrexate, azathioprine, leflunomide, and mycophenolate mofetil should be considered in chronic/refractory disease or in patients with high risk of steroid-related complications [25, 26]. Limited data exist comparing the effectiveness between these steroid-sparing therapies. Choice of treatment depends on clinician familiarity, patient preferences, and the presence of comorbidities. Currently, methotrexate is the most well studied. If there is disease progression or toxic effects, escalation of therapy with infliximab or adalimumab may be necessary [27] (Fig. 1).

Family/Community Problems

Often patients with sarcoidosis are being managed by specialists, particularly if they have chronic or refractive disease. The family physicians hold a unique role in the initial evaluation and more importantly monitoring appropriate healthcare maintenance issues for those on long-term steroids such as appropriate vaccinations, *Pneumocystis* pneumonia prophylaxis if needed, osteoporosis evaluation/management, etc.

Vaping-Induced Pulmonary Injury

E-cigarette or vaping product use-associated lung injury (EVALI) is characterized by pulmonary injury linked to the use of e-cigarette products.

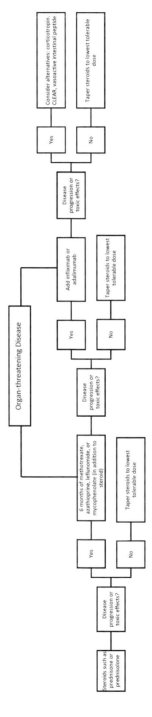

Fig. 1   Treatment strategies for patients with pulmonary sarcoidosis. (Adapted from [27])

The initial outbreak of EVALI was identified in July 2019; since then over 2500 hospitalized cases have been reported. Patients commonly present with symptoms including cough, shortness of breath, and chest pain. Unfortunately, progression to acute respiratory failure is common [28].

While information about the exact etiology of EVALI is limited, one case series compared bronchoalveolar lavage specimens from patients with EVALI to healthy participants and found vitamin E acetate was found in the EVALI specimens. This suggests that vitamin E acetate-containing products may be related to the development of EVALI [29].

Diagnosis

Given the recent identification of the disease process, there is not yet an agreed-upon diagnostic criteria. For the purpose of clinical surveillance, the following diagnostic criteria have been proposed. Probable cases have been defined by a patient use of an e-cigarette 90 days prior to symptom onset, presence of pulmonary infiltrates on imaging, respiratory infection not believed to be the cause of the patient's symptoms, and no existing alternative plausible diagnosis. Confirmed cases were defined with the same criteria as probable except that pulmonary infection had been definitively ruled out with various infectious disease testing modalities [30].

Management

Management of EVALI is based on observational studies. Supportive care is the mainstay of treatment. In one case series, 95% of patients who presented with EVALI symptoms required hospitalization. Respiratory support is crucial to management with 53% of patients requiring ICU care and 26% requiring intubation. Many patients received glucocorticoids at the time of hospitalization and clinical teams reported improvement in their symptoms with steroid treatments [28].

Prognosis

Long-term prognosis data for EVALI are lacking. Of the 2409 cases reported to the US Center for Disease Control (CDC) since the summer of 2019, there were 52 deaths, 31 rehospitalizations (median 4 days after discharge), and 7 deaths after discharge (median 3 days after discharge). E-cigarette avoidance is the most important aspect of post hospital care [31].

Primary care physicians should regularly screen for e-cigarette and engage in targeted cessation counseling. The US Food and Drug Administration is currently engaged in efforts to reduce e-cigarette use in children by removing flavored e-cigarette products from the market. The CDC currently recommends against e-cigarettes [30].

References

1. Hoeper MM, Bogaard HJ, Condliffe R, Frantz R, Khanna D, Kurzyna M, et al. Definitions and diagnosis of pulmonary hypertension. J Am Coll Cardiol. 2013;62(25):D42.
2. Strange G, Playford D, Stewart S, Deague JA, Nelson H, Kent A, et al. Pulmonary hypertension: prevalence and mortality in the Armadale echocardiography cohort. Heart. 2012;98(24):1805–11.
3. Galiè N, Humbert M, Vachiery J-L, Gibbs S, Lang I, Torbicki A, Simonneau G, Peacock A, Noordegraaf AV, Beghetti M, Ghofrani A, Sanchez MAG, Hansmann G, Klepetko W, Lancellotti P, Matucci M, McDonagh T, Pierard LA, Trindade PT, Zompatori M, Hoeper M. 2015 ESC/ERS guidelines for the diagnosis and treatment of pulmonary hypertension. The Joint Task Force for the Diagnosis and Treatment of Pulmonary Hypertension of the European Society of Cardiology (ESC) and the European Respiratory Society (ERS). Eur Respir J. 2015;46:903–75. Eur Respir J. 2015;46(6):1855–6.
4. Frost A, Badesch D, Gibbs JSR, Gopalan D, Khanna D, Manes A, et al. Diagnosis of pulmonary hypertension. Eur Respir J. 2019;53(1):1801904.
5. Braganza M, Shaw J, Solverson K, Vis D, Janovcik J, Varughese RA, et al. A prospective evaluation of the diagnostic accuracy of the physical examination for pulmonary hypertension. Chest. 2019;155(5):982–90.
6. Noppen M, Keukeleire TD. Pneumothorax. Respiration. 2008;76(2):121–7.
7. Tschopp J-M, Marquette C-H. Spontaneous pneumothorax: stop chest tube as first-line therapy. Eur Respir J. 2017;49(4):1700306.

8. Tschopp J-M, Bintcliffe O, Astoul P, Canalis E, Driesen P, Janssen J, et al. ERS task force statement: diagnosis and treatment of primary spontaneous pneumothorax. Eur Respir J. 2015;46(2):321–35.

9. Roberts DJ, Leigh-Smith S, Faris PD, Blackmore C, Ball CG, Robertson HL, et al. Clinical presentation of patients with tension pneumothorax. Ann Surg. 2015;261(6):1068–78.

10. Sahn SA, Huggins JT, Jose ES, Alvarez-Dobano JM, Valdes L. The art of pleural fluid analysis. Clin Pulm Med. 2013;20(2):77–96.

11. Light RW. The light criteria. Clin Chest Med. 2013;34 (1):21–6.

12. Kummerfeldt CE, Chiuzan CC, Huggins JT, Divietro ML, Nestor JE, Sahn SA, et al. Improving the predictive accuracy of identifying exudative effusions. Chest. 2014;145(3):586–92.

13. Kreuter M, Herth FJF, Wacker M, Leidl R, Hellmann A, Pfeifer M, et al. Exploring clinical and epidemiological characteristics of interstitial lung diseases: rationale, aims, and design of a Nationwide Prospective Registry – The EXCITING-ILD Registry. Biomed Res Int. 2015;2015:1–9.

14. Vos T, et al. Global, regional, and national incidence, prevalence, and years lived with disability for 310 diseases and injuries, 1990–2015: systematic analysis for the Global Burden of Disease Study 2015. Lancet. 2016;388:1545.

15. Wells AU, Hirani N. Interstitial lung disease guideline. Thorax. 2008;63(Suppl 5):v1–v58.

16. King TE. Approach to the adult with interstitial lung disease: clinical evaluation. In: UpToDate, Flaherty KR, editors. UpToDate, Waltham. Accessed 12 Apr 2020.

17. Mittoo S, Gelber AC, Christopher-Stine L, Horton MR, Lechtzin N, Danoff SK. Ascertainment of collagen vascular disease in patients presenting with interstitial lung disease. Respir Med. 2009;103(8):1152–8.

18. Siegel RL, Miller KD, Jemal A. Cancer statistics, 2019. CA Cancer J Clin. 2019;69(1):7–34.

19. Alberg AJ, Samet JM. Epidemiology of lung cancer*. Chest. 2003;123(1):21s.

20. Ost DE, Yeung S-CJ, Tanoue LT, Gould MK. Clinical and organizational factors in the initial evaluation of patients with lung cancer. Chest. 2013;143(5):e121S.

21. The National Lung Screening Trial Research Team. Reduced lung-cancer mortality with low-dose computed tomographic screening. N Engl J Med. 2011;365(5):395–409.

22. Rivera MP, Mehta AC, Wahidi MM. Establishing the diagnosis of lung cancer. Chest. 2013;143(5):e142S.

23. Ungprasert P, Carmona EM, Utz JP, Ryu JH, Crowson CS, Matteson EL. Epidemiology of sarcoidosis 1946–2013. Mayo Clin Proc. 2016;91 (2):183–8.

24. Judson M, Boan A, Lackland D. The clinical course of sarcoidosis: presentation, diagnosis, and treatment in a large white and black cohort in the United States. Sarcoidosis vasculitis and diffuse lung disease. Mattioli 1885 J. 2012;29(2):119–27.

25. Costabel U, Hunninghake G. On behalf of the sarcoidosis statement committee. ATS/ERS/WASOG statement on sarcoidosis. Eur Respir J. 1999;14(4):735.

26. Wijsenbeek MS, Culver DA. Treatment of sarcoidosis. Clin Chest Med. 2015;36(4):751–67.

27. Baughman RP, Grutters JC. New treatment strategies for pulmonary sarcoidosis: antimetabolites, biological drugs, and other treatment approaches. Lancet Respir Med. 2015;3(10):813–22.

28. Layden JE, Ghinai I, Pray I, Kimball A, Layer M, Tenforde MW, et al. Pulmonary illness related to e-cigarette use in Illinois and Wisconsin – final report. N Engl J Med. 2020;382(10):903–16.

29. Blount BC, Karwowski MP, Shields PG, Morel-Espinosa M, Valentin-Blasini L, Gardner M, et al. Vitamin E acetate in bronchoalveolar-lavage fluid associated with EVALI. N Engl J Med. 2020;382(8): 697–705.

30. Schier JG, et al. Severe pulmonary disease associated with electronic-cigarette–product use – interim guidance [Internet]. Centers for Disease Control and Prevention. Centers for Disease Control and Prevention; 2019 [cited 2020 Mar 26].

31. Mikosz CA, Danielson M, Anderson KN, Pollack LA, Currie DW, Njai R, et al. Characteristics of patients experiencing rehospitalization or death after hospital discharge in a nationwide outbreak of e-cigarette, or vaping, product use–associated lung injury – United States, 2019. MMWR Morb Mortal Wkly Rep. 2020;68(5152):1183–8.

Part XIX

The Digestive System

Gastritis, Esophagitis, and Peptic Ulcer Disease

91

Jennifer L. Grana, Christopher R. Heron, and Alan M. Adelman

Contents

Dyspepsia/Epigastric Pain

Gastritis, esophagitis, and peptic ulcer disease (PUD) present commonly with epigastric pain or dyspepsia. Dyspepsia is defined as "a predominant epigastric pain lasting at least 1 month" and "can be associated with any other upper gastrointestinal symptoms such as epigastric fullness, nausea, vomiting, or heartburn, provided epigastric pain is the patient's primary concern." [1]. The

J. L. Grana · C. R. Heron · A. M. Adelman (✉)
Family and Community Medicine, Penn State University
College of Medicine, Hershey, PA, USA
e-mail: aadelman@pennstatehealth.psu.edu

© Springer Nature Switzerland AG 2022
P. M. Paulman et al. (eds.), *Family Medicine*,
https://doi.org/10.1007/978-3-030-54441-6_94

recent Rome IV criteria for functional dyspepsia is the presence of at least one of the following: post-prandial fullness, early satiety, epigastric pain or epigastric burning [2]. Dyspepsia is a common problem. Most patients have no organic cause and are defined as having functional dyspepsia.

Epidemiology

Dyspepsia is a common problem, with an annual incidence of 1–2% in the general population and a prevalence that may reach 20–40%. The four major causes of dyspepsia are functional dyspepsia (FD), PUD, gastroesophageal reflux disease (GERD), and gastritis. FD accounts for 70% of all causes of dyspepsia. Less common causes of dyspepsia are symptomatic cholelithiasis, irritable bowel disease, esophageal or gastric cancer, pancreatitis, pancreatic cancer, Zollinger-Ellison syndrome, and abdominal angina. Rarely, patients with coronary artery disease present with dyspepsia. Patients who seek medical attention for dyspepsia are more likely to be concerned about the seriousness of the symptom, worried about cancer or heart disease, and experiencing more stress than individuals who do not seek medical attention for dyspepsia.

Presentation

No single symptom is helpful for distinguishing between the different causes of dyspepsia, but some patient characteristics are suggestive of serious disease. For example, as single symptoms, nocturnal pain, relief of pain by antacids, worsening of pain by food, anorexia, nausea, and food intolerance are not helpful for determining the cause of dyspepsia. Patients older than 50–60 years or with alarm "red flag" symptoms (i.e., weight loss, anemia, dysphagia, persistent vomiting, gastrointestinal bleeding, hematemesis, and melena) are more likely to have a serious underlying disorder. With the possible exceptions of PUD and duodenitis, there is no clinically meaningful association between endoscopic findings and dyspeptic symptoms. It is important to inquire about the use of nonsteroidal anti-inflammatory drugs (NSAIDs), as their use is a frequent cause of PUD. Alcohol is a frequent cause of gastritis, esophagitis, and chronic liver disease/cirrhosis which may lead to portal hypertension and esophageal varices with risk of life-threatening gastrointestinal bleeding.

General Approach

Individuals with evidence of complications or alarm symptoms should be promptly evaluated with endoscopy and, as needed, hospitalized [1–3]. Because age is the strongest predictor of finding "organic" disease on endoscopy, individuals over the age of 50–60 years should also be evaluated with endoscopy. For the remaining patients, a test and treat strategy is recommended. Test for *Helicobacter pylori* by either urea breath test or stool antigen and if positive *Helicobacter pylori* eradication should by undertaken (see section on PUD). If negative, the patient should be treated with a proton-pump inhibitor (PPI).

If *Helicobacter* pylori negative, empiric treatment for functional dyspepsia consists of proton-pump inhibitors (PPIs), available over the counter or by prescription (Table 1). If a PPI fails to relieve symptoms, there are several options. Prokinetic agents such as metoclopramide may be tried. Tricyclic antidepressants are another option. If still without improvement, referral for psychotherapy should be considered [1, 3].

Gastroesophageal Reflux Disease

Gastroesophageal reflux disease (GERD) is a common problem with a prevalence of reflux of around 18% in North America, which can reach

Table 1 Usual daily dosage of antacid medications

Proton-pump inhibitors	
Omeprazole (Prilosec)	20–40 mg qd
Lansoprazole (Prevacid)	15–30 mg qd
Rabeprazole (Aciphex)	20 mg qd
Esomeprazole (Nexium)	20–40 mg qd
Pantoprazole (Protonix)	40 mg qd

25–35% over a lifetime in the US population [4]. Around 5–10% of patients with GERD experience symptoms daily and nearly 44% on a monthly basis. The incidence of GERD increases during pregnancy, with obesity and tobacco use. GERD occurs when injurious gastric contents breech the esophageal-gastric (EG) junction with impaired luminal clearance but exact pathophysiology is unknown [5]. Exposure to excessive acid or pepsin can lead to damage of the esophageal mucosa, resulting in inflammation and ultimately scarring and stricture formation. Several factors may lead to GERD including hiatal hernia, incompetence of the lower esophageal sphincter (LES), inappropriate LES relaxation, impaired esophageal peristalsis and acid clearance, impaired gastric emptying, and repeated vomiting. Multiple prescription and over the counter medications lead to an increased risk of GERD. These include NSAIDS (most common), bisphosphonates, SSRI therapy, sirolimus, anti-platelets, chemotherapeutic agents, as well as certain anticholinergics, nitrates, narcotics, estrogens, diazepam, alpha-antagonists, theophylline, and beta-agonists. GERD may occur as an isolated entity or as part of a systemic disorder such as scleroderma. GERD is a risk factor for gastric ulcerations, esophageal strictures, Barrett's esophagitis, and esophageal adenocarcinoma, one of the fastest-growing cancers in the United States.

Presentation

The most reliable symptom of GERD is heartburn, a retrosternal burning sensation that may radiate from the epigastrium to the throat. Patients may also complain of pyrosis or water brash, the regurgitation of bitter-tasting material into the mouth. Belching is frequently described. Symptoms may be worse after eating, bending over, or lying down. Nocturnal symptoms may awaken the patient. GERD can cause respiratory problems including laryngitis, chronic cough, aspiration pneumonia, and wheezing. Atypical chest pain can also be caused by GERD. Finally, patients may complain of hoarseness, a globus sensation, odynophagia (pain with swallowing), or

dysphagia. Red flag symptoms indicating a more serious etiology may include persistent nausea and vomiting, weight loss, bleeding, mass or iron deficiency anemia and would warrant further workup.

Diagnosis

A young patient with no evidence of systemic illness typically requires no further workup and can be treated empirically with a trial of PPI therapy and removal of insulting medications or lifestyle risks. This is both proven clinically and cost effective. Older patients greater than age 50 with new onset of symptoms, particularly those with above mentioned red flag symptoms, may warrant further evaluation. Upper endoscopy is the evaluation of choice [6]. Ambulatory 24-h pH monitoring is the most sensitive test for demonstrating reflux if endoscopy is negative although poorly tolerated by most patients. A barium swallow study or esophageal manometry may be necessary if a motility disorder is suspected, as endoscopy is often normal in patients with this problem and may point to a diagnosis of function dyspepsia.

Management

GERD is treated by both non-pharmacologic and pharmacologic means [6, 7]. Whereas patients with mild disease may respond to non-pharmacologic treatment, patients with moderate to severe symptoms or recurrent disease usually require medication therapy added or intensified, in addition to continuation of lifestyle changes.

All patients with GERD should be advised to reduce weight (if over their ideal body weight), avoid large meals (especially several hours before going to sleep), refrain from lying down after meals, and refrain from wearing tight clothing around the waist. Avoidance of certain food triggers such as alcohol, caffeine, chocolates, fatty and spicy foods, citrus fruits, and tomato-based foods can help with the symptoms. This treatment method has also demonstrated benefit in overall cardiovascular risk factors as well as the reduction of certain cancer risks. Patients who experience nocturnal symptoms often find relief by putting the head of the bed on blocks 4–6 inches in height. Sleeping on more pillows or on a wedge may be less effective because of nocturnal movements. Because nicotine lowers LES pressure, smoking cessation is recommended [8].

Patients who do not respond to lifestyle changes alone are treated with pharmacologic agents. H2 Receptor Antagonist (H2RA) suppress acid secretion by competing with histamine, thereby blocking its effect on parietal cells of the stomach. H2RAs are effective, but both daytime and nocturnal acid production may be necessary to sufficiently inhibited acid production. PPIs irreversibly block the final step in parietal cell acid secretion and are the most potent antisecretory agents available. The pharmacologic treatment of GERD can be approached in a stepwise process. For mild, intermittent symptoms, antacids or over the counter H2RAs can be used, in twice daily divided dosing. For persistent or severe symptoms, PPIs are the mainstay of treatment. Studies done with omeprazole 40 mg daily have been proven effective and there has not been found to be a difference in different brand PPIs with respect to therapeutic efficacy [9]. PPIs are less effective when taken on an as-needed basis. They are effective when dosed daily before breakfast, although some patients may require twice daily (before meals) dosing to achieve symptom control and/or esophageal healing. Once a patient's symptoms are controlled, a trial of decreasing the dose of medication (e.g., from twice daily to once daily).

PPI do come with risk. This includes multiple drug interactions such as Plavix. They cause risk for fracture due to decreased bone mineralization; this was not observed with H2RA [10]. Other long-term risks have included community-acquired pneumonia, dementia, and nutrient deficiencies [11]. For those patients with GERD who require maintenance medication, periodic examination coupled with efforts to try to reduce medication is warranted. Clinicians should avoid inappropriate prescribing of PPIs and other medications in the treatment of GERD and seek to decrease and "de-prescribe" medications where appropriate and tolerated. Patients often reach for over the counter antacids as initial treatment with possible long-term side effects which, at high doses, can cause constipation, diarrhea, osteomalacia (rare), milk-alkali syndrome, and rebound symptoms.

A concern in patients with chronic GERD is Barrett's esophagus. Barrett's esophagus is metaplasia of the cells of the distal esophagus and is considered a precancerous lesion. The risk of development of adenocarcinoma of the esophagus following a diagnosis of Barrett's esophagus may be as high as 2%. Unfortunately, neither aggressive medical therapy nor surgical therapy for GERD has been shown to alter the progression between Barrett's esophagus and esophageal adenocarcinoma. There is uncertainty as to the efficacy and optimal frequency of endoscopic surveillance of patients with Barrett's esophagus. When dysplasia, the stage between metaplasia and adenocarcinoma, is identified, the recommended frequency of surveillance with esophagogastroduodenoscopy (EGD) and repeat biopsy varies, depending on the severity of dysplasia.

For severe or refractory GERD, the initial approach should be to ensure that the patient is on maximal PPI therapy. If symptoms continue, the addition of a prokinetic agent such as metoclopramide should be considered. Metoclopramide can increase esophageal contraction amplitude, increase LES pressure, and accelerate gastric emptying, three of the most significant motility problems in the pathogenesis of GERD. Metoclopramide is a dopamine antagonist that can cause extrapyramidal symptoms and, rarely, tardive dyskinesia. This may limit its use.

Individuals who are intolerant or unresponsive to optimal medical therapy or non-adherent to medical therapy are suitable operative candidates. Laparoscopic fundoplication surgery has been shown to be effective, at least in the short term [12]. Bariatric surgery for obesity may also be helpful [6].

Peptic Ulcer Disease

Peptic ulcer disease is defined by EGD as a break in the gastric or duodenal mucosal of greater than 5 mm. Those mucosal breaks noted to be less than 5 mm are defined by the term erosion. Peptic ulcer disease carries a 5–10% overall prevalence with as high as approximately 8.4% in the US population. This has led to PPI drugs being 2 of the top 5 medications sold in the United States. Most peptic ulcers are caused by either *H. pylori* or NSAIDs. Although infection with *H. pylori* appears to be common, most individuals with *H. pylori* do not develop ulcers. Peptic ulcers may involve any portion of the UGI tract, but ulcers are most often found in the stomach and duodenum. Duodenal ulcers are approximately three times as common as gastric ulcers and nearly 95% of patients with a duodenal ulcer are colonized with *H. pylori*. In the past, PUD was marked by periods of healing and recurrence. Successful treatment of ulcers associated with *H. pylori* infection greatly diminishes recurrences and may also decrease the risk of gastric ulcerations leading to gastric cancers, such as gastric adenoma as well as mucosal associated lymphoid tissue (MALT).

Presentation

Epigastric pain is the most common presenting symptom of both duodenal and gastric ulcer disease. The pain may be described as gnawing, burning, boring, aching, or severe hunger pains. Patients with duodenal ulcers typically experience pain within a few hours after meals and complete or partial relief of pain with ingestion of food or antacids. Pain related to gastric ulcers is more variable and may be characterized by pain that worsens with eating. Both duodenal and gastric ulcers may occur and recur in the absence of pain. Pain is variable among patients with both kinds of ulceration and correlates poorly with ulcer healing as documented by endoscopy. Older individuals often present with less pain and may present acutely in nearly 50% of patients with a three times higher mortality rate. Children often present

with less localized symptoms but have a much lower rate of perforation or penetration. Physical examination may reveal epigastric tenderness midway between the xiphoid process and umbilicus, but maximal tenderness may sometimes be to the right of the abdominal midline. Abdominal rigidity is a "red flag" sign that can be associated with ulcer perforation and is an indication for prompt hospitalization and urgent surgical consultation. For other red flag symptoms, see the section on "Dyspepsia." Patients at higher risk include those patients with an BMI >25, tobacco, cocaine or alcohol uses, those on high-risk medications, an underlying hypersecretory disease state such as Zollinger-Ellison syndrome, systemic mastocytosis, vasculitis or carcinoid syndromes, CMV infections, or a history of radiation therapy. High-risk medications are similar to those which increase risks for GERD and esophagitis. NSAIDS are the most common of these medications and aspirin use is also a common trigger. Both of these medications should be discontinued as initial management, if appropriate. In those patients where this is not possible, they should be used in conjunction a PPI or transitioning to a COX-2 inhibitor. PPI do appear to reduce the risk of recurrent ulcers and time to next ulcer in patients on long-term aspirin therapy.

Diagnosis

There are two ways that PUD may be diagnosed. Unless the patient has red flag symptoms, a test and treat strategy for H. pylori is recommended as outlined in the "General Approach" section for "Dyspepsia" [13]. The use of proton-pump inhibitors, bismuth preparations, and antibiotics can suppress *H. pylori* and lead to false-negative results and should be discontinued at least 2 weeks prior to testing using urea breath testing. This is not required for stool antigen testing. Stool antigen testing is the less expensive of two options. An ulcer may also be diagnosed by either radiographic studies or endoscopy. Although duodenal and gastric ulcers can be diagnosed by UGI studies, upper endoscopy is the investigation of first choice. Gastric ulcers more than 3 cm in diameter or without radiating mucosal folds are more likely to be malignant. In addition to the indications listed earlier in the chapter, endoscopy should be considered in patients with persistent and refractory symptoms even in the presence of negative radiographic studies, those with a history of deformed duodenal bulbs (thus making radiographic examination difficult), and in patients with suspected or confirmed upper GI bleeding. If an ulcer is diagnosed endoscopically, a rapid *Campylobacter*-like organism urease test (CLO test) is a quick, sensitive test for determining the presence of *H. pylori*. False positives are uncommon while false negatives occur in approximately 5–10% of cases. The presence of *H. pylori* can also be determined histologically and by culture following biopsy at the time of endoscopy.

Most patients, especially those who are asymptomatic posttreatment, do not require documentation of eradication of *H. pylori*. If one wishes to test for cure, a urea breath test (4 weeks after therapy) or stool antigen test can be performed. Test of cure has been found to be neither cost effective nor practical.

Treatment

All patients with PUD who smoke should be advised to stop smoking as continued smoking can delay the rate of ulcer healing. Higher risk of ulcerations occurs with NSAID use due to submucosal erosions and inhibition of prostaglandins and COX-2 pathways, which stimulates bicarb production and mucosal blood flow. Whether or not a patient's PUD is associated with the use of an NSAID, existing NSAIDs should be discontinued and future NSAID use should be avoided and traditional antiulcer therapy begun with a PPI. For patients who test positive for *H. pylori*, antibiotic treatment should be given. A number of drug regimens have been shown to be effective [13, 14]. A PPI is part of every antibiotic regimen. Patients with *H. pylori*-negative ulcers are treated with traditional antacid agents without antibiotics for 4–6 weeks. In areas with high

clarithromycin and metronidazole resistance, amoxicillin can be utilized as an option.

Treatments for the eradication of *Helicobacter pylori* are for 10–14 days and include the following options:

- PPI plus clarithromycin 500 mg BID, and amoxicillin 1 g BID or metronidazole 500 mg BID (Do not use in areas where clarithromycin resistance >15%).
- PPI plus bismuth subsalicylate 525 mg QID, metronidazole 250 mg QID, tetracycline 500 mg QID.
- PPI plus levofloxacin 500 mg daily, amoxicillin 1 gm BID.

In all of the above treatments, the PPI typically recommended is Omeprazole 20 mg orally twice daily. The first two options are considered the primary treatments for eradication of *H. pylori*.

There are a number of problems with the current antibiotic regimens. First, patient adherence may be a problem because of cost, duration of therapy, and side effects. GI side effects can occur with metronidazole, amoxicillin, and clarithromycin. Probiotics may reduce side effects during *H. pylori* eradication therapy. There is no difference in outcome between a 10- and 14-day course of therapy. A second problem is the emergence of antibiotic resistance involving both metronidazole and clarithromycin, which favors the use of the triple-antibiotic regimen or the levofloxacin containing regimen.

For patients with PUD and no documented *H. pylori*, all PPIs effectively heal ulcers in equipotent doses (Table 1). About 75–90% of ulcers are healed after 4–6 weeks of therapy. The PPIs heal ulcers more quickly than H$_2$RAs, but healing rates at 6 weeks are not significantly improved over those with H$_2$RAs. PPIs should be considered first-line medication therapy.

Dietary therapy should be limited to the elimination of foods that exacerbate symptoms and the avoidance of alcohol and coffee (with or without caffeine) because alcohol and coffee increase gastric acid secretion.

Refractory Ulcers and Maintenance Therapy

Most duodenal ulcers heal within 4–8 weeks of the start of pharmacologic therapy. Gastric ulcers heal more slowly than duodenal ulcers, but 90% are healed after 12 weeks. Higher doses of H_2RAs (e.g., ranitidine 600–1200 mg/day) or PPIs may be used in an effort to heal refractory ulcers with an extended treatment course of 6–8 weeks [15].

Individuals with persistent or recurrent symptoms after completing a full course of pharmacologic therapy should be reevaluated. Adherence with previous treatment recommendations, as well as smoking cessation and avoidance of NSAID use, should be reviewed [16]. If no overt cause of treatment failure is identified, endoscopy should be performed to document ulcer healing. Antibiotic drug resistance may be a factor in persistence of ulcers secondary to H. pylori. Gastric cancer should be excluded by biopsy if a gastric ulcer remains unhealed (see section on "Gastric Cancer" below). Zollinger-Ellison syndrome should also be considered in the case of refractory ulcers.

In patients successfully treated for H. pylori or who have discontinued the use of NSAIDs, maintenance treatment with H_2RAs or PPIs should not be needed. Patients with ulcers in the absence of H. pylori, complicated PUD (e.g., bleeding or perforation), a history of refractory ulceration, aged greater than 60 years, or a deformed duodenum are candidates for maintenance therapy with H_2RAs or PPIs.

Gastritis/Gastropathy

Gastritis represents a group of entities characterized by histologic evidence of inflammation. Gastropathy is characterized by the absence of histologic evidence of inflammation of the gastric mucosa. Both gastritis and gastropathy may be either acute or chronic. It may be difficult to distinguish the two entities by clinical, radiographic, and endoscopic examinations. Gastritis and gastropathy may occur simultaneously and/or overlap with conditions such as GERD or PUD or may be a manifestation of less common conditions such as Crohn's, celiac disease, or sarcoidosis.

Acute gastritis may be due to infections (mainly H. pylori; less commonly viral, fungal, mycobacterial, or parasitic etiologies) and autoimmune conditions (e.g., pernicious anemia, eosinophilic gastritis). Histologic variants of uncertain cause include lymphocytic and eosinophilic gastritis. Gastropathy is commonly due to medications (e.g., NSAIDs including aspirin and cyclooxygenase-2 (COX-2) inhibitors, bisphosphonates, potassium, and iron), alcohol, refluxed bile, ischemia ("stress," as is seen in patients with shock, sepsis, trauma, or burns), or vascular congestion (as in portal hypertension or congestive heart failure).

Chronic gastritis may be preceded by episodes of symptomatic acute gastritis (e.g., that due to H. pylori) or present without prior warning with dyspepsia and constitutional symptoms. H. pylori is the most common cause of chronic gastritis; this association may be accentuated in patients receiving chronic PPI therapy. Pernicious anemia may be associated with chronic gastritis.

These conditions range in presentation from asymptomatic to life-threatening. Of particular interest to the clinician are acute and chronic erosive changes that may be complicated by symptomatic anemia or frank hemorrhage (presenting with melena or hematemesis – see section "Upper Gastrointestinal Bleed" below) and chronic atrophic changes that may progress to gastric cancer. Treatment consists of managing the underlying disease and removing gastric irritants.

Upper Gastrointestinal Bleed

Upper gastrointestinal bleed is defined as GI blood loss above the ligament of Treitz [11]. If the bleeding is clinically evident, it may present in one of three ways. Hematemesis may be bright-red or coffee ground-appearing material and usually is indicative of active bleeding. Melena signifies that the blood has transited through the GI tract, digestion of the blood resulting in dark coloration and sticky texture and is also found in lower GI bleeding. And finally, although uncommon, a UGI bleed may present as hematochezia if bleeding is brisk. If subacute or chronic, the UGI bleed may be discovered during the workup of iron-deficiency anemia or hemoccult-positive stools.

Causes

The four most common causes of UGI bleeding are: peptic ulceration, gastritis/gastropathy, esophageal varices, and esophagogastric mucosal tear (Mallory-Weiss syndrome). The causes of gastritis/gastropathy are described above. Bleeding due to varices is usually abrupt and massive. Varices may be due to alcohol cirrhosis, portal vein thrombosis, or any other cause of cirrhosis/portal hypertension. This includes nonalcoholic steatohepatitis, or NASH/"fatty liver" – an increasingly common condition and frequently associated with obesity and the metabolic syndrome. Mallory-Weiss syndrome classically presents with retching followed by hematemesis. Other causes of UGI bleeding include gastric carcinoma, lymphoma, polyps, and diverticula.

Diagnosis and Management

The diagnosis and management of the patient with UGI bleeding depends on the site and extent of bleeding. Vomitus and stool should be tested to confirm the presence of blood. Initial management for all patients includes assessment of vital signs including orthostatic changes. Patients with significant blood loss should be hospitalized and typed and matched for blood replacement and large-bore intravenous lines placed for fluid and blood replacement.

Though a nasogastric tube can be placed to evaluate gastric aspirate for resolution of intragastric bleeding and clearance of clots and particulate, the routine placing of a nasogastric tube for diagnosis or therapeutic effect is not required [18, 19].

Once the patient is hemodynamically stable, upper endoscopy can be performed. Rapid upper endoscopy upon presentation of patients in stable condition may hasten diagnosis and limit hospitalization. Endoscopy may not reveal an obvious source of bleeding when bleeding has ceased. Massive hemorrhage from varices can make endoscopy impractical. The other more common causes of upper GI bleeding will be readily apparent with use of endoscopy. If the patient continues to bleed and a source has not been identified, angiography may be used to identify the source of bleeding. Upper endoscopy can be therapeutic as well as diagnostic; sclerotherapy or ligation of esophageal varices can be performed through the endoscope. A variety of endoscopic treatments are available for bleeding peptic ulcers.

When bleeding is refractory to medical and endoscopically administered therapies, transcatheter arterial embolization or surgery (resection or shunting) should be considered. Though only 2.5–5% of upper GI bleeding cases require operative intervention, early surgical consultation is advised.

There are two additional therapies for bleeding varices [20]. Peripherally administered vasopressin or somatostatin or balloon tamponade are effective alternative treatments for bleeding varices.

Prevention of GI bleeding is more effective than treatment. Smoking and alcohol cessation should be recommended and NSAIDs avoided. Treatment of *H. pylori*-positive PUD or maintenance therapy for *H. pylori*-negative PUD may decrease subsequent bleeding episodes. Nonselective beta-blockers (propranolol or nadolol) can be used to prevent a first-time episode of bleeding in patients with known varices who have never bled [21].

Gastric Cancer

The overall incidence of gastric cancer has declined significantly in the United States since the 1930s. There has been a shift in prominence from distal to proximal stomach cancers. Individuals moving from Japan to the United States lower their risk of gastric cancer, suggesting that dietary and environmental factors play roles in the pathogenesis of this disorder. Additional risk factors include *H. pylori* infection, gastric polyps, and chronic gastritis.

The majority of gastric cancers are adenocarcinomas. Early gastric cancers are usually asymptomatic. As the cancer grows, patients may complain of anorexia or early satiety, vague discomfort, or steady pain. Weight loss, nausea and vomiting, and dysphagia (more common with proximal cancers) may also be present. Rarely, paraneoplastic manifestations occur. The physical examination is usually normal in patients with early disease, but a palpable abdominal mass or supraclavicular nodes, enlarged liver, or ascites may be present with advanced or metastatic disease. Patients with gastric cancer may present with GI bleeding, overt or otherwise occult, although this represents a minority of presentations.

Upper endoscopy is the preferred test when gastric cancer is suspected. Upper gastrointestinal (UGI) X-ray studies can detect gastric cancer, but it is not as accurate, and biopsy of suspicious lesions can be obtained during upper endoscopy. If an ulcer is suspicious in appearance, alarming symptoms are present, or if the patient is >45 years of age, EGD with biopsy is the preferred procedure. If the initial biopsies are benign, then endoscopy should be repeated at 12 weeks to ensure that the ulcer has healed completely. Benign gastric ulcers should heal within 6–12 weeks.

Prognosis for gastric cancer is generally poor, with a 5-year overall survival rate of < 5% [22]. Surgical treatment is the only chance for definitive cure. Perioperative or postoperative adjuvant chemotherapy is considered standard of care. The addition of postoperative radiation therapy has not been shown to offer survival benefit [23].

References

1. Moayyedi PM, Lacy BE, Andrews CN, Enns RA, Howden CW, Vakil N. ACG and CAG linical guideline: management of dyspepsia. Am J Gastroenterol. 2017;112:988–1013.
2. Drossman DA, Hasler WL. Rome IV-functional GI disorders: disorders of gut-brain interaction. Gastroenterology. 2016 May;150(6):1257–61.
3. Mounsey A, Barzin A, Rietz A. Functional dyspepsia: evaluation and management. Am Fam Physician. 2020;101(2):84–8.
4. El-Serag HB, Sweet S, Winchester CC, Dent J. Update on the epidemiology of gastro-oesophageal reflux disease: a systematic review. Gut. 2014;63:871–80.
5. Sandlers RS, Everhart JE, Donowitz M, et al. The burden of selected digestive diseases in the United States. Gastroenterology. 2002;122(5):1500–11.
6. Katz PO, Gerson LB, Vela MF. Guidelines for the diagnosis and treatment of gastroesophageal reflux disease. Am J Gastroenterol. 2013;108:308–28.
7. Gikas A, Triantafillidis JK. The role of primary care physicians in early diagnosis and treatment of chronic gastrointestinal diseases. Int J Gen Med. 2014;7:159–73.
8. Ling-Zhi Y, Ping Y, Gang-Shi W, et al. Lifestyle intervention for gastroesophageal reflux disease: a national multicenter survey of lifestyle factor effects on gastroesophageal reflux disease in China. Ther Adv Gastroenterol. 2019;12:1–12.
9. Sigterman KE, van Pinxteren B, Bonis PA, et al. Short-term treatment with proton pump inhibitors, H2-receptor antagonists and prokinetics for gastro-oesophageal reflux disease-like symptoms and endoscopy negative reflux disease. Cochrane Database Syst Rev. 2013;2013(5):CD002095.
10. Poly TN, Islam MM, Yang HC, Wu CC, Li YJ. Proton pump inhibitors and risk of hip fracture: a meta-analysis of observational studies. Osteoporos Int. 2019 Jan;30(1):103–14.
11. Jaynes M, Kumar A. The risks of long term proton pump inhibitors: a critical review. Ther Adv Drug Saf. 2019;10:1–13.
12. Wileman SM, McCann S, Grant AM, Krukowski ZH, Bruce J. Medical versus surgical management for gastro-oesophageal reflux disease (GORD) in adults. Cochrane Database Syst Rev. 2010;(3):CD003243. https://doi.org/10.1002/14651858.CD003243.pub2.
13. Fashner J, Gitu AC. Diagnosis and treatment of peptic ulcer disease and *H. pylori* infection. Am Fam Physician. 2015;91:236–42.
14. Ford AC, Gurusamy KS, Delaney B, Forman D, Moayyedi P. Eradication therapy for peptic ulcer disease in Helicobacter pylori-positive people. Cochrane Database Syst Rev. 2016;2016(4):CD003840.
15. Heung Up K. Diagnostic and treatment approaches for refractory peptic ulcers. Clin Endosc. 2015;48(4):285–90.
16. Rantanen T, Udd M, Honkanen T, et al. Effect of omeprazole dose, nonsteroidal anti-inflammatory agents, and smoking on repair mechanisms in acute peptic ulcer bleeding. Dig Dis Sci. 2014;59:2666–74.
17. Laine L, Jensen DM. Management of patients with ulcer bleeding. Am J Gastroenterol. 2012;107:345–60. https://doi.org/10.1038/ajg.2011.480. Published online 7 Feb 2012
18. Rockey DC, Ahn C, de Melo SW Jr. Randomized pragmatic trial of nasogastric tube placement in patients with upper gastrointestinal tract bleeding. J Investig Med. 2017;65:759.

19. Stanley AJ, Laine L. Management of acute upper gastrointestinal bleeding. BMJ. 2019;364:l536.
20. Wilkins T, Wheeler B, Carpenter C. Upper gastrointestinal bleeding in adults: evaluation and management. Am Fam Physician. 2020 Mar 1;101(5):294–300.
21. Smith A, Baumgartner K, Bositis C. Cirrhosis: diagnosis and management. Am Fam Physician. 2019 Dec 15;100(12):759–70.
22. Charalampakis N, Economopoulou P, Kotsantis I, et al. Medical management of gastric cancer: a 2017 update. Cancer Med. 2018 Jan;7(1):123–33.
23. Cats A, Jansen EP, van Grieken NC, et al. Chemotherapy versus chemoradiotherapy after surgery and preoperative chemotherapy for resectable gastric cancer (CRITICS): an international, open-label, randomized phase 3 trial. Lancet Oncol. 2018;19:616–28.

Corin Archuleta, Matthew Wright, Anne Marie Kennedy, and Sara DeSpain

Contents

C. Archuleta · M. Wright · A. M. Kennedy ·
S. DeSpain (✉)
UNMC Family Medicine Residency Program,
Omaha, NE, USA

© Springer Nature Switzerland AG 2022
P. M. Paulman et al. (eds.), *Family Medicine*,
https://doi.org/10.1007/978-3-030-54441-6_181

Infectious Diarrhea

There are approximately 179 million cases of acute diarrhea illness in the United States each year. Worldwide, gastroenteritis accounts for two to three million deaths per year, most frequently at the extremes of age in developing countries. Diarrhea is defined as the passage of three or more unformed stools per day or the passage of more than 250 g of unformed stool per day. Acute diarrhea lasts less than 14 days. Diarrhea that persists for more than 3 weeks is considered chronic. A general approach to these patients involves defining the diarrhea to include volume and blood or mucus content, assessing for risk factors, assessing for invasive disease, determining the level of dehydration, and performing testing when indicated [1, 2].

Viral Gastroenteritis

Viral pathogens are the most common cause of gastroenteritis in the United States. Presentation is sudden onset, with copious amount of diarrhea frequently associated with nausea and vomiting. The disease is a self-limited process. The incubation period averages 24–48 h and symptoms between 24 and 60 h. Before the advent of the rotavirus vaccine, this was the most prevalent. Now *Norovirus* and, to a lesser extent, *Calicivirus* and *Sapovirus* are the most common agents. Viral gastroenteritis (VGE) typically arises in one of three settings: sporadically in infants/young children, as outbreaks on cruise ships or military barracks and healthcare facilities, and occasionally sporadically in adults. *Norovirus* is highly contagious, with an inoculum of as few as ten viral particles needed to infect patients. Routine testing is not useful in VGE. Symptomatic treatment with Zofran from 4 to 8 mg every 4–6 h can be safely offered to most patients. Most will recover spontaneously without medical intervention, though for the young and old, close monitoring of hydration status to prevent more severe outcomes may be necessary [2, 3].

Bacterial Infections

Bacterial infections typically cause inflammatory diarrhea illness. The bacteria are invasive or produce toxins, which lead to a more severe diarrheal presentation. *Escherichia coli*, *Salmonella*, *Campylobacter jejuni*, *Yersinia*, and *Shigella* are the most relevant organisms implicated.

E. coli is acquired by ingestion of raw or undercooked meat/poultry or unpasteurized dairy products. The bacteria are divided into two types: Shiga toxin-producing and non-Shiga toxin-producing. Of the Shiga toxin-producing strains (STEC), *E. coli* O157:H7 is the most well-studied. Other strains of *E. coli* are enteropathogenic, enteroinvasive, and enteroaggregative. The enterotoxigenic strain is associated with traveler's diarrhea, discussed further below. Shiga toxin-producing strains present with abdominal pain, cramps, and severe, often bloody diarrhea. Renal failure is a possible severe complication. A stool test for the presence of Shiga toxin should be completed before treatment with antibiotics, as this could precipitate hemolytic uremic syndrome [4, 5].

Salmonella infection arises from ingestion of contaminated eggs or dairy products. *Salmonella* usually causes gastroenteritis but can also cause typhoid fever, localized infection in bones/joints/meninges, and an asymptomatic carrier state. Up to 75% of *Salmonella* gastroenteritis cases follow the typical course of a bacterial diarrhea illness, with the resolution of fever, diarrhea, and nausea/vomiting after 2–4 days. Infection is diagnosed by stool culture. Typical mild infections do not warrant treatment. In chronic carriers, a course of ciprofloxacin 750 mg twice a day for 4–6 weeks may be used for treatment [4].

Campylobacter jejuni is typically found in contaminated water, milk, or meat and poultry. Domestic pets can also be carriers of the bacteria. Typically, the clinical syndrome begins with 24 h of fever and malaise, followed by the usual gastrointestinal symptoms: abdominal pain, nausea, vomiting, and diarrhea. Guillain-Barre syndrome has been reported to develop within 2 months in 1–2 of 10,000 cases. A stool culture is required for diagnosis. Treatment should be initiated if the clinical course lasts longer than 7 days. Erythromycin is the agent of choice dosed at 500 mg twice daily for 5 days [5].

Yersinia produces a clinical syndrome that typically lasts longer (10–14 days) than the other bacterial pathogens. It may cause mesenteric adenitis that mimics acute appendicitis. Additionally, the bowel wall nodularity and mucosal thickening on imaging can appear similar to Crohn's colitis features. Critical illness is treated with TMP-SMX one to two tablets twice a day.

Shigella can cause severe invasive diarrhea with blood and mucus production. Stool culture is necessary for diagnosis. Treatment is with ciprofloxacin 500 mg two times a day for 3 days.

Traveler's Diarrhea

Traveler's diarrhea is the most commonly identified post-travel diagnosis according to the global travel surveillance project by the GeoSentinel Surveillance System. The CDC states 30–70% of travelers are affected. In contrast to the most infectious diarrhea, TD is most often attributed to a bacterial agent. Globally, enterotoxigenic *Escherichia coli* (ETEC) is the most common, followed by *Campylobacter jejuni*, *Shigella* spp., and *Salmonella* spp. The counseling provided to the patient in a travel or family physician's clinic is crucial to the appropriate recognition and treatment of TD [6–8].

TD is defined as three or more stools with or without associated fevers, abdominal cramps, and vomiting within 24 h. The International Society of Travel Medicine adds a functional classification, which practitioners might find helpful in discussing TD with patients (Table 1).

Rates of TD have persisted despite the adage for prevention of "boil it, cook it, peel it, or forget it." Preventive measures for patients include proper food and beverage selection, handwashing recommendations, and prophylactic medications. Expressly, travelers should be advised to drink only sealed beverages with no ice, avoid consuming salads or uncooked vegetables, peel fruits themselves if possible, only consume pasteurized milk and milk products, and avoid undercooked meat. Additionally, poor hygiene practices in

local restaurants pose a significant risk factor for the development of TD [1, 6, 7, 9].

A strategy that relies solely on risk avoidance is often at odds with patients' goals of travel being to immerse themselves in the destination local culture. Therefore, thorough counseling on region-specific risks, endemic viruses, recommended vaccines, and prophylactic medicine is of paramount importance. It is also crucial to counsel about recognition of dysentery, acute versus chronic diarrhea, and when to seek medical care.

Commercially available vaccines against *Salmonella enterica* (typhoid fever) and *Vibrio cholerae* (cholera) exist, but are not recommended, primarily due to a lack of efficacy. Options for prophylactic medications include bismuth subsalicylate (BSS) and antibiotics. BSS can bind to bacterial toxins and protects the gut mucosa. It is recommended because of the effectiveness in reducing the incidence of TD by up to 50% and its safety profile. Adverse effects are mild and include black discoloration of tongue and stools, tinnitus, and constipation. It should be avoided in those who are allergic to aspirin, have renal insufficiency, are pregnant, or are on anticoagulants. Studied effective doses of BSS are 2.1 g/day or 4.2 g/day in four divided doses (meals and bedtime) [7, 9].

It is recommended to avoid prophylactic antibiotics unless the patient is at high risk of complications if they develop TD or if the traveler has essential duties and jobs to perform. When indicated, rifaximin in doses of 200–1100 mg daily can be used. This poorly absorbed antibiotic has fewer adverse effects than the previously recommended fluoroquinolones. *Campylobacter* spp. are resistant to rifaximin, so if travel is to South or Southeast Asia, another prophylactic agent should be used. There is insufficient data to recommend probiotics in the prevention of TD [6].

Treatment of TD depends on severity of disease and includes the management of fluid and electrolyte status, antimotility agents, and antibiotics. In mild to moderate cases, when the patient can tolerate oral intake, oral rehydration solutions (ORS) are strongly recommended. Packets of

Table 1 Adapted from *Journal of Travel Medicine* consensus statement

Mild	Tolerable and not distressing Does not interfere with planned activities
Moderate	Interferes with planned activities
Severe	Incapacitating Includes all dysentery
Persistent	Symptoms last longer than 14 days

World Health Organization ORS are widely available in the developing world and involve dissolving one salt packet in 1 liter of boiled or treated water. There is strong evidence for the use of BSS or the antimotility agent loperamide for symptom control. Loperamide has an FDA indication for use in TD and can reach therapeutic effect within 1 to 2 h of the first dose. Loperamide (starting dose of 4 mg) is taken at the onset of symptoms. With each additional stool, another 2 mg can be taken. Travelers should be cautioned about the time to effectiveness, as rebound constipation can develop. Do not use loperamide if fever, bloody diarrhea, or severe abdominal pain is present [1, 7, 9].

In severe cases, when the patient cannot maintain hydration status orally, intravenous fluids should be used. Antibiotics can reduce the duration of symptoms to about a day and a half. Treatment is ciprofloxacin 500–750 mg for 1–3 days. The FDA warning cautioning against use of fluoroquinolones (FQs) in patients with aortic aneurysms and the rare risk of tendon rupture is reduced by newer one-dose regimens. There is widespread *Campylobacter* spp. resistance to FQs in Southeast Asia. Azithromycin is an alternative treatment for moderate TD and should be the first-line agent for severe cases or dysentery. A single 1 gram dose of azithromycin has been proven effective but is better tolerated with divided 500 mg dosing [1, 9].

Thorough counseling, in a travel or primary care clinic, prepares travelers with avoidance and management strategies for TD. Upon return from travel, if the patient is experiencing persistent or refractory diarrhea, antibiotic-resistant bacteria, *Clostridium difficile*, or protozoal parasite infection should be suspected and tested for with a stool sample.

Clostridioides difficile Infection (CDI)

Clostridioides difficile is a gram-positive spore-producing anaerobic bacillus. Bacterial virulence is the result of cytotoxin (A and B) release, which causes colitis. Disruption of gut microbiome with the overgrowth of *C. difficile* results in severe watery diarrhea and significant morbidity and mortality. Transmission is by the fecal-oral route or from direct exposure to a contaminated environment. The spores formed are heat, acid, and antibiotic resistant and can survive outside the colon. Infection control and patient contact precautions are a crucial part of disease control [10].

The most well-established risk factor for CDI is antibiotic use, specifically clindamycin followed by cephalosporins and FQs. Other risk factors include age over 70, enteral feeding, inflammatory bowel disease, or chronic kidney disease. CDI is now the most commonly reported nosocomial pathogen in the United States and is associated with an estimated 4.8 billion dollars in healthcare costs [10, 11].

CDI should be suspected in patients who present with profuse watery diarrhea (particularly with mucus or small amounts of blood), mild abdominal pain or cramping, fever, or malaise especially with recent antibiotic use or hospitalization. The Infectious Diseases Society of America (IDSA) recommends reserving testing for patients with acute, unexplained diarrheal illness with >3 stools in 24 h. They additionally discourage testing on infants younger than 12 months, given the high rates of normal colonization in that demographic.

Diagnosis is established by stool testing for the *C. difficile* toxin or genes that encode them. Most labs will not accept formed stool samples for analysis. Available lab tests include enzyme immunoassays (EIAs) for toxins A and B or glutamate dehydrogenase (GDH) and nucleic acid amplification testing (NAAT) to detect genes that encode the toxins. Clinical suspicion should drive the decision of which test to order. If clinical suspicion is high, a NAAT can establish the diagnosis. In cases of low clinical suspicion, the high sensitivity of EIA testing for toxin and GDH make it a useful screening tool. Concordant results confirm the diagnosis of *C. difficile*. Incongruent results can be followed up with NAAT [10–12].

The following ancillary laboratory testing assists in qualifying severity of disease and patient disposition: complete blood count (CBC) for peripheral leukocytosis and lactate and complete metabolic panel (CMP) for hypoalbuminemia and

Table 2 CDI classification

Non-severe	WBC count of <15,000 per mL Serum creatinine level <1.5 mg per dL
Severe	WBC count >15,000 per mL Serum creatinine level >1.5 mg per dL
Fulminant	Hypotension Shock Ileus Megacolon

renal injury. Diagnostic imaging augments laboratory findings of disease severity. Plain radiographs can show ileus or distention >10 cm. Computed tomography (CT) findings include wall thickening, signs of mucosal/submucosal edema, peri-colonic stranding, and ascites [12].

Treatment of CDI involves fluid and electrolyte management, stopping the offending antibiotic agent, initiating treatment antibiotics, and possibly surgical intervention. The classification of disease into non-severe, severe, and fulminant, as outlined in Table 2, can help guide treatment. Oral vancomycin and fidaxomicin, in fixed or pulse/taper dosing, are the mainstays of treatment. For initial non-severe or severe episodes, the preferred agent is vancomycin 125 mg orally four times a day for 10 days. Fidaxomicin 200 mg orally twice a day for 10 days is equally efficacious but cost prohibitive. The regimen for fulminant CDI is vancomycin 500 mg orally or via nasogastric tube four times a day plus metronidazole 500 mg IV every 8 h. Recurrence occurs in up to 25% of cases; for those with recurrent infection, a pulse/taper regimen is recommended. The proposed mechanism of pulsed dosing is the spores are allowed to germinate and enter a vegetative form, thus rendering them susceptible to the antibiotics [10, 11].

For patients with disease refractory to conventional treatment, fecal microbiota transplantation (FMT) can be considered. FMT is low cost, with high apparent safety and a cure rate of 90%. FMT utilizes stool from a healthy donor, prescreened for communicable diseases. After donor selection and collection, the distillate is transplanted into the donor via NG tube, oral capsules, enema, or colonoscope. FMT introduces healthy flora from the donor to grow and replace the disrupted flora of the affected patient [13].

Surgical consultation is indicated in severe CDI or CDI complicated by ileus or toxic megacolon and should be considered early. Delayed operative treatment >3 days after admission is associated with higher mortality rates [11].

Parasitic Infections

Parasitic infections have a high worldwide prevalence, with a significant morbidity and, occasionally, mortality burden. They are mainly associated with poor sanitation in poverty-stricken areas. The signs and symptoms of parasitic infections include abdominal pain, diarrhea, and potentially weight loss. Parasitic infections can be further divided into two categories: protozoa and helminths. Protozoa are single-celled organisms that multiply in their hosts and include *Giardia*, *Cryptosporidium*, and *Entamoeba histolytica*. The helminths are a group of roundworms and flatworms with more complex life cycles.

Protozoa

Giardia intestinalis is the most common intestinal parasite in the United States. Outbreaks occur from ingesting contaminated water. *Giardia* cysts are ingested and, in the neutral environment of the small bowel, transform into its trophozoite form, enabling replication. Symptoms of infection include diarrhea, flatulence, and steatorrhea. Diagnosis is made by the presence of cysts in stool culture or antigen testing using enzyme-linked immunoassays. Treatment is metronidazole 500 mg orally three times a day for 5 days [14, 15].

Cryptosporidium is spread via contaminated water or from person-to-person. The protozoan can complete its entire life cycle in one human host's small intestine epithelia. This intestinal parasite has a self-limited course in immunocompetent hosts. It is characterized by 2 weeks of voluminous watery or mucus-containing diarrhea occasionally with nausea, vomiting, abdominal pain, and fever. In immunocompromised patients, especially those with acquired immunodeficiency syndrome (AIDS), the most common presentation is chronic diarrhea, lasting months or more. Most patients with AIDS never clear the infection, resulting in profound weight loss and extra-intestinal manifestations (biliary cryptosporidiosis). Diagnosis is confirmed by oocyst detection on microscopic examination of the stool with acid-fast staining. There are no effective treatments [14–16].

Amoebiasis caused by *Entamoeba histolytica* is a severe form of protozoal infection. The organism is ingested in feces-contaminated food and water and is endemic to Mexico, Central and South America, Asia, and Africa. Sexual transmission is possible, particularly in men who have sex with men. Virulent strains produce the proteinase histolysain and facilitate an invasion of the bowel wall and sometimes liver abscess formation. Treatment is with metronidazole and diloxanide for 10 days [17, 18].

Helminths

Helminths are further divided into three categories: cestodes (tapeworms), nematodes (roundworms), and trematodes (flukes). As with protozoal infections, these are mostly associated with contaminated water supplies, undercooked meats, and poor sanitation and are endemic in developing countries.

Cestodes, or tapeworms, have a complex life cycle that starts with the ingestion of eggs by an intermediate (often animal) host. Consumption of undercooked meat from an infected animal leads to human infection. Thoroughly cooking the meat before consumption will kill any cysticerci. The parasite develops into its adult form in the definitive host's small intestine, completing its life cycle. The cestodes of clinical significance in humans are *Taenia saginata* (beef tapeworm) and *Taenia solium* (pork tapeworm). Symptoms of *T. saginata* are usually mild and might only be noticed by passing segments of the cestode in the stool. Conversely, *T. solium* eggs can implant in various tissues, including the brain, causing serious harm. This condition, known as neurocysticercosis, causes seizures and results in 50,000 deaths annually worldwide. Treatment is with albendazole or praziquantel [14, 15, 19].

Nematodes include *Ascaris lumbricoides*, *Necator americanus*, or *Ancylostoma duodenale* (hookworms), *Strongyloides stercoralis*, and *Enterobius vermicularis* (pinworms). There are multiple routes of infection, including fecal-oral, direct contact with infected soil or water, and ingestion of infected meat. The nematode life cycle requires a human host to ingest an egg. It then invades the vasculature of the small intestine and migrates to the lungs. Larvae develop in the alveolar spaces, ascend the airway, and are subsequently swallowed. The larvae mature in the small intestine and lay eggs into the bowel lumen, which are then expelled in feces [19].

Enterobius vermicularis, or pinworms, is the most common helminth infection and is equally prevalent among all socioeconomic levels. After defecation, gravid females migrate to the perianal and perineal regions to deposit their eggs. The eggs cause a pruritus, relieved by itching, but resulting in egg transfer underneath fingernails and subsequent reingestion. Infection can also be sexually transmitted. The most common presentation is perianal and perineal pruritus with restless sleep. Diagnosis is made clinically, with the "tape test." An adhesive is applied to the perianal region early in the morning and examined for eggs. A single dose of albendazole 400 mg is sufficient treatment, but given the high occurrence of reinfection, a second dose should be given 2 weeks later.

Ascaris lumbricoides infects up to a fourth of the world's population and causes 20,000 deaths a year. Most infections are initially asymptomatic, but after approximately 3 months, the worm burden is high enough to produce symptoms: abdominal discomfort, dyspepsia, loss of appetite, or nausea. A large worm burden can cause small bowel obstruction or rarely invade the hepatobiliary system causing biliary colic, cholecystitis, acute pancreatitis, or hepatic abscess. In some patients, larval migration causes Loeffler's syndrome, characterized by pleuritic chest pain, wheezing, fevers, and occasionally hemoptysis. This typically presents 1–2 weeks after the initial infection. In children, recurrent ascariasis can cause stunted linear growth, malnutrition, and reduced cognitive function. Diagnosis is established by the presence of *Ascaris* eggs in the feces. Early infection results in eosinophilia on CBC. Worms in gas-filled areas of the bowel can occasionally be seen on radiographs. Treatment is with oral albendazole in a 400 mg single dose, alternatively with mebendazole 500 mg single dose or pyrantel pamoate 11 mg/kg single dose [14, 19].

Hookworm infections are caused by two organisms, *Necator americanus* and *Ancylostoma duodenale*. Hookworms require warm weather and a moist environment to survive and are endemic in sub-Saharan Africa and Asia. Transmission is through direct contact with human skin. Once inoculated, hookworms migrate to the small bowel. The clinical presentation is mild with epigastric pain, diarrhea, and loss of appetite. A pruritic maculopapular rash at the site of entry is a clinical clue of infectious source on physical exam. Hookworms attach to the intestinal wall and secrete anticoagulants and inhibitors of platelet activators potentially resulting in a clinically significant iron deficiency anemia. Presence of hookworms on a fecal smear examination makes the diagnosis. Treatment is with a single 400 mg dose of albendazole [19].

Strongyloides stercoralis is the only nematode that can complete its entire life cycle in one human host. It is endemic throughout the tropics and subtropics. In the United States, it is found among migrant workers and endemic in the Appalachia region. The clinical presentation is usually mild, with nonspecific gastrointestinal or pulmonary symptoms and a maculopapular rash. A life-threatening hyperinfection syndrome has been associated with strongyloides, characterized by fever, chills, and anorexia with progression to multiorgan failure with ARDS. Diagnosis is via stool examination for ova or enzyme-linked immunosorbent assay (ELISA) testing. Treatment with thiabendazole or ivermectin is effective [14, 19].

Structural Diseases

Diverticular Disease

General Principles
Diverticulosis is the outpouching or herniation of the colonic wall. Colonic diverticula commonly form at vulnerable regions throughout the colon, usually in areas where the vasa recta penetrate the colonic wall. Although the exact cause is unknown, diverticulosis is thought to occur as a result of a low-fiber diet. Low fiber results in diminished stool volumes, which in turn alters the motility of the colon, thus creating higher pressures within the lumen. Diverticulosis, particularly of the sigmoid colon, is common in Western countries and has been discovered in up to 60% of patients over the age of 70. In contrast diverticulosis is less common in Asian countries and occurs predominately in the proximal colon [20].

A patient with symptomatic diverticular inflammation is said to have the diverticular disease [21]. Approximately 20% of diverticulosis patients will develop the acute diverticular disease, diverticulitis. Diverticulitis is thought to occur as a result of diverticular obstruction from colonic debris, such as a fecalith or food particle. The obstruction allows for bacterial infiltration and accumulation in the diverticula, causing inflammation [20].

Clinical Presentation
The clinical presentation of patients with diverticular disease depends on the severity of the inflammation and the presence of complications. Signs and symptoms range from colicky abdominal pain relieved with bowel movements to acute abdominal pain, fever, and leukocytosis. Other symptoms include nausea, vomiting, diarrhea, or constipation. On exam, the patient may have left lower quadrant tenderness and/or fullness [21].

Currently, there is no universally accepted clinical classification of diverticular disease; however, it can be divided into acute or chronic; acute diverticulitis can be additionally classified as uncomplicated, recurrent, and complicated [20, 21]. The classic presentation of acute diverticulitis is fever, left lower quadrant pain, and leukocytosis [20]. Recurrent diverticular disease is defined as more than one episode of diverticulitis per year [21].

Complications of diverticulitis include phlegmon, perforation, abscess, fistula, peritonitis, strictures, small bowel obstruction, and hemorrhage [20, 21].

Diverticular disease may develop into chronic diverticular disease as a result of ongoing mucosal inflammation, and symptoms can include left lower quadrant pain, bloating, and diarrhea [20].

Diagnosis

The diagnosis of acute diverticulitis is usually made clinically; however, an abdominal computed tomography (CT) scan with IV contrast helps confirm the diagnosis if there is uncertainty [20]. Additionally, a CT scan can identify complications of diverticulitis, which would determine if a patient requires early surgical intervention [20, 21].

Laboratory studies such as a complete blood count (CBC) and basic metabolic panel (BMP) should be obtained to assess for leukocytosis and renal function/electrolyte abnormalities, respectfully [22].

Management

In general, asymptomatic diverticulosis does not require treatment; however, these patients may benefit from making certain lifestyle changes, such as increasing physical activity and adopting a high-fiber low-fat diet [21].

Antibiotic therapy is generally indicated for acute diverticulitis. Typically, broad-spectrum antibiotics with aerobic and anaerobic coverage are prescribed; and the route of administration and duration of treatment depend on disease severity [20, 21].

In patients with mild or moderate diverticulitis without signs of complicated disease (i.e., fever, peritonitis), patients can generally be treated with oral antibiotics for 7–10 days in the outpatient setting with close follow-up. Hospitalization, IV antibiotics, and bowel rest are indicated if a patient has severe diverticulitis and/or fails to improve with outpatient therapy. IV antibiotics are typically administered for 7–10 days, and oral antibiotics are recommended for an additional 7–10 days after discharge [21].

In addition to the above treatment, patients with complicated diverticulitis may require more invasive treatments, such as surgery or percutaneous drainage of an abscess [21] (Table 3).

Microscopic Colitis

General Principles

Microscopic colitis (MC) is a general term for patients with otherwise unexplained chronic watery diarrhea. Colonoscopy in these patients will reveal grossly normal mucosa; however, inflammatory changes are seen on biopsy [23, 24].

MC has two major subgroups: collagenous colitis (CC) and lymphocytic colitis (LC) [24]. These subgroups share symptoms and respond to the same treatment; however, they differ in histologic appearance; CC demonstrates thickening of the subepithelial collagen band (≥ 10 μm), while an increased number of intraepithelial lymphocytes (IEL) is the hallmark characteristic of LC (≥ 20 IELs/100 epithelial cells) [23].

Etiology, Risk Factors, and Associated Diseases

The etiology of MC is generally unknown; however, the development and/or severity of the disease is linked with several risk factors and certain medications. Medications associated with the development of MC include NSAIDs, PPIs (notably lansoprazole and omeprazole), ASA, lisinopril, simvastatin, paroxetine, sertraline, carbamazepine, acarbose, ranitidine, and ticlopidine [24, 25].

Risk factors for MC include female gender, increased age (average age at diagnosis is between 50 and 60), certain autoimmune diseases, malignancy (either past or present), and solid organ transplant. While it is generally unknown why females are affected more than males, some speculate MC may have a hormonal component [24].

MC also has a strong association with autoimmune disorders. Up to 30–50% of patients diagnosed with MC have at least one preexisting autoimmune disease, such as celiac disease or thyroid disease. As for other associations, a well-documented environmental risk factor for MC is cigarette smoking. It has been demonstrated that MC develops approximately 10 years earlier in active smokers [23, 24].

Clinical Presentation and Diagnosis

Patients with MC typically present with chronic, watery, non-bloody diarrhea. Other symptoms

Table 3 Diverticulitis treatment options [20–22]

Uncomplicated diverticulitis	**Mild to moderate disease**
	Outpatient management with close follow-up
	Oral antibiotics (7–10 days)
	    Possible combinations:
	        Trimethoprim/sulfamethoxazole (160/800 mg po q12 hours)
	        OR
	        Ciprofloxacin (750 mg po q12 hours) + metronidazole (500 mg po q6 hours)
	        OR
	        Amoxicillin + clavulanate ER (two 1000/62.5 mg tablets po q12 hours)
	        OR
	        Moxifloxacin (400 mg po q24 hours)
	Severe disease:
	Hospitalization
	Bowel rest
	IV antibiotics (7–10 days)
	    Possible combinations:
	        Piperacillin/tazobactam (3.375 g IV q6 hours or 4.5 g IV q8 hours)
	        OR
	        Ciprofloxacin (400 mg IV q12 hours + metronidazole (500 mg IV q6 hours or 1 g IV q12 hours)
	        OR
	        Moxifloxacin (400 mg IV q24 hours)
	Oral antibiotics at discharge (7–10 days) (see above)

Complicated diverticulitis	**Abscess:**
	  <4 cm = same as severe disease (see above)
	  >4 cm = percutaneous drainage in addition to above
	Perforation, fistulas:
	  Surgical intervention
	Bleeding:
	  Colonoscopy
	  Surgical intervention

Recurrent diverticulitis	Surgical intervention

include crampy/dull abdominal pain (common), fatigue (present in 50–60% of patients), weight loss, and fecal incontinence. The clinical presentation of MC mimics that of irritable bowel syndrome; however, MC has some additional features: nocturnal bowel movements, arthralgias, and fecal incontinence [23, 24].

A diagnosis of MC cannot be definitively made clinically. If MC is suspected, a colonoscopy with biopsy is the next step to make the diagnosis. Given that the microscopic lesions are not always continuous in MC, it is recommended that random biopsies be taken in all areas of the colon. Furthermore, to make the correct diagnosis, the biopsies should be examined by a pathologist with specialized training [24].

Treatment

Treatment is patient-dependent and should be modified based on disease severity and clinical response. Budesonide is considered first-line treatment and is highly effective at inducing clinical remission. In contrast to other glucocorticoids, budesonide undergoes high first-pass metabolism in the liver resulting in low systemic absorption. If the disease is refractory to treatment, a differential diagnosis should be reconsidered, and concurrent celiac disease or bile-acid malabsorption should be appropriately managed [23, 25] (Fig. 1).

Inflammatory Bowel Disease

General Principles

Inflammatory bowel disease (IBD) encompasses the diseases ulcerative colitis (UC), Crohn's disease (CD), and indeterminate colitis. The incidence of IBD has increased in almost every industrialized country over the twenty-first

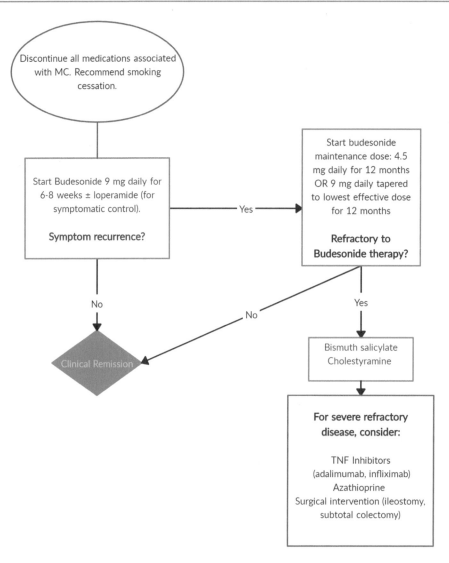

Fig. 1 Approach to MC management [23–25]

century. IBD is more common in North America and northern Europe than the rest of the world. Approximately 1.6 million Americans have been diagnosed with IBD. Disease onset is most likely between the second and fourth generations of life. It affects both men and women equally.

Although the etiology is still widely not understood, it seems to be multifactorial with genetics, host immunity, and environmental-related factors. All these factors lead to an increase in intestinal inflammation manifesting as IBD. The genetic link associated with IBD has been extensively studied over the last decade. Twin studies have shown a positive concordance of both UC and CD, and positive family history of IBD in a first-degree relative shows five times increased likelihood of developing the disease. There are several genes identified in IBD, concluding the disease is likely polygenic. Mutations in genes involved in host immunity, specifically in response to the intestinal bacterial microbiome, have been implicated, most of which lead to an abhorrent immune response. The incidence of IBD has increased in parts of Africa and Asia, where IBD used to be rare. Industrialization and the introduction of diets higher in saturated fats, processed meats, and

Table 4 Extraintestinal manifestations of CD

Organ system	Manifestation	Incidence (%)
Bone	Peripheral arthropathy	20
Dermatologic	Erythema nodosum, oral aphthous ulcers, Sweet's syndrome	15, 10
Ocular	Episcleritis, uveitis	3–6, 0.5–3

lower fiber (especially for CD) are thought to contribute to the development of IBD. Dietary and industrialization changes may lead to a decrease in the diversity of the microbiome and overgrowth of certain bacteria leading to the development of IBD, specifically a decrease in Firmicutes and an increase in Proteobacteria and Bacteroidetes. Lastly, certain common medications have been shown to alter the microbiome: antibiotics, NSAIDs, contraceptives, and statins. The combination of environmental and host immunity factors may lead to the development of IBD in an already genetically predisposed individual [26].

Clinical Presentation

Symptoms of IBD often vary based on the location of the intestinal tract affected. The symptoms can be nonspecific but include:

- Irregular bowel habits and predominantly diarrhea, occasionally with blood or mucus
- Abdominal pain and intestinal cramping
- Fevers
- Fatigue and progressive weight loss

Crohn's Disease

CD produces transmural inflammation of the gastrointestinal tract anywhere from the mouth to the anus. The presentation can vary based on the location and severity of the disease. Classic symptoms include abdominal pain (improved with defecation), watery diarrhea, and progressive weight loss due to malabsorption. CD commonly involves the terminal ileum leading to pain in the right lower quadrant of the abdomen. Abdominal pain can be colicky, coinciding with flares and remission. These symptoms may persist for years before diagnosis. The chronic inflammatory state associated with CD can lead to penetrating fistulas or fibrostenotic obstructions due to

adhesions. Fistulas are eventually present in 20–40% of patients. Enteroenteric fistulas are the most common, followed by enterovaginal fistulas in females. Intestinal strictures most commonly occur in the small bowel and may present with obstructive symptoms like postprandial nausea and vomiting. Up to one-third of patients present with perianal involvement, which indicates more severe disease and often involves more complex medical management and possible surgical interventions [26].

Up to 50% with CD will have extraintestinal manifestations (EIM) (Table 4). The pathogenesis of EIM is not well understood; however, it is hypothesized that the affected gut lining may trigger an altered immune response at extraintestinal sites. It is proposed that bacteria translocating across the leaky intestinal barrier trigger an autoimmune response, unable to differentiate bacterial epitopes from the host synovial tissue (i.e., joints and skin). There may also be a genetic predisposition to EIM based on studies examining IBD and patients with abnormal HLA complexes [27].

Ulcerative Colitis

Ulcerative colitis is characterized by inflammation of the mucosa and submucosa and is confined to the colon. Symptom severity correlates to the extent of the affected colon. Hallmark symptoms include abdominal pain, diarrhea (often with blood and mucus), and tenesmus. Symptom onset is usually acute and can be severe; therefore, a diagnosis is made in weeks, as opposed to years in CD. Complications of UC include fulminant colitis and toxic megacolon, which affects approximately 15% of patients and requires urgent evaluation and management [26]. Up to 7.5% of patients with UC are diagnosed with primary sclerosing cholangitis (PSC) during their disease. PSC is an independent risk factor for the development of colorectal malignancy in patients with IBD, necessitating the recommendation for annual surveillance colonoscopies once diagnosed [27].

Workup

If a physician suspects IBD, the first step is to take a good history and physical exam. A personal medical history should include the assessment of intestinal symptoms as well as extraintestinal symptoms. Nocturnal symptoms can help distinguish IBD from functional abdominal syndromes. Smoking history should be assessed, and signs/symptoms suggestive of malignancy ruled out. A family history of malignancies and IBD should be noted.

On physical exam, patients may have non-specific tenderness to palpation of the abdomen. Clinicians may be able to palpate a mass that can indicate an intestinal abscess, phlegmon, or adhesion. A rectal exam should be performed for the identification of fissures, abscesses, fistulas, and skin tags [26].

Laboratory

Initial laboratory workup should include a CBC, CMP, vitamin D, vitamin B12, and stool studies (heme occult, microscopic examination, and stool culture). Results may reveal mild microcytic anemia, thrombocytosis, hypoalbuminemia, and vitamin D and B12 deficiencies. Stool samples are often heme positive with the presence of neutrophils and eosinophils. Stool cultures can rule out the presence of ova and parasites and *C. difficile* as infectious causes.

Inflammatory biomarkers such as C-reactive protein (CRP) and erythrocyte sedimentation rate (ESR) are nonspecific to IBD and are better for assessing disease remission rather than diagnosis. Fecal calprotectin is an inflammatory marker specific to the intestinal system; however, it can also be positive in diverticulitis, certain malignancies, cirrhosis, and with the use of NSAIDs and proton pump inhibitors (PPIs). It has a high negative predictive value and can be a useful screening tool in the assessment of chronic diarrhea, especially in the adolescent to young adult population. Recent evidence suggests peri-nuclear anti-neutrophil cytoplasmic antibody (p-ANCA) can distinguish UC from CD, whereas anti-*Saccharomyces cerevisiae* antibody (ASCA) may help distinguish CD from UC. IBD laboratory panels exist; however, these tests are expensive and are not well-validated, and positive results still require direct visualization diagnosis [26, 28].

Diagnosis

Colonoscopy, with intubation of the terminal ileum, is the primary diagnostic modality of choice in IBD. Esophagogastroduodenoscopy (EGD) is not initially recommended in asymptomatic patients. To assess for small bowel involvement, magnetic resonance imaging/magnetic resonance enterography (MRI/MRE) or computed tomography/computed tomography enteropathy (CT/CTE) is recommended. Capsule pill endoscopy can be used to aid in the diagnosis of suspected small bowel disease in CD when EGD or cross-sectional imaging is equivocal, but luminal strictures must be ruled out beforehand. Patients with IBD are likely to require numerous imaging studies throughout their lifetime; thus, several gastroenterologists prefer MRI or US (performed at specialty centers) over CT to decrease radiation risk [28].

Management

IBD is a lifelong disease characterized by periods of flare and remission. The best treatment strategies come from team-based care with frequent collaboration between primary care physicians, gastroenterologists, and surgical specialists. Most patients will require both medical and surgical interventions over their lifetimes. With advances in pharmacologic options for IBD, treatment has shifted away from symptom-based to target mucosal healing. This is especially true in CD, where chronic subclinical inflammation is present and leads to possible fistulas and stenosis, which frequently require surgical correction. Delays in diagnosis and achieving remission result in cumulative bowel intestinal damage, which can progress to fibrosis and an increase in disability and function. In UC early diagnosis and treatment can reduce the need for surgery and reduce the risk of colorectal cancer [29].

A Stepwise Approach to Treatment

The goal of treating IBD is to prevent ongoing inflammation and promote gut healing by inducing and maintaining remission (prevent flares). Evidence shows a reduction of intestinal mucosal wall inflammation (<3 months) can reduce intestinal damage. Treatment strategies are aimed at inducing remission and objectively measuring remission maintenance.

Corticosteroids

Corticosteroids are the most effective treatment option to induce remission, but they must never be used alone. For patients with mild to moderate IBD, budesonide 9 g orally daily for 6–10 weeks is recommended. For patients with mild to severe colonic CD, prednisolone prescribed at a dose of 40–60 mg per day tapered over 4–8 weeks is appropriate. Failure to induce remission should be followed by the prompt addition of an immunomodulator [28].

5-Aminosalicylic Acids

In patients with UC and mild disease, aminosalicylates (5-ASA) are the mainstay of treatment for remission induction of active disease and flare prevention. Of the drugs available, sulfasalazine and mesalazine are equally effective and safe, though mesalazine may be better tolerated and can be used in those allergic to sulfasalazine. The dose for remission induction is 2–3 g orally per day (depending on the formulation), whereas doses of 1 g orally per day are effective in maintaining quiescence of disease activity. Rectal 5-ASA formulations are effective for left-sided colitis or proctitis and can be used alone or in conjunction with oral 5-ASA drugs. Unlike in UC, 5-ASA-based drugs are modest at best in maintaining remission in CD. Specifically, mesalazine is not recommended for induction or maintenance of remission in CD. An immunomodulator should be added to the treatment regimen if properly dosed 5-ASA medications do not achieve remission [29].

Immunomodulators

Immunomodulators, including thiopurines (azathioprine and 6-mercaptopurine) and methotrexate 15 mg (subcutaneously or orally) weekly, are the treatment of choice for moderate to severe UC and CD. Due to their prolonged onset of action (2–3 months), they should not be used to induce remission. Methotrexate is indicated for use in CD and should be reserved for patients who fail to respond to or are intolerant of thiopurines. Methotrexate is contraindicated in pregnancy and breastfeeding. Upon starting these medications, patients will require serial monitoring with a complete blood count (CBC) and liver function test (LFT). Adverse reactions include leukopenia, increased risk of infection (especially viral), and a rare, but significant risk of lymphoma and non-melanoma skin cancer. Before initiating therapy with an immunomodulator or biologic agent, patients require screening for tuberculosis (with anti-TNF therapy), hepatitis, HIV, and the presence of intra-abdominal abscesses, as treatment can reactivate these disease processes. Primary care physicians should consider concurrent consultation with a gastroenterologist if initiating treatment with an immunomodulator for IBD [29].

Biologicals

It is reasonable to consider the addition of a biological agent if disease remission is not maintained with the use of an immunomodulator alone. Monoclonal antibody (MAB) agents targeting tumor necrosis factor alpha (TNFα) and integrin have been shown to control intestinal wall inflammation. MAB therapy is indicated for moderate to severe luminal CD (adalimumab and infliximab) and moderate to severe UC (adalimumab, infliximab, and golimumab). It is also indicated in patients with debilitating EIM. Combination therapy with an immunomodulator appears to be superior to MAB monotherapy. A significant loss of response (20–40%) during the first year of anti-TNFα use is thought to be due to immunogenicity. The use of TNFα antagonists is associated with hepatosplenic T-cell lymphoma, a rare, but potentially fatal disease in young males [29].

Microbiome Therapies

Much like the concept of using fecal transplants as a treatment for *C. difficile*, researchers are investigating the use of microbiome fecal transplants in patients with IBD; however, this therapy is in its infancy. Preliminary studies have shown it may be helpful in the induction, but not the maintenance, of remission in UC [29].

Surgery

Surgery can be curative for patients with UC; however, because CD can affect anywhere along the alimentary tract from mouth to anus, surgery may only be a temporizing measure. It can lead to complications of obstruction from adhesions and short bowel syndrome development in the future. In UC, surgery is indicated in patients who fail or are intolerant to medical management, develop colonic perforation or toxic megacolon, or have precancerous lesions found on screening colonoscopy. Surgical options include resection of the entire colon with or without the rectum. Restorative proctocolectomy with ileal pouch-anal anastomosis and total abdominal colectomy with ileorectal anastomosis (TAC-IRA) both preserve fecal continence and do not result in permanent end ileostomy; however, the latter is infrequently performed because it preserves the rectum; therefore, the potential for persistent inflammatory symptoms and the risk of malignancy remain. TAC-IRA may be the preferred surgical option in women who wish to preserve their fertility.

In CD laparoscopic resection can be considered in patients with localized ileocecal disease who fail or relapse on medical management. Surgery may also be necessary for intra-abdominal abscesses or fistulas, once medically optimized, and if percutaneous drainage is not feasible [28].

Additional Primary Care Considerations

IBD is a lifelong disease, which requires frequent monitoring of remission and flare status. During all disease states, it is essential to encourage healthy lifestyle behaviors, optimize nutrition, ensure updated vaccination status, and monitor for drug side effects. Smoking cessation should be emphasized at every visit as smoking tobacco is strongly associated with adverse outcomes in CD and postsurgical resections. Vitamin B12, vitamin D, folate, and an iron panel should be ordered every 6 months to assess for malabsorption and supplementation as

appropriate. Diets should be rich in variety, including high fiber, low processed meats, and foods. Low-fiber diets should only be advised for patients with stricturing CD. Patients who have been on prolonged or repeated doses of corticosteroids should be screened for osteoporosis with a dual-energy X-ray absorptiometry (DXA) scan and be encouraged to supplement with calcium/vitamin D. Hepatitis A and B, tetanus, diphtheria, pertussis, human papillomavirus (HPV), pneumococcal, and influenza vaccines are all recommended. Live vaccines are not to be given while patients are on immunosuppressive therapy. Patients on thiopurine medications should be advised about regular sunscreen use and should have regular skin checks. Regular endoscopy helps assess disease status but is especially crucial for dysplasia surveillance in UC [28]. Preconception counseling is especially important in women with IBD because the best pregnancy outcomes are seen in patients with disease remission at the time of conception and control of the disease throughout the pregnancy. Most medications, except methotrexate, are safe during pregnancy, while the risk of disease flare is associated with increased risk of spontaneous abortion, preterm birth, and low birth weight [30].

Malabsorption

General Principles

The term "malabsorption syndrome" has been used in the past to encompass malabsorption and maldigestion or the inability to absorb or digest nutrient or electrolytes. However, it is not a single disease, diagnosis, or process. Subclassifications include global, selective, primary, and acquired, each one specific in its pathogenesis, diagnosis, and treatment (see Table 5).

Presentation and Workup

Chronic diarrhea, due to high osmotic load, is the most common clinical manifestation of malabsorption. Diarrhea can be watery, pale, foul-

Table 5 Malabsorption classification table

Type	Process and example
Global	Distributed mucosal involvement, multiple nutrients affected; celiac sprue
Selective	Single or limited number of nutrients involved; pernicious anemia
Primary	Secondary to congenital defects in transport systems; cystic fibrosis
Acquired	Usually surgical in nature; resections or bypass

Table 6 Malabsorption: nutrient deficiency with correlated labs with features

Common nutrients	Presentation	Lab work/imaging
Carbohydrates	Watery diarrhea, flatulence, dairy intolerance	Increased breath hydrogen, stool osmotic gap, acidic stool pH
Fat	Steatorrhea, pale and voluminous stools, limited flatulence, dermatitis, poor wound healing	Increased fractional fat excretion ($>7\%$)
Protein	Edema, muscle wasting	Hyperproteinemia, hypoalbuminemia
Vitamin B12/Folate	Fatigue, pallor, SOB, paresthesia	Macrocytic anemia, elevated homocysteine levels, decreased B12/folate
Iron	Fatigue, pallor, chest pain, SOB, pica, tachycardia	Low serum iron and ferritin
Calcium and vitamin D	Tetany, paresthesia, pathologic fractures, fatigue	Decreased calcium, elevated alkaline phosphatase, decreased vitamin D

smelling, greasy, and of varying volume depending on the severity and classification. Other presentations can include weight loss, fatigue, flatulence, anorexia, abdominal distention, and, more rarely, abdominal pain. Workup includes a detailed history to narrow possible etiologies, including clarifying the duration of symptoms, nature of stool, type of foods causing symptoms, timing of symptoms with foods, medical history, surgical history, family history (especially in relation to celiac disease), alcohol use, and other associated symptoms.

Lab tests and imaging should be focused and based on the patient's presentation. Routine lab tests can include complete blood count, calcium, albumin, magnesium, iron studies (serum iron and TIBC specifically), vitamin B12, 25-hydroxyvitamin D, and folate. Although these are not considered diagnostic, they provide more auxiliary evidence for your diagnosis. By using the patient's clinical presentation, in combination with the laboratory findings, a specific nutrient deficiency may be isolated (see Table 6).

Some etiologies of malabsorption are clear (e.g., cystic fibrosis which can be diagnosed at birth or early in childhood), while others are not. When initial lab work and history are not sufficient to make a diagnosis, other more specific tests should be employed. The most common tests include tissue transglutaminase-IgA antibody and total IgA levels for celiac disease (sprue), fecal elastase for pancreatic insufficiency, and carbohydrate breath test for small intestinal bacterial overgrowth. Imaging and further evaluation can be warranted to confirm diagnosis and determine the extent of the disease.

Procedures and Imaging

In patients where history and lab work are inadequate to limit the diagnosis or identify the underlying cause, the physician should order/perform an upper endoscopy and colonoscopy. During these procedures the overall state of the mucosal lining is evaluated, and multiple biopsies are performed. Histologic studies are helpful in ruling out multiple conditions including Crohn's disease and ulcerative colitis. If the endoscopies are unremarkable, proceeding with specific imaging is indicated. Computed tomography (CT), magnetic resonance enterography (MRE), or an upper gastrointestinal series with small bowel follow through are all viable options. While wireless

Table 7 Directed therapies based on diagnosis

Diagnosis	Treatments	Diagnosis	Treatments
Bile acid deficiency	Exogenous acids	Zollinger-Ellison syndrome	High-dose PPI
Small intestine bacterial overgrowth	Antibiotics (rifaximin, TMP-SMX, ciprofloxacin)	Carbohydrate intolerance (lactose deficiency)	Avoidance or exogenous enzymes
Exocrine pancreatic insufficiency/cystic fibrosis	Exogenous enzymes, managed fat intake	Ileal resection/short bowel	Cholestyramine and vitamin supplementation, small meals, and antidiarrheals
Celiac disease	Gluten-free diet		

capsule endoscopy is also available, its role is limited and should be employed by gastroenterologists for specific circumstances.

Treatment

In malabsorptive disorders the goal is to identify the deficiency and then treat the underlying cause. When treatments are not curative, the goal should be to increase the patient's quality of life with symptomatic control. Treatments for each individual etiology vary greatly, and therapies should be directed for each condition as diagnosed (see Table 7).

Diet and medication recommendations for patients with undifferentiated malabsorption and chronic diarrhea are general and based on improving quality of life. Advise patients to decrease their osmotic load with decreased sugar and sorbitol intake, especially in shortened colons. Limit diuretics use, including caffeine. When underlying disease management and diet modification are not sufficient, loperamide can be prescribed to prolong transit time and increase absorption. A tincture of opium can be utilized if loperamide is ineffective. However, care must be used as its side effects include sedation and addiction [31–34].

Irritable Bowel Syndrome

General Principles

Irritable bowel syndrome (IBS) is a common chronic functional gastrointestinal disorder occurring in approximately 9%–23% of the population worldwide. IBS is typically found in young or middle-aged adults, with a prevalence of 14% in women and 9% in men. Patients normally present with abdominal pain (usually characterized as cramping), altered bowel habits (diarrhea, constipation, or alternating between the two), bowel frequency, flatus, bowel urgency, and pain relief with defecation. The cause of IBS and its pathophysiology is still unclear. There is no identified underlying anatomic or inflammatory pathology. IBS is a clinical diagnosis and can be divided into four different subtypes. Patients commonly have psychosocial complications that may perturb gastrointestinal function and propagate symptoms. These associated psychiatric disorders include anxiety, depression, and somatization. Conditions such as fibromyalgia, functional dyspepsia, chronic fatigue syndrome, and noncardiac chest pain are also closely related to patients diagnosed with IBS.

Clinical Presentation

Patients with the hallmark symptoms of chronic bowel pain (especially if relieved by defecation) and altered bowel habits should be suspected to have IBS. Patients may also experience lack of appetite, nausea, excessive flatus, bowel urgency, and food intolerance. Symptoms such as weight loss, fever, nocturnal symptoms, age of onset >50, melena, progressive pain, and cachexia are less likely to be indicators of IBS. The physical exam is typically normal although some may exhibit mild abdominal tenderness to palpation and some stool burden may be felt in IBS-C patients.

Diagnosis

IBS is a diagnosis of exclusion, and a thorough elimination of organic causes should be performed. Lab work should include obtaining a CBC, CMP, TSH, fecal calprotectin (or lactoferrin), stool testing for *C. difficile* toxin, giardia, ova and parasites with culture, and serologic testing for celiac disease. It is also important to complete age-appropriate colorectal cancer screening and, if presenting with constipation, an abdominal radiograph. Colonoscopy, outside of age-related screening, is reserved for patients with normal lab work but a family history of inflammatory bowel disease and/or colon cancer. Patients with abnormal lab work (anemia, elevated inflammatory markers, or electrolyte disturbances) and concerning symptoms such as hematochezia, melena, and weight loss should also be considered for colonoscopy. The most widely accepted diagnostic standard is currently the Rome criteria (Table 8).

When possible, subclassification is helpful for determining treatment. The most commonly accepted subtypes are IBS-D (diarrhea predominant), IBS-C (constipation predominant), IBS-M (mixed diarrhea and constipation), and IBS-A (alternating diarrhea and constipation). There are currently arguments to include a pain predominant subtype as well.

Management

The foundation of successful management of IBS is a strong relationship between patient and physician. It is also key in setting realistic expectations. After diagnosis, the patient should be reassured that although the disease is chronic, it does not increase risk of malignancy and does not have a serious pathological course. Treatment should be individualized and based on subtype if possible. A comprehensive diet history should be examined to identify trigger foods. Patients may benefit from adherence to a low FODMAP diet along with avoidance of gas-producing food. Data support the intake of additional dietary fiber in patients with IBS-C, although it may increase bloating and gas. Probiotics and regular exercise may also be beneficial in overall IBS symptom reduction. Complementary and alternate medicine (CAM) such as cognitive behavioral therapy, mind-body therapies, acupuncture, and hypnotherapy should be explored. However, the current CAM research leaves a void for more robust and significant studies evaluating those modalities.

Pharmacological therapies are broad, and benefits may vary greatly between patients. Treatment should be based on predominant symptoms, and changes should occur over 2–4-week intervals. General medications include anticholinergics (dicyclomine and hyoscyamine), tricyclic antidepressants (amitriptyline, imipramine), serotonin 5-HT3 receptor antagonists (alosetron), guanylate cyclase C agonists (linaclotide), and antispasmodics (peppermint oil, pinaverium, trimebutine, cimetropium/dicyclomine). IBS-C can be directed toward chloride channel activators (lubiprostone) when symptoms are resistant toward osmotic laxatives. In IBS-D antidiarrheals (loperamide, diphenoxylate) are used as the initial treatment with bile acid sequestrants as second-line therapy. Treatment should be based on the predominant symptom, and changes should occur over 2–4-week intervals. In IBS without constipation, with significant bloating, a 2-week trial of rifaximin can be used; however antibiotics are not routinely recommended [34–37].

Table 8 Rome criteria

Recurrent abdominal pain for at least 1 day per week in the last 3 months, as an average, and association with two or more of the following:	1) Related to defecation 2) Associated with a change in stool frequency 3) Associated with a change in stool form (appearance)

References

1. Steffen R, Hill DR, DuPont HL. Traveler's diarrhea: a clinical review. JAMA. 2015;313(1):71–80.
2. Dennehy PH. Viral gastroenteritis in children. Pediatr Infect Dis J. 2011;30(1):63–4.
3. Blacklow NR, Cukor G. Viral gastroenteritis. N Engl J Med. 1981;304(7):397–406.
4. DuPont HL. Acute infectious diarrhea in immunocompetent adults. N Engl J Med. 2014;370(16):1532–40.
5. Switaj TL, Winter KJ, Christensen SR. Diagnosis and management of foodborne illness. Am Fam Physician. 2015;92(5):358–65.
6. Zaidi D, Wine E. An update on travelers' diarrhea. Curr Opin Gastroenterol. 2015;31(1):7–13.
7. Travelers' Diarrhea – Chapter 2–2020 Yellow Book | Travelers' Health | CDC [Internet]. [cited 2020 May 26]. Available from: https://wwwnc.cdc.gov/travel/yellowbook/2020/preparing-international-travelers/travelers-diarrhea
8. Guerrant RL, Bobak DA. Bacterial and protozoal gastroenteritis. N Engl J Med. 1991;325(5):327–40.
9. Riddle MS, Connor BA, Beeching NJ, DuPont HL, Hamer DH, Kozarsky P, et al. Guidelines for the prevention and treatment of travelers' diarrhea: a graded expert panel report. J Travel Med. 2017;24(Suppl_1):S57–74.
10. Mounsey A, Lacy Smith K, Reddy VC, Nickolich S. Clostridioides difficile infection: update on management. Am Fam Physician. 2020;101(3):168–75.
11. Napolitano LM, Edmiston CE. *Clostridium difficile* disease: diagnosis, pathogenesis, and treatment update. Surgery. 2017;162(2):325–48.
12. McDonald LC, Gerding DN, Johnson S, Bakken JS, Carroll KC, Coffin SE, et al. Clinical practice guidelines for *Clostridium difficile* infection in adults and children: 2017 update by the Infectious Diseases Society of America (IDSA) and Society for Healthcare Epidemiology of America (SHEA). Clin Infect Dis. 2018;66(7):e1–e48.
13. Rohlke F, Stollman N. Fecal microbiota transplantation in relapsing *Clostridium difficile* infection. Ther Adv Gastroenterol. 2012;5(6):403–20.
14. Schafer TW, Skopic A. Parasites of the small intestine. Curr Gastroenterol Rep. 2006;8(4):312–20.
15. Jernigan J, Guerrant RL, Pearson RD. Parasitic infections of the small intestine. Gut. 1994;35(3):289–93.
16. Chen X-M, Keithly JS, Paya CV, LaRusso NF. Cryptosporidiosis. N Engl J Med. 2002;346(22):1723–31.
17. Marie C, Petri WA. Regulation of virulence of *Entamoeba histolytica*. Annu Rev Microbiol. 2014;68:493–520.
18. Luaces AL. A new test for infection by *Entamoeba histolyticia*. Parasitology Today 1993;9:69–71.
19. Maguire JH. Intestinal nematodes (roundworms). In: Mandell, Douglas, and Bennett's principles and practice of infectious diseases: Elsevier; 2010. p. 3577–86.
20. Sheth AA, Longo W, Floch MH. Diverticular disease and diverticulitis. Am J Gastroenterol. 2008;103(6):1550–6.
21. Tursi A. Diverticular disease: a therapeutic overview. World J Gastrointest Pharmacol Ther. 2010;1(1):27–35.
22. Wilkins T, Embry K, George R. Diagnosis and management of acute diverticulitis. Am Fam Physician. 2013;87(9):612.
23. Bohr J, Wickbom A, Hegedus A, Nyhlin N, Hultgren Hörnquist E, Tysk C. Diagnosis and management of microscopic colitis: current perspectives. Clin Exp Gastroenterol. 2014;7:273–84.
24. Storr MA. Microscopic colitis: epidemiology, pathophysiology, diagnosis and current management-an update 2013. ISRN Gastroenterol. 2013;2013:352718.
25. Shor J, Churrango G, Hosseini N, Marshall C. Management of microscopic colitis: challenges and solutions. Clin Exp Gastroenterol. 2019;12:111–20.
26. Flynn S, Eisenstein S. Inflammatory bowel disease presentation and diagnosis. Surg Clin North Am. 2019;99(6):1051–62.
27. Vavricka SR, Schoepfer A, Scharl M, Lakatos PL, Navarini A, Rogler G. Extraintestinal manifestations of inflammatory bowel disease. Inflamm Bowel Dis. 2015;21(8):1982–92.
28. Lamb CA, Kennedy NA, Raine T, Hendy PA, Smith PJ, Limdi JK, et al. British Society of Gastroenterology consensus guidelines on the management of inflammatory bowel disease in adults. Gut. 2019;68(Suppl 3):s1–s106.
29. Wright EK, Ding NS, Niewiadomski O. Management of inflammatory bowel disease. Med J Aust. 2018;209(7):318–23.
30. Bell SJ, Flanagan EK. Updates in the management of inflammatory bowel disease during pregnancy. Med J Aust. 2019;210(6):276–80.
31. Högenauer C, Hammer HF. Maldigestion and malabsorption. In: Sleisenger and Fordtran's gastrointestinal and liver disease: Elsevier; 2010. p. 1735–1767.e7.
32. Garcia-Naveiro R, Udall JN. Maldigestion and malabsorption. In: Pediatric gastrointestinal and liver disease: Elsevier; 2011. p. 337–349.e2.
33. Bo-Linn GW, Fordtran JS. Fecal fat concentration in patients with steatorrhea. Gastroenterology. 1984;87(2):319–22.
34. James D. Diseases of the small and large bowel. In: Paulman PM, Taylor RB, Paulman AA, Nasir LS, editors. Family medicine. Cham: Springer International Publishing; 2017. p. 1141–56.
35. Eswaran SL, Chey WD, Han-Markey T, Ball S, Jackson K. A randomized controlled trial comparing the low FODMAP diet vs. modified NICE guidelines in US adults with IBS-D. Am J Gastroenterol. 2016;111(12):1824–32.
36. Whitehead WE, Drossman DA. Validation of symptom-based diagnostic criteria for irritable bowel syndrome: a critical review. Am J Gastroenterol. 2010;105(4):814–20; quiz 813, 821.
37. Saha L. Irritable bowel syndrome: pathogenesis, diagnosis, treatment, and evidence-based medicine. World J Gastroenterol. 2014;20(22):6759–73.

Diseases of the Pancreas

Douglas J. Inciarte and Daniel Ramon

Contents

D. J. Inciarte (✉) · D. Ramon
West Kendall Baptist Health/Florida International
University, Herbert Wertheim College of Medicine,
Family Medicine Residency Program, Florida, SW, USA
e-mail: douglasI@baptisthealth.net;
danielramI@baptisthealth.net

© Springer Nature Switzerland AG 2022
P. M. Paulman et al. (eds.), *Family Medicine*,
https://doi.org/10.1007/978-3-030-54441-6_175

Pancreatic disease causes significant health issues ranging from pancreatitis and pancreatic cysts to cancer. To reduce this burden, family physicians need a systematic approach to evaluation and treatment.

Acute Pancreatitis

Background

Acute pancreatitis, an inflammatory disease of the pancreas, is one of the most common gastrointestinal disorders requiring hospitalization. It has a reported annual incidence of 13–45 cases per 100,000 persons [1]. Acute pancreatitis is hypothesized to be caused by unregulated activation of trypsin within pancreatic acinar cells, leading to the autodigestion of the gland and local inflammation [2].

Etiology

The most common causes are gallstones (40–70%) and alcohol use (25–35%) [3]. In patients greater than 40 years of age, a pancreatic tumor can be considered as a possible cause. For the remainder of patients for whom no etiology is established (15–25%), this is referred to as idiopathic acute pancreatitis.

Diagnosis

Acute pancreatitis is diagnosed when two out of three of the following criteria are present: (1) abdominal pain consistent with the disease, (2) serum amylase and/or lipase greater than three times the upper limit of normal, and (3) characteristic findings from abdominal imaging [3].

Clinical Features

Patients with acute pancreatitis typically describe a history of constant epigastric or upper quadrant pain, with radiation to the back, chest, or flanks. On examination, the upper abdomen can be tender, and bruising caused by bleeding due to pancreatic necrosis can be seen in the periumbilical region (Cullen's sign) and flanks (Grey Turner's sign). Also, extension of inflammatory exudates to the diaphragm may result in shallow respiration [2].

Laboratory Tests

For initial laboratory studies, serum amylase alone cannot be used reliably for the diagnosis. Serum lipase is more specific for acute pancreatitis and remains elevated longer than amylase. However, serum amylase and lipase may be high in the absence of acute pancreatitis. Another important laboratory marker in assessing severity is C-reactive protein (CRP), an acute phase reactant that reaches a peak concentration 72–96 hours after symptom onset. It is significantly higher in patients with necrotizing disease [4]. Genetic testing may also be considered in young patients (less than 30 years old) if no cause is evident and a family history of pancreatic disease is present [3].

Imaging

A transabdominal ultrasound should be performed in all patients with acute pancreatitis to assess for gallstones. While a contrast-enhanced CT (CECT) provides greater than 90% sensitivity and specificity for the diagnosis of acute pancreatitis, its routine use is not needed. Magnetic resonance imaging (MRI) is comparable to CECT in the early assessment of acute pancreatitis, and MRI employing magnetic resonance cholangiopancreatography (MRCP) has the additional advantage of diagnosing choledocholithiasis and pancreatic duct disruption. MRI can be substituted for CECT in patients with contrast allergy and renal insufficiency (can perform without gadolinium contrast and still diagnose pancreatic necrosis). Either follow-up CECT or MRI is useful for patients lacking clinical improvement, with clinical deterioration, or when invasive intervention is considered [3, 5].

Differential Diagnosis

The differential includes cholecystitis, cholelithiasis, cholangitis, choledocholithiasis, peptic ulcer disease, gastritis, chronic pancreatitis, acute or chronic alcohol consumption, perforated ulcer, early appendicitis, bowel obstruction, mesenteric ischemia, gastroenteritis, post-traumatic injury, or malignancy [6].

Treatment

Severity Prediction

Most episodes of acute pancreatitis are mild and self-limited, requiring brief hospitalization. Approximately 20% of patients develop severe disease with local and extrapancreatic complications involving hypovolemia and multiple organ dysfunction. Therefore, risk stratification of acute pancreatitis is important. The revised Atlanta classification now divides acute pancreatitis into three categories: (1) mild, no organ failure or local complications; (2) moderate, local complications and/or transient organ failure (less than 48 hours), the presence of shock, gastrointestinal bleeding, pulmonary insufficiency, or renal failure; and (3) severe, persistent organ failure (greater than 48 hours). Various scales can assess injury to extrapancreatic organs – the greater the number of organs injured, the greater the score [2, 3].

Fluid Therapy

Early aggressive intravenous hydration is most beneficial during the first 12–24 hours to correct third spacing and maintain an adequate intravascular volume. Fluid requirements should be reassessed at frequent intervals – within 6 hours of admission and for the next 24–48 hours – using caution in patients with cardiovascular, renal diseases, or other comorbidities [3].

Nutrition

Patients with mild-to-moderate acute pancreatitis do not require nutritional support and can start oral feeding once abdominal pain decreases and inflammatory markers improve. For patients with severe acute pancreatitis, necrotic pancreas, or organ failure, enteral nutrition should be started within 48 hours: [5] nasogastric or nasojejunal feeding is comparable in efficacy and safety [7]. Avoid parenteral nutrition due to risk of infections and other line-related complications, unless the enteral route is not available, not tolerated, or not meeting caloric requirements [3].

Pain Management

Adequate analgesia is important for patients with acute pancreatitis. For mild cases, non-opioid drugs may be enough to manage pain. Narcotic agents are often needed for severe cases [8].

Antibiotics

Intravenous antibiotic prophylaxis is not recommended for the prevention of complications in acute pancreatitis. In severe pancreatitis with infected necrosis, coverage for gram-negative organisms (using carbapenems, quinolones, and metronidazole) is strongly recommended as soon as possible after a severe attack [5].

Causative Therapy

Early endoscopic retrograde cholangiopancreatography (ERCP), preferably within 24 hours, is indicated for concomitant cholangitis, significant persistent biliary obstruction, or severe biliary pancreatitis without biliary sepsis or obstruction. It is not indicated in mild pancreatitis of suspected or proven biliary etiology in the absence of biliary obstruction [3]. For mild gallstone-associated acute pancreatitis, early cholecystectomy (preferably during the same hospitalization) is recommended, and no later than 2–4 weeks after discharge. In patients with severe gallstone-associated acute pancreatitis, cholecystectomy should be delayed until there is sufficient resolution of the inflammatory response and clinical recovery [3].

Complication Management

Pancreatic necrosis is the most severe complication as it is frequently associated with pancreatic infections. It occurs when a local area of nonviable parenchyma becomes infected with bacteria originating from the gut, leading to infected necrosis, pancreatic abscess, or infected pseudocysts. A pseudocyst is a pancreatic fluid collection that has been enclosed by a wall of granulation tissue that results from pancreatic duct leakage [2]. In acute necrotizing pancreatitis, the findings of necrosis on CECT and a persistent severe inflammatory response syndrome (SIRS) should prompt fine needle aspiration (FNA) with gram stain and culture to differentiate sterile and infected necrosis. For patients with sterile necrosis in the first week, mortality is between 10% and 40%. Surgery is indicated for the presence of massive pancreatic necrosis (greater than 50%) with a deteriorating clinical course and in patients with progression of organ dysfunction or no signs of improvement. In infected necrosis, after 3 weeks, mortality ranges between 20% and 70%. Antibiotics should be used for treatment first, and if patients remain ill and infected necrosis has not resolved, then minimally invasive necrosectomy is recommended [3].

Chronic Pancreatitis

Background

Chronic pancreatitis is a progressive inflammatory change of the pancreas that results in permanent structural damage, leading to impairment of exocrine and endocrine function [9]. It has a reported annual incidence of 5–12 cases per 100,000 persons, which accounts for more than 120,000 outpatient visits and 50,000 hospitalizations annually [10].

Etiology

Most cases are due to alcohol abuse, ductal obstruction, genetic mutations, systemic disease, autoimmune pancreatitis, tropical pancreatitis, and idiopathic pancreatitis [11, 12]. Cigarette smoking has been found to be an independent, dose-dependent risk factor for acute and chronic pancreatitis [13].

Diagnosis

Clinical Features

The primary clinical manifestations are abdominal pain and pancreatic insufficiency. The abdominal pain is typically epigastric, radiates to the back, worsens postprandially, and may be alleviated with leaning forward. This pain may occur sporadically but become more continuous as the condition progresses. Clinically significant fat and protein deficiencies do not occur until over 90% of pancreatic function is lost [14]. At variable states of progression, this may result in steatorrhea, indigestion, weight loss, and malaise. While the classic triad of pancreatic calcifications, steatorrhea, and diabetes mellitus strongly suggests the diagnosis of chronic pancreatitis, most cases are challenging to identify given the potential absence of symptoms and normal laboratory or imaging studies in over 20% of cases [15].

Laboratory Tests

Since chronic pancreatitis is a patchy, focal disease that leads to minimal increase in pancreatic enzymes in the blood, serum concentrations of amylase and lipase are usually normal or may be slightly elevated. Significant fibrosis can also result in decreased abundance of these enzymes within the pancreas. Thus, pancreatic enzyme levels should only be used when suspecting acute pancreatitis and not chronic pancreatitis. While complete blood counts, electrolytes, and liver function tests tend to be normal, elevations of serum bilirubin and alkaline phosphatase may suggest intrapancreatic compression of the bile duct. Markers of autoimmune chronic pancreatitis include an elevated ESR, IGG4, rheumatoid factor, ANA, and anti-smooth muscle antibody titer [16]. Direct pancreatic function testing for secretin with suggestive clinical features can also be used to diagnose chronic pancreatitis. However, this test is invasive, usually done under fluoroscopy, and not readily available [17]. Fecal elastase is also thought to suggest exocrine deficiency and may be used to evaluate steatorrhea [18].

Imaging

Diagnosis can be confirmed by pancreatic calcifications on imaging (abdominal plain film or CT) or a pancreatogram revealing beading or ecstatic branching of the main pancreatic duct [14]. When comparing imaging studies, the sensitivity and specificity of ultrasound for the diagnosis of chronic pancreatitis are 60–70% and 80–90%, respectively, which is slightly less than corresponding values for CT, which are 75–90% and 85%, respectively [19]. These values drop in early disease for both forms of imaging. Magnetic resonance cholangiopancreatography (MRCP) is becoming the diagnostic test of choice since it can demonstrate calcifications and pancreatic duct obstruction while avoiding risks of radiation without the invasiveness of the prior test of choice, endoscopic retrograde cholangiopancreatography (ERCP). Endoscopic ultrasonography (EUS) may also be as sensitive as ERCP when done by a highly skilled gastroenterologist [15] and provide additional procedures that may detect earlier disease missed by approaches aforementioned [20].

Classification

The Cambridge classification system divides severity of disease into category I equivocal changes, category II mild to moderate, and category III considerable changes based on ERCP findings [21].

Differential Diagnosis

Due to its nonspecific presentation, it is important to differentiate from other diseases such as pancreatic cancer, acute pancreatitis, pancreatic endocrine tumors, pancreatic duct stones, pseudocysts, hepatobiliary disease, systemic autoimmune disease, or lymphoma [14].

Treatment

Treatment for chronic pancreatitis focuses on pain management, correction of pancreatic insufficiency, and management of complications. Recommendations begin with alcohol and tobacco cessation and consumption of small low-fat meals [22]. If pain is persistent, pancreatic enzyme supplements can be initiated. Oral intake should be avoided to minimize pancreatic stimulation. Analgesics with opioids and/or NSAIDs can be used. Adjuvant therapy with neuropathic agents (i.e., gabapentin or pregabalin) and tricyclic antidepressants (i.e., amitriptyline and nortriptyline) may provide additional pain control [23, 24]. Pancreatic enzyme supplementation is based on suppression of pancreatic exocrine secretion, and while several studies do show benefit from placebo effect, it has also been shown with some evidence as a reasonable addition to measures above for patients with persistent pain [25]. In cases of refractory pain, EUS may be diagnostic and therapeutic, with procedures such as celiac plexus block and celiac plexus neurolysis and EUS-guided drainage of pancreatic fluid collections [20]. Extracorporeal shock wave lithotripsy in conjunction with EUS can help remove larger or impacted pancreatic ductal stones [26]. Finally, surgery is reserved for refractory pain. Although medical treatment and endoscopic interventions are primarily offered to patients with chronic pancreatitis, approximately 40–75% will ultimately require surgery. Although pancreaticoduodenectomy has been considered the standard surgical procedure, its high postoperative complication and pancreatic exocrine and/or endocrine dysfunction rates have led to a growing popularity for duodenal-preserving pancreatic head resection such as the Frey procedure [27]. Nutritional deficiencies have been documented in advanced disease, including fat-soluble vitamins, vitamin B12, zinc, calcium, magnesium, thiamine, and folic acid [28]. Monitoring levels and supplementing accordingly along with screening for diseases or symptoms associated with these deficiencies are also important.

Pancreatic Cysts

Background

In the past two decades, the prevalence of pancreatic cysts diagnosed in US adults has dramatically increased [29]. In the USA, 20% of patients who undergo MRI for nonpancreatic diseases are found to have a pancreatic cyst [30]. The most common include pseudocysts, serous cystadenomas (SCA), mucinous cystic neoplasms (MCN), and intraductal papillary mucinous neoplasms (IPMN) [31]. Distinguishing SCA from MCN and IPMN is key as SCA is benign while MCN and IPMN are potentially or overtly malignant lesions.

Clinical Features

There is no typical presentation or physical exam findings. IPMNs are more likely to be found in males while SCA and MCN are mostly seen in women. There is no alcohol abuse or history of pancreatitis in SCA, MCN, or IPMN. Malignancy potential is rare in SCA, moderate to high in MCN, and low to high in IPMN [31].

Diagnosis

Transabdominal ultrasound has difficulty visualizing the entire pancreas and is highly operator dependent. The preferred imaging options are CT, MRI, and endoscopic ultrasound. ERCP can be used but it can only help diagnose IPMN and is an invasive test. MRI has been considered superior to CT for characterizing morphological features of pancreatic cysts [32]. However, CT was shown to have an accuracy rate of 80% for discriminating between mucinous and non-mucinous cysts [33], while MRI had less interobserver agreement [32]. EUS provides another option if CT and MRI imaging are not diagnostic, particularly in showing internal septa, mural nodules, solid masses, vascular invasion, and lymph node metastases. EUS can be combined with FNA of the lesion for collection and analysis of fluid and solid components. Cyst fluid with elevated carcinoembryonic antigen distinguishes mucinous from non-mucinous cysts but cannot determine malignancy potential [34]. Cyst fluid cytology can be helpful, but the fluid often has low cellularity. Because expertise in this procedure and technique is not readily available, consult with a local radiologist and endoscopist to determine the best locally available imaging approach.

Management

The initial steps are to assess patient symptoms and determine the cyst size, location, and presence of main branch involvement. If the patient has no symptoms, cyst <1 cm with no solid components or thickened cyst walls, main duct <5 mm with no abrupt caliber changes, and no mural nodule, then imaging surveillance in 2–3 years is recommended. Further EUS is not needed. If the patient has obstructive jaundice with a cystic lesion in the head of the pancreas, enhancing solid component within the cyst, or main pancreatic duct >10 mm, then surgical resection should be considered. If the cyst is >3 cm, there are thickened cyst walls, the main duct is 5–9 mm, a mural nodule is present, or the main duct has abrupt caliber changes with distal pancreatic atrophy, then the patient should undergo EUS to further define the lesion [34].

Intraductal Papillary Mucinous Neoplasm

First described in the mid-1980s, IPMN is a cystic neoplasm of the pancreas – a slow growing tumor with malignant potential. There are three types of IPMN: main duct, branch duct, and mixed type. Main duct IPMN features segmental or diffuse dilation of the main pancreatic duct of >5 mm without other causes of obstruction. Because the rate of malignancy is very high (up to 70% in reported surgical series), in surgically fit patients, the recommendation is for surgical removal of the affected portion of the pancreas or entire pancreas (total pancreatectomy) if the entire duct is involved [33]. Branch duct IPMNs may be found in various locations throughout the gland and are seen with equal frequency in both genders. Their management is challenging and lifetime risk of malignancy is not entirely known. There is no medication to treat these cysts – only options are surveillance and surgical removal. Important factors to consider include the patient's age, symptoms, the size of the cyst, and whether or not there is a solid component or mural nodule.

Mucinous Cystic Neoplasm

MCNs are defined by the presence of ovarian stroma and are usually located in the pancreatic body and tail. Cancer is very rare in MCN <4 cm without mural nodules [31, 34]. It is most commonly diagnosed in middle-aged women. In surgically fit patients resection is routinely recommended, while observation is recommended for elderly frail patients. Surgical resections should be done at high-volume institutions, generally those that perform 15 or more pancreatic resections annually. These institutions have reported decreased mortality, hospital length of stay, and overall cost compared to low-volume institutions [35].

Pancreatic Cancer

Background

Pancreatic cancer is the fourth leading cause of cancer-related deaths in the USA [36]. The incidence is equal in both genders but slightly higher in African Americans compared to Caucasians [37]. Over 90% of these cancers are pancreatic ductal adenocarcinomas (PDAC). There are several risk factors associated with the development of PDAC: tobacco use, alcohol use, obesity, and type 2 diabetes for five or more years. Routine screening for pancreatic cancer in asymptomatic adults who are at average risk is not recommended due to lack of mortality benefit [35]. However, in the office a clinician can consider screening individuals from families with known genetic defects predisposing them to pancreatic cancer or with familial pancreatic cancer. Although, there is insufficient evidence to assess benefits or harms of surgical intervention for screen-detected pancreatic adenocarcinoma. The US Preventive Service Task Force recommends against screening for pancreatic cancer in asymptomatic adults [38].

Clinical Features

Abdominal pain, jaundice, pruritus, dark urine, and acholic stools may all be presenting symptoms because of obstruction within the biliary tree [39]. Nonspecific findings from cancers of the pancreatic body or tail include unexplained weight loss, anorexia, early satiety, dyspepsia, nausea, and depression [40]. Also, a sudden onset of atypical type 2 diabetes (a thin adult 50 years or older) that is difficult to control suggests pancreatic cancer [41]. Patients may present in early stages with normal exams or advanced disease with manifestations of liver involvement such as abdominal tenderness, jaundice, and cachexia. A nontender, distended, palpable gallbladder in a jaundiced patient (Courvoisier's sign) is 83–90% specific but is only 26–55% sensitive for a biliary obstruction due to malignancy [39]. Advanced pancreatic cancer, like other abdominal malignancies, can be associated with recurring superficial thrombophlebitis (Trousseau's sign) or left supraclavicular lymphadenopathy (Virchow's node). Subcutaneous areas of nodular fat necrosis (pancreatic panniculitis) may be evident in rare cases [42].

Diagnosis

CT is the gold standard for diagnosing and staging patients with pancreatic cancer [43]. A pancreas protocol CT involves triphasic (i.e., arterial phase, late phase, and venous phase) cross-sectional imaging that allows for enhancement between the parenchyma and adenocarcinoma. When CT is not possible (i.e., not available, contrast allergy, etc.), MRI with contrast can be used for diagnosis and staging. If a pancreatic mass is identified, subsequent EUS and FNA are indicated. If no mass is identified and no evidence of metastatic disease is present, further EUS or ERCP is indicated [35]. The most common serum tumor marker used for PDAC is carbohydrate antigen (CA) 19-9, which is expressed in pancreatic and hepatobiliary disease. In symptomatic patients, it can help confirm the diagnosis and predict prognosis and recurrence after resection [35]. However, CA 19-9 is not tumor specific and therefore is not a sufficient individual screening tool for asymptomatic patients [44].

Staging

Once a mass is identified and FNA confirms tissue diagnosis, EUS can determine the tumor size and extent of lymph node metastases and assess for portal venous system involvement to complete the staging [35]. In addition to EUS, chest CT and serum liver enzyme tests are useful to determine surgical candidacy [35]. A multidisciplinary team with expertise from surgery, diagnostic imaging, pathology, interventional endoscopy, and medical and radiation oncology is highly recommended to define surgical candidates [35].

Management

Surgical resection is the only potentially curative treatment for PDAC. Around 15–20% of patients are candidates for pancreatic resection, but only around 20% of those who undergo surgery survive to 5 years [35]. Although postoperative mortality is less than 5%, the median survival is still only 12–19 months [35]. Pancreatic resections should be done at high-volume institutions, generally those that perform 15 or more pancreatic resections annually [35]. The classic operation for resection of a carcinoma of the head of the pancreas is a pancreaticoduodenectomy (Whipple procedure). For surveillance in patients with resected pancreatic cancer, expert consensus recommends history and physical examination every 3–6 months for 2 years and then annually [45]. Monitoring for recurrence with CA 19-9 levels, CT scans, and EUS every 3–6 months can also be considered, although evidence is limited that earlier treatment improves patient outcomes [46]. Over 80% of patients present with unresectable disease. Some studies have addressed the use of chemoradiation with or without chemotherapy to convert unresectable disease status to resectable. Post-resection, these patients have similar survival rates as those initially determined to be resectable [35]. The primary treatment for advanced pancreatic cancers is palliative care (i.e., adequate nutrition and pain control), which may have some effect on survival.

Exocrine Pancreatic Insufficiency

Background

Exocrine pancreatic insufficiency (EPI) is a disease characterized by deficiency of the exocrine pancreatic enzymes, resulting in maldigestion. The pathophysiological mechanism for EPI involves pancreatic parenchymal damage, pancreatic duct obstruction, or loss of sites of secretin and cholecystokinin secretion in the gastrointestinal tract [48].

Etiology

The most common causes of EPI are chronic pancreatitis, cystic fibrosis, pancreatic cancer, pancreatic resection, gastric or small bowel resection, inflammatory bowel disease, celiac disease, and diabetes mellitus [47]. The prevalence of EPI is higher in type 1 diabetes (26–57%) compared with type 2 diabetes (20–36%).

Clinical Features

Clinical symptoms associated with EPI include steatorrhea (greasy, foul-smelling stools), weight loss, increased flatulence, and abdominal pain. Deficiency of the fat-soluble vitamins (e.g., vitamins A, D, E, and K) can lead to impaired night vision, decreased bone mineralization, coagulation problems, and ataxia and peripheral neuropathy [48]. Because the exocrine pancreas has a large functional reserve capacity, clinical symptoms may not manifest until exocrine pancreatic function is <10% of normal.

Diagnosis

No single widely available test allows diagnosing EPI accurately. Diagnosis of EPI requires the evaluation of symptoms, nutritional markers, and a pancreatic function test [49]. Early diagnostic studies relied on direct pancreatic function tests (i.e., those involving collection and analysis of secretions directly from the duodenum or pancreatic duct), including the secretin-pancreozymin and Lundh tests, which remain the most sensitive and specific methods for assessing exocrine pancreatic function. Direct tests, however, are limited by their cost, duration, and invasive nature, which involve endoscopic aspiration or tube aspiration of secretions from the duodenum for several hours [48]. During the past 20 years, the use of noninvasive indirect methods, such as fecal elastase, has become more common. Evidence suggests the fecal elastase-1 (FE-1) test is reliable for the evaluation of pancreatic function in many pancreatic and nonpancreatic disorders. Fecal elastase, measured by enzyme-linked immunosorbent assay, has a good sensitivity for moderate EPI (75%) and high sensitivity for severe EPI (95%), and has a higher specificity (79–96%) compared with the direct tests [50].

Treatment

Patients with abnormal fecal fat excretion, steatorrhea, and/or weight loss are considered candidates for pancreatic enzyme replacement therapy (PERT). Although there is a lack of long-term trials assessing the effect of PERT on patient survival, PERT has been shown to improve digestion, symptoms, nutritional status, and quality of life of patients with EPI [49].

References

1. Yadav D, Lowenfels AB. The epidemiology of pancreatitis and pancreatic cancer. Gastroenterology. 2013;144:1252–61.
2. Frossard JL, Steer ML, Pastor CM. Acute pancreatitis. Lancet. 2008;371:143–52.
3. Tenner S, Baillie J, DeWitt J, Vege SS. American College of Gastroenterology. American College of Gastroenterology guideline: management of acute pancreatitis. Am J Gastroenterol. 2013;108:1400–15, 16
4. Schutte K, Malfertheiner P. Markers for predicting severity and progression of acute pancreatitis. Best Pract Res Clin Gastroenterol. 2008;22:75–90.
5. Working Group IAP/APA Acute Pancreatitis Guidelines. IAP/APA evidence-based guidelines for the management of acute pancreatitis. Pancreatology. 2013;13:e1–15.
6. Carroll JK, Herrick B, Gipson T, Lee SP. Acute pancreatitis: diagnosis, prognosis, and treatment. Am Fam Physician. 2007;75:1513–20.
7. Eatock FC, Chong P, Menezes N, et al. A randomized study of early nasogastric versus nasojejunal feeding in severe acute pancreatitis. Am J Gastroenterol. 2005;100:432–9.
8. Phillip V, Steiner JM, Algul H. Early phase of acute pancreatitis: assessment and management. World J Gastrointest Pathophysiol. 2014;5:158–68.
9. Steer ML, Waxman I, Freedman S. Chronic pancreatitis. N Engl J Med. 1995;332:1482–90.
10. Peery AF, Dellon ES, Lund J, et al. Burden of gastrointestinal disease in the United States: 2012 update. Gastroenterology. 2012;143:1179–87, e1–3
11. Yadav D, Hawes RH, Brand RE, et al. Alcohol consumption, cigarette smoking, and the risk of recurrent acute and chronic pancreatitis. Arch Intern Med. 2009;169:1035–45.
12. Etemad B, Whitcomb DC. Chronic pancreatitis: diagnosis, classification, and new genetic developments. Gastroenterology. 2001;120:682–707.
13. Cote GA, Yadav D, Slivka A, et al. Alcohol and smoking as risk factors in an epidemiology study of patients with chronic pancreatitis. Clin Gastroenterol Hepatol. 2011;9:266–73; quiz e27.
14. Conwell DL, Wu BU. Chronic pancreatitis: making the diagnosis. Clin Gastroenterol Hepatol. 2012;10:1088–95.
15. Gupte AR, Forsmark CE. Chronic pancreatitis. Curr Opin Gastroenterol. 2014;30:500–5.
16. O'Reilly DA, Malde DJ, Duncan T, Rao M, Filobbos R. Review of the diagnosis, classification and management of autoimmune pancreatitis. World J Gastrointest Pathophysiol. 2014;5:71–81.
17. Chey WY, Chang TM. Secretin: historical perspective and current status. Pancreas. 2014;43:162–82.
18. Benini L, Amodio A, Campagnola P, et al. Fecal elastase-1 is useful in the detection of steatorrhea in patients with pancreatic diseases but not after pancreatic resection. Pancreatology. 2013;13:38–42.
19. Choueiri NE, Balci NC, Alkaade S, Burton FR. Advanced imaging of chronic pancreatitis. Curr Gastroenterol Rep. 2010;12:114–20.
20. Teshima CW, Sandha GS. Endoscopic ultrasound in the diagnosis and treatment of pancreatic disease. World J Gastroenterol. 2014;20:9976–89.
21. Schreyer AG, Jung M, Riemann JF, et al. S3 guideline for chronic pancreatitis – diagnosis, classification and therapy for the radiologist. Rofo. 2014;186:1002–8.
22. Forsmark CE. Management of chronic pancreatitis. Gastroenterology. 2013;144:1282–91.e3
23. Gilron I, Bailey JM, Tu D, Holden RR, Jackson AC, Houlden RL. Nortriptyline and gabapentin, alone and in combination for neuropathic pain: a double-blind, randomised controlled crossover trial. Lancet. 2009;374:1252–61.
24. Olesen SS, Bouwense SA, Wilder-Smith OH, van Goor H, Drewes AM. Pregabalin reduces pain in patients with chronic pancreatitis in a randomized, controlled trial. Gastroenterology. 2011;141:536–43.

25. Trang T, Chan J, Graham DY. Pancreatic enzyme replacement therapy for pancreatic exocrine insufficiency in the 21(st) century. World J Gastroenterol. 2014;20:11467–85.

26. Kim YH, Jang SI, Rhee K, Lee DK. Endoscopic treatment of pancreatic calculi. Clin Endosc. 2014;47:227–35.

27. Roch A, Teyssedou J, Mutter D, Marescaux J, Pessaux P. Chronic pancreatitis: a surgical disease? Role of the Frey procedure. World J Gastrointest Surg. 2014;6:129–35.

28. Afghani E, Sinha A, Singh VK. An overview of the diagnosis and management of nutrition in chronic pancreatitis. Nutr Clin Pract. 2014;29:295–311.

29. Laffan TA, Horton KM, Klein AP, et al. Prevalence of unsuspected pancreatic cysts on MDCT. AJR Am J Roentgenol. 2008;191:802–7.

30. Zhang XM, Mitchell DG, Dohke M, Holland GA, Parker L. Pancreatic cysts: depiction on single-shot fast spin-echo MR images. Radiology. 2002;223:547–53.

31. Oh HC, Kim MH, Hwang CY, et al. Cystic lesions of the pancreas: challenging issues in clinical practice. Am J Gastroenterol. 2008;103:229–39; quiz 8, 40

32. de Jong K, Nio CY, Mearadji B, et al. Disappointing interobserver agreement among radiologists for a classifying diagnosis of pancreatic cysts using magnetic resonance imaging. Pancreas. 2012;41:278–82.

33. Sahani DV, Lin DJ, Venkatesan AM, et al. Multidisciplinary approach to diagnosis and management of intraductal papillary mucinous neoplasms of the pancreas. Clin GastroenterolHepatol. 2009;7:259–69.

34. Tanaka M, Fernandez-del Castillo C, Adsay V, et al. International consensus guidelines 2012 for the management of IPMN and MCN of the pancreas. Pancreatology. 2012;12:183–97.

35. National Comprehensive Cancer Network, Inc. (NCCN). Clinical practice guidelines in oncology (NCCN Guidelines TM): Pancreatic Adenocarcinoma (Version 1.2012). http://www.nccn.org/professionals/physician_gls/f_guidelines.asp-pancreatic. Accessed 12 Mar 2012.

36. Siegel R, Naishadham D, Jemal A. Cancer statistics, 2012. CA Cancer J Clin. 2012;62:10–29.

37. Cancer Facts & Figures. 2011. http://www.cancer.org/Research/CancerFactsFigures/CancerFactsFigures/cancer-facts-figures-2011. Accessed 16 Mar 2012.

38. Screening for Pancreatic Cancer: A Systematic Evidence Review for the U.S. Preventive Services Task Force. Rockville (MD): Agency for Healthcare Research and Quality (US); 2019 Aug. Report No.: 19-05250-EF-1.

39. American Gastroenterological Association medical position statement: epidemiology, diagnosis, and treatment of pancreatic ductal adenocarcinoma. Gastroenterology. 1999;117:1463–84.

40. Krech RL, Walsh D. Symptoms of pancreatic cancer. J Pain Symptom Manag. 1991;6:360–7.

41. Girelli CM, Reguzzoni G, Limido E, Savastano A, Rocca F. Pancreatic carcinoma: differences between patients with or without diabetes mellitus. Recenti Prog Med. 1995;86:143–6.

42. Mcgee SR. Palpation and percussion of the abdomen. In: Evidence-based physical diagnosis. Philadelphia: Saunders; 2001. p. 1–4.

43. Klauss M, Schobinger M, Wolf I, et al. Value of three dimensional reconstructions in pancreatic carcinoma using multidetector CT: initial results. World J Gastroenterol. 2009;15:5827–32.

44. Safi F, Roscher R, Bittner R, Schenkluhn B, Dopfer HP, Beger HG. High sensitivity and specificity of CA 19–9 for pancreatic carcinoma in comparison to chronic pancreatitis. Serological and immunohistochemical findings. Pancreas. 1987;2:398–403.

45. Tempero MA, Arnoletti JP, Behrman S, et al. Pancreatic adenocarcinoma. J Natl Compr Cancer Netw. 2010;8:972–1017.

46. Sheffield K, Crowell K, Lin Y-L, Djukom C, Goodwin J, Riall T. Surveillance of pancreatic cancer patients after surgical resection. Ann Surg Oncol. 2012;19:1670–7.

47. Vujasinovic M, Valente R, Del Chiaro M, Permert J, Löhr JM. Pancreatic exocrine insufficiency in pancreatic cancer. Nutrients. 2017;9(3):183.

48. Singh VK, Haupt ME, Geller DE, Hall JA, Quintana Diez PM. Less common etiologies of exocrine pancreatic insufficiency. World J Gastroenterol. 2017;23(39):7059–76.

49. Dominguez-Muñoz JE. Diagnosis and treatment of pancreatic exocrine insufficiency. Curr Opin Gastroenterol. 2018;34(5):349–54.

50. Chronic Pancreatitis German Society of Digestive and Metabolic Diseases (DGVS), Hoffmeister A, et al. S3-Consensus guidelines on definition, etiology, diagnosis and medical, endoscopic and surgical management of chronic pancreatitis. German Society of Digestive and Metabolic Diseases (DGVS). Z Gastroenterol. 2012;50:1176–224.

Diseases of the Liver

David T. O'Gurek

Contents

The liver as the largest solid organ in the body carries out a large number of critical functions, including the manufacture of essential proteins, metabolism of fats and carbohydrates, and elimination of harmful waste products, alcohol, certain medications, and environmental toxins. Therefore, diseases of the liver encompass a wide variety of clinical conditions with intrahepatic and extrahepatic manifestations and complications. These also range from acute, self-limited presentations to fulminant disease with rapid liver failure to chronic, low-level disease and also to chronic liver disease that progresses slowly over time. While the history and physical signs of this broad range of clinical disorders are quite similar, often with nonspecific findings with broad-range differentials, laboratory evaluation is critical to sorting through these disease processes. It is critical for family physicians to have an understanding of liver pathology and the laboratory assessment of the hepatic system.

The term "liver function test" is often a misnomer used to describe a variety of tests that assess hepatic synthetic function (e.g., serum albumin, prothrombin time), excretory function (e.g., serum bilirubin, direct bilirubin), necroinflammatory activity (e.g., alanine aminotransferase or ALT/SGPT, aspartate aminotransferase or AST/

D. T. O'Gurek (✉)
Department of Family and Community Medicine, Lewis Katz School of Medicine at Temple University, Philadelphia, PA, USA
e-mail: David.OGurek@tuhs.temple.edus

© Springer Nature Switzerland AG 2022
P. M. Paulman et al. (eds.), *Family Medicine*,
https://doi.org/10.1007/978-3-030-54441-6_97

Table 1 Uncommon causes of chronic liver disease and cirrhosis

Disease	Description	Diagnostic testing
Autoimmune hepatitis	Hepatic inflammation of unclear cause with hepatitis: hypergammaglobulinemia, and liver-associated autoantibodies; 2 subtypes of the disease; treatment usually with immunosuppression	Antinuclear antibody (ANA); anti-smooth muscle antibody
Alpha-1 antitripsin deficiency	Genetic disorder causing metabolic liver disorder in children; affects both hepatic and pulmonary systems	Alpha-1 antitripsin activity
Cystic fibrosis	Autosomal recessive disorder most commonly affecting Caucasian population; cirrhosis with portal hypertension common	Sweat chloride testing
Hemochromatosis	Autosomal recessive disorder resulting in dysregulation of iron absorption and resulting in iron toxicity to liver and other tissues; "bronze diabetes"	Transferrin saturation
Primary biliary cirrhosis	Female predominance; often asymptomatic; diagnosed with persistently elevated signs of cholestasis, normal biliary imaging and presence anti-mitochondrial antibody	Anti-mitochondrial antibody
Wilson's disease	Genetic disorder disrupting copper attachment to ceruloplasmin and resultant defective biliary secretion; Kayser-Fleischer rings on ophthalmologic exam; treatment with D-penicillamine	Ceruloplasmin

SGOT, and γ-glutamyltransferase or GGT), and cholestasis (alkaline phosphatase). While these tests can aid in the correct identification of liver disease, a single elevation must be confirmed with subsequent testing. Furthermore, normal or minimally abnormal tests do not preclude the presence of significant liver disease or possibly advanced disease or cirrhosis. While these tests will demonstrate liver disease, they are nonspecific and require specific testing based on risk assessment, history, and laboratory evaluation directed at specific etiologies.

The major causes of liver disease include infectious hepatitis, excessive alcohol usage, and toxic hepatopathy from drugs or other substances; however, less common metabolic abnormalities can also result in chronic liver disease and cirrhosis (see Table 1). This chapter will review the more common causes and their associated complications.

Viral, Alcoholic, and Drug-Induced Liver Disease

Hepatitis A

Hepatitis A virus (HAV) is an enveloped RNA agent classified as a picornovirus that is a common worldwide disease affecting the liver, spread through fecal-oral contamination with occasional outbreaks through food sources or within communities with specific risk factors. It can range in severity from an asymptomatic infection to a severe illness lasting several months; however, it is most commonly an acute, self-limited disease. Those at risk for worsening disease include the elderly as well those with chronic hepatitis B or hepatitis C with cirrhosis [1].

Clinical Presentation and Diagnosis

History should be targeted at collecting the chronology of symptomatology. The manifestations of HAV vary by age. While the manifestation in children is typically silent or subclinical, adults often present with signs and symptoms. With an average incubation period of about 30 days, HAV causes a prodrome of generalized fatigue, anorexia, nausea, vomiting, and fever which typically abate with the onset several days to a week later of jaundice with dark urine, acholic stools, and diffuse pruritis [2]. Clinical suspicion particularly for HAV infection is increased if there are specific risk factors by history including exposure to HAV in the household or close contact, exposure to raw vegetables or fruit or other uncooked or undercooked foods, exposure to drinking water that is not sanitized, or travel to areas endemic for HAV [3].

Despite clinical suspicion, the symptoms are indistinguishable from other forms of viral hepatitis and other possible liver or biliary conditions, and therefore, laboratory evaluation is necessary for diagnosis. Laboratory findings often demonstrate transaminitis followed by elevated total and direct bilirubin and elevated alkaline phosphatase levels. With any type of viral hepatitis, alanine transaminase (ALT) is typically higher than the aspartate transaminase (AST), and the range for both in HAV infection is typically between 500 and 5000 U/L [4]. Diagnosis is confirmed with detection of serum immunoglobulin M (IgM) anti-HAV antibodies, which typically becomes positive within 5–10 days of infection, concurrently with onset of jaundice. This will remain positive for 4–6 months following acute infection and therefore can be used to determine whether illness which has resolved was related to HAV. Total anti-HAV (IgM and immunoglobulin G) or immunoglobulin G (IgG) levels are checked to confirm immunity or past exposure and will remain positive for a patient's lifetime.

Management

The treatment of HAV infection is solely supportive, and hospitalization is reserved for patients with significant dehydration requiring parenteral fluid resuscitation or those with complications. Patients should be advised not to return to school or work until fever and jaundice have subsided, and hepatotoxic agents such as alcohol or medications should be avoided during the acute illness. The best treatment strategy for HAV infection remains a preventive strategy with immunization.

Prevention

The prevention of HAV infection begins with the practice of sanitary practices such as hand washing, heating foods appropriately, and avoiding water and foods from endemic areas. Preexposure prophylaxis with vaccination is the most widely used prevention strategy with the recommendation that all children should receive the hepatitis A vaccine as part of routine childhood immunizations, beginning the series between 12 and 23 months of age which includes a two-vaccine series with one immunization and a repeat dose 6 months later. Additionally, those at increased

risk including those traveling to endemic areas (available at http://www.cdc.gov/travel), men who have sex with men (MSM), people who inject drugs (PWID), people with chronic liver disease such as hepatitis B or hepatitis C, people experiencing homelessness, people treated with clotting-factor concentrates, parents adopting children from endemic areas, and those that work with HAV-infected animals or in HAV research labs should also receive vaccination [5–7].

Postexposure prophylaxis is available if a healthy individual has been exposed to HAV within the past 2 weeks as prophylaxis efficacy beyond this time is not well known. Hepatitis A vaccine is recommended for persons aged $\geq$ 12 months for PEP, and providers may also administer immunoglobulin (IG) to adults aged $>$ 40 years, if indicated [8]. Infants aged $<$ 12 months and persons for whom the vaccine is contraindicated should receive IG. Indications for postexposure prophylaxis include previously unvaccinated household or sexual contacts with confirmed disease; unvaccinated staff and attendees of child care centers with one or more cases in the center or two or more household cases of attendees; food handlers in facility with confirmed case; and immunocompromised persons (congenital or acquired, HIV infection, chronic renal failure, transplant recipients, persons on immunosuppressive drugs or biologics; and those with chronic liver disease) [5, 8].

Hepatitis B

Hepatitis B virus (HBV) is an incompletely double-stranded DNA virus belonging to the family of hepadnaviruses that is spread through contact with blood, semen, or other bodily fluid of an individual infected with HBV. The HBV has 10 genotypes (A through J) and more than 30 subtypes. Dissimilar to HAV, HBV causes both an acute illness as well as a chronic disease state. Although anyone can become infected with HBV, those at greater risk include individuals with multiple sexual partners, individuals with other sexually transmitted infections, MSMs, PWID, those living with someone with chronic HBV, infants born to infected mothers, individuals exposed to blood through their work, patients on hemodialysis, and those traveling to countries with moderate to high rates of HBV infection.

Clinical Presentation and Diagnosis

The history and presenting symptoms may vary depending upon the current state of the disease process whether in its acute phase or chronic phase. Most cases of acute hepatitis B are asymptomatic, and those with symptoms are more likely to be adults or over the age of 5. The average incubation period of HBV is 75 days, longer than that of HAV, and then patients proceed to have a prodrome with symptoms similar to that of HAV with fever, malaise, anorexia, and nausea followed by jaundice, darkening of the urine, and right upper quadrant pain.

During acute infection, elevations occur in the transaminases, both ALT and AST, with a typically higher elevation in ALT compared to AST. The alkaline phosphatase and total and direct serum bilirubin levels may be normal in someone presenting with anicteric hepatitis. As these tests are nonspecific markers for HBV infection, specific HBV testing must be obtained. Hepatitis B surface antigen (HBsAg) and hepatitis B e antigen (HBeAg) can be detected in the serum as well as high levels of IgM antibodies to the viral core antigen (IgM anti-HBc) during the acute phase [9]. An immune response targeted to clear the virus would clear the HBeAg and subsequently the HBsAg resulting in development of antibody to HBeAg and HBsAg with the appearance of antibodies to HBsAg indicating recovery from acute infection [10].

From acute infection, patients can go on to develop chronic hepatitis. Chronic HBV (CHB) infection is defined as presence of disease defined by HBsAg for at least 6 months. The risk of development of CHB infection is lowest in adults (<5%) and highest in neonates whose mothers are HBeAg positive (>90%) [11]. Most patients with CHB are asymptomatic unless they develop complications from their CHB either intrinsic to the liver or extrahepatic manifestations. History may not reveal a prior history of acute hepatitis given that acute episodes are often characterized by nonspecific symptoms and can be asymptomatic. Nonspecific symptoms of CHB may include fatigue or develop subacute symptoms of hepatitis. Evaluation should be directed at evaluating for signs and symptoms of cirrhosis, evaluation of alcohol intake and metabolic risks, family history of hepatocellular carcinoma (HCC), and HAV and HBV vaccination status.

There are five distinct phases of CHB infection including an immune tolerant phase, immune reactive HBeAg positive phase, inactive HBV carrier state, HBeAg-negative CHB, and occult CHB [12]. Laboratory findings associated with CHB infection is dependent upon the status of the chronic infection (see Table 2). Not all patients experience every phase, and the duration of phases can be variable; moreover, reversion or reactivation can occur between different phases without warning [12]. Family physicians must be comfortable interpreting HBV serologies (see Table 3) to determine the status of the disease not necessarily for the particular phase in the CHB disease process but more so for overall management and prevention of complications and spread of disease.

Management

The role of the family physician in the management of HBV, both acute and chronic, is correct

Table 2 Laboratory evaluation of phases of chronic HBV infection

	Immune tolerant	Immune reactant	Inactive HBV carrier	HBeAg-negative CHB	HBsAg negative
ALT	Normal	High	Normal	Normal or high	Normal
HBsAg	Positive	Positive	Positive	Positive	Negative
HBV DNA	High	High	Low or undetectable	High	Undetectable
HBeAg	Positive	Positive	Positive	Positive	Negative

Table 3   Evaluating the HBY panel

Test	Result	Interpretation
HBsAg	Negative	Susceptible (no immunity)
Anti-HBc	Negative	
Anti-HBs	Negative	
HBsAg	Negative	Immune (due to infection)
Anti-HBc	Positive	
Anti-HBs	Positive	
HBsAg	Negative	Immune (due to vaccination)
Anti-HBc	Negative	
Anti-HBs	Positive	
HBsAg	Positive	Acute infection
Anti-HBc	Positive	
IgM anti-HBc	Positive	
Anti-HBs	Negative	
HBsAg	Positive	Chronic infection
Anti-HBc	Positive	
IgM anti-HBc	Negative	
Anti-HBs	Negative	
HBsAg	Negative	Four possible
Anti-HBc	Positive	Interpretations[a]
Anti-HBs	Negative	

Source: Immunization Action Coalition publication "Needle Tips," available at www.immunize.org
[a]Possible Interpretations
   1. May be recovering from acute HBV infection
   2. May be distantly immune and test is not sensitive enough to detect low level anti-HBs
   3. May be susceptible with false-positive anti-HBc
   4. May be chronically infected and have an undetectable level of HBsAg

identification and diagnosis of the disease as well as its status and severity. There is no specific treatment for acute HBV infection; however, with identification of CHB infection, family physicians must complete a thorough evaluation on patients with special emphasis on risk factors for complications (coinfection with hepatitis C virus or HIV, alcohol use, and family history of HBV infection and liver malignancy). Laboratory evaluation on the status of CHB infection including assessment of liver disease, markers for HBV replication (HBeAg, anti-HBe, HBV DNA), and tests for coinfection should be performed. While screening for hepatocellular carcinoma with alpha-fetoprotein levels and ultrasounds are recommended as part of the pretreatment and management algorithms, screening remains largely controversial [13]. A liver biopsy to determine the extent and severity of disease is no longer necessary in the process of deciding upon treatment. Individuals should also be vaccinated for hepatitis A.

The role of treatment is prevention of complications from CHB infection including cirrhosis, hepatic failure, and hepatocellular carcinoma. Goals that correlate with improvements in patient-oriented outcomes include HBV DNA suppression, HBeAg loss/seroconversion, ALT normalization, and HBsAg loss [12]. Current treatments include conventional interferon alpha, pegylated interferon alpha, and nucleoside/nucleotide analogues (NUCs), with pegylated interferon alfa-2a (Pegasys), entecavir (Baraclude), and tenofovir being first-line treatment options. Treatment regimens with specifications on criteria, drug regimen, and laboratory monitoring have been developed, most notably by the American Association for the Study of Liver Diseases (AASLD) [14] and the European Association for the Study of the Liver (EASL) [12].

Prevention

Vaccination remains a significant mechanism of prevention of HBV infection. Vaccination is recommended for all children and adolescents, adults in certain ethnic groups, health care workers, and high-risk groups [15]. Postvaccination testing is recommended for individuals who may not elicit a complete response with anti-HBs performed 1–2 months following completion of the series. This should be performed in certain populations (persons on hemodialysis, persons who are immunocompromised, sex partners of persons positive for HBsAg, and health care personnel with revaccination indicated if the anti-HBs level is less than 10 mIU per mL) [15]. No more than two complete HBV vaccine series should be administered unless a patient is on dialysis where annual anti-HBs testing should be performed [15].

Routine screening for HBV infection is recommended for all pregnant women, which should be done through HBsAg at the first pregnancy visit. Screening is beneficial due to the significant benefit of postexposure prophylaxis in reducing the mother-to-child vertical transmission of HBV [15] accomplished through administration of HBV immune globulin and HBV vaccine to the infant within 12 h of birth. HBV is not an indication for a cesarean section as no current evidence suggests it to reduce transmission, and it is important to note that CHB infection is not a contraindication to breastfeeding.

Other screening can be performed on individuals at risk for HBV; however, routine universal screening is not recommended. Preventive strategies that also target these at-risk individuals that are part of a comprehensive public health strategy at risk reduction include screening of blood and blood products, needle exchange programs, and routine condom use. Postexposure prophylaxis is also available for health care workers and others exposed to bodily fluids from an individual with known or confirmed HBV infection.

Hepatitis C

Hepatitis C virus (HCV) is a single-stranded RNA virus transmitted through percutaneous exposure to infected blood and blood products as well as through sexual transmission; however, sexual transmission is less common. It can lead to both acute as well as chronic infections. HCV is likely responsible for the majority of hepatitis caused by what was formerly known as "non-A, non-B hepatitis" [16]. Risk factors for HCV infection include using IV or intranasal (IN) illicit drugs; HIV; recipients of blood transfusion, blood products, or organs before 1992; hemodialysis; sexual contact with those with HCV infection; piercings and tattoos; maternal-to-child transmission at birth; and sharing common household products such as razors or toothbrushes with someone infected with HCV.

Clinical Presentation and Diagnosis

In comparison to HBV and HAV infections, the acute phase of HCV hepatitis is much less likely to be symptomatic; if symptoms do develop, they are similar to the prodrome associated with HAV and HBV with nonspecific symptoms such as fatigue, nausea, anorexia, myalgias, arthralgias, weakness, and weight loss. Due to the largely asymptomatic presentation, it is unusual to perform diagnostic and laboratory evaluation unless an individual has a confirmed acute exposure. In this situation, a hepatitis viral load PCR test should be ordered to assess for possible transmission as antibody development is delayed.

HCV acute infection is much more likely than that of HBV infection to progress to a chronic infection. The definition of chronic HCV infection is the presence of virus for at least 6 months. Despite variations in data and studies, on average approximately 80% of individuals with acute HCV infection will progress to chronic infection, [17, 18] with 20% of those patients going on to develop cirrhosis (see Fig. 1) [18]. Therefore, it is clear that much more so than HBV, the chronic disease burden of liver disease secondary to HCV is significant. Symptoms of chronic HCV infection tend to be infrequent and again are nonspecific and typically mild, similar to that of acute infection. With acute infection being frequently asymptomatic, targeted history at risk factors is important in deciding to perform further

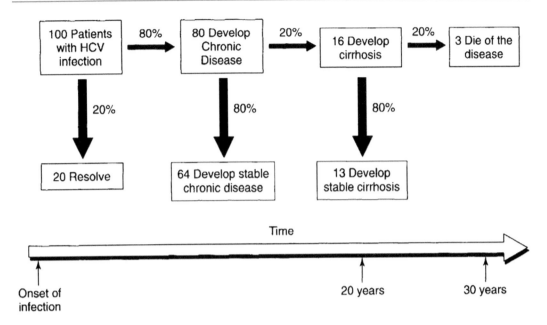

Fig. 1   The natural history of HCV infection is said to follow the "80/20 rule." While this is representative of population data, the percentages are approximate and vary based on several cofactors

clinical evaluation. Physical examination, similar to that of HBV, should be directed at evaluating for underlying signs of chronic liver disease or extrahepatic involvement with signs of cirrhosis and portal hypertension.

Laboratory evaluation with transaminases is not typically reliable to assist in the diagnosis of chronic HCV infection. The transaminases are typically normal and are only above 2 times that of normal in about 25% of patients and are rarely 10 times that of normal [19] and cannot be correlated with liver pathology. Formal diagnosis requires evaluation of the presence of antibody (HCAb) to HCV in the blood. Formerly, the initial test was an enzyme-linked immunoassay (ELISA) with the need for a recombinant immunoblot assay (RIBA) test performed for confirmation; however, newer third-generation ELISA testing enables a single antibody test with confirmation through further testing with a molecular assay that detect and/or quantify HCV RNA. The presence of HCV RNA for 6 months confirms chronic infection while a positive HCAb and negative HCV RNA suggests previous exposure to HCV with spontaneous clearance.

Management

Similar to HBV infection, the role of the family physician in the management of HCV is correct identification and diagnosis of chronic HCV infection. However, newer options for treatment facilitate this occurring in primary care with the CDC encouraging family physicians to treat HCV [20] with outcomes comparable to that of subspecialists [21]. Once diagnosed, patients should also be screened for HIV, as well as adequate immunity to HAV and HBV should be determined and provided if no immunity is apparent. In addition to making the diagnosis, the family physician should identify patients who qualify for treatment which includes assessment of fibrosis as the HCV viral load is not a sign of disease severity and fibrosis remains the most reliable prognostic factor to predict progression, morbidity, and mortality [22]. A number of methods are available to determine the degree of fibrosis with liver biopsy previously serving as the diagnostic standard; however, noninvasive tests using serum biomarkers or imaging such as serum fibrosis marker panels and transient elastography allow for accurate diagnosis of cirrhosis in most individuals [22, 23].

The goal for HCV treatment is virological cure or sustained virological response (SVR), defined as the absence of detectable HCV RNA for at least 12 weeks. However, due to exposure, HCAb will remain positive for the patient's lifetime. SVR results in reduction of symptoms as well as both intrahepatic and extrahepatic complications of chronic HCV infection. While immediate therapy is reserved for patients with advanced fibrosis, compensated cirrhosis, liver transplant recipients, or severe extrahepatic complications, therapy should be considered earlier in the course given that SVR has significant benefits at reducing the overall complications. Treatments are determined based on the genotype and subtype of HCV infection as they have varying responses to different therapies. Genotype 1 is the most common form of chronic HCV seen in the United States and with previous drug therapies was known to be the most resistant to treatment.

The American Association for the Study of Liver Diseases (AASLD) and the Infectious Disease Society of America (IDSA) developed a guideline for the recommended treatments of chronic HCV infection directed at each individual genotype and subtype (found at http://www.hcvguidelines.org) [24]. Whereas most patients formerly received a regimen including interferon and ribavirin, recent years have brought newer antivirals to the scene including boceprevir (Victrelis) and telaprevir (Incivek) that reduced the use of interferon, yet side effects remained significant. Advancements and drug approvals led to even newer therapies, potentially removing the need for ribavirin use as well, including sofosbuvir/velpatasvir (Epclusa) and glecaprevir/pibrentasvir (Mavyret) for all genotypes, elbasvir/grazoprevir (Zepatier) for genotypes 1 and 4, and sofosbuvir/ledipasvir (Harvoni) for genotypes 1a, 1b, 4, 5, and 6. The AASLD and IDSA guideline is viewed as a living document during this time of significant advancements in the field of HCV treatment and also provides information on monitoring both prior to and after treatment.

Prevention

It is in large part due to the number of genotypes and subtypes of HCV that vaccine development against HCV has been difficult. Primary prevention should be targeted at reducing risk factors for transmission. Such strategies include screening of blood and blood products, needle exchange programs, and routine condom use. Education on these topics should not be reserved solely for those in contact with those infected with HCV but for all to ensure an appropriate public health strategy. Based on risk factors, individuals should be appropriately screened for HCV infection with an HCAb. This is recommended by the USPSTF as well as an additional recommendation that one-time screening for adults aged 18–79 [25].

Despite maternal-to-child transmission being the largest cause of HCV infection in children, routine testing of all pregnant women is not recommended. Additionally, inconclusive evidence remains on whether specific labor management strategies are effective at reducing transmission. Most practice involves limiting internal fetal monitoring, rupture of membranes, and instrumented deliveries. It is important to note that HCV infection is not a contraindication to breastfeeding. Newborns of mothers infected with HCV should be tested for HCV transmission; however, this is complicated by passage of maternal HCAb through the placenta. While diagnosis can be made earlier with two positive HCV RNA between 2 and 6 months of age in an infant, [26], the American Academy of Pediatrics (AAP) recommends testing with an HCAb at 18 months or later since HCV treatment is not recommended for infants less than 3 months [27].

Other Viral Agents

Hepatitis D and E are far less common viral hepatitides that have been demonstrated to cause infection. Hepatitis D virus, previously known as delta hepatitis, is an incomplete virus which is structurally an RNA virus that requires helper function of HBV to replicate and cause both an acute and chronic hepatitis. It is transmitted similarly to HBV and either occurs as coinfection or superinfection in an individual with chronic HBV. Hepatitis E virus is rare in the United States. It is similar to HAV such that it is transmitted via the fecal-oral route and only causes a self-limited acute infection. There are no vaccines or treatments currently available for hepatitis D or E viruses; however, hepatitis D can be prevented in an individual without HBV infection through the HBV vaccine.

Alcoholic Hepatitis

Alcoholic liver disease (ALD) is a serious health problem worldwide that encompasses several disease processes including alcoholic fatty liver disease (with or without steatohepatitis), alcoholic hepatitis, and cirrhosis. Excessive alcohol consumption can result in both short-term and long-term liver damage. Regular alcohol use, even for several days, results in fat deposition in the liver hepatocytes or steatosis (fatty liver). While abstinence reverses the process, steatosis places individuals who continue to drink at increased risk of progression to fibrosis and cirrhosis. Cirrhosis only develops, however, in a small number of patients with ALD [28]. While the mean intake of regular alcohol to result in liver disease is approximated to be around 100 g/day for more than 20 years, lesser amounts can potentially result in ALD as regular consumption of 30 g/day increases the risk for development of cirrhosis [29].

Clinical Presentation and Diagnosis

Given that excessive, regular alcohol consumption is necessary, most patients with ALD are often between 40 and 50 years old [30]. Careful history should be obtained from patients as they often will cease drinking with onset of symptoms due to disease severity. Excessive, regular alcohol consumption may not represent daily drinking as patterns of drinking can vary to include weekends or intermittent heavy drinking behaviors that family members are unaware. While long-term drinking (more than 20 years) is typically the overall course, individuals can present with ALD who have been drinking for shorter duration.

The individual will usually present with similar symptoms to that of viral hepatitis including fatigue, anorexia, jaundice, fever, right upper quadrant or epigastric pain, abdominal fullness, or bloating. Physical examination can demonstrate jaundice, icteric sclera, hepatomegaly, as well as possible findings of more chronic liver disease with cirrhosis including muscle wasting, ascites, or sequelae of portal hypertension. A bruit may be heard over the liver, a feature of more severe alcoholic hepatitis, has been demonstrated in over 50% with ALD [30]. While history can suggest that alcohol is the etiology for symptoms, one cannot completely rule out other causes of liver injury, and therefore, history and laboratory evaluation is needed to rule out other etiologies.

Laboratory findings associated with alcoholic hepatitis include transaminitis with AST-to-ALT ratio of 2:1 (levels are typically less than 300 IU/L and rarely higher than 500 IU/L), elevated serum bilirubin, elevated gamma-glutamyltransferase (GGT), and a leukocytosis with neutrophil predominance. Other laboratory findings can suggest severity of disease such as moderate to severe disease that would result in an elevated international normalized ratio (INR), anemia secondary to thiamine or folate deficiencies, low albumin and prealbumin in the setting of malnutrition, and thrombocytopenia from bone marrow suppression from alcohol or related to portal hypertension. Abdominal imaging (ultrasound, computed tomography, or magnetic resonance imaging) can also be utilized to assess for degree of steatosis, ascites, and cirrhosis. Liver biopsy is often helpful in assessing the severity of hepatocellular damage; however, it is not required for diagnosis.

Management

The overall management of alcoholic hepatitis for the family physician is targeted at patient education and safe cessation of alcohol. The potential complications due to alcohol use as well as a result of the alcoholic hepatitis such as ascites, hepatic encephalopathy, malnutrition, and alcohol withdrawal with or without delirium tremens should be treated as supportive care. Lifetime cessation of alcohol is critical to prevent the progression of disease, and patients should be supported through the process. Family physicians are poised to lead or be part of the multidisciplinary approach that may need to address comorbid alcohol use disorder (AUD). Relapse prevention medications can be utilized by family physicians. However, only baclofen has been studied in patients with alcoholic liver disease [31]. Acamprosate can be utilized as it is not metabolized by the liver; however, there are no studies regarding its efficacy for alcohol cessation in a population with alcoholic hepatitis.

While a number of therapies and treatments have been studied or suggested in the use of treatment of alcoholic hepatitis including psychotherapy, corticosteroids, pentoxifylline, infliximab, etanercept, nutritional support, oxandrolone, vitamin E, and silymarin (milk thistle extract), only corticosteroids have been shown to demonstrate improvements on mortality in specific populations with disease [32]. Liver transplantation may be necessary in severe cases; however, due to alcohol use being the etiology of their underlying disease process, patients often need to demonstrate sobriety for 6 months prior to consideration, and patients who might qualify for liver transplant may suffer significant complications during this time period.

Prevention

As ALD results from prolonged excessive alcohol intake, there is certainly a window of time for both screening and intervention to occur to combat alcohol misuse. The public health approach to the problem of alcohol use is screening, brief intervention, and referral to treatment (SBIRT). Family physicians play a critical role in screening individuals for alcohol use and misuse. The United States Preventive Services Task Force (USPSTF) recommends that "clinicians screen adults aged 18 or older for alcohol misuse and provide persons engaged in risky or hazardous drinking with brief behavioral counseling interventions to reduce alcohol misuse" [33].

Drug-Induced Liver Disease

Due to its role in clearing and metabolizing chemicals, the liver is a particular target for damage from drugs. The cellular damage that occurs as part of drug-induced liver disease is typically a result of the drug or metabolite having a direct toxic effect on the liver or an immune-mediated response that causes liver injury. While liver damage from drugs and medications is common except in rare cases of drug-induced hepatitis, the majority of damage is reversible with cessation of the substance with a return to normal function [34]. One of the most frequent causes of hepatic injury due to a drug is from acetaminophen, which can be either acute or chronic use. It has been shown that over 1000 drugs have caused liver disease on more than one occasion [35] and therefore a comprehensive list is not easily developed. Table 4 lists some of the more common drugs that can induce liver damage.

HIV Liver Disease

Despite advancements in treatment that has made HIV infection a chronic illness, it remains a major global health issue. While HIV does not result in a direct injury or primary disease process in the liver, data demonstrates the burden of liver disease in patients with HIV is large, with liver disease being second only to AIDS-related complications in causing mortality [36]. Due to similarities in transmission routes, patients with HIV may also be coinfected with HBV and/or HCV. In fact, of liver-related deaths in patients with HIV, 66% were secondary to complications of HCV and 17% secondary to complications of HBV [36]. This is largely secondary to fibrosis and complication rates in patients coinfected with HIV and either HBV or HCV being much higher [37]. Patients with HIV are also at risk of developing opportunistic infections that may also cause liver damage including mycobacterium tuberculosis (Tb), mycobacterium avium complex (MAC), and cytomegalovirus (CMV).

In addition to infectious etiologies, increasing recognition of highly active antiretroviral therapy (HAART) as a source of liver damage

Table 4 Common potential hepatotoxic medication agents

Over the counter (OTC) agents	Acetaminophen (Tylenol)
	NSAIDs (ibuprofen, naproxen, etc.)
Anti-arrhythmics	Amiodarone
	Diltiazem
Antibiotics	Isoniazid
	Nitrofurantoin
	Amoxicillin/clavulonic acid
	Rifampin
	Tetracycline (minocycline, tetracycline)
Antiepileptics	Phenytoin
	Carbamazepine
	Valproic acid
Antifungals	Azoles (ketonazole, fluconazole)
	Amphoteracin
	Terbinafine (systemic)
Anti-hyperglycemics	Sulfonylureas (glipizide, glyburide)
	Thiazolidinediones (pioglitazone)
Anti-hyperlipidemics	Statins (rosuvastatin, simvastatin, etc.)
	Nicotinic acid (niacin)
	Fibrates (gemfibrozole, fenofibrate)
Endocrinologic agents	Methimazole
Hormonal agents	Anabolic steroids
	Estrogen and oral contraceptives
	Testosterone
Rheumatolic agents	Methotrexate
	Quinadine
Psychiatric agents	Atypical antipsychotics (quetiapine, etc.)
	Nefazodone
	Trazodone
	Venlafaxine

Table 5 Risks of HAART on liver disease

NRTIs		
Caution	Didanosine (ddl)	
	Stavudine (d4T)	
	Zidovudine (ZDV/AZT)	
	Zalcitabine (ddC)	
Safer	Abacavir (ABC)	
	Tenofovir (TDF)	
	Lamivudine (3TC)	
	Emtricitabine (FTC)	
Integrate inhibitors		
Safer	Raltegravir (RAL)	
	Elvitagravir (EVG)	
	Dolutegravir (DTG)	
Entry inhibitors		
	Maraviroc (MVC)	
	Enfuvirtide (INN;T20)	
NNRTIs		
Caution	Nevirapine (NVP)	
	Efavirenz (EFV)	
Safer	Etravirine (ETV)	
	Rilphirine (RPV)	
Protease inhibitors (Pi's)		
Caution	Ritonavir (RTV)	
	Telapravir (TPV)	
Safer	Indinavir (IDV)	
	Atazanavir (ATAZ)	
	Saquinavir (SQV)	
	Lopinavir (LPV)	
	Darunavir (DRV)	
	Amprenavir (APV)	
	Nelfinavir (NFV)	
Enhancer		
Safer	Cobicistat (COBI)	

is also occurring. Monitoring transaminases is recommended for newly diagnosed and newly treated patients as HIV infection with high viremia alone may result in transaminase elevation with reduction as HAART is initiated [38]. Additionally, many patients with HIV whose liver enzymes are elevated are asymptomatic during this time [39]. Due to combination therapies, it can be difficult to determine the culprit drug resulting in liver damage. Table 5 lists drugs from HAART regimens with documented liver toxicity [40].

Patients with HIV should also be appropriately screened for other potential etiologies of liver disease including alcohol-induced disease, drug-induced liver disease, and nonalcoholic fatty liver disease (NAFLD). NAFLD is the hepatic manifestation of metabolic syndrome and is noted to have significantly higher rates in those infected with HIV compared to the general population [41].

Hepatocellular Carcinoma

Despite most malignancy involving the liver being due to metastatic disease commonly from colorectal cancer, hepatocellular carcinoma (HCC) remains a significant cause of morbidity and mortality worldwide. Most of the disease burden remains in developing countries where HBV infection is endemic; however, HCC secondary to HCV infection is a significant cause of cancer-related death in the United States [42], with the incidence tripling and the 5-year survival rate remaining below 12% [43]. While significant risk factors are largely infection with HBV or HCV, preexisting cirrhosis is found in more than 80% of individuals diagnosed with HCC [44]. Therefore, any etiology that would result in chronic liver injury resulting in cirrhosis should be considered a risk factor for HCC. HCC is rarely seen in individuals younger than 40 years of age, and peak incidence occurs around age 70 with a predilection for males as the rates are two to four times higher in males than females [45].

Clinical Presentation and Diagnosis

Given that a large majority of patients with HCC have underlying cirrhosis, the presentation of HCC is almost indistinguishable other than typical signs of cirrhosis including fatigue, upper abdominal pain, weight loss, early satiety, encephalopathy, and potentially jaundice. HCC can be suspected in a patient who develops acute decompensated cirrhosis who has previously been stable. Solid liver lesions are often noted with screening in patients at risk for HCC through ultrasound screening, which according to the AASLD should be performed in high-risk patients every 6 months [46]. As previously noted, it is increasingly recognized that alpha-fetoprotein lacks adequate sensitivity and specificity to be utilized as a screening or diagnostic aid [47]. Ultrasound findings are monitored based on their size with testing and diagnosis becoming

increasingly possible with the use of noninvasive imaging techniques. Biopsy, although reassuring, cannot completely rule out the presence of HCC, and lesions, despite normal biopsy, need to be followed until disappearance or progression to malignant disease [48].

Management

Based on the staging at diagnosis (Barcelona Clinic Liver Cancer (BCLC) staging system) [49], there are several potentially curative or palliative approaches to treatment [50] including resection, radiofrequency ablation, chemoembolization, medication therapy, and liver transplantation. While family physicians should be aware of the potential treatment options for HCC and remain supportive in the care, treatment of HCC is typically performed in conjunction with hepatologist or gastroenterologist management.

Prevention

Prevention of HCC is targeted at modification of the underlying risk factors for HCC. HBV vaccination remains an effective prevention strategy for avoiding HBV viral infection and resultant cirrhosis. Primary prevention seems to be the most effective strategy at prevention. While treatment of HBV infection and HCV infection does reduce the risk of development of HCC, it does not completely eliminate this risk.

Family Issues of Diseases of the Liver

The family physician is challenged with being on the front lines of prevention, patient education, risk factor assessment, diagnosis, management, and monitoring of patients and families afflicted with liver diseases. Advances in treatment have expanded the role of family physicians in addressing diseases of the liver. As many common medications can cause liver damage, family physicians must be aware of the pharmacological properties of the medications they are prescribing and use caution in patients to avoid drug-drug interactions as well as use safe medications in patients with liver disease. Additionally, as family physicians care for patients across the age spectrum, diagnosis of viral hepatitides as well as appropriate testing and treatment targeting at reducing maternal-to-child transmission is important information for the practicing family physician. While the family physician has a duty to respect the privacy of the patient with regard to possible diagnosis of HBV and HCV chronic infections, he also cares for their family members and has the unique role to protect privacy but also protect his patients from transmission. Furthermore, as alcohol-related disorders cause not only physical damage but also rifts in relationships and connections with family and friends, the family physician has a critical role in coordinating care as well as a comprehensive addiction treatment program including patient and family. Poised with an effective role in public health, family physicians ensure appropriate education and counseling occurs for patients and family members on risk reduction as well as discussion of typical course and prognosis for chronic liver diseases. While the complications of chronic liver disease are often managed by a multidisciplinary team, the intrinsic value of the family physician in this process due to the above cannot be understated.

Conclusion

Diseases of the liver represent a variety of conditions that vary in chronicity, complications, and management strategies. With viral hepatitides, alcoholic liver disease, and drug-induced liver disease being some of the most common forms of both acute and chronic liver disease, the family physician plays a critical role in the diagnosis and management. Due to the significant family issues associated with liver disease and the family physician's role in diagnosis and management, it is critical that the practicing family physician have an awareness of the diagnosis, management, and prevention strategies and approach them with an evidence-based perspective.

References

1. Vento S, Garofano T, Renzini C, et al. Fulminant hepatitis associated with hepatitis A virus superinfection in patients with chronic hepatitis C. N Engl J Med. 1998;338:286. CrossRef PubMed
2. Kojaoglanian T. Hepatitis A. Pediatr Rev. 2010;31(8): 348–50. CrossRef PubMed
3. Matheny SC, Kingery JE. Hepatitis A. Am Fam Physician. 2012;86(11):1027–34. PubMed
4. Johnston DE. Special considerations in interpreting liver function tests. Am Fam Physician. 1999;59(8): 2223–30. PubMed
5. CDC. Prevention of hepatitis A through active or passive immunization: recommendations of the Advisory Committee on Immunization Practices (ACIP). MMWR. 1999;48:1–37.
6. CDC. Updated recommendations from the ACIP for use of hepatitis A vaccine in close contacts of newly arriving international adoptees. MMWR. 2009;58:1–36.
7. Doshani M, Weng M, Moore KL, Romero JR, Nelson NP. Recommendations of the Advisory Committee on Immunization Practices for the use of hepatitis A vaccine for persons experiencing homelessness. MMWR Morb Mortal Wkly Rep. 2019;68:153–6.
8. Nelson NP, Link-Gelles R, Hofmeister MG, et al. Update: recommendations of the Advisory Committee on Immunization Practices for the use of hepatitis a vaccines for Postexposure prophylaxis and for Pre-exposure prophylaxis for international travel. MMWR Morb Moral Wkly Rep. 2018;67:1216–20.
9. Raimondo G, Pollicino T, Squadrito G. Clinical virology of hepatitis B virus infection. J Hepatol. 2003;39: S26–30. CrossRef PubMed
10. Lok AS, McMahon BJ. Chronic hepatitis B. Hepatology. 2001;34:1225–41. CrossRef PubMed
11. Trépo C, Chan HL, Lok A. Hepatitis B virus infection. Lancet. 2014;384(9959):2053–63.
12. European Association for the Study of the Liver. EASL 2017 clinical practice guidelines on the management of hepatitis B virus infection. J Hepatol. 2017;67(2):370–98.
13. Aghoram R, Cai P, Dickinson JA. Alpha-foetoprotein and/or liver ultrasonography for screening of hepatocellular carcinoma in patients with chronic hepatitis B. Cochrane Database Syst Rev. 2012;2012(9):CD002799.
14. Terrault NA, Lok A, McMahon BJ, et al. Update on prevention, diagnosis, and treatment of chronic hepatitis B: AASLD 2018 hepatitis B guidance. Hepatology. 2018;67(4):1560–99.
15. Schillie S, Vellozzi C, Reingold A, et al. Prevention of hepatitis B virus infection in the United States: recommendations of the advisory committee on immunization practices. MMWR Recomm Rep. 2018;67(RR-1):1–31.
16. Gitnick G. Non-A, non-B hepatitis: etiology and clinical course. Annu Rev Med. 1984;35:265–78. CrossRef PubMed
17. Nelson PK, Mathers BM, Cowie B, Hagan H, Des Jarlais D, Horyniak D, Degenhardt L. Global

epidemiology of hepatitis B and hepatitis C in people who inject drugs: results of systematic reviews. Lancet. 2011;378(9791):571–83. CrossRef PubMed PubMedCentral

18. Seef LB. Natural history of hepatitis C. Hepatology. 1997;26(Suppl 1):21S–8. CrossRef

19. Barrera JM, Bruguera M, Ercilla MG, Gil C, Celis R, Gil MP, del Valle Onorato M, Rodes J, Ordinas A. Persistent hepatitis C viremia after acute self-limiting posttransfusion hepatitis C. Hepatology. 1995;21(3):639. CrossRef PubMed

20. Mitruka K, Thornton K, Cusick S, Centers for Disease Control and Prevention, et al. Expanding primary care capacity to treat hepatitis C virus infection through an evidence-based model – Arizona and Utah, 2012–2014. MMWR Morb Mortal Wkly Rep. 2014;63(18):393–8.

21. Tran TT. Hepatitis C: who should treat hepatitis C virus? The role of the primary care provider. Clin Liver Dis. 2018;11(3):66–8.

22. AASLD/IDSA HCV Guidance Panel. Hepatitis C guidance: AASLD-IDSA recommendations for testing, managing, and treating adults infected with hepatitis C virus. Hepatology. 2015;62:932–54.

23. Boursier J, de Ledinghen V, Zarski JP, et al. Comparison of eight diagnostic algorithms for liver fibrosis in hepatitis C: new algorithms are more precise and entirely noninvasive. Hepatology. 2012;55(1):58–67. CrossRef PubMed

24. AASLD/ISDA/IAS-USA. Recommendations for testing, managing, and treating hepatitis C. http://www.hcvguidelines.org. Accessed 20 Mar 2020.

25. USPSTF. Screening for hepatitis C virus infection in adolescents and adults: US preventive services task force recommendation statement. JAMA. 2020;323(10): 970–5.

26. National Institutes of Health. Management of hepatitis C: 2002. National Institutes of Health consensus conference statement. 10–12 June 2002. http://consensus.nih/gov/2002/2002HepatitisC2002116PDF.pdf. Accessed 20 Mar 2020.

27. Hepatitis C virus infection. American Academy of Pediatrics. Committee on Infectious Diseases. Pediatrics. 1998;101(3 Pt1):481–5.

28. Bellentani S, Saccoccio G, Costa G, et al. Drinking habits as cofactors of risk for alcohol induced liver damage. Gut. 1997;41:845–50. CrossRef PubMed PubMedCentral

29. Cohen SM, Ahn J. Review article: the diagnosis and management of alcoholic hepatitis. Aliment Pharmacol Ther. 2009;30(1):3–13. CrossRef PubMed

30. Dugum MF, McCullough AJ. Acute alcoholic hepatitis, the clinical aspects. Clin Liver Dis. 2016;20(3): 499–508.

31. Yamini D, Lee SH, Avanesyan A, Walter M, Runyon B. Utilization of baclofen in maintenance of alcohol abstinence in patients with alcohol dependence and alcoholic hepatitis with or without cirrhosis. Alcohol Alcohol. 2014;49:453–6.

32. Crabb DW, Im GY, Szabo G, Mellinger JL, Lucey MR. Diagnosis and treatment of alcohol-associated liver diseases: 2019 practice guidance from the American Association for the Study of Liver Diseases. Hepatology. 2020;71(1):306–33.

33. Moyer VA, Preventive Services Task Force. Screening and behavioral counseling interventions in primary care to reduce alcohol misuse: U.S. preventive services task force recommendation statement. Ann Intern Med. 2013;159(3):210–8. PubMed

34. Kaplowitz N. Drug-induced liver injury. Clin Infect Dis. 2004;38(Suppl 2):S44–8. CrossRef PubMed

35. Kaplowitz N. Drug-induced liver disorders: implications for drug development and regulation. Drug Saf. 2001;24:483–90. CrossRef PubMed

36. Weber R, Sabin CA, Friis-Moller N, et al. Liver-related deaths in persons infected with the human immunodeficiency virus: the D:A:D study. Arch Intern Med. 2006;166:1632–41. CrossRef PubMed

37. Benhamou Y, Bochet M, Di Martino V, et al. Liver fibrosis progression in human immunodeficiency virus and hepatitis C virus coinfected patients. The Multivirc Group. Hepatology. 1999;30:1054–8.

38. Joshi D, O'Grady J, Dieterich D, Gazzard B, Agarwal K. Increasing burden of liver disease in patients with HIV infection. Lancet. 2011;377:1198–209. CrossRef PubMed

39. Aranzabal L, Casado JL, Moya J, et al. Influence of liver fibrosis on highly active antiretroviral therapy-associated hepatotoxicity in patients with HIV and hepatitis C coinfection. Clin Infect Dis. 2005;40:588–93. CrossRef PubMed

40. Soriano V, Puoti M, Garcia-Gasco P, et al. Antiretroviral drugs and liver injury. AIDS. 2008;22:1–13. CrossRef PubMed

41. Crum-Cianflone N, Dilay A, Collins G, et al. Nonalcoholic fatty liver disease among HIV-infected persons. J Acquir Immune Defic Syndr. 2009;50:464–73. CrossRef PubMed PubMedCentral

42. Angulo P. GI epidemiology: nonalcoholic fatty liver disease. Aliment Pharmacol Ther. 2007;25:883–9. CrossRef PubMed

43. Marrero JA, Kulik LM, Sirlin CB, et al. Diagnosis, staging, and management of hepatocellular carcinoma: 2018 practice guidance by the American Association for the Study of Liver Diseases. Hepatology. 2018;68(2): 723–50.

44. Surveillance, Epidemiology, and End Results (SEER) Program. SEER*Stat database: incidence – SEER 9 Regs research data, Nov 2009 Sub (1973–2007). Bethesda: National Cancer Institute; 2010 April.

45. Bruix J, Sherman M. Management of hepatocellular carcinoma: an update. Hepatology. 2011;53(3):1020–2. CrossRef PubMed PubMedCentral

46. El-Serag HB. Hepatocellular carcinoma. N Engl J Med. 2011;365:1118–27. CrossRef PubMed

47. Lok AS, Sterling RK, Everhart JE, HALT-C Trial Group, et al. Des-gamma-carboxy prothrombin and alpha-fetoprotein as biomarkers for the early detection of hepatocellular carcinoma. Gastroenterology. 2010;138:493–502. CrossRef PubMed
48. Bruix J, Sherman M. Management of hepatocellular carcinoma. Hepatology. 2005;42:1208–36. CrossRef PubMed
49. Forner A, Reig ME, de Lope CR, Bruix J. Current strategy for staging and treatment: the BCLC update and future prospects. Semin Liver Dis. 2010;30:61–74. CrossRef PubMed
50. El Serag HB, Marrero JA, Rudolph L, Reddy KR. Diagnosis and treatment of hepatocellular carcinoma. Gastroenterology. 2008;134:1752–63. CrossRef PubMed

Kalyanakrishnan Ramakrishnan

Contents

K. Ramakrishnan (✉)
Department of Family and Preventive Medicine,
University of Oklahoma Health Sciences Center,
Oklahoma, OK, USA
e-mail: kramakrishnan@ouhsc.edu

© Springer Nature Switzerland AG 2022
P. M. Paulman et al. (eds.), *Family Medicine*,
https://doi.org/10.1007/978-3-030-54441-6_98

Anatomy of the Rectum and Anal Canal

The rectum extends from the rectosigmoid to the anorectal junction (about 15 cm); the anal canal measures about 5 cm, extending from the lower border of the anal crypts at the dentate line to the anal verge [1]. The rectum and the anal canal above the undulating dentate line are lined by columnar epithelium and below by stratified squamous epithelium that transitions to the skin at the anal verge [1]. Innervation above the dentate line is sympathetic (L-1 to L-3) and insensate; below is somatic (pudendal nerves, S2–S4) [1]. The vascular supply of the anorectal region is through the superior, middle, and inferior hemorrhoidal vessels.

Hemorrhoids followed by anal fissures, anorectal abscesses and fistulas, fecal incontinence, rectal prolapse, pruritus ani, proctitis, hidradenitis suppurativa, condyloma acuminatum, and anorectal cancer are common problems pertaining to the anorectal region.

Hemorrhoids

Background

Hemorrhoids represent the enlarged normally observed fibrovascular cushions (hemorrhoidal cushions) lining the anal canal [2]. Hemorrhoidal cushions help exercise bowel control by sustaining a resting pressure; vascular engorgement associated with increasing intra-abdominal pressure (as in laughing, coughing, sneezing) closes the anal canal, helping maintain continence. The innervation feedback from the hemorrhoidal cushions helps differentiate between flatus, liquid, and solid stool [2]. Aging and continual straining associated with constipation cause degeneration and weakening of the securing fibrous tissue, detachment of the cushions from the internal sphincter, and prolapse. The overlying mucosa also becomes loose, bulges into the anal canal, and becomes thin and friable due to sustained trauma by feces and ulcerates, sometimes causing bright red rectal bleeding.

Epidemiology

Hemorrhoids are most common among men and women between 45 and 65 years of age with hemorrhoid-related symptoms being experienced by nearly one in two Americans over 50 [3]. Predisposing factors include older age, irregular bowel habits, decreased fiber intake, obesity, pregnancy, ascites, positive family history, and absent valves within the hemorrhoidal veins. Hepatic cirrhosis, portal hypertension, and portal vein thrombosis also predispose to development of hemorrhoids.

Classification

Hemorrhoids may be located above (internal) or below the dentate line (external) or both above and below (intero-external) [4, 5]. Based on symptoms of bleeding and prolapse, hemorrhoids are classified as grade 1 or first degree (bleeding with prominent hemorrhoidal veins, without mucosal prolapse), grade 2 or second degree (bleeding and mucosal prolapse on straining reducing spontaneously), grade 3 or third degree (bleeding and mucosal prolapse on straining, requiring manual reduction), and grade 4 or fourth degree, representing persistent prolapsed hemorrhoids with or without complications (strangulation, ulceration, fibrosis, gangrene, sepsis) [4–6].

Diagnosis

History

Patients with hemorrhoids experience painless bright red bleeding during or after stooling. Constipation and straining may be present. With second-degree or more advanced hemorrhoids, mucus discharge, a sense of incomplete defecation, pruritus ani, and a perianal rash are noticed. Thrombosis or ulceration leads to perianal pain and swelling, bleeding, and a bloodstained discharge [7]. Blood from more proximal sources (polyps, diverticula, angiodysplasia, ischemic colitis) is usually darker or clotted blood mixed with stool. Fever, throbbing pain, redness, swelling, and inability to sit indicate perianal sepsis. Abdominal discomfort and distention, anorexia, weight loss, and worsening constipation or persisting diarrhea should suggest cancer, ischemic colitis, or inflammatory bowel disease (IBD).

Examination, Special Testing

Physical examination usually yields little information in healthy patients. Presence of anemia indicates a different pathology. Jaundice, hepatosplenomegaly, and enlarged abdominal wall collaterals characterize hepatic cirrhosis and portal hypertension. A palpable abdominal mass suggests possible colon cancer and, if tender, a peridiverticular mass. Perianal inspection, digital rectal examination (DRE), and anoscopy in the left lateral (Sims') or the knee chest position complete the initial patient assessment. Perianal inspection may reveal skin tags, prolapsed and thrombosed hemorrhoids, anal fissure or abscess, excoriation, fistula, cancer, or condyloma. Bearing down during DRE or anoscopy relaxes the sphincter and causes second- and third-degree hemorrhoids to prolapse. Uncomplicated hemorrhoids are impalpable and non-tender; when thrombosed or fibrosed, hemorrhoids are palpable; and prolapsed and strangulated hemorrhoids are tender. Insertion of a side-viewing anoscope causes hemorrhoids to bulge into the lumen. When examining a patient in the Sims' position, the anal cushions (internal hemorrhoids) are usually located at the 11 o'clock (left anterior), 3 o'clock (right lateral), and 7 o'clock (left posterior) positions. Prolapsed hemorrhoids should be reduced to minimize risk of strangulation and ulceration. Patients over 50 years with rectal bleeding should undergo a colonoscopy, even though hemorrhoids are detected [4, 5, 6].

Treatment: Non-operative

Adequate fluid and fiber intake (20–35 G daily) is the primary first-line non-operative therapy for patients with symptomatic hemorrhoids of all grades [4, 5]. Many symptoms associated with hemorrhoids (bleeding, prolapse, and pain) improve on increasing fiber intake. Sitz baths (a warm water bath in which the patient squats or sits), analgesics, and anti-inflammatory medications relieve pain and decrease tissue edema and sphincter spasm in patients with thrombosed hemorrhoids and following hemorrhoidectomy [8]. Oral flavonoids and topical preparations such as Preparation H, glyceryl trinitrate 0.2% ointment applied three times daily for 14 days, and nifedipine 0.3% with lidocaine 1.5% ointment applied twice daily for 14 days also decrease symptoms associated with hemorrhoids and their complications [9, 10]. Exercising and losing excess weight are also beneficial.

Office Procedures

The rubber band ligation (RBL) technique is useful in treating grade I through III internal hemorrhoids. A small rubber band is loaded onto a hollow applicator, the hemorrhoid is grasped 1 cm or more above the dentate line and pulled inside the applicator, and the rubber band is released at the base of the hemorrhoid, which sloughs off over 5–7 days. Moderate pain can follow RBL. One or more hemorrhoids can be banded at the same or subsequent office visits [5]. RBL is successful in most (93%) patients with grade II and III hemorrhoids, though 11% symptomatic recurrence is observed over 2 years [11]. Suction ligation, in which an anoscope/ligator is attached to the wall suction (vacuum suction ligation), is associated with less bleeding and post-procedure pain. Complications following RBL are rare (<1%) and include band placement at or near the dentate line (requires removal and reapplication), urinary retention, rectal bleeding (post-procedure or 7–10 days later, usually self-limiting), extrusion of the band, pain, ulceration, thrombosis, and perineal infection [3].

Sclerotherapy involves injection of an irritant (5 ml sodium morrhuate, 5% phenol in oil, hypertonic saline) through the anoscope into the submucosa at the apex of the hemorrhoid, causing ischemia and fibrosis, fixing the hemorrhoid to the rectal wall, decreasing bleeding and prolapse. Though effective in grade I, II, and III hemorrhoids, the majority of patients over time experience recurrence, especially in grade III hemorrhoids [12]. Complications include mucosal sloughing, thrombosis, abscess formation, and bacteremia. Sclerotherapy using Polidocanol 2% with or without foam is efficacious in I, II, and III hemorrhoids with improvement observed in most cases [13].

Infrared photocoagulation (direct application of infrared waves through the anoscope) produces superficial tissue destruction, reducing blood flow and tethering the hemorrhoid to the underlying tissues. It is most useful in grade I and II hemorrhoids [5].

In-Hospital Surgery

Hemorrhoidectomy is indicated in patients with intero-external hemorrhoids and grade III and IV hemorrhoids, in hemorrhoids recurring after office procedures, or in patients intolerant of office procedures [5]. The surgery, performed under general or regional anesthesia, requires distal bowel preparation to minimize soiling during and after the procedure. Preoperative antibiotic administration is unnecessary. In open hemorrhoidectomy, the hemorrhoid is excised after ligating the pedicle, and the raw area is allowed to granulate. In closed hemorrhoidectomy, the raw area is closed primarily. The LigaSure procedure involves sealing of the hemorrhoidal tissue between the LigaSure forceps during dissection, minimizing tissue destruction, blood loss, and post-procedure pain [14]. Using an ultrasonic scalpel for dissection is an advance found to result in less post-procedure pain and complications and earlier return to work [5]. Bleeding, urinary retention, wound infection, fecal incontinence, and anal stricture may follow surgery (all uncommon). In the "stapled hemorrhoidopexy" (hemorrhoidectomy), a ring of anal mucosa with the underlying fibrovascular cushions is removed using a modified, circular anastomotic stapler. Though bleeding, wound complications, constipation, and pruritus are decreased, recurrence rates and prolapse are higher than in conventional hemorrhoidectomy [15]. The Doppler-guided trans-anal hemorrhoidal ligation involves suture ligation of the hemorrhoidal vessels after localizing them with Doppler ultrasound. This procedure, best applicable to grade II and III hemorrhoids, allows most patients to be discharged at 24 h and return to work in 2–3 days. Complication rates are low, though pooled recurrence rates of 17.5% were observed, higher in grade IV hemorrhoids [16].

External Hemorrhoids

Most patients with thrombosed external hemorrhoids (perianal hematoma) improve with sitz baths twice daily, stool softeners, and analgesics. Patients presenting within 72 h of onset of symptoms benefit from evacuation of the clot [5]. This is usually performed under local anesthesia using lidocaine (1–2%). Following clot clearance, bleeding from the base and edges is managed with sutures, packing, or electrocautery, and analgesics, stool softeners, and sitz baths are continued until healing is complete. Perianal skin tags may cause irritation or interfere with hygiene but rarely require excision.

Prolapsed and strangulated hemorrhoids are best managed with stool softeners, analgesics, rest, warm soaks, and ice packs to decrease pain and swelling, minimizing constipation and tissue ischemia. Swelling and pain resolve over several days; the residual hemorrhoid may then be managed by RBL or hemorrhoidectomy. Immediate excision leads to excess tissue removal, anal canal narrowing, and infection. Spreading perianal infection and tissue necrosis occur occasionally, requiring immediate debridement and broad-spectrum antibiotics [3].

Nonhemorrhoidal Anorectal Diseases

Anal Fissure

Epidemiology and Classification
Anal fissures are painful linear cracks in the anal mucosa distal to the dentate line. They may be acute (<8 weeks) or chronic (symptoms persisting >8 weeks) [17]. Anal fissures are more common in younger adults and have an equal sex distribution. The majority (>90% in men; 75% in women) are posterior; anterior fissures have a female preponderance. Lateral or multiple fissures may follow

trauma, infections (syphilis, tuberculosis, anorectal abscesses, herpes, or human immunodeficiency virus – HIV – infection), cancer, and IBD [17, 18]. Low fiber intake, chronic diarrhea or constipation, excessive laxative use, and anal trauma (including surgery) also predispose to anal fissures [18]. Fiber increases stool volume and bulk minimizing anorectal trauma during defecation. Anal surgery predisposes to tissue ischemia through fibrosis, increasing the risk of non-healing fissures.

Diagnosis
Diagnosis is clinical. Severe pain initiated by and persisting for several hours after defecation is characteristic of acute fissures [17]. Bright red blood is often seen in the toilet paper, stool, or toilet bowl. Constipation (due to painful evacuation and unwillingness to defecate), perianal discharge, pruritus, and a perianal mass may also be present.

Acute fissures usually appear as midline tears, with a skin tag extending distally from the base of the tear (the "sentinel pile"). There is significant perianal spasm; DRE or anoscopy is painful. Chronic fissures are less painful and tender and evidence more scarring and raised edges, the floor exposing the white horizontal fibers of the internal sphincter.

Perianal tenderness and induration or lateral, multiple, or recurrent fissures should prompt a search for a more definitive cause. Dark-field microscopy of perianal discharge may demonstrate spirochetes. Serum antibody testing may detect treponemal or HIV antibodies. Imaging studies (endoanal ultrasound, computed tomography (CT), magnetic resonance imaging (MRI)) are useful in revealing the extent of anal involvement and perianal/extra-anal extension of infection or malignancy. Endoscopy is valuable in detecting proximal bowel pathology (IBD, malignancy) associated with chronic or multiple fissures; biopsies confirm IBD or cancer.

Treatment
Non-operative treatment measures improve pain and bleeding, heal fissures in nearly 50% of patients, and are advocated initially in both acute and chronic fissures [17]. These include fiber

Table 1 Treatment options in acute and chronic anal fissures (text from multiple sources)

[a]Nonsurgical measures – in acute and chronic fissures	
Dietary fiber/fiber supplements	Increase dietary fiber to 20G–35G daily Fiber supplements (psyllium, Citrucel, FiberCon) Increase intake gradually over 6 weeks. Bloating a side effect
Sitz baths	Patient sits in a shallow tub of warm water, to which some salt is added, for 15–20 min. Relieves pain and itching, relaxes perianal spasm, removes discharge, and assists with healing of raw areas
Medicated gels/ointments (all applied twice daily for 6–8 weeks)	Nitroglycerin 0.2–0.4% ointment Diltiazem gel or ointment 2% Nifedipine 0.3% with lidocaine 1.5% ointment Relieves pain and spasm and assists with healing
Botulinum toxin	Twenty units injected into the internal sphincter muscle on both sides. Relieves pain and spasm and assists healing
Surgical measures – In acute fissures not responding to non-operative measures and in chronic fissures	
Lateral internal sphincterotomy (LIS)	Full thickness of internal sphincter divided distal to the dentate line away from fissure (usually lateral). Relieves spasm and assists healing
Tailored LIS	Sphincterotomy stops at the apex of the fissure. Relieves spasm and lessens risk of incontinence compared to LIS
Subcutaneous fissurotomy, anal advancement flap	In patients with preexisting continence problems or in those with normal sphincter tone (postpartum women) Sphincter not divided Less risk of postoperative incontinence

[a]Usually continued for 6 weeks

supplementation, bulk laxatives, sitz baths, topical corticosteroid, local anesthetic, or medicated creams (nitroglycerin ointment, diltiazem gel, and nifedipine with lidocaine ointment) (Table 1). They relieve constipation and minimize sphincter spasm and pain, hastening healing, and should probably be continued for 6 weeks in acute fissures before surgery is considered. Injecting botulinum toxin (Botox) relaxes the internal sphincter hastening cure. Topical nifedipine with Botox injection induces lasting healing in chronic fissures [19]. Surgery is, however, consistently superior to medical therapy in chronic fissures and may be offered without initial conservative treatment failure [17].

Lateral internal sphincterotomy (open or closed) is the recommended surgical treatment for acute anal fissures not responding to conservative treatment and in chronic fissures (Table 1) [17]. The internal sphincter muscle distal to the dentate line is incised laterally (as most fissures are anteroposterior), decreasing sphincter pressure and promoting healing. The upper third of the sphincter and the anal mucosa remains intact, maintaining continence. The sentinel pile may be resected at the same sitting. Sphincterotomy

relieves pain (95%) and results in healing in most (93.3%) patients with chronic fissures [20]. Resulting incontinence to flatus and liquid stool is potentially minimized by halting the sphincterotomy at the apex of the fissure (tailored sphincterotomy) rather than extending it to the dentate line [17]. Patients with preexisting continence problems or normal sphincter tone may benefit from techniques that preserve the internal anal sphincter (anal advancement flap and subcutaneous fissurotomy). Combining sphincterotomy or anal advancement flap with Botox injection decreases post-procedure pain, enhances healing, and minimizes fecal incontinence [17].

Anorectal Abscess

Pathogenesis and Classification

Anorectal abscesses originate from cryptoglandular infections at the dentate line (occluded anal gland duct with superimposed bacterial overgrowth and suppuration) [21, 22]. Anorectal abscesses may be perianal, ischiorectal, intersphincteric, or supralevator. A perianal abscess (most common) is a collection of pus in the perianal tissues. The abscess may extend into the ischiorectal fossa (ischiorectal abscess – unilateral or bilateral), forming a horseshoe-shaped collection, or, more rarely, tracks upwards between the sphincters (intersphincteric) and through the levator ani musculature (supralevator). The infection is generally polymicrobial, involving both gram-negative organisms and anaerobes, indigenous to the gut.

Diagnosis

Patients with perianal abscess present with perianal swelling and throbbing pain, aggravated by pressure and defecation. Systemic symptoms (fever, chills, vomiting, and diaphoresis) characterizing sepsis are generally absent. Ischiorectal and higher-level suppurations often result in dull throbbing perianal or pelvic pain, low back or buttock pain, and systemic symptoms [22, 23]. Physical examination reveals a brawny red, extremely tender, indurated perianal mass. DRE is extremely uncomfortable but might reveal induration extending along the lateral anorectal wall in an intersphincteric or ischiorectal abscess. Supralevator abscesses usually have few local physical findings. Associated anal fistulas may be observed in over half of patients (30–70%) [22].

Treatment

Incision and drainage (under local anesthesia with or without conscious sedation) is the treatment of choice in perianal abscess [21, 22]. The incision is deepened to enter the abscess cavity; any slough is removed, the cavity is irrigated with saline and a drain left in, or the cavity is packed loosely; the raw area heals by secondary intention. Antibiotics, unnecessary in uncomplicated perianal infections, do not decrease recurrences or healing times [21, 22]. Antibiotics effective against both aerobes and anaerobes are a consideration in diabetics, in those immunosuppressed, in those with extensive perianal cellulitis or prosthetic devices, and in those with systemic sepsis. Over a third of patients may have

recurrent perianal infection or a fistula following drainage, more frequent in those under 40 years of age [24]. Patients with ischiorectal or intersphincteric abscesses may require a more formal drainage procedure under general anesthesia; any associated fistulous tract is laid open at the time of abscess drainage, or a seton (suture, rubber band, Silastic vessel loop) is left in the fistulous tract, and the abscess cavity is allowed to heal. Internal sphincterotomy is useful in draining intersphincteric abscesses into the anal canal. Concomitant simple fistulas may be laid at the time of abscess drainage.

The diagnosis of supralevator (pelvic) abscess usually requires initial confirmation by imaging (US or CT) to delineate its extent and determine the underlying cause (IBD, appendicitis, cancer) [25]. These patients usually require a combination of broad-spectrum antibiotics, imaging-assisted drainage, and treatment of the underlying cause. A temporary colostomy for fecal diversion may be necessary to enable resolution of distal (anorectal) infection.

Anorectal Fistula

Pathogenesis and Classification

Anorectal fistula (fistula-in-ano) is an abnormal tract connecting the anorectum to the perianal skin lined with granulation tissue and producing a mucopurulent or feculent perianal discharge. Most follow cryptoglandular infection and spontaneous rupture or drainage of a perianal abscess and denote continued perianal infection and/or formation of an epithelialized tract [22]. Anorectal fistulas may also complicate IBD, radiation, cancer, actinomycosis, lymphogranuloma venereum (LGV), tuberculosis, trauma including obstetrical injuries, and foreign body. It is twice as common in adult males; among infants it is seen solely in boys.

Anorectal fistulas are classified into intersphincteric (type 1, fistulous tract in the intersphincteric plane, most common, 45%), transsphincteric (type 2, tract passing from the anal canal through the external sphincter to the ischiorectal fossa, 30%), suprasphincteric (type 3, tract passing from the anal canal along the intersphincteric plane and over the puborectalis muscle into the ischiorectal fossa, 20%), and extrasphincteric (type 4, tract outside the sphincter complex passing through the ischiorectal fat and levator ani muscles connecting the rectum and the skin, least common, 5%) [26]. Fistulas may also be designated as simple (most common, usually intersphincteric and low transsphincteric fistulas) or complex (high transsphincteric, extrasphincteric, or suprasphincteric fistulas) based on the risk of fecal incontinence following surgery. Anterior fistulas in women and fistulas associated with IBD (Crohn's disease) and cancer or following radiation are also considered complex [27].

Diagnosis

Symptoms include perianal pain and swelling followed by purulent or bloodstained perianal drainage and dyschezia. Passing bowel contents through the perianal opening indicates a high (rectal) internal opening. History of abscess drainage (in 50% of patients), other anorectal surgery, radiation, or pelvic trauma may be present. Perianal examination and DRE may reveal redness, swelling, induration, fluctuance, and external openings of fistulas with drainage or granulations. "Goodsall's rule" states that all fistulous tracts posterior to a line, drawn between the ischial spines with external openings within 3 cm of the anal margin, have a curvilinear course to the posterior midline of the anal canal. Tracks with anterior external openings originate from the nearest crypt and have a straight course to the anal canal.

Proctosigmoidoscopy is useful in visualizing the internal opening(s) and may show other mucosal abnormalities such as proctitis [27]. Imaging studies (endoanal ultrasound, CT, MRI) are useful in defining anatomy and guiding management in patients with complex fistulas.

Treatment

The goal of treatment is to obliterate the fistulous tract and openings while causing negligible sphincter disruption and maintaining continence. Treatment is determined by the etiology and anatomy of the fistula, degree of symptoms, and patient comorbidities [27]. Asymptomatic fistulas associated with Crohn's disease do not need treatment. Fistulotomy (fistulous tract laid open and allowed to heal) is highly successful, maintains continence, and is recommended for simple perianal fistulas, including Crohn's fistulas; marsupialization (suturing mucocutaneous edges) may further enhance wound healing [22, 27]. Coexisting abscesses are drained. Complex or recurrent fistulas, prior surgery, female sex, preexisting incontinence, and Crohn's disease increase risk of persisting or recurrent infection and postsurgical incontinence. Ligation of the intersphincteric tract (LIFT procedure) is an effective treatment option in simple and complex transsphincteric fistulas with little morbidity and high success [22]. Fistulectomy (complete excision of the tract and surrounding tissue in one block) results in larger tissue defects, requires longer healing times, and produces more incontinence while not improving recurrence rates. Anal fistulas in infants and children respond well to abscess drainage and antibiotics; immediate fistulotomy is avoided.

Debridement of the fistulous tract and injection of fibrin glue is an option in both simple and complex anal fistulas, especially in patients at risk for incontinence [22, 27]. A bioprosthetic anal fistula plug closing the internal opening, endoanal advancement flaps, and passing a seton (suture, rubber band, Silastic vessel loop) through the fistula tract to initiate a foreign body reaction and scarring are other options in treating complex fistulas. The seton is gradually tightened to cut through the fistula; fibrosis maintains sphincter integrity. Both fibrin glue and the fistula plug have been found to be relatively ineffective in recent studies with healing rates under 50% [22].

Perianal involvement including fistulas may be seen in over half of patients with Crohn's disease. Medical measures result in healing in many patients [27]. Surgical approaches, though less effective with higher recurrence rates, are useful. Permanent fecal diversion or proctectomy is rarely required for severe persisting disease [27].

Initial non-operative treatment of rectovaginal fistulas following obstetric injuries for 3–6 months (treating infection, wound care) promotes healing in over half of patients [22]. Using a seton results in symptomatic relief and encourages resolution of infection. Endorectal advancement flap with or without sphincteroplasty is optimal for most simple rectovaginal fistulas. More complex or high rectovaginal fistulas associated with fecal incontinence may require extensive excisional and reconstructive procedures (episioproctotomy, proctectomy with coloanal anastomosis, gracilis or bulbocavernosus muscle flap reconstruction).

Anal Incontinence

Background

Anal incontinence is the inability to control the evacuation of bowel contents (flatus or feces) or recurrent uncontrolled passage of fecal material [28]. It is frequently seen among the elderly (over 65) and approaches 50% among nursing home residents, many of whom are also incontinent of urine. Fecal incontinence is twice as common among Caucasian as in African-American women. Functional limitations, hypertension, neurological disorders, obesity, physical inactivity, pregnancy, smoking, and type 2 diabetes mellitus also increase its prevalence [29]. Fecal incontinence may also follow anatomical or physiological changes resulting from trauma, surgery or disease, changes in stool characteristics, cognitive deficits, malabsorption, medications, or underlying psychiatric conditions (Table 2) [28]. Congenital anomalies, developmental disorders, encopresis (fecal retention), and mental retardation are the predominant causes among children [28]. Incontinence causes significant limitations in social interactions and loss of self-esteem and increases health-care costs.

Diagnosis

A problem-specific history should be obtained [28, 30]. Examination should address the patient's general well-being with particular focus on neurological disorders and deficits and abdominal and anorectal pathology. Generalized weakness, balance and gait disturbances, and need for ambulatory aids imply functional incontinence. A speculum and a digital rectovaginal examination may detect perineal and anal hypotonia and intrarectal pathology. Contracting the perianal muscles over the palpating digit also helps assess pelvic floor integrity. Pelvic organ prolapse is best evaluated by asking the squatting patient to strain (Valsalva). Proctosigmoidoscopy detects rectal ulcers associated with prolapse, IBD, and neoplasms. Colonoscopy is recommended in patients ≥50 years.

Imaging and physiologic studies complement clinical evaluation. Endoanal ultrasound (EUS) identifies sphincter defects in suspected sphincter injury. Anal manometry evaluates maximum resting and squeeze pressures in the anal canal, the rectoanal inhibitory reflex, and the rectal sensation and compliance. Most patients with fecal incontinence have manometric abnormalities. Electromyography (EMG) identifies injury to the sphincter muscles. Pudendal nerve terminal motor latency (PNTML) measures intactness of the pudendal nerve-anal sphincter neuromuscular unit; PNTML abnormalities correlate well with poor surgical outcomes. Scoring systems incorporating the patient's subjective experience of fecal incontinence as well as its effect on quality of life help select patient for treatment and evaluate treatment results [30].

Treatment

Goals of treatment are to reestablish normal evacuation, improve lifestyle, and restore functional capacity. Conservative measures improve continence, quality of life, psychological well-being, anal sphincter function, and patient coping strategies. Mucocutaneous and soft tissue complications (skin excoriations, decubitus ulcers, abscesses) should be handled through judicious drainage, antibiotics, antifungals and barrier creams, or, in extreme cases, temporary or permanent fecal diversion until healing is complete.

Table 2 Common causes and mechanisms of fecal incontinence (Modified from text in Ref. [28])

Enumeration of causes	Mechanism
Congenital Anorectal anomalies – Rectal agenesis, imperforate anus Spina bifida – Meningocele, meningomyelocele	Sphincter weakness, impaired anorectal sensation, loss of stool awareness, pudendal neuropathy
Trauma (including surgery) to pelvic floor muscles, pudendal nerve, and the spinal cord Anorectal surgery Colon resection Pelvic and anorectal trauma, spinal trauma Vaginal delivery – Spontaneous or assisted	Possible sphincter weakness, pudendal neuropathy, impaired rectal accommodation
Neurological impairment Cerebrovascular accident Dementia (Alzheimer's disease, multi-infarct dementia, normal pressure hydrocephalus) Diabetes mellitus Intracranial injury Meningoencephalitis Multiple sclerosis Neoplasm (brain, spinal cord) Pudendal neuropathy due to trauma or traction injury Spina bifida (meningocele, meningomyelocele)	Impaired anorectal sensation, pelvic floor dysfunction, loss of stool awareness, impaired rectal accommodation
Miscellaneous Anorectal prolapse Fecal impaction Malabsorption Medications (anticholinergic agents, antidepressants, caffeine, laxatives, muscle relaxants) Physical disabilities (due to aging, disease, or trauma) Proctitis (inflammatory bowel disease, radiation) Psychiatric disorders	Pelvic floor dysfunction, altered stool characteristics, anorectal hypersensitivity, wilful soiling, functional incontinence

Underlying IBD, diabetes mellitus, or malabsorption should be treated [28]. Agents precipitating inappropriate stooling (laxatives) are avoided. Increasing dietary fiber improves stool consistency; antidiarrheal agents reduce frequency and urgency in stooling [30]. Patients with fecal impaction benefit from disimpaction through suppositories, enemas, or manual evacuation, followed by using stool softeners and laxatives (polyethylene glycol), bowel retraining (regular toilet use after meals), and treating underlying behavioral problems.

Biofeedback (neuromuscular training) is a first-line treatment option in motivated patients with some preserved sphincter tone and impaired rectal sensation not responding to conservative measures [30]. It is often combined with pelvic floor muscle exercises and stimulation to enhance pelvic floor strength.

Disposable anal plugs alleviate fecal leak and seepage but are difficult to tolerate. Injecting biocompatible material into the anorectal submucosa or the intersphincteric space augments the perianal/perirectal tissue and approximates the anal mucosa, thereby closing the anal canal and/or raising the anorectal pressure to avert fecal incontinence [30]. Short-term improvement is noticed in over half of patients [31].

Surgery should be considered in patients who have failed conservative measures and neuromuscular training. Patients with significant symptoms and a defined defect of the external anal sphincter benefit from sphincteroplasty by plication or imbrication (85% good to excellent short-term results; 10–14% sustained improvement at 5 years) [30]. Those with more extensive sphincter damage may need an autologous gracilis or gluteus muscle transfer (dynamic graciloplasty) or implantation of an artificial bowel sphincter. Both procedures have significant potential complications, and long-term outcomes are not encouraging. Sacral nerve stimulation, in which electrodes are implanted in the second and third sacral nerve roots, stimulating the muscles of the pelvic floor appears to achieve greater than 50% improvement in most (89%) patients and full continence in over a third (36%) of patients [30, 32]. Children and patients with neurological disorders benefit from an antegrade continent enema procedure that offers periodic colon washout through an appendicostomy or a cecostomy. Permanent fecal diversion is another alternative in paralyzed, immobile patients with non-healing decubitus ulcers.

Rectal Prolapse

Background

Rectal prolapse is defined as protrusion of the layers of the rectal wall through the anal canal. The prolapse may be mucosal (partial), when only the mucosal and submucosal layers protrude, or full thickness (complete), when all layers overhang the anal canal [33]. It is seen more often among older women (sixfold increase compared to men); men tend to present at younger ages. Rectal prolapse is thought to commence as an intussusception from the rectosigmoid region at the level of the peritoneal reflection, progressing distally through the anal canal on continued exertion. Multiple factors predispose to rectal prolapse (Table 3).

Diagnosis

Patients present with dull perianal pain, rectal bleeding or mucorrhea, and fecal/urinary incontinence. Irreducibility and strangulation of the prolapsed segment cause severe and persistent perianal and abdominal pain and distention, fever, vomiting, and diaphoresis; gangrene may supervene. Perianal inspection is best accomplished with the patient sitting or squatting, and it assists in differentiating full-thickness prolapse from mucosal prolapse or prolapsed hemorrhoids [34]. Mucosal prolapse is thin and often segmental; full-thickness prolapse may be segmental or circumferential, plum colored with concentric mucosal folds. Prolapse longer than 5 cm usually contains a fold of peritoneum; larger prolapses contain small bowel. DRE identifies anal sphincter hypotonia; anoscopy may reveal a solitary rectal ulcer, present usually on the anterior rectal wall in 10–15% of patients [34]. Imaging studies, colonoscopy, and urodynamic studies are useful in further defining the diagnosis and identifying coexisting cystocele or colorectal pathology [34]. Physiologic tests (anorectal manometry, electromyography, and pudendal nerve testing) help identify and evaluate associated pelvic floor dysfunction and colonic inactivity [34].

Treatment

Non-operative approach yields poor results [34]. Increased fiber intake, fiber supplements, and stool softeners improve constipation, minimize straining, and may help heal rectal ulcers. Biofeedback is useful in retraining and enhancing sphincter function and improves continence and constipation following surgery [35]. Rubber band ligation or trans-anal excision is beneficial in patients with second–/third-degree mucosal prolapse without ulceration [36].

Transabdominal rectopexy is the procedure of choice in patients with full-thickness rectal prolapse, considered suitable for laparotomy [34, 37]. Laparoscopic approach has fewer postoperative complications and a shorter hospital course when compared with open rectopexy. Prosthetic meshes (polypropylene, polytetrafluoroethylene) are used to reinforce attachment of the mobilized rectum to the sacral promontory, inducing fibrosis and minimizing risk of recurrent prolapse and fecal incontinence. Rectopexy also helps heal

Table 3 Common causes of rectal prolapse in infants/children and adults

Infants/ children	Cystic fibrosis Disturbances in bowel function (chronic diarrhea, constipation) Hirschsprung's disease Parasitic infestations Poor nutritional status Neoplasms (polyps) Neurological disorders (spina bifida, meningocele, meningomyelocele)
Adults	Aging (age-related tissue degeneration, weakness, and intercurrent illness) Cerebrovascular accident Dementia Increased intra-abdominal pressure (chronic constipation, chronic cough, heavy lifting, obesity) Multiparity (direct injury to pelvic floor muscles, nerves, and connective tissues caused by maternal expulsive forces). Large fetus, prolonged second stage of labor, episiotomy, anal sphincter laceration, epidural analgesia, operative deliveries, and oxytocin use are also considered risk factors Pelvic floor muscle weakness following spinal or pelvic trauma including surgery Psychiatric illness Pudendal neuropathy

Information from multiple sources

rectal ulcers. Coexisting uterovaginal prolapse may also be corrected (rectocolpopexy).

Perineal procedures (mucosal sleeve resection, Delorme procedure (mucosal sleeve resection and imbrication of the muscularis mucosa), perineal proctosigmoidectomy (Altemeier procedure involving trans-anal full-thickness resection of the prolapsed rectum and coloanal anastomosis)) are useful in older patients with multiple comorbidities unfit for laparotomy. Patients with short, full-thickness rectal prolapse may undergo the Delorme procedure; longer-segment prolapses require a proctosigmoidectomy.

Pruritus Ani

Background

Intense perianal itching (pruritus ani) is experienced by 1–5% of people, more often by men (2–4 times more common) between 30 and 60 years of age [38, 39]. The long-standing itch-scratch cycle eventually causes dryness and hyperpigmentation, infection, ulceration, and scarring of the involved skin. Irritability and depression often coexist [39]. Pruritus ani may be idiopathic; though in up to three-fourths of patients, an underlying local or systemic cause may be identified [40].

Causes

Hemorrhoids (20%), anal fissure (12%), idiopathic proctitis (6%), and condyloma/ulcerative proctitis (5%) are the predominant causes [38]. All these pathologies produce mucus or fecal soiling, initiating or aggravating the pruritus. Other causes include atopic and contact dermatitis, bacterial and fungal skin infections, clothing (retains moisture), medications (antibiotics, colchicine, laxatives, steroids), other dermatologic pathology (psoriasis, lichen planus, lichen sclerosis), parasitic infestations, systemic diseases (diabetes mellitus, hepatorenal disease, anemia, hyperthyroidism, and underlying anxiety), and various foods (alcohol, caffeinated drinks, chocolate, citrus fruits, milk products, peanuts, spices) [40].

Diagnosis

Diagnosis is usually based on history and examination focusing on the gastrointestinal tract and skin, including nails. The perianal region is closely inspected for primary perianal pathology and skin changes. Bacterial/fungal cultures and patch or Scotch tape testing establish the diagnosis of infections, parasitic infestations, or contact dermatitis. Endoscopy and biopsy are useful in diagnosing colitis. Manometric studies help diagnose motility disorders. Perianal skin biopsies may be required when the diagnosis is obscure or if a premalignant or cancerous lesion is suspected.

Treatment

The principles of management include ruling out secondary causes, eliminating all irritants (soaps, talcum powders, certain foods and fluids), avoiding trauma (scratching, vigorous scrubbing, using toilet paper), keeping the perianal skin clean and dry (cotton underclothes changed daily to minimize moisture accumulation, washing with water after stooling, and drying the skin), and ensuring regular bowel movements and normal consistency stool (increasing dietary fiber and adequate fluid intake) [41]. Using white, undyed, unscented toilet tissue minimizes allergic skin reactions. Those with diurnal hyperhidrosis should be encouraged to change their underclothes frequently to restrict perianal moisture accumulation. Low-potency steroids may help break the itch-scratch cycle. Underlying psychiatric issues (anxiety, obsessive-compulsive disorder) need treatment. Mittens or socks over hands may reduce nocturnal scratching. Vaseline may be applied locally if the skin is dry and thickened.

Topical capsaicin cream diluted in paraffin applied three times daily over 4 weeks relieves intractable perianal pruritus in over 70% of patients [42]. Perianal intradermal injection of methylene blue (15 ml of a 1% solution diluted with 0.5% lidocaine) also eases symptoms in a majority (60%) of patients with intractable pruritus, the improvement persisting over 4 years [43]. Tacrolimus ointment (0.035–0.1% applied 1–2 times daily) has also been shown to improve symptoms [41].

Infectious Proctitis

Background

Proctitis is defined as an inflammation of the anorectal mucosa, usually seen in adult males. Causes include sexually transmitted diseases (STDs – gonorrhea, chlamydia, syphilis, genital herpes), chemical irritation, IBD, ischemia, radiation, trauma, and miscellaneous causes (immune deficiency, vasculitis, other infections – amebiasis, *Clostridium difficile* infection, campylobacter infection) [44]. Radiation proctitis may be acute or chronic, and its incidence is probably related to radiation dosage, area of exposure, method of delivery, and use of cytoprotective agents [45].

Diagnosis

Patients usually present with perianal or lower abdominal pain, blood or mucus per rectum, change in bowel habits (diarrhea or constipation), sense of incomplete defecation, and tenesmus. Abdominal examination may show lower abdominal fullness and tenderness. Proctosigmoidoscopy may reveal mucosal edema, erythema, friability, bleeding, ulceration, inflammatory exudate, or herpetic vesicles limited to the anorectum. In chronic radiation proctitis, mucosal pallor, changes in vascularity, strictures, ulcerations, and fistulas may be seen [45]. The anal discharge can be analyzed (gram stain, nucleic acid detection and DNA amplification tests, and bacterial, fungal, or viral cultures) to identify specific infections. Stool studies (ova, cysts, parasites, *Clostridium difficile* toxin, and antigen) also help diagnose bacterial infections and parasitic infestations [46]. Endoscopy is useful in detecting proximal bowel involvement, especially in IBD; biopsies may be obtained for confirmation. Contrast imaging assists in detecting obstruction and fistula formation – consequences of IBD and radiation.

Treatment

The principles of management include providing symptomatic relief and addressing primary causes (Table 4). Antispasmodics and a low-residue diet relieve diarrhea and tenesmus. Steroid or mesalamine enemas are useful in patients with IBD. Antibiotics and antivirals administered appropriately help resolve specific infections [46]. Campylobacter proctitis and acute radiation

Table 4 Treatment options in proctitis Refs. [44–48]

General measures	Hydration, analgesics, and antidiarrheals in acute proctitis Low-residue diet Antispasmodics
Cause-specific treatment	
Campylobacter infection	Erythromycin 500 mg twice daily for 5 days
Chlamydia infection	Doxycycline 100 mg orally twice daily for 7 days. Three-week therapy in men intimate with men and if HIV+
Crohn's colitis/proctitis	5-ASA (foam, gel, suppository, enema) Oral mesalamine 2.4 G daily in divided doses Topical steroids (enemas, foam, suppositories) In patients failing to respond to topicals – Oral 5-ASA/mesalamine Oral prednisone (20 to 60 mg daily) – In patients not responding to topical steroids Azathioprine 1.5–2.5 mg/kg/day orally – Patients not responding to or dependent on steroids. Used as steroid-sparing therapy
Giardiasis	Metronidazole 750 mg orally three times daily for 10 days followed by paromomycin 25–30 mg/kg per day three times daily for 7 days for eradication of cysts in bowel lumen
Gonococcal proctitis	Ceftriaxone 250 mg IM once + doxycycline 100 mg orally twice daily for 7 days
Herpes simplex proctitis	Acyclovir 400 mg three times daily for 7–10 days Famciclovir 250 mg three times daily for 7–10 days Valacyclovir 1G orally twice daily for 7–10 days
Shigella infection	Ciprofloxacin 500 mg orally twice daily for 7 days
Radiation proctitis	
Grade 1 [a]	Watchful waiting
Grades 2 and 3	Anti-inflammatory agents (oral sulfasalazine or mesalamine, steroid enemas, oral steroids, oral metronidazole) Antioxidants (vitamins A, C, E)
Grades 2 and 3 (no response to anti-inflammatories)	Rectal sucralfate or pentosan polysulfate Short-chain fatty acid enemas Hyperbaric oxygen at 2 atm for 90 min
Grade 3 (no response to above measures)	Chemical cauterization – Formaldehyde 10% applied for 2–3 min Endoscopic coagulation Argon or YAG laser photocoagulation
Grade 4	Surgery (fecal/urinary diversion, local excision, stricturoplasty, pelvic exenteration). Often requires reconstruction using vascularized flaps

[a]Grading based on intensity of symptoms, degree of ulceration and stricture, and presence of complications (hemorrhage, fistula, perforation, obstruction). Grade 0, no symptoms; grades 1–3, increasing intensity of symptoms; grade 4, uncontrollable pain/urgency or development of complications; grade 5, sepsis, multiple organ failure usually resulting in demise

proctitis are usually self-limiting; the latter resolves with discontinuing radiation for short periods. Chronic radiation proctitis may require more intensive management depending on its extent (grade) and symptomatology and may involve the use of anti-inflammatory agents (oral sulfasalazine with steroid enemas), sucralfate enemas, short chain fatty acid, or pentosan polysulfate enemas or oral metronidazole. Antioxidants (vitamins A, C, and E) reduce diarrhea and tenesmus and supplement the beneficial effects of other treatment measures [45]. Hyperbaric oxygen, administered at 2 atm daily five times a week, improves symptoms probably by enhancing tissue oxygenation, impeding bacterial overgrowth and toxin production, and stimulating angiogenesis [47]. Topical formalin (10%) applied during proctosigmoidoscopy cauterizes and seals the fragile vessels in radiation-damaged tissues. Endoscopic electrocoagulation and laser photocoagulation are other options to control refractory bleeding. Surgery is reserved for patients with uncontrollable pain, fistula, bleeding, fecal incontinence, and obstruction and may involve a diverting colostomy, stricturoplasty, or pelvic exenteration [45, 48].

Hidradenitis Suppurativa

Background

Hidradenitis suppurativa is a chronic recurrent inflammatory skin disorder affecting the hair and areas containing apocrine sweat glands and adjacent connective tissue; perineal involvement occurs more often in men [49]. Pathophysiology involves occlusion of the ducts of the hair follicles, stasis and dilatation of the apocrine glands, secondary bacterial infection, abscess formation, development of sinuses and fistulas, and ultimately fibrosis and hypertrophic scarring. Cryptoglandular infections or Crohn's disease may coexist.

Diagnosis

Diagnosis is clinical and based on the characteristic history and physical findings of chronically draining sinuses with malodorous discharge and hypertrophic skin [7]. Proctosigmoidoscopy may show evidence of anal gland infections or IBD. Incontinence, lymphedema, and malignant transformation to squamous cell carcinoma (rare) are all possible sequelae.

Treatment

Treatment is usually prolonged and unsatisfactory in advanced stages. Broad-spectrum antibiotics (clindamycin, tetracyclines, rifampin) administered orally or applied topically reduce pain, redness, and discharge. Abscesses need drainage and sinus tracts may be de-roofed or marsupialized. Isotretinoin is useful, though contraindicated in women of childbearing age due to potential teratogenicity. Immunosuppressants (steroids, cyclosporine, infliximab, etanercept) also show promise but increase risk of concurrent infections and malignancy. Radiation, cryotherapy, and laser surgery are other options. Wide excision of the involved skin and underlying connective tissue followed by skin grafting or flap closure may be necessary in recalcitrant disease and, rarely, may also require temporary fecal diversion [49].

Condyloma Acuminatum

Background

Anal condyloma acuminatum (warts) is caused by sexual (usual) or nonsexual transmission of the human papillomavirus (HPV); most (>95%) are caused by types 6 and 11 [50]. These warts are more frequent in men who have sex with men and practicing receptive anal intercourse, in those with multiple sexual partners, and in the immunosuppressed, in whom the warts are more aggressive, relapse earlier, and are more often dysplastic [7]. Buschke-Löwenstein tumor (giant condyloma acuminata) is a rare and rapidly progressing variant, locally invasive, causing extensive destruction of surrounding tissue [7].

Diagnosis

Perianal warts are typically asymptomatic, but depending on the size and location of the warts, they may cause pain, itching, drainage, foul odor, bleeding, or dyschezia. Patients may also exhibit anxiety, guilt, anger, and loss of self-esteem [50]. Anal warts may be perianal or intra-anal; the diagnosis is made by visual inspection [46]. The lesions are usually found over sites traumatized during intercourse, vary from 5 to 15 in number, and, occasionally, coalesce into plaques (more common in diabetics and the immunosuppressed) [50]. Proctoscopy displays the intra-anal condyloma, usually confined below the dentate line. Biopsy confirms the diagnosis and rules out malignancy, and HPV typing categorizes the lesion as pertaining to low- and high-risk subtypes. Biopsy is, however, required only in failure of response to usual treatment measures, if dysplasia or malignancy is suspected, or in immunosuppressed patients. Complete genital examination should be performed to check for penile, scrotal, and cervicovaginal lesions; women should be offered a Papanicolaou (PAP) smear. Anal warts in children should arouse suspicion of sexual abuse, though vertical transmission at birth is possible.

Screening, Prevention, and Treatment

Current sexual partners as well as partners within the last 6 months should be screened for warts and other STDs. Condom use should be encouraged to minimize recurrence and infecting partners. Smoking cessation measures should be implemented. Both sexes between 9 and 26 years of age should be offered the quadrivalent HPV vaccine (Gardasil) to prevent infection by high-risk strains 6, 11, 16, and 18 [7, 50].

Multiple patient-applied local therapies (podofilox 0.5% solution or gel applied twice daily for 3 days a week (four such cycles), imiquimod 5% cream applied daily at bedtime for 16 weeks, sinecatechin 15% ointment applied three times daily for 16 weeks) are available [7, 46, 50]. They may all cause local redness, burning, induration, and ulceration. Both sinecatechin and podofilox are not yet considered safe for use during pregnancy. Clearance rates of 40–70% have been noticed with these treatment modalities [50]. Office therapies include application of acetic acid solutions, cryotherapy and electrosurgery, laser surgery, or scissor excision. Trichloro- or bichloroacetic acid 80–90% solution applied weekly works by coagulating proteins and is safe for use during pregnancy. Cryotherapy using liquid nitrogen is also safe during pregnancy but may also need to be repeated at regular intervals. Pain, irritation, and drainage are side effects of the treatment. Response rates parallel that of patient-applied therapies. Electrosurgical excision and destruction (fulguration) are also effective for removing condyloma. The smoke plume generated during destruction carries HPV particles; hence, there should be appropriate smoke evacuation techniques, and both patients and healthcare providers should wear masks to prevent inhalation of the particles. Scissor excision under local anesthesia using lidocaine with epinephrine to minimize pain and bleeding is useful where smaller numbers of lesions are involved. Both electrosurgery and sharp excision have high success rates (90–100%). Larger warts, especially in children, intra-anal warts, and Buschke-Löwenstein lesions require excision under general anesthesia. Recombinant interferon alpha may be injected under lesions or used as adjuvant therapy after surgical excision or fulguration [46, 50–51].

Anal Canal Cancers

Squamous cell carcinoma (SCC) is the most common type of malignancy in the anal canal (80%) followed by adenocarcinomas (16%) [7]. A strong causal relationship (86–100%) exists between oncogenic strains of HPV (types 16 and 18), immunosuppressive states (HIV, autoimmune diseases, transplant recipients), and SCC. Anal intraepithelial neoplasias (high grade, low grade) are precursors of SCC; the risk is higher in HIV-positive individuals, males in mutual conjugal relationships, and women with history of cervical dysplasia [51]. Screening high-risk populations with anal cytology or high-resolution anoscopy is a consideration. Universal vaccination against HPV in both sexes under 26 years of age is strongly recommended for primary prevention of premalignant lesions.

Half of patients with SCC manifest localized disease, the rest with regional nodal or distant metastases. Most patients with anal canal cancers present with a slow-growing intra-anal or perianal mass, bleeding (most common symptom – 45%), discharge, pain, and occasionally inguinal lymph node or intra-abdominal masses due to hepatic metastases. The diagnosis is evident in most patients on examination of the perianal region, DRE, and anoscopy. Biopsies from the primary and enlarged inguinal nodes should be taken for confirmation of the diagnosis and spread. The extent of thoracoabdominal spread should be evaluated by imaging of the chest, abdomen, and pelvis; endoanal ultrasound and MRI delineate the extent of local spread into the sphincters and perirectal lymph nodes. Chemotherapy (mitomycin-C and 5-fluorouracil) and radiation are the recommended treatment modalities for both the anal canal primary and inguinal disease (80% complete response rates); small superficial node-negative localized lesions may be excised with a 1 cm margin. Cisplatin may be substituted for 5-fluorouracil. Abdominoperineal resection of the rectum and anal canal is an option in recurrent or persisting disease (seen in 20–30% of patients) and has a 50% cure rate [7]. Presence of distant metastases denotes poor prognosis with median survivals under 1 year. Continued surveillance after chemoradiation or surgery is recommended with history, physical examination including DRE and anoscopy, and imaging at regular intervals for 5 years. Systemic chemotherapy, metastasectomy, and epidermal growth factor inhibitors are treatment options in those with widespread disease.

Melanoma of the anal canal usually has a poor outcome as most patients have widespread metastases at the time of diagnosis. Wide excision or abdominoperineal resection may be offered for local control in patients with disseminated disease.

References

1. Barleben A, Mills S. Anorectal anatomy and physiology. Surg Clin North Am. 2010;90(1):1–15.
2. Sneider EB, Maykel JA. Diagnosis and management of symptomatic hemorrhoids. Surg Clin North Am. 2010;90(1):17–32.
3. Johanson JF, Sonnenberg A. Temporal changes in the occurrence of hemorrhoids in the United States and England. Dis Colon Rectum. 1991;34(7):585–93.
4. Rivadeneira DE, Steele SR, Ternent C, Chalasani S, Buie WD, Rafferty JL. Standards practice task force of the American society of colon and rectal surgeons. Practice parameters for the management of hemorrhoids (revised 2010). Dis Colon Rectum. 2011;54(9):1059–64.
5. Davis BR, Lee-Kong SA, Migaly J, Feingold DL, Steele SR. The American Society of Colon and Rectal Surgeons clinical practice guidelines for the management of hemorrhoids. Dis Colon Rectum. 2018;61(3):284–92.
6. Billingham RP, Isler JT, Kimmins MH, Nelson JM, Schweitzer J, Murphy MM. The diagnosis and management of common anorectal disorders. Curr Probl Surg. 2004;41(7):586–645.
7. Abdelnaby A, Marcus DJ. Chapter 129: Diseases of the anorectum. In: Feldman M, editor. Sleisenger and Fordtran's gastrointestinal and liver disease. 10th ed. Philadelphia: Saunders/Elsevier; 2016. p. 2316–36.
8. Alonso-Coello P, Castillejo MM. Office evaluation and treatment of hemorrhoids. J Fam Pract. 2003;52(5):366–74.
9. Tjandra JJ, Tan JJ, Lim JF, Murray-Green C, Kennedy ML, Lubowski DZ. Rectogesic (glyceryl trinitrate 0.2%) ointment relieves symptoms of haemorrhoids associated with high resting anal canal pressures. Color Dis. 2007;9(5):457–63.
10. Perrotti P, Dominici P, Grossi E, Cerruti R, Antropoli C. Topical nifedipine with lidocaine ointment versus active control for pain after hemorrhoidectomy: results of a multicentre, prospective, randomized, double-blind study. Can J Surg. 2010;53(1):17–24.
11. El Nakeeb AM, Fikry AA, Omar WH, Fouda EM, El Metwally TA, Ghazy HE, et al. Rubber band ligation for 750 cases of symptomatic hemorrhoids out of 2200 cases. World J Gastroenterol. 2008;14(42):6525–30.
12. Kanellos I, Goulimaris I, Vakalis I, Dadoukis I. Long-term evaluation of sclerotherapy for haemorrhoids. A prospective study. Int J Surg Investig. 2000;2(4):295–8.
13. Rajesh Kumar Rathore. Comparative study of management of second and third degree hemorrhoids with injection Sclerotherapy using Polidocanol. Int J Surg Sci 2019; 3(2): 145–147. https://doi.org/10.33545/surgery.2019.v3.i2c.30. Accessed 11 Nov 2019.
14. Xu L, Chen H, Lin G, Ge Q. Ligasure versus Ferguson hemorrhoidectomy in the treatment of hemorrhoids: a meta-analysis of randomized control trials. Surg Laparosc Endosc Percutan Tech. 2015;25(2):106–10.
15. Watson AJ, Hudson J, Wood J, Kilonzo M, Brown SR, McDonald A, et al. eTHoS study group. Comparison of stapled haemorrhoidopexy with traditional excisional surgery for haemorrhoidal disease (eTHoS): a pragmatic, multicenter, randomized control trial. Lancet. 2016;388(10058):2375–85.
16. Pucher PH, Sodergren MH, Lord AC, Darzi A, Ziprin P. Clinical outcome following Doppler-guided hemorrhoidal artery ligation: a systematic review. Color Dis. 2013;15(6):e284–94.
17. Stewart DB, Gaertner W, Glasgow S, Migaly J, Feingold D, Steele SR. Clinical practice guideline for the management of anal fissures. Dis Colon Rectum. 2017;60(1):7–14.
18. Herzig DO, Lu KC. Anal fissure. Surg Clin North Am. 2010;90(1):33–44.
19. Tranqui P, Trottier DC, Victor C, Freeman JB. Nonsurgical treatment of chronic anal fissure: nitroglycerin and dilatation versus nifedipine and botulinum toxin. Can J Surg. 2006;49(1):41–5.
20. Karamanlis E, Michalopoulos A, Papadopoulos V, Mekras A, Panagiotou D, Ioannidis A, et al. Prospective clinical trial comparing sphincterotomy, nitroglycerin ointment and xylocaine/lactulose combination for the treatment of anal fissure. Tech Coloproctol. 2010;14(Suppl 1):S21–3.

21. Whiteford MH, Kilkenny J 3rd, Hyman N, Buie WD, Cohen J, Orsay C. Standards practice task force. American society of colon and rectal surgeons. Practice parameters for the treatment of perianal abscess and fistula-in-ano (revised). Dis Colon Rectum. 2005; 48(7):1337–42.

22. Vogel JD, Johnson EK, Morris AM, Paquette IA, Saclarides TJ, Feingold DL, Steele SR. Clinical practice guideline for the management of anorectal abscess, fistula-in-ano, and rectovaginal fistula. Dis Colon Rectum. 2016;59(12):1117–33.

23. Rickard MJ. Anal abscesses and fistulas. ANZ J Surg. 2005;75(1):64–72.

24. Hamadani A, Haigh PI, Liu IL, Abbas MA. Who is at risk for developing chronic anal fistula or recurrent anal sepsis after initial perianal abscess? Dis Colon Rectum. 2009;52(2):217–21.

25. Ommer A, Herold A, Berg E, Furst A, Sailer M, Schiedeck T. German S3 guideline: anal abscess. Int J Colorectal Dis. 2012;27(6): 831–7.

26. Parks AG, Gordon PH, Hardcastle JD. A classification of fistula-in-ano. Br J Surg. 1976;63(1):1–12.

27. Steele SR, Kumar R, Feingold DL, Rafferty JL, Buie WD. Standards practice task force of the American Society of Colon and Rectal Surgeons. Practice parameters for the management of perianal abscess and fistula-in-ano. Dis Colon Rectum. 2011;54(12):1465–74.

28. Rao SSC. Chapter 18: Fecal incontinence. In: Feldman M, Friedman LS, Brandt LJ, editors. Feldman: Sleisenger and Fordtran's gastrointestinal and liver disease. 10th ed. Philadelphia: Saunders; 2016. p. 251–70.

29. Townsend MK, Matthews CA, Whitehead WE, Grodstein F. Risk factors for fecal incontinence in older women. Am J Gastroenterol. 2013;108(1):113–9.

30. Paquette IM, Varma MG, Kaiser AM, Steele SR, Rafferty JF. The American society of colon and rectal surgeons' clinical practice guideline for the treatment of fecal incontinence. Dis Colon Rectum. 2015;58(7): 623–36.

31. Maeda Y, Laurberg S, Norton C. Perianal injectable bulking agents as treatment for faecal incontinence in adults. Cochrane Database Syst Rev. 2013;2:CD007959.

32. Hull T, Giese C, Wexner SD, Mellgren A, Devroede G, Madoff RD, Stromberg K, Coller JA, SNS Study Group. Dis Colon Rectum. 2013;56(2):234–45.

33. Felt-Bersma E, Stella MTE, Cuesta MA. Rectal prolapse, rectal intussusceptions, rectocele, solitary rectal ulcer syndrome and enterocele. Gastroenterol Clin N Am. 2008;37(3):645–68.

34. Bordeianou L, Paquette I, Johnson E, Holubar SD, Gaertner W, Feingold DL, Steele SR. Clinical practice guidelines for the treatment of rectal prolapse. Dis Colon Rectum. 2017;60(11):1121–31.

35. Kairaluoma M, Raivio P, Kupila J, Aarino M, Kellokumpu I. The role of biofeedback therapy in functional proctologic disorders. Scand J Surg. 2004;93(3):184–90.

36. Pescatori M, Quondamarcio C. A new grading of rectal internal mucosal prolapse and its correlation with diagnosis and treatment. Int J Color Dis. 1999;14(4–5):245–9.

37. Brown AJ, Anderson JH, McKee RF, Finlay IG. Strategy for selection of type of operation for rectal prolapse based on clinical criteria. Dis Colon Rectum. 2004;47(1):103–7.

38. Daniel GL, Longo WE, Vernava AM 3rd. Pruritus ani. Causes and concerns. Dis Colon Rectum. 1994;37(7): 670–4.

39. Chaudhry V, Bastawrous A. Idiopathic pruritus ani. Semin Colon Rectal Surg. 2003;14(4):196–202.

40. Siddiqi S, Vijay V, Ward M, Mahendran R, Warren S. Pruritus ani. Ann R Coll Surg Engl. 2008;90(6): 457–63.

41. Siddika A. A review of the therapeutic interventions in the management of pruritus ani. Invest Dermatol Venerol Res. 2017;3(1):91–102.

42. Lysy J, Sistiery-Ittah M, Israelit Y, et al. Topical capsaicin – a novel and effective treatment for idiopathic intractable pruritus ani: a randomized, placebo controlled, crossover study. Gut. 2003;52(9):1323–6.

43. Samalavicius NE, Poskus T, Gupta RK, Lunevicius R. Long-term results of single intradermal 1% methylene blue injection for intractable idiopathic pruritus ani: a prospective study. Tech Coloproctol. 2012;16(4): 295–9.

44. Irizarry L. Acute proctitis. Medscape. 2018. http://emedicine.medscape.com/article/775952. Accessed 24 Dec 2019.

45. Do NL, Nagle D, Poylin VY. Radiation proctitis: current strategies in management. Gastroenterol Res Pract 2011. http://www.hindawi.com/journals/grp/2011/917941/. Accessed 23 Dec 2019.

46. Workowski KA, Bolan GA. Sexually transmitted diseases treatment guidelines 2015. MMWR 2015; 64(3): 1–138. https://www.cdc.gov/std/tg2015/tg-2015-print. pdf. Accessed 24 Dec 2019.

47. Paquette IM, Vogel JD, Abbas MA, Feingold DL, Steele SR. The American society of colon and rectal surgeons clinical practice guidelines for the treatment of chronic radiation proctitis. Dis Colon Rectum. 2018;61(10):1135–40.

48. Tabaja L, Sidani SM. Management of radiation proctitis. Did Dis Sci. 2018;63(10):2180–8.

49. Asgeirsson T, Nunoo R, Luchtefeld MA. Hidradenitis suppurativa and pruritus ani. Clin Colon Rectal Surg. 2011;24(1):71–80.

50. Gilson R, Nugent D, Werner RN, Ballesteros J, Ross J. 2019. European guidelines for the management of anogenital warts. https://www.iusti.org/regions/europe/pdf/2019/IUSTIguidelinesHPV2019.pdf. Accessed 23 Dec 2019.

51. Stewart DB, Gaertner WB, Glasgow SC, Herzig DO, Feingold D, Steele SR. The American society of colon and rectal surgeons clinical practice guidelines for anal squamous cell cancer (revised 2018). Dis Colon Rectum. 2018;61(7):755–74.

Colorectal Cancer

Thad Wilkins, Jillian Soto, Temitope I. Afon, and
Dean A. Seehusen

Contents

T. Wilkins (✉) · J. Soto · T. I. Afon · D. A. Seehusen
Department of Family Medicine, Medical College of
Georgia, Augusta University, Augusta, GA, USA
e-mail: jwilkins@augusta.edu; JSOTO@augusta.edu;
TAFON@augusta.edu; DSEEHUSEN@augusta.edu

© Springer Nature Switzerland AG 2022
P. M. Paulman et al. (eds.), *Family Medicine*,
https://doi.org/10.1007/978-3-030-54441-6_183

General Principles

Colorectal cancer (CRC) is the third most common cancer in men after lung and prostate cancer and women after breast and lung cancer [1]. In 2019, the American Cancer Society estimated that 101,420 cases of colon cancer and 44,180 cases of rectal cancer would be diagnosed, and 27,640 men and 23,380 women would die from CRC [1]. The mortality from CRC has been decreasing for several decades due to improved CRC screening, risk factor modification, and better treatments. Over the last 15 years, the incidence of CRC in adults 55 years and older decreased by 3.7% per year, while the incidence in adults less than 55 years old decreased by 1.8% [1].

The majority (70%) of CRC cases are sporadic disease, i.e., no family history of CRC, while only 30% of CRCs have a genetic predisposition. The multistep progression from normal colonic epithelium to invasive cancer involves an intermediate precursor, the adenomatous polyp. CRC screening may detect and remove this adenomatous polyp and detect early CRCs when treatment is most successful. Most organizations recommend that CRC screening starts between ages 45–50 and continue up to ages 75–85 [1].

Adenomatous polyps are typically asymptomatic. As the polyp to carcinoma cycle progresses, it is more likely to cause rectal bleeding, change in bowel habits, weight loss, anorexia, abdominal pain, or anemia, which may result in fatigue and weakness [1]. For most patients with localized CRC, surgery is the most common treatment. When CRC has local or distant metastasis, treatment may involve surgery, chemotherapy, targeted immunotherapy, and radiation.

Risk Factors

There are known risk factors that increase the chances of developing CRC. Modifiable factors include obesity and smoking, while genetic factors include hereditary conditions, personal or family history of CRC (Table 1).

Polyps

Polyps are fleshy growths that occur in the lining of the colon (Fig. 1). Polyps represent the most significant single risk factor for developing CRC. Polyps are classified as hyperplastic, neoplastic (adenomatous and malignant), hamartomatous, and inflammatory. The malignant potential of neoplastic polyps depends on the type and degree of dysplasia and the polyp's size.

Polyps with malignancy risk include adenomatous polyps, which have three histologic variants (Table 2) and sessile serrated adenomas (SSAs). SSAs may progress to dysplastic lesions, leading to unstable microsatellite carcinomas [2]. Polyps more than 2 cm in size have more than a 40% chance of malignancy [3].

Table 1 Factors that increase the risk of colorectal cancer

Modifiable factors	Hereditary and medical factors
Obesity	Personal or family history of CRC or adenomatous polyps
Physical inactivity	Certain genetic conditions
Long-term smoking	Personal history of inflammatory bowel disease
High consumption of red or processed meat	Type 2 diabetes
Low calcium intake	
Moderate to heavy alcohol consumption	
Very low intake of fruits and vegetables	
Low intake of whole-grain fiber	

Source: [1]

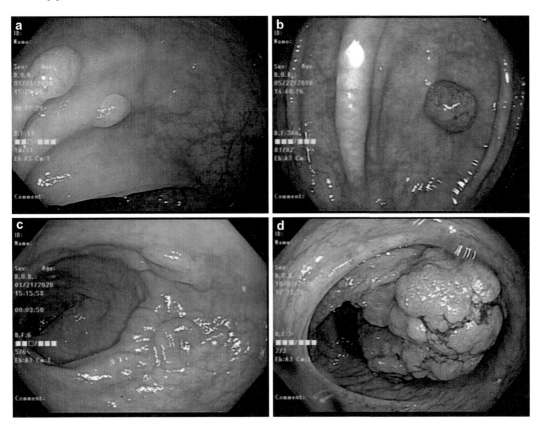

Fig. 1 Colonoscopy images showing colonic polyps and adenocarcinoma. (**a**) Hyperplastic polyps. (**b**) Tubular adenoma. (**c**) Sessile serrated adenomas. (**d**) Invasive adenocarcinoma. (Source: Original)

Genetics

Lynch Syndrome

Hereditary CRC syndromes contribute to about 5% of all CRCs [4]. At least one-fourth of CRC patients have a positive family history for CRC [4]. Lynch syndrome is the most common cause of hereditary CRC, accounting for 2–4% of all CRC cases. Lynch syndrome is an autosomal dominant syndrome caused by a mutation in one of five genes that results in interference with DNA repair. The lifetime risk of CRC in Lynch syndrome is estimated to be 40–60%. It is also associated with an increased risk of several other cancers,

Table 2 Types of adenomatous polyps and malignant potential

Adenoma type	Prevalence (%)	Risk of malignancy (%)
Tubular	75–85	<5
Tubulovillous	10–15	20–25
Villous	5–10	35–40

Source: [3]

including endometrial, ovarian, gastric, hepatobiliary, and urinary tract malignancies [4].

Familial Adenomatous Polyposis

Familial adenomatous polyposis (FAP) is the second most common underlying cause of hereditary CRC, causing around 1% of all CRC. It is also an autosomal dominant condition. FAP is caused by germline mutations in the APC tumor suppressor gene and results in hundreds or thousands of adenomatous polyps throughout the colon. Approximately 25% of FAP patients are the result of de novo mutations rather than familial inheritance [4].

Other Hereditary Syndromes

MUTYH associated polyposis (MAP) is an autosomal recessive defect in DNA oxidative injury repair. Patients with MAP develop numerous colonic polyps, but many fewer than in FAP. Hamartomatous polyposis syndrome and serrated polyposis syndrome are hereditary conditions that increase the risk for CRC [4].

Tobacco

Smoking increases the risk of adenomas. A meta-analysis of 42 observational studies found pooled risk estimates for current, former, and ever smokers compared with never smokers for the development of adenomatous polyps were 2.1, 1.5, and 1.8, respectively. This study found that the association was stronger for high-risk compared to low-risk adenomas

and concluded that smoking is associated with the formation and aggressiveness of adenomas [5].

Alcohol

Alcohol consumption of 2 or more drinks per day (> 30 g/d) is associated with increased risk for colorectal cancer. Compared with nondrinkers, the relative risk for colorectal cancer is 1.2 for persons consuming 30 to 45 g/d and 1.4 for persons consuming 45 g/d or greater [6]. A retrospective cohort analysis of 1448 patients found that significant alcohol consumption increased the risk of adenoma formation (adjusted hazard ratio of 1.86) [7].

Comorbidities

Obesity

Obesity (body mass index (BMI) exceeding 30 kg/m^2) and being overweight (BMI 25–29.9 kg/m^2) are modifiable risk factors for CRC. A systematic review and meta-analysis of prospective studies, including 12,837 CRC cases among 1,343,560 participants, found that waist circumference (RR 1.42) and waist-to-hip ratio (RR 1.39) were significantly associated with CRC [8]. A case-control study of 693 patients referred to a colonoscopy unit found that the incidence of overweight and obesity was significantly higher in adenoma patients than controls (49.9% versus 0.9%, p-value = 0.04) [9].

Diabetes Mellitus

A case-control study of 693 individuals found a significant association between diabetes and adenomatous polyps (OR 1.83, p-value = 0.023) [9]. A meta-analysis of case-control and cohort studies found that diabetes was associated with an increased risk of colon cancer (RR 1.4) and rectal cancer (RR 1.20) [10].

Pathogenesis

There are three main pathways by which cancers arise in the colon: chromosomal instability (CIN), CpG island methylator phenotype (CIMP), and microsatellite instability (MSI) [11]. These mechanisms overlap in the carcinogenesis of CRC. With CIN, there is a mutation in the adenomatous polyposis coli (APC), then the activation of oncogene KRAS and inactivation of tumor suppressor gene, TP53. About 85% of the sporadic tumors and the gemline APC gene mutation seen in FAP involve aneuploidy and loss of heterozygosity. The CIMP pathway involves the hypermethylation of tumor suppressor genes, particularly MGMT and MLH1. BRAF mutation and microsatellite instability are involved with this process of hypermethylation. With the MSI pathway, there is a disruption in the activation of genetic alterations, where there had been a DNA mismatch requiring a mismatch repair. Familial Lynch syndrome is an example of the MSI pathway. The hypermethylation of the MMR gene can also lead to MSI. MSI tumors are often poorly differentiated, though with better prognosis, and are often located in the proximal colon [11].

Approach to the Patient

Choosing a Screening Modality

There are several widely accepted modalities to screen for CRC. The choice of screening tests depends upon availability, patient preference, cost, and individual patient risk. A US Multi-Society Task Force on CRC concluded that a risk-stratifying strategy, offering multiple options and allowing the patient to choose, and sequentially offering tests beginning with a preferred test are all acceptable strategies for selecting a screening modality [12]. There are three broad categories of screening modalities: stool-based, radiographic imaging, and endoscopy [13].

Stool-Based Screening

Stool-based screening modalities considered acceptable by the USPSTF include annual Guaiac fecal occult blood tests (gFOBT), annual fecal immunochemical tests (FIT), and FIT-DNA every 1–3 years [14]. gFOBTs have a sensitivity of over 70% and a specificity of over 90%. However, they require dietary restrictions and multiple samples to be turned in. FIT do not require dietary restriction, and only one sample is needed. Sensitivity is around 80%, and specificity is as high as 94% [15]. FIT-DNA combines occult blood testing with testing for DNA alterations known to be associated with CRC. FIT-DNA is more sensitive than FIT for detecting CRC and precancerous lesions [15]. FIT-DNA is considerably more expensive than FIT or gFOBT [12].

Radiographic-Based Screening

The USPSTF also approves CT colonography every 5 years [14]. The American College of Radiology has given CT colonography every 5 years an Appropriateness Category of "Usually Appropriate" for CRC screening of both average and moderate-risk individuals [15]. CT colonography has a 93% sensitivity and a 97% specificity for polyps 10 mm or greater [15]. A barium enema is not recommended for CRC screening.

Endoscopic-Based Screening

Colonoscopy every 10 years, flexible sigmoidoscopy every 5 years, and a combined strategy of sigmoidoscopy every 10 years plus annual FIT are endoscopic modalities considered acceptable by the USPSTF [14, 16]. Colonoscopy is regarded as the ideal screening method. Compared to colonoscopy, the disadvantage of flexible sigmoidoscopy is that proximal lesions may be missed. Capsule endoscopy is not FDA approved for screening average-risk individuals for CRC [12].

Serum-Based Screening

The Septin9 assay is an FDA-approved serum test for CRC screening [12]. Septin9 has a sensitivity for CRC of 48%, but no sensitivity for polyps [17]. It is also relatively expensive compared to FIT [17]. In 2017, a US Multi-Society Task Force recommended against using Septin9 for CRC screening [12].

Average Risk Screening

For average-risk patients, patient preference, financial considerations, and test availability should be factored into the choice of which screening method to use [18]. As an alternative to universal screening, risk calculators (https://qcancer.org/15yr/colorectal/) are available to help clinicians and patients understand their risk to decide whether or not to screen for CRC. Using such a calculator, some experts suggest using a three percent 15-year risk as to the cutoff for screening [19].

Many organizations have produced screening guidelines for patients at average risk for CRC (Table 3). There are some notable differences in these recommendations. Most major authorities recommend screening from age 50–75, with several screening modalities being acceptable [19].

Table 3 Colorectal cancer screening recommendations by organization

Organization	Year of most recent update	Screening age	Recommended Test and Timing
American College of Gastroenterology	2009	Start at age 50	Colonoscopy every 10 years
US preventive services task Force	2016	Screening for ages 50–75; for ages 76–85, an individualized discussion	gFOBT or FIT every year
			FIT-DNA every 1–3 years
			FIT every year and sigmoidoscopy every 10 years
			Sigmoidoscopy every 5 years
			Colonoscopy every 10 years
			CT colonography every 5 years
American college of physicians	2019	Ages 50–75; beyond age 75 with a life expectancy of 10 years or greater	High sensitivity gFOBT or FIT every 2 years
			Colonoscopy every 10 years
			Sigmoidoscopy every 10 years and FIT every 2 years
American Cancer Society	2018	Ages 45–75; for ages 76–85, an individual decision based on preference, life expectancy, and overall health	High sensitivity gFOBT or FIT every year
			FIT-DNA every 3 years
			Colonoscopy every 10 years
			CT colonography every 5 years
			Sigmoidoscopy every 5 years

Sources: [18, 45–47]

Increased Risk Screening

Patients with a known genetic predisposition and those with at least one first degree relative with CRC are at increased risk and should be screened more aggressively. The US Multi-Specialty Task Force recommends that patients with a single first-degree relative diagnosed at age 60 or above begin screening at age 40. For these patients, the modality and frequency of testing are the same as average-risk individuals. However, for patients with more than one first-degree relative, or any first-degree relative diagnosed below age 60, it is recommended that screening starts at age 40 or 10 years earlier than the youngest relative at their age of diagnosis, whichever is earlier. Colonoscopy is the recommended modality for these patients [12].

Overview of Colonoscopy Procedure

Colonoscopy is the most widely used direct visualization screening method for CRC in the United States. It is usually performed in an ambulatory or hospital-based endoscopy suite. Colonoscopy can cause serious risks to include cardiopulmonary complications (0.9%), bowel perforation (less than 0.1%), hemorrhage (0.1% to 0.6%), infection (less than 0.1%), and post-polypectomy syndrome (2.9%) [20].

Bowel Preparations

Most patients must undergo bowel preparation for 1–2 days before colonoscopy. Diagnostic accuracy is dependent on the quality of colonic preparation and the skill of the endoscopist. Inadequate bowel preparation can lead to an inability to detect neoplastic lesions and increases the risk of adverse events during the procedure. A clear liquid diet is recommended 24–48 h before starting the bowel prep and using a colon cleansing agent. On the day of the procedure, the patient should be made "NPO" or take nothing by mouth. There are many commercial agents available, and suggested use is usually per provider preference

and patient history (Table 4). If a patient has had unsuccessful and inadequate bowel preparation on one agent, it can be switched to another of a different class or used for a more extended period before a colonoscopy in the future. A split-dose prep involves giving half of the bowel preparation dose the day before the colonoscopy and the remaining dose on the morning of the procedure. There is evidence that split-dose prep results in a higher-quality colonoscopy examination than the ingestion of the entire preparation on the day or evening before colonoscopy [21].

Colonoscopy Overview

Patients should inform their provider of all prior conditions and medications before the colonoscopy. Aspirin and anticoagulants may need to be stopped before undergoing the procedure. Warfarin should be stopped 5–7 days before the procedure. New oral anticoagulants such as dabigatran (Pradaxa), rivaroxaban (Xarelto), apixaban (Eliquis), and edoxaban (Savaysa) should be held 48 h before the procedure; clopidogrel (Plavix) should be held 5 days before the procedure. If the patient has a high risk of a cardiac condition such as recent cardiac stenting, non-emergent colonoscopies should be postponed. Low-dose aspirin, i.e., 81 mg, can be continued prior to and after the procedure. Antibiotics are not recommended before colonoscopy. Colonoscopy is usually performed with the patient under conscious sedation for analgesic and anxiolytic control. Deep sedation, i.e., propofol administered by anesthesia personnel, may be considered if available but increases the cost of the procedure.

Quality Metrics for Colonoscopy

Adenoma detection rate (ADR) is the percentage of colonoscopies in which one or more adenomas were detected. ADR is dependent on the skill of the provider, positioning of the patient, withdrawal time, and bowel preparation, all affecting the ability to visualize the haustral folds completely. A ten times higher hazard ratio for

Table 4 Common bowel preparations for colonoscopy

Brand	Composition	Recommended dosing	Additional fluid	Split dosing	Warnings
GoLYTELY	PEG, sodium sulfate, sodium, bicarbonate, sodium chloride, potassium chloride	4 l	None	2–3 l day before and 1–2 l day of procedure	
NuLYTELY; Trilyte	PEG, sodium bicarbonate, sodium chloride, potassium chloride	4 l	None	2–3 l day before and 1–2 l day of procedure	
Moviprep	PEG-3350, sodium sulfate, sodium chloride, ascorbic acid	2 l	1 l clear liquids	1 l day before and 1 l day of procedure	Avoid in patients with glucose-6-phosphate dehydrogenase deficiency
Suprep	Sodium sulfate, potassium sulfate, magnesium sulfate	12 oz	2.5 l water	6 oz. OSS with 10 oz. of water +32 oz. water day before and 6 oz. OSS with 10 oz. of water +32 oz. water day of procedure	
Suclear	Sodium sulfate, potassium sulfate, magnesium sulfate, PEG-3350	6 oz. oral sodium sulfate/ 2 l PEG-ELS	1.25 l water	6 oz. OSS with 10 oz. of water +32 oz. water day before and 2 l PEG-ELS day of procedure	
Prepopik	Sodium picosulfate, magnesium sulfate, anhydric citric acid	10 oz	2 l water	5 oz. Prepopik day before +40 oz. clear liquids and 5 oz. Prepopik +24 oz. clear liquids the day of the procedure	Avoid in patients with renal insufficiency
Osmoprep	Monobasic and dibasic NaP tablets	32 tablets	2 l water	20 tablets day before and 12 tablets the day of the procedure	Avoid in patients with renal insufficiency or risk factors for acute phosphate nephropathy; not recommended for routine use

Source: [21]

PEG polyethylene glycol, *ELS* electrolyte solution, *NaP* sodium phosphate, *l* liter, *oz.* ounces

interval cancer has been noted for colonoscopists with an ADR <20% compared to that for colonoscopists with an ADR >20% [22]. Providers aim to have a high ADR to increase CRC detection and reduce the risk of interval cancer. A low ADR is associated with increased rates of post-colonoscopy CRC. Recent guidelines suggest that colonoscopists should have an overall ADR of more than 25% (for men ≥30%, for women ≥20%) [22].

The cecum is identified once the colonoscope has reached the ileocecal valve and the entire medial wall of the cecum between the ileocecal valve and appendiceal orifice is visible. The cecal intubation rate (CIR) is the ratio of the number of screening colonoscopies that the cecum was visualized divided by the total number of screening colonoscopies. The CIR is a frequently used indicator for colonoscopy competency and an important quality metric. Guidelines suggest that the CIR of competent colonoscopists should be higher than 95% [22].

ADR and CIR are directly affected by bowel preparation. Complications associated with inadequate bowel preparation include incomplete colonoscopy, prolonged colonoscopy time, and reduced diagnostic yield [22]. The bowel preparation should be documented thoroughly and described at each part of the colon. Providers may use validated preparation scores such as the Boston Bowel Preparation Scale (BBPS) or the Ottawa Bowel Preparation Scale (OPBS) [23]. If bowel preparation is inadequate, then the procedure must be repeated within 6–12 months.

Workup of Individual Suspected of Colorectal Cancer

In individuals suspected or newly diagnosed with CRC, the next step in evaluating these patients is preoperative clinical staging. A complete history and examination should be completed looking for ascites, hepatomegaly, or lymphadenopathy. Helpful labs include carcinoembryonic antigen (CEA), a colon cancer tumor marker, complete blood count, BUN, creatinine, and liver enzymes. Computed tomography (CT) of the abdomen and pelvis is often obtained before surgery, as the results could influence the surgical approach. Chest imaging may be considered to exclude lung metastases, but its use is controversial. Positron emission tomography (PET) scans do not appear to be helpful in preoperative staging. PET scans are often not obtained except as an adjunct to other imaging in particular circumstances, i.e.,

in patients thought to be candidates for resection of liver metastasis of CRC.

TMN and Anatomic Stage

CRCs may spread by four methods: lymphatic, hematogenous, continuous, and transperitoneal. CRCs most commonly spread to lymph nodes, the liver, and lungs but may also spread to bone and brain. The tumor, node, and metastasis (TMN) staging system is the preferred staging system for CRC and older staging systems, i.e., Astler-Coller modifications of the Duke's classification are discouraged (Tables 5 and 6) [24].

Treatment

Endoscopic Therapy

Endoscopic polypectomy is a standard treatment option for colorectal neoplasia and decreases mortality from CRC. The aim of polypectomy is the complete removal of the polyp and prevention of further developing CRC. Polypectomy is performed using forceps, cold snare, and hot snare. The majority (80%) of all polyps recognized during colonoscopy are 1–5 mm in size, known as diminutive polyps, representing the majority of colorectal polyps [25]. The American Society for Gastrointestinal Endoscopy (ASGE) recommends the use of cold snare polypectomy for most diminutive polyps. Hot snare polypectomy is associated with the additional risk of thermal injury and a possible increase in bleeding. If necessary, cold forceps resection should be limited to small polyps (≤2 mm) and only to those anticipated to be resected in a single bite. For complex or excessively large polyps, i.e., >20 mm, endoscopic mucosal resection is recommended.

Surgery

Surgical resection is another treatment option for complex polyps not amenable to conventional

Table 5 The TNM staging system

	Definition	Score
T	Tumor	Tx – Cannot be measured
		T0 – No evidence of a primary tumor
		Tis – Carcinoma in situ
		T1 – Cancer has grown through the muscularis mucosa into the submucosa
		T2 – Cancer has grown into the muscularis propria
		T3 – Cancer has grown into the outermost layers of the colon or rectum but has not gone through them
		T4a – Cancer has grown through the wall of the colon or rectum but has not grown into other nearby tissues or organs
		T4b – Cancer has grown through the wall of the colon or rectum and is attached to or has grown into other nearby tissues or organs
N	Nodes	Nx – Cannot be measured
		N0 – Nearby nodes do not contain cancer
		N1 – Has spread to 1–3 nearby lymph nodes
		N1c – Has spread into areas of fat near the lymph nodes but not the nodes themselves
		N2a – Has spread to 4–6 nearby lymph nodes
		N2b – Has spread to 7 or more nearby lymph nodes
		N3 – Metastasis in 7 or more regional lymph nodes
M	Metastasis	M0 – No distant cancer found
		M1 – Cancer has spread to distant organs or tissues

Source: [24]

Table 6 The American Joint Committee on Cancer (AJCC) and the TNM system

AJCC stage	TNM grouping
0	Tis, N0, M0
I	T1 or T2, N0, M0
IIA	T4a, N0, M0
IIB	T4b, N0, M0
IIIA	T1 or T2, N1/N1c, M0 **OR** T1, N2a, M0
IIIB	T3 or T4a, N1/N1c, M0 **OR** T2 or T3, N2a, M0 OR T1 or T2, N2b, M0
IIIC	T4, N2a, M0 **OR** T3 or T4a, N2b, M0 **OR** T4b, N1 or N2, M0
IVA	Any T, any N, M1a
IVB	Any T, any N, M1b
IVC	Any T, any N, M1c

Source: [24]

polypectomy and is the primary curative method of CRC. Polyps with characteristics of deep submucosal invasion, which have been proven by advanced endoscopic imaging techniques, should be referred for surgery [25]. In patients with CRC, resection of the affected colon or rectum is recommended. To ensure that the tumor and its principal zone of lymphatic spread are removed, the dissection should ideally follow the embryological anatomical planes with special attention given to the circumferential resection margins [26]. Local lymph node metastasis can also be removed during laparoscopic surgery in most cases [25]. Surgery may be done either laparoscopically or open. Laparoscopic resection of CRC is as safe as open surgery [26]. Surgical success rates are highly dependent on preoperative staging, patient age, and comorbidities. CEA should be obtained before the surgery to serve as a baseline value for postoperative surveillance.

Chemotherapy and Radiation

Patients with stage 0 or I rectal or colon cancer do not typically require chemotherapy. Chemotherapy is controversial for stage II colon cancer but is frequently used in stage III colon cancer and is the mainstay of stage IV colon cancer therapy. 5-FU or capecitabine may be used in stage II rectal cancer, and these agents may be part of a regime for stage III or IV rectal cancer. Radiation therapy is considered in patients with stage III or IV colon cancer for those not considered surgical candidates or to treat symptoms, i.e., pain. Radiation therapy is typically used in combination with chemotherapy in patients with stage II–IV rectal cancers. Hepatic artery infusion or infusion of immunotherapy drugs may be considered in patients with stage IV colon or rectal cancer for treatment of metastases, i.e., liver metastases.

Postoperative Surveillance

The American Cancer Society recommends intensive postoperative surveillance, beginning 4–6 weeks after surgery, then every 3–6 months for the first 2–3 years, then every 6 months for 5 years. CEA testing is recommended at each visit. Routine testing other than CEA to monitor for recurrent disease is not recommended. Surveillance colonoscopy is recommended 1 year after initial treatment. If advanced adenoma (>1 cm with a villous component or high-grade dysplasia) is found, then colonoscopy should be repeated in 1 year. Otherwise, repeat surveillance colonoscopy in 3 years, then every 5 years. Patients with a higher risk of recurrence should be offered annual CT of chest, abdomen, and pelvis for 5 years after curative treatment for CRC. Routine CEA testing or CT scans after 5 years of initial treatment is not recommended [27].

Prognosis

The most important factor in the prognosis of CRC is the stage at presentation. Other important prognostic factors include the presence of extramural tumor, lymphovascular and perineural invasion, histologic grade, the preoperative level of CEA, microsatellite instability (MSI), and the RAS and BRAF mutations. There is a difference regarding the prognosis in the location of CRC, as left-sided (distal colon and rectal) CRCs versus right-sided (proximal colon) CRCs are associated with a better prognosis [28].

Prevention

Prevention of CRC can be approached from primary, secondary, and tertiary prevention. Primary prevention includes smoking cessation, reduction in alcohol usage, regular physical activity, and dietary modification. Secondary prevention aims to detect early disease by screening and to excise precancerous lesions. Individuals at high risk for CRC such as a family history of CRC, a personal history of ulcerative colitis or previous adenomas should have regular screening colonoscopies. Tertiary prevention is directed to the needed care post-CRC treatment, with the goal of improved outcomes and reduced risk of recurrence of CRC. Individuals may inquire about prevention strategies for CRC and polyps (Table 7).

Diet

There is good evidence that moderate daily intake of cow's milk reduces the risk of CRC [29]. There is no direct evidence that decreasing cholesterol, fat, or red meat intake reduces the risk for CRC or polyps. There is conflicting evidence for coffee intake, and there is strong evidence that increasing fiber intake does not reduce the risk of CRC or polyps [30, 31].

Lifestyle

There is good evidence that increasing physical activity decreases the risk of CRC, and there is indirect evidence that weight loss decreases the risk of CRC [32, 33]. There is fair to moderate evidence that moderate or higher alcohol intake and cigarette smoking increase the risk of CRC and polyps [5, 34, 35].

Medications

There is strong evidence that daily calcium use for 3–4 years decreases the risk of polyps and CRC [36, 37]. There is good evidence that daily statin use for at least 5 years decreases the risk of CRC and polyps [38]. Aspirin, nonsteroidal anti-inflammatory drugs, cyclooxygenase-2 inhibitors decrease the risk of CRC or polyps; however, these medications are not recommended in the average-risk population due to the risk of GI

Table 7 Summary of dietary, lifestyle, and medications to prevent colorectal cancer and polyps

Factor	Effect	Comment	Evidence
Diet			
Cholesterol and fat intake	Increased risk of CRC with increased cholesterol intake, and increased risk of serrated polyps with increased fat intake	There is no evidence that reduction in cholesterol or fat intake lowers risk of CRC or serrated polyps	One meta-analysis, one RCT, and one prospective study
Coffee consumption	Conflicting evidence	More research is needed from high-quality trials	One case-control study, one RCT, and one meta-analysis of prospective cohort studies
Dairy intake	Reduced risk of CRC with more than 8 oz. of cow's milk per day	Moderate daily intake of cow's milk reduced risk of CRC	Meta-analysis of 10 cohort studies
Fiber	No evidence for reduced risk of CRC or polyps with increasing fiber intake	Fiber from different sources was used	Two Cochrane reviews and 1 meta-analysis of 13 prospective studies
Red meat intake	Increased risk of CRC with increasing red meat and processed meat intake	There is no direct evidence that decreasing red meat and processed meat intake reduces risk of CRC and polyps	Meta-analysis of 13 prospective studies and meta-analysis of 34 case-control studies and 14 cohort studies
Lifestyle			
Alcohol intake	Increased risk of CRC and increased risk of serrated polyps	Evaluated effect of >15 g per day of beer, wine, or spirits	Large cohort study (CRC) and meta-analysis of 10 observational studies (serrated polyps)
Cigarette smoking	Increased risk of high-risk adenomatous polyps and CRC in current smokers	Strong association between smoking and high-risk adenomatous polyps and CRC; no direct evidence that smoking cessation decreases risk	Meta-analysis of 42 observational studies
Obesity	Bariatric surgery associated with reduced risk of CRC	Indirect evidence	Meta-analysis of four observational studies and a systematic review of 15 cohort studies
Physical activity	Decreased risk of colorectal cancer for occupational and recreational physical activity	Demonstrated benefit of increasing occupational and recreational physical activity for reducing the risk of colon and rectal cancers	Meta-analysis of 17 cohort studies and 21 case-control studies
Medications			
Antioxidants	No benefit for beta carotene; vitamins A, C, or E; or selenium	Not recommended to decrease the risk of CRC or adenomatous polyps	Meta-analysis of 20 RCTs
Aspirin	Reduced risk of CRC	Not recommended in the average-risk population because of the risk of GI bleeding and hemorrhagic stroke	Review of three RCTs
Calcium	Reduced risk of adenomatous polyps and reduced risk of CRC; no effect for serrated polyps	Calcium use for 3–4 years is recommended to decrease risk of CRC or adenomatous polyps but not serrated polyps	Cochrane review and meta-analysis

(continued)

Table 7 (continued)

Factor	Effect	Comment	Evidence
Cyclooxygenase-2 inhibitors	Reduced risk of adenomatous polyps	Not recommended secondary to increased risk of GI and cardiovascular events	Two RCTs
Folic acid	Did not decrease risk of adenomatous polyps	Not recommended secondary to no benefit, more study needed	Single RCT
Hormone therapy	Reduced risk of CRC but no decreased risk of serrated polyps	Harms outweigh potential benefits, and routine use is not recommended at this time	Meta-analysis of four studies and one case-control study
Nonsteroidal anti-inflammatory drugs	Decreased risk of CRC	Not recommended secondary to increased risk of GI and cardiovascular events	Meta-analysis of 15 RCTs
Statins	Statin use associated with decreased risk of advanced adenomatous polyps and decreased risk of CRC	Effect observed in individuals who had used a statin for at least 5 years	Meta-analysis of six studies and one case-control study
Vitamin D	Conflicting evidence	More research is needed from high-quality trials	Guideline based on 3 RCTs and 28 observational studies, and meta-analysis of 18 observational studies

Source: [20]

bleeding, hemorrhagic stroke, and cardiovascular events [39–41]. Hormone therapy reduces the risk of CRC but is not recommended because the harms outweigh the benefits [42]. There is good evidence that beta carotene, vitamins A, C, or E, selenium, and folate are not effective for decreasing the risk of CRC or polyps [20].

Family and Community Issues

CRC has a better prognosis with early detection; therefore, screening should be recommended to all age-eligible individuals. State and national initiatives address public health strategies that promote primary prevention, cancer screening, early diagnosis, and access to effective evidence-based treatment and survivorship care [43]. Family physicians often play a key role in communities by encouraging the routine use of CRC screening and education. Individuals may fear undergoing a colonoscopy due to stigmatism or misconceptions about the procedure. Other screening modalities, such as fecal studies, should be offered when individuals decline screening colonoscopy. Educational pamphlets distributed or available at routine doctor's visits, community awareness events, support groups, and media campaigns can all contribute to promoting screening. For individuals diagnosed with CRC, social integration, and community support are essential. Research has established that strong social relationships predict lower all-cause mortality. The health risks associated with social isolation are comparable to traditional risk factors, such as smoking, blood pressure, and obesity. Large social networks may improve survival through increased support, including assistance in getting to medical appointments, reminders to take medications, and help with nutrition and mobility [44].

References

1. Siegel RL, Miller KD, Jemal A. Cancer statistics, 2019. CA Cancer J Clin. 2019;69(1):7–34.
2. Salaria SN, Streppel MM, Lee LA, Iacobuzio-Donahue CA, Montgomery EA. Sessile serrated adenomas: high-risk lesions? Hum Pathol. 2012;43(11):1808–14.
3. Amersi F, Agustin M, Ko CY. Colorectal cancer: epidemiology, risk factors, and health services. Clin Colon Rectal Surg. 2005;18(3):133–40.

4. Kanth P, Grimmett J, Champine M, Burt R, Samadder NJ. Hereditary colorectal polyposis and cancer syndromes: a primer on diagnosis and management. Am J Gastroenterol. 2017;112(10):1509–25.

5. Botteri E, Iodice S, Raimondi S, Maisonneuve P, Lowenfels AB. Cigarette smoking and adenomatous polyps: a meta-analysis. Gastroenterology. 2008;134(2):388–95.

6. Durko L, Malecka-Panas E. Lifestyle modifications and colorectal cancer. Curr Colorectal Cancer Rep. 2014;10:45–54.

7. Yang YJ, Bang CS, Choi JH, Lee JJ, Shin SP, Suk KT, et al. Alcohol consumption is associated with the risk of developing colorectal neoplasia: propensity score matching analysis. Sci Rep. 2019;9(1):8253.

8. Dong Y, Zhou J, Zhu Y, Luo L, He T, Hu H, et al. Abdominal obesity and colorectal cancer risk: systematic review and meta-analysis of prospective studies. Biosci Rep. 2017;37(6):1–12. chrome-extension://oemmndcbldboiebfnladdacbdfmadadm/https://www.ncbi.nlm.nih.gov/pmc/articles/PMC5725611/pdf/bsr-37-bsr20170945.pdf

9. Soltani G, Poursheikhani A, Yassi M, Hayatbakhsh A, Kerachian M, Kerachian MA. Obesity, diabetes and the risk of colorectal adenoma and cancer. BMC Endocr Disord. 2019;19(1):113.

10. Yuhara H, Steinmaus C, Cohen SE, Corley DA, Tei Y, Buffler PA. Is diabetes mellitus an independent risk factor for colon cancer and rectal cancer? Am J Gastroenterol. 2011;106(11):1911–21; quiz 22

11. Tariq K, Ghias K. Colorectal cancer carcinogenesis: a review of mechanisms. Cancer Biol Med. 2016;13(1):120–35.

12. Rex DK, Boland CR, Dominitz JA, Giardiello FM, Johnson DA, Kaltenbach T, et al. Colorectal cancer screening: recommendations for physicians and patients from the U.S. multi-society task Force on colorectal cancer. Am J Gastroenterol. 2017;112(7):1016–30.

13. Hadjipetrou A, Anyfantakis D, Galanakis CG, Kastanakis M, Kastanakis S. Colorectal cancer, screening and primary care: a mini literature review. World J Gastroenterol. 2017;23(33):6049–58.

14. Lin JS, Piper MA, Perdue LA, Rutter CM, Webber EM, O'Connor E, et al. Screening for colorectal cancer: updated evidence report and systematic review for the US preventive services task Force. JAMA. 2016;315(23):2576–94.

15. Expert Panel on Gastrointestinal I, Moreno C, Kim DH, Bartel TB, Cash BD, Chang KJ, et al. ACR appropriateness criteria(R) colorectal cancer screening. J Am Coll Radiol. 2018;15(5S):S56–68.

16. Force USPST, Bibbins-Domingo K, Grossman DC, Curry SJ, Davidson KW, Epling JW Jr, et al. Screening for colorectal cancer: US preventive services task Force recommendation statement. JAMA. 2016;315(23):2564–75.

17. Rex DK, Boland CR, Dominitz JA, Giardiello FM, Johnson DA, Kaltenbach T, et al. Colorectal cancer screening: recommendations for physicians and patients from the U.S. multi-society task force on colorectal cancer. Gastrointest Endosc. 2017;86(1):18–33.

18. Wolf AMD, Fontham ETH, Church TR, Flowers CR, Guerra CE, LaMonte SJ, et al. Colorectal cancer screening for average-risk adults: 2018 guideline update from the American Cancer Society. CA Cancer J Clin. 2018;68(4):250–81.

19. Helsingen LM, Vandvik PO, Jodal HC, Agoritsas T, Lytvyn L, Anderson JC, et al. Colorectal cancer screening with faecal immunochemical testing, sigmoidoscopy or colonoscopy: a clinical practice guideline. BMJ. 2019;367:l5515.

20. Wilkins T, McMechan D, Talukder A. Colorectal cancer screening and prevention. Am Fam Physician. 2018;97(10):658–65.

21. Committee ASoP, Saltzman JR, Cash BD, Pasha SF, Early DS, Muthusamy VR, et al. Bowel preparation before colonoscopy. Gastrointest Endosc. 2015;81(4):781–94.

22. Jang HJ. Training in endoscopy: colonoscopy. Clin Endosc. 2017;50(4):322–7.

23. Kastenberg D, Bertiger G, Brogadir S. Bowel preparation quality scales for colonoscopy. World J Gastroenterol. 2018;24(26):2833–43.

24. Jessup JM, Goldberg R, Aware EA, et al. Colon and rectum. In: AJCC Cancer Staging Manual. 8th ed.; 2017. 251p.

25. Herszenyi L. The "difficult" colorectal polyps and adenomas: practical aspects. Dig Dis. 2019;37(5):394–9.

26. Kuipers EJ, Grady WM, Lieberman D, Seufferlein T, Sung JJ, Boelens PG, et al. Colorectal cancer. Nat Rev Dis Primers. 2015;1:15065.

27. Burgers K, Moore C, Bednash L. Care of the colorectal cancer survivor. Am Fam Physician. 2018;97(5):331–6.

28. Dekker E, Tanis PJ, Vleugels JLA, Kasi PM, Wallace MB. Colorectal cancer. Lancet. 2019;394(10207):1467–80.

29. Cho E, Smith-Warner SA, Spiegelman D, Beeson WL, van den Brandt PA, Colditz GA, et al. Dairy foods, calcium, and colorectal cancer: a pooled analysis of 10 cohort studies. J Natl Cancer Inst. 2004;96(13):1015–22.

30. Schmit SL, Rennert HS, Rennert G, Gruber SB. Coffee consumption and the risk of colorectal cancer. Cancer Epidemiol Biomark Prev. 2016;25(4):634–9.

31. Yao Y, Suo T, Andersson R, Cao Y, Wang C, Lu J, et al. Dietary fibre for the prevention of recurrent colorectal adenomas and carcinomas. Cochrane Database Syst Rev. 2017;1:CD003430.

32. Dai Z, Xu YC, Niu L. Obesity and colorectal cancer risk: a meta-analysis of cohort studies. World J Gastroenterol. 2007;13(31):4199–206.

33. Afshar S, Kelly SB, Seymour K, Lara J, Woodcock S, Mathers JC. The effects of bariatric surgery on colorectal cancer risk: systematic review and meta-analysis. Obes Surg. 2014;24(10):1793–9.

34. Ferrari P, Jenab M, Norat T, Moskal A, Slimani N, Olsen A, et al. Lifetime and baseline alcohol intake and risk of colon and rectal cancers in the European prospective investigation into cancer and nutrition (EPIC). Int J Cancer. 2007;121(9):2065–72.

35. Wang YM, Zhou QY, Zhu JZ, Zhu KF, Yu CH, Li YM. Systematic review with meta-analysis: alcohol

consumption and risk of colorectal serrated polyp. Dig Dis Sci. 2015;60(7):1889–902.

36. Weingarten MA, Zalmanovici A, Yaphe J. Dietary calcium supplementation for preventing colorectal cancer and adenomatous polyps. Cochrane Database Syst Rev. 2005;3:CD003548.

37. Zhang X, Keum N, Wu K, Smith-Warner SA, Ogino S, Chan AT, et al. Calcium intake and colorectal cancer risk: results from the nurses' health study and health professionals follow-up study. Int J Cancer. 2016;139(10):2232–42.

38. Jung YS, Park CH, Eun CS, Park DI, Han DS. Statin use and the risk of colorectal adenoma: a meta-analysis. J Gastroenterol Hepatol. 2016;31(11):1823–30.

39. Bibbins-Domingo K, Force USPST. Aspirin use for the primary prevention of cardiovascular disease and colorectal cancer: U.S. preventive services task force recommendation statement. Ann Intern Med. 2016;164(12):836–45.

40. Bertagnolli MM, Eagle CJ, Zauber AG, Redston M, Solomon SD, Kim K, et al. Celecoxib for the prevention of sporadic colorectal adenomas. N Engl J Med. 2006;355(9):873–84.

41. Dulai PS, Singh S, Marquez E, Khera R, Prokop LJ, Limburg PJ, et al. Chemoprevention of colorectal cancer in individuals with previous colorectal neoplasia: systematic review and network meta-analysis. BMJ. 2016;355:i6188.

42. Rennert G, Rennert HS, Pinchev M, Lavie O, Gruber SB. Use of hormone replacement therapy and the risk of colorectal cancer. J Clin Oncol. 2009;27(27):4542–7.

43. Weir HK, Stewart SL, Allemani C, White MC, Thomas CC, White A, et al. Population-based cancer survival (2001 to 2009) in the United States: findings from the CONCORD-2 study. Cancer. 2017;123 (Suppl 24):4963–8.

44. Sarma EA, Kawachi I, Poole EM, Tworoger SS, Giovannucci EL, Fuchs CS, et al. Social integration and survival after diagnosis of colorectal cancer. Cancer. 2018;124(4):833–40.

45. Dominic OG, McGarrity T, Dignan M, Lengerich EJ. American College of Gastroenterology guidelines for colorectal cancer screening 2008. Am J Gastroenterol. 2009;104(10):2626–7; author reply 8–9

46. Lin JS, Piper MA, Perdue LA, Rutter C, Webber EM, O'Connor E, et al. Screening for Colorectal Cancer: A Systematic Review for the US Preventive Services Task Force. U.S. Preventive Services Task Force Evidence Syntheses, formerly Systematic Evidence Reviews, Rockville; 2016.

47. Qaseem A, Crandall CJ, Mustafa RA, Hicks LA, Wilt TJ. Clinical guidelines committee of the American College of P. Screening for colorectal cancer in asymptomatic average-risk adults: a guidance statement from the American College of Physicians. Ann Intern Med. 2019;171(9):643–54.

Surgical Problems of the Digestive System

97

Brian Coleman and Kalyanakrishnan Ramakrishnan

Contents

B. Coleman · K. Ramakrishnan (✉)
Department of Family and Preventive Medicine,
University of Oklahoma Health Sciences Center,
Oklahoma, OK, USA
e-mail: brian-coleman@ouhsc.edu;
Kalyanakrishnan-Ramakrishnan@ouhsc.edu;
kramakrishnan@ouhsc.edu

© Springer Nature Switzerland AG 2022
P. M. Paulman et al. (eds.), *Family Medicine*,
https://doi.org/10.1007/978-3-030-54441-6_100

Recent developments in the field of general surgery have generated significant innovations in the management of patients with abdominal pathology. Advances in imaging (FAST – focused assessment with sonography in trauma, computed tomography (CT) angiography) have enabled earlier and a more precise diagnosis to be made and minimized the role of exploratory surgeries for trauma. Minimally invasive (keyhole) and "robotic" surgeries have also provided greater precision in treatment while minimizing surgical trauma, enabling maximal postsurgical preservation of organ function and earlier patient return to normal activity. However, the cardinal surgical principles (judicious preoperative assessment, meticulous operative technique, and prevention of postoperative complications) remain unchanged.

Abdominal Pathology

The abdomen has long been considered a "Pandora's box," a cavity within which many varied and undetected pathologies may progress unchecked. Diseases of the digestive system comprised nearly eight million (6.1%) emergency room visits in 2010; over ten million patients (8%) sought emergency care for abdominal pain [1]. Apart from problems related to the abdomen and pelvis, pain from vertebral pathology radiating anteriorly may present with abdominal pain. Patients with cardiopulmonary diseases (pneumonia, pulmonary embolism, pneumothorax, acute coronary syndrome) may also present with upper abdominal pain, mimicking abdominal pathology. Abdominal wall pathology (Herpes Zoster, rectus sheath hematoma) and systemic diseases (diabetic ketoacidosis, porphyria, and sickle cell disease) may also present with abdominal symptoms [2, 3].

Some Key Terms and Maneuvers

Abdominal pain is the cardinal-presenting symptom, and the most confounding and potentially life-threatening complaint evaluated by an emergency room or family physician. Abdominal pain may be *acute* (lasting a week or less) or *chronic*. It may also be *parietal* (sharp, well-defined and localized, and usually due to inflammation of the parietal peritoneum) or *visceral* (ill-defined, dull and gnawing pain arising from the abdominopelvic viscera often associated with parasympathetic overdrive producing bradycardia, diaphoresis, and nausea). *Referred pain*, pain experienced at a site distant from the focus of involvement, follows nerve roots subserving intra-abdominal and other (usually cutaneous) regions converging at the same levels in the spinal cord. An *"acute abdomen"* is an intra-abdominal process (inflammation, infection, posttraumatic) producing acute abdominal pain and other symptoms requiring urgent evaluation, hospitalization, and often surgical intervention. *Guarding* is voluntary contraction of the abdominal wall muscles in response to underlying peritoneal/visceral irritation. It may be reduced by distraction techniques such as using a stethoscope to palpate the abdomen, and by administering analgesics. *Rigidity* is the involuntary contraction of abdominal wall muscles that resolves only after anesthesia. *"Rebound tenderness"* is worsening abdominal pain following sudden release of pressure of the palpating hand. It indicates peritoneal irritation. *Rebound tenderness* may also be elicited by abdominal percussion, patient coughing or jolting the bed, or having the standing patient rock back on his heels [4]. Examination techniques eliciting characteristic responses as well as classic sites for referred pain will be discussed under the sections on individual abdominal pathologies.

Evaluation of Patients with Abdominal Pathology

History

Careful history and examination is crucial in diagnosing abdominal pathology. Initial history and examination should be focused to rule out life-threatening causes, which if found, mandates immediate specialist consultation for corrective action. The principal symptoms of abdominal pathology are abdominal pain, nausea, vomiting, diarrhea or constipation, hematemesis/melena, dysuria/hematuria, abdominal distention, anorexia, weight loss, menstrual irregularities, and jaundice. Fever reflects inflammatory/infective states. Characteristics of abdominal pain that need to be elicited in history include duration, nature (colicky, persistent, burning, sharp), location, onset, intensity, radiation, migration, and provoking/relieving factors. Nausea and vomiting may follow vagal response to pain, peritoneal irritation, toxemia, or abdominal distention. Feeding often precipitates pain and emesis. Repeated retching or gastroduodenal irritation/ulceration may produce hematemesis or melena (passage of black, smelly, sticky, slimy stool). Diarrhea is a feature of irritation (infection/inflammation) involving the small or large bowel; constipation may indicate mechanical bowel obstruction or ileus. Anorexia usually accompanies significant abdominal pathology. Urinary symptoms (oliguria, dysuria, frequency, hesitancy, urgency, and hematuria) indicate genitourinary pathology. Jaundice denotes hepatobiliary or pancreatic involvement [2, 3]. Fever reflects inflammatory/infective states. Back pain may indicate retroperitoneal organ involvement (renal colic, pyelonephritis, abdominal aortic aneurysm).

History of trauma, especially prior surgery, is significant. Postoperative adhesions cause over three-fourths of all episodes of bowel obstruction. Embolism from a mural thrombus associated with atrial fibrillation and low flow states secondary to congestive heart failure may cause mesenteric ischemia and bowel infarction. Diabetic ketoacidosis (edema of the mesentery), sickle cell crises (infarction of liver, spleen, or kidney), acute intermittent porphyria (possible visceral ischemia), and renal insufficiency may all cause abdominal pain, confirming the association with cardiorespiratory and systemic illnesses [2, 5].

History of amenorrhea in women of childbearing age may indicate pregnancy. Many features of abdominal pathology (nausea, vomiting, constipation, dysuria, pelvic/abdominal discomfort) are characteristics of normal pregnancy. Medications (antiarrhythmics, nonsteroidal anti-inflammatory agents – NSAIDs, steroids, beta-blockers, anticoagulants, and over-the-counter medications and supplements) often contribute to abdominal crises and interfere with assessment by causing abdominal pain, bleeding, arrhythmias, bradycardia, and hypotension. Alcohol and recreational drug use/abuse also promote or worsen abdominal pathology [6]. In evaluating infants and young children, history is obtained from the parent or caregiver; older children often provide a coherent history, though clarification should be sought from the caregiver. Menstrual and sexual histories are important in adolescents and older age-groups [7].

Abdominal pathology in elderly patients is more difficult to evaluate. Cognitive impairment and poor pain perception complicate assessment of pain. Increased intestinal transit time predisposes to constipation and ileus. Immunosenescence of B and T cells result in inadequate febrile and leukocytic response, increasing risk of infections. Decreased renal function delays clearance of medications. Chronic diseases and prior abdominal surgery, more frequent in older people, also impact pain perception and disease progression. Elderly patients are usually on multiple medications (beta-blockers, NSAIDs, anticoagulants, narcotics, antidepressants) all of which alter perception and progression of abdominal pathology, and influence its prognosis [6, 8].

Physical Examination

Presence of shock (hemodynamic compromise) suggests systemic sepsis, significant intra-abdominal bleeding or peritonitis. Signs of trauma (closed head injury, chest, pelvis, long bones) should be identified. Cardiorespiratory, pelvic/rectal examination, and examination of the back complement abdominal examination in evaluating the acute abdomen.

A systematic approach (inspection, auscultation, palpation, and percussion) is recommended. All hernial orifices (umbilical, inguinal femoral) and abdominal incisions should be palpated for masses (possible hernia). Presence of guarding, rigidity and rebound tenderness on abdominal palpation suggests ischemic bowel or peritonitis. Recent increase in size, tenseness, tenderness, or absent cough impulse over a hernia suggests

ischemia of contents (entrapped bowel or omentum). Re-examination enables the provider to detect evolving pathology. Organ-specific palpatory signs consistent with specific pathology (Murphy's sign in cholecystitis or Rovsing's sign in appendicitis) may be present. Percussion is useful in detecting free fluid, gaseous distention, and rebound tenderness. Auscultation detects abnormal bruits and borborygmi (peristaltic sounds); hyperactive bowel sounds indicate mechanical bowel obstruction, whereas decreased or absent sounds denote adynamic ileus.

Peritoneal signs are often absent in pregnancy. Lifting and stretching of the abdominal wall prevents underlying inflamed organs from abutting and involving the parietal peritoneum, minimizing guarding. In the later stages of pregnancy, women should be examined in the lateral decubitus position to palpate organs obscured by the gravid uterus. In recumbent patients, the right hip should be elevated slightly in the later stages of pregnancy to avoid compressing the inferior vena cava, which may produce supine hypotension syndrome [9].

Additional Testing: Laboratory Tests

Initial tests include a complete blood count, urinalysis, and analysis of liver and kidney functions. Other specific tests reflecting inflammation/change in organ function are useful in disorders of the pancreas, and in ischemic bowel. Most acute abdominal pathology initiates an inflammatory response and also impacts the function of the involved viscera, which is reflected in changes in body fluid composition. Patient symptoms (gastrointestinal bleeding, vomiting, diarrhea, or hematuria) also influence laboratory values. Some changes seen in acute abdominal pathology include anemia (bleeding), leukocytosis (inflammatory response), hematuria, pyuria, bacteriuria (urinary tract infection, renal trauma), elevation of blood urea nitrogen (BUN) and creatinine (dehydration, poor renal perfusion), elevation of bilirubin and liver enzymes (hemolysis, poor hepatic perfusion, biliary obstruction), elevation of amylase and lipase (pancreatic inflammation), and increased lactic acid (hypotension and shock, bowel ischemia and gangrene). Women of child-bearing age should have a pregnancy test. Cardiorespiratory pathology (pneumonia, pulmonary embolism, myocardial ischemia) presenting with abdominal symptoms need to be ruled out by thoracic imaging, measuring cardiac biomarkers, or D-dimer levels.

Age, pregnant state, medications, and pre-existing disease states can affect laboratory values and their utility in diagnosis. The white cell count and alkaline phosphatase may be elevated during normal pregnancy; fever and leukocytosis may be absent in acute abdomen in the elderly [8, 9].

Additional Testing: Imaging

Ultrasonography (US) is useful in suspected pathology of the gall bladder, spleen, and pelvic organs (diagnosis of cholelithiasis and its complications, splenic trauma, ectopic gestation, pelvic inflammatory disease) – Table 1 [10]. It is also recommended in children and in pregnant women. Computed tomography (CT) has greater sensitivity and specificity for bowel (diverticulitis, appendicitis), pancreatic and retroperitoneal (kidney and abdominal aorta) pathology, and is the imaging modality of choice in suspected bowel ischemia. Magnetic resonance imaging (MRI) is useful in patients with iodine allergy or renal dysfunction, and in pregnant women. Other special and focused diagnostic tests are outlined in Table 2 [11, 12]. FAST (focused abdominal sonography in trauma) or E-FAST (extended focused abdominal sonography in trauma) and EMBU (emergency bed-side ultrasound) are both rapid, reliable, performed bedside, and do not interfere with continued resuscitation.

Limited radiation exposure (<5 rad) during pregnancy is safe; greatest fetal risk is between 8 and 15 weeks gestation. Most imaging studies in this generally young and healthy subset involves exposure well below this threshold. If considered necessary, the abdomen should be shielded during diagnostic imaging in pregnancy and patients should be counseled on risk of miscarriage, genetic disease, congenital anomalies, and growth restriction. Both US and MRI are safe during pregnancy [13].

Children are more radiosensitive and have more opportunities to develop radiation-induced cancers (estimated as 1.5–2% of all cancers in the United States) [7]. Hence radiation exposure should be selective and minimized in this age-group.

Preparing the Patient for Surgery

Preoperative Testing

Once the diagnosis and/or the decision to operate is made, further preoperative testing should be based on the need to clarify and optimize the

Table 1 Recommended imaging studies based on location of acute abdominal pain/organ

Epigastrium	Acute abdominal series [a] (erect chest, erect and supine abdominal x-rays), CT (stomach, pancreas)
Right upper quadrant	US+, CT [b] (liver, gall bladder, hepatic flexure)
Left upper quadrant	US, CT (spleen, splenic flexure, pancreas)
Umbilicus	US, CT (pancreas, abdominal aorta, transverse colon)
Right/left lumbar	US/CT (kidney, ascending/descending colon)
Right iliac fossa	US/CT (cecum, appendix, right tube and ovary)
Left iliac fossa	US/CT (sigmoid colon, left tube and ovary)
Hypogastrium	US/CT (urinary bladder, uterus, prostate, seminal vesicles)
External genitalia (males)	US (testes, appendages)

Text from Ref. [10]

+ Ultrasonography

[a]Plain x-rays useful in detecting bowel perforation (free peritoneal air), bowel obstruction (distended bowel, air-fluid levels), and ischemic bowel (pneumatosis intestinalis)

[b]Computed tomography – using oral/rectal and intravenous contrast

Table 2 Special diagnostic studies in patients presenting with an acute abdomen

FAST/E-FAST	Rapid, reliable, performed bedside in unstable patients. In suspected trauma to solid organs, mesentery. AAA leak
Angiography	Mesenteric ischemia, vascular abdominal emergencies (AAA leak), solid organ trauma (diagnostic and therapeutic embolization)
DPL	Bedside in unstable patients. Saline infused into peritoneal cavity and return analyzed for bowel contents, bile, blood and pus cells. Useful in detecting intraperitoneal bleeding, perforation, peritonitis
Magnetic resonance imaging	If CT contraindicated (iodine allergy, poor renal function). Useful in pregnancy
Helical (spiral) CT	Suspected pulmonary embolism, abdominal trauma
Saline/air/barium enema	In diagnosis and non-operative reduction of intussusception
Non-stress test	Detects fetal well-being. Useful in decision making regarding delivery at later stages of pregnancy at time of laparotomy

Text from Refs. [7, 9, 11]

AAA abdominal aortic aneurysm, *CT* computed tomography, *DPL* diagnostic peritoneal lavage, *FAST* focused assessment with sonography in trauma

patient's physical status and monitor resuscitation and recovery. Patients who have been evaluated and determined to have no preoperative indication for laboratory testing can safely undergo surgery with tests ordered only as needed during or after surgery. Tests should be ordered only when the initial assessment would have indicated a need even if surgery had not been planned.

Resuscitation

Resuscitation commences with assessment and optimization of airway, breathing and circulation, and should precede diagnostic imaging. Cerebral hypoperfusion and mental status changes increase risk of aspiration. Pallor, cyanosis, mottling, prostration, hypotension, tachycardia, and confusion suggest sepsis and dehydration, or ongoing bleeding. Multiple studies have shown that early administration of analgesics does not interfere with subsequent ability to diagnose and treat acute abdominal pathology, nor does it impact patient outcomes [2]. Antibiotics are not administered in stable and immunocompetent patients unless an infective source is evident or identified; immunocompromised patients require early and preoperative broad-spectrum antibiotic administration [11]. Fluid and electrolyte imbalances due to vomiting and third-space sequestration should be corrected, any hypotension reversed, renal

perfusion optimized and adequate urine output ensured prior to operative intervention, unless emergent surgery is mandated for continued bleeding or progressing sepsis. It is important to recognize ongoing transfusion requirements, identify and treat life-threatening causes of abdominal pain and monitor patients closely until recovery.

Perioperative Glucose Control

Patients with diabetes mellitus have poorer surgical outcomes, higher perioperative morbidity (coronary events, renal failure, infections), and longer postoperative hospital stays [14]. In critically ill patients requiring intensive care, a lower glycemic target (80–110 mg/dL) is recommended; a fasting glucose under 110 mg/dL and a random glucose under 180 mg/dL are considered desirable in patients less critically ill. Glucose, insulin, and potassium are infused judiciously in the perioperative period to maintain these parameters. Hydration should be maintained and acidosis (ketosis), hypoglycemia, and hypokalemia avoided. Oral agents are withheld on day of surgery. Preoperative medication regime is restored in stable patients in whom oral intake is tolerated. Metformin is usually held for 48–72 h following surgery or contrast-enhanced imaging and restarted after normal renal function is reestablished.

Laparoscopic Surgery

Evidence-based guidelines recommend laparoscopic surgery in patients with perforated peptic ulcer, acute cholecystitis, acute appendicitis, for adhesiolysis in patients with bowel obstruction caused by adhesions, gynecological disorders, and following abdominal trauma. Diagnostic laparoscopy is useful for assessing peritoneal intactness and avoiding laparotomy in stable patients with penetrating abdominal trauma. It is also valuable in stable patients with blunt abdominal trauma to exclude intra-abdominal injury requiring laporotomy. Laparoscopy results in decreased hospital stay, earlier return of bowel function, less postoperative pain, earlier ambulation, and less incidence of wound infection and incisional hernia. Optimal gestational age at which to perform laparoscopic surgery during pregnancy is unclear, but an upper limit of 26–28 weeks is advocated [13, 15]. Complications include visceral and vascular trauma during entry and dissection, pneumothorax, air embolism, carbon-dioxide narcosis, and low cardiac output.

Etiology of Acute Abdominal Pain in Patients Seeking Emergency Care

Mid-gut volvulus, intestinal atresia, and meconium ileus occur in newborns and infants; intussusception and Meckel's diverticulitis occur in infants and children; appendicitis and acute urogenital pathology are seen in children, adolescents, and young adults (Table 3). Incidence of bowel obstruction, diverticulitis, and consequences of atherosclerosis (aneurysm and bowel ischemia) increase with age [7, 8, 11]. Unusual causes of emergency room visit due to abdominal pain in children include constipation, Henoch-Schonlein purpura, pneumonia, streptococcal tonsillitis (tonsil tummy), gastroenteritis, and functional abdominal pain [7]. Both pregnancy-related causes (miscarriage, ectopic gestation, placental abruption, uterine rupture) and unrelated causes (appendicitis, cholecystitis) may cause acute abdominal pain requiring surgical intervention during pregnancy [13] .

Life-Threatening Causes

Early recognition and management of continued bleeding, bowel ischemia, and infarction minimizes the high associated mortality. History of amenorrhea should be obtained from women of child-bearing age. Myocardial ischemia is a consideration in elderly patients with upper abdominal pain (Table 4).

Abdominal Trauma

Background

Abdominal trauma accounts for over one-eighth of all traumatic injuries. The majority (75%) follow blunt trauma, mainly motor vehicle and auto-pedestrian accidents (50–75%), and direct blows to the abdomen (15%) [16–18]. As blunt injuries

Table 3 Etiology of acute abdominal pain in patients seeking emergency care

In children/adolescents	In adults/elderly
Acute appendicitis/cholecystitis	Acute appendicitis/cholecystitis
Small/large bowel obstruction (intussusception, volvulus, hernia, atresia, meconium ileus)	Small/large bowel obstruction, bowel perforation
Ectopic gestation	Acute pancreatitis
Twisted ovarian cyst, testicular torsion	Diverticulitis
Renal/ureteric colic	Mesenteric vascular occlusion
Pelvic inflammatory disease	Ischemic colitis
Meckel's diverticulitis	Renal/ureteric colic
	Ectopic gestation

Text from Refs. [7, 9, 11]

Table 4 Life-threatening causes of abdominal pain

Cause	Features
Ruptured abdominal aortic aneurysm	Hypotension, pulsatile abdominal mass, abdominal/low back pain. CT diagnostic
Rupture liver/spleen	Secondary to trauma, mononucleosis, rarely malaria, hematologic conditions. Abdominal pain, hypotension
Ruptured ectopic pregnancy	Amenorrhea, lower abdominal pain, hypotension
Hollow viscus perforation	Sudden severe initially localized then spreading abdominal pain, vomiting, abdominal distention, possible history of trauma including surgery and endoscopy
Intestinal ischemia/infarction	History of CAD, atrial fibrillation. Sudden severe abdominal pain out of proportion to physical findings, hypotension, prostration
Myocardial infarction	Upper abdominal pain, tachycardia, hypotension, minimal abdominal findings

Text from multiple sources

usually involve multiple viscera within and outside the abdomen and pose diagnostic challenges, they have a higher mortality compared with penetrating injuries [18]. Abdominal organs are especially vulnerable to lower chest wall, back, buttock, or pelvic trauma. The spleen, followed by the liver, is the most common solid organ involved; the bowel is the most common hollow viscus injured. Penetrating injuries usually involve the bowel and liver. Stab wounds to the abdomen are three times more common than gunshot wounds, though gunshot wounds account for almost all (90%) mortality due to penetrating injuries.

Abdominal trauma, also the second leading cause of death among physically abused children, accounts for nearly 10% of children admitted to pediatric trauma centers; most (85%) follow blunt abdominal trauma (BAT). Children under 2 years of age are at greatest risk of abuse [17, 19]. The thin abdominal wall in children and larger proportional size of solid organs compared with adults place them at higher risk for abdominal injuries after BAT. The liver, spleen, and kidney followed by the gastrointestinal tract are most commonly traumatized in children [17].

Diagnosis

Patients with BAT may pose a complex diagnostic challenge. Nearly half of patients may have no localizing features on admission. History may not always be available due to associated injuries,

lack of witnesses, altered mental status, and drug and alcohol use. Physical examination should encompass whole body evaluation including the cranium and cervical spine, chest, abdomen, pelvis and long bones. In penetrating injuries, entry and exit wounds should be carefully assessed as they predict nature and extent of injury. Hypotension, most often caused by solid viscus or vascular injury has high specificity for abdominal trauma [18, 20]. Abdominal distention, guarding, rebound tenderness and rigidity, presence of a seat-belt sign, and concomitant femoral fracture also have high specificity for intra-abdominal injuries [20]. However, physical examination has low sensitivity (55–65%) in BAT [17].

Management

Initial management should optimize patient's airway, breathing, and circulation. Laboratory analysis should focus on evaluating patient's clinical status and stability, and the need to detect and correct ongoing bleeding, fluid, electrolyte and acid–base imbalance, and renal and tissue hypoperfusion. Serial measurements help direct resuscitative efforts and monitor patient response. A complete blood count, urinalysis, a comprehensive metabolic panel (evaluating liver and kidney function), serum amylase and arterial blood gases are obtained initially. Patient is also typed and cross-matched as preparation for possible packed cell transfusions. Acidosis, hematuria, and anemia have high specificities for intra-abdominal injury [20]. Adequate intravenous access (two large-bore peripheral lines or a central line) is obtained, a nasogastric tube is inserted to decompress the proximal bowel and a Foley catheter is placed to monitor urine output.

In hemodynamically unstable patients (systolic blood pressure $\leq$ 90 mmHg) with BAT, bedside ultrasound (FAST –focused assessment with sonography in trauma or E-FAST- extended focused assessment with sonography in trauma), when available, should be the initial diagnostic modality performed to identify the need for emergent laparotomy [16, 21]. FAST has lower sensitivity (79%) but higher specificity (95%) for BAT. FAST is quick, performed bedside, identifies the presence of free fluid but not its etiology or the injury, and may be absent when performed early before enough fluid (400 mL) accumulates. Accuracy of FAST is extremely operator-dependent [16, 21].

Diagnostic peritoneal lavage (DPL) involves introducing an infra-umbilical catheter by an open, semi-open, or closed technique under local anesthesia with or without conscious sedation, after decompressing the stomach and urinary bladder [22]. Aspiration of 10 mL of blood is considered positive. If none is aspirated, 1 L of normal saline or lactated Ringer's solution is infused into the peritoneal cavity, allowed to drain out and examined for red blood cells ($>$100,000/mm^3 considered positive), white blood cells ($>$500/mm^3 considered positive), amylase, bile, food particles, and bacteria [22]. The presence of lavage fluid in an intercostal chest tube or Foley catheter is also documented (suggesting diaphragmatic or bladder rupture). DPL is useful in both blunt and penetrating injuries in patients with altered mental status or hemodynamic instability when FAST is not available. It is also indicated in patients with significant trauma to other systems (thorax, cranium, pelvis, long bones) requiring surgical intervention with equivocal abdominal findings. DPL does not identify the source of bleed, or retroperitoneal injuries. Prior abdominal surgery, obesity, hepatic cirrhosis, pregnancy, and coagulopathy are contraindications. DPL has largely been superseded

by FAST in unstable patients and by helical CT in stable patients.

Helical CT has both high sensitivity and specificity (97–99%) for intra-abdominal injury though less than one-fifth of CTs are positive for trauma and fewer patients (3%) end up requiring surgery [20]. CT is expensive, time-consuming, needs expertise for interpretation, and involves infusion of contrast and radiation, with risks of contrast-induced nephropathy and radiation-induced cancer. Clinical prediction rules have been developed to minimize its use and optimize its value. One rule consisting of seven variables (hypotension, Glasgow coma scale $<$14, costal margin tenderness, abdominal tenderness, femur fracture, hematuria $\geq$25 RBC/hpf, hematocrit $<$30 and chest x-ray showing rib fracture or pneumothorax) has high sensitivity; patients without any of these variables have negligible risk of intra-abdominal injury and are unlikely to benefit from abdominal CT scans [23]. CT may be performed with only intravenous contrast; ingesting oral contrast is unnecessary even when bowel injury is a concern [16].

Intravenous pyelography and cystourethrography are of value when damage to the urinary tract is suspected by the presence of lower abdominal, retroperitoneal or perineal trauma, hematuria or urinary retention. Laparoscopy is most useful for assessing penetrating injuries to the thoracoabdominal region in stable patients (especially the diaphragm). It has little value in BAT, assessing hollow viscus or retroperitoneal injuries, or evaluating the extent of injury to solid organs like the liver or spleen [18].

Surgery involves laparotomy, identifying the injury, staunching bleeding sources, repairing rents in hollow or solid viscera, excising organs injured beyond repair (spleen, kidney, bowel segments), peritoneal washout, and closing the incision either primarily or secondarily based on the degree of wound contamination and need for re-exploration. Resuscitation with fluids, packed cells, and blood products are continued. Invasive monitoring and ventilation in an intensive care unit may be necessary in critically ill patients until recovery.

Appendicitis

Background

Inflammation of the appendix follows luminal obstruction by fecoliths, Peyer's patches, foreign bodies, worms, and rarely tumors (carcinoid, carcinoma). The resultant rising intraluminal pressure causes distention, ischemia, and perforation. The parietal peritoneum, surrounding bowel and omentum attempt to localize the infection, on occasion, forming an appendicular mass. Perforation is more common among patients at extremes of age and in pregnant women.

Over 250,000 cases of appendicitis are diagnosed annually; the peak incidence occurs in the second decade of life (median age at diagnosis – 10–11 years) [24]. There is a slight male predominance (1.4:1). Appendicitis is also the most common non-obstetric surgical emergency during pregnancy.

Diagnosis: History and Examination

Classic symptoms of appendicitis (seen in <50% of children) include dull periumbilical pain migrating to the right lower abdomen, nausea, vomiting, anorexia, and low-grade fever [24]. Urinary frequency and urgency, diarrhea, and tenesmus are more common in pelvic appendicitis. In adults, right lower abdominal pain and migration of pain best predict appendicitis; absence of fever or pain before vomiting greatly reduces its likelihood. Pain may shift to the right lumbar area and even to the right upper quadrant of the abdomen in the later stages of pregnancy.

Guarding and tenderness in the right lower abdomen (McBurney's sign – most specific), and rebound tenderness (elicited on palpation/percussion) predict appendicitis. The inflamed appendix causes spasm of the adjacent abdominal wall and retroperitoneal musculotendinous structures resulting in overlying rigidity, and pain on ipsilateral hip hyperextension or internal rotation (psoas sign, obturator sign). Increase in intra-abdominal pressure as in coughing reproduces pain (Dunphy's sign). Palpation of the left iliac fossa shifts the bowel and intracolonic air producing greater pressure over the inflamed appendix, worsening the pain (Rovsing's sign) as does dropping from tiptoe to heel with a jarring landing (Markle sign- jar tenderness). Vomiting, rectal tenderness, rebound tenderness, and fever have greater positive predictive value in children than in adults, whereas right lower quadrant tenderness is less helpful [24–26].

Diagnosis: Investigations

Leukocytosis with a left shift and an elevated C-reactive protein (CRP) characterize appendicitis. Ultrasound shows appendiceal thickening, periappendiceal edema, increased peritoneal fluid, hypervascularity (on Doppler US), and the "sonographic McBurney's sign" – tenderness in response to pressure from the US probe. CT also shows the enlarged and thickened appendix and periappendiceal stranding. If both guarding and leukocytosis (>10,000/mm^3) are present – probability of appendicitis is high (>90%); elevated white count and C-reactive protein also increases likelihood of appendicitis (~90%). CT has high sensitivity and specificity (>90%) for appendicitis. US with graded compression has slightly lower sensitivity (85–90%) but high specificity (>90%). Initial US, followed by CT in patients with ambiguous findings on US, minimize radiation; preferred in children [7, 11, 26, 27].

Scoring systems (Alvarado, Pediatric appendicitis and Ohmann scores) incorporate several features in history, examination and laboratory tests to predict likelihood of disease. Knowledge of the pretest probability is important to maximize utility of scoring systems. When pretest probability is low, a higher score is required to rule in the diagnosis. Patients with a high likelihood of appendicitis should undergo appendectomy; those with a low probability should be discharged or treated for other pathology; those with an intermediate probability should be imaged, and based on the information, should undergo surgery, or observation until the clinical picture becomes clearer [28].

Appendicitis: Differential Diagnosis

Inflammatory, ischemic or other pathology in the right lower abdomen (Cecal diverticulitis, ectopic gestation, mesenteric adenitis, pyelonephritis, ureteric calculus, terminal ileitis) may all mimic appendicitis.

Appendicitis: Treatment

Appendectomy is usually performed through a low transverse (Lanz) or the classic McBurney muscle-splitting incision. Laparoscopic appendectomy is safer and causes fewer complications; these patients have shorter postoperative stays and return to work earlier.

Antibiotic choices in appendicitis include piperacillin-tazobactam and cefoxitin, which are effective against the *E.coli, streptococcus* species, *anerobes,* and *pseudomonas*, commonly found in appendicitis. Antibiotics are continued until features of infection resolve [24]. Whereas, a single-dose is sufficient in uncomplicated appendicitis, longer (5–7 day) courses are indicated in perforated appendicitis [24].

Wound infection, the most common complication, is minimized by intraoperative peritoneal lavage, which reduces bacterial contamination. Intra-abdominal collections (pelvic, subphrenic, right paracolic gutter) are rare, could follow ruptured appendicitis, and may need open or imaging-guided drainage. Urinary retention, urinary tract infections, and pneumonia are more common in the elderly, the debilitated and the immunosuppressed. Involvement of the fallopian tubes in the inflammatory mass may cause infertility. Appendicitis during pregnancy may cause miscarriage or preterm labor.

Patients presenting late (after 72 h, with localized infection, appendicular mass on examination or on imaging, absent systemic sepsis and peritonitis) may be managed nonoperatively with broad-spectrum antibiotics and image-guided drainage of fluid collections. Those with appendicoliths appear to have a higher likelihood of recurrent infections and merit consideration for interval appendectomy [24].

Cholelithiasis and Cholecystitis

Background

Cholelithiasis is a significant problem among adults and the elderly in the United States (6.3 million men, 14.2 million women aged 20–74 years) [29]. The female predominance persists across ethnicities (non-Hispanic whites, African-Americans and Mexican-Americans), and is five-fold among 20–29 year olds, though less among older age groups. The highest incidence of cholelithiasis appears to be among North American Indians over 30 years (nearly three-fourths). Gallstones are also associated with obesity (sevenfold increase in obese women), physical inactivity, parity, rapid weight loss, tobacco use, diabetes mellitus, lower alcohol consumption, and lower serum cholesterol [29, 30]. Other contributing factors and associations include Crohn's disease, ileal resection, medications (ceftriaxone, clofibrate, estrogens, octreotide, steroids), spinal cord injuries, and total parenteral nutrition [31].

Pathophysiology

Gallstones develop as a result of precipitation of cholesterol and calcium salts in supersaturated bile [32]. In addition, impaired gall bladder motility, increased biliary nucleation, presence of excess pronucleating proteins, and increased mucin production appear to promote gallstone formation [33]. Gallstones are classified as either cholesterol stones (commonest, nearly 80%) or pigment stones (usually associated with hemolytic disorders – hereditary spherocytosis, sickle cell disease). Black pigment stones containing calcium bilirubinate, form in sterile bile and are rare below 50 years of age; brown pigment stones are formed in the bile ducts and result from chronic bacterial or parasitic infection [33]. Though the majority (80%) of patients with gallstones are asymptomatic (silent gallstones), the rest present with symptoms and complications necessitating intervention.

Gallstones may cause functional dyspepsia, biliary colic, acute cholecystitis, mucocele of the gallbladder, gallbladder perforation and biliary peritonitis, choledocholithiasis, obstructive jaundice, cholangitis, acute and chronic pancreatitis, and gall stone ileus. Acute cholecystitis is inflammation of the gallbladder wall most often (90%) following cystic duct obstruction due to gallstones or biliary sludge; it develops in 1–3% of patients with gallstones [30, 32]. Following cystic duct obstruction, continued mucus production causes gallbladder distention, ischemia, and release of inflammatory mediators, necrosis, and perforation, either at the neck or the fundus that has the least blood supply, leading to biliary peritonitis. Secondary polymicrobial infection (*gram-negative bacilli, anerobes, enterococci*) may complicate cholecystitis and overgrowth of gas-forming bacteria (*clostridium species, E.coli*) within the gallbladder leads to emphysematous cholecystitis.

Diagnosis: History and Examination

Acute cholecystitis has a female preponderance (threefold) and presents with a rapid onset of severe, cramping right upper abdominal (RUQ) pain initially radiating to the back, then localizing to the RUQ. Abdominal pain lasting over 6 h indicates cholecystitis and not biliary colic [31]. Low-grade fever, chills, malaise, nausea, vomiting, and anorexia coexist [30, 32]. Almost three-fourths of patients report prior episodes of biliary colic. Occasionally the pain may localize in the chest or back [31]. Though vomiting and poor oral intake may lead to oliguria and high-colored urine, orange-colored urine, and clay-colored stools suggest complete biliary obstruction due to choledocholithiasis or pancreatobiliary tumors. Mirizzi syndrome refers to a gallstone impacted in the gallbladder neck or cystic duct compressing the common hepatic duct, causing varying degrees of biliary obstruction and jaundice. Elderly and immunocompromised patients may have milder symptoms.

Physical findings include low-grade fever (high fevers suggest gangrene or perforation), tachycardia, scleral icterus (more common in the elderly), and RUQ guarding and tenderness [31]. Murphy's sign (cessation of inspiration in response to pain on RUQ palpation) is characteristic of cholecystitis, has high sensitivity (97.2%), though less reliable in the elderly [34]. The gallbladder may be palpable in up to 33% of patients, especially those with first episodes [31]. Hypotension and mental status changes suggest sepsis, more commonly in the elderly, the debilitated and the immunosuppressed.

Diagnosis: Investigations

No solitary or combination of laboratory abnormalities is sufficiently sensitive or specific for cholecystitis. Leukocytosis with bandemia, and elevations of serum bilirubin and liver enzymes are observed, though serum bilirubin levels over 4 mg/dL or elevated amylase and lipase suggest choledocholithiasis [31].

Abdominal radiographs may rarely show gallstones or biliary air and seldom help diagnose cholecystitis, but may exclude other conditions such as bowel obstruction or perforation. US is both sensitive (82%) and specific (81%) for cholecystitis. Sonographic Murphy's sign (RUQ tenderness induced by the US probe) has a positive predictive value over 90% in detecting acute calculous cholecystitis. Presence of pericholecystic fluid and gallbladder wall thickening over 4 mm on US are other findings suggesting acute cholecystitis [31]. MRI has comparable sensitivity (86%) and specificity (82%) [35]. CT is less sensitive (75%) than US, has higher specificity (93%) and is more useful for identifying other abdominal (especially solid organ) pathology, and in detecting emphysematous cholecystitis, abscess, gallbladder perforation, and peritonitis. CT and MRI findings in cholecystitis are the same as that in US. HIDA (hepatobiliary iminodiacetic acid) scan, performed after injecting technetium-labeled derivatives of iminodiacetic acid, usually visualizes the gallbladder in 30 min and the small bowel in 60 min. Non-filling of the gallbladder within 60 min in patient with acute upper abdominal pain is highly suggestive of acute cholecystitis. HIDA scan has the highest diagnostic accuracy of all imaging modalities in detecting acute cholecystitis (sensitivity 96%, specificity 90%) [35] .

Differential Diagnosis

This includes other inflammatory intra-abdominal or pulmonary pathologies (peptic ulcer disease, pancreatitis, appendicitis, renal colic, pyelonephritis, pneumonia, liver abscess, liver tumors, and gonococcal perihepatitis) [31]. Most of these can be ruled in or out by a combination of clinical assessment, laboratory analysis and imaging.

Cholecystitis: Treatment

Treatment involves hospital admission, intravenous hydration, bowel rest, pain relief, and intravenous broad-spectrum antibiotics (ampicillin and gentamicin, ampicillin-sulbactam, piperacillin – tazobactam, a third-generation cephalosporin such as ceftriaxone, or a fluoroquinolone such as levofloxacin) [32]. Early cholecystectomy (within 24–48 h) is recommended. Earlier cholecystectomy within 12–24 h is a consideration in older patients, diabetics, and the immunosuppressed, more prone to develop rapid disease progression and complications (gangrene, emphysematous cholecystitis, empyema, or rupture) [32]. Early cholecystectomy is safe, highly successful, feasible with the laparoscope, has a low conversion rate to the open procedure, and associated with decreased hospital stay and earlier return to usual activities [30]. Delayed cholecystectomy (4–8 weeks after the acute episode) is not recommended as it does not reduce morbidity or conversion to open cholecystectomy, and increases risk of recurrent cholecystitis in the interim [30]. Ailing patients with comorbidities, who are poor surgical candidates, benefit from antibiotics and supportive care, and a percutaneous cholecystostomy under US or CT guidance.

Laparoscopic cholecystectomy is the gold standard for uncomplicated acute cholecystitis. Open cholecystectomy is preferred in patients with complications such as pancreatitis, gallbladder perforation and peritonitis, sepsis, suspected gallbladder cancer, or cholecystoenteric fistulas. Emergency surgery, dependent functional status, male gender, worsening American Society of Anesthesiology (ASA) class (3 through 5), older age, and presence of comorbidities or laboratory abnormalities (ascites, bleeding diathesis, pneumonia, decreased serum sodium or albumin, elevated white count, BUN, alkaline phosphatase or international normalized ratio (INR)) are all predictive of an initial decision to perform open cholecystectomy or a greater rate of conversion to the open procedure[36].

Acalculous Cholecystitis

Acalculous cholecystitis usually follows major trauma or surgery, resuscitation from cardiac arrest, systemic sepsis or presence of major comorbidities such as congestive heart failure, end-stage renal disease, and cancer [37]. Delayed diagnosis, poor patient status, and increased complication rate (gangrene, perforation, and peritonitis) associated with acalculous cholecystitis escalate mortality (around 30%). Bile stasis, gallbladder ischemia, and release of multiple vasoactive and inflammatory mediators are responsible for the cellular hypoxia and mucosal injury initiating this process. Unreliable clinical features, paucity of physical signs and confusing laboratory findings, make early diagnosis a challenge. US is diagnostic – features include wall thickness ≥ 3.5 mm (sensitivity 80%, specificity 98.5%), gallbladder distention, sonographic Murphy sign, pericholecystic fluid, intramural gas and a "halo" indicating intramural edema. CT is more accurate (sensitivity and specificity 95%); findings parallel that on US. HIDA scan is marginally less accurate than CT (sensitivity 80–90%, specificity 90–100%) [38]. Treatment includes intravenous hydration, bowel rest, broad-spectrum antibiotics as in calculous cholecystitis, and continued treatment of the primary pathology precipitating this event. Cholecystectomy (laparoscopic or open) is curative; percutaneous cholecystostomy controls the infection in most (85–90%) patients [37].

Special Situations

Conservative management of acute cholecystitis is recommended in pregnancy unless pancreatitis, ascending cholangitis, or common bile duct obstruction develops. Surgery is indicated in treatment failure. Laparoscopic cholecystectomy is the most common laparoscopic procedure during pregnancy, ideally performed in the second trimester [13].

Nearly a third of elderly patients with cholecystitis present with minimal abdominal pain and peritoneal signs, not correlating with severity of infection. Empyema of the gallbladder, gangrenous cholecystitis, biliary peritonitis, subphrenic or hepatic abscess may all occur in the elderly with minimal symptoms, little fever or elevated white counts. Emphysematous cholecystitis due to gas-producing organisms is also more common among the elderly, especially in men and diabetics [8].

Oral Dissolution of Cholelithiasis

This is an option in symptomatic patients with small ($\leq$5 mm) cholesterol stones in a functioning gallbladder and a patent cystic duct ($<10\%$ of cholesterol stones), who are unfit for surgery [39]. Options include chenodeoxycholic acid and ursodeoxycholic acid administered for 6–12 months. Recurrence is seen in nearly 50% of patients with multiple gallstones. Oral dissolution combined with lithotripsy is another treatment option avoiding open cholecystectomy but may also involve endoscopic sphincterotomy and removal of stones from the common bile duct and, in many cases, subsequent open cholecystectomy.

Inguinal Hernia

Background

A hernia is a protrusion of a viscus or tissue through an anatomical opening or an abnormal weakness in the wall of its containing cavity. Abdominal wall hernias develop in one in 20 patients; inguinal hernias constitute the majority (75%) [40]. Other commonly occurring hernias include umbilical, paraumbilical, and incisional hernias; the rest (femoral, epigastric,

spigelian, lumbar, gluteal, sciatic hernias) are uncommon. Multiple causes predispose to the development of hernias either by increasing intra-abdominal pressure or stretching and weakening of the abdominal wall (ascites, aging, chronic cough, constipation, heavy lifting, obesity, obstructive uropathy, pregnancy, prior lower abdominal surgery, smoking, and weight loss). Existence of an anatomical defect (inguinal canal, umbilicus, femoral canal) also predisposes to its development [40–42]. Inguinal hernias have a male predominance and are more common on the right.

Hernia- Anatomy

A hernia comprises of the hernial sac, the coverings of the sac and its contents. The "neck" of the sac is the narrow area usually located at its junction with the peritoneal cavity. The hernia contents can be diverse – extraperitoneal fat or omentum (omentocele), intestinal loops (enterocele), bladder diverticulum, or ovary and fallopian tube. The composition and types of hernia are outlined in Table 5.

The superficial inguinal ring is an opening in the external oblique aponeurosis just above and lateral to the pubic tubercle. The deep inguinal ring is a defect in the transversalis fascia just above the mid-point of the inguinal ligament. The inguinal canal traverses the two rings and contains the spermatic cord in men (round ligament in women), the ilioinguinal nerve, and the genital branch of the genitofemoral nerve. The inguinal canal is bounded anteriorly by the external oblique aponeurosis, posteriorly by the transversalis fascia, inferiorly by the inguinal ligament, and superiorly by the arched fibers of the conjoint tendon. Whereas in infants, the two rings are adjacent and the canal is short; in adults, the canal is oblique, directed downwards and medially, running from deep to superficial. Hesselbach's triangle, which forms the floor of the inguinal canal, is bounded superiorly and laterally by the inferior epigastric vessels, medially by the rectus sheath and inferiorly by the inguinal and pectineal ligaments [40].

Table 5 Types of hernia

Type	Nature
Reducible hernia	Hernial contents can be reduced into the peritoneal cavity usually be the patient or the surgeon (taxis). Omentum has a doughy consistency and is difficult to reduce. Bowel loops reduce with a gurgle
Irreducible hernia	Inability to reduce hernial contents-usually due to adhesions between sac and contents or between contents. Predisposes to obstruction and strangulation. Attempts at reduction may reduce the sac with its contents
Obstructed hernia	Bowel obstruction without features of bowel ischemia
Strangulated hernia	Hernial contents become ischemic and gangrenous. May involve omentum or intestine
Sliding hernia (hernia en glissade)	Type of inguinal hernia in which the posterior wall of the hernia sac is comprised of cecum or sigmoid colon, peritoneum and occasionally a part of the urinary bladder
Richter's hernia	Hernial sac contains only part of the bowel
Littre's hernia	Hernial sac containing a Meckel's diverticulum
Maydl's hernia	Hernial sac contains two loops of intestine with an intraperitoneal central loop that may develop ischemia
Pantaloon hernia	Inguinal hernia with indirect and direct components

Text from multiple sources

Inguinal Hernia: Types, Diagnosis, and Complications

Inguinal hernias pass either through the inguinal canal in their entirety (through the internal to the external ring, lateral to the Hasselbach's triangle – *indirect* – two-thirds of inguinal hernias) or through the weakened floor of the canal, through the Hasselbach's triangle (*direct*). The neck of an indirect hernia is thus lateral to the inferior epigastric vessels, whereas that of a direct hernia is medial [40].

In infants, and children inguinal hernias usually result from a persistent processus vaginalis, present at birth or shortly thereafter. Most children (90%) with cryptorchidism (maldescended testis) have an associated patent processus vaginalis and may present with an asymptomatic, irreducible, or strangulated inguinal hernia. Adults usually have a more insidious presentation, though a rapid onset may be precipitated by unusual straining or exertion. Patients may complain of a pulling sensation, discomfort, pain, or an increasing groin bulge. Occasional soreness or burning along the distribution of the ilioinguinal nerve (scrotum, medial upper thigh) may be noticed. Standing, coughing, and straining makes the hernia more noticeable; hence patients are usually examined in the upright position and asked to cough or strain.

The skin over the base of the scrotum can be invaginated to feel the superficial ring (*invagination test*). If the patient is asked to cough, the impulse from an indirect hernia is felt at the tip of the finger, whereas one from a direct hernia is felt at its pulp. The internal ring can be occluded by pressure after reducing the hernia (*internal ring occlusion test*); if the patient is asked to strain, an indirect hernia will remain reduced whereas a direct hernia will pouch. In the *Zieman's* technique, the index, middle, and ring fingers are placed over the deep, superficial, and femoral rings and the patient asked to cough, thereby helping to distinguish indirect and direct, inguinal, and femoral hernias. An omentocele has a doughy consistency; an enterocele gurgles on palpation and attempted reduction, and the initial portion of the reduction is more difficult. Bowel sounds can be heard on auscultation over an enterocele.

Irreducibility is diagnosed when the hernia does not reduce spontaneously in the recumbent position, or on attempts at reduction. Patients with obstructed hernias present with features of bowel obstruction (colicky abdominal pain, vomiting, abdominal distention, and constipation). Absent cough impulse, recent increase in size, a tense and tender swelling, and a tender distended abdomen indicate strangulation of the hernial contents (rare – 0.55% of asymptomatic hernias followed over 4 years) [43]. Imaging studies (US, CT) are useful in confirming the diagnosis of hernia and recognizing coexisting problems (cryptorchidism). Abdominal radiographs help diagnose bowel obstruction (distended bowel, air-fluid levels).

Differential Diagnosis

The differential diagnosis includes other inguinoscrotal pathology mimicking a hernia (vaginal hydrocele, spermatocele, undescended testis, an encysted hydrocele or lipoma of the spermatic cord, or a femoral hernia) [44].

Inguinal Hernia: Treatment

Watchful waiting is an option in patients with small hernias and minimal or no symptoms [45]. Most patients, over time, will develop discomfort enough to require surgery. In infants and children, a *herniotomy* – reduction of the hernial contents and ligation of the patent processus vaginalis (hernial sac) at the level of the deep ring – is sufficient. In adults, the posterior wall of the inguinal canal is strengthened either by approximation or imbrication using non-absorbable sutures (*herniorrhaphy*) or by using prosthetic material (*hernioplasty*). The traditional *Bassini* repair involves approximating the conjoint tendon to the inguinal ligament. The *Shouldice* repair involves a more extensive dissection of the inguinal region to define the layers of the abdominal wall and imbricating the posterior wall of the inguinal canal using stainless steel wire or polypropylene. It is considered the best non-mesh technique for inguinal hernia repair (recurrence 3.6%) [46]. In the "Lichtenstein tension-free hernia repair," the posterior wall is reinforced with a polypropylene mesh, placed preperitoneally and sutured in position. This acts as scaffolding in which tissue forms, further buttressing the abdominal wall, and significantly reducing the risk of recurrence (0.8%) [46]. The *plug and patch* technique uses two layers of polypropylene mesh to plug the defect (deep ring or the posterior wall defect) followed by buttressing the posterior wall further with a polypropylene mesh. The mesh may also be placed intra- or extraperitoneally, through laparoscopy. Advantages of laparoscopy include confirming the diagnosis of hernia, visualization of the defect and hernial sac, small incisions, and rapid return to work [41]. Disadvantages include need for general anesthesia and mesh, contributing to increased costs. Antibiotics are not indicated in elective hernia repairs.

Surgical techniques in irreducible and obstructed hernias are no different though patients with bowel obstruction need bowel rest, nasogastric suction, and replacement of fluids and electrolytes, continued until return of bowel function. Strangulated hernias with ischemic contents require resection of the contents (omentum, bowel resection followed by anastomosis); concomitant mesh repair increases risk of infection and rejection.

Complications

Operative complications include hemorrhage, hematoma, wound infection, and injury to the adjacent structures (bowel, bladder, spermatic cord structures, and nerves) and mesh rejection. Attention to detail and meticulous technique minimize complications. Long-term complications include recurrence (least in the Shouldice and mesh repairs), pain, and infertility (injury to the vasa deferentia in bilateral hernia repairs). Over half of patients may experience some degree of pain following surgery; less after the mesh or laparoscopic procedures. Pain may follow injury to the pubic tubercle, spermatic cord, the iliohypogastric or ilioinguinal nerves, or the lateral cutaneous nerve of the thigh. Though pain improves over time, some patients may require trigger point injections, medications, or surgical neurolysis for pain relief. Chronic pain is more common after recurrent hernia repair and in patients experiencing severe pain soon after surgery [41, 47].

Bowel Obstruction

Background

Intestinal obstruction may be divided into two types – dynamic (mechanical) obstruction of the bowel lumen with continued proximal peristalsis and progressive bowel distention, and adynamic (functional) obstruction with absent or inadequate peristalsis [48]. Obstruction may involve any part of the bowel including the esophagus, stomach, small and large bowel (Table 6). Adhesions, neoplasms, and hernias account for most (>90%) small bowel obstructions, with adhesions accounting for over three-fourths. Malignancy, volvulus, and diverticulitis cause most large bowel obstructions (>80%) [5]. Proximal to the site of obstruction the bowel distends with air (swallowed air, luminal gas) and fluid (impaired absorption, increased secretion) leading to bowel wall edema, loss of fluids and electrolytes, and dehydration [49]. In *closed loop obstruction* (bowel obstructed both proximally and distally due to adhesions or volvulus) the intermediate segment distends rapidly, with initially venous followed by arterial occlusion that progresses rapidly to ischemia, gangrene and perforation, and supervening infection, making it a surgical emergency.

Diagnosis: History and Examination

Symptoms of bowel obstruction depend on the site of the obstruction. Patients with esophageal obstruction may present with dysphagia, odynophagia, retrosternal discomfort or pain, retching, vomiting, regurgitation, and anorexia. Patients with gastric outlet obstruction (GOO) experience upper abdominal discomfort and vomiting, anorexia, and early satiety. Associated gastritis may cause hematemesis. Fetor is common in both esophageal and GOO. Patients with small bowel obstruction (SBO) generally experience pain, vomiting, abdominal distention, and constipation, in that order, whereas those with large bowel obstruction (LBO) experience initial constipation followed by abdominal distention, pain, and vomiting (the exception is in closed loop obstructions such as cecal or sigmoid volvulus, in which patients experience severe colicky followed by persistent abdominal pain out of proportion to physical findings, abdominal distention, and vomiting) [49]. Abdominal pain is usually colicky, though it becomes persistent in the presence of ischemic bowel or peritonitis; frequency and intensity diminishes with prolonged obstruction. The vomitus is usually clear or contains altered blood in GOO, contains bile in high SBO, is yellow in low SBO, and feculent in LBO. Abdominal distention is minimal or absent

Table 6 Site and causes of bowel obstruction

Site of obstruction	Cause of obstruction (mechanical)	Cause of obstruction (adynamic)
Esophagus	Atresia, Zenker's diverticulum, esophageal webs, goiter, foreign body impaction (food bolus), thoracic aortic aneurysm, benign and malignant strictures, Schatzki's ring, hiatal hernia	Scleroderma, achalasia, pharyngo-esophageal dysmotility (following stroke)
Gastric	Peptic ulcer disease, bezoars, gallstones, carcinoma, caustic injury, gastric volvulus	Diabetic gastroparesis
Small bowel	Annular pancreas, superior mesenteric artery syndrome, midgut volvulus, meconium ileus, adhesions, neoplasms, hernia, strictures, gallstone ileus	Mesenteric vascular occlusion, adynamic ileus (secondary to trauma, shock, peritonitis, metabolic/electrolyte imbalance, medications)
Large bowel	Carcinoma, volvulus (sigmoid, cecal), stricture (diverticular disease, ischemic colitis, radiation), intussusception	Constipation, pseudo-obstruction (trauma, shock, peritonitis, metabolic/electrolyte imbalance, sepsis, medications)

Text from multiple sources

in esophageal, gastric outlet and high SBO, central in low SBO, and generalized in LBO [49, 50]. Constipation may be absent initially in bowel obstruction due to continued peristaltic activity distal to the obstruction [50]. It may also be absent in partial bowel obstructions (adhesions, Richter's hernia), gall stone ileus, mesenteric vascular occlusion, and in ileus duplex. Continued vomiting, anorexia, and sequestration of fluid in the proximal bowel leads to dehydration, which manifests as fatigue, weakness, dizziness, and syncope.

Physical examination may reveal fever, tachycardia, hypotension, and mental status changes suggesting shock and sepsis (present in ischemic bowel or perforation). Abdominal distention, visible intestinal peristalsis, and hyperactive bowel sounds may be present. Abdominal scars indicating prior surgery is characteristic of adhesion-related obstruction. Guarding and rebound tenderness on palpation or percussion suggests ischemic bowel or peritonitis. Mass over a hernial orifice (inguinal, femoral, umbilical, incisional) is consistent with an irreducible and possibly obstructed hernia. A tense or tender hernia with a history of recent increase in size and absent cough impulse is characteristic of strangulated contents. The rectal examination shows an empty and ballooned rectum.

Investigations

Laboratory studies may show leukocytosis, hypochloremic, hypokalemic metabolic alkalosis (due to vomiting), elevated BUN, and serum creatinine (reflecting dehydration and poor renal perfusion). Elevated lactic acid and metabolic acidosis suggest gangrene, peritonitis, and sepsis [51]. Increased levels of intestinal fatty acid binding protein (I-FABP) has been detected in intestinal ischemia.

Plain abdominal x-rays (low sensitivity – 66%) may confirm both presence and level of bowel obstruction. In patients with high complete SBO, there is little air in the bowel, whereas more distal obstructions produce a "stepladder" pattern of air-fluid levels within bowel loops on erect abdominal x-rays. Presence of 2 or more air-fluid levels, differential air-fluid levels in the same loop of bowel and a mean air-fluid level width of at least 25 mm is very characteristic of high-grade SBO [52]. On supine abdominal x-rays, distended jejunal (identified by mucosal folds traversing the breadth of the lumen – valvulae conniventes) and ileal loops (featureless) are seen. With colonic obstruction, distended colon (identified by haustral folds, not traversing the width of the bowel) is seen. Using contrast (barium or diatrizoate meglumine – gastrografin) to outline the bowel helps delineate the site of obstruction and the transition zone. The contrast can be ingested orally or infused into the duodenum (enteroclysis); it can also be combined with CT (CT enteroclysis – specificity 100%; sensitivity 88% in SBO) [52]. Oral contrast is avoided in suspected bowel ischemia or perforation. Barium, diatrizoate, or air enemas are successful in reducing intussusception in the majority of children (70–84%) [7]. Diatrizoate, though safer than barium, does not provide mucosal detail, and its hygroscopic effect may exacerbate intravascular hypovolemia and electrolyte imbalance.

CT has high sensitivity (90–95%) and specificity (96%) in identifying high-grade bowel obstruction (distended proximal and collapsed distal bowel), locates transition zone and also diagnoses volvulus, ischemia (bowel thickening, poor IV contrast filling), perforation, and gangrene (pneumatosis intestinalis, pneumoperitoneum, mesenteric fat edema, ascites) [49]. CT also helps identify those patients without initial clear indications for emergent surgery, likely to fail conservative management and benefit from early intervention. Schwenter et al. devised a scoring system incorporating multiple variables (clinical, laboratory, and CT parameters) into a model (pain ≥ 4 days, guarding, C-reactive protein ≥ 75 mg/L, white cell count $\geq 10 \times 10^9$/L, ascitic fluid volume ≥ 500 mL on CT, reduced CT small bowel wall contrast enhancement), and found that the risk of intestinal ischemia was 6% in patients with score ≤ 1. Scores ≥ 3 are highly suggestive of ischemia (sensitivity 67.7%, specificity 90.8%) making surgery more likely to be considered in these patients [53]. Bedside US is an option in unstable patients and during pregnancy. US is extremely sensitive (98–100%) and specific (88–100%) in diagnosing intussusception. It is noninvasive, rapid, involves no radiation, identifies the apex of the intussusception, provides information regarding reducibility, and monitors reduction; it also identifies alternative diagnoses [7]. MRI also has both high sensitivity (95%) and specificity (100%) for SBO and LBO [54]. Colonoscopy is useful in confirming the diagnosis of LBO when in doubt, obtaining biopsies of obstructing lesions, derotating sigmoid volvulus, decompressing pseudo-obstruction, stenting strictures, and avoiding unnecessary surgery [55] .

Bowel Obstruction: Treatment

Principles of treatment include intravenous hydration, bowel rest, bowel decompression by nasogastric suction, correction of fluid and electrolyte imbalance, ascertaining the level and cause of obstruction, and determining need for emergent surgery. Prompt surgery is essential after resuscitation in patients with frank peritonitis, suspected ischemic/necrotic bowel, closed loop obstructions, in patients with obstructed/irreducible hernias, and in patients with volvulus or intussusception not responding to endoscopic derotation or hydrostatic reduction respectively. Surgery is also indicated if conservative measures do not result in clinical improvement (optimal duration of conservative management is controversial) and if progressive hemodynamic instability and acidosis point to worsening ischemia or sepsis. Fever, leukocytosis, acidosis and hemodynamic instability, or clinical evidence of peritonitis or bowel ischemia also indicates initiation of broad-spectrum antibiotic therapy (effective against gram-negative organisms and anaerobes).

Surgery may involve laparotomy or laparoscopy, release of adhesions, segmental resection of ischemic or obstructing segments of small/large bowel, and primary anastomosis in the absence of infection or peritoneal contamination. In the presence of active peritoneal sepsis or spillage of bowel contents, the healthy bowel ends are sutured to the skin (jejunostomy, ileostomy, colostomy); the ends re-anastomosed

after patient recovery a few weeks later. Antibiotics are continued until infection resolves. Patient characteristics predicting increased postoperative morbidity (12–47%) include older age, comorbid illness (cerebrovascular accident with neurological deficit, CHF, chronic obstructive pulmonary disease), leukopenia ($<4500/mm^3$), renal dysfunction (creatinine >1.2 mg/dL), and poor functional status. Wound contamination or infection and resection of bowel also predict increased postoperative morbidity [56]. Advanced age, higher ASA class (≥ 3), chronic illness, treatment delay, and bowel ischemia predict higher mortality [49].

Complications of surgery include hemorrhage, wound infection, intra-abdominal collections, inadvertent trauma to bowel, nerves, vessels, ureter or solid organs (liver, spleen, kidney), recurrent obstruction, atelectasis, pneumonia, respiratory failure requiring ventilator support, urinary tract infection, and renal failure.

Surgical Problems of the Digestive System: Prevention

Lifestyle changes including seat belt use, defensive driving, minimizing alcohol use, and avoiding recreational drug use will decrease abdominal trauma associated with motor vehicle accidents. Incidental appendectomy, though an option and generally safe, is not recommended but may have some value in women presenting with undiagnosed abdominal/pelvic pain as part of laparoscopic evaluation [57] Incidental cholecystectomy is recommended in patients prone to develop cholelithiasis and cholecystitis (hemolytic disorders, gall bladder polyps, and cholesterolosis, Porcelain gallbladder and those with large gall stones- over 3 cm) [58] Maintaining ideal body weight, exercising, repairing symptomatic hernias, and meticulous operative technique and postoperative care will reduce risk of hernia-related complications and recurrence. No surgical technique has been found to reduce the risk of adhesions causing bowel obstruction significantly, though minimal manual trauma to the intra-abdominal structures, omental interposition between the abdominal wall and intra-abdominal organs, and excluding foreign materials in the peritoneal cavity (sutures) help.

References

1. National Hospital Ambulatory Medical Care Survey: 2016 Emergency department summary tables. https://www.cdc.gov/nchs/data/nhamcs/web_tables/2016_ed_web_tables.pdf. Accessed 24 Oct 2019.
2. McNamara R, Dean AJ. Approach to acute abdominal pain. Emerg Med Clin North Am. 2011;29(2):159–73.
3. Smith KA. Abdominal pain. In: Walls RM, editor. Rosen's emergency medicine – concepts and clinical practice. Philadelphia: Saunders Elsevier; 2018. p. 213–24. Ch 24.
4. Mangione S. The abdomen. In: Physical diagnosis secrets. 2nd ed. Philadelphia: Mosby Elsevier; 2008. p. 445–87. Ch 15.
5. Hayden GE, Sprouse KL. Bowel obstruction and hernia. Emerg Med Clin North Am. 2011;29(2):319–45.
6. Duncan KO, Leffell DJ. Preoperative assessment of the elderly patient. Dermatol Clin. 1997;15(4):583–93.
7. Marin JR, Alpern ER. Abdominal pain in children. Emerg Med Clin North Am. 2011;29(2):401–28.
8. Ragsdale L, Southerland L. Acute abdominal pain in the older adult. Emerg Med Clin North Am. 2011;29(2):429–48.
9. Cappell MS, Friedel D. Abdominal pain during pregnancy. Gastroenterol Clin N Am. 2003;32(1):1–58.
10. Cartwright SL, Knudson MP. Evaluation of acute abdominal pain in adults. Am Fam Physician. 2008;77(7):971–8.
11. Millham FH. Acute abdominal pain. In: Feldman M, editor. Sleisenger and Fordtran's gastrointestinal and liver disease. 9th ed. Philadelphia: Saunders Elsevier; 2010. p. 151–62. Ch 10.
12. Stoker J, van Randen A, Lameris W, Boermeester MA. Imaging patients with acute abdominal pain. Radiology. 2009;253(1):31–46.
13. Kilpatrick CC, Monga M. Approach to the acute abdomen in pregnancy. Obstet Gynecol Clin N Am. 2007;34(3):389–402.
14. Smiley DD, Umpierrez GE. Perioperative glucose control in the diabetic or nondiabetic patient. South Med J. 2006;99(6):580–9.
15. Sauerland S, Agresta F, Bergamaschi R, et al. Laparoscopy for abdominal emergencies. Evidence-based guidelines of the European Association of Endoscopic Surgery. Surg Endosc. 2006;20(1):14–29.
16. Diercks DB, Mehrotra A, Nazarian DJ, Promes SB, Decker WW, Fesmire FM. American College of Emergency Physicians. Clinical policy: critical issues in the evaluation of adult patients presenting to the emergency department with acute blunt abdominal trauma. Ann Emerg Med. 2011;57(4):387–404.
17. Isenhour JL, Marx J. Advances in abdominal trauma. Emerg Med Clin North Am. 2007;25(3):713–33.
18. Nichols JR, Puskarich MA. Abdominal trauma. In: Walls RM, editor. Rosen's emergency medicine – concepts and clinical practice. 9th ed. Philadelphia: Saunders Elsevier; 2018. p. 404–19. Ch 39.
19. Lane WG, Dubowitz H, Langenberg P. Screening for occult abdominal trauma in children with suspected physical abuse. Pediatrics. 2009;124(6):1595–602.
20. Nishijima DK, Simel DL, Wisner DH, Holmes JF. Does this adult patient have a blunt intra-abdominal injury? JAMA. 2012;307(14):1517–27.
21. Williams SR, Perera P, Gharahbaghian L. The FAST and E-FAST in 2013: trauma ultrasonography: overview, practical techniques, controversies, and new frontiers. Crit Care Clin. 2014;30(1):119–50.
22. Whitehouse JS, Weigelt JA. Diagnostic peritoneal lavage: a review of indications, technique, and interpretation. Scand J Trauma Resusc Emerg Med. 2009;17:13.
23. Holmes JF, Wisner DH, McGahan JP, Mower WR, Kuppermann N. Clinical prediction rules for identifying adults at very low risk for intra-abdominal injuries after blunt trauma. Ann Emerg Med. 2009;54(4):575–84.
24. Pepper VK, Stanfill AB, Pearl RH. Diagnosis and management of pediatric appendicitis, intussusception and Meckel's diverticulum. Surg Clin North Am. 2012;92(3):505–26.
25. Bundy DG, Byerley JS, Liles EA, Perrin EM, Katznelson J, Rice HE. Does this child have appendicitis? JAMA. 2007;298(4):438–51.
26. Andersson RE. Meta-analysis of the clinical and laboratory diagnosis of appendicitis. Br J Surg. 2004;91(1):28–37.
27. Doria AS, Moineddin R, Kellenberger CJ, et al. US or CT for diagnosis of appendicitis in children and adults? A meta-analysis. Radiology. 2006;241(1):83–94.
28. Ebell MH. Diagnosis of appendicitis: part I. History and physical examination. Am Fam Physician. 2008;77(6):828–30.
29. Everhart JE, Khare M, Hill M, Maurer KR. Prevalence and ethnic differences in gallbladder disease in the United States. Gastroenterology. 1999;117(3):632–9.
30. Knab LM, Bohler A, Mahvi DM. Cholecystitis. Surg Clin North Am. 2014;94(2):455–70.
31. Wang DQH, Afdahl NH. Gallstone disease. In: Feldman M, editor. Sleisenger and Fordtran's gastrointestinal and liver disease. 9th ed. Philadelphia: Saunders Elsevier; 2010. p. 1089–120. Ch 65.
32. Elwood DR. Cholecystitis. Surg Clin North Am. 2008;88(6):1241–52.
33. Venneman NG, van Erpecum KJ. Pathogenesis of gallstones. Gastroenterol Clin N Am. 2010;39(2):171–83.
34. Privette TW Jr, Carlisle MC, Palma JK. Emergencies of the liver, gall bladder and pancreas. Emerg Med Clin North Am. 2011;29(2):293–317.
35. Kiewiet JJ, Leeuwenburgh MM, Bipat S, Bossuyt PM, Stoker J, Boermeester MA. A systematic review and meta-analysis of diagnostic performance of imaging in acute cholecystitis. Radiology. 2012;264(3):708–20.
36. Kaafarani HM, Smith TS, Neumayer L, Berger DH, Depalma RG, Itani KM. Trends, outcomes, and

predictors of open and conversion to open cholecystectomy in veterans health administration hospitals. Am J Surg. 2010;200(1):32–40.

37. Barie PS, Eachempati SR. Acute acalculous cholecystitis. Gastroenterol Clin N Am. 2010;39(2):343–57.

38. Lane JD. Acalculous cholecystitis imaging; 2017. http://emedicine.medscape.com/article/365553-overview#showall. Accessed 15 May 2020.

39. Portincasa P, Di Ciaula A, Bonfrate L, Wang DQ. Therapy of gallstone disease: what it was, what it is, what it will be. World J Gastrointest Pharmacol Ther. 2012;3(2):7–20.

40. Malangoni MA, Rosen MJ. Hernias. In: Townsend CM, editor. Sabiston textbook of surgery. 20th ed. Philadelphia: Saunders Elsevier; 2017. p. 1092–120. Ch 44.

41. Matthews RD, Neumayer L. Inguinal hernia in the 21st century. An evidence-based review. Curr Probl Surg. 2008;45(4):261–312.

42. Holzheimer RG. Inguinal hernia: classification, diagnosis and treatment – classis, traumatic and sportsman's hernia. Eur J Med Res. 2005;10(3):121–34.

43. Mizrahi H, Parker MC. Management of asymptomatic inguinal hernia. Arch Surg. 2012;147(3):277–81.

44. Tulloh B, Nixon SJ. Abdominal wall, hernia and umbilicus. In: Bailey and love's short practice of surgery. 27th ed. London: Hodder Arnold; 2018. p. 1022–47. Ch 60. https://www.academia.edu/37780581/Bailey_and_Loves_Short_Practice_of_Surgery_27th_Edition.pdf. Accessed 27 Nov 2019.

45. Turaga K, Fitzgibbons RJ, Puri V. Inguinal hernias: should we repair? Surg Clin North Am. 2008;88(1):127–38.

46. Amato B, Moja L, Panico S, Persico G, Rispoli C, Rocco N, Moschetti I. Shouldice technique versus other open techniques for inguinal hernia repair. Cochrane Database Syst Rev. 2012;4:CD001543.

47. Poobalan AS, Bruce J, Smith WC, King PM, Krukowski ZH, Chambers WA. A review of chronic pain after inguinal herniorrhaphy. Clin J Pain. 2003;19(1):48–54.

48. Winslet MC. Intestinal obstruction. In: Bailey and love's short practice of surgery. 27th ed. Florida: Taylor and Francis Group; 2017. p. 1280–98. Ch 71. https://www.academia.edu/37780581/Bailey_and_Loves_Short_Practice_of_Surgery_27th_Edition.pdf. Accessed 26 Nov 2019.

49. Turnage RH, Heldman M. Intestinal obstruction. In: Feldman M, editor. Sleisenger and Fordtran's gastrointestinal and liver disease. 9th ed. Philadelphia: Saunders Elsevier; 2010. p. 2105–20. Ch 119.

50. Hayanga AJ, Bass-Wilkins K, Bulkley GB. Current management of small-bowel obstruction. Adv Surg. 2005;39:1–33.

51. Jackson PG, Raiji M. Evaluation and management of intestinal obstruction. Am Fam Physician. 2011;83(2):159–65.

52. Maglinte DD, Heitkamp DE, Howard TJ, Kelvin FM, Lappas JC. Current concepts in imaging of small bowel obstruction. Radiol Clin N Am. 2003;41(2):263–83.

53. Schwenter F, Poletti PA, Platon A, Perneger T, Morel P, Gervaz P. Clinicoradiological score for predicting the risk of strangulated small bowel obstruction. Br J Surg. 2010;97(7):1119–25.

54. Beall DP, Fortman BJ, Lawler BC, et al. Imaging bowel obstruction: a comparison between fast magnetic resonance imaging and helical computed tomography. Clin Radiol. 2002;57(8):719–24.

55. Katsanos KH, Maliouki M, Tatsioni A, Ignatiadou E, Christodoulou DK, Fatouros M, Tsianos EV. The role of colonoscopy in the management of intestinal obstruction: a 20-year retrospective study. BMC Gastroenterol. 2010;10:130.

56. Margenthaler JA, Longo WE, Virgo KS, Johnson FE, Grossmann EM, Schifftner TL, Henderson WG, Khuri SF. Risk factors for adverse outcomes following surgery for small bowel obstruction. Ann Surg. 2006;243(4):456–64.

57. Song JY, Yordan E, Rotman C. Incidental appendectomy during endoscopic surgery. J Soc Laparoendosc Surg. 2009;13(3):376–83.

58. Zakko SF, Afdhal NH. Approach to patients with gall stones. Up To Date 2019. www.uptodate.com. Accessed 25 Oct 2019.

Selected Disorders of the Digestive System

98

Jason Domagalski

Contents

J. Domagalski (✉)
Medical College of Wisconsin, Menomonee Falls, WI,
USA
e-mail: jason.domagalski@froedtert.com

© Springer Nature Switzerland AG 2022
P. M. Paulman et al. (eds.), *Family Medicine*,
https://doi.org/10.1007/978-3-030-54441-6_101

Acute Diarrheal Illness

General Principles

Acute diarrheal illness is a common presenting condition in primary care with the majority of cases attributed to viral gastroenteritis. Acute gastroenteritis in children under the age of five leads to 300 deaths, over 1.5 million outpatient visits, and 200,000 hospitalizations in the United States every year [1]. Annual deaths attributed to diarrheal illness are estimated to be 2.5 million worldwide [2].

Acute diarrhea is defined as increased stool frequency as well as increased water content and volume lasting less than 14 days [3]. Viral infections are the most common etiology of acute diarrhea, with rotavirus attributing to 75–90% of cases in children [1]. Bacterial pathogens are more likely with recent travel, foodborne illness, or immunocompromised states. The most common bacterial causes of acute diarrhea in the US include enterohemorrhagic *E. coli*, *Clostridioides (formerly clostridium) difficile*, *Shigella*, *Salmonella*, and *Campylobacter* [4].

Approach to Patient

The initial approach to a patient presenting with acute diarrheal illness should include a thorough history and physical exam evaluating the following questions:

1. What is the onset, duration, and consistency of the stool (i.e., bloody, watery, bilious)?
2. Is the patient showing signs of dehydration (i.e., thirst, decreased urine output, dizziness)?
3. Has there been any recent travel?
4. Is the patient vomiting (suggestive of a viral illness or foodborne illness)?
5. Is the patient showing signs of invasive bacterial diarrhea (i.e., fever, tenesmus, and grossly bloody stool)?
6. Is the patient pregnant (pregnant women are 12 times more likely to contract listeriosis)?
7. Is there any history of other gastroenterologic disease or surgery (i.e., partial colectomy or celiac disease)?
8. Any risk factors for immunosuppression? (i.e., human immunodeficiency virus, long-term steroid use, chemotherapy).

Diagnosis

Diagnostic testing is not typically indicated for acute diarrheal illnesses; however, further investigation is warranted for patients with longer duration of illness, signs of dehydration, history of being immunocompromised, or historical features indicating a serious bacterial infection. Common characteristic features and management of the covered pathogens are summarized in Table 1.

Lactoferrin is the preferred test for identifying leukocytes in the stool as a marker of inflammation. Fecal leukocytes lack the sensitivity and specificity

Table 1 Clinical features and management of acute diarrheal illness

Pathogen	Historical features	Symptoms	Management
Viral (*Norovirus, Rotavirus*)	Variable, increased risk in day care centers, group living	+/− fever, abdominal pain, nausea/vomiting	Hydration, antipyretics, antispasmodics, loperamide/Lomotil
Salmonella	Consumption of raw milk, undercooked meat, fecal-oral sexual contact	Fever, abdominal pain, +/− nausea, +/− bloody stool	Hydration, antipyretics, antispasmodics
Clostridioides difficile	Hospital admission, antibiotics within past 3 months	+/− fever, +/− abdominal pain, +/− bloody stools	Oral vancomycin 125 mg qid × 10 days, fidaxomicin 200 mg bid for 10 days
EHEC	Consumption of raw beef, seed sprouts, raw milk	No fever, abdominal pain, bloody stool	Oral/intravenous hydration

compared to lactoferrin which is >90% and >70%, respectively [5]. Positive occult blood in combination with lactoferrin increases the likelihood of an inflammatory diarrhea. Stool cultures are rather expensive and should only be reserved to use in patients with grossly bloody diarrhea, severe dehydration, history of immunosuppression, or signs of inflammatory disease [6]. Testing for *Clostridioides difficile* toxins A and B is indicated in any patient that develops diarrhea after 3 days of hospitalization, during any antibiotic course or up to 3 months after an antibiotic course is discontinued. Testing for ova and parasites is indicated in patients with diarrheal illnesses exceeding 7 days along with one or more features: patients with AIDs, men who have sex with men (MSM), bloody diarrhea with few fecal leukocytes, community waterborne outbreaks, children attending daycare, or recent travel to mountainous regions [7]. Endoscopic evaluation is often of limited use and should be reserved for those patients with unclear diagnosis after routine blood and stool tests are negative, if empiric therapy is ineffective or if symptoms persist [8].

Treatment

Viral Infections

Viral gastroenteritis accounts for the majority of diarrheal illnesses with the most common causative viruses being *Rotavirus*, adenoviruses, echoviruses, and reoviruses. Ambulatory management generally involves avoidance of solid foods for the first 24–48 h and fluid replacement with oral rehydration with commercially available products (Pedialyte) or following the 2002 World Health Organization-endorsed reduced osmolarity oral rehydration solution by combining 1 l of water, six teaspoons of sugar, and half teaspoon of salt [8]. Antidiarrheal agents such as loperamide (Imodium) or diphenoxylate/atropine (Lomotil) may also be used to reduce duration of illness in patients with nonbloody stool.

Bacterial Infections

Salmonella

Typically associated with *typhimurium* serotype, *Salmonella* induces mild enteritis associated with fever, nausea, and vomiting which is self-limited to less than 4 days duration. Management is usually supportive in nature with oral rehydration and antispasmodics. Antibiotics are not generally indicated as they will prolong the carrier status [8].

Enterohemorrhagic *Escherichia coli* (EHEC)

Typically associated with the consumption of raw seed sprouts, unpasteurized juice, and undercooked poultry or hamburger meat, EHEC may produce severe symptoms to include bloody diarrhea and multisystem organ failure in the very young or old. Also commonly known as Shiga toxin producing *E. coli* (STEC), EHEC typically is managed with supportive care and IV hydration when necessary. Antibiotics are often cautioned against as their use may increase risk of developing hemolytic uremic syndrome (HUS) in which the patient develops thrombocytopenia, hemolytic anemia, and renal failure [8].

Clostridioides Difficile

Clostridioides (formerly clostridium) difficile infections are commonly associated with nosocomial-induced diarrhea as well as diarrhea that develops during or soon after antibiotic exposure. *C. difficile* infection is 7–10 times more likely during any point of an antibiotic course [8]. Major complications include fulminant colitis, toxic megacolon, intestinal perforation, and even septic shock. First-line management for nonsevere disease is oral vancomycin 125 mg qid for 10 days or oral fidaxomicin 200 mg bid for 10 days. Metronidazole 500 mg qid for 10 days is an acceptable alternative if the other two agents are unavailable, but should be avoided in patients who are elderly, infirmed, or who have developed the infection in association with inflammatory bowel disease. Oral vancomycin or oral fidaxomicin are more appropriate for severe infections. Although both are effective, recurrence with *Clostridium difficile* is as high as 15–25%. For recurrent or severe infections, fecal transplant from a healthy donor is a viable treatment strategy [9].

Prevention/Family and Community Issues

General hygiene and hand washing can prevent the majority of diarrheal illnesses. Certain populations should avoid high-risk behaviors. Patients with heavy alcohol use or people with chronic liver disease consuming shellfish as they are at risk for contracting *Vibrio vulnificus*. Pregnant women are at risk for being infected with *Listeria monocytogenes* from soft cheeses and unheated deli meats. Vaccines currently available include those to prevent *Rotavirus* in small infants and typhoid fever for travelers [3].

Ischemic Bowel Syndromes

General Principles

The colon can tolerate significantly reduced blood flow with up to 80% of capillaries not perfusing during bowel rest without sacrificing adequate oxygen delivery [10]. Compromise of blood flow to the colon can present as an acute or chronic process and is always secondary to an underlying disease process ranging from trauma to a hypercoaguable state. Acute mesenteric ischemia is a rare but fatal condition with an incidence of only 12.9 per 100,000 person-years and a mortality rate greater than 50% [10, 11]. The four major conditions that cause acute mesenteric ischemia include acute superior mesenteric artery (SMA) thromboembolic occlusion, mesenteric arterial thrombosis, mesenteric venous thrombosis, and nonocclusive mesenteric ischemia.

Approach to Patient

The common clinical triad of acute bowel ischemia includes severe abdominal pain out of proportion to physical exam, bowel emptying, and a source of occlusion or decreased blood flow [10]. Chronic ischemia will typically present with a history of postprandial pain (intestinal angina), fear of food, and weight loss. Prompt diagnosis requires a high index of clinical suspicion, focused history and physical exam, and prompt ordering of a high-resolution CT [11]. Common conditions associated with mesenteric ischemia include atrial fibrillation, congestive heart failure, hypovolemia, hyper-coaguable states, portal hypertension, and major trauma [11].

Diagnosis

There is no one single plasma marker sensitive enough to make an early diagnosis [10]. Signs of metabolic acidosis on arterial blood gas and metabolic panels are often a late finding indicating bowel infarction. Other lab markers of early bowel ischemia include elevated levels of amylase and lipase [11]. An elevated white blood cell count or left shift may indicate a full-thickness injury or ischemia with bacterial translocation [12].

Diagnosis typically requires early ordering of abdominal CT with contrast. This allows complete evaluation of both the mesenteric arterial and venous patency. The use of mesenteric vessel angiography has diminished due to the efficiency and availability of CT scans for acute ischemia but still may have high utility in the workup of chronic mesenteric ischemia [11]. Magnetic Resonance Angiography is another option, but is limited due to duration of test, lacks necessary resolution, and can overestimate degree of stenosis [12].

Treatment

Acute Mesenteric Ischemia

The approach to management of acute bowel ischemia relies on three essential principles: the cause of the ischemia, severity of presentation, and duration of compromised blood flow. Another key aspect in management is the availability of therapeutic procedures in interventional radiology as well as vascular surgery.

Acute SMA Occlusion

Initial treatment in stable patients includes aggressive parenteral fluid replacement, bowel decompression with nasogastric tube, and/or broad-spectrum antibiotics if sepsis is suspected. In patients with suspected bowel infarction, immediate exploratory laparotomy is warranted. Embolic obstructions require surgical embolectomy of the superior mesenteric artery as the occlusions are typically secondary to a cardiac thrombus and not amenable to thrombolysis due to the high risk of fragmentation and distal embolization [11]. Mesenteric arterial thrombosis due to chronic atherosclerotic occlusive disease of the SMA however is more amenable to endovascular techniques with stenting when possible. Despite this less-invasive approach, exploratory laparotomy may still be necessary to assess the recovery of the ischemic bowel. In more severe cases, aorto-mesenteric bypass may be necessary [11].

Acute Mesenteric Venous Thrombosis

Mesenteric venous thrombosis is best treated medically with anticoagulation using continuous infusion of unfractionated heparin and restoration of circulating blood volume with parenteral fluid replacement. Nonsurgical management has been documented to have as high as 80% 30-day survival rate [10]. Surgical management is reserved for patients with signs of bowel infarction requiring resection of necrotic bowel [11]. Necrosis typically occurs when venous engorgement obstructs arterial blood flow. When surgery is performed, it often requires extensive removal of affected bowel, and prognosis is typically poor. Patients who do recover often undergo extensive bowel removal and subsequently suffer from short gut syndrome [11].

Nonocclusive Disease

Almost always secondary to critical illness, non-occlusive ischemia is often associated with cardiopulmonary insufficiency and treatment of septic shock. Management is limited to replenishing mesenteric circulation and observing for early signs of infarction. Ischemic colitis, a type of nonocclusive ischemia, typically responds to medical management with bowel rest, broad-spectrum antibiotics, and fluid replacement in up to 60% of cases. Exploratory laparotomy is warranted with any type of nonocclusive ischemia if patients begin to develop signs of peritonitis or clinical decompensation indicating possible bowel infarction [11].

Chronic Mesenteric Ischemia

Chronic mesenteric ischemia is an uncommon condition and more than 90% of cases are related to progressive atherosclerotic stenosis of one or more mesenteric arteries [13]. The goals of management are to resolve patient symptoms, improve nutritional status, and prevent possible infarction. When attempted, revascularization with angioplasty and possible stent placement should be as complete as possible. Stent placement is typically warranted when post-angioplasty residual stenosis is 30% or greater, the area of involvement has a high-pressure gradient or the patient has a history of dissection with prior angioplasty attempts. Open surgical revascularization can be considered if endovascular approach failed, contraindications to radiation or contrast exist or if endovascular technique is not technically possible due to extensive occlusion [13].

Prevention and Family and Community Issues

Patients at risk for developing atherosclerotic disease should be managed for maximal risk reduction with smoking cessation as well as management of hypertension and hyperlipidemia. Patients with hypercoaguable states or strong family history of hypercoagulability should be advised on risks of medications that may increase the risk of thrombosis. Any patients with the above risk factors should be made aware of the signs and symptoms of bowel ischemia and advised to seek immediate medical attention if symptoms develop.

Food Allergy

General Principles

The exact prevalence of food allergy is unknown; however, recent studies indicate that it affects anywhere from 2% to 10% of the population with approximately 8% of children in the United States having one food allergy, 2.4% having multiple, and approximately 3% having a history of severe reactions. The most common offenders are cow's milk, peanuts, and tree nuts in children while shellfish, fruits, and vegetables being the most common in adults. Although somewhat unclear, epidemiologic studies are indicating a potential rise in food allergies among children in the United States over the last 2–3 decades [14].

Multiple risk factors are associated with food allergy development as listed in Table 2 and may provide areas of intervention to prevent food allergies. Resolution of childhood allergies to milk, eggs, wheat, and soy is common whereas allergies to peanut, tree nuts, fish, and shellfish tend to persist.

Table 2 Risk factors for food allergy

Modifiable risk factors	Nonmodifiable risk factors
Reduced consumption of dietary fat	Male gender (in children)
Reduced consumption of antioxidants	Black ethnicity
Obesity	Asian ethnicity
Vitamin D deficiency	Atopic dermatitis
Increased hygiene	

Approach to Patient

Common assessment for potential food allergies should include the following historical clinical questions:

1. What symptoms does the patient develop (urticaria versus more severe symptoms such as airway compromise)?
2. Does the patient suffer from other signs of atopic disease (eczema or asthma)?
3. Does the patient have any history of difficulty swallowing or choking with known food exposure (indicating possible underlying eosinophilic esophagitis)?
4. Does the patient suffer from an underlying metabolic disorder (lactose intolerance versus true milk allergy)?

Diagnosis

Identifying an underlying food allergy requires careful review of clinical history and familiarization with common clinical manifestations. It is also necessary to be aware of common conditions that appear similar to but are not true food allergies. Examples include gustatory rhinitis in which spicy foods induce rhinorrhea, scombroid fish poisoning where spoiled dark meat fish release histamine-like toxins, and aurico-temporal syndrome where foods that trigger salivation may also induce vasodilation in the capillaries of the lower cheek [14].

General approaches to diagnosis include elimination diets, skin prick testing, serologic IgE measurements, and oral food challenges [15]. Although commonly avoided, oral food challenges can be very beneficial as many food triggers may not be true allergies allowing for significant expansion of the affected patient's diet. There is also a low risk of severe reaction, but up to 3% can have reactions to the food later despite tolerating it during testing [14].

Treatment

The first-line approach to management is avoidance of the offending agent(s) and preparation to respond to allergic responses. This requires education on prehospital treatment, appropriate use of subcutaneous epinephrine, label reading, and when to seek medical attention.

Prevention/Family and Community Issues

Previous recommendations of allergen avoidance both in pregnancy and early childhood have for the most part been rescinded in general guidelines for food allergy prevention [15]. Newer studies have shown regular exposure to common allergens such as peanuts during pregnancy may actually reduce the likelihood of atopic disease [16]. Studies have also shown that delayed introduction of common food allergens is also not protective and may even increase risk of developing food allergies [14]. In one large study, introduction of peanuts to high-risk infants (severe eczema and or known egg allergy) had only a 10% rate of peanut allergy when peanuts were introduced at 4–6 months compared to 35% when peanut introduction was avoided until 5 years of age [14].

Lactose Intolerance

General Principles
Lactose is digested primarily in the small intestine where it is broken down by the enzyme lactase into glucose and galactose. In lactase-deficient individuals, lactose is passed to the colon where gut flora break it down to small-chain fatty acids

Table 3 Conditions that may contribute to lactose malabsorption

Acquired	Disease related
Gastrointestinal surgery	Systemic sclerosis
Small bowel bacterial overgrowth (SBBO)	Celiac disease
Infectious enteritis (giardiasis)	Inflammatory bowel disease
Medications	Short bowel syndrome
Radiation enteritis	

and gas by-products of hydrogen, methane, and carbon dioxide. The main cause of lactose intolerance is downregulation of lactase resulting in lactose malabsorption. Lactose intolerance is defined as a constellation of symptoms to include abdominal pain, bloating, and/or diarrhea secondary to lactose malabsorption. The worldwide prevalence of lactose malabsorption is 68% with the lowest occurrence in Nordic countries ($<5\%$ in Denmark) and highest in Korea and Han Chinese populations (close to 100%) [17]. It is also important to point out that lactase deficiency may be secondary to another condition such as those listed in Table 3.

Approach to Patient
Common complaints of a patient with lactose intolerance may include diarrhea, flatulence, bloating, abdominal pain, and borborygmi. Systemic findings may include failure to thrive in children, skin disease, chronic fatigue, and rheumatologic complaints in adults [17].

Diagnosis

Lactose intolerance was recently defined by the NIH as "the onset of gastrointestinal symptoms following a blinded, single dose challenge of ingested lactose by an individual with lactose malabsorption along with absence of symptoms when the person ingests an indistinguishable placebo" [18]. Despite this recognized definition, this test is not currently performed in clinical practice. Objective testing for lactose intolerance includes duodenal biopsies, genetic testing, lactose tolerance test, serum gaxilose test, urine galactose test, and H2 breath test.

Although being the reference standard and offering the advantage of ruling out other conditions that may affect the small intestine such as celiac disease, mucosal biopsies of the duodenum hold the highest expense, and are the most invasive of all other testing. Genetic testing for the $-13,910$: C/T genotype, which evaluates for lactase nonpersistence in Caucasian patients, had a high correlation with other tests for lactose malabsorption within European countries. The test, however, is of limited use in other ethnic groups and would have false-negative results in individuals with secondary causes for clinical lactose intolerance. The lactose tolerance test and H2 breath test are both performed after an oral challenge with a standard dose of lactose. The lactose tolerance test measures change in serum glucose while the breath test measures the hydrogen gas produced by intestinal bacteria in expired air. The serum gaxilose and urine galactose test are detection of D-xylose in the serum or galactose in the urine after given gaxilose orally [17].

Treatment

General reduction of lactose intake instead of complete exclusion should be advocated as the majority of patients can tolerate a minimum of 12 g of lactose, which is equivalent to 8 oz. of milk, without symptoms. Patients with symptoms in smaller amounts should bring into question the possibility of a cow's milk protein allergy. Lactase enzyme replacement is another option, but it does cause a change in flavor due to the breakdown of lactose to the much sweeter sugars glucose and galactose. Probiotics may also offer improvement in patients with concomitant IBS by altering gut flora. Studies have also shown potential for prebiotics by way of manipulating microbiota with one study showing over 20% improvement in lactose tolerance after only 1 month worth of treatment [17]. Tolerance may also be improved by successive increases in lactose ingestion [19].

Prevention/Family and Community Issues

Dietary education for populations at risk and adapting modified menus for broad population dietary programs such as school lunches or adult care facilities are the main modes of prevention.

Marine Poisoning

General Principles

Although more common in coastal rural communities of the Pacific with an annual incidence of 1200 per 100,000, marine poisoning is being seen in rising numbers after consumption of imported seafood or by travelers to these areas [20]. The three major clinical syndromes that may present with neurologic sequelae include ciguatera, shellfish poisoning, and tetrodotoxin poisoning.

Approach to Patient

Key factors to identify and evaluate for in the workup of a patient with possible marine poisoning include:

1. Type of seafood consumed and timing of ingestion (reef fish associated with ciguatera and puffer fish with tetrodotoxin).
2. Severity of gastrointestinal symptoms (severe in ciguatera while mild with tetrodotoxin poisoning).
3. What are the neurologic symptoms (paresthesia more common with ciguatera while paralysis common with tetrodotoxin and shellfish poisoning)?

Diagnosis

Diagnostic tests are not clinically available in primary care settings; hence, diagnosis is based on clinical symptoms and consumption of offending marine agent within the preceding 24 h. Clinical characteristics of the most common marine poisoning syndromes are outlined in Table 4.

Table 4 Common marine poisoning syndrome characteristics

Syndrome	Toxin	Source	Symptoms	Onset (hours)	Geographic origin
Puffer fish poisoning	Tetrodotoxin	Puffer fish, toadfish	Mild GI effects, descending paralysis, rapid progression to respiratory failure when severe	0.5–3	Southeast Asia, China, and Japan
Ciguatera	Ciguatoxins	Reef fish	Severe GI effects, myalgia, paresthesia, ataxia, rarely fatal	1–48	All tropical areas
Paralytic shellfish poisoning	Saxitoxin and gonyautoxin	Bivalve shellfish (mussels, oysters, clams)	Descending paralysis, respiratory failure when severe	0.5–4	NW/NE US, southern Chile, North Sea, Japan
Neurotoxic shellfish poisoning	Brevetoxin	Shellfish	Severe GI effects, paresthesia, "temperature reversal," vertigo	3–6	West Florida, Caribbean
Amnesic shellfish poisoning	Domoic acid (diatom algae)	Shellfish	Moderate GI effects, amnesia, CN palsies, seizures	GI <24; neuro <48	East Canada, NE and West USA

Treatment

As there are no clinically available antidotes, management is restricted to supportive care and mechanical ventilation when indicated [20]. Although an accepted treatment for ciguatera poisoning includes the use of IV mannitol, recent double-blinded studies have shown no significant clinical outcomes when compared to infusion of normal saline [21].

Prevention/Family and Community Issues

To prevent potentially fatal poisoning, travelers should use caution when consuming exotic seafood and consult medical travel resources and season-specific information. Shellfish harvesting is quarantined in areas of the United States and Canada at times when toxic sources such as dinoflagellates are the highest in concentration.

Botulism

General Principles
First described in the eighteenth century, botulism is a neurologic disorder induced by an anaerobic,

gram-positive, spore-forming bacterium, *Clostridium botulinum*. Contraction of the infection typically follows consumption of honey in the case of infant botulism or affected foodstuffs such as home-canned foods and fermented uncooked dishes in foodborne botulism [22].

Approach to Patient/Diagnosis

The onset of symptoms after consumption of contaminated food often occurs within 12–36 h of ingestion. Presentation can vary with an onset of gastrointestinal symptoms (nausea, vomiting, diarrhea) followed by neurologic symptoms. Neurologic complaints of blurred vision and diplopia occur first followed by findings of slurred speech, dysphonia, and difficulty swallowing. Descending paralysis is a late finding leading to compromised diaphragm and intercostal muscles inducing respiratory failure [22].

Diagnosis is based on clinical suspicion, history of ingested food source, and physical exam findings. Definitive diagnosis can be made with toxin detection in serum, stool, or gastric aspirate; however, this should not delay treatment as clinical assays for detection may take days.

Treatment

Management of suspected clinical botulism involves supportive care to include the use of mechanical ventilation as well as administration of the heptavalent antitoxin. The antitoxin is targeted against free toxin molecules to prevent paralysis and has little clinical effect on already paralyzed musculature [23].

Prevention/Family and Community Issues

Widespread education for parents of infants to avoid honey consumption for the first year of life as well as education on the risks of improperly home-canned and cured items is essential. Commercial canneries take special precautions to prevent clinical botulism by heating prepared foods to high temperatures or adding acidifying agents to prevent spore formation. Spores have shown to be destroyed by heating to 121 °C for a minimum of 2.5 min [22].

References

1. Hartman S, Brown E, Loomis E, Russel HA. Gastroenteritis in children. Am Fam Physician. 2019;99(3):159–65.
2. Kosek M, Bern C, Guerrant RL. The global burden of diarrheal disease, as estimated from studies published between 1992 and 2000. Bull World Health Organ. 2003;81(3):197–204.
3. Guerrant RL, Van Gilder T, Steiner TS, et al. Infectious disease Society of America practice guidelines for the management of infectious diarrhea. Clin Infect Dis. 2001;32(3):331–51.
4. Centers for Disease Control and Prevention. Preliminary FoodNet data on the incidence of infection with pathogens transmitted commonly through food-10 states. MMWR Morb Mortal Wkly Rep. 2010;59 (14):418–22.
5. Choi SW, Park CH, Silva TM, et al. To culture or not to culture: fecal lactoferrin screening for inflammatory bacterial diarrhea. J Clin Microbiol. 1996;34(4):928–32.
6. Bauer TM, Lalvani A, et al. Derivation and validation of guidelines for stool cultures for enteropathogenic

bacteria other than *Clostridium difficile* in hospitalized adults. JAMA. 2001;285(3):313–9.
7. Siegel DL, Edelstein PH, Nachamkin I. Inappropriate testing for diarrheal diseases in the hospital. JAMA. 1990;263(7):979–82.
8. Barr W, Smith A. Acute diarrhea in adults. Am Fam Physician. 2014;89(3):180–9.
9. McDonald LC, Gerding DN, et al. Clinical practice guidelines for Clostridium difficile infection in adults and children: 2017 update by the Infectious Diseases Society of America (IDSA) and Society for Healthcare Epidemiology of America (SHEA). Clin Infect Dis. 2018;66(7):e1.
10. Acosta S, Bjorck M. Modern treatment of acute mesenteric ischaemia. Br J Surg. 2014;101:e101–8.
11. Sise M. Acute mesenteric ischemia. Surg Clin N Am. 2014;94:165–81.
12. Clair DG, Beach BM. Mesenteric ischemia. N Engl J Med. 2016;374:959–68.
13. Van Dijk LJ, van Noord D, et al. Clinical management of chronic mesenteric ischemia. United European Gastroenterol J. 2019;7(2):179–88.
14. Sicherer SH, Sampson HA. Food allergy: a review and update on epidemiology, pathogenesis, diagnosis, prevention and management. J Allergy Clin Immunol. 2018;141(1):41–58.
15. Boyce JA, Assa'ad A, et al. Guidelines for the diagnosis and management of food allergy in the United States: report of the NIAID-sponsored expert panel. J Allergy Clin Immunol. 2010;126(Supp):S1–58.
16. Maslova E, Granstrom C, et al. Peanut and tree nut consumption during pregnancy and allergic disease in children-should mothers decrease their intake? Longitudinal evidence from the Danish National Birth Cohort. J Allergy Clin Immunol. 2012;130:724–32.
17. Misselwitz B, Butter M, et al. Update on lactose malabsorption and intolerance:pathogenesis, diagnosis and clinical management. Gut. 2019;68(11):2080–91.
18. Brannon PM, Carpenter TO, et al. NIH consensus development conference statement: lactose intolerance and health. NIH Consens Statement. 2010;27:1–27.
19. Shaukat A, Levitt M, et al. Systematic review: effective management strategies for lactose intolerance. Ann Intern Med. 2010;152:797–803.
20. Isbister G, Kiernan M. Neurotoxic marine poisoning. Lancet Neurol. 2005;4:219–28.
21. Schnorf H, Taurarii M, et al. Ciguatera fish poisoning: a double-blind randomized trial of mannitol therapy. Neurology. 2002;58:873–80.
22. Zhang J, Sun L, et al. Botulism, where are we now? Clin Toxicol. 2010;48:867–79.
23. Centers for Disease Control and Prevention (CDC). Investigational heptavalent botulinum antitoxin (HBAT) to replace licensed botulinum antitoxin AB and investigational botulinum antitoxin E. MMWR Morb Mortal Wkly Rep. 2010;59:299.

Part XX

The Renal, Urinary, and Male Genital Systems

Urinary Tract Infections

Mindy J. Lacey

Contents

M. J. Lacey (✉)
College of Medicine, University of Nebraska, Omaha, NE, USA
e-mail: mlacey@unmc.edu

© Springer Nature Switzerland AG 2022
P. M. Paulman et al. (eds.), *Family Medicine*,
https://doi.org/10.1007/978-3-030-54441-6_102

Urinary tract infections (UTIs) are defined as the presence of a significant number of pathogenic bacteria in appropriately collected urine and result in over seven million office visits with an estimated one million episodes annually of UTI-related illness requiring hospitalizations. Among children, 1 in 20 girls and 1 in 50 boys have a UTI each year [1]. The primary goal of UTI diagnosis and management is the prevention of long-term complications of progressive events that affect later-life morbidity or mortality. Major risk groups include school-age girls, young women in their sexually active years, pregnant women, males with prostate obstruction, and the elderly [2].

This chapter discusses important clinical issues in the following categories: UTI in children, UTI in pregnancy, acute uncomplicated lower UTI in young women, recurrent infection in women, acute uncomplicated pyelonephritis in young women, complicated UTIs, UTIs in younger men, catheter-associated UTIs, chronic UTIs in the elderly, UTIs with spinal cord injuries, and fungal UTIs.

Asymptomatic Bacteriuria

Except for pregnancy and prior to urologic surgery, screening for asymptomatic bacteriuria has no apparent value, and if incidentally found treatment is not necessary. Even among the elderly where there may be an association between asymptomatic bacteriuria and mortality, a causal link has not been demonstrated [3].

UTI in Children

For boys and girls, the incidence of symptomatic infection during the first 6 months of life is similar, but after 6 months to a year it falls off rapidly for boys. Among girls, the first-year incidence is more evenly distributed through the year. During the first 3 months of life, boys are more likely to be infected presumably related to not being circumcised. In neonates, the prevalence is threefold higher among premature infants [4]. In girls, the incidence steadily rises with a small transient increase at preschool period and remains level until sexual activity

becomes a factor. Asymptomatic bacteriuria is not observed in boys until later in adult life when obstructive problems occur. In girls, asymptomatic bacteriuria is present early in infancy and remains fairly constant throughout the late teens [5].

The primary host-related factors that lead to the development of UTI include infancy, female sex, abnormal defense mechanisms, the presence of urinary tract abnormalities, sexual activity, lack of circumcision, and prior instrumentation [4]. In children without urinary tract abnormalities, periurethral bacterial colonization is a risk factor for UTI [6].

Escherichia coli accounts for as many as 80% of UTI [7, 8]. In neonates, *Proteus mirabilis* (mainly in boys), *Klebsiella pneumoniae, Pseudomonas aeruginosa, Enterobacter* species, *Staphylococcus aureus* (mainly in older children), *Streptococcus viridans*, enterococci, and *Candida albicans* should be considered [7].

Diagnosis

Urinalysis and Culture

In any febrile infant or child, the differential diagnosis should include UTI. Screening by urinalysis is first line in diagnosis; however, due to its relatively low sensitivity (approximately 90%), a negative urinalysis should be confirmed with culture. In a properly collected specimen (urethral catheterization or suprapubic aspiration in infants), a presumptive diagnosis can be made with the presence of any bacteria and five leukocytes per high-power field (hpf) [9].

Imaging Evaluation

Imaging should be conducted after the first episode of UTI in girls younger than 5 years, boys of any age, older sexually inactive girls with recurrent UTI, and any child with pyelonephritis [9]. Debate continues about the best radiologic approach for evaluation [10]. The issue centers around the role of radionuclide scans and how these methods may replace or be used in conjunction with traditional ultrasonography (US), voiding cystourethrography (VCUG), intravenous pyelography (IVP), and spiral computer-assisted tomography (CT).

Scintigraphic studies using 99 m-technetium dimercaptosuccinic acid (DMSA) has become a leading choice for gauging renal function, identifying renal cortical defects, and is the gold standard for diagnosis of acute pyelonephritis. However, it should not be used in routine evaluation of the child with a first UTI due to exposure to radiation [10–12]. When applied at 6–12 months after cortical defects have first developed, the DMSA scan may be the best test for renal scarring. US has the obvious advantage of being a noninvasive test that may rule out obstruction. Spiral CT is the first choice for the presence of obstructive stone disease. VCUG gives comprehensive lower tract information and allows grading the severity of reflux [10].

An imaging strategy can be summarized this way: use renal/bladder US to look for obstruction; use a DMSA scan to identify cortical defects and assess differential kidney function; use a VCUG to detect bladder anomalies, neurogenic defects, residual urine, and urethral abnormalities such as posterior valves, urethral strictures, and the presence of vesicoureteral reflux; and use spiral CT to determine the presence of stones [10].

Management

Early diagnosis and prompt treatment of UTI in infants and young children are crucial. With vesicoureteral reflux or other urinary tract abnormalities, immediate treatment reduces the risk of renal scarring. In the history, inquire about the defecation pattern. Physical examination should include a rectal examination to detect a large fecal reservoir, as fecal impaction can obstruct urine flow [13].

Symptomatic neonates should be treated for 7–10 days with a parenteral combination of ampicillin and gentamicin. Young infants with UTI, children with clinical evidence of acute pyelonephritis, and children with upper tract infection associated with urologic abnormalities or surgical procedures can be treated with a combination of an aminoglycoside and ampicillin, or an aminoglycoside and a third- or fourth-generation cephalosporin [4]. For complicated and uncomplicated infection, 7–14 days and 3–5 days of therapy recommended, respectively [10].

For uncomplicated UTI, first-line oral agents are cephalosporins. Alternatives include amoxicillin, trimethoprim-sulfamethoxazole or nitrofurantoin. Antibiotic treatment of asymptomatic bacteriuria in children is controversial. There is limited evidence that renal damage is prevented, or loss of function reduced, replacement of a low-virulence organism with a more virulent one may occur, and the child may experience long-term side effects from antibiotics [4]. A reasonable approach with asymptomatic bacteriuria is to treat children younger than 5 years or those who have urinary tract structural abnormalities.

UTI in Pregnancy

Pregnant women with UTIs are at greater risk for preterm birth and delivering infants with low birth weight or that are small for gestational age. There is strong evidence that UTI causes low birth weight through premature delivery rather than growth retardation [14]. In addition, there is increased risk of premature labor, hypertension/preeclampsia, anemia, and chorioamnionitis.

The risk of pyelonephritis from antepartum asymptomatic bacteriuria may be as high as 30%. Identification and eradication reduce this risk to less than 5%. Antepartum bacteriuria has an estimated prevalence of 2–7% [15, 16].

An optimal time for screening all pregnancies is at the first prenatal visit and urinalysis with culture should be obtained. If negative, no further studies are necessary unless there is a history of prior UTI or the patient becomes symptomatic. If the screening culture result is 10^5 colony-forming units (CFU)/mL or higher, treatment for asymptomatic bacteriuria should be undertaken.

Similar to nonpregnant females, *E. coli* is the most common cause of UTI and asymptomatic bacteriuria during pregnancy. Other organisms include *Enterobacter* species, *Klebsiella* species, *Proteus* species, and *Group B Streptococcus* [17].

The first concern regarding treatment during pregnancy is the safety of antibiotics. Considered reasonably safe are penicillins, cephalosporins, and nitrofurantoin.

For asymptomatic bacteriuria, a regimen of 7–10 days is used; there is little support for single-dose therapy. Pyelonephritis is managed the same as in nonpregnant females.

Acute Uncomplicated Lower UTI in Young Women

Acute uncomplicated UTIs (cystitis and urethritis) are confined to the bladder and have no signs of systemic infection [3]. The risk is increased by sexual intercourse, delayed postcoital voiding, use of a diaphragm or spermicidal gel, and history of recurrent infections [18].

Cystitis pathogens include *E. coli*, *S. saprophyticus*, *Proteus* species, or *Klebsiella* species. Symptoms are abrupt in onset and include dysuria, increased frequency, and urgency. Suprapubic pain and low back pain may also occur, and pyuria and hematuria can be present.

Urethritis pathogens include *Chlamydia trachomatis*, *N. gonorrhoeae*, and herpes simplex virus. Symptoms are more likely to be gradual in onset and mild (including dysuria and possibly vaginal discharge and bleeding from a concomitant cervicitis) and include lower abdominal pain. Suspicion is raised if the patient has a new sexual partner or evidence of cervicitis on examination. Pyuria is also usually present.

With no multidrug resistance (MDR) in the community, reasonable empiric treatment prior to organism identification includes nitrofurantoin, trimethoprim-sulfamethoxazole (TMP-SMX), or fosfomycin.

Acute Uncomplicated Pyelonephritis in Young Women

Findings suggestive of uncomplicated upper tract parenchymal involvement can include fever and flank pain. Urine culture and sensitivity should be performed in all patients with known or possible acute pyelonephritis. This process allows for alteration of empiric treatment.

Characteristic pathogens in acute uncomplicated pyelonephritis in young women include *E. coli*, *Proteus mirabilis*, *K. pneumoniae*, and *S. saprophyticus*. Outpatient management is reasonable for mild to moderate illness without nausea and vomiting. A 10–14-day regimen of the following is appropriate: oral TMP-SMX, ciprofloxacin, and levofloxacin are first line until an organism and sensitivities are available. For severe illness requiring hospitalization, the following regimen can be followed: parenteral fluoroquinolone, aminoglycoside with or without ampicillin, extended-spectrum cephalosporin, an extended-spectrum penicillin, or a carbapenem [19].

Complicated UTIs

Complicated UTIs may present in the same way as uncomplicated but extends beyond the bladder. They occur in urinary tracts that have a functional, metabolic, or anatomic derangement predisposing to an infection that is more resistant to typical therapeutic measures. This infection should be suspected in patients with systemic symptoms such as fever, chills, malaise, flank pain, costovertebral tenderness, as well as pelvic/perineal pain in men.

Characteristic organisms include *E. coli*, *Proteus* species, *Klebsiella* species, *Pseudomonas* species, *Serratia* species, enterococci, and staphylococci.

Antibiotic selection includes levofloxacin or ciprofloxacin if MDR is low. For severe illness requiring hospitalization, intravenous ceftriaxone is an appropriate first line choice. If MDR is high, then pipercillin/tazobactam should be used. This regimen should be continued until that patient is afebrile and then may be changed to oral therapy with either TMP-SMX, amoxicillin-clavulanic acid, or cefdinir for a total of 14–21 days [3]. Results of urine culture sensitivities and susceptibilities should be followed to be certain the antibiotic is appropriate.

Recurrent Infections (Cystitis) in Women

Recurrent cystitis is defined as recurrence of symptoms within 2 weeks of completing therapy with the same pathogen, or if more than two infections in 6 months or three annually.

For fewer than two incidents of UTI per year, therapy can be started based on symptoms using either single-dose or 3-day therapy. For three or more UTIs per year, the relation to coitus must be considered. If the UTI is not related to coitus, a low-dose antibiotic daily or three times weekly is recommended, and treatment is commonly continued for 3–6 months [20]. If related to coitus, a single low-dose postcoital treatment may be preferable.

UTIs in Younger Men

Without underlying structural urologic abnormalities, risk factors for UTIs in young men include lack of circumcision, intercourse with other men and a sexual partner colonized with uropathogens [3, 21]. Symptoms include dysuria, urinary frequency/urgency +/− suprapubic pain or perineal pain. Pyuria and bacteriuria are typically present.

Management of symptomatic cystitis without obvious complicating factors requires urinalysis and urine culture to establish the pathogen. This step establishes sensitivity and helps in the event of recurrence. Once the culture is obtained, antibiotic choices include nitrofurantoin, TMP-SMX, or fosfomycin.

The traditional approach of undertaking a thorough post-UTI evaluation to rule out a urologic abnormality has been disputed [22, 23]. If pursued in young men who have responded to treatment, the probability of finding a urinary tract defect is low [24].

Catheter-Associated UTIs

Catheter-associated UTI (CAUTI) is the most common acquired infection in long-term-care facilities, and in the intensive care setting, with 95% of nosocomial UTIs being catheter-associated [25]. The presence of an indwelling catheter for at least 3 days has been identified as a risk factor with a 3–10% incidence of UTI per day of catheterization. CAUTI is a significant cause of morbidity and mortality in this population [26, 27].

Causative organisms are like those of complicated UTIs. E. coli and Enterbacteriaceae are the most common. Other pathogens include Pseudomonas aeruginosa, K. pneumoniae, enterococci, and candida species [28, 29]. Yeast may become an isolated pathogen when antibiotics are in use [25, 28].

Treatment in this setting depends on the clinical presentation: baseline prevention, antimicrobials for asymptomatic bacteriuria, symptomatic lower UTI and symptomatic (complicated) upper UTI. Treatment is typically 7–14 days. Prevention focuses on avoiding catheterization if possible. If catheterization is mandatory, the duration should be minimized, and a closed drainage system used.

Chronic UTIs in the Elderly

UTI is the most common infectious illness in adults aged 65 and older [39, 40]. Age-related physiologic changes play a role in UTI development including lack of estrogen in women, diminished prostatic secretion in men [30], and altered bacterial adhesion factors in both sexes.

Whereas E. coli and S. saprophyticus are the most common cause of UTI in young adults, some significant shifts in causative organism occur with the elderly. E. coli remains the most common causative organism with Enterococcus faecalis and Klebsiella species following [31].

The presentation of UTIs among the elderly can be similar to that of younger patients. However, these signs and symptoms can be absent with patients presenting as fever of unknown origin, altered mental status (lethargy), gastrointestinal complaints, incontinence, or respiratory symptoms [32]. Pharmacologic therapy and duration of treatment are similar to that in other age groups [33].

UTI in Patients with Spinal Cord Injuries

UTI is the most frequent infection in patients with spinal cord injuries and occurs at a rate of 2.5 episodes/patient/year [34]. Special considerations for increased risk of UTI with spinal cord injuries include bladder overdistention, vesicoureteral reflux, high-pressure voiding, large postvoid residuals, stones in the urinary tract, and outlet obstruction [35]. Management focuses primarily on proper drainage of the bladder with intermittent catheterization reducing the risk of significant bacteriuria. Development of bacteriuria is common with indwelling and suprapubic catheters [36]. Asymptomatic UTIs are generally not treated and in general there is no role for prophylactic antibiotics as they may result in emergence of resistant bacteria [37].

Fungal UTIs

Fungal UTIs are common in hospitalized patients and are typically asymptomatic [38, 39]. Risk factors include urinary tract drainage devices, prior antibiotic therapy, diabetes, urinary tract pathology, and malignancy [40]. Common pathogens include *Candida albicans, Cryptococcus neoformans,* or *Aspergillus* species.

For asymptomatic colonization with *Candida,* no specific antifungal therapy is required unless there is a high risk of dissemination (neutropenia and very low birthweight (<1500 g)) or urinary tract manipulation [41]. Symptomatic patients should be treated, and fluconazole is the preferred agent if there is no resistance.

Treatment of asymptomatic infections is no longer mandatory in renal transplant patients. Therapy is considered on a case by case basis and undertaken only if there is a high risk of graft involvement or if the patient has ureteral stents [42].

Laboratory Guides and Interpretation

Pyuria

From a practical standpoint, pyuria represents measurable evidence of host injury. The most accurate method of defining significant pyuria is the leukocyte excretion rate and there is evidence that 400,000 white blood cells (WBC)/h is significant [43]. This measurement is cumbersome – hence the popularity of quicker, simpler, but less accurate screening tests. Those screening tests include microscopic examination of unspun urine in a counting chamber (WBC/mm^3), spun urine under a coverslip (WBC/hpf), and leukocyte esterase [44]. Diagnostic information related to these tests is displayed in Table 1.

Bacteriuria

Urine culture is considered the gold standard for defining significant bacteriuria. All other tests are simply screening devices chosen to balance immediacy of results and ease of performance with accuracy. The most common tests are direct microscopy and the urine dipstick (nitrite and leukocyte esterase). Commonly used screening tests with approximated diagnostic information are shown in Table 1.

Urine Culture

Urine cultures are not 100% sensitive or specific. The colony count that represents significant bacteriuria varies with age, sex, anatomic location of the infection, and symptoms. Colony counts of what can currently be considered as significant bacteriuria for infection are shown in Table 2.

Table 1 Diagnostic value of the positivity of commonly used urine screening tests, individually and in various combinations

Screening test	Sensitivity	Specificity	Positive likelihood ratio	Negative likelihood ratio
Nitrite (present or absent)	0.5	0.95	10.00	0.53
Bacteria				
Unstained, spun (2+ on scale of 4+)	0.75	0.8	3.75	0.31
Gram stain, unspun (1/hpf)	0.8	0.85	5.33	0.24
Microscopic pyuria				
Spun (5 WBCs/hpf)	0.6	0.85	4.00	0.47
Unspun (50 WBC/mm^3)	0.65	0.9	6.50	0.39
WBCs + bacteria				
Standard spun[a]	0.66	0.99	66.00	0.34
Enhanced unspun[b]	0.85	0.98	42.50	0.15
Leukocyte esterase (present or absent)	0.2	0.95	4.00	0.84
Leukocyte esterase + nitrite	0.5	0.98	25.00	0.51
Methylene blue	0.6	0.98	30.00	0.41
Uriscreen	0.9	0.9	9.00	0.11
Bac-T-Screen	0.9	0.7	3.00	0.14
Chemstrip LN	0.9	0.7	3.00	0.14

hpf high-power field, *WBC* white blood cell count
[a]5 WBCs/hpf + any bacteria in spun urinalysis
[b]10 WBCs/mm^3 + any bacteria by Gram stain

Table 2 Suggested culture colony count thresholds for significant bacteriuria

Various clinical settings	Significant bacteriuria (CFU/mL)
Infants and children	
Voided	$\geq 10^3$
Catheter	$\geq 10^3$
Suprapubic aspirate (SPA)	$\geq 10^3$
External collection devices	$\geq 10^4$
Adult	
Midstream, clean-catch	
Female	
Asymptomatic	$\geq 10^5$
Symptomatic	$\geq 10^2$
Male	$\geq 10^3$
In-and-out (straight) catheterization	$\geq 10^2$
Chronic indwelling catheter	$\geq 10^2$
Indwelling catheter or SPA in spinal injuries	Any detectable colony count
External collection devices	$\geq 10^5$
Condom collection device in spinal injuries	$\geq 10^4$

Sources: Data are from Cardenas and Hooton [35] and Eisenstadt and Washington [45]

References

1. Stull TL, LiPuma JJ. Epidemiology and natural history of urinary infections in children. Med Clin North Am. 1991;75(2):287–98.
2. Stamm WE, Hooton TM, Johnson JR, et al. Urinary tract infections: from pathogenesis to treatment. J Infect Dis. 1989;159(3):400–6.
3. Stamm WE, Hooton TM. Management of urinary tract infections in adults. N Engl J Med. 1993;329:1328.
4. Zelikovic I, Adelman RD, Nancarrow PA. Urinary tract infections in children. An update. West J Med. 1992;157(5):554–61.
5. Warren JW. Clinical presentations and epidemiology of urinary tract infections. In: Mobley LT, Warren JW, editors. Urinary tract infections: molecular pathogenesis and clinical management. Washington, DC: ASM Press; 1996. p. 3–28.
6. Shortliffe LM. The management of urinary tract infections in children without urinary tract abnormalities. Urol Clin North Am. 1995;22(1):67–73.
7. Edlin RS, Shapiro DJ, Hersh AL, Copp HL. Antibiotic resistance patterns of outpatient pediatric urinary tract infections. J Urol. 2013;190(1):222–7.
8. Yakubov R, van den Akker M, Machamad K, et al. Antimicrobial resistance among uropathogens that cause childhood community-acquired urinary tract infections in central Israel. Pediatr Infect Dis J. 2017;36:113.
9. Carmack MA, Arvin AM. Urinary tract infections – navigating complex currents [editorial]. West J Med. 1992;157(5):587–8.
10. Linshaw MA. Controversies in childhood urinary tract infections. World J Urol. 1999;17(6):383–95.
11. Conway JJ, Cohn RA. Evolving role of nuclear medicine for the diagnosis and management of urinary tract infection [editorial comment]. J Pediatr. 1994;124(1):87–90.
12. Roberts KB. Urinary tract infection: clinical practice guideline for the diagnosis and management of the initial UTI in febrile infants and children 2 to 24 months. Pediatrics. 2011;128(3):595.
13. Hellerstein S. Urinary tract infections in children: why they occur and how to prevent them. Am Fam Physician. 1998;57(10):2440–6.
14. Schieve LA, Handler A, Hershow R, et al. Urinary tract infection during pregnancy: its association with maternal morbidity and perinatal outcome. Am J Public Health. 1994;84(3):405–10.
15. Patterson TF, Andriole VT. Detection, significance, and therapy of bacteriuria in pregnancy. Update in the managed healthcare era. Infect Dis Clin North Am. 1997;11(3):593.
16. Nicolle LE, Gupta K, Bradley SF, et al. Clinical practice guidline for the management of asymptomatic bacteriuria: 2019 update by the Infectious Diseases Society of America. Clin Infect Dis. 2019;68:e83.
17. Hill JB, Sheffield JS, McIntire DD, Wendel GD Jr. Acute pyelonephritis in pregnancy. Obstet Gynecol. 2005;105:18.
18. Hooton TM, Hillier S, Johnson C, et al. *Escherichia coli* bacteriuria and contraceptive method. JAMA. 1991;265(1):64–9.
19. Hooton TM. Clinical practice. Uncomplicated urinary tract infection. N Engl J Med. 2012;366(11):1028.
20. Madersbacher S, Thalhammer F, Marberger M. Pathogenesis and management of recurrent urinary tract infection in women. Curr Opin Urol. 2000;10(1):29–33.
21. Spach DH, Stapleton AE, Stamm WE. Lack of circumcision increases the risk of urinary tract infection in young men. JAMA. 1992;267:679.
22. Krieger JN, Ross SO, Simonsen JM. Urinary tract infections in healthy university men. J Urol. 1993;149(5):1046–8.
23. Pfau A. Re: urinary tract infections in healthy university men [letter]. J Urol. 1994;151(3):705–6.
24. Johnson JR. Treatment and prevention of urinary tract infections. In: Mobley LT, Warren JW, editors. Urinary tract infections: molecular pathogenesis and clinical management. Washington, DC: ASM Press; 1996. p. 95–118.
25. Burrows LL, Khoury AE. Issues surrounding the prevention and management of device-related infections. World J Urol. 1999;17(6):402–9.
26. Warren JW, Platt R, Thomas RJ, et al. Antibiotic irrigation and catheter-associated urinary-tract infections. N Engl J Med. 1978;299:570.
27. Haley RW, Hooton TM, Culver DH, et al. Nosocomial infections in U.S. hospitals, 1975-1976: estimated frequency by selected characteristics of patients. Am J Med. 1981;70:947.
28. Warren JW. The catheter and urinary tract infection. Med Clin North Am. 1991;75:481–95.
29. Weiner LM, Webb AK, Limbago B, et al. Antimicrobial-resistant pathogens associated with healthcare-associated infections: summary of data reported to the National Healthcare Safety Network at the Centers for Disease Control and Prevention, 2011–2014. Infect Control Hosp Epidemiol. 2016;37:1288.
30. Nicolle LE. Urinary tract infections in long-term care facilities. Infect Control Hosp Epidemiol. 1993;14(4):220–5.
31. Cardone S, Petruzziello C, Migneco A, et al. Age-related trends in adults with urinary tract infections presenting to the emergency department: a 5-year experience. Rev Recent Clin Trials. 2019;14:147.
32. Baldassarre JS, Kaye D. Special problems in urinary tract infection in the elderly. Med Clin North Am. 1991;75(2):375–90.
33. Saint S, Veenstra DL, Sullivan SD, Chenoweth C, Fendrick AM. The potential clinical and economic benefits of silver alloy urinary catheters in preventing urinary tract infection. Arch Intern Med. 2000;160(17):2670–5.
34. Salameh A, Al Mohajer M, Darouiche RO. Prevention of urinary tract infections in patients with spinal cord injury. CMAJ. 2015 Aug 11;187(11):807–11.

35. Cardenas DD, Hooton TM. Urinary tract infection in persons with spinal cord injury. Arch Phys Med Rehabil. 1995;76(3):272–80.

36. Bakke A, Vollset SE. Risk factors for bacteriuria and clinical urinary tract infection in patients treated with clean intermittent catheterization. J Urol. 1993;149:527.

37. Nicolle L, Bradley S, Colgan R, et al. Infectious Diseases Society of America guidelines for the diagnosis and treatment of asymptomatic bacteriuria in adults. Clin Infect Dis. 2005;40:643–54.

38. Sobel JD, Fisher JF, Kauffman CA, Newman CA. Candida urinary tract infections – epidemiology. Clin Infect Dis. 2011;52(Suppl 6):S433.

39. Kauffman CA. Diagnosis and management of fungal urinary tract infection. Infect Dis Clin N Am. 2014;28:61.

40. Kauffman CA, Vazquez JA, Sobel JD, et al. Prospective multicenter surveillance study of funguria in hospitalized patients. The National Institute for Allergy and Infectious Diseases (NIAID) Mycoses Study Group. Clin Infect Dis. 2000;30:14.

41. Pappas PG, Kauffman CA, Andes DR, et al. Clinical practice guideline for the management of candidiasis: 2016 update by the Infectious Diseases Society of America. Clin Infect Dis. 2016;62:e1.

42. Safdar N, Slattery WR, Knasinski V, et al. Predictors and outcomes of candiduria in renal transplant recipients. Clin Infect Dis. 2005;40:1413.

43. Stamm WE. Measurement of pyuria and its relation to bacteriuria. Am J Med. 1983;75.(1B:53–8.

44. Pappas PG. Laboratory in the diagnosis and management of urinary tract infections. Med Clin North Am. 1991;75(2):313–26.

45. Eisenstadt J, Washington JA. Diagnostic microbiology for bacteria and yeasts causing urinary tract infections. In: Mobley LT, Warren JW, editors. Urinary tract infections: molecular pathogenesis and clinical management. Washington, DC: ASM Press; 1996. p. 29–68.

Fluid, Electrolyte, and Acid–Base Disorders

100

KelliAnn Leli, Gwendolyn Warren, Stephen Horras, Jennifer Bepko, and Nicholas Longstreet

Contents

K. Leli (✉) · G. Warren · S. Horras · N. Longstreet
David Grant Family Medicine Residency Program, David Grant Medical Center, Travis AFB, CA, USA
e-mail: KelliAnn.Leli@gmail.com; Gwendolyn.Warren.mil@mail.mil; stephen.horras.1@us.af.mil; nicholas.longstreet.1@us.af.mil

J. Bepko
David Grant Family Medicine Residency Program, David Grant Medical Center, Fairfield, CA, USA
e-mail: jennifer.bepko@us.af.mil

© Springer Nature Switzerland AG 2022
P. M. Paulman et al. (eds.), *Family Medicine*,
https://doi.org/10.1007/978-3-030-54441-6_103

Volume Overview

Volume distribution in the body is comprised of extracellular fluid and intracellular fluid. Most volume, approximately two-thirds, is found in the intracellular compartments. One-third is extracellular water, which accounts for extravascular (interstitial space) and intravascular. Water is able to cross membranes to freely move between compartments through aquaporin channels [1]. Thus, fluid distribution is dictated by effective solutes, largely sodium, to maintain osmolality via osmotic pressures. Given the kidney regulates sodium hemostasis, it is responsible for maintaining volume balance. In discussing volume status, it is important to remember that intravascular volume status, accounted for in our extracellular water hemostasis, is of most clinical significance.

Volume Depletion

Intravascular volume depletion can occur from actual volume loss or due to a fluid redistribution to another compartment, often the extravascular or interstitial compartment often clinically referred to as "third spacing." Actual volume loss occurs through various losses: hemorrhage, the gastrointestinal (GI) tract (i.e., poor intake, vomiting, diarrhea), kidneys (urination), and evaporation (through sweating and breathing). Relative volume loss results in decreased intravascular volume without a decrease of total fluid in the body. Third spacing refers to the redistribution of intravascular fluids to the interstitial space between skin and fascia, which is not normally perfused with fluids. Third spacing is commonly seen clinically as it can occur with increased fluid volume (fluid replacement, renal dysfunction), increased capillary hydrostatic pressure (CHF), decreased sodium level (due to sodium loss), lowered albumin (malnutrition, liver disease, protein-losing enteropathy), increased capillary permeability (burns, trauma, disseminated intravascular coagulation, infections), or lymphatic obstruction (iatrogenic removal).

Hypovolemia can be difficult to determine clinically, often requiring a thorough history and physical exam. In clinical scenarios of actual volume loss, patients can have clinical exam findings of hypovolemia including increased time to capillary refill, pallor of skin, dry mucous membranes, or positive orthostatic vital signs (i.e., postural blood pressure and pulse changes). However, volume status is particularly difficult to assess when patients appear fluid overloaded or edematous, but are instead intravascularly depleted, such as is seen in common clinical scenarios (e.g., congestive heart failure [CHF], cirrhosis, and nephrosis).

Laboratory data can often be helpful to determine fluid status in clinical cases where history and physical exam do not lead to obvious findings. Measurements such as serum osmolality (SOSM), blood urea nitrogen (BUN), urine osmolality (UOSM), urine specific gravity, kidney function, and blood counts can all be a part of your clinical evaluation. Signs of volume depletion include high urine specific gravity and UOSM (i.e., >1.015 and >350 mOsm/kg, respectively) as a result of ADH-induced renal water conservation leading to concentrated urine [1]. Renal hypoperfusion results in prerenal azotemia and functional renal injury causing BUN to be retained such that the normal 10:1 BUN/creatinine ratio is elevated (e.g., to >20:1) and may also lead to an increase in creatinine or decrease in GFR. When volume loss is due to hemorrhage, a hematocrit/hemoglobin can be low. However, hemoconcentration can occur with significant third spacing. Generally with hypovolemia, an increased SOSM, increased serum sodium, and corresponding decreased urine sodium (UNa) is seen; however, inappropriate responses can be seen with certain comorbidities.

Whether actual or relative, volume depletion results in decreased "effective circulating volume" (ECV) causing a cascade of multiple compensatory mechanisms. In response to a decreased ECV, cardiac and cerebral blood flow is compromised. Accordingly, cardiac and arterial baroreceptors sense the change in mean arterial pressure. This drop in mean arterial pressure triggers a norepinephrine-induced increase in heart rate and heart contractility with peripheral arterial vasoconstriction. Concurrently, decreased renal blood flow due to decreased ECV triggers antidiuretic hormone (ADH) release and activates the renin–angiotensin–aldosterone system (RAAS) [2].

Once activated, renal sodium is retained and vasoconstriction further promoted. ADH secretion contributes to vasoconstriction and decreased renal water clearance in an attempt to restore the

ECV. Intrarenal prostaglandins are released with ADH stimulation and activation of RAAS. These prostaglandins blunt the hypovolemia-induced vasoconstriction in the renal vasculature, thereby disproportionately preserving renal blood flow and glomerular filtration. This physiological response to volume depletion is illustrated in Fig. 1. These vasoconstrictor mechanisms are triggered by volume depletion to protect cardiac and cerebral blood flow, while sacrificing blood flow to less critical organ systems [3].

Volume depletion is treated according to the clinical situation and etiology. Treatment for mild volume depletion occurs with slow restoration of the ECV such as using oral electrolyte solutions. Treatment escalates to infusion of isotonic fluid in more severe settings. In addition to replacing excess fluid loss, volume repletion must also include the replacement of daily obligate fluid losses. The rate of volume replacement depends on the clinical situation. Restoration of ECV results in normalization of orthostatic vital signs, improvement in tachycardia, and normalization of urinary excretion of sodium [3]. Once the volume status has been restored, treatment can be directed to restoring electrolyte loss and imbalances.

Volume Excess

Volume excess, or hypervolemia, can be caused by excessive fluid intake, excessive sodium intake, chronic hepatic or renal failure, steroid therapy, transfusion reaction, decreased cardiac output, head injury, medications, malnutrition, and mineralocorticoid excess. Volume overload can also be caused by decreased ECV, as discussed previously, which results in renal sodium and water conservation and edema formation (e.g., hypoalbuminemia and left ventricular dysfunction).

Total body volume excess caused by decreased ECV and edema formation may cause symptoms of vital organ hypoperfusion (e.g., syncope, unstable angina, decreased urine output, mental status changes). Depending on the etiology of volume excess, physical findings of CHF, hepatic cirrhosis, and nephrosis might be present. Weight gain

may reflect the quantity of the volume retention, and monitoring weight gain can be clinically useful. Evidence of hypervolemia on exam could include edema, typically seen in the lower extremities or presacral area, pulmonary edema, elevated jugular venous pressure, or prolonged hepatojugular reflux in CHF [1]. However, exam findings of volume excess are not always evident, such as seen in a patient with anasarca or bowel wall edema. Hypervolemia associated with increased ECV causes urine sodium (UNa) wasting (UNa >20 mEq/L) and no excessive water retention (assuming normal osmolality).

Treating volume excess involves recognition and treatment of the underlying cause. For example, if caused by heart failure, increasing cardiac output. Furthermore, it would require restoring intravascular oncotic forces in patients with cirrhosis and hypoalbuminemia. Removal of some edema by loop diuretics may be required, especially if the retained fluid compromises ventilation. When third-spaced fluid is significant, it should be removed with caution, as removal of large amounts can cause rapid re-accumulations extracted from the circulating volume, resulting in hypotension [1]. With states of aldosterone excess, an aldosterone antagonist (i.e., spironolactone, eplerenone) is used to decrease sodium reabsorption and edema, but ideally the source of the hyperaldosteronism is removed. In renal failure, diuresis with potent loop diuretics may be required to remove excess volume that may be causing renal hypoperfusion, and in some cases, dialysis will be required to remove excess fluid in conjunction with a nephrology specialist.

Sodium Disorders

Appreciating a patient's fluid status is crucial when assessing and treating disorders of sodium concentration. Hyponatremia ($[Na^+] < 136$ mEq/L) and hypernatremia ($[Na^+] > 145$ mEq/L) should be approached in term of free water status. A firm understanding of tonicity is required when approaching sodium disorders.

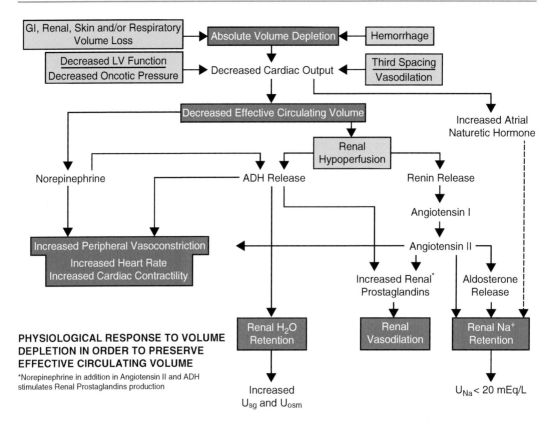

Fig. 1 Physiological response to volume depletion. *GI* gastrointestinal, *LV* left ventricle, U_{Na} urine sodium concentration, U_{osm} urine osmolality, U_{sg} urine specific gravity, *ADH* antidiuretic hormone, *SIADH* syndrome of inappropriate ADH secretion. (Originally appeared in: Taylor R, David A, Fields S, Phillips M, Scherger J, editors. Family medicine (Taylor). New York: Springer; 2003)

Tonicity is the measure of the osmotic pressure gradient between the intracellular fluid compartment (ICF) and extracellular compartment (ECF). Tonicity is affected only by solutes that cannot cross a membrane while osmolality is the property of a particular solution. These compartmentalized solutes create an osmotic gradient across the cellular membrane [4]. Tonicity is the effective plasma osmolality with a normal range of 275–300 mOsm/kg H_2O. Only solutes that do not pass between the ECF and ICF contribute to creating osmotic gradients and effect the flow of water between the ECF and ICF. Sodium is a major plasma solute that cannot cross freely between the ECF and ICF, and is therefore important when evaluating plasma osmolality.

The plasma osmolality (POSM) is the total osmolality of the solutes in the plasma and can be calculated as:

$$P_{osm} = 2[Na^+] + \frac{[glucose]}{18} + \frac{[BUN]}{2.8}$$

Calculating the osmolality gap, the difference between effective POSM and measured osmolality can indicate the presence of unmeasured solutes that can be toxic such as ethanol, methanol, isopropanol, ethylene glycol, propylene glycol, or acetone. Therefore, evaluating plasma osmolality, effective and measured, would be the first step when approaching sodium disorders, with hyponatremia being the most common electrolyte abnormality [5]. Determining osmolality is also needed when approaching metabolic acidosis disorders which will be discussed later.

Hyponatremia

Hyponatremia is defined as $[Na^+] < 136$ mEq/L. Hypotonic, or hypoosmolar, hyponatremia (i.e., plasma osmolality <275 mOsm/kg) indicates excess water content relative to sodium caused by renal retention of ingested water such as hypovolemic-induced ADH release, SIADH, or excess water ingestion greater than renal free water clearance (Table 2). Pseudohyponatremia, which is hyponatremia with normal plasma osmolality between 275 and 300 mOsm/kg H_2O, occurs in the presence of severe hyperlipidemia, hyperproteinemia, or hyperglycemia as these cause relatively lower proportions of sodium in the plasma. When evaluating hyperglycemia, the correct sodium should be calculated [6].

Corrected sodium = Measured sodium +0.024 × (serum glucose – 100) [7]

Hyperglycemia causes an osmotic diuresis leading both to salt and water losses, total body volume depletion, or decreased renal perfusion.

Clinically, hypotonic hyponatremia can be further categorized by determining volume status [1]; there are three types of hyponatremia: hypovolemic, euvolemic, and hypervolemic.

Common causes for hyponatremia are shown in Table 1.

Hypovolemic hyponatremia occurs in relation of solute to total body water, and sodium loss is mediated either by the kidneys or via extrarenal loss of sodium [4]. UNa concentration can be a helpful to measure to determine the etiology of hyponatremia, as UNa >20 mEq/L represents sodium loss through the kidneys [1].

Renal losses of sodium include diuretics, mineralocorticoid deficiency, cerebral salt wasting, salt wasting nephropathy, and renal tubular acidosis (RTA). Diuretic usage typically enhances urinary excretion of sodium-rich fluid by inhibiting sodium reabsorption in the nephron [1]. Mineralocorticoid deficiency from adrenal insufficiency leads to renal sodium wasting, causing a hypovolemic state and activating vasopressin to further concentrate urine sodium. Elevated serum potassium with hypovolemic hyponatremia should lead to further investigation of mineralocorticoid insufficiency. Cerebral salt wasting can occur after neurological surgery or head injury. A baroreceptor-mediated vasopressin release is activated by urine sodium and chloride loss, though etiology of this process is not well established [1, 2].

Medication side effects (beyond diuretic use) are another common cause of hyponatremia. Common medication classes associated with this

Table 1 Main causes of hyponatremia

Hypovolemic states	Euvolemic states	Hypervolemic states
Osmotic (e.g., glucosuria, bicarbonaturia, ketonuria)	Hypothyroidism	Congestive heart failure
Diuretics	SIADH (see Table 2)	Renal failure
Mineralocorticoid deficiency	Severe pain and/or stress	Cirrhosis
Salt-losing nephropathies	Glucocorticoid deficiency	Nephrosis
Cerebral salt wasting	Primary polydipsia	Decreased vascular integrity (e.g., sepsis, anaphylaxis)
GI volume losses (e.g., diarrhea, vomiting)	Beer potomania	Acute or chronic renal failure
Sweat losses	Dilute formula intake	
Third-space sequestration	Dilute tube feeding	

References used: [2]
ADH antidiuretic hormone, *GI* gastrointestinal, *SIADH* syndrome of inappropriate secretion of ADH, *ECV* effective circulating volume, UNa urine sodium concentration

Table 2 Causes of syndrome of inappropriate antidiuretic hormone secretion

Central nervous system disorders causing increased hypothalamic production of antidiuretic hormone	Ectopic production of antidiuretic hormone (e.g., bronchogenic carcinoma, oat cell carcinoma of the lung, pancreatic carcinoma)
Infections (e.g., meningitis, HIV infection)	Pancreatic carcinoma
Vascular problems (e.g., subdural hemorrhage)	Prolactinoma
Primary and metastatic cancers	Others
Psychosis	Postoperative patient
Post pituitary surgery	Severe nausea
Hypothalamic infiltrative disease (e.g., sarcoidosis)	Pulmonary disorders causing increased antidiuretic hormone production
Others (e.g., Guillain-Barré syndrome)	Pneumonias
Pharmacologic agents	Tuberculosis
Stimulants of hypothalamic antidiuretic hormone secretion – haloperidol, amitriptyline, thioridazine, thiothixene, carbamazepine, fluoxetine and sertraline, monoamine oxidase inhibitors, and others	Acute respiratory failure
Potentiators of antidiuretic hormone effect – chlorpropamide, tolbutamide, carbamazepine	Others (e.g., asthma, pneumothorax)
Exogenous antidiuretic hormone preparations – vasopressin, oxytocin	

Adapted from: [2, 8]

change include proton pump inhibitors (PPIs), serotonin selection reuptake inhibitors (SSRIs), and antiepileptic medications. Although the mechanism is not clear for all medication classes, most often medication side effects leading to hyponatremia are related to SIADH or sodium-losing nephropathy [8].

Extrarenal losses leading to hypovolemic hyponatremia can be differentiated by a urine sodium concentration of <20 mEq/L and include GI losses (i.e., vomiting and diarrhea) and third-space sequestration (i.e., bowel obstruction, pancreatitis, peritonitis, ascites, massive tissue injury, venous congestion).

Euvolemic hyponatremia can be thought of as dilutional hyponatremia and is related to fluid intake above the kidneys' ability to excrete water (Table 1, Fig. 2) [5]. SIADH is the most common form of euvolemic hyponatremia (UNa usually >40 mEq/L) and occurs when excess ADH is secreted in the absence of volume or osmotic stimuli, resulting in water excess and hyponatremia. This can be caused by a variety of disorders including central nervous system and pulmonary diseases (Table 2). In addition, medications, hypothyroidism, and stress can all be common culprits of euvolemic hyponatremia [1].

Hypervolemic hyponatremia can commonly be seen with congestive heart failure (CHF), cirrhosis, nephrotic syndrome, and severe renal insufficiency are diseases that increase ECF volume through elevated ADH. Although total body sodium and water are increased in these states, the amount of water to sodium ratio is increased, leading to a lower sodium concentration. ADH secretion increases in left heart function and decreases due to baroreceptor mechanisms. If U[Na] > 20, this indicates an advanced renal disease such as acute or chronic renal failure. If U[Na] is low, this is more indicative of nonrenal causes such as congestive heart failure, cirrhosis, or nephrotic syndrome [1].

Symptoms of hyponatremia vary depending on the cause, severity, and rapidity of decline. Patients may be asymptomatic or mildly symptomatic with symptoms such as gait disturbance or mild cognitive deficits if hyponatremia is more chronic and less severe. However, if hyponatremia is more acute or sever, often below 125 mEq/L symptoms can be more profound. The spectrum of symptoms could range from mild headache, nausea, or confusion to severe features such as seizures, coma, or death [6].

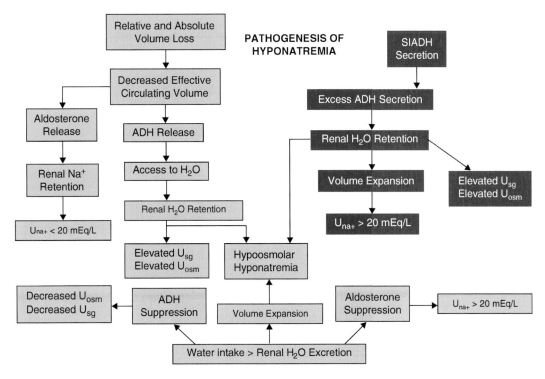

Fig. 2 Pathogenesis of hyponatremia. U_{Na} urine sodium concentration, U_{osm} urine osmolality, U_{sg} urine specific gravity, *ADH* antidiuretic hormone, *SIADH* syndrome of inappropriate ADH secretion. (Originally appeared in: Taylor R, David A, Fields S, Phillips M, Scherger J, editors. Family medicine (Taylor). New York: Springer; 2003)

Treatment of hyponatremia is dependent on the expected cause. In hypotonic hypovolemic hyponatremia, sodium replacement should almost always be with oral or intravenous isotonic volume repletion. Both normal saline 0.9% (NS) and Lactated Ringer's Solution (LR) are considered isotonic. In NS, the sodium concentration is 154 mmol/L with an osmolarity of 286 mmol/kg. In LR, the sodium concentration is 130 mmol/L with an osmolarity of 273 mmol/kg. For patients with euvolemic hyponatremia, often caused by SIADH, re-equilibrating plasma osmolality is done via fluid restriction. Identifying and removing the source of SIADH secretion is also key. If hyponatremia cannot be corrected via fluid restriction and removal of inciting source in SIADH, oral tolvaptin can be considered [1]. In hypervolemic hyponatremia, the mainstay of treatment is at correcting the underlying condition, which is often done with diuretic therapy and fluid restriction [6]. In patients with severe hyponatremia symptomatic hyponatremia, infusion of hypertonic saline or hemodialysis can sometimes be required. Physicians comfortable with intensive or emergent medicine should direct this treatment. Goal of treatment in these cases is to restore ECV and normalize plasma osmolality. The sodium level should not be corrected more quickly than 9–12 mmol/L in the first 24 h [1].

Hypernatremia

Hypernatremia, serum sodium concentration > 145 mmol/L (Fig. 3), is caused by increased hypotonic fluid loss. Similar to hyponatremia, hypernatremia can occur in hypovolemic, euvolemic, or hypervolemic states [6]. Since hypernatremia is related to water status, thirst and access to water with an intact sensorium to drink when thirsty is crucial to not developing hypernatremia. However, excessive oral intake of

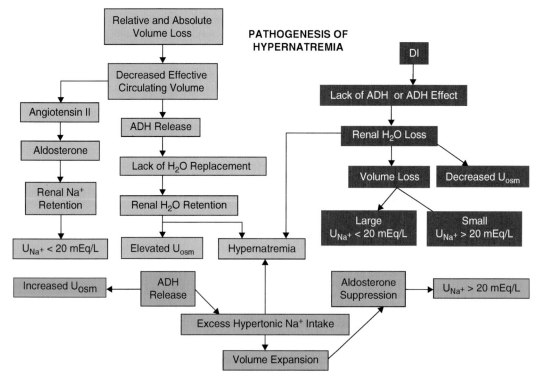

Fig. 3 Pathogenesis of hypernatremia. *DI* diabetes insipidus. (See Fig. 2 for other abbreviations). (Originally appeared in: Taylor R, David A, Fields S, Phillips M, Scherger J, editors. Family medicine (Taylor). New York: Springer; 2003)

Table 3 Causes of hypernatremia

Causes	Examples
Primary hypodipsia (defect of thirst)	Primary or metastatic tumor, granulomatous disease, vascular disease, trauma
Diabetes insipidus	Central, nephrogenic
Pure hypertonic solute gain	Ingestion of hypertonic solutions, ingestion of salt tablets
Inadequate fluid intake with increased free water loss	Increase sweating, fever, GI losses, osmotic diuresis, diuretics

sodium salts and hypertonic volume expansion can also be a cause of hypernatremia [6, 9] (Table 3).

In hypernatremia, plasma osmolality is >300 mOsm/kg. Urine sodium concentration of <20 mEq/L can be seen in a hypernatremic patient with GI or insensible losses with inadequate hypotonic volume replacement. Additionally, high urine osmolality (e.g., >600 mOsm/kg) is observed in these patients as the kidneys attempt to maintain stable fluid and sodium balance through renal water conservation. When hypernatremia is caused by renal volume losses from diuretics or osmotic diuresis with inadequate hypotonic volume replacement, urine sodium concentration is >20 mEq/L, while urine osmolality may be <350 mOsm/kg and is less than plasma osmolality. With the addition of sodium salts for volume expansion, hypernatremia is associated with urine osmolality >350 mOsm/kg and urine sodium concentration > 20 mEq/L. Patients with severe hypernatremia (serum sodium concentration >155 mEq/L) without maximum concentrated urine (i.e., 800–1200 mOsm/kg) suggests diabetes insipidus, intrinsic renal disease, osmotic diuresis, or diuretic use [9, 10].

The symptoms of hypernatremia occur due to primarily to hypertonicity of ECF, which results in volume shifting out of cells. This primarily leads to neurologic symptoms ranging from confusion to coma depending on severity. Other clinically encountered neurologic disorders can include seizures, focal neurologic deficits, and intracerebral hemorrhage [1]. Polyuria can be seen depending on etiology of hypernatremia and reveal a renal loss of pure water (e.g., diabetes insipidus), osmotic diuresis (e.g., glycosuria), or diuretic use, especially in medications altering ADH function.

Treating hypernatremia depends on the cause. Correction of asymptomatic or chronic hypernatremia that develops over greater than 48 h or previously unknown hypernatremia must proceed slowly (i.e., [Na$^+$] reduction of 0.5 mEq/L/h) to avoid cerebral edema and resultant neurological dysfunction [11]. In cases when hypernatremia has developed in less than 48 h, or acute hypernatremia, correction can proceed at up to 1 mEq/L/h [11]. Hypernatremia correction that is too slow can also cause complications [12]. When ECV is diminished by hypotonic volume loss, volume expansion with isotonic saline is initially used until signs of hypovolemia have resolved. An added benefit of isotonic saline infusion is that it can contribute to equilibrating plasma osmolality in patients with hyperosmolality. Once euvolemia is re-established, hypotonic fluids (e.g., 0.45% normal saline or dextrose 5% in water [D$_5$W]) can be administered in order to decrease plasma osmolality in pure water losses from the skin or kidneys [12]. Hypernatremia caused by the addition of Na$^+$ salts is treated with D$_5$W and diuretics. Calculating free water deficit can be helpful for management; however, total body water and free water loss are grossly underestimated with the most commonly used equation: total body water deficit = correction factor x premorbid weight × (1–140/Na$^+$) [13]. Hypernatremia caused by diabetes insipidus is often treated with vasopressin (V2) agonists, such as desmopressin, with possible use of thiazide diuretics and a low sodium diet [6].

Potassium Disorders

Hypokalemia

Plasma potassium levels are typically maintained at 3.5–5.0 mmol/L, with hypokalemia described by potassium levels <3.5 mmol/L. Hypokalemia can be caused by a variety of nonrenal causes, where urine potassium (UK) <25 mEq/L, and due to renal causes with UK >25 mEq/L (e.g., sodium-losing nephropathies, mineralocorticoid excess, vomiting, diuretics, and hypomagnesemia) (Table 4). Hypokalemia is a common electrolyte abnormality that can be found, and is a common side effect of medications, such as non-potassium sparing diuretics.

Potassium is typically passively reabsorbed in the proximal tubule of the kidney with the movement of sodium and chloride, while being actively reabsorbed in the thick ascending loop of Henle in the medulla via Na-K-2Cl (NKCC2) cotransporter. Increased flow to the distal nephron that occurs in diuretics that are effective more proximally (e.g., loop and thiazide diuretics) lead to increased potassium loss. Additionally, volume depletion activates RAAS causing an increase in potassium excretion. In fact, anything that leads to increases in mineralocorticoid activity and subsequent aldosterone activity will also lead to renal potassium loss.

Aldosterone can directly increase the activity of the Na-K-ATPase pump, shifting potassium intracellularly. In addition, it can facilitate secretion of potassium into the tubular lumen. This can be seen in any condition or medication that leads to increased aldosteronism. If the amount of potassium transported to the distal lumen increases, it will lead to increased excretion. High urine output will also lead to increased potassium excretion. The increase in delivery of potassium to the distal lumen and the higher urine output are methods by which diuretic use can lead to low potassium. Metabolic alkalosis can also lead to an increase in potassium excretion [6].

Symptoms associated with hypokalemia can include generalized weakness, musculoskeletal complaints (muscle cramps, muscle tenderness), GI complaints (anorexia, nausea, vomiting,

Table 4 Causes of hypokalemia

Renal potassium loss	Gastrointestinal loss	Intracellular K + sequestration	Pseudohypokalemia
Diuretics, current use	Diarrhea	Metabolic and respiratory alkalosis	Prolonged standing of collected blood with extremely high WBC count
Vomiting and nasogastric tube drainage	Excess sweating	Excess insulin	Blood specimen collected immediately after insulin administration
Magnesium depletion	Intestinal fistulas	Treatment of megaloblastic anemias	Decreased K+ intake
Mineralocorticoid excess (e.g., primary and secondary hyperaldosteronism, Cushing's disease, licorice ingestion, hyperreninism, Bartter syndrome, adrenal adenoma)	Rectal villous adenoma	Granulocyte-macrophage colony-stimulating factor (GM-CSF)	Starvation
Diabetic ketoacidosis	Geophagia (i.e., clay ingestion)	β-adrenergic agonist	
Renal tubular acidosis	Laxative abuse	Hypothermia	
Ureterosigmoidostomy	Chloride-losing diarrhea	Catecholamine excess	
Polyuria		Hypokalemic periodic paralysis	
Osmotic diuresis			
Correction of chronic hypercapnia			

Adapted from Taylor R, David A, Fields S, Phillips M, Scherger J, editors. Family medicine (Taylor). New York: Springer; 2003

constipation), polyuria, polydipsia, and cardiac complaints (palpitations, syncope). In skeletal muscle injury and rhabdomyolysis, potassium release from contracting skeletal muscle that would normally cause vasodilation and improved blood flow regionally is blunted in severe hypokalemia [14]. Potassium is also involved in cardiac muscle repolarization allowing for appropriate cardiac muscle relaxation and diastolic filling. With hypokalemia, cardiac repolarization is prolonged leading to classic electrocardiogram (EKG) changes. First noted is decreased magnitude of T waves, then U wave formation, and finally ST segment depression on EKG.

Oral replacement with potassium chloride or potassium bicarbonate and underlying correction of the cause are the mainstays of initial treatment. Oral therapy is less likely to have side effects and less likely to lead to over correction, and thus is the method of choice for repletion.

However, intravenous repletion can be used for patient's unable to tolerate oral potassium, of it hypokalemia is severe (<3.0 mEq/L). Typically, 10 mEq of potassium supplementation will increase plasma potassium level by about 0.1 mEq/L. Potassium levels should be monitored every 2–3 h during repletion to avoid an overcorrection [6]. Low magnesium must be corrected to ensure potassium is not lost renally during repletion [15]. Diuretics that work in the distal convoluted tubule and antagonize aldosterone receptors (i.e.,spironolactone) can decrease urine excretion of potassium.

Hyperkalemia

Hyperkalemia (see Table 5) is less well tolerated by the body than hypokalemia and occurs when extracellular potassium levels are elevated beyond the ability of kidneys, skin, and GI tract to excrete

Table 5 Causes of hyperkalemia

Increased K+ intake	Intracellular K+ extrusion	Measurement error
Dietary intake, medication intake	Metabolic and respiratory acidosis	Thrombocytosis
Decreased K+ excretion	Tissue injury (e.g., crush, rhabdomyolysis, hematoma resorption)	Leukocytosis
Acute and chronic renal failure	Insulin deficiency in diabetic ketoacidosis, prolonged fasting; hyperosmolality from hyperglycemia	Hemolysis of blood sample (i.e., delay after blood draw, cell destruction from vigorous sample shaking
Decreased effective circulating volume	Drugs (e.g., digitalis intoxication, succinylcholine, and arginine HCl, β-adrenergic blockers)	Blood collection from ischemic extremity
Hypoaldosteronism – K^+-sparing diuretics, hyporenin hypoaldosteronism in mild renal disease, NSAIDs, ACE inhibitors, adrenal insufficiency	Hyperkalemic periodic paralysis (from excessive exercise, fasting)	

References used [2, 19–22]

potassium. Extracellular potassium concentration can be affected by potassium shift from intracellular space to extracellular, potassium intake, and potassium excretion [16]. The kidneys perform most potassium excretion. Many medications can lead to hyperkalemia. Spironolactone, ACE-I, ARBs decrease aldosterone production, which can lead to hyperkalemia. Medications such as triamterene, amiloride, and the antibiotic trimethoprim decrease potassium excretion by blocking sodium channels. Other medications (e.g., nonselective beta-blockers, NSAIDs) can increase extracellular potassium by inhibiting Na-K ATPase pump, causing potassium to remain in extracellular fluid space and decreasing aldosterone production [17]. Avoiding a combination of these medications in patients with coexistent renal failure is important [17]. Kidney dysfunction (RTA type 4, CHF, and other causes of hypoaldosteronism) can inhibit potassium excretion [16].

Additional conditions and ingestions affect transcellular movement of potassium leading to hyperkalemia such as metabolic acidosis (0.2–1.7 mEq/L increase in $[K^+]$ for every 0.1 decrease in pH), hypertonicity from hyperglycemia or hypernatremia, insulin deficiency in diabetes mellitus or from starvation, rhabdomyolysis and hematoma resorption or other forms of cellular destruction, digitalis intoxication, and

hyperkalemic periodic paralysis from intense exercise or fasting. Hyperkalemia due to measurement error is also quite common and can be caused by hemolysis of red blood cells as a result of collection (i.e., prolonged tourniquet use, fist clenching leading to minor ischemia) [18] or storage, release of K^+ during coagulation of blood samples with increased WBCs (e.g., WBCs >100,000/mm^2 in leukemia) (or increased platelets (i.e., >1,000,000/mm^2) [18–20].

Hyperkalemia can cause nonspecific symptoms such as muscle weakness, fatigue, malaise, nausea, vomiting, and paresthesias. Peaked T waves are hallmark EKG findings in hyperkalemia, though flattened P waves, increased PR interval, prolonged QRS duration with shortened QT interval may also be present. Uncorrected hyperkalemia can lead to sine wave development with resultant ventricular fibrillation and asystole. Bradycardia, dysrhythmias, and paralysis can also occur.

Treatment of acute hyperkalemia can be done by enhancing potassium cellular entry using insulin, glucose, and inhaled beta-agonists (i.e., albuterol or levalbuterol) [21]. If hyperkalemia is associated with life-threatening dysrhythmias, calcium is used to decrease the threshold of myocardial tissue excitability induced by hyperkalemia, thereby minimizing risk of serious cardiac events. Calcium chloride has more elemental calcium and greater bioavailability than calcium gluconate but is typically associated with tissue necrosis and therefore cannot be infused as rapidly; however, one salt has not been proven more effective over the other [22]. Sodium bicarbonate has not shown to be more effective than placebo [22]. Loop diuretics are effective for excreting total body potassium in patients who make urine and kayexalate. Sodium polystyrene was previously shown to be effective [16], but new data shows no difference compared to stool softeners alone and is associated with increased risk of intestinal necrosis [21, 23, 24]. In patients refractory to these treatments, hemodialysis may prove necessary [22].

Acid–Base Disorders

Normal acid–base status is defined as a pH 7.35–7.45. This homeostasis is maintained by renal and respiratory compensatory mechanisms. Acidosis is defined as pH <7.35. If the pH > 7.45, it would be an alkalosis. These abnormalities can either be metabolic, from renal dysfunction, or respiratory in nature.

Metabolic Acidosis

Metabolic acidosis is a primary reduction in plasma bicarbonate concentration leading to hypobicarbonatemia (Table 6), which stimulates compensatory hyperventilation and hypocapnia (i.e., decreased pCO_2). In metabolic acidosis, the compensatory hyperventilation can be determined with the following formula. Full compensation may take several hours.

$$\text{Calculation for expected } pCO_2$$
$$pCO_2 = 1.5 \times [HCO_3] + 8$$

The limit of compensatory hyperventilation in metabolic acidosis is 10 mmHg that may be more difficult to achieve in acute versus acute process. If the rate of the pCO_2 decrease is less or more than predicted, a mixed acid–base disturbance occurs [25–28]. If the actual pCO_2 is too high,

then an additional respiratory acidosis is present; conversely, if the pCO_2 is too low, then an additional respiratory alkalosis is present.

The clinical scenario must be taken into account when approaching acid–base disorders. The etiology for the bicarbonate loss must be determined. Losses can occur with GI bicarbonate loss (e.g., diarrhea), renal bicarbonate loss (e.g., renal tubular acidosis), or bicarbonate titration with fixed endogenous acids (e.g., ketoacidosis) and exogenous acids (e.g., salicylate intoxication). Metabolic acidosis caused by pure bicarbonate loss is characterized by hyperchloremia and a normal anion gap. However, when metabolic acidosis is caused by the addition (e.g., methanol ingestion), retention (e.g., renal failure) [29], or excess production (e.g., lactic acidosis) of fixed acids that titrate bicarbonate, acidic anions remaining in extracellular body fluids cause expansion of the anion gap and a normal chloride concentration [30–32].

In reference to a calculated anion gap, a result of 20–30 has a high chance of metabolic acidosis, while a result >30 reflects metabolic acidosis. The anion gap is calculated using serum values with the following formula:

$$\text{Anion Gap} = [\text{Sodium}] -- [\text{Chloride}] - [HCO3]$$

Metabolic acidosis can be divided into three categories: increased anion gap, normal anion gap, and decreased anion gap. Increased anion gap metabolic acidosis is caused by ingestion of organic acids (salicylates, methanol, ethylene glycol, paraldehyde, propylene glycol), increased organic acid production (lactic acidosis, ketoacidosis), renal failure (phosphates, sulfates), or errors of metabolism (lipid metabolism errors, urea cycle disorders). Normal anion gap metabolic acidosis is due to intake of chloride salts (total parental nutrition, normal saline infusion), GI bicarbonate loss (diarrhea, colostomy, ileostomy, enteric fistula), urological procedures (ureterosigmoidostomy, ureteroileal conduit), ingestions (acetazolamide, magnesium sulfate), and renal bicarbonate loss (RTA, tubulointerstitial renal disease, hyperparathyroidism).

Table 6 Causes of hypobicarbonatemia[a]

Hyperchloremia, normal anion gap	Normochloremia, large anion gap (urine pH < 5.5)	Increased CNS stimulation
Bicarbonate loss (hypokalemia and urine pH < 5.5)	Excessive production of endogenously generated organic acids	Physiologic and psychogenic hyperventilation
GI tract bicarbonate loss (e.g., diarrhea, ureterosigmoidostomy, fistulas, tube drainage)	Diabetic ketoacidosis (i.e., excessive β-hydroxybutyrate and acetoacetate)	CNS disease (e.g., infectious, trauma, infarct, bleeding, tumors, heat stroke)
Renal bicarbonate loss and production failure (e.g., RTA type 2, RTA type 1, RTA type 4, carbonic anhydrase inhibitors)	Starvation ketosis	Pregnancy
HCl addition (e.g., NH_3Cl and some hyperalimentation fluids)	Alcoholic ketosis	Progesterone-producing tumors
Hypoaldosteronism (hyperkalemia, submaximal urinary acidification)	Lactic acidosis	Hepatic encephalopathy
Primary adrenal insufficiency	Muscle necrosis	Methylxanthines, nicotine, salicylates
Hyporeninemic hypoaldosteronism (e.g., during early chronic renal failure, acute renal failure interstitial nephritis, angiotensin-converting enzyme inhibition, and nonsteroidal anti-inflammatory drug use)	Decreased excretion of endogenous acid metabolites	Sepsis
Aldosterone resistance (e.g., spironolactone, amiloride, triamterene)	Renal failure	Hypoxia
Intestinal nephritis	Ingestion of exogenous agents causing organic acidosis	High altitude
Early renal failure	Methanol	Anemia, severe
Acute renal failure	Ethylene glycol	
Initial recovery from organic acidosis (variable $[K^+]$ and urine pH)	Paraldehyde	
	Salicylates	
	Respiratory alkalosis (i.e., increased pH, decreased $[HCO_3^-]$[c] and decreased pCO_2[b])	

Originally appeared in: Taylor R, David A, Fields S, Phillips M, Scherger J, editors. Family medicine (Taylor). New York: Springer; 2003
[a]Hypobicarbonatemia = decreased $[HCO_3^-]$
[b]Primary acid–base event
[c]Secondary or compensatory acid–base event

Metabolic acidosis causes extracellular hyperkalemia due to cellular buffering of hydrogen ions (failure of acidosis-induced hyperkalemia suggests total body potassium depletion), but because significant volume loss is a frequent complication (e.g., diabetic ketoacidosis), total body hypokalemia must always be expected (chronic renal failure and hypoaldosteronism may be an exception) [18]. The ingestion of acid toxins (e.g., paraldehyde, methanol, ethylene glycol, and salicylates) is associated not only with the distinct acid metabolite but also lactic acid as vascular collapse ensues [33].

Generally, compensatory responses will not be able to restore pH back to the normal value. Some of the most dangerous effects of acidosis on the body include hyperventilation, depression of myocardial contractility, sympathetic over activity, peripheral arteriolar vasodilation, hyperkalemia, and cerebral vasodilation with resultant increased intracranial pressure. Many of these conditions can be deleterious and deadly. Therapy for metabolic acidosis is initially directed at restoration of the systemic pH to levels that do not compromise cardiac function or predispose to cardiac dysrhythmias. Dangerous pH levels differ depending on the etiology of the acidosis; in general, however, safe systemic pH exists at 7.2. The use of sodium bicarbonate to increase pH has been controversial. Although useful in disorders associated with sodium loss, such as diarrhea or rental tubular acidosis, it has not been proven to be useful in all clinical setting. Specifically, it has not improved outcomes or mortality in common causes of metabolic acidosis, such as sepsis, lactic acidosis, and diabetic ketoacidosis [89]. Severe forms of metabolic acidosis requiring administration of sodium bicarbonate should be undertaken with care taken to avoid volume excess and post-treatment metabolic alkalosis by overaggressive alkali therapy [34]. If the metabolic acidosis is severe enough to warrant consideration of alkali therapy, a specialist consult would be warranted [33, 34].

Metabolic Alkalosis

Metabolic alkalosis is a primary increase in plasma bicarbonate concentration (i.e., hyper-bicarbonatemia) that causes a compensatory reduction in ventilation and relative hypercapnia (i.e., increased pCO_2) [2]. The bicarbonate accumulation is due to acid loss, alkali administration, intracellular shifts, or bicarbonate retention. With primary metabolic alkalosis, the compensatory hypoventilation occurs at a rate of 0.7 mmHg increase in the pCO_2 for every 1.0 mEq/L increase in the bicarbonate concentration. The limit of this compensatory hypoventilation is 55 mmHg because of hypoxia-induced ventilation. If the rate of pCO_2 increase is less or more than predicted, a mixed acid–base disturbance consisting of metabolic alkalosis and respiratory alkalosis or acidosis is present. The list of potential causes for metabolic alkalosis is extensive, but most common reasons include loss of gastric acid, renal acid loss, hypovolemia, hypokalemia, and diuretic use (Table 7).

Signs and symptoms associated with metabolic alkalosis relate to underlying cause. Metabolic alkalosis caused by volume depletion is characterized by a urinary chloride concentration of less than 10 mEq/L (i.e., saline-responsive), whereas metabolic alkalosis due to a primary increase in distal renal tubule activity (e.g., mineralocorticoid excess) and increased alkali ingestion is characterized by a urinary chloride concentration higher than 10 mEq/L (i.e., saline-resistant). Paradoxically, the urinary pH is usually acidic except when the disorder is caused by excessive alkali ingestion.

Treatment of saline-responsive metabolic alkalosis requires volume repletion with isotonic normal saline, which inhibits the volume depletion-induced retention of bicarbonate, resulting in an alkaline diuresis. With saline-resistant metabolic alkalosis, the source of the excess alkali ingestion must be removed or inhibited. Potassium deficits should also be replete using potassium chloride.

Respiratory Acidosis

Respiratory acidosis is a primary increase in the pCO_2 (i.e., hypercapnia), which stimulates compensatory cellular and renal retention of bicarbonate [2]. With primary acute and chronic respiratory acidosis, the compensatory bicarbonate retention occurs at a rate of 1.0 mEq/L or 4.0 mEq/L for every 10 mmHg increase in the pCO_2. The limits of the metabolic compensations during acute and chronic respiratory acidosis are 30 and 45 mEq/L, respectively. If the rate of compensatory bicarbonate retention is less or more than predicted, a mixed acid–base disturbance consisting of respiratory acidosis and metabolic acidosis or alkalosis is present. Respiratory acidosis occurs through three mechanisms: (1) excess CO_2 in the inhaled gas, (2) decreased alveolar ventilation, and (3) increased production of CO_2. The most likely cause is inadequate alveolar ventilation. A list of etiologics is provided in Table 7.

Symptoms of respiratory acidosis include shortness of breath and the mental status changes associated with progressive acute and chronic

Table 7 Causes of hyperbicarbonatemia[a]

Acid–base disorder	Etiology	Example
Metabolic alkalosis (i.e., increased [HCO$_3$⁻][b], increased pCO$_2$, increased pH)	Hypervolemia (i.e., hypochloremia, hypokalemia; urine Na⁺ > 10 mEq/L, Cl⁻ > 10 mEq/L, pH < 6.0)	Mineralocorticoid excess, renal artery stenosis, primary aldosteronism, adrenal hyperplasia
	Hypovolemia and chloride depletion (i.e., hypochloremia, hypokalemia: urine Na⁺ < 10 mEq/L, Cl⁻ < 10 mEq/L, pH < 6, K⁺ < 10 mEq/L	Vomiting, post-diuretic use, congenital chloride diarrhea, Bartter syndrome, acute correction of hypercapnia in hypovolemia
	Excessive alkali (hypochloremia, hypokalemia; urine Na⁺ > 10 mEq/L, Cl⁻ > 10 mEq/L, pH > 7.0)	Excessive exogenous alkali (e.g., absorbable antacids, milk-alkali syndrome, excessive infusion of NaHCO$_3$), excessive endogenous alkali (NaHCO$_3$), acute correction of chronic hypercapnia in euvolemia, metabolism of β-hydroxybutyrate, acetoacetate, lactate, and citrate
	Severe hypokalemia	
	Hypercalcemia (e.g., primary hyperparathyroidism)	
Respiratory acidosis (i.e., lactate, increased pCO$_2$,[b] increased [HCO$_3$⁻]	Suppression of CNS respiratory center	Oxygen-induced acute pCO$_2$ retention in chronic obstructive pulmonary disease (COPD), sedating medications, sleep apnea
	Disorders of respiratory muscles	
	Obstructed airway	Laryngeal edema or spasm, extrinsic foreign body, aspiration, bronchospasm
	Disturbances of gas exchange across alveolar membrane	Pulmonary edema, adult respiratory distress syndrome, diffuse pneumonia, COPD
	Loss of ventilatory volume	Hemothorax, pneumothorax, pleural effusions

Originally appeared in: Taylor R, David A, Fields S, Phillips M, Scherger J, editors. Family medicine (Taylor). New York: Springer; 2003
[a]Hyperbicarbonatemia = increased [HCO$_3$⁻]
[b]Primary acid–base event

hypercapnia. The treatment of respiratory acidosis is directed to the primary cause to increase the effectiveness of ventilation and pulmonary gas exchange.

Respiratory Alkalosis

Respiratory alkalosis is a primary reduction in the pCO$_2$ (i.e., hypocapnia), which stimulates a compensatory cellular and renal reduction in bicarbonate concentration [2]. With primary acute and chronic respiratory alkalosis, the compensatory bicarbonate loss occurs at a rate of 2.0 mEq/L or 5.0 mEq/L for every 10 mmHg decrease in the pCO$_2$. The limits of these metabolic compensations in acute and chronic respiratory alkalosis are 18 and 12 mEq/L, respectively. If the rate of compensatory bicarbonate loss is less or more than predicted, a mixed acid–base disturbance is present which is discussed later. Respiratory alkalosis is caused by central causes, hypoxia, pulmonary causes, and iatrogenically (excessive controlled ventilation) (Table 6).

Acute hypocapnia may be associated with circumoral and digital paresthesias, lightheadedness, carpopedal spasm, and tetany. The associated hyperventilation is obvious, as it is mostly rate driven. With chronic hypocapnia, the respiratory rate may be normal, and the depth of respiration may predominate as the mechanism of pCO_2 removal. Treatment is directed to the underlying cause.

Mixed Acid–Base Disturbances

The presence of a mixed acid–base disturbance is usually detected when a primary acid–base event fails to demonstrate the expected compensation. This failure of compensation can predict the presence of a respiratory and metabolic acid–base event occurring concurrently but does not predict the presence of mixed metabolic events or mixed respiratory events. Acid–base maps have similar diagnostic limitations. The mixture of more than two events can be determined by other laboratory evidence but is best detected when historical evaluations suggest multiple acid–base events. Although laboratory data may be the first evidence of acid–base disturbances, utilization of these tools to predict primary and mixed acid–base disturbances must be related with clinical data to ensure that the information is appropriately interpreted (Table 8).

The presence of a mixed acid–base disturbance is best detected by anticipating its presence in clinical settings, although some laboratory findings can be helpful. The compensation in acid–base disturbances minimizes changes in systemic pH but never totally corrects the pH (the possible exception is chronic hypocapnia in persons living at high altitudes). Therefore, the presence of a normal pH with normal $[HCO_3^-]$ and pCO_2 indicates the presence of a mixed acid–base disturbance. Likewise, with primary acid–base

Table 8 Common mixed acid–base disturbances

Disorder	Examples
Predicted by rules of compensation	
Metabolic acidosis and respiratory alkalosis (partial pressure of carbon dioxide reduction greater than predicted for metabolic acidosis)	Chronic renal failure and septicemia
Metabolic alkalosis and respiratory acidosis (partial pressure of carbon dioxide reduction less than predicted for metabolic acidosis)	Lactic acidosis and chronic obstructive pulmonary disease
Metabolic and respiratory alkalosis (partial pressure of carbon dioxide elevation less than predicted for metabolic alkalosis)	Diuretic overuse and psychogenic hyperventilation
Metabolic alkalosis and respiratory acidosis (partial pressure of carbon dioxide elevation greater than predicted for metabolic alkalosis)	Vomiting and adult respiratory distress syndrome
Not predicted by rules of compensation	
Hyperchloremia and large anion gap metabolic acidosis (nonequivalent changes in chloride and bicarbonate concentrations and an elevated anion gap)	Diarrhea and chronic renal disease
Metabolic alkalosis and large anion gap acidosis (nonequivalent changes in chloride bicarbonate concentrations and an elevated anion gap)	Vomiting and chronic renal failure
Acute and chronic respiratory alkalosis ($[HCO_3^-]$ reduction greater than predicted for acute respiratory alkalosis and less than predicted for chronic respiratory alkalosis)	Septicemia and psychogenic hyperventilation
Acute and chronic respiratory acidosis ($[HCO_3^-]$ elevation greater than predicted for acute respiratory acidosis and less than predicted for chronic respiratory acidosis)	Acute respiratory failure and COPD
Chronic respiratory acidosis and acute respiratory alkalosis ($[HCO_3^-]$ elevation or reduction inconsistent with expected pCO_2 elevation or reduction for either of these disorders, respectively)	COPD and pulmonary embolus
Metabolic alkalosis and nonanion gap metabolic acidosis (difficult to recognize because $[Cl^-]$ and $[HCO_3^-]$ changes depend on which disorder predominates; if each disorder is of equal magnitude, then $[Cl^-]$, $[HCO_3^-]$, pCO_2, and pH are normal)	Chronic diuretic overuse and diarrhea

Originally appeared in: Taylor R, David A, Fields S, Phillips M, Scherger J, editors. Family medicine (Taylor). New York: Springer; 2003

COPD chronic obstructive pulmonary disease

disturbances, the compensatory event is in the same direction as the primary event; therefore, acid–base disturbances where the compensatory event and the primary event are in opposite directions also indicate the presence of a mixed acid–base disturbance. A large anion gap metabolic acidosis occurring concurrently with a hyperchloremia metabolic acidosis (e.g., a patient with diabetic ketoacidosis and diarrhea) is detected when the anion gap does not account for the amount of $[HCO_3^-]$ concentration reduction. An example of this mixed disturbance is a sign of recovery during the appropriate treatment of diabetic ketoacidosis as β-hydroxybutyrate and acetoacetate (ketone bodies) are hepatically converted to $[HCO_3^-]$, resulting in a transition from the original large anion gap metabolic acidosis to a hyperchloremia metabolic acidosis with less severe systemic pH reductions. The presence of a large anion gap, regardless of the systemic pH, indicates the presence of metabolic acidosis. For example, a patient with plasma metabolic alkalosis caused by diuretic use may have a $[HCO_3^-]$ of 36 mEq/L, and if the hypovolemia becomes severe enough, lactic acidosis may ensue. However, an 8 mEq/L drop in $[HCO_3^-]$ caused by titration of lactic acid would result in a $[HCO_3^-]$ of 28 mEq/L, essentially no change in $[Cl^-]$, and an appropriate pCO_2 response with the pH still slightly alkalemic. This process can be detected early based on the concurrent increase in the anion gap as $[HCO_3^-]$ is consumed in the titration with lactic acid and elevated plasma lactic acid – if the potential for this disorder had been anticipated clinically.

The limits of compensation are important factors to consider especially when suspecting respiratory acidosis in a patient with metabolic alkalosis. Although the compensation for metabolic alkalosis is pCO_2 retention, pCO_2 values higher than 55 mmHg do not occur because the resulting hypoxia stimulates ventilation. Therefore, in patients with metabolic alkalosis and a pCO_2 higher than 55 mmHg, primary impairment of ventilation causing respiratory acidosis must also be present. Because the limits of compensation in chronic respiratory alkalosis is a $[HCO_3^-]$ of 14 mEq/L, $[HCO_3^-]$ less than that implies the additional presence of metabolic acidosis. Likewise, the limits of compensation for chronic respiratory acidosis is renal HCO_3 retention to 45 mEq/L, and higher $[HCO_3^-]$ concentrations imply the additional presence of metabolic alkalosis. Because chronic renal disease in its end stages results in a $[HCO_3^-]$ of 12–14 mEq/L, greater $[HCO_3^-]$ reductions would suggest additional causes of metabolic acidosis (e.g., vomiting).

Mixtures of acute and chronic respiratory acidosis as well as acute and chronic respiratory alkalosis can be detected using the rules of compensation for primary acid–base disorders and by plotting pCO_2 and $[HCO_3^-]$ on acid–base maps. Points that define mixtures of acute and chronic respiratory alkalosis or respiratory acidosis may also be consistent with a mixture of acute respiratory and metabolic alkalosis or acute respiratory acidosis and metabolic alkalosis. Mixtures of respiratory acidosis and respiratory alkalosis pose special problems. The more profound event may alter the pCO_2 enough to leave the respiratory-induced metabolic compensation unopposed for hours to days (e.g., a patient with chronic obstructive pulmonary disease who is mechanically hyperventilated, thereby decreasing the pCO_2 and leaving the pCO_2-induced $[HCO_3^-]$ elevation until renal $[HCO_3^-]$ excretion occurs over the following hours to days).

Miscellaneous Electrolyte Disturbances

Magnesium

Hypomagnesemia ($Mg^{2+} < 1.5$ mEq/L) associated with urinary magnesium (UMg) conservation (UMg < 10 mg/day) can be caused by decreased magnesium intake (e.g., protein calorie malnutrition), decreased magnesium absorption, and extrarenal magnesium loss [2]. Hypomagnesemia associated with urinary magnesium excretion (UMg > 10 mg/day) can be caused by excessive renal magnesium loss (e.g., diuretic use, hypokalemia, hypercalciuria, hypervolemia, and hyperthyroidism). Hypomagnesemia is also caused by chronic magnesium wasting and treatment-induced intracellular magnesium redistribution (e.g., diabetic ketoacidosis and alcoholism). Hypomagensium is commonly seen concurrently with hypokalemia. In these instances, it is best to replete magnesium prior to repleting potassium, as hypomagnesemia can lead to renal potassium wasting [1].

Hypermagnesemia is often transient and related to increased dietary magnesium intake. However, the kidney has a large capacity to excrete magnesium. When hypermagnesemia is persistent, it is most often due to chronic renal insufficiency in conjunction with taking excessive amounts of magnesium medications or supplementation. When magnesium reaches levels above 4-6 mg/dL, it can be toxic and lead to grave effects including hypotension, urinary retention, and ileus. At levels above 8–12 mg/dL, hyporeflexia, paralysis, bradyarrythemias, and death from respiratory depression or cardiac arrest is possible [1].

Phosphate

Hypophosphatemia (plasma phosphorus <2.5 mg/dL) is caused by increased phosphate renal excretion (i.e., UPO4 > 100 mg/24 h) in diabetic ketoacidosis, hypokalemia, and phosphate deficiency (UPO4 < 100 mg/24 h) in hypoparathyroidism and decreased phosphate intake (e.g., alcoholism, vitamin D deficiency, and use of phosphate binders), as well as intracellular phosphate shifts (UPO4 < 100 mg/24 h) in metabolic and respiratory alkalosis [2]. Hyperphosphatemia (phosphorus >4.8 mg/dL) associated with UPO4 > 1500 mg/24 h is caused by increased release of phosphates into the extracellular fluid by cell lysis (e.g., rhabdomyolysis) and initial anionic redistribution of metabolic acidosis (e.g., diabetic ketoacidosis and lactic acidosis).

Hyperphosphatemia associated with UPO4 < 1500 mg/24 h is caused by decreased renal phosphate excretion (e.g., volume depletion, acute and chronic renal failure, and hyperparathyroidism). Clinical manifestations vary depending on time course and mechanism. Symptom presentation is more severe with acute versus chronic. Symptoms may be mild if from intracellular shift as intracellular phosphate levels are enough for ATP production. Clinically patients may develop respiratory muscle dysfunction, decreased contractility of heart, hemolysis, insulin resistance, myopathy, rhabdomyolysis, and seizures. These symptoms are largely caused by adenosine triphosphate depletion in hypophosphatemia. Treatment is phosphate repletion and may be done either orally or intravenously.

Calcium

Hypocalcemia (Ca^{2+} < 8.5 mg/dL or ionized Ca^{2+} < 4.1 mg/dL) associated with normal or subnormal parathyroid hormone (PTH) is caused by PTH-deficient hypoparathyroidism and severe hypomagnesemia. Since 40% of Ca is bound to plasma proteins, it is important to adjust for low albumin by adding 0.8 mg/dL for every 10 g/L decrease in normal albumin [1]. Calcium is regulated by parathyroid hormone. When levels of Ca^{2+} are low, PTH is secreted from the parathyroid resulting in increased renal reabsorption as well as increased renal vitamin D production, which stimulates increased intestinal absorption of calcium. Hypocalcemia associated with elevated PTH is caused by chronic renal failure, vitamin D deficiency, malabsorption, drug-induced microsomal enzyme induction (e.g., mithramycin and phenytoin), osteomalacia, and causes of severe acute hyperphosphatemia such as acute pancreatitis, hepatic failure, and other causes of massive tissue necrosis.

Hypercalcemia (total $[Ca^{2+}]$ > 10.5 mg/DL or ionized $[Ca^{2+}]$ > 5.1) with elevated PTH is caused by primary hyperparathyroidism (i.e., excessive production of PTH) and severe secondary hyperparathyroidism of chronic renal failure. Hypercalcemia associated with normal PTH is caused by vitamin D excess, sarcoidosis, hyperthyroidism, increased bone calcium release (e.g., immobilization and bony metastasis), extracellular fluid depletion, thiazides, or milk-alkali syndrome. Clinical manifestations include nephrolithiasis, bone pain, abdominal pain from constipation, nausea, vomiting, and psychiatric symptoms. Asymptomatic patients with mild hypercalcemia do not need treatment; however, if >14 mg/DL or if >12 mg/DL with symptoms should be treated with aggressive saline rehydration followed by furosemide diuresis, calcitonin, and bisphosphonates. Surgery would be indicated for primary hyperparathyroidism.

References

1. Goldman L, Schafer A. Goldman-Cecil medicine. 25th ed. Philadelphia: Elsevier; 2016.
2. Fluid HJ. Electrolyte, and acid–base disorders. In: Taylor R, David A, Fields S, Phillips M, Scherger J, editors. Family medicine (Taylor). New York: Springer; 2003.
3. Rose BD. Regulation of the effective circulating volume. In: Rose BD, editor. Clinical physiology of acid–base and electrolyte disturbances. 5th ed. - New York: McGraw-Hill; 2001. p. 258–84.
4. Verbalis JG, Goldsmith SR, Greenberg A, Schrier RW, Sterns RH. Hyponatremia treatment guidelines 2007: expert panel recommendations. Am J Med. 2007;120(11 Suppl 1):S1.
5. Upadhyay A, Jaber BL, Madias NE. Incidence and prevalence of hyponatremia. Am J Med. 2006;119 (7 Suppl 1):S30–5.
6. Gilbert S, Weiner D, Gipson D, Perazella M, Tonelli M. National kidney foundation's primer on kidney diseases. 6th ed. Philadelphia: Elsevier; 2014.
7. Hillier TA, Abbott RD, Barrett EJ. Hyponatremia: evaluating the correction factor for hyperglycemia. Am J Med. 1999;106(4):399.
8. Liamis G, Milionis H, Elisaf M. A review of drug-induced hyponatremia. Am J Kidney Dis. 2008;52 (1):144–53.
9. Rose BD. Hyperosmolal states – hypernatremia. In: Rose BD, editor. Clinical physiology of acid–base and electrolytes disorders. 5th ed. New York: McGraw-Hill; 2001. p. 746–93.
10. Briggs JP, Singh IIJ, Sawaya BE, Schnermann J. Disorders of salt balance. In: Kokko JP, Tannen RL, editors. Fluids and electrolytes. 3rd ed. Philadelphia: WB Saunders; 1996. p. 3–62.
11. Alshayeb HM, Showkat A, Babar F, Mangold T, Wall BM. Severe hypernatremia correction rate and mortality in hospitalized patients. Am J Med Sci. 2011;341 (5):356–60.
12. Bataille S, Baralla C, Torro D, Buffat C, Berland Y, Alazia M, Vacher-Coponat H. Undercorrection of hypernatremia is frequent and associated with mortality. BMC Nephrol. 2014;15:37.
13. Cheuvront SN, Kenefick R, Sollanek KJ, Ely BR, Sawka MN. Water-deficit equation: systematic analysis and improvement. Am J Clin Nutr. 2013;97(1):79.
14. Knochel JP, Schlein EM. On the mechanism of rhabdomyolysis in potassium depletion. J Clin Invest. 1972;51(7):1750.
15. Medford-Davis RZ. Derangements of potassium. Emerg Med Clin North Am. 2014;32(2):329–47.
16. Alfonzo AVM, Isles C, Deighan C, Geddes C. Potassium disorders–clinical spectrum and emergency management. Resuscitation. 2006;70(1):10.
17. Mount DB, Zandi-Nejad K. Disorders of potassium balance. In: Brenner BM, Levine SA, editors. Brenner and Rector's the kidney. 8th ed. Philadelphia: Saunders Elsevier; 2007. p. 547–87.
18. Adrogue HJ, Madias NE. Changes in plasma potassium concentration during acute acid–base disturbances. Am J Med. 1981;71:456.
19. Tannen RL. Potassium disorders. In: Kokko JP, Tannen RL, editors. Fluids and electrolytes. 3rd ed. Philadelphia: WB Saunders; 1996. p. 111–99.
20. Hobbs J. Acid–base, fluid and electrolyte disorders. In: Rakel RE, editor. Textbook of family practice. 4th ed. Philadelphia: WB Saunders; 1990.
21. Mahoney BA, Smith WAD, Lo DS, Tsoi K, Tonelli M, Clase CM. Emergency interventions for hyperkalaemia. Cochrane Database Syst Rev. 2005;(2)CD003235. https://doi.org/10.1002/14651858.CD003235.pub2
22. Putcha N, Allon M. Management of hyperkalemia in dialysis patients. Semin Dial. 2007;20(5):431–9.
23. McGowan CE, Saha S, Chu G, Resnick MB, Moss SF. Intestinal necrosis due to sodium polystyrene sulfonate (Kayexalate) in sorbitol. South Med J. 2009;102 (5):493–7.
24. Weisberg LS. Management of severe hyperkalemia. Crit Care Med. 2008;36(12):3246–51.
25. Narins RG, Jones ER, Stom MC, Rudnick MR, Bastl CP. Diagnostic strategies in disorders of fluid, electrolyte and acid–base homeostasis. Am J Med. 1982;72:496–504.
26. Narins RG, Emmett M. Simple and mixed acid–base disorders: a practical approach. Medicine. 1980;59:161–87.
27. Rose BD. Introduction to simple and mixed acid–base disorders. In: Rose BD, editor. Clinical physiology of acid–base and electrolytes disorders. 5th ed. New York: McGraw-Hill; 2001. p. 535–50.
28. Rose BD. Metabolic acidosis. In: Rose BD, editor. Clinical physiology of acid–base and electrolytes disorders. 5th ed. New York: McGraw-Hill; 2001. p. 578–646.
29. Prough DS. Physiologic acid–base and electrolyte changes in acute and chronic renal failure patients. Anesthesiol Clin North Am. 2000;18(4):809–33.. ix
30. Oster JR, Perez GO, Materson BJ. Use of the anion gap in clinical medicine. South Med J. 1988;81:225–37.
31. Emmett M, Narins RG. Clinical use of the anion gap. Medicine. 1977;56:38.
32. Gabow PA, Kaehny WD, Fennessey PV, Goodman MD, Gross P, Schrier RW. Diagnostic importance of an increased anion gap. N Engl J Med. 1980;303:854.
33. Rice M, Ismail B, Pillow MT. Approach to metabolic acidosis in the emergency department. Emerg Med Clin North Am. 2014;32(2):403–20.
34. Fidkowski C, Helstrom J. Diagnosing metabolic acidosis in the critically ill: bridging the anion gap and base excess methods. Can J Anaesth. 2009;56:247–56.

Diseases of the Kidney

Margaret Baumgarten, Todd W. B. Gehr,
Niraj R. Kothari, and Daniel Carl

Contents

M. Baumgarten (✉)
Family and Community Medicine, Eastern Virginia
Medical School, Norfolk, VA, USA
e-mail: baumgamy@evms.edu

T. W. B. Gehr · N. R. Kothari
Division of Nephrology/Department of Internal Medicine,
Virginia Commonwealth University Medical College of
Virginia Campus, Richmond, VA, USA
e-mail: todd.gehr@vcuhealth.org; niraj.
kothari@vcuhealth.org

D. Carl
Salmon Creek Medical Office, Nephrology, Vancouver,
WA, USA

Medical College of Virginia Campus, Virginia
Commonwealth University, Richmond, VA, USA
e-mail: dcarl@mcvh-vcu.edu

© Springer Nature Switzerland AG 2022
P. M. Paulman et al. (eds.), *Family Medicine*,
https://doi.org/10.1007/978-3-030-54441-6_104

Glomerulonephritis

The nephritic syndrome is acute in onset and associated with oliguria, azotemia, hypertension, and proteinuria of variable quantity. Hematuria (usually dysmorphic) and RBC casts are the hallmark of glomerular inflammation and glomerular basement membrane disruption. A diverse group of diseases cause the syndrome and the presentation is often dramatic and can be life threatening.

Acute Proliferative Glomerulonephritis/Poststreptococcal Glomerulonephritis

This condition is characterized by diffuse proliferation within the glomerulus and the prototypical disease is poststreptococcal glomerulonephritis. The disease occurs 1–2 weeks after a skin infection or sore throat and may occur in as many as 25% of patients affected by Group A streptococci, M-type stains [1, 5, 13]. The condition usually develops in children but can occur at any age. Serum complement is typically low; anti-streptolysin O and DNAase B titers are high. These patients usually have a dramatic presentation with nephrotic syndrome, gross hematuria with dark and smoky urine, RBC casts, hypertension, and acute kidney failure. Milder manifestations with non-nephrotic proteinuria and microscopic hematuria without renal failure can

also be seen. Most patients recover spontaneously although persistent urinary abnormalities may persist and a small subset of patients may develop chronic kidney disease (CKD) [1, 2].

Immunoglobulin A Nephropathy

IgA nephropathy is the most common form of glomerulonephritis worldwide. IgG-IgA1 immune complexes are deposited in the mesangium of the glomerulus and incite an inflammatory reaction. IgA levels in the blood do not correlate with disease although the pathogenesis may involve a decrease in galactosylation of IgA1 making it susceptible to an antibody response. Primary care physicians are often the first providers who evaluate these patients for gross hematuria following an upper respiratory infection in adolescence or as young adults. Although the condition is often benign, a more aggressive form of the disease can occur which can lead to End-Stage Kidney Disease (ESKD). IgA nephropathy often accompanies Henoch-Schönlein purpura which is a condition appearing earlier in life (mean age 6–7 years) and associated with a purpuric rash usually involving the legs and buttocks, abdominal pain, arthritis and arthralgias. The condition, including IgA nephropathy, usually resolves spontaneously with conservative management. IgA deposits with or without associated nephropathy can accompany a variety of diseases including sarcoidosis, HIV infection, liver disease, and inflammatory bowel disease. The significance of these deposits remains unclear. Therapy for typical IgA nephropathy includes omega-3-fatty acids and/or angiotensin-converting enzyme inhibitors, both of which have shown promise in slowing the progression of disease; glucocorticoids may be of benefit in the setting of persistent proteinuria [3].

Lupus Nephritis

Patients with systemic lupus erythematosus commonly have renal involvement, although the extent of involvement is highly variable. Lupus nephritis is an immune complex mediated glomerular disease with autoantibodies to a variety of antigens (nuclear, double-stranded DNA). These autoantibodies are deposited in the glomerulus, activate complement and elicit an inflammatory response that damages the kidney. Six histologically distinct classes of renal involvement have been described with class 4, diffuse proliferative glomerulonephritis being the most severe. It is not uncommon for glomerular histology to change in a single patient necessitating very close follow-up. Besides following renal function and urinalysis, complement activity and anti-double-stranded DNA titers fluctuate with disease activity. Therapy is best described for class 4 diffuse proliferative lupus nephritis. Treatment with high doses of intravenous and oral steroids and intravenous or oral cyclophosphamide have been successfully employed. Oral mycophenolate mofetil has been shown to be equally effective and has fewer side effects. Recently, intravenous rituximab has also been used as a second-line agent [4].

Rapidly Progressive Glomerulonephritis (RPGN)

RPGN, also known as crescentic glomerulonephritis, is a dramatic condition causing a rapid, often irreversible, decline in renal function.

Prompt diagnosis is required, if left untreated it uniformly leads to ESKD or death. Crescents are cellular elements that follow the contour of Bowman's capsule, crowding out the capillary loops in the glomerulus. Crescents are not specific to any particular type of RPGN but the extent of their presence (>60% glomerular involvement) denotes the severity of the inflammatory response within the glomerulus. There are three types of RPGN based on distinct pathogenic mechanisms.

Type 1 RPGN

Although rare, this type of RPGN is often the best known of the types of RPGN. It is known as anti-GBM disease when the disorder is confined to the kidney, but if there is cross-reactivity to alveolar basement membrane leading to pulmonary hemorrhage it is known as Goodpasture syndrome. Early initiation of therapy is critical in this disorder in order to prevent ESRD. Anti-GBM antibody titers can be followed to monitor therapeutic effectiveness, but results are often delayed; for more expedient results a kidney biopsy is often required. Intravenous steroids, cyclophosphamide, and plasmapheresis are usually effective in improving renal function and controlling pulmonary hemorrhage if used early in the course of the disease. As this is an antibody mediated disorder, use of the anti-CD20 agent, rituximab, has also shown promise in controlling the disorder. In most instances, maintenance therapy with cyclophosphamide, mycophenolate mofetil, or azathioprine is necessary to control the disease [5].

Type 2 RPGN

Type 2 RPGN can be produced by any immune complex–mediated glomerulonephritis. The immune complexes can be virtually anywhere within the glomerular structure: mesangial, subendothelial, intramembranous, or subepithelial. The presence of crescents is a result of the intense inflammatory response. Although IgA nephropathy is usually a benign glomerular disease, it can present as Type 2 RPGN leading to ESKD. Therapy consists of intravenous steroids and cytotoxic drugs with less reliance on plasmapheresis.

Again, early initiation of therapy is critical if ESKD is to be avoided.

Type 3 RPGN

Type 3 RPGN is also known as pauci-immune complex glomerulonephritis owing to the lack of immune complexes demonstrated in the glomerulus. However, circulating antineutrophil cytoplasmic antibodies (ANCA) are usually present and are thought to be critical in the pathogenesis of the disease. Most of these patients will have an underlying small vessel vasculitis such as microscopic polyangiitis (MPA), granulomatosis with polyangiitis (GPA), or eosinophilic granulomatosis with polyangiitis (EGPA). Asthma is frequently the most prominent symptom, but these disorders often affect multiple organ systems simultaneously. Flu-like symptoms often occur for weeks in affected individuals. Rash (usually purpuric), arthralgias, symptoms of a peripheral neuropathy, and nonspecific pulmonary symptoms including pulmonary hemorrhage and chronic sinusitis may be present. Eosinophilia is usually present but not specific for EGPA. With MPA and GPA circulating ANCA is usually present. Two major classes of ANCA are reported. Antibodies with a cytoplasmic pattern of staining, c-ANCA, are directed toward proteinase-3 whereas antibodies with perinuclear staining, p-ANCA, are directed toward myeloperoxidase. Over 75% of patients will have some pattern of positive ANCA with c-ANCA being more common with GPA and p-ANCA positive in MPA. There is considerable overlap in ANCA patterns, however, with some patients even demonstrating a negative ANCA or positivity to both c- and p-ANCA. As with the other types of RPGN, early diagnosis and therapy is essential in order to avoid ESKD. Dramatic response to intravenous steroids and cyclophosphamide is often seen, with an overall response rate exceeding 90%. For patients with aggressive pulmonary disease, plasmapheresis should also be employed. Rituximab has also been shown to be of benefit, particularly as maintenance therapy which is necessary for up to 1 or 2 years. Relapse can occur after many years: close, regular follow-up is essential [6].

Nephrotic Syndrome

Nephrotic syndrome is characterized by heavy proteinuria (greater than 3.5 g in a 24 h urine collection, protein to creatinine ratio greater than 3 g of protein per g of creatinine) in association with hypoalbuminemia, edema, and hyperlipidemia. In contrast to nephritic sediment, cellular casts and hematuria are uncommonly encountered in nephrotic syndrome.

Clinical and Laboratory Features

Heavy proteinuria is the hallmark of nephrotic syndrome, and nephrotic-range proteinuria is defined as greater than 3.5 g of proteinuria in a 24 h urine collection. Not all patients with nephrotic-range proteinuria have nephrotic syndrome, which is accompanied by edema, hypoalbuminemia, and hyperlipidemia. The typical presenting symptom of nephrotic syndrome is progressive edema. Edema generally starts in the lower extremities; periorbital edema, genital edema, ascites, pleural and pericardial effusions can be seen in advanced disease. Nephrotic syndrome should be suspected in patients with these findings in the absence of cirrhosis or congestive heart failure. The decrease in oncotic pressure from albumin loss, with a resultant movement of fluid from the intravascular space to the interstitial space, contributes to the edema. Recent studies have suggested the presence of increased renal sodium reabsorption in nephrotic syndrome, which may occur from both glomerular and tubulointerstitial factors. Severe tubulointerstitial inflammation in nephrotic syndrome has been theorized to increase vasoconstrictive agents (e.g., angiotensin II) while decreasing vasodilatory agents (e.g., nitric oxide) [7]. The 24 h urine collection remains the gold standard for quantifying proteinuria, although it has limitations in routine screening for proteinuria. Proteinuria evaluated by a urinalysis dipstick is a semiquantitative screening tool available to most physicians. In addition, the spot urine protein to creatinine ratio is easy to use in the clinic setting, and provides a quantitative value that accurately estimates the 24 h urine value. The value obtained from the spot urine (in mg/mg) will correlate to the protein excretion in grams per m^2 body surface area. Hypoalbuminemia is often less than 3 g/dL in patients with nephrotic syndrome, although the pathophysiology behind this remains incompletely understood. Most patients with nephrotic syndrome have hyperlipidemia, which may manifest as elevated total and low-density lipoprotein cholesterol, lipoprotein (a), and hypertriglyceridemia. The pathophysiological mechanism of hyperlipidemia likely occurs from increased hepatic synthesis, which is stimulated by decreased plasma oncotic pressure. In addition to these clinical symptoms of nephrotic syndrome, there are multiple additional potential complications encountered. Patients with marked proteinuria and hypoalbuminemia have a prothrombotic tendency, and experience increased risk of venous thromboembolism. Moreover, patients with membranous nephropathy as well as those with severe disease (albumin levels less than 2 mg/dL or proteinuria greater than 10 g in 24 h) appear to experience the highest risk of thromboembolic disease. In general, patients with nephrotic syndrome have a 1.7 relative risk increase in developing DVT compared to patients without it [8]. The cause of increased thrombosis is likely multifactorial, including increased fibrinogen levels, enhanced platelet aggregation, and loss of anticoagulants (such as antithrombin III) in the urine. Patients with nephrotic syndrome have increased susceptibility to infection, especially cellulitis and pneumococcal infection. Children and patients with frequent relapsing disease are at the highest risk. The pathophysiology is not completely understood, but urinary loss of IgG may play a role [9]. Finally, nephrotic syndrome can confer a negative protein balance, which can predispose patients to protein malnutrition. Decreased gastrointestinal absorption of protein from severe edema may play a role in this as well.

Etiology and Work Up

Heavy proteinuria and the nephrotic syndrome can occur from both primary kidney injury as well as secondary systemic diseases. In children, minimal change disease remains the most frequent cause of nephrotic syndrome. The two most commonly encountered primary or idiopathic causes of nephrotic syndrome are focal segmental glomerulosclerosis (FSGS) and membranous nephropathy, both of which can affect up to 30% of adults. In fact, in African-American adults, FSGS accounts for up to 50% of cases. Table 1 lists the most commonly encountered primary causes of nephrotic syndrome. Systemic diseases frequently lead to nephrotic syndrome in adults, with diabetes and systemic lupus erythematosus (SLE) the most common causes of secondary nephrotic syndrome (see list below). Accordingly, additional studies are often necessary to further investigate the possibility of a secondary etiology, which include but are not limited to: hemoglobin A1C complement, HIV screening test, hepatitis serologies (to investigate for hepatitis B and C), rapid plasma reagin (RPR) to evaluate for syphilis, serum and urine protein electrophoresis (to screen for multiple myeloma and amyloidosis), and antinuclear antibodies (for SLE evaluation). Although important to evaluate for hydronephrosis and cystic renal diseases, renal imaging will yield little in differentiating between the different causes of nephrotic syndrome, with the exception of enlarged kidney sizes in diabetes and infiltrative disease states. A kidney biopsy is often indicated to help

Table 1 Causes of primary nephrotic syndrome in adults

Idiopathic or primary nephrotic syndrome	Incidence (%)
Minimal change disease	10–15
Focal segmental glomerulosclerosis	20–30
Membranous nephropathy	25–40
Membranoproliferative glomerulonephritis	5
Other forms of glomerulonephritis	10–20

diagnose the type of glomerular disease, identify subtype of disease, as well as to evaluate for activity and chronicity of illness. The results can help clinicians identify who will benefit from treatment. However, not all patients require a kidney biopsy, for example a patient with long standing diabetes with high clinical suspicion for diabetic nephropathy.

Causes of secondary nephrotic syndrome

- **Systemic Diseases**
  - Diabetes mellitus
  - Systemic lupus erythematous
  - Sarcoidosis
  - Rheumatoid arthritis
  - Amyloidosis (can be associated with AA or AL amyloid)
  - Vasculitis (cryoglobulinemia, Henoch-Schönlein purpura, etc.)
  - Celiac disease
  - Scleroderma
- **Infections**
  - Viral (hepatitis B, hepatitis C, HIV, mononucleosis)
  - Bacterial (streptococcal, syphilis, sub-acute bacterial endocarditis, shunt nephritis)
  - Parasitic (malaria, schistosomiasis)
- **Medications**
  - Nonsteroidal anti-inflammatory drugs
  - Gold, heavy metals
  - Lithium
  - Penicillamine
  - Captopril
  - Antibiotics (ampicillin, rifampin, etc.)
  - Bisphosphonates (pamidronate)
  - Anabolic steroids
  - Interferon
- **Neoplastic/malignancies**
  - Leukemia and lymphomas (typically minimal change disease)
  - Solid tumors (membranous)
- **Hereditary diseases**
  - Sickle cell disease
  - Fabry's disease
  - Alport's syndrome
  - Partial lipodystrophy
  - Nail-patella syndrome
  - Familial nephrotic syndrome
- **Others**
  - Pregnancy associated (pre-eclampsia)
  - Serum sickness
  - Obesity
  - Reflux nephropathy
  - Allergies (food, pollen, bee stings)

Minimal Change Disease

Minimal change disease (MCD) accounts for up to 90% of idiopathic nephrotic syndrome in children, and 10–15% in adults. MCD often presents suddenly, and can be associated with medications (nonsteroidal anti-inflammatory drugs) and hematological malignancies (leukemia and lymphomas). Treatment with high dose prednisone usually leads to remission. Because of the high rate of remission with steroids, kidney biopsies are generally not performed in children with new onset nephrotic syndrome until after a trial of prednisone. However, MCD can follow a course of remission and relapses; up to 50% of adults can relapse after 1 year. Alternative agents, including cyclophosphamide and cyclosporine, can be considered in patients with frequent relapses to decrease steroid exposure.

Focal Segmental Glomerulosclerosis

FSGS is the most common cause of nephrotic syndrome in African-Americans and accounts for up to 30% of lesions seen on kidney biopsies. FSGS can be idiopathic as well as seen secondary to HIV, obesity, and sickle cell disease, amongst others. Up to 40% of patients with FSGS have hypertension, hematuria, and decreased glomerular filtration rate upon presentation. Spontaneous remission is uncommon, and untreated patients with nephrotic range proteinuria often progress to ESKD within 5–10 years. Accordingly, patients with nephrotic range proteinuria are typically started on immunosuppressive agents, with prednisone being the most common initial agent. Response to therapy can preserve long-term renal function in FSGS, and glucocorticoids can lead to partial or complete remission of proteinuria in up to 60% of patients. Other immunosuppressive medications used in the treatment of FSGS include cyclosporine and mycophenolate mofetil, specifically in patients who relapse or to attenuate steroid exposure.

Membranous Nephropathy

Membranous nephropathy is the most common cause of idiopathic nephrotic syndrome in adults, occurring in up to 40% of cases in some biopsy series. Membranous nephropathy can be idiopathic or occur secondarily to systemic disease (SLE), medications, malignancies (solid tumors), and infections (hepatitis B and C). Recent studies have demonstrated an association between idiopathic membranous nephropathy with antibodies against phospholipase A2 receptors found on podocytes [10]. Membranous nephropathy is the most common type of nephrotic syndrome associated with prothrombotic events, including DVT and renal vein thrombosis. Spontaneous remission occurs in one third of patients, while one third have stable renal function longitudinally; the remaining third develop progressive renal failure. Because one third of patients do spontaneously remit, immunosuppressive treatment is generally reserved for patients who are at moderate to high risk for progressive renal failure. Factors associated with increased risk for progression include male gender, increased age, a decline in GFR over 3 months, and greater than 8 g of proteinuria. The most common initial immunosuppressive regimen includes 6 months of therapy with cyclophosphamide alternating with glucocorticoids on a monthly basis [11]. Alternatively, cyclosporine can be used as an induction agent, with increased rates of relapse once discontinued. More recently, rituximab can be used, primarily in patients with positive anti phospholipase A2 receptor status [12, 13].

Membranoproliferative Glomerulonephritis

Membranoproliferative glomerulonephritis is a rare type of nephrotic syndrome, accounting for approximately 5% of lesions seen on biopsy registries. There are two major types of MPGN. Type I is immune mediated and often associated with hepatitis C and/or cryoglobulins. Treatment usually centers on targeting the hepatitis virus. Type II MPGN, also called dense deposit disease, is rare and complement mediated.

Treatment

There are few placebo-controlled double-blind studies investigating the impact of immunosuppressive regimens on the different primary types of nephrotic syndrome, with commonly employed agents including glucocorticoids. Nonimmunosuppressive treatment modalities can be implemented for the nephrotic syndrome, regardless of the lesion seen on biopsy. It is important to limit sodium intake, often to less than 3 g/day. Furthermore, diuretics are frequently necessary to facilitate a negative sodium balance. Loop diuretics (furosemide and bumetanide) are first-line agents, and may be required to be administered via the intravenous route if there is a concern for intestinal edema in severe cases. In addition, patients may require a second thiazide-type diuretic (metolazone) in severe cases.

In addition to treating the edema associated with nephrotic syndrome, treatment should also target attenuating proteinuria. In addition to their antihypertensive effects, angiotensin-converting enzyme inhibitors (ACE inhibitors) or angiotensin receptor blockers (ARBs) reduce intraglomerular pressure; this in turn can reduce proteinuria [14]. The hyperlipidemia associated with nephrotic syndrome often resolves with treatment of the nephrotic syndrome. However, statin medications are often implemented to assist in controlling the lipid derangements.

Complications of nephrotic syndrome, specifically hypercoagulable disorders, are managed on an individual basis. Heparin, followed by warfarin, is used once a clot is detected. The use of prophylactic warfarin in patients at high risk remains controversial, but may carry greater benefit in patients with membranous nephropathy. Decision analysis tools such as GNTools have been developed to assist clinicians with risk-benefit analyses for anticoagulation in patients with membranous nephropathy [15].

Tubulointerstitial Diseases of the Kidney

Tubulointerstitial injury of the kidney may occur with any of the primary kidney disorders but also may be the principal manifestation of a diverse array of genetic, toxic, infectious, and metabolic diseases. Features usually include non-nephrotic range proteinuria, hematuria, pyuria, and a variety of tubular disorders such as renal tubular acidosis and nephrogenic diabetes insipidus. Cystic kidney diseases are the most common abnormality that the primary care physician first discovers. Cysts may be single or multiple and may be acquired, developmental, or genetic in origin. Cysts may be benign in nature but also may confer an increased risk of cancer. Table 3 details the different types of cystic kidney disease [16].

Autosomal Dominant Polycystic Kidney Disease (ADPKD)

ADPKD is the most common inherited kidney disease and accounts for 10% of the ESKD population. Genetic mutations occur on either the short arm of chromosome 16 (PKD1) (85% of patients) or on chromosome 4 (PKD2) (15% of patients). Cysts usually arise from the distal tubules and may only affect a fraction of the tubules. These cysts enlarge and crowd out normal nephrons resulting in progressive kidney failure. There is great variability in this process which translates in a variable phenotype for a particular family. The diagnosis of ADPKD is usually confirmed with imaging studies and is age dependent. In patients with a family history and age < 40 years, more than 3 cysts in one or both kidneys establishes the diagnosis. In patients over 60 years, more than 4 cysts in both kidneys are required to establish the diagnosis. Progressive kidney disease is the norm for patients with ADPKD although the occurrence of ESKD is variable. Risk factors for a more rapid progression include

family history, childhood onset, male gender, hypertension, urinary tract infection, kidney stones, black race, and sickle cell disease. Hypertension is very common and is sometimes used as a clinical marker for the disease especially when it occurs at a young age. Drugs that disrupt the renin–angiotensin axis are preferred as initial therapy although multiple drugs may be necessary as CKD progresses. Flank pain is the most common manifestation of the disorder and may be debilitating. Gross hematuria associated with cyst rupture, non-nephrotic range proteinuria, urinary tract infection, and kidney stones occur with increasing frequency. Several extrarenal manifestations of ADPKD often occur. Cysts can occur in other organs besides the kidney with the liver being most commonly involved. These cysts rarely produce organ failure but hemorrhage or infection can occur. Infections in any cyst may be difficult to treat as antibiotic penetration into the cyst fluid may be variable—recommended treatment includes antibiotics capable of penetrating the cyst wall such as trimethoprim-sulfamethoxazole, fluoroquinolones, erythromycin, tetracyclines, or metronidazole. Cyst drainage may be necessary to successfully eradicate the infection. The most devastating complication of ADPKD is rupture of an intracerebral aneurysm. Up to 4% of patients with ADPKD will have this complication, with a potential familial predilection. Patients with a family history of sudden noncardiac death or aneurysm should undergo screening. MRI angiography and preemptive repair may be indicated. Other complications of ADPKD include colonic diverticuli (80%) and cardiac valvular abnormalities (25%). Vasopressin V2 receptor antagonists (tolvaptan), mTor pathway inhibitors (sirolimus/everolimus), somatostatin analogs (octreotide, lantreotide), and statins (pravastatin) have all shown promise in slowing the progression of ADPKD. Large clinical trials are underway testing the benefits of these therapies that will alter the natural course of this devastating genetic disease [17]. Of the aforementioned therapies, tolvaptan has been most clearly demonstrated to slow progression of ADPKD, but careful monitoring of liver function is required [18].

Table 3 Types of cystic kidney disease

Type of cystic kidney disease	Occurrence	Genetics	Radiographic appearance	Progression and complications	Risk of cancer
Simple cysts	Increase with age	Unknown	Solitary, multiple, round, smooth fluid filled	Usually none, no calcifications or hemorrhage	<1%
Complex cysts	Increase with age	Unknown	Solitary, multiple, septa, calcification, enhancement, irregular borders	Usually none, hemorrhage, infection	Increase with greater Bosniak category 5–90%
Acquired cystic disease ESRD	Increase with length of dialysis	Unknown	Similar to simple cysts	Similar to simple cysts unless malignant transformation	5–10%
ADPKD	>1:1,000 live births	PKD1 and PKD2 genes	Enlarged kidneys with numerous cysts	May progress to ESRD, bleeding, infection, kidney stones	Unknown
ARPKD	1:20,000 live births	PKHD1 gene	Enlarged kidneys with numerous, uniform cysts	Progressive loss of kidney function, hepatic fibrosis prominent feature	0
Medullary sponge kidney	Unknown	Unknown	Dilated collecting ducts	Usually none, kidney stones more common	0
Nephronophthisis	1:50,000 live births	Nine genes (ciliopathy)	Corticomedullary cysts with severe atrophy and scarring of cortex, small kidneys	Tubular dysfunction, sodium wasting, DI, RTA, ESRD by age 20	0

Chronic Interstitial Nephritis (CIN)

CIN includes a diverse group of diseases that culminate in prominent interstitial fibrosis and tubular atrophy. A similar disease, reflux nephropathy, affects the lower urinary track initially but invariably gives rise to chronic pyelonephritis and is usually discovered in childhood. Diseases in this group include urinary tract obstruction, prolonged ingestion of non-narcotic analgesics, urate nephropathy, hyperoxaluria, heavy metal poisoning with lead, cadmium or mercury, and infiltrative disorders such as lymphoma or sarcoidosis. Drugs that affect the interstitium include lithium, cisplatin, and calcineurin inhibitors such as cyclosporine. The clinical manifestations of CIN are often overlooked as they are often indolent. CKD occurs but progression is usually measured over a number of years. Renal tubular acidosis, nephrogenic diabetes insipidus, or Fanconi syndrome may be the predominant manifestation. Non-nephrotic range proteinuria with minimal albuminuria is often present. Renal sonography reveals shrunken, hyperechoic kidneys and a kidney biopsy is usually not helpful. There is no specific treatment for CIN except for treatment of the underlying disorder.

Acute Kidney Injury

Acute Kidney Injury (AKI) could be defined as abrupt (within 7 days) and sustained (over 24 h) decrease in glomerular filtration, urine output, or both. AKI is a common condition, which occurs in significant number of hospitalized patients and affects up to 50% of patients admitted to the ICU [19]. Importantly, community based cases comprise at least one third of all AKI cases [20]. Early stages of AKI might be difficult to recognize, as it does not have any specific symptoms. Detection might be particularly difficult in edematous

Table 4 Stages of AKI

| Stage | Assessment | |
	Serum creatinine	Urine output
1	1.5–1.9× baseline or ≥ 0.3 mg/dl above baseline	<0.5 ml/kg/h for 6–12 h
2	2.0–2.9× baseline	<0.5 ml/kg/h for 12 h
3	≥3.0 baseline, ≥ 4.0 mg/dl[a], or initiation of renal replacement therapy	<0.3 ml/kg/h for ≥24 h or anuria for ≥12 h

[a]with an acute increase of at least 0.5 mg/dl

patients with fluid overload as they might have falsely lower levels of serum creatinine (SCr). AKI typically develops in the setting of another illness and is associated with high mortality, especially in patients requiring renal replacement therapy (RRT). Current guidelines define AKI as an elevation in SCr by ≥0.3 mg/dl within 48 h or urine output <0.5 ml/kg/h for 6 h. Stages of AKI are based on the severity of the impairment (Table 4).

The causes of AKI historically have been categorized into three groups: prerenal (caused by abnormal perfusion of the kidney), renal (due to intrinsic kidney damage), and postrenal (caused by obstruction of the urinary tract). AKI is a syndrome, it is important to determine the cause of it whenever possible. However, most of the AKI cases in the hospital are multifactorial in etiology.

Prerenal AKI accounts for 70% of AKI in the outpatient setting [21] and for 21% of AKI in the hospital [22]. Prerenal AKI is often reversible, but can lead to ischemic AKI if it is not timely addressed. Common causes include poor perfusion of the kidney due to hypovolemia, which could be caused by GI, renal or cutaneous losses or by blood loss. Decreased effective volume in patients with congestive heart failure or liver disease may cause prerenal AKI despite the total fluid overload and edematous state. ACE inhibitors and ARBs, nonsteroidal anti-inflammatory medications (NSAIDs) affect renal perfusion and glomerular filtration and can further promote prerenal AKI by impairing renal auto regulation in the setting of hypo volemia. Patients with CKD are especially susceptible to developing AKI [23]. Fractional Excretion of Sodium (FeNa) and Fractional Excretion of Urea (FeUr) are often used to differentiate between prerenal and renal causes of AKI. FeNa could be calculated using formula:

$$\text{FENa (\%)} = \left[\frac{(\text{NaU(mEq/L)}/\text{Na}^+(\text{mEq/L}))/}{(\text{CrU (mg/dL)}/\text{SCr (mg/dL)})} \right] \times 100$$

FeNa <1% is usually consistent with a prerenal cause of AKI, but it should be interpreted carefully. FeNa might be low in AKI patients with contrast nephropathy, rhabdomyolysis, and urinary tract obstruction [24] while diuretic use could be associated with FeNa >1%. In might be useful in evaluation of hepatorenal syndrome. Given limitations of FeNa FeUr is often used to distinguish prerenal and renal AKI. FeUr could be calculated using formula:

$$\text{FEUr (\%)} = \left[\frac{(\text{UrU (mg/dL)}/\text{urea (mg/dL)})/}{(\text{CrU (mg/dL)}/\text{SCr (mg/dL)})} \right] \times 100$$

A low FeUr (<35%) is usually indicative of prerenal AKI, but aging and sepsis may effect it. Urine fractional excretion indices might be helpful in AKI evaluation; a comprehensive clinical assessment should be used to determine volume status and guide therapy.

A blood urea nitrogen to creatinine ratio > 20 is often used to differentiate between prerenal and renal AKI. Recent data does not support its use as a marker for prerenal AKI [25, 26]. Evaluation of urine sediment could offer an additional information and urine microscopy should not be overlooked. Several biomarkers of AKI have been identified (IL-18, NGAL, LFABP and KIM-1, but their clinical applicability is limited [27].

Intrinsic Renal AKI

Intrinsic renal causes could be further subdivided into tubular, glomerular, interstitial, or vascular based on the anatomical structure of the kidney. Acute tubular necrosis (ATN) is the most common cause of AKI in hospitalized patients. It is often a result of ischemia or exposure to nephrotoxins including antibiotics or radiocontrast medications. Muddy brown granular casts could be seen on urine microscopy. ATN often occurs with patients with predisposing conditions, it is usually reversible, but may require RRT. Glomerular causes include different types of glomerulonephritis like acute post infectious nephritis, lupus nephritis and RPGN among other types. In the presence of active urinary sediment showing proteinuria, hematuria or casts a prompt serological assessment is indicated. Rapid recognition and initiation of appropriate immunosuppressive agent is important to reduce the risk of complications and delay the progression of the disease. Interstitial causes included acute interstitial nephritis which could be caused by an allergic reaction to medications. It is often resolved with supportive treatment and withdrawal of the affecting agent. Eosinophiluria and white blood cell casts might be found on urine microscopy in some patients. Clinical symptoms may include maculopapular rash, fever, and arthralgias. Corticosteroids have a role in treatment of acute interstitial nephritis. Vascular causes of AKI comprise occlusion of the renal artery or disease of the abdominal aorta. Microvascular diseases include microangiopathic anemia due to thrombotic thrombocytopenic purpura, hemolytic uremic syndrome, HELLP (*H*emolysis, *E*levated *L*iver enzymes, and *L*ow *p*latelets) and may require use of plasmopheresis for treatment. Atheroembolic disease as a cause of AKI should be suspected in a patient with recent arterial intervention or after vascular surgery.

Contrast Induced AKI (CI-AKI)

CI-AKI is one of the most common types of AKI found in a hospital setting. CI-AKI is often defined as an increase in serum creatinine of 0.5 mg/dL or 25% from baseline. It typically occurs within 48–72 h of exposure to iodinated contrast and often resolves over the following 1–3 weeks. It might be associated with the development of CKD in some cases. Patients with normal kidney function have minimal risk for CI-AKI. Patients with an estimated GFR < 60 mls/min/1.73 m^2, diabetes related CKD, congestive heart failure, vascular disease hadvanced age and hypotension are at increased risk. Critically ill patients are more vulnerable to CI-AKI. Medications altering renal perfusions like diuretics, ACEi, ARBs and NSAIDs should be held in the morning of procedure if possible and not restarted back until 48 h after contrast administration if creatinine is stable. Unenhanced scanning, low or iso-osmolar iodinated contrast medium should be considered for those who are at risk for developing CI-AKI. Intravenous volume expansion with either 0.9% sodium chloride or isotonic sodium bicarbonate is recommended in patients identified as at risk of CI-AKI [28]. Common regimen includes infusion at a rate of 1 ml/kg given for 12 h before and after the contrast. Shorter regimen at a rate of 3 ml/kg per h for 1 h before the contrast administration and 1 ml/kg per h for 6 h after may be used if needed. *N*-Acetylcysteine is commonly used for CI-AKI prevention due to low cost and lack of the harm data, however recent data does not support its benefits [29].

Postrenal AKI

Postrenal AKI accounts for up to 10% of the hospital and 17% of the community AKI cases respectively and results from an obstruction of urine flow at different levels. Both urinary tracts need to be obstructed for AKI to develop unless the patient has a single functioning kidney. Obstruction could be mechanical (prostate hypertrophy, prostate and cervical cancer, retroperitoneal fibrosis) or functional (neurogenic bladder). Papillary necrosis can cause intrarenal obstruction and lead to AKI. Relieving obstruction is the ultimate treatment and should be done promptly to improve the chance of recovery.

AKI Risk Factors

A number of chronic diseases including diabetes mellitus and cardiovascular disease are associated with AKI development. CKD and proteinuria [30] are proven to be risk factors for AKI as well as older age, female gender, volume contraction, solitary kidney, septic shock, obesity, use of the nephrotoxic drugs [31] (see list below), blood product transfusion, and underlying chronic heart, lung, and liver disease [32].

Drugs that contribute to AKI

- Radiocontrast agents
- Aminoglycosides
- Amphotericin
- Nonsteroidal anti-inflammatory drugs
- β-lactam antibiotics (specifically contribute to interstitial nephropathy)
- Sulphonamides
- Aciclovir
- Methotrexate
- Cisplatin
- Ciclosporin
- Tacrolimus
- Angiotensin-converting-enzyme inhibitors
- Angiotensin-receptor blockers

Diagnostic Evaluation

Careful interpretation of clinical history, physical exam findings, and laboratory values is very important (Fig. 1). SCr is affected by a number of different factors including nutrition, muscle mass, steroid use, presence of gastrointestinal bleeding, age, sex, and muscle injury. SCr may not change until glomerular filtration decreases by 50%. Measurement of creatine kinase might be helpful in suspected cases of rhabdomyolysis, while the measurement of inflammatory markers and assays that detect specific antibodies (anti-GBM, ANCA anti-DNA) is helpful to diagnose vasculitis or glomerulonephritis. Haptoglobin, lactic dehydrogenase, bilirubin, and free hemoglobin should be measured if the diagnosis of thrombotic thrombocytopenic purpura is considered. Peripheral smear with the finding of schistocytes may support the diagnosis of microangiopathic hemolysis. Finding monoclonal proteins in serum and/or urine might provide diagnostic clues and point towards multiple myeloma and amyloidosis. In some cases, when clinical history, diagnosis and imaging tests are not sufficient, renal biopsy might be needed to establish the diagnosis. Renal ultrasound should be considered in most patients, specifically in older men. Finding of >50–100 ml on the bladder scan in a patient with AKI should raise suspicion for postrenal causes.

Prevention and Treatment of AKI

Prevention of AKI relies on an earlier recognition of its potential causes, avoidance of possible renal insults whenever possible, and treatment of suspected AKI triggers to minimize damage. Most of the patients with AKI will require comanagement between primary care physicians, hospitalists, nephrologists, and other subspecialists depending on the underlying disease process. Treatment of AKI should include thorough assessment and is mainly supportive. It includes monitoring of volume status, SCr, urine output and management and treatment of underlying cause. Renal doses of medications should be used and nephrotoxic medications should be avoided. Drug monitoring should be used, whenever possible, to guide the therapy, specifically for vancomycin, aminoglycosides, and other medications. When fluid resuscitation is required, isotonic crystalloid solutions are preferred. Small boluses (500 ml over 30 min) can given followed by an assessment of cardiac output. Urine output should be carefully charted and fluids should be discontinued if oliguria persists. In patients with fluid overload and those who present with acute decompensated heart failure and cardiorenal syndrome, loop diuretics either as continuous infusion or intermediate dose boluses could be used with close monitoring of serum electrolytes [33]. Patients who present with severe hyperkalemia or have EKG changes should be treated with intravenous calcium gluconate (10 mL of 10% solution infused over 5 min) to stabilize the cardiac cell membrane. IV insulin (5–10 units with 12.5 or 25 g of dextrose) with or without a β_2-Adrenergic agonist

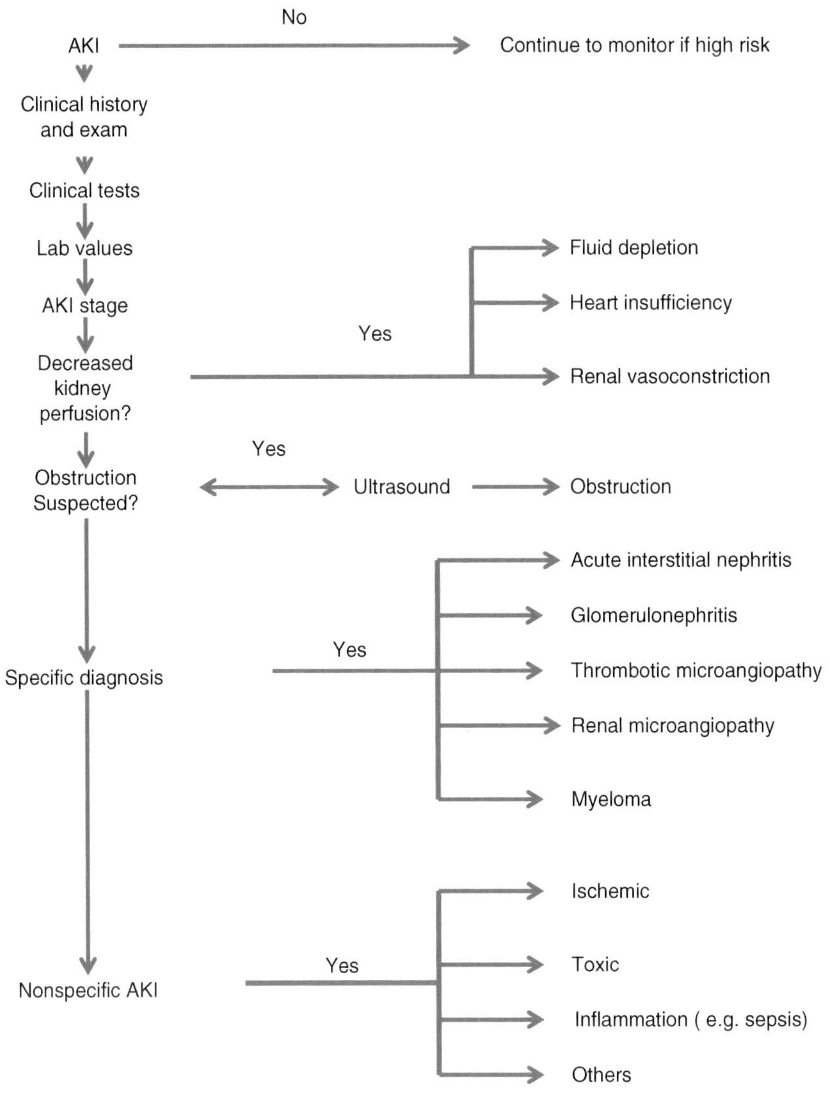

Fig. 1 Evaluation of AKI

could be used to lower potassium by causing intracellular shift. When administered together they work better than either medication alone; rebound occurs in about 1–2 h. Delivery of caloric intake at 20–30 kcal/kg/day in patients with any stage of AKI is recommended [28], enteral nutrition is preferred. After nephrology consult is obtained, consideration might be given to a renal biopsy and disease specific treatment (steroids, plasmapheresis, immunosuppressive therapy) might be initiated. For patients who do not improve with conservative management or exhibit uremic complications like difficult to control hyperkalemia, metabolic acidosis or volume overload, RRT might be required.

Follow Up Care

AKI is an important risk factor for CKD even among patients who recovered completely from this condition. Severity and number of AKI episodes are risks for development of CKD [34]. Patients with history of AKI should be reevaluated in 3 months for AKI resolution, new onset, or worsening of CKD [28].

CKD

CKD is a worldwide problem and is associated with increased mortality, morbidity, and health care costs. Disease affects an estimated 15% or approximately 37 million adults in the United States and it is the 9th leading cause of death. One out of three patients with diabetes and one out of five patients with hypertension might have CKD [35]. CKD is more common in patients aged 65 years or older and seen more frequently in women. Patients with CKD are at significantly increased risk for cardiovascular disease and stroke [36, 37]. Incidence and prevalence of CKD has continued to rise which might be explained by the increasing prevalence of diabetes mellitus and hypertension, the leading risk factors for CKD. The incidence of CKD stage 5 requiring dialysis or transplantation is the US is the highest in the world, but might be on the decline due to improvements in the prevention and treatment of CKD. About 1% of CKD patients are treated with dialysis and/or kidney transplantation, primary care physicians manage most of the nondialysis CKD patients.

CKD Definition and Detection

CKD is defined as abnormality of kidney structure or function with or without an accompanying reduction in Glomerular Filtration Rate (GFR), present for over 3 months, with implications for health.

Markers of kidney damage include presence of albuminuria, urine sediment abnormalities, electrolyte abnormalities due to tubular disorders, abnormalities detected by histology, structural abnormalities found on imaging and history of kidney transplant. Patients with CKD may have decreased estimated GFR (eGFR). eGFR of less than 60 mL per minute per 1.73 m^2 for at least 3 months is indicative of CKD. CKD is classified into five stages on the basis of eGFR. Normal GFR in young adults is around 125 mL/min per 1.73 m^2; eGFR <15 mL/min per 1.73 m ^{2} is defined as kidney failure. Presence of albuminuria even with normal eGFR signifies CKD. Patients with eGFR <45 ml/min per 1.73 m ^{2} experience faster disease progression [38]. Proteinuria affects CKD evolution and influences mortality [39]. Table 6 outlines prognosis of CKD by eGFR and albuminuria categories [39].

It is now recognized that CKD and AKI are closely connected: AKI can lead to CKD, if duration of the abnormal GFR is unknown, the possibility of AKI should be considered and a timely appropriate evaluation should performed to identify reversible causes. CKD is a risk factor for developing AKI, patients with CKD are 10 times more likely to develop AKI than those without CKD [40]. Patients who are older, have diabetes, hypertension, obese, and those with cardiovascular disease are at risk for CKD. CKD is often asymptomatic until advanced stages. It makes screening and early identification with two simple tests: eGFR and urine albumin to creatinine ratio very important. When symptoms are present, they include fatigue, hypertension, edema, shortness of breath, leg cramps, poor appetite, and abnormal urination pattern. Annual CKD screening for patients at risk (patients with diabetes, hypertension, cardiovascular disease) is recommended by several professional organizations [41, 42]. The

Table 6 Prognosis of CKD by eGFR and albuminuria categories

Persistent albuminuria categories				
Stage	GFR ml/min/1.73 m ^{2}	<30 mg/g	30–300 mg/g	>300 mg/g
1	≥90 normal or high	Low risk	Moderate risk	High risk
2	60–89 mildly decreased	Low risk	Moderate risk	High risk
3A	45–59 mildly to moderately decreased	Moderate risk	High risk	Very high risk
3B	30–44 moderately to severely decreased	High risk	Very high risk	Very high risk
4	15–29 severely decreased	Very high risk	Very high risk	Very high risk
5	<15 kidney failure	Very high risk	Very high risk	Very high risk

evidence to support CKD screening in asymptomatic adults without risk factors or family history of CKD is lacking.

Etiology

Although the most common causes of CKD are diabetes and hypertension, which account for over two thirds of all CKD cases, CKD can be caused by many other conditions (Table 7). Diabetic kidney disease develops in 20–40% of diabetic patients and characterized by slowly progressing albuminuria associated with eGFR decline, elevated blood pressure and increased cardiovascular morbidity and mortality. Untreated albuminuria progresses from microalbuminuria (30–300 mg/g creatinine, albuminuria grade A2) to clinical albuminuria ($>$ 300 mg/g creatinine, albuminuria grade A3) over 5–15 years and can reach "nephrotic range." "Nephrotic range "proteinuria is diagnosed when albumin to creatinine ratio is over 2,200 mg/g or protein to creatinine ration is over 3,000 m/g, Nephrotic range proteinuria in the presence of hypoalbuminemia and edema defines nephrotic syndrome. Hypertensive kidney disease might be associated with albuminuria that develops after eGFR decline. Black patients are at much higher risk for developing hypertension induced end stage kidney disease. Urinalysis might be helpful as it can provide diagnostic clues to detection of glomerulonephritis, tubulointerstitial disease, vasculitis, hereditary nephritis, and lupus nephritis.

A thorough investigation is important in assessing CKD and includes determining etiology and type of CKD whenever possible and evaluating for comorbidities. Proteinuria refers to an increased excretion of any urinary proteins, including albumin and other serum proteins (tubular proteins). A normal urinary protein-to-creatinine ratio is less than 200 mg per g; proteinuria is predictor of total mortality and CKD progression and can help determine the type of CKD. Albuminuria is an abnormal excretion of albumin when albumin-to-creatinine ratio exceeds 30 mg per g. Albuminuria on a random nontimed urine should be confirmed with subsequent early morning urine sample. If significant, nonalbumin proteinuria is suspected, assays for detection of Bence Jones proteins should be used. Albuminuria and eGFR should be assessed annually for patients with CKD [39] and small variations in eGFR are common and might not indicate progression. Rapid progression is defined as drop of 5 ml/min/1.73 m^2 per year. At the time of CKD diagnosis all patients should be assessed to identify the risk factors for progression that include: cause of CKD, stage of CKD using eGFR and albuminuria (lower GFR levels and higher degree of albuminuria are associated with CKD progression). Other factors contributing to CKD progression include age, race/ethnicity, elevated blood pressure, hyperglycemia, dyslipidemia, smoking, and exposure to nephrotoxic drugs.

Table 7 Etiology of CKD

Diabetic kidney disease	Diabetes Mellitus Type 2
	Diabetes Mellitus Type 1
Nondiabetic kidney disease	
Vascular diseases	Hypertension, ischemic renal disease
Glomerular diseases	*Primary*: Lupus nephritis, vasculitis, membranous nephropathy, minimal change disease, focal segmental glomerulosclerosis, immunoglobulin A nephropathy
	Secondary: Infections (e.g., hepatitis B and C, human immunodeficiency virus–associated bacterial endocarditis), amyloidosis, heroin use, malignancy (e.g., leukemia, Hodgkin lymphoma, carcinoma)
Cystic diseases	Polycystic kidney disease
Tubulointerstitial disease	Urinary tract infections, nephrolithiasis, obstruction, sarcoidosis, multiple myeloma, drug toxicity (e.g., proton pump inhibitors, lithium, nonsteroidal anti-inflammatory drugs)

Treatment

The goals of CKD treatment is to slow progression of CKD, reduce compilations of decreased eGFR, reduce risk of cardiovascular disease, and improve survival and quality of life. Death is more likely than progression to dialysis in any stage of CKD [42]; an assessment of cardiovascular risk factors including smoking status, and dyslipidemia is very important. Salt intake should be reduced to less than 2 g of sodium a day (less than 5 g of sodium chloride). Patients with CKD should be encouraged to participate in physical activity 30 min, five times a week. Target for Hg A1C in diabetic patients is about 7% or less to prevent or slow down the progression of kidney disease. For patients with comorbidities, reduced life expectancy, and those who are at risk for hypoglycemia HgA1c goals should be loose and increased to closer to 8% [34]. Best HgA1c attainable should be achieved whenever possible. Metformin may be continued in people with diabetic kidney disease and eGFR $\geq$45 ml/min/1.73 m^2. Its use should be reviewed in patients with GFR 30–45 ml/min/1.73 m^2 and it should be stopped when GFR is 30 ml/min/1.73 m^2 or less [39]. The sodium glucose transporter-2 (SGLT2) inhibitors, a new class of diabetic medications, might offer renal protection, slow down eGFR decline and reduce the degree of albuminuria [43].

Therapeutic strategies that have been shown to prevent cardiovascular events in patients with CKD include BP control, statins, and use of angiotensin-converting enzyme inhibitors and angiotensin receptor blockers. The optimal blood pressure goal is the area of controversy. JNC 8 recommends blood pressure goal of less than 140/90 for patients with diabetes and nondiabetic CKD [44]. The American College of Cardiology/ American Heart Association 2017 Hypertension Guidelines set a BP goal of <130/80 mm Hg for patients with CKD [45].

Use of ACE inhibitors and ARBs in CKD patients is associated with delaying CKD progression including in patients with advanced disease stages and, importantly, offers a greater survival. Medications could be stopped temporarily in the setting of AKI and should be restarted when creatinine stabilizes. In patients with cardiovascular disease and CKD, levels of cardiac biomarkers like BNP and troponin could be used for prognostication and cardiovascular risk stratification, but diagnostic utility is unclear. Patients with eGFR of less than 60 mL per minute per 1.73 m^2 require further evaluation to assess for CKD complications. Evaluation for anemia is recommended in women with hemoglobin levels less than 12 g per dL (120 g per L) and in men with levels less than 13.5 g per dL (135 g per L), in addition to nutritional assessment and evaluation for bone disease. Hemoglobin goals should not exceed 11 g per dL (110 g per L) in patients receiving erythropoiesis-stimulating agents due to the risk of major cardiovascular events. Referral to a nephrologist is recommended for patients with CKD stage 4 and for patients who meet other criteria for referral including albuminuria (ACR ratio > 300 mg/g), nephrotic range proteinuria, resistant hypertension, hyperkalemia, hereditary kidney disease and hematuria not secondary to urologic conditions. Doses of medications should be adjusted; decreased eGFR affects pharmacokinetics and pharmacodynamics of many medications, increasing the risk of toxicity. Multispecialty team including nephrologist should manage patients with advanced stages of CKD. Renal replacement therapy when eGFR falls below 10 ml/min/1.73 m^2 might need to be initiated to manage symptoms of kidney failure (serositis), acid-based and electrolyte abnormalities, control volume status, and blood pressure. Preemptive renal transplantation should be considered for patients with eGFR less than 20 ml/min/1.73 m^2 with evidence of progressive and irreversible decline over the preceding 6–12 months. Advanced planning should be offered to all patients with CKD and end of life care discussion should be cared on with those choosing conservative care for CKD.

Renal Cell Carcinoma

Renal-cell carcinomas account for approximately 3% of adult malignancies and for 90–95% of kidney cancers and originate from renal epithelium. Genetic and environmental factors influence disease development. Established risk factors include active and passive smoking, hypertension and obesity. Acquired renal cystic disease, ESKD, duration of dialysis and tuberous sclerosis are all associated with increased risk for developing renal cell carcinoma. Males have higher predominance than females and disease peaks in sixties and seventies. Clear cell carcinomas account for 70–85% of renal cell carcinomas followed by papillary type that accounts for 7–15%: approximately 2–3% of the cases are genetic. Von Hippel-Lindau syndrome (occurring 1 in 36,000 births) is an autosomal dominant cancer disorder and is associated with retinal angiomas, hemangioblastomas of the central nervous system and clear cell type renal cell carcinomas. The gene responsible for that syndrome is located on chromosome 3 (3p25–26) [46]. Patients with this syndrome develop multifocal and often bilateral renal tumors earlier in life; they require monitoring of lesions size. Only about 10% of all patients present with classic triad of symptoms: flank pain, palpable abdominal mass and hematuria and over 50% of the tumors are found on the unrelated imaging studies [47] Some patients might present with nonspecific symptoms like fatigue, weight loss, anemia, and micro or gross hematuria. Hematuria should always be promptly evaluated by computed tomography (CT) to rule out a renal mass and patients older than 35 or with risk factors may require cystoscopy to rule our bladder carcinoma as well. The paraneoplastic syndromes seen in patients with renal cell carcinoma include polycythemia from abnormal erythropoietin production, unexplained fever, hypercalcemia, and Stauffer syndrome: cholestatic jaundice and organomegaly in the absence of liver metastasis. For smaller tumors detected early consideration can be given to nephron sparing surgery, thermal ablation or surveillance as treatment options. Nephrectomy (partial or total) is indicated for larger and central tumors. Radio frequency or cryoablative treatments are alternative approaches, especially in patients with small cortical tumors, hereditary RCC, and multiple bilateral tumors. Prognosis depends on the stage and histological subtype. Approach and type of the surgery depends on the size, location, TNM classification, and other anatomical considerations. About one -third of the patients who undergo surgical treatment for localized disease will have recurrence. Median survival varies from 8.8 to 27 months based on the number of risk factors present.

Transitional Cell Carcinoma

Renal transitional cell carcinoma or renal urothelial carcinoma is a rear type of kidney cancer arising from the transitional (urothelial) cell lining of the urinary tract and accounts for approximately 7% of all kidney tumors. It is the most common cancer of the renal pelvis. Risks factors include smoking, carcinogens exposure, and analgesic use. Most of the patients present with microscopic or macroscopic hematuria. Patients with upper urinary tract urothelial cancer are at risk for the development of bladder urothelial cancer. Men are affected more frequently. Over 90% of patients with superficial and confined disease to the renal pelvis or ureter could be cured. The cure rate drops to 10–15% for those with deeply invasive tumors that are still limited to the renal pelvis or ureter. Patients with cancer spread through the uroepithelial wall or with distant metastases have poor prognosis. The main prognostic factor is the degree of the invasion into or through the uroepithelial wall. Tumor grade is another prognostic factor, stage and grade correlate in over 80% of cases. Surgical treatment (laparoscopic or open) varies from conservative to total excision of the ureter with a bladder cuff, renal pelvis, and kidney in an attempt to offer the best chance for cure. Chemotherapy with cisplatin-based taxanes and/or gemcitabine agents could be used as an adjuvant to a surgical treatment, for those who are not candidates due to advanced disease or poor general condition or for patients with metastatic disease [48]. The role of radiation treatment is not well stated, but might be beneficial to patients with stages T3/T4 cancer [48].

Bladder Cancer

Bladder cancer is the fourth most common cancer in men. The chance men will acquire it during their life is about 1 in 26; for women, the chance is about 1 in 90 [48]. Over 90% of the bladder cancer is transitional (urothelial) cell carcinomas. Squamous cell carcinoma accounts for about 5% of bladder cancers in US and less than 2% are adenocarcinomas. On initial presentation 55–60% of patients have low grade non-invasive disease that can be treated conservatively and 4% present with distant metastasis. The incidence of bladder cancer increases with age peaking between 50 and 70 years, average age at the time of the diagnosis is 73 years of age. Risk factors for bladder cancer include smoking, environmental and chemical exposures, chronic irritation and infections, and genetic and molecular abnormalities. Patients treated with long-term cyclophosphamide are also at risk. The main symptom is gross painless hematuria; other symptoms like increased frequency, urgency and feeling irritation with voiding should raise a concern for bladder cancer. Evaluation includes urine cytology, cystoscopy, and imaging studies [49]. Several urine tumor markers are commercially available, they have high false-positive and false-negative rates and their role in detection and surveillance of the bladder cancer is controversial [50]. The diagnosis and stage is established by transurethral resection with several options available for urinary diversion. Because of the high recurrence rate regular surveillance is critical in management of bladder cancer. After transurethral resection of the tumor, patients need cystoscopy and voided urine cytology every 3 months for 2 years, then 6 months for 2 years, and then once yearly, indefinitely [49]. Imaging to the upper urinary tract every 12–24 months is also recommended to monitor for cancer occurrence. Intravesicular treatment with the BCG and interferon alfa, mitomycin, doxorubicin, thiotepa or gemcitabine could be used to reduce the recurrence.

Wilms' Tumor

Wilms' tumor or nephroblastoma amounts for about 7% of all cancers in children, and it is the most common renal neoplasm in pediatric patients. Boys and girls are evenly affected by this disease. 10% of the children with this disease have other congenital abnormalities. Wilms'-tumor is usually unilateral, but 5% of the patients develop lesions in the second kidney or have bilateral disease. The mean age for the genetic type is 2 years of age and for sporadic cases is 3 years of age. Some patients may present with abdominal pain and hematuria, but most commonly, patients present with abdominal mass found by caregivers or pediatricians. About one fourth of the patients have hypertension due to an excessive renal secretion of renin secondary to renal ischemia produced by the mechanical effect of the tumor. CT or MRI of the abdomen is used for diagnosis and staging. Wilms' tumor metastasizes to the abdominal lymph nodes, lungs, and liver. Wilms' tumor has a favorable prognosis. It is a curable disease and nearly 90% of the patients with Wilms' tumor have over 5 years survival rate. Prognosis depends on a number of factors including tumor size, stage of the disease, histopathologic type, and on presence of biological markers of poor prognosis including mutations of *WT1*, 1q gain, alterations at 17p, LOH at 4p and 14q, *MYCN* amplification, and LOH at 11q. Overall, patients with anaplastic Wilms tumor have a worse prognosis. All patients with this tumor should be considered for entry into clinical trials.

References

1. Van De Voorde RG 3rd. Acute poststreptococcal glomerulonephritis: the most common acute glomerulonephritis. Pediatr Rev. 2015;36:3–13.
2. Brodsky SV, Nadasdy T. Acute Poststreptococcal glomerulonephritis. Bacterial infections and the kidney. Cham: Springer International AG; 2017. p. 1–36.
3. Wyatt RJ, Julian BA. IgA nephropathy. N Engl J Med. 2013;368:2402–14.
4. Ortega LM, Schultz DR, Lenz O, Pardo V, Contreras GN. Review: lupus nephritis: pathologic

features, epidemiology and a guide to therapeutic decisions. Lupus. 2010;19:557–74.

5. Hellmark T, Segelmark M. Diagnosis and classification of Goodpasture's disease (anti-GBM). J Autoimmun. 2014;48–49:108–12.

6. Falk RS, Jennette CJ. ANCA disease; where is this field heading? J Am Soc Nephrol. 2010;21:745–52.

7. Rodríguez-Iturbe B, Herrera-Acosta J, Johnson RJ. Interstitial inflammation, sodium retention, and the pathogenesis of nephrotic edema: a unifying hypothesis. Kidney Int. 2002;62(4):1379–84.

8. Mahmoodi BK, ten Kate MK, Waanders F, Veeger NJ, Brouwer JL, Vogt L, Navis G, van der Meer J. High absolute risks and predictors of venous and arterial thromboembolic events in patients with nephrotic syndrome: results from a large retrospective cohort study. Circulation. 2008;117(2):224–30.

9. Hull RP, Goldsmith DJA. Nephrotic syndrome in adults. BMJ. 2008;336(7654):1185–9.

10. Beck LH Jr, Bonegio RG, Lambeau G, Beck DM, Powell DW, Cummins TD, Klein JB, Salant DJ. M-type phospholipase A2 receptor as target antigen in idiopathic membranous nephropathy. N Engl J Med. 2009;361(1):11–21.

11. Ponticelli C, Passerini P. Treatment of the nephrotic syndrome associated with primary glomerulonephritis. Kidney Int. 1994;46:595–604.

12. Beck LH Jr, Fervenza FC, Beck DM, Bonegio RG, Malik FA, Erickson SB, Cosio FG, Cattran DC, Salant DJ. Rituximab-induced depletion of anti-PLA2R autoantibodies predicts response in membranous nephropathy. J Am Soc Nephrol. 2011;22(8):1543–50.

13. Ruggenenti P, Cravedi P, Chianca A, Perna A, Ruggiero B, Gaspari F, Rambaldi A, Marasà M, Remuzzi G. Rituximab in idiopathic membranous nephropathy. J Am Soc Nephrol. 2012;23(8):1416–25.

14. Maschio G, Alberti D, Janin G, Locatelli F, Mann JF, Motolese M, Ponticelli C, Ritz E, Zucchelli P. Effect of the angiotensin-converting-enzyme inhibitor benazepril on the progression of chronic renal insufficiency. The angiotensin-converting-enzyme inhibition in progressive renal insufficiency study group. N Engl J Med. 1996;334:939–45.

15. Lee T, Biddle AK, Lionaki S, Derebail VK, Barbour SJ, Tannous S, Hladunewich MA, Hu Y, Poulton CJ, Mahoney SL, Jennette JC, Hogan SL, Falk RJ, Cattran DC, Reich HN, Nachman PH. Personalized prophylactic anticoagulation decision analysis in patients with membranous nephropathy. Kidney Int. 2014;85(6):1412–20.

16. Schmitz PG. Renal: an integrated approach to disease. New York: McGraw Hill-Lange; 2012.

17. Mahnensmith RL. Novel treatments of autosomal dominant polycystic kidney disease. Clin J Am Soc Nephrol. 2014;9:831–6.

18. Torres VE, Chapman AB, Devuyst O, Gansevoort RT, Grantham JJ, Higashihara E, Perrone RD, Krasa HB, Ouyang J, Czerwiec FS. Tolvaptan in patients with autosomal dominant polycystic kidney disease. N Engl J Med. 2012;367:2407–18.

19. Case J, Khan S, Khalid R, Khan A. Epidemiology of acute kidney injury in the intensive care unit. Crit Care Res Pract. 2013;2013:479730. https://doi.org/10.1155/2013/479730.. Epub 2013 Mar 21

20. Hackworth LA, Wen X, Clermont G, et al. Hospital versus community acquired acute kidney injury in the critically ill: differences in epidemiology (abstr). J Am Soc Nephrol. 2009;20:115A.

21. Kaufman J, Dhakal M, Patel B, Hamburger R. Community-acquired acute renal failure. Am J Kidney Dis. 1991;17(2):191–8.

22. Liaño F, Pascual J, The Madrid Acute Renal Failure Study Group. Epidemiology of acute renal failure: a prospective, multicenter, community-based study. Kidney Int. 1996;50:811–8. https://doi.org/10.1038/ki.1996.380.

23. Christensen PK, Hansen HP, Parving HH. Impaired autoregulation of GFR in hypertensive non-insulin dependent diabetic patients. Kidney Int. 1997;52 (5):1369–74.

24. Nguyen MT, Maynard SE, Kimmel PL. Misapplications of commonly used kidney equations: renal physiology in practice. Clin J Am Soc Nephrol. 2009;4:528–34. https://doi.org/10.2215/CJN.05731108.

25. Uchino S, Bellomo R, Goldsmith D. The meaning of the blood urea nitrogen/creatinine ratio in acute kidney injury. Clin Kidney J. 2012;5:187–91.

26. Manoeuvrier G, Bach-Ngohou K, Batard E, et al. Diagnostic performance of serum blood urea nitrogen to creatinine ratio for distinguishing prerenal from intrinsic acute kidney injury in the emergency department. BMC Nephrol. 2017;18:173. https://doi.org/10.1186/s12882-017-0591-9.

27. Parikh CR, Mansour SG. Perspective on clinical application of biomarkers in AKI. JASN. 2017;28(6):1677–85. https://doi.org/10.1681/ASN.2016101127.

28. Kidney Disease: Improving Global Outcomes (KDIGO) Acute Kidney Injury Work Group. KDIGO clinical practice guideline for acute kidney injury. Kidney Int. 2012;2:1–138.

29. Weisbord SD, Gallagher M, Jneid H, Garcia S, Cass A, Thwin SS, Conner TA, Chertow GM, Bhatt DL, Shunk K, Parikh CR, McFalls EO, Brophy M, Ferguson R, Wu H, Androsenko M, Myles J, Kaufman J, Palevsky PM, PRESERVE Trial Group. Outcomes after angiography with sodium bicarbonate and acetylcysteine. N Engl J Med. 2018;378(7):603–14.

30. Hsu RK, Hsu CY. Proteinuria and reduced glomerular filtration rate as risk factors for acute kidney injury. Curr Opin Nephrol Hypertens. 2011;20:211–7.

31. Bellomo R, Kellum JA, Ronco C. Acute kidney injury. Lancet. 2012;380:756–66. https://doi.org/10.1016/S0140-6736(11)61454-2).

32. Cartin-Ceba R, Kashiouris M, Plataki M, Kor DJ, Gajic O, Casey ET. Factors for development of acute kidney injury in critically ill patients: a systematic review and meta-analysis of observational studies. Crit Care Res Pract. 2012;2012:691013, 15 Risk

33. Murray PT, Liu KD (co-editors), Goldfarb S (editor-in-chief), Townsend RR (deputy editor). Acute kidney injury and critical care nephrology. Nephrol Self-Assessment Program 2013;2(2):106–111.

34. Thakar CV, Christianson A, Himmelfarb J, Leonard AC. Acute kidney injury episodes and chronic kidney disease risk in diabetes mellitus. Clin J Am Soc Nephrol. 2011;6:2567–72.

35. Centers for Disease Control and Prevention. Chronic Kidney Disease Surveillance System website. https://nccd.cdc.gov/CKD. Accessed 19 April, 2020.

36. Keith DS, Nicols GA, Gullion CM, Brown JB, Smith DH. Longitudinal follow-up and outcomes among a population with chronic kidney disease in a large managed care organization. Arch Intern Med. 2004;164(6):659–63.

37. Abramson JL, Jurkovitz CT, Vaccarino V, Weintraub WS, McClellan W. Chronic kidney disease, anemia and incident of stroke in a middle-aged, community-based population: the ARIC study. Kidney Int. 2003;64(2):610–5.

38. O'Hare AM, Choi AI, Bertenthal D, et al. Age affects outcomes in chronic kidney disease. J Am Soc Nephrol. 2007;18:2758–65.

39. Kidney Disease: Improving Global Outcomes (KDIGO) CKD Work Group. KDIGO 2012 clinical practice guideline for the evaluation and management of chronic kidney disease. Kidney Int. 2013;3:1–150.

40. Chawla LS, Eggers PW, Star RA, Kimmel PL. Acute kidney injury and chronic kidney disease as interconnected syndromes. N Engl J Med. 2014;371:58.

41. American Diabetes Association. Standards of medical care in diabetes-2014. Diabetes Care. 2014;37(Supplement 1):S14–80.

42. National Kidney Foundation. K/DOQI clinical practice guiudelines for chronic kidney disease: evaluation, classification and stratification. Am J Kidney Dis. 2002;39(2 suppl 1):S1–266.

43. de Boer IH, Kahn SE. SGLT2 inhibitors—sweet success for diabetic kidney disease? JASN. 2017;28 (1):7–10.

44. Paul AJ, Suzanne O, Barry LC, William CC, Cheryl D-H, Joel H, Daniel TL, Michael LL, Thomas DM, Olugbenga O, Sidney CS, Laura PS, Sandra JT, Raymond RT, Jackson TW, Andrew SN, Eduardo O. Evidence-based guideline for the management of high blood pressure in adults report from the panel members apointed to the eighth joint national committee (JNC 8). JAMA. 2014;311 (5):507–20.

45. Whelton PK, Carey RM, Aronow WS, et al. 2017 ACC/AHA/AAPA/ABC/ACPM/AGS/APhA/ASH/ASPC/NMA/PCNA guideline for the prevention, detection, evaluation, and management of high blood pressure in adults: executive summary: a report of the American College of Cardiology/American Heart Association task force on clinical practice guidelines. J Am Coll Cardiol. 2018;71:2199–269.

46. Latif F, Tory K, Gnarra J, et al. Identification of the von Hippel-Lindau disease tumor suppressor gene. Science. 1993;260:1317–20.

47. Cohen HT, McGovern FJ. Renal-cell carcinoma. N Engl J Med. 2005;353:2477–90. https://doi.org/10.1056/NEJMra043172.

48. Chen B, Zeng Z-C, Wang G-M, Zhang L, Lin Z-M, Sun L-A, Zhu T-Y, Wu L-L, Zhang J-Y, Ji Y. Radiotherapy may improve overall survival of patients with T3/T4 transitional cell carcinoma of the renal pelvis or ureter and delay bladder tumour relapse. BMC Cancer. 2011;11:297. https://doi.org/10.1186/1471-2407-11-297.

49. Kaufman DS, Shipley WU, Feldman AS. Bladder cancer. Lancet. 2009;374:239–49.

50. Miyake M, Goodison S, Rizwani W, Ross S, Bart Grossman H, Rosser CJ. Urinary BTA: indicator of bladder cancer or of hematuria. World J Urol. 2012;30(6):869–73.

Karl T. Rew

Contents

Lower Urinary Tract Symptoms

Lower urinary tract symptoms (LUTS) encompasses a range of bladder storage and voiding symptoms that can include urinary frequency, urgency, nocturia, weak stream, hesitancy, intermittency (starting and stopping), and a sense of incomplete emptying. Dysuria, pain, or discomfort in the bladder and genital areas, hematuria, and urinary incontinence are other symptoms that can be associated with the infectious, inflammatory, and neoplastic prostate conditions that cause LUTS. Many men experience these types of urinary symptoms. A study of 30,000 patients over age 40 in the USA, UK, and Sweden showed that 72.3% of the men had LUTS at least "sometimes," and 47.9% had LUTS at least "often" [1].

Three of the most important potential causes of LUTS in men are prostatic hyperplasia, prostatitis, and prostate cancer, but other causes also need to be considered. For example, medical problems that increase urine volume may present with LUTS, such as poorly controlled diabetes mellitus, heart failure, or use of diuretic medicines. Some medications, particularly those with anticholinergic effects, can lead to urinary retention, which may cause or exacerbate LUTS. Infectious causes of LUTS include urinary tract infections, sexually transmitted infections, and other problems such as epididymitis. Kidney and bladder stones can cause LUTS, as can other serious problems that may present with microscopic or gross hematuria, such as bladder cancer and kidney cancer. Men with pelvic floor muscle dysfunction may have LUTS from overactive bladder or they may experience urinary incontinence.

K. T. Rew (✉)
Departments of Family Medicine and Urology, University of Michigan Medical School, Ann Arbor, MI, USA
e-mail: karlr@med.umich.edu

© Springer Nature Switzerland AG 2022
P. M. Paulman et al. (eds.), *Family Medicine*,
https://doi.org/10.1007/978-3-030-54441-6_185

International Prostate Symptom Score (I-PSS)

Patient Name: _____ Date of birth: _____ Date completed _____

In the past month:	Not at all	Less than 1 in 5 times	Less than half the time	About half the time	More than half the time	Almost always	Your score
1. Incomplete emptying How often have you had the sensation of not emptying your bladder?	0	1	2	3	4	5	
2. Frequency How often have you had to urinate less than every two hours?	0	1	2	3	4	5	
3. Intermittency How often have you found you stopped and started again several times when you urinated?	0	1	2	3	4	5	
4. Urgency How often have you found it difficult to postpone urination?	0	1	2	3	4	5	
5. Weak stream How often have you had a weak urinary stream?	0	1	2	3	4	5	
6. Straining How often have you had to strain to start urination?	0	1	2	3	4	5	
	None	**1 Time**	**2 Times**	**3 Times**	**4 Times**	**5 Times**	
7. Nocturia How many times did you typically get up at night to urinate?	0	1	2	3	4	5	
Total I-PSS score							

Score   1–7: *Mild*   8–19: *Moderate*   20–35: *Severe*

Quality of life due to urinary symptoms	Delighted	Pleased	Mostly satisfied	Mixed	Mostly dissatisfied	Unhappy	Terrible
If you were to spend the rest of your life with your urinary condition just the way it is now, how would you feel about that?	0	1	2	3	4	5	6

Fig. 1 International Prostate Symptom Score (IPSS). Found at: https://musculoskeletalkey.com/benign-prostatic-hyperplasia/. (From Kellerman R, Rakel R. Conn's current therapy 2020, Saunders 2020. International Prostate Symptom Score (IPSS) questionnaire, available from the urological Sciences Research Foundation at www.usrf.org/questionnaires/UA_SymptomScore.html)

The severity of LUTS can be quantified using a self-administered patient questionnaire called the International Prostate Symptom Score (IPSS) (Fig. 1). To complete it, the patient ranks each of 7 symptoms on a 1–5 scale [2], with an additional question to assess the impact on quality of life. This questionnaire has been well studied in men. Scores from 0 to 7 indicate mild symptoms, 8 to 19 indicate moderate symptoms, and 20 to 35 indicate severe symptoms. Printable versions of the IPSS questionnaire can readily be found online. The IPSS does not directly assess dysuria, pain, hematuria, or incontinence, so clinicians will want to also ask about these symptoms.

The initial approach to a male patient with LUTS is to obtain a thorough history and quantify the symptoms and their impact using the IPSS. Ask about dysuria, fever, chills, penile discharge, suprapubic or genital pain, gross hematuria, urinary incontinence, and any risk factors for sexually transmitted infections. Assess tobacco use history, because smoking increases the risk of bladder and kidney cancers. Ask about other medical problems, such as diabetes or kidney stones. Review the patient's current medications and consider if they might affect urination. Ask if there is any family history of urinary problems, such as kidney stones or prostate cancer.

The approach to the physical exam for patients with LUTS is guided by the history. Palpate the abdomen for masses or tenderness, and percuss the kidneys to check for costovertebral angle tenderness that may indicate pyelonephritis or kidney stones. Palpate the scrotum to assess for epididymitis, orchitis, and testicular masses. Examine the penis for balanitis, skin lesions such as herpes simplex, and anatomic abnormalities like hypospadias that can increase risk of urinary tract infection. Look for urethral discharge that might indicate urethritis. Digital rectal exam of the prostate is helpful to evaluate for evidence of prostatic hyperplasia, prostatitis, and prostate cancer.

The initial laboratory and diagnostic evaluation for a male with LUTS is guided by the history and physical examination. If a sexually transmitted infection is possible, the first step is to collect an initial first-catch urine sample (without cleansing the tip of the penis) to send for gonorrhea and Chlamydia testing. For all patients with LUTS, also collect a mid-stream clean-catch urine sample and do a urinalysis (UA). If the UA appears to show hematuria, also do a urine microscopic evaluation to confirm this (at least three to five RBC/HPF is considered positive). When a urinary tract infection is suspected, send the clean-catch urine sample for culture.

After the patient has urinated, measure the bladder post-void residual volume (PVR) with ultrasound to evaluate for urinary retention. Ultrasound measurement of PVR is more reliable than physical examination and less invasive than catheterization, and it can easily be done using a dedicated portable bladder-scan machine. With proper documentation, this is a billable procedure under CPT 51798. Normal PVR volumes vary, but about 60% of men will completely empty their bladders (PVR ≤ 10 mL) [3]. A PVR over 180 mL has been associated with an increased risk of bacteriuria. Elevated PVR volume can be due to bladder outlet obstruction, bladder detrusor dysfunction, or both. Some specialized tests that are typically done by urologists and can be useful in diagnosing patients with LUTS include measuring urine flow rate and testing bladder function with urodynamic studies.

Blood tests can be useful for some men with LUTS. Prostate specific antigen (PSA) results can help determine if the patient needs further evaluation for prostate cancer. Check PSA for symptomatic men age ≥ 50 years, or men age ≥ 40 years who are at increased risk of prostate cancer due to their family history or African-American ethnicity. Also check PSA for all men with a palpable prostate nodule. Be aware that the PSA will almost always be elevated in a man with an acute febrile urinary tract infection, and it will typically remain elevated for several months after the infection resolves, so the result must be interpreted in clinical context [4]. It is also reasonable to evaluate men with LUTS for diabetes, using A1c or fasting glucose, and to assess their renal function with a metabolic panel.

Management of LUTS depends on the cause. Approaches to prostatic hyperplasia and prostatitis are detailed below, and prostate cancer is addressed in a separate chapter. The initial evaluation and treatment of most causes of LUTS is generally done by the patient's family physician. Consult a urologist when the diagnosis is unclear, the patient is not improving, or if a procedure such as cystoscopy or prostate biopsy may be indicated.

Prostatic Hyperplasia

The prostate gets bigger as a man ages. This growth process is called benign prostatic hyperplasia (BPH). ("Hyperplasia" means that the number of prostate cells is increasing, as opposed to the older term "hypertrophy" which implied that the cells were just getting bigger.) Autopsy studies show that BPH is present in about 20% of men in their 40s, 40% of men in their 50s, 70% of men in their 60s, and 80–90% of men age 70 or older [5].

Although a prostate that is over 30 mL in volume is often considered to be "enlarged," prostate size does not correlate well with symptoms [6]. When prostatic enlargement is associated with symptoms, the most common reason is that the prostate has caused some degree of bladder outlet obstruction. Hyperplasia of the transitional zone of the prostate can press on the urethra at the bladder outlet, and the resulting obstruction can cause a slow urinary stream, hesitancy, intermittency, and incomplete emptying. Men with bladder outlet obstruction are at increased risk of acute and chronic urinary retention, as well as urinary tract infections and bladder stones. If ongoing bladder outlet obstruction causes the bladder smooth muscle to become overactive, symptoms can include urinary urgency, frequency, and nocturia. However, men with slowly progressive obstructive disease may be asymptomatic. Longstanding bladder outlet obstruction can lead to bladder distention, urinary incontinence, hydronephrosis, hypertension, and chronic kidney disease.

Additionally, BPH can cause gross or microscopic hematuria, but other causes of blood in the urine need to be ruled out. An evaluation of an adult with hematuria should include imaging of the kidneys and upper urinary tracts, usually using CT urogram (performed with and without contrast), to assess for both renal cell carcinoma and kidney stones, plus a cystoscopy to look for bladder cancer or bladder stones.

The causes of BPH, which occurs mostly after age 40, are not fully understood, but exposure to androgens is a major factor. Testosterone stimulates prostate growth, and testosterone is itself converted by the enzyme 5-alpha-reductase into dihydrotestosterone, which is another androgen five to ten times more active than testosterone in stimulating prostate growth. Other factors also appear to stimulate BPH, such as the inflammation associated with problems such as obesity, diabetes, and metabolic syndrome.

The approach to a patient with suspected BPH starts with history gathering and administration of the IPSS questionnaire (Fig. 1). The severity of symptoms and their effects on quality of life are key factors when choosing treatment options. Ask about the time frame over which symptoms occurred. BPH symptoms tend to progress gradually over years. Key elements of the physical exam include the abdominal exam, genital exam, and a digital rectal exam of the prostate. An enlarged prostate that is symmetric and smooth supports a diagnosis of BPH. Urinalysis and measurement of bladder post-void residual volume are helpful tests. Check PSA whenever prostatic hyperplasia is suspected. Although BPH is not a risk factor for prostate cancer, BPH and prostate cancer occur in the same patient population. When the PSA is elevated above the normal range for the patient's age, urology consultation is indicated, and prostate biopsy may be needed.

Lifestyle changes are a reasonable initial approach to managing BPH, and they may be sufficient for some men with mild BPH symptoms. Recommend avoidance of bladder irritants such as caffeine, weight loss as needed to maintain a body mass index (BMI) below 25 kg/m^2, and regular exercise.

Consider prescribing medicine to treat BPH when symptoms have become bothersome, when urinary retention is present, or if the patient has had other complications of BPH, such as a urinary tract infection. Initial medication treatment is usually with an alpha blocker, such as tamsulosin (Flomax) 0.4 mg daily, alfuzosin (Uroxatral) 10 mg daily, or silodosin (Rapaflo) 8 mg daily. Older alpha blockers such as terazosin (Hytrin) or doxazosin (Cardura) can be used, but they are more likely to cause orthostatic hypotension, so the dose should be titrated up slowly. Symptom relief is often noted within the first few days of treatment with an alpha blocker. The most common side effect of alpha blockers is hypotension. Some men may note retrograde ejaculations, also called dry ejaculations.

A second category of medicines useful for treating moderate to severe symptomatic BPH in men with prostates larger than 40 mL size is the 5-alpha reductase inhibitors, which inhibit the conversion of testosterone to dihydrotestosterone. Typical dosing for BPH is finasteride (Proscar) 5 mg daily or dutasteride (Avodart) 0.5 mg daily. These medicines work slowly to decrease prostate size, with the resulting effect of also artificially lowering PSA by about 50% after 6–12 months of treatment [7]. This decrease in PSA can obscure PSA changes due to prostate cancer, so be sure to obtain a baseline PSA before prescribing a 5-alpha reductase inhibitor, and continue to monitor PSA at least annually for patients taking these medicines. Adverse effects in some men may include decreased libido or erectile dysfunction. Gynecomastia also can occur.

The US Food and Drug Administration (FDA) has also approved the use of tadalafil (Cialis), a phosphodiesterase type 5 inhibitor, for treating symptomatic BPH. For men with BPH, tadalafil dosing is 5 mg daily. Tadalafil is a long-acting medication that is also used for erectile dysfunction. When prescribed for erectile dysfunction, typical tadalafil dosing is 10–20 mg by mouth up to once daily as needed, prior to sexual activity. However, even at the lower 5 mg daily dose used for BPH, tadalafil may also be beneficial for erectile dysfunction. Headache and myalgias are the most common adverse effects. Nitrates, such as nitroglycerin or isosorbide dinitrate (Dilatrate-SR, Isordil), are strictly contraindicated in patients taking tadalafil, due to the risk of a drug-drug interaction causing severe hypotension, syncope, and myocardial infarction.

Combination treatment of BPH with both an alpha blocker and a 5-alpha reductase inhibitor can be more effective than either treatment alone. Tadalafil also can be used together with other BPH medications. However, the combination of tadalafil plus an alpha blocker increases the risk of hypotension. Phytotherapy is commonly tried by men with BPH, but no plant extract has been shown to reduce prostate size, improve bladder outlet obstruction, or slow disease progression [7].

Some men who have an overactive bladder due to BPH and obtain only partial symptom relief with the treatments listed above may benefit from the addition of an antimuscarinic medication. Examples include oxybutynin (Ditropan XL), solifenacin (Vesicare), tolterodine (Detrol), and trospium (Sanctura). However, this category of medications can cause urinary retention in men with BPH. They should therefore be used with caution, while closely monitoring symptoms and regularly measuring bladder post-void residual volume. Another medication used for overactive bladder is the beta-3 agonist mirabegron (Myrbetriq).

When a patient with suspected BPH is not improving with pharmacotherapy, consultation with a urologist is recommended. A variety of procedural treatments for BPH can be considered. Prostate size and other factors need to be taken into account. Holmium laser enucleation of the prostate (HoLEP) can be used for prostates of all sizes, even for very large prostates (>100 mL size), so it is gradually replacing the older standard treatment, transurethral resection of the prostate (TURP) [8]. Another advantage of laser technique such as HoLEP and photoselective vaporization of the prostate (PVP) is that they often can be used even in patients at increased risk of bleeding [9].

Prostatitis

Prostatitis is inflammation of the prostate, and it has three main clinical types: acute bacterial prostatitis, chronic bacterial prostatitis, and urologic chronic pelvic pain syndrome (also known as chronic nonbacterial prostatitis). Many patients (and clinicians) think of prostatitis as a prostate infection, but actually less than 10% of prostatitis is due to acute or chronic bacterial infection. Most cases of prostatitis are nonbacterial. A fourth (also uncommon) category is asymptomatic prostatitis, diagnosed when histologic evidence of inflammation is found on prostate biopsy or prostatectomy. Symptomatic prostatitis is common, occurring in 35–50% of men at some time in their lives. A 2015 population study of 10,617 men showed 8.2% had prostatitis symptoms [10].

Acute Bacterial Prostatitis

Acute bacterial prostatitis is essentially an acute bacterial urinary tract infection (UTI) that affects the prostate. It can occur in males of any age but is most typical in adult men, with an increased frequency in men age ≥65. Less than 1% of cases of prostatitis are acute bacterial prostatitis [11]. Most occur after a bladder catheterization, transrectal prostate biopsy, or other urinary tract instrumentation. Other factors that increase the risk for bacterial prostatitis include diabetes and the presence of BPH with urine retention.

Typical symptoms of acute bacterial prostatitis are fever, dysuria, urinary urgency and frequency, slow urinary stream, a sense of incomplete bladder emptying, hematuria, chills, pain in the suprapubic or groin areas (which may radiate to the testes or penis), nausea, and vomiting. Physical exam findings commonly include fever and an enlarged and tender boggy prostate. Do not perform an aggressive prostate examination or prostate massage; it can trigger acute clinical decompensation. The differential diagnosis includes sexually transmitted infections and pyelonephritis. Be sure to assess men with fever and dysuria for kidney tenderness; if they do not have pyelonephritis, 90% of these men will have bacterial prostatitis [12].

Urinalysis usually shows leukocyte esterase, and depending on the bacterial cause, may be nitrite positive. (*E. coli* and other members of the Enterobacteriaceae family are the bacteria most likely to be able to convert urinary nitrate to nitrite.) Urine microscopic evaluation may show white blood cells, bacteria, and/or red blood cells. Send a urine culture before starting antibiotics. Remember to also test for sexually transmitted infections when indicated by history or physical findings. The most common bacterial causes of acute prostatitis are uropathogenic strains of *E. coli* (causing 65–80% of cases), Klebsiella and other Enterobacteriaceae, Pseudomonas, and Enterococci. Acute prostatitis can be caused by *Staphylococcus saprophyticus*; this usually occurs in older men. Avoid checking PSA in men who have bacterial prostatitis; the PSA will usually be elevated and remain so for several months, but this elevation just reflects the presence of prostate inflammation and is not helpful in the acute setting. Measure bladder PVR volume with ultrasound; acute urinary retention may be present.

Other imaging is usually not needed for men with an initial episode of acute prostatitis that responds to treatment.

Treat bacterial prostatitis with an antibiotic that penetrates the prostate, such as ciprofloxacin (Cipro) 500 mg twice daily, levofloxacin (Levaquin) 750 mg once daily, or trimethoprim/sulfamethoxazole (Bactrim) DS twice daily. Nitrofurantoin (Macrobid) does not penetrate the prostate and should not be used. Treatment duration for acute bacterial prostatitis is usually at least 14 days, although some experts recommend treating for 4–6 weeks [13]. Patients with urinary retention may require catheterization. Adjust the antibiotic choice based on urine culture results. Some patients will be acutely ill and need inpatient management and parenteral antibiotics. Potential complications of acute prostatitis include urosepsis and prostate abscess. Sepsis is more likely in men who are elderly, immunocompromised, or have diabetes or urolithiasis.

Chronic Bacterial Prostatitis

Some men will develop chronic bacterial prostatitis, which is characterized by repeated episodes of UTI symptoms associated with positive urine cultures, usually growing the same bacterial strain each time. Chronic bacterial prostatitis is uncommon, occurring in about 5% of those men who have an initial episode of acute bacterial prostatitis [14]. Symptoms may be similar to acute prostatitis or may be subacute; some patients may present without fever. On digital rectal exam, the prostate is typically enlarged, tender, and boggy. Urine test results will be similar to the details listed above for acute prostatitis. Uropathogenic strains of *E. coli* are the most common bacteria isolated. Imaging tests useful in men with chronic bacterial prostatitis include ultrasound measurement of bladder PVR volume to assess for urine retention, and CT imaging of the abdomen and pelvis to rule out urolithiasis; these problems can cause recurrent infections.

Treat chronic bacterial prostatitis with antibiotics that penetrate the prostate, such as ciprofloxacin, levofloxacin, or trimethoprim/sulfamethoxazole, similar to the treatment for acute prostatitis. Use the urine culture to guide antibiotic selection. Most experts recommend a prolonged course (4–6 weeks) of antibiotic therapy for men with documented chronic bacterial prostatitis, and some recommend treating for up to 12 weeks in an attempt to eradicate the infection. Management of comorbid conditions such as urine retention and diabetes can reduce the risk of recurrent infections. When the urine cultures are negative, the patient likely has chronic nonbacterial prostatitis (see below), and antibiotics are not indicated.

For men who have recurrent urinary tract infections, consider consultation and further evaluation by a urologist. Cystoscopy may be needed to assess for problems such as a bladder stone or bladder diverticula. When urine cultures repeatedly show mixed bacterial infections, or when each infection presents with a different type of bacteria, consider if there might be a fistula between the colon and the bladder; diverticulitis is the most common cause.

Chronic Nonbacterial Prostatitis

The most common type of prostatitis is nonbacterial, accounting for 90–95% of cases. The current terminology for this entity is chronic nonbacterial prostatitis/chronic pelvic pain syndrome (CNP/CPPS). CNP/CPPS is often considered together with interstitial cystitis/bladder pain syndrome, under the umbrella term urologic chronic pelvic pain syndrome (UCPPS). The etiology is unclear, but affected patients often have a lower pain threshold than healthy individuals. They typically experience both voiding symptoms and pain, although these are only somewhat correlated. Symptom flares are common and vary in intensity, duration, and impact on quality of life [15].

The evaluation for chronic nonbacterial prostatitis is the same as described above for bacterial prostatitis. However, antibiotics should not be used if urine cultures are negative. Treatment is focused on symptom relief, and satisfaction may be difficult to achieve. Alpha blockers (as described above in the section on "Lower Urinary Tract Symptoms") may improve voiding

symptoms. Analgesics such as ibuprofen and other nonsteroidal anti-inflammatory drugs are often used to manage the pain. Some patients respond to centrally acting pain medications such as amitriptyline (Elavil) and pregabalin (Lyrica). Counseling may help with the psychosocial aspects of chronic pain. Nonpharmacologic approaches such as pelvic floor physical therapy, regular exercise, and acupuncture can provide relief for some patients. Consultation with a urologist or chronic pain specialist is recommended for patients with persistent symptoms [16].

References

1. Coyne KS, Sexton CC, Thompson CL, Milsom I, Irwin D, Kopp ZS, Chapple CR, Kaplan S, Tubaro A, Aiyer LP, Wein AJ. The prevalence of lower urinary tract symptoms (LUTS) in the USA, the UK and Sweden: results from the Epidemiology of LUTS (EpiLUTS) study. BJU Int. 2009;104(3):352–60.
2. Barry MJ, Fowler FJ, O'Leary MP, Bruskewitz RC, Holtgrewe HL, Mebust WK, Cockett AT, Measurement Committee of the American Urological Association. The American Urological Association symptom index for benign prostatic hyperplasia. J Urol. 1992;148(5 Part 1):1549–57.
3. May M, Brookman-Amissah S, Hoschke B, Gilfrich C, Braun KP, Kendel F. Post-void residual urine as a predictor of urinary tract infection – is there a cutoff value in asymptomatic men? J Urol. 2009;181 (6):2540–4.
4. Wagenlehner FM, Weidner W, Pilatz A, Naber KG. Urinary tract infections and bacterial prostatitis in men. Curr Opin Infect Dis. 2014;27(1):97–101.
5. Berry SJ, Coffey DS, Walsh PC, Ewing LL. The development of human benign prostatic hyperplasia with age. J Urol. 1984;132(3):474–9.
6. Chughtai B, Forde JC, Thomas DD, Laor L, Hossack T, Woo HH, Te AE, Kaplan SA. Benign prostatic hyperplasia. Nat Rev Dis Primers. 2016;2(1):1–5.
7. Gravas S, Bach T, Bachmann A, Drake M, Gacci M, Gratzke C. Guidelines on the management of non-neurogenic male lower urinary tract symptoms (LUTS), incl. benign prostatic obstruction (BPO) [internet]. Arnhem: European Association of Urology; 2015.
8. Michalak J, Tzou D, Funk J. HoLEP: the gold standard for the surgical management of BPH in the 21st century. Am J Clin Exp Urol. 2015;3(1):36.
9. Foster HE, Dahm P, Kohler TS, Lerner LB, Parsons JK, Wilt TJ, McVary KT. Surgical management of lower urinary tract symptoms attributed to benign prostatic hyperplasia: AUA guideline amendment 2019. J Urol. 2019;202(3):592–8.

10. Rees J, Abrahams M, Doble A, Cooper A, Prostatitis Expert Reference Group (PERG). Diagnosis and treatment of chronic bacterial prostatitis and chronic prostatitis/chronic pelvic pain syndrome: a consensus guideline. BJU Int. 2015;116(4):509–25.
11. Lipsky BA, Byren I, Hoey CT. Treatment of bacterial prostatitis. Clin Infect Dis. 2010;50:1641–52.
12. Gill BC, Shoskes DA. Bacterial prostatitis. Curr Opin Infect Dis. 2016;29(1):86–91.
13. Dietrich EA, Davis K. Antibiotics for acute bacterial prostatitis: which agent, and for how long. Consultant. 2017;57(9):564–5.
14. Khan FU, Ihsan AU, Khan HU, Jana R, Wazir J, Khongorzul P, Waqar M, Zhou X. Comprehensive overview of prostatitis. Biomed Pharmacother. 2017;94:1064–76.
15. Clemens JQ, Mullins C, Ackerman AL, Bavendam T, van Bokhoven A, Ellingson BM, Harte SE, Kutch JJ, Lai HH, Martucci KT, Moldwin R. Urologic chronic pelvic pain syndrome: insights from the MAPP Research Network. Nat Rev Urol. 2019;16(3):187–200.
16. Doiron RC, Shoskes DA, Nickel JC. Male CP/CPPS: where do we stand? World J Urol. 2019;37(6):1015–22.

Prostate Cancer

Bumsoo Park

Contents

Introduction

Prostate cancer is the third most common cancer in the United States, and the most common cancer in American men, with an estimated 1,600,000 cases and 29,000 deaths in 2018 [1]. It is an adenocarcinoma that grows in the glandular tissue of the prostate, mostly in the peripheral zone. Prostate cancer has no specific symptoms. Patients may

B. Park (✉)
Departments of Family Medicine and Urology, University of Michigan Medical School, Ann Arbor, MI, USA
e-mail: pbumsoo@med.umich.edu

© Springer Nature Switzerland AG 2022
P. M. Paulman et al. (eds.), *Family Medicine*,
https://doi.org/10.1007/978-3-030-54441-6_140

present with lower urinary tract symptoms, gross or microscopic hematuria, or hematospermia, but these symptoms and signs also occur in benign conditions. Most cases of prostate cancer are diagnosed using prostate-specific antigen (PSA)-based screening.

Screening

Using PSA to screen for prostate cancer has been controversial for many years due to the risks of both overdiagnoses, resulting in unnecessary invasive or expensive procedures such as prostate biopsy or magnetic resonance imaging (MRI) and overtreatment, resulting in significant quality of life issues such as urinary incontinence, erectile dysfunction, or gastrointestinal complications. Since 2012 the United States Preventive Services Task Force (USPSTF) had recommended against prostate cancer screening using PSA for those reasons, giving it a Grade D recommendation. However, in 2018 their recommendation shifted to Grade C [2], largely influenced by the 13-year follow-up results of the European Randomized Study of Screening for Prostate Cancer (ERSPC), which confirmed a substantial reduction in prostate cancer mortality attributable to PSA screening [3].

The USPSTF recommends PSA-based screening for men age 55 to 69 years after a careful decision-making process but still advises against it for men age 70 years or older [2]. The American Urological Association (AUA) has the same recommendations as USPSTF in terms of age range, and they recommend screening every 2 years, rather than annually, to reduce harms [4]. The American Cancer Society (ACS) recommends routine PSA screening starting at age 50 and starting at age 45 for African-American men and men who have a first-degree relative diagnosed with prostate cancer at an early age (younger than age 65) [5].

Routine PSA screening requires a thorough shared decision-making process. African-American men are at higher-than-average risk for prostate cancer, as are men whose family members have had prostate cancer.

African-American Men

The USPSTF currently does not specify a screening guideline for African-American men due to a lack of direct evidence, but clinicians may consider screening using shared decision-making for this group [2]. The AUA guideline states that clinicians may consider PSA screening for African-American men age 40 to 55 years after discussing the potential benefits and harms [4]. The ACS recommends clinicians discuss PSA screening with African-American men at age 45 years [5].

Family History of Prostate Cancer

The USPSTF currently does not specify a screening guideline for patients with a family history of prostate cancer due to a lack of direct evidence, but clinicians may consider screening using shared decision-making for this group [2]. The AUA has the same recommendations for patients with a family history of prostate cancer as for African-American men [4]. Interestingly, the ACS further specifies a screening guideline for this group. ACS recommends clinicians discuss PSA screening from age 45 for men with a first-degree relative (father or brother) diagnosed with prostate cancer at an early age (younger than age 65) and from age 40 for men at appreciably higher risk (multiple family members diagnosed before age 65 years) [5]. Researchers currently are investigating the role of prostate cancer screening for patients with familial cancer syndromes such as BRCA1, BRCA2, and mismatch-repair mutations, as in Lynch syndrome.

Interpreting Prostate-Specific Antigen

PSA is a "prostate-specific" marker, but it is not "prostate cancer specific." Please see Table 1 that summarizes the benign conditions and procedures that are associated with PSA elevation. A threshold PSA value of 4.0 ng/mL has been most widely accepted standard cutoff between normal and abnormal. There have been studies of lowering the PSA cutoff down to 3.0 ng/mL or 2.5 ng/mL

Table 1 Benign conditions and procedures associated with PSA elevation

| Acute or chronic bacterial prostatitis |
| Acute urinary retention |
| Aging |
| Benign prostatic hyperplasia |
| Chronic prostatitis/chronic pelvic pain syndrome |
| Digital rectal examination |
| Ejaculation |
| Prostate biopsy |
| Prostatic massage |
| Rigid cystoscopy |
| Transurethral resection of the prostate |
| *No association* |
| Non-traumatic urethral catheterization |
| Diagnostic flexible cystoscopy |

for early detection, but doing so increases the risks of overdiagnosis and overtreatment of clinically insignificant prostate cancers [6]. The AUA does not recommend a single threshold PSA value to prompt a prostate biopsy, noting that risks exist at any PSA level [7].

Family physicians should be careful in interpreting PSA when a patient is on a 5-alpha reductase inhibitor such as finasteride or dutasteride, because these medications lower the PSA by about 50% when used over 12 months [8]. Therefore, it is suggested that measured PSA values need to be doubled when interpreting the level for a patient who has been on a 5-alpha reductase inhibitor for more than 12 months.

There also have been suggested PSA derivatives to help prostate cancer detection, such as age-specific PSA, free/total PSA ratio, complex PSA, PSA density, and PSA velocity. It is still unclear if these PSA derivatives are of clinical significance. It is helpful to know that a typical cutoff for PSA velocity (rise in PSA over time) is 0.75 ng/mL/year. The AUA guideline states that PSA derivatives should be considered secondary tests, not primary screening tests with potential utility for determining prostate biopsy [9].

Role of Digital Rectal Examination

Digital rectal examination (DRE) looking for a hard prostate nodule used to be the traditional method for screening for prostate cancer. The USPSTF does not recommend DRE as a screening tool due to lack of evidence [2]. The AUA guideline states that DRE should be considered as a secondary test, not a primary screening test with potential utility for determining prostate biopsy [9]. A 2018 systematic review and meta-analysis concluded that routine DRE as a prostate cancer screening test in the primary care setting should be discouraged, given the considerable lack of evidence [10]. On the other hand, there is evidence that DRE in conjunction with PSA testing enhances the prostate cancer detection rate [11]. Therefore, even though DRE is not a routine screening method, it should be considered as a secondary tool if prostate cancer is clinically suspected.

Diagnosis

Prostate Biopsy

If prostate cancer is suspected, patients should be referred for a core needle prostate biopsy, which is typically an outpatient procedure done with local or regional anesthesia. A 12-core transrectal ultrasound (TRUS)-guided biopsy is the most commonly performed standard approach. Another method is fusion biopsy, which uses computer software to electronically fuse magnetic resonance images of the prostate with ultrasound images to guide the biopsy; fusion biopsy has been used to further enhance the prostate cancer detection rate [12]. In some centers, transperineal prostate biopsy is increasingly used due to lower rates of infection and better access to the anterior prostate than the transrectal approach.

Staging and Risk Stratification

Family physicians are encouraged to be familiar with prostate cancer staging and risk stratification, which are based on the number of positive biopsy cores, the PSA level, clinical stage, and the Gleason score. All of these factors are fundamental for choosing treatment options. Gleason scores range from 6 to 10, with higher numbers indicating a more aggressive cancer; the score is determined by the pathologist who examines the biopsy samples. Grade Group is a related method that scores prostate cancer aggressiveness from 1 to 5, with 5 being the most aggressive. Please see below for summaries of the clinical tumor-nodes-metastases (TNM) staging and risk stratification methods [13, 14] (Tables 2 and 3).

Role of Magnetic Resonance Imaging

Family physicians may be asked by patients about the role of MRI in prostate cancer.

Table 2 Clinical TNM staging of prostate cancer

Primary tumor (T)
TX: Primary tumor cannot be assessed
T0: No evidence of primary tumor
T1: Clinically inapparent tumor neither palpable nor visible by imaging
T1a: Tumor incidental histologic finding in 5% or less of tissue resected
T1b: Tumor incidental histologic finding in more than 5% of tissue resected
T1c: Tumor identified by needle biopsy (e.g., because of elevated PSA)
T2: Tumor confined within prostate
T2a: Tumor involves one-half of one lobe or less
T2b: Tumor involves more than one-half of one lobe but not both lobes
T2c: Tumor involves both lobes
T3: Tumor extends through the prostate capsule
T3a: Extracapsular extension (unilateral or bilateral)
T3b: Tumor invades seminal vesicle(s)
T4: Tumor is fixed or invades adjacent structures other than seminal vesicles, such as external sphincter, rectum, bladder, levator muscles, and/or pelvic wall

Regional lymph nodes (N)
NX: Regional lymph nodes were not assessed
N0: No regional lymph node metastasis
N1: Metastasis in regional lymph node(s)

Distant metastasis (M)
M0: No distant metastasis
M1: Distant metastasis
M1a: Nonregional lymph node(s)
M1b: Bone(s)
M1c: Other site(s) with or without bone disease

Source: American Joint Committee on Cancer: Prostate Cancer Staging, 7th Edition. Available at: https://cancerstaging.org/references-tools/quickreferences/Documents/ProstateSmall.pdf. Accessed 2/29/2020

Prostate MRI is primarily and conventionally used when staging unfavorable intermediate risk to very high risk biopsy-proven prostate cancer. The AUA guideline states that MRI should not be performed for very low risk or low-risk disease [15]. However, multi-parametric MRI (mpMRI) of the prostate has had an increasingly important role. It consists of conventional T1 and T2 MRI sequences, supplemented by diffusion-weighted, dynamic contrast-enhanced, and spectroscopic imaging. Given the evidence that MRI/ultrasound fusion biopsy increases the prostate cancer detection rate [12], the mpMRI is increasingly used as a tool for doing fusion biopsies for patients with a previous negative biopsy but a persistently elevated PSA and for patients who are on active surveillance to look for high-grade prostate cancer. However, prostate MRI should not be used for routine primary screening for prostate cancer. The AUA guideline states that MRI can be considered as a secondary test with potential utility for determining prostate biopsy [9].

Atypical Lesions on Biopsy

Sometimes atypical lesions are found on prostate biopsy which are not fully confirmed malignant. Two commonly encountered atypical lesions are high-grade prostatic intraepithelial neoplasia (HGPIN) and atypical small acinar proliferation (ASAP). Given that the risk of prostate cancer following the diagnosis of HGPIN is 20–30%, which is not significantly higher than that after a benign biopsy, and most of the cancers found after previous HGPIN are Gleason 6 (grade group 1), men with single-core HGPIN do not need a routine repeat prostate biopsy [16]. If HGPIN is multifocal, monitoring with serum and urine markers and/or imaging such as mpMRI may be warranted. In contrast, ASAP has about 20% risk of higher Gleason score (>7) prostate cancer, which mandates careful monitoring and may warrant repeat prostate biopsy in selected patients [16].

Table 3 Risk stratification of clinically localized prostate cancer

Very low risk
Clinical stage of T1c *AND*
Grade group 1 *AND*
PSA < 10 ng/mL *AND*
Fewer than 3 biopsy fragments/cores positive, ≤ 50% cancer in each fragment/core *AND*
PSA density < 0.15 ng/mL/g
Low risk
Clinical stage of T1 to T2a *AND*
Grade group 1 *AND*
PSA < 10 ng/mL
Intermediate risk
Clinical stage of T2b to T2c *OR*
Grade group 2 (favorable) or group 3 (unfavorable) *OR*
PSA 10–20 ng/mL
High risk
Clinical stage of T3a *OR*
Grade group 4 or 5 *OR*
PSA > 20 ng/mL
Very high risk
Clinical stage of T3b to T4 *OR*
Primary Gleason pattern 5 *OR*
> 4 cores with grade group 4 or 5
Grade group 1: Any Gleason score ≤ 6
Grade group 2: Gleason score 3 + 4 = 7
Grade group 3: Gleason score 4 + 3 = 7
Grade group 4: Any Gleason score 8 (3 + 5, 4 + 4, or 5 + 3)
Grade group 5: Any Gleason score 9 or 10 (4 + 5, 5 + 4, or 5 + 5)-

Source: NCCN Clinical Practice Guidelines in Oncology: Prostate Cancer, Version 4.2019. Available at: https://www.nccn.org/professionals/physician_gls/pdf/prostate.pdf. Accessed 3/10/2020

Treatment

Treatment of prostate cancer largely depends on risk stratification, as summarized in the Risk Stratification of Clinically Localized Prostate Cancer above. The AUA guideline states that patients with very low-risk or low-risk prostate cancer should be offered active surveillance as an initial option. Definitive treatment such as radical prostatectomy or radiotherapy can be considered for selected low-risk patients who have a risk of disease progression. Androgen-deprivation therapy should not be recommended to very low-risk or low-risk patients. For those who have intermediate-risk prostate cancer, either radical prostatectomy or radiotherapy (combined with androgen-deprivation therapy) should be considered as an initial treatment modality. For high-risk disease, either radical prostatectomy or radiotherapy (combined with androgen-deprivation therapy) should be the standard initial treatment option. Focal therapy such as cryotherapy or high-intensity focused ultrasound (HIFU) should not be offered for high-risk disease. Also, either radiotherapy alone or androgen-deprivation therapy alone should not be the choice for high-risk disease [15]. More advanced or metastatic prostate cancer should be treated with different anti-androgen or chemotherapeutic regimens, depending on the clinical stage and decision-making [17]. It is important to offer supplemental calcium and vitamin D to help maintain bone health for patients who have metastatic bone diseases. The AUA guideline states that clinicians may choose either denosumab (Prolia, Xgeva) or zoledronic acid (Reclast) when considering preventive measures for skeletal-related events to patients with metastatic bone disease [17].

Survivorship

Active Surveillance Vs. Watchful Waiting

Family physicians are encouraged to be familiar with both active surveillance and watchful waiting as these approaches to prostate cancer can be performed in a primary care setting. Active surveillance and watchful waiting may appear similar, but their treatment goals are completely different. Active surveillance focuses on early detection of cases that require definitive treatment such as radical prostatectomy or radiotherapy. However, watchful waiting is mainly intended to maintain quality of life by avoiding unnecessary definitive treatment when prostate cancer is not likely to cause mortality or significant morbidity. Watchful waiting is waiting until the disease progresses or causes symptoms, when appropriate palliative treatment can be performed. Watchful waiting should therefore be offered to patients who have significantly reduced life expectancy.

Protocols for active surveillance and watchful waiting may vary depending on physician preference or health system policy. The National Comprehensive Cancer Network (NCCN) guideline recommends that active surveillance include PSA no more often than every 6 months unless clinically indicated, DRE no more often than every 12 months unless clinically indicated, repeat prostate biopsy no more often than every 12 months unless clinically indicated, and repeat mpMRI no more often than every 12 months unless clinically indicated [14]. Regarding watchful waiting, NCCN recommends both PSA and physical examination no more often than every 6 months, without surveillance biopsies or radiographic imaging. When symptoms develop or are imminent, patients can begin palliative androgen-deprivation therapy [14].

Monitoring after Prostate Cancer Treatment

The American Society of Clinical Oncology (ASCO) recommends measuring serum PSA every 6 to 12 months for the first 5 years after definitive prostate cancer treatment and then annually [18]. Family physicians are encouraged to become familiar with the definition of biochemical recurrence (also called biochemical failure), as explained below. Patients who have a biochemical recurrence after definitive treatment need to be referred back to their original treatment team in a timely manner. Sometimes clinicians miss the diagnosis of biochemical recurrence, misinterpreting the rise in PSA as being within the normal range.

There are important differences between biochemical recurrences in patients who are post-prostatectomy and post-radiotherapy. The AUA defines biochemical recurrence after radical prostatectomy as an initial PSA value ≥ 0.2 ng/mL, followed by a subsequent confirmatory PSA value ≥ 0.2 ng/mL [19]. However, after radiotherapy, AUA uses the 2005 Consensus Committee conclusion in their guideline to define post-radiotherapy biochemical recurrence as a serum PSA ≥ 2.0 ng/mL above nadir or 3 consecutive rises in PSA level [20]. (The term "nadir" refers to the lowest PSA attained after radiotherapy.) This definition can be applied to both external beam radiation therapy and interstitial brachytherapy, regardless of whether the radiotherapy was accompanied by androgen-deprivation therapy [20, 21].

In addition, family physicians should be familiar with how to interpret PSA values for patients on androgen-deprivation therapy for metastatic prostate cancer. For these patients, a failure to achieve a PSA nadir of <4.0 ng/mL 7 months after androgen-deprivation therapy initiation suggests very poor prognosis, whereas patients with a PSA nadir of <0.2 ng/mL have a relatively good prognosis [22].

Quality of Life

Quality of life is a key focus of treatment for patients who have undergone prostate cancer treatment. Erectile dysfunction (ED) occurs in 30–60%

of patients after radical prostatectomy or radiotherapy. Patients who had radical prostatectomy and lose erectile function may regain it during the 2 years following surgery, whereas radiotherapy typically causes a gradual decline in erectile function during the first 24–36 months after treatment, followed by stabilization or partial recovery. Primary care physicians can offer phosphodiesterase-5 inhibitors such as avanafil (Stendra), sildenafil (Viagra), tadalafil (Cialis), or vardenafil (Levitra, Staxyn) as the initial treatment for patients with ED. Patients with persistent sexual dysfunction should be referred to a urologist, sexual health specialist, or psychotherapist [18]. Other treatment options for ED include intracavernosal alprostadil injections (Caverject, Edex), intraurethral alprostadil (Muse), vacuum erectile devices, or penile prosthesis placement.

Most men who undergo radical prostatectomy experience urinary incontinence for the first few months after the surgery. The incontinence usually subsides to become small to no bother by 1 year after radical prostatectomy [15]. Family physicians can refer patients with incontinence to physical therapy for pelvic floor rehabilitation and should instruct such patients on Kegel exercises [18]. For persistent and bothersome incontinence, patients should be referred to a urologist for evaluation and consideration of possible procedures such as male urethral sling or artificial urinary sphincter placement.

Proctitis occurs in less than 10% of patients after radiotherapy for prostate cancer, but it can cause rectal frequency, urgency, loose stools, or rectal bleeding [15]. Primary care physicians can offer these patients stool softeners, topical steroids, or anti-inflammatories as an initial measure but should refer to specialists for persistent symptoms [18].

Mood issues including anxiety and depression should be monitored in prostate cancer survivors. The ASCO recommends managing survivors' distress and depression using in-office counseling resources or pharmacotherapy as appropriate [18]. A 2018 systematic review showed that exercise is effective at improving cardiorespiratory fitness, muscle strength, fatigue, incontinence, physical activity levels, and quality of life [23], so prostate cancer survivors should be encouraged to exercise.

Prevention

Risk Factors

It is important to understand prostate cancer risk factors so that clinicians can better plan preventive strategies. Both genetics and environmental factors are known to play a role in carcinogenesis. The most well-known risk factors are advanced age, African-American ethnicity, and genetic factors (such as BRCA). Obesity, hormonal factors, and a variety of dietary factors have been studied, but their role in carcinogenesis is inconclusive. Currently, there is no evidence that prostatitis, benign prostatic hyperplasia, or vasectomy is associated with prostate cancer.

Chemoprevention

Two key trials have studied the role of 5-alpha reductase inhibitors (finasteride, dutasteride) on prostate cancer prevention: Prostate Cancer Prevention Trial (PCPT) and Reduction by Dutasteride of Prostate Cancer Events (REDUCE). The PCPT trial concluded that finasteride reduced prostate cancer prevalence by 24.8% over a 7-year period compared to placebo [24]. The REDUCE trial showed that dutasteride reduced prostate cancer risk by 22.8% over a 4-year period compared to placebo [25]. However, both trials found a significantly higher rate of aggressive cancers (those with high Gleason scores) in the 5-alpha reductase inhibitor groups compared to placebo, which was problematic. There currently is no standardized guideline for using 5-alpha reductase inhibitors for prostate cancer chemoprevention.

Dietary factors including soy, lycopene, and green tea have not shown any proven efficacy in prostate cancer prevention. The roles of vitamin E and selenium have been studied, but the Selenium and Vitamin E Cancer Prevention Trial (SELECT) showed that neither one prevents prostate cancer, and it showed that vitamin E significantly increased the risk of prostate cancer among healthy men [26].

When to Refer to Urology

Patients with any of the following findings should be referred to a urologist:

- Screening PSA $\geq$ 4.0 ng/mL on two or more occasions.
- Screening PSA $\geq$ 2.0 ng/mL on two or more occasions in a patient who has been on a 5-alpha reductase inhibitor (finasteride or dutasteride) for at least 6 months.
- Screening PSA velocity (rise over time) $\geq$ 0.75 ng/mL/year.
- DRE showing a hard prostate nodule.
- PSA $\geq$ 0.2 ng/mL after radical prostatectomy.
- PSA $\geq$ 2.0 ng/mL above nadir after radiotherapy.

References

1. Siegel RL, Miller KD, Jemal A. Cancer statistics, 2018. CA Cancer J Clin. 2018;68(1):7–30.
2. US Preventive Services Task Force, Grossman DC, Curry SJ, et al. Screening for prostate cancer: US preventive services task force recommendation statement. JAMA. 2018;319(18):1901–13.
3. Schröder FH, Hugosson J, Roobol MJ, et al. Screening and prostate cancer mortality: results of the European randomised study of screening for prostate cancer (ERSPC) at 13 years of follow-up. Lancet. 2014;384(9959):2027–35.
4. Carter HB, Albertsen PC, Barry MJ, et al. Early detection of prostate cancer: AUA guideline. J Urol. 2013;190(2):419–26.
5. Wolf AM, Wender RC, Etzioni RB, et al. American Cancer Society guideline for the early detection of prostate cancer: update 2010. CA Cancer J Clin. 2010;60(2):70–98.
6. Welch HG, Schwartz LM, Woloshin S. Prostate-specific antigen levels in the United States: implications of various definitions for abnormal. J Natl Cancer Inst. 2005;97(15):1132–7.
7. American Urological Association Guideline: Optimal techniques of prostate biopsy and specimen handling. Available at: https://www.auanet.org/guidelines/prostate-biopsy-and-specimen-handling. Accessed 29 Feb 2020.
8. Pannek J, Marks LS, Pearson JD, et al. Influence of finasteride on free and total serum prostate specific antigen levels in men with benign prostatic hyperplasia. J Urol. 1998;159(2):449–53.
9. American Urological Association Guideline: Early detection of prostate cancer. Available at: https://www.auanet.org/guidelines/prostate-cancer-early-detection-guideline. Accessed 29 Feb 2020.
10. Naji L, Randhawa H, Sohani Z, et al. Digital rectal examination for prostate cancer screening in primary care: a systemic review and meta-analysis. Ann Fam Med. 2018;16(2):149–54.
11. Catalona WJ, Richie JP, Ahmann FR, et al. Comparison of digital rectal examination and serum prostate specific antigen in the early detection of prostate cancer: results of a multicenter clinical trial of 6,630 men. J Urol. 1994;151(5):1283–90.
12. Siddiqui MM, Rais-Bahrami S, Truong H, et al. Magnetic resonance imaging/ultrasound-fusion biopsy significantly upgrades prostate cancer versus systemic 12-core transrectal ultrasound biopsy. Eur Urol. 2013;64(5):713–9.
13. American Joint Committee on Cancer: Prostate Cancer Staging. 7th edition. Available at: https://cancerstaging.org/references-tools/quickreferences/Documents/ProstateSmall.pdf. Accessed 29 Feb 2020.
14. NCCN Clinical Practice Guidelines in Oncology: Prostate Cancer, version 4.2019. Available at: https://www.nccn.org/professionals/physician_gls/pdf/prostate.pdf. Accessed 10 Mar 2020.
15. American Urological Association Guideline: Clinically localized prostate cancer: AUA/ASTRO/SUO guideline. Available at: https://www.auanet.org/guidelines/prostate-cancer-clinically-localized-guideline. Accessed 29 Feb 2020.
16. Tosoian JJ, Alam R, Ball MW, Carter HB, Epstein JI. Managing high-grade prostatic intraepithelial neoplasia (HGPIN) and atypical glands on prostate biopsy. Nat Rev Urol. 2018;15(1):55–66.
17. American Urological Association Guideline: Castration-Resistant Prostate Cancer. Available at: https://www.auanet.org/guidelines/prostate-cancer-castration-resistant-guideline. Accessed 10 Mar 2020.
18. Resnick MJ, Lacchetti C, Bergman J, et al. Prostate cancer survivorship care guideline: American Society of Clinical Oncology clinical practice guideline endorsement. J Clin Oncol. 2015;33(9):1078–85.
19. Cookson MS, Aus G, Burnett AL, et al. Variation in the definition of biochemical recurrence in patients treated for localized prostate cancer: the American urological association prostate guidelines for localized prostate Cancer update panel report and recommendations for a standard in the reporting of surgical outcomes. J Urol. 2007;177(2):540–5.
20. Horwitz EM, Thames HD, Kuban DA, et al. Definitions of biochemical failure that best predict clinical failure in patients with prostate cancer treated with external beam radiation alone: a multi-institutional pooled analysis. J Urol. 2005;173(3):797–802.

21. Kuban DA, Levy LB, Potters L, et al. Comparison of biochemical failure definitions for permanent prostate brachytherapy. Int J Radiat Oncol Biol Phys. 2006;65(5):1487–93.

22. Hussain M, Tangen CM, Higano C, et al. Absolute prostate-specific antigen value after androgen deprivation is a strong independent predictor of survival in new metastatic prostate cancer: data from southwest oncology group trial 9346 (INT-0162). J Clin Oncol. 2006;24(24):3984–90.

23. Crawford-Williams F, March S, Goodwin BC, et al. Interventions for prostate cancer survivorship: a systematic review of reviews. Psychooncology. 2018;27(10):2339–48.

24. Thompson IM, Goodman PJ, Tangen CM, et al. The influence of finasteride on the development of prostate cancer. N Engl J Med. 2003;349(3):215–24.

25. Andriole GL, Bostwick DG, Brawley OW, et al. Effect of dutasteride on the risk of prostate cancer. N Engl J Med. 2010;362(13):1192–202.

26. Klein EA, Thompson IM Jr, Tangen CM, et al. Vitamin E and the risk of prostate cancer: the Selenium and Vitamin E Cancer Prevention Trial (SELECT). JAMA. 2011;306(14):1549–56.

Karl T. Rew

Contents

Neonatal Circumcision

Neonatal circumcision is controversial, and family physicians should make an effort to fully understand the religious, cultural, medical, and ethical arguments on both sides of the debate in order to provide parents with accurate and unbiased information. Questions to consider include: Should circumcision be done, and if so, when, how, and by whom?

Religious and cultural norms are the primary motivation for most neonatal circumcisions. Ritual circumcision remains nearly universal among Jews and Muslims. In the USA, non-ritual (secular) neonatal circumcision is common, although it is not common in most of the rest of the world. Rates of neonatal circumcision in the USA decreased from 64.5% to 58.3% between 1979 and 2010, with significant regional, ethnic, and racial variation. Circumcision rates are highest in the US Midwest and lowest in the West [1].

Potential medical benefits of circumcision include a reduction in urinary tract infections during the first year of life. There also is evidence that circumcision reduces the subsequent risk of heterosexual acquisition of HIV for those living in high-risk areas and may reduce the transmission of other sexually transmitted infections. Potential harms of circumcision include acute complications such as pain, bleeding, infection, and injury to the glans of the penis, as well as later complications that may need surgical management, such as meatal stenosis, skin bridges, or redundant foreskin leading to an uncircumcised appearance. The effects of circumcision on adult penile sensation and sexual satisfaction are unclear but vigorously debated.

Ethical issues related to circumcision include the patient's autonomy and right to bodily integrity. This consideration advocates for decisions

K. T. Rew (✉)
Departments of Family Medicine and Urology, University of Michigan Medical School, Ann Arbor, MI, USA
e-mail: karlr@med.umich.edu

© Springer Nature Switzerland AG 2022
P. M. Paulman et al. (eds.), *Family Medicine*,
https://doi.org/10.1007/978-3-030-54441-6_141

regarding circumcision to be made by the person undergoing the procedure when he is old enough to give consent, rather than by his parents. In much of the world outside the USA, neonatal male circumcision is increasingly seen as a needless and harmful human rights violation, just as is female genital cutting [2]. However, in the USA, weighing the risks and benefits of this decision is generally left up to the parents.

An influential 2012 policy statement from the American Academy of Pediatrics recognizes some of the controversy surrounding circumcision, pointing out that, "Although health benefits are not great enough to recommend routine circumcision for all male newborns, the benefits of circumcision are sufficient to justify access to this procedure for families choosing it." [3] The American Academy of Family Physicians 2018 policy statement on neonatal circumcision uses similar but somewhat less supportive language [4]. Outside the USA, support for non-ritual neonatal circumcision is uncommon. In the United Kingdom, circumcision is considered to have essentially no medical benefit and is not covered by insurance. In the Netherlands, circumcision is not only considered to have no medical benefit but also is seen as causing physical and psychological trauma [5].

About half of circumcisions in the USA are performed during the neonatal period, defined as the first 30 days of life. At this age, the cost of the procedure is lower because most circumcisions can be done under local anesthesia, and suturing is typically not needed. Most non-ritual neonatal circumcisions in the USA are performed by the physicians immediately involved in the birthing process, including family physicians, pediatricians, and obstetricians. After the neonatal period, urologists perform the majority of circumcisions [6].

Physicians have a duty to provide clear, accurate, and unbiased information for parents who are considering circumcising their newborn son, and physicians should respect the parents' decision. It is worthwhile having this discussion even before the child is born. Informed consent must be obtained prior to the procedure. For families who choose a natural penis, advise them that a tight foreskin (physiological phimosis) is normal

in young boys and instruct them to avoid forceful retraction of the foreskin, especially in the first year of life.

When evaluating a newborn male whose parents are requesting circumcision, the next important element is to assess for contraindications. Candidates for neonatal circumcision should be healthy, at least 12 h old, and have urinated at least once. Examine the genitalia carefully. Micropenis (stretched length ≤1.9 cm), concealed penis, and ambiguous genitalia are contraindications. Premature infants are often not candidates due to small penis size. Infants with anatomic abnormalities that may require surgical repair should not undergo neonatal circumcision. These conditions include hypospadias, epispadias, chordee, and webbed or buried penis. Sometimes hypospadias or another abnormality is discovered after a dorsal slit is performed during circumcision; in that situation, the procedure should be stopped and the patient referred for a urology consultation. Infants with bleeding disorders such as hemophilia or thrombocytopenia should not undergo neonatal circumcision [7].

Circumcision at any age is an invasive and painful procedure, so anesthesia is necessary. Local anesthesia is usually sufficient for neonatal circumcision. Ring block or dorsal penile nerve block using lidocaine are the preferred approaches. Lidocaine with epinephrine should never be used because the vasoconstrictive properties of epinephrine increase the risk of ischemia and tissue necrosis. Topical anesthesia with EMLA cream (a eutectic mixture of lidocaine 2.5% and prilocaine 2.5%) is less effective alone but improves pain relief when used in combination with a ring block or dorsal penile nerve block [8].

The most common instruments used for neonatal circumcision in the USA are the Gomco clamp, the PlastiBell device, and the Mogen clamp. The choice depends on the clinician's training and preference. Outcomes are similar, with some variation in risk of complications. The most important element is the skill of the operator. The Gomco and Mogen clamps are reusable metal devices. The PlastiBell device is disposable, comes in a range of sizes (the correct size must be selected), and is left in place after the procedure. The Gomco clamp and PlastiBell device require a dorsal slit. Detailed procedural guidelines are beyond the scope of this chapter but can be found elsewhere [9]. In some cases, absorbable sutures may be needed to control bleeding. If suturing ventrally, take care to avoid the urethra. If bleeding persists, clotting studies are indicated.

Instruct parents to watch for bleeding or evidence of infection. Provide them with printed postprocedural instructions. Parents should apply petrolatum jelly (Vaseline) to the front of the diaper to help prevent the healing area from sticking to the diaper. Acetaminophen can be used for pain relief if needed. The PlastiBell device, if used, should fall off within a week. Surgical follow-up can generally be done at the next well-child visit.

Undescended Testis

Before birth, the testes of a male fetus develop along the posterior abdominal wall near the kidneys, and they later descend from the abdomen, eventually moving through the inguinal canal and then into the scrotum around 25–30 weeks of gestation. At the time of birth, undescended testis, or cryptorchidism, is present in 2–4% of full-term newborn males; in preterm males, the rate is 20–30%. In about a third of cases, both testes are undescended. The etiology is unclear but probably multifactorial. Male infants whose father or brother had an undescended testis are at higher risk, and other genetic, hormonal, and environmental factors likely contribute to the risk. Spontaneous resolution is common during the first few months of life, so that by age 12 months, the prevalence of undescended testis has decreased to about 1% [10].

The potential complications associated with undescended testis include infertility and testicular cancer. The risk of testicular torsion is also increased; torsion is discussed in more detail later in this chapter. One reason males with a history of undescended testis are at risk for infertility or subfertility appears to be that an undescended testis is exposed to an environment that is too warm. Abdominal temperature is higher than scrotal temperature, and for optimal testicular germ cell development and successful spermatogenesis, an ambient temperature that is lower than abdominal temperature is needed. Fertility is most likely to be affected in males with bilateral undescended testes, or if treatment is delayed. For the best results regarding future fertility, the undescended testis should be brought into the scrotum between ages 6 and 18 months. Undescended testis is also the most important known risk factor for testicular germ cell tumors. The cause for this association is unclear. Definitive early treatment of undescended testis appears to provide the most effective reduction in the patient's future risk of testicular cancer [11]. The American Urological Association (AUA) recommends urology consultation at age 6 months and surgical treatment by age 18 months [12].

Physical exam is the most reliable method of diagnosing undescended testis. Ultrasound or other imaging is not necessary. Examine the genitalia at each well-child visit. An effective approach is to place the patient in a supine frog leg position. Inspect the penis and urethral opening. Palpate the scrotum on each side. If a testis is not palpable in the scrotum, palpate the inguinal canal. If the testis is still not palpable, start at the anterior superior iliac spine and use fingers to sweep the inguinal area down towards the scrotum. About 70% of undescended testes are palpable, and most will be in the inguinal canal [12]. Testes that are descended but retractile can be delivered into the scrotum by gradually stretching the cremasteric muscle [13]. Retractile testes typically do not require surgical intervention but should be monitored annually with a physical exam for possible secondary ascent. If the diagnosis is unclear on physical exam, consult a urologist. If bilateral undescended testes are noted on a newborn exam, look for hypospadias or other genital abnormalities; when present, promptly refer the patient to a pediatric urologist. Genital ambiguity with bilateral undescended testes could indicate a genetic female with virilization, which can occur with congenital adrenal hyperplasia or a disorder of sexual differentiation, such as intersex.

If the genitalia of a newborn male with undescended testis otherwise appear normal, the recommended initial management is 6 months of watchful waiting. If one or both testes remain undescended by age 6 months, refer the patient to a pediatric urologist so that definitive treatment can be accomplished before age 18 months. (For preterm infants, use corrected age, rather than chronological age. For example, a 6-month-old infant who was born 2 months early has a corrected age of 4 months.)

In the USA, the recommended treatment for a palpable undescended testis is orchiopexy (an alternative spelling is orchidopexy), which is a surgical repositioning of the testis and fixing it in the scrotum [13]. Approaches to treatment that use hormonal manipulation via repeated injections in an attempt to induce testicular descent are not recommended due to low response rates and lack of evidence for long-term efficacy [12].

If an undescended testis is not palpable, it might be in the abdomen, or it might be atrophic (typically due to prenatal torsion), or absent (anorchia). When a testis is not palpable, exploration and orchiopexy are usually performed laparoscopically. If a nonpalpable undescended testis not found in the abdomen, it is generally assumed to have undergone prenatal torsion; orchiopexy is then typically done on the contralateral testes to minimize the future risk of torsion on that side. An undescended testis is often associated with a patent processus vaginalis, so most patients have an inguinal hernia or hydrocele that will need to be repaired at the time of orchiopexy.

A history of undescended testis increases the risk of testicular cancer, even after prepubertal orchiopexy. Compared to other cancers, testicular cancer is not common, accounting for about 1% of cancers in men and occurring in about 1 in 250 males at some point during their lifetimes. Treatment is very effective at all stages [14]. Evidence does not support screening for testicular cancer in the general population. However, because males who had an undescended testis are at increased risk of testicular cancer, the American Urological Association recommends instructing them to do monthly testicular self-exams beginning at puberty to facilitate early detection [12].

Testicular Torsion

Testicular torsion occurs when the spermatic cord twists, blocking blood flow to the testis. This is a surgical emergency for which rapid recognition and treatment are essential. Irreversible changes due to ischemia in the affected testis start within hours. Testicular salvage rates are 90–100% if surgery is done within 6 h of symptom onset, but fall to about 50% after 12 h, and are less than 10% after 24 h [15].

Torsion can occur at any age but is more common in younger males, with two peaks in incidence: one during the first year of life and another around age 12–13 years that is thought to be associated with the increase in testicular size at puberty [16]. Males with undescended testis are at increased risk for torsion, as are with those a family history of torsion. In some patients, torsion occurs after trauma. Infant perinatal torsion may be extravaginal, but postnatal and later (adolescent) torsion is usually intravaginal, which means that the twisting occurs within the tunica vaginalis. A common finding on surgical exploration is the bell-clapper deformity, where the testicular attachment to the tunica vaginalis is abnormal, allowing easier rotation of the testis [17]. The bell-clapper deformity may be bilateral, and in some patients, it can lead to intermittent torsion with episodic testicular pain.

Torsion is diagnosed by history and physical exam. Classic symptoms include sudden severe unilateral scrotal pain, often with nausea and vomiting, but without dysuria or other urinary symptoms. On exam, the affected testis is usually high-lying. About half of affected testes will have a transverse (horizontal) lie, where the normal position would be vertical. An absent cremasteric reflex means torsion is likely. Scrotal swelling and erythema may be present. Torsion of the appendix testis causes pain and focal tenderness in the upper pole of testis, and a tender blue dot may be visible through the scrotal skin; this problem does not require surgical treatment [18]. The differential diagnosis for acute scrotal pain includes infectious causes such as epididymitis and orchitis, where pain and tenderness are common, urinary symptoms and fever may be present, but the cremasteric reflex is usually normal. If the diagnosis is unclear, consult a urologist. Color Doppler ultrasound can confirm a diagnosis of torsion, but clinicians should never postpone surgical treatment to wait for ultrasound. Laboratory tests are rarely needed.

If the physical exam is consistent with torsion and surgical management will be delayed, manual detorsion can be considered. With the patient lying in a supine frog leg position and the examiner at the patient's feet, manual detorsion is traditionally attempted clockwise for the left testis (on the examiner's right) and counterclockwise for the right testis (on the examiner's left). These directions of motion, often described as "opening a book," will only be correct for reversing torsion in about two-thirds of cases, and in the other one-third will make it worse. Manual detorsion causes significant discomfort; however, success results in prompt pain relief that confirms the diagnosis. The number of twists present in a torsed testis ranges from a half twist (180°) to 3 full twists (1080°), although the most common is 1 full twist (360°) to 1.5 twists (540°). Residual torsion is present in about 27% of cases after attempted manual detorsion [19].

In all cases, whether an attempted detorsion appears successful or not, urology consultation is required for immediate surgical exploration, detorsion, and bilateral orchiopexy. Completing an orchiopexy on the unaffected contralateral testis helps minimize the risk of future torsion on that side. A midline transscrotal approach is usually adequate for this type of surgery. Orchiectomy will be needed if the affected testis is not viable. Testicular salvage rates are minimal for patients with neonatal torsion. For patients who require orchiectomy, later placement of a testicular prosthesis is an option for cosmetic purposes. After torsion, the affected testis may become atrophic, even when the patient has received timely surgical treatment. Additionally, future fertility can be impaired, [20] although testicular hormonal function is likely to remain intact. Because testicular injury due to sports participation is rare, males with a single testis can participate in contact sports. However, it is reasonable to counsel them to use a scrotal protective cup [21].

Vasectomy

Vasectomy is the most effective form of contraception available for men. For couples in the USA, it is currently the fifth most popular method after oral contraceptives, tubal ligation, condoms, and long-acting reversible contraceptive methods such as intrauterine devices and hormonal implants [22]. Vasectomy is safer, less expensive, and more effective than tubal ligation. However, it is less widely used: about 6.6% of US men ages 18–45 years have had a vasectomy, while 16.4% of women in the same age range have undergone tubal ligation [23]. Approximately 525,000 vasectomies were performed in the USA in 2015, about 82% of them by urologists [24].

Pre-vasectomy counseling is important. Although vasectomy should be seen as a permanent form of contraception, about 20% of men who have had vasectomy express a desire for more children, and 1.9% will undergo vasectomy reversal [23]. Men considering vasectomy should therefore be advised to think carefully about whether they might want to have children in the future, particularly if their circumstances were to change. Men who chose to have a vasectomy in their 20s are significantly more likely to later undergo vasectomy reversal than men who were 30 years or older at the time of their vasectomies [25]. About 10% of couples will express regret after sterilization [23]. For men who have had a vasectomy, regret is most common when they are in a new relationship after separation, divorce, or death of a former partner [26].

The AUA vasectomy guideline [27] recommends that pre-vasectomy counseling cover the following topics:

- Vasectomy is intended to be permanent.
- Other permanent and nonpermanent alternatives are available.

- Options for fertility after vasectomy include surgical reversal and sperm retrieval, but these approaches are expensive and are not always successful.
- Vasectomy does not produce immediate sterility.
- After vasectomy, another form of contraception is necessary until successful vas occlusion is confirmed with a post-vasectomy semen analysis.
- Even when vas occlusion is confirmed, vasectomy is not 100% reliable in preventing pregnancy.
- The risk of pregnancy after vasectomy is 1 in 2000 if the post-vasectomy semen analysis is negative (showing zero sperm or rare non-motile sperm).
- Repeat vasectomy is occasionally necessary (in less than 1% of cases).
- Chronic scrotal pain occurs in 1–2% of men after vasectomy.
- The surgical complication rate is 1–2%; the most common complications include symptomatic hematoma and infection.
- Patients should refrain from ejaculation for approximately 1 week after vasectomy.

During the pre-vasectomy visit, assess for contraindications. Men who have uncontrolled coagulation disorders should not undergo vasectomy. A bacterial infection of the scrotum is also a contraindication. Before the procedure, make sure the patient has reasonable expectations and does not expect the vasectomy to resolve conflict in a relationship or cure sexual problems. Obtain informed consent.

When examining a patient who is considering vasectomy, perform a thorough genital exam. Palpate the scrotum, making sure both testes are normal and that the vas deferens is clearly palpable on both sides and can be elevated. Assess for inguinal hernia, hydrocele, and varicocele. Do not proceed if the patient is too anxious, has excessive scrotal sensitivity, or otherwise cannot tolerate the exam.

For most men, no laboratory testing is needed prior to vasectomy. Antiplatelet medications and warfarin (Coumadin) should be stopped 5–7 days prior to vasectomy and not restarted for 2–3 days afterward. Most direct oral anticoagulants should be stopped 2 days before the procedure and can usually be restarted after adequate hemostasis is attained. If in doubt, consult a coagulation specialist.

Detailed procedural guidance is beyond the scope of this chapter but can be found elsewhere [27, 28]. Local anesthesia administered either using a jet injector or a syringe and small gauge (25–32 gauge) needle is appropriate for most patients. The no-scalpel technique (which uses a sharp pointed hemostat) or a similar minimally invasive technique is recommended for accessing and isolating each vas. A single scrotal incision is usually sufficient. Three main approaches to occluding the vas have been shown to be effective and are commonly used in the USA.

1. Mucosal cautery with fascial interposition.
2. Mucosal cautery without fascial interposition.
3. Open ended vasectomy, which leaves the testicular end of the vas unoccluded, and uses mucosal cautery and fascial interposition on the abdominal end.

There are many variations on these methods. Clips and ligatures are used by some surgeons but are not required. Some surgeons routinely excise a short (about 1 cm) section of the vas, but this is also not required. The surgeon's training and experience with the selected method are the keys to consistent and satisfactory results [27].

Sending an excised portion of the vas for routine histologic analysis adds additional expense and is not necessary. Instead, a single post-vasectomy semen analysis is typically sufficient to ensure effectiveness. Motile sperm are usually cleared from the semen by 6 weeks after vasectomy. Perform the semen analysis 8–16 weeks after the vasectomy. Although a routine post-procedural physical examination is not usually needed, scheduling an appointment for the semen analysis improves the likelihood it will be completed. Instruct the patient to collect a fresh specimen via masturbation. Analyze the undiluted, uncentrifuged specimen within 2 h of collection, examining at least 50 high-power fields looking for motile or nonmotile sperm. A negative semen analysis is defined as no motile sperm and rare nonmotile sperm (meaning $\leq 100,000$ nonmotile sperm per mL). If the semen analysis is negative, it does not need to be repeated. If it is positive, instruct the patient to continue to use another method of contraception, and repeat the semen analysis at intervals of 4–6 weeks. If motile sperm are still present 6 months after vasectomy, the vasectomy has failed; this result may represent recanalization. Repeat vasectomy should be considered [27].

Swelling, bruising, and discomfort are common adverse effects of vasectomy that usually resolve without intervention. The main potential acute complications of vasectomy include hematoma, scrotal infection, and abscess formation. These occur in 1–2% of patients. Additionally, about 1–2% of patients will develop post-vasectomy pain syndrome, with chronic scrotal or pelvic pain; however, surgical management is rarely necessary. Initial treatment options include nonsteroidal anti-inflammatory drugs, tricyclic antidepressants, nerve blocks, gabapentin (Neurontin), as well as acupuncture and other complementary approaches. Surgical vasectomy reversal is used in some cases to manage post-vasectomy pain syndrome due to epididymal congestion, but it is not always successful in resolving the pain, and may restore fertility [29]. Another treatment for post-vasectomy pain is surgical removal of the epididymis (epididymectomy); this is technically easier than vasectomy reversal and leaves the patient sterile.

Although vasectomy is a simple and effective procedure, vasectomy reversal (vasovasostomy or vasoepididymostomy) is a technically challenging procedure usually not covered by insurance, and it is only 30–76% effective at restoring fertility [25]. Another option for post-vasectomy men who desire fertility is in vitro fertilization via intra-cytoplasmic sperm injection, which can use sperm harvested from the testis or epididymis. This approach to restoring fertility also is complex, expensive, and may not be covered by insurance. Pre-vasectomy sperm cryopreservation is a less costly option, although annual storage fees will add up over time. Men who are uncertain about their future plans for having children should not undergo vasectomy and should use an alternate form of contraception.

References

1. Owings M, Uddin S, Williams S. Trends in circumcision for male newborns in US hospitals. NCHS Health Notes: Citeseer. 2013. p. 1–5.
2. Svoboda JS. Circumcision of male infants as a human rights violation. J Med Ethics. 2013;39(7):469–74.
3. Task Force on Circumcision. Circumcision policy statement. Pediatrics. 2012;130(3):585–6.
4. American Academy of Family Physicians. Neonatal Circumcision. 2018. Congress of delegates. Accessed April 30, 2020, and available at: https://www.aafp.org/about/policies/all/neonatal-circumcision.html
5. Jacobs M, Grady R, Bolnick DA. Current circumcision trends and guidelines. In: Surgical guide to circumcision. London: Springer; 2012. p. 3–8.
6. Many BT, Rizeq YK, Vacek J, Cheon EC, Johnson E, Hu YY, Raval MV, Abdullah F, Goldstein SD. A contemporary snapshot of circumcision in US children's hospitals. J Pediatr Surg. 2020;55(6):1134–1138. https://doi.org/10.1016/j.jpedsurg.2020.02.031. Epub 2020 Feb 27.
7. Simpson E, Carstensen J, Murphy P. Neonatal circumcision: new recommendations & implications for practice. Mo Med. 2014;111(3):222.
8. Sharara-Chami R, Lakissian Z, Charafeddine L, Milad N, El-Hout Y. Combination analgesia for neonatal circumcision: a randomized controlled trial. Pediatrics. 2017;140(6):e20171935.
9. Fowler GC. Chapter 167: Newborn circumcision and office Meatotomy. In: Pfenninger and fowler's procedures for primary care fourth edition, E-book. Philadelphia: Elsevier Health Sciences; 2020.
10. Berkowitz GS, Lapinski RH, Gazella JG, Dolgin SE, Bodian CA, Holzman IR. Prevalence and natural history of cryptorchidism. Pediatrics. 1993;92(1):44–9.
11. Pettersson A, Richiardi L, Nordenskjold A, Kaijser M, Akre O. Age at surgery for undescended testis and risk of testicular cancer. N Engl J Med. 2007;356(18):1835–41.
12. Kolon TF, Herndon CA, Baker LA, Baskin LS, Baxter CG, Cheng EY, Diaz M, Lee PA, Seashore CJ, Tasian GE, Barthold JS. Evaluation and treatment of cryptorchidism: AUA guideline. J Urol. 2014;192(2):337–45.
13. Kolon TF, Patel RP, Huff DS. Cryptorchidism: diagnosis, treatment, and long-term prognosis. Urol Clin North Am. 2004;31(3):469–80.
14. PDQ Screening and Prevention Editorial Board. Testicular Cancer Screening (PDQ®), Health Professional Version. In PDQ Cancer Information Summaries [Internet] 2019 Mar 6. National Cancer Institute (US). Accessed April 27, 2020, and available at: https://www.ncbi.nlm.nih.gov/books/NBK65967/

15. Sharp VJ, Kieran K, Arlen AM. Testicular torsion: diagnosis, evaluation, and management. Am Fam Physician. 2013;88(12):835–40.

16. Zhao LC, Lautz TB, Meeks JJ, Maizels M. Pediatric testicular torsion epidemiology using a national database: incidence, risk of orchiectomy and possible measures toward improving the quality of care. J Urol. 2011;186(5):2009–13.

17. Fehér ÁM, Bajory Z. A review of main controversial aspects of acute testicular torsion. J Acute Dis. 2016;5 (1):1–8.

18. Bowlin PR, Gatti JM, Murphy JP. Pediatric testicular torsion. Surg Clin. 2017;97(1):161–72.

19. Sessions AE, Rabinowitz R, Hulbert WC, Goldstein MM, Mevorach RA. Testicular torsion: direction, degree, duration and disinformation. J Urol. 2003;169 (2):663–5.

20. Kapoor S. Testicular torsion: a race against time. Int J Clin Pract. 2008;62(5):821–7.

21. Styn NR, Wan J. Urologic sports injuries in children. Curr Urol Rep. 2010;11(2):114–21.

22. Kavanaugh ML, Jerman J. Contraceptive method use in the United States: trends and characteristics between 2008, 2012 and 2014. Contraception. 2018;97(1):14–21.

23. Sharma V, Le BV, Sheth KR, Zargaroff S, Dupree JM, Cashy J, Brannigan RE. Vasectomy demographics and postvasectomy desire for future children: results from a contemporary national survey. Fertil Steril. 2013;99 (7):1880–5.

24. Ostrowski KA, Holt SK, Haynes B, Davies BJ, Fuchs EF, Walsh TJ. Evaluation of vasectomy trends in the United States. Urology. 2018;118:76–9.

25. Potts JM, Pasqualotto FF, Nelson D, Thomas AJ Jr, Agarwal A. Patient characteristics associated with vasectomy reversal. J Urol. 1999;161(6):1835–9.

26. Sandlow JI, Westefeld JS, Maples MR, Scheel KR. Psychological correlates of vasectomy. Fertil Steril. 2001;75(3):544–8.

27. Sharlip ID, Belker AM, Honig S, Labrecque M, Marmar JL, Ross LS, Sandlow JI, Sokal DC. Vasectomy: AUA guideline. J Urol. 2012;188(6):2482–91.

28. Fowler GC. Chapter 111: Vasectomy. In: Pfenninger and Fowler's procedures for primary care fourth edition, E-book. Philadelphia: Elsevier Health Sciences; 2020.

29. Smith-Harrison LI, Smith RP. Vasectomy reversal for post-vasectomy pain syndrome. Transl Androl Urol. 2017;6(Suppl 1):S10.

Diane Holden and Paul Crawford

Contents

D. Holden
Nellis Family Medicine Residency, Las Vegas, NV, USA

P. Crawford (✉)
Department of Family Medicine, Uniformed Services
University of the Health Sciences, Bethesda, MD, USA
e-mail: paul.crawford@usuhs.edu

© Crown 2022
P. M. Paulman et al. (eds.), *Family Medicine*,
https://doi.org/10.1007/978-3-030-54441-6_107

Scrotal Mass

Some genitourinary (GU) disorders present as a scrotal mass and are commonly seen by family physicians for initial evaluation and management. These nontesticular masses include hydrocele, varicocele, indirect hernia, spermatocele, and epididymitis and testicular masses such as testicular cancer. A clinically useful distinction can be made between painful and painless scrotal masses. Although painless masses are not uniformly benign, painful masses are much more likely to require urgent intervention.

Normal testes are firm but not hard, nearly equal in size, smooth, and ovoid. Normal testicular length ranges from 1.5 to 2 cm before puberty and from 4 to 5 cm after puberty. The epididymis is posterolateral to the testicle; the epididymis and testicle are separate but attached. The vas deferens emanates from the tail of the epididymis and joins the vascular pedicle of the testicle to form the spermatic cord. The spermatic cord travels superiorly to the inguinal canal.

Nontesticular Masses

Hydrocele and Indirect Inguinal Hernia

Hydroceles can be differentiated from other testicular masses by transillumination of the fluid with a penlight. Patients with hydroceles also have a palpably normal spermatic cord and inguinal ring above the swollen area. In an upright position or during Valsalva maneuver, hernia and noncommunicating hydrocele enlarge. Scrotal ultrasonography may be helpful in making the diagnosis [1].

Hydroceles are caused by incomplete obliteration of the processus vaginalis allowing a collection of peritoneal fluid between the parietal and visceral layers of the tunica vaginalis surrounding the testicle. Communicating hydroceles have freely flowing fluid between the peritoneal cavity and the tunica vaginalis while noncommunicating hydroceles do not. Hydroceles occur more frequently on the right and are often bilateral [1, 2].

Pediatric hernias are present in 0.1–0.2% of live births. Risk factors include prematurity and low birth weight. Sudden presentation in an adult of a noncommunicating hydrocele may be secondary to torsion, neoplasm, injury, or infection. Adult hydroceles require no treatment unless they are uncomfortable [1].

Inguinal hernia and communicating hydrocele are indications for surgery in children.

Noncommunicating hydroceles often spontaneously close by 1–2 years of age and should not be repaired until that time. Repair by high ligation of the patent processus vaginalis is the same for both hydrocele and inguinal hernia.

Varicocele

A varicocele is a dilation of the venous pampiniform plexus of the spermatic cord, which coalesces into a single testicular vein. The majority are left sided resulting from higher pressures on the left compared to the right. Varicoceles are classically described as feeling like a bag of worms; this feeling increases with Valsalva maneuvers. Varicoceles occur in 15% of males and usually first appear in adolescence. There is conflicting evidence about the association between varicoceles and male infertility [1]. A meta-analysis of 12 randomized controlled trials found some increases in testicular volume and sperm concentration from surgical treatment of varicoceles in children and adolescents; however, long-term outcomes for paternity and fertility remain unknown [3]. Sudden adult left-sided varicocele may indicate renal tumor, and right-sided varicocele could indicate obstruction of the vena cava.

In adolescent boys, evaluation of testicular size is important to determine the need for surgical correction. Sonography, a comparative orchidometer, or punched-out elliptical rings can be used to determine size. A volume difference between the testicles of greater than 2 cm^3 is the minimal requirement for surgical repair (Figs. 1 and 2).

Spermatocele and Epididymal Cyst

A spermatocele or epididymal cyst presents as a painless mass superior and posterior to the testicle and is completely separate from the testicle (cysts of the rete testes, epididymis, or ductuli efferentes). Enlarged and symptomatic cysts should be removed.

Epididymitis

Epididymitis is the most common cause of scrotal pain in adults and is characterized by acute unilateral pain and swelling [1]. The pain usually begins at the epididymis and can spread to the

Fig. 1 Anatomy of scrotal contents

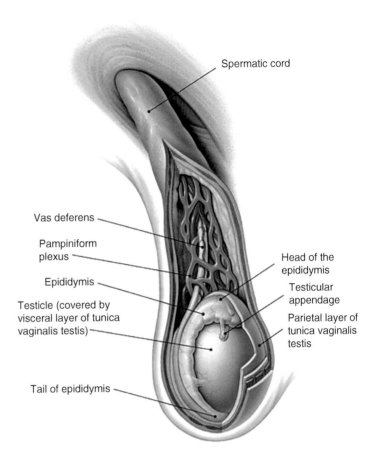

Spermatic cord

Vas deferens

Pampiniform plexus

Epididymis

Testicle (covered by visceral layer of tunica vaginalis testis)

Head of the epididymis

Testicular appendage

Parietal layer of tunica vaginalis testis

Tail of epididymis

entire testicle (epididymo-orchitis). Other symptoms include fever, erythema of the scrotal skin, and dysuria. It is associated with a C-reactive protein level of more than 24 mg per L (228.6 nmol per L) (96% sensitive and 85% specific for epididymitis/orchitis) [4] and increased blood flow on ultrasonography. *Chlamydia trachomatis* and *Neisseria gonorrhoeae* are the most common organisms responsible for bacterial epididymitis in males younger than 35 years [5]. Guidelines recommend empiric ceftriaxone (Rocephin) and doxycycline for treatment of suspected epididymitis in males younger than 35 years [6]. Epididymitis may cause a painful swelling of the testicle and is a common cause of a painful testicle in postpubertal males. Presentation is usually of increasing testicular pain and discomfort and can be accompanied by urethral discharge. On exam, the epididymis is enlarged and

may be indistinguishable from the testicle. The epididymis is tender and may be indurated [7].

Treatment should be directed at the most likely cause. For suspected UTI, levofloxacin (Levaquin) 500 mg orally twice daily for 10 days is usually adequate. In prepubertal boys, an evaluation of the GU system to include urinary system sonography and a voiding cystourethrogram should be considered.

Testicular Masses

Testicular Torsion

Testicular torsion or torsion of the testicular appendages presents as a painful testicle that is often enlarged or demonstrates a mass. These topics are covered in ▸ Chap. 104, "Surgery of the Male Genital Tract."

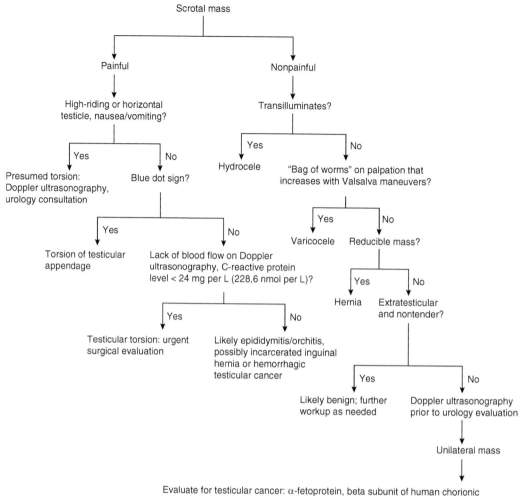

Fig. 2 Algorithm for evaluation of a scrotal mass

Acute Orchitis

Acute orchitis presents with sudden onset of testicular pain and high fever, usually with nausea and vomiting. On exam the testicle is tender, enlarged, and may be indurated. The most common causes are bacterial and viral infections. Mumps orchitis occurs in 20–35% of cases of mumps parotitis and presents 3–4 days after onset of parotid symptoms. Management of acute orchitis includes bed rest, scrotal support, ice, and analgesics. Antibiotics are important if a bacterial cause is suspected. Since only 15% of cases are bilateral, infertility is rare.

Testicular Cancer

Epidemiology and Risk Factors

Although only occurring in 6 out of 100,000 men annually in the United States, testicular cancer is the most common solid tumor among men between the ages of 20 and 34 years old and accounts for approximately 1% of all cancers in men [8, 11]. The most important risk factor for testicular cancer is cryptorchidism – 10% of cancer cases have a history of cryptorchidism. Cryptorchidism increases testicular cancer risk 3- to 17-fold. Early orchidopexy (before 1 year of age) reduces, but does not eliminate, this increased risk. Orchidopexy later in life is not as effective at reducing rates of cancer. Other risk factors include family history, infertility, tobacco use, white race, and a history of testicular cancer [9].

Screening

The US Preventive Services Task Force does not recommend screening for testicular cancer with either self- or physician examination [11].

Pathology

Germ cell tumors account for more than 90% of all testes tumors, the majority of which are classified as pure seminomas or nonseminomas. Most nonseminomatous germ cell tumors are composed of a combination of the following histological patterns: embryonal carcinoma, teratoma, teratocarcinoma, and choriocarcinoma [9].

The most common non-germ cell testicular tumors are Sertoli and Leydig cell tumors. The majority of these tumors are benign. Leydig cell tumors can present with sequelae of increased androgen production such as precocious puberty in boys and virilization in girls [9].

Diagnosis and Evaluation

Patients with testicular cancer are usually asymptomatic, but they may present with acute pain in the testicle or scrotum, dull ache in the scrotum or abdomen, scrotal heaviness, firmness of the testicle, infertility, intratesticular mass, or painless swelling/redness. Five percent of patients present with symptoms of metastasis to include gastrointestinal symptoms, gynecomastia, lumbar back pain, neck mass, and respiratory symptoms (e.g., cough, hemoptysis, dyspnea) [8].

All intratesticular masses should be considered a malignancy until proven otherwise. Patients with testicular masses should have a scrotal ultrasound to confirm the presence of a solid intratesticular mass and to evaluate the contralateral testicle. When cancer is a concern in a patient with a testicular mass, laboratory testing includes α-fetoprotein (AFP), beta subunit of human chorionic gonadotropin (β-HCG), and lactate dehydrogenase levels since >90% of patients with a

nonseminomatous germ cell tumor have elevated levels of one or all of these [8]. Urgent referral to a urologist is indicated for patients with intratesticular masses, even though smaller masses are less likely to be cancerous. Patients with intratesticular masses should generally undergo radical orchiectomy through an inguinal approach; however, there is some evidence that more conservative testicular sparing surgery may be curative, though it is generally not considered first-line treatment at this time. For small tumors, active surveillance is a recommended option in compliant patients who are amenable to frequent follow-up and monitoring [10]. There is no role for needle biopsy. Once diagnosed with a germ cell tumor, patients should be staged with an abdominal computed tomography (CT) scan and chest radiographs.

Treatment

Clinical stage and histology determine appropriate therapy. Typical chemotherapy agents include bleomycin (Blenoxane), etoposide (VePesid), cisplatin (Platinol AQ), EP (etoposide, cisplatin), and VIP (etoposide, ifosfamide (Ifex), cisplatin).

Seminoma [8, 9]

- Stage I – active surveillance is preferred; however, single-agent carboplatin or radiotherapy is an alternative.
- Stage IIA is treated with radiation to the regional lymph nodes; however, chemotherapy with four cycles of etoposide (EP) or three cycles of bleomycin (BEP) is an alternative.
- Stage IIB is treated with chemotherapy with four cycles of EP or three cycles of BEP; however, radiotherapy of regional lymph nodes is an alternative.
- Stage IIC is treated with chemotherapy with four cycles of EP or three cycles of BEP.
- Stage III is treated with four cycles of EP or three cycles of BEP.

Nonseminoma [8, 9]

- Stage IA – active surveillance is preferred; however, retroperitoneal lymph node dissection (RPLND) is an alternative.

- Stage IB – active surveillance is preferred; however, RPLND or one or two cycles of BEP are options.
- Stage IIA is treated with RPLND or chemotherapy with four cycles of EP or three cycles of BEP.
- Stage IIB is treated with chemotherapy with four cycles of EP or three cycles of BEP; RPLND can be considered in select cases.
- Stage IIC is treated with chemotherapy with four cycles of EP or three cycles of BEP.
- Stage IIIA is treated with chemotherapy with four cycles of EP or three cycles of BEP.
- Stage IIIB is treated with chemotherapy with four cycles of BEP.
- Stage IIIC is treated with chemotherapy with four cycles of BEP or VIP in select patients.

Complications of Treatment

Complications can result from chemotherapy, radiation, surgery, or the disease process. Chemotherapy-specific complications include azoospermia, lung disease (with bleomycin use), neuropathy (with etoposide use), renal or otologic injury (with cisplatin use), increased risk of cardiovascular disease, infertility, recurrence, cardiac mortality after radiation, and second malignancy (e.g., leukemia) after radiation or chemotherapy [8, 9].

Urothelial Tumors (Bladder Cancer)

Epidemiology and Risk Factors

Bladder cancer is the sixth most prevalent malignancy in the United States, accounting for approximately 7% of cancers in men and 3% of cancers in women. Annually in the United States, about 62,000 men and 19,000 women are diagnosed with this disease, while 18,000 die from it annually. The incidence of bladder cancer increases with age in men and women. Ninety percent of cases occur in those over 55 years of age [12].

The most significant risk factor for bladder cancer is cigarette smoking, which accounts for approximately 50% of all bladder cancer cases. It increases bladder cancer risk by four- to seven-fold. Other established risk factors include male sex, older age, white race, occupational exposure to certain chemicals, pelvic radiation, use of medications such as cyclophosphamide, chronic bladder infections/irritation, and personal or family history of bladder cancer. Bladder cancers may be associated with diabetes mellitus, obesity, and HPV [12]. The diabetes medication pioglitazone (Actos) has been independently associated with a slightly increased risk of bladder cancer.

Pathology

About 90% of bladder cancers diagnosed in the United States are urothelial, formerly known as transitional cell, carcinomas.

Squamous cell carcinoma accounts for about 7% of bladder cancers in the United States. Adenocarcinoma of the bladder is rare, accounting for fewer than 2% of all bladder cancers. Adenocarcinomas of the bladder are more common in patients with a urachal remnant or in patients who were born with bladder exstrophy [12]. In areas of the world with endemic schistosomiasis, squamous cell adenocarcinoma actually accounts for up to 81% of bladder cancers.

Location

About 96% of urothelial malignancies occur in the bladder. Upper tract (ureters and collecting system) tumors occur in 2–3% of patients with bladder tumors, while 30–75% of patients with upper tract tumors have associated bladder tumors. Bilateral involvement occurs in 2–5% of all patients with upper tract transitional cell carcinomas.

Screening

Screening for bladder cancer is not recommended [13].

Diagnosis and Staging

Painless hematuria is the most common presenting sign or symptom of bladder cancer. The incidence of bladder cancer in a patient with gross hematuria is 20% and with microscopic hematuria is 2% [12]. Other less common signs include urinary frequency, irritability, and dysuria. Although the vast majority of bladder cancers are associated with microscopic hematuria, the hematuria frequently is intermittent, and a negative urinalysis does not exclude bladder cancer. All patients with hematuria should be evaluated with a urine cytology, cystoscopy, intravenous, CT, or MRI. Those with gross hematuria should be further evaluated with a renal ultrasound or CT.

Urine cytology has a high sensitivity (>90%) for the detection of high-grade urothelial cancers; however, renal calculi and urinary tract infections can lead to false-positive results [12]. Urine cytology is a helpful adjunct for surveillance in those with known urothelial carcinoma and the evaluation of patients at high risk of urothelial tumors due to its positive predictive value.

Cystoscopy is the primary diagnostic tool for bladder cancer. Once a tumor is identified, transurethral resection is performed to confirm the diagnosis and to determine the tumor stage. The primary goal of staging is to determine if the cancer is superficial or invasive. TNM staging of bladder cancer is very complex with 14 types of T, 5 types of N, and 4 types of M. Since transurethral resection can frequently understage patients, frequently patients with high-grade Tl disease are treated as if they had muscle-invasive disease [12, 14].

CT examination of the abdomen and pelvis is obtained in patients with muscle-invasive bladder cancer (T2 or higher) and/or high-grade disease to evaluate the perivesical soft tissue, pelvic and retroperitoneal lymph nodes, as well as the liver and adrenal glands. CT scans are relatively unreliable in determining depth of tumor invasion and may fail to detect lymph node metastasis in up to 40% of patients with them [12].

CT, MRI, or intravenous urograms or retrograde ureteropyelograms should be obtained in all patients with bladder cancer to exclude the presence of an upper tract transitional cell carcinoma.

Treatment

Treatment of bladder cancer is different for each stage. Low-grade Ta through high-grade T1 cancer is generally treated with transurethral resection and intravesical *Bacillus Calmette-Guerin* (BCG) or mitomycin. T2a through T3b are treated with radical cystectomy and bilateral pelvic lymphadenectomy followed by either chemotherapy or adjuvant chemotherapy. T4a through metastatic disease is treated with chemotherapy alone or in combination with radiation therapy [12].

Urinary reconstruction following cystectomy is an important component in the management of patients with invasive bladder cancer. Various modalities to restore a semblance of normal urinary function using cutaneous diversions (both catheterizable and noncatheterizable) are in use currently. Other options in which a reservoir is connected directly to the native urethra lessen the impact of cystectomy on quality of life. These diversions can be performed successfully in men and women.

Additionally, radical cystectomy can preserve the neurovascular bundles in men and the vagina in women. Thus, normal urinary and sexual function can be retained despite curative therapy for invasive bladder cancer. Anastomotic strictures can be common, so patients must be followed closely for the development of hydronephrosis and deterioration of renal function.

Urolithiasis

Urolithiasis is common. Family physicians must distinguish it from other causes of abdominal and flank pain. Urolithiasis causes pain when a stone partially or completely obstructs the collecting system or ureter while it migrates. Distal ureteral stones may be associated with dysuria, frequency, and penile or labial pain, while stones in the renal collecting system may be painless. Classically, the patient presents with severe, colicky, unilateral flank, or lower abdominal pain. The pain may radiate to the groin, scrotum, or labia and be associated with nausea and vomiting, dysuria, gross hematuria, urinary frequency, or fever. Fever is present when associated with UTI. Conditions that may be similar to or mimic renal colic include pyelonephritis, urethritis, prostatitis, vaginitis, pelvic inflammatory disease, pelvic pain syndrome, gallbladder disease, various gastrointestinal diseases, dissecting abdominal aortic aneurysm, ovarian or testicular pathology, ectopic pregnancy, and ureteral tumors [15].

Table 1 Causes of urolithiasis [15–18]

Obesity	Hypomagnesuria
Diabetes	Hyperoxaluria
Hypercalciuria	Increased dietary fructose intake
Idiopathic (absorptive types I and II)	Medications and supplements
Renal	Allopurinol
Unclassified	Antibiotics (sulfonamides, ampicillin, amoxicillin, ceftriaxone (Rocephin), quinolones, furans, pyridines)
Primary hyperparathyroidism	Carbonic anhydrase inhibitors (acetazolamide, topiramate (Topamax))
Hyperuricosuria	Ephedra alkaloids
Cystinuria	HAART (highly active antiretroviral therapy)
Gouty crystal deposits	Laxatives
Stones secondary to urinary infection	Potassium channel blockers (amiodarone, sotalol)
Renal tubular acidosis type 1	Potassium-sparing diuretics (triamterene)
Hypocitraturia	Sulfonylureas

Epidemiology

Lifetime risk of developing urolithiasis is 10–15% with higher prevalence in the southeastern United States. It is two to three times more common in males than females and affects Caucasians more than Asians and Blacks. Incidence peaks between 30 and 50 years old, and recurrence rates are as high as 40–75% over 25 years. Frequency of different stone types varies greatly with the population studied. In the United States, calcium stones are by far the most common, with calcium oxalate stones accounting for 56–61% and calcium phosphate stones accounting for 8–18%. Less common (in descending order) are uric acid, magnesium ammonium phosphate (struvite), and cystine stones. Children have more struvite than uric acid stones [15, 16]. Chronic medical conditions can increase the risk of developing certain times of stones. For example, patients with Crohn's disease and ulcerative colitis, pancreatic insufficiency, and a history of bariatric surgery are more likely to develop calcium oxalate stones [19].

Etiology

In modern times, obesity and diabetes are common causes of urolithiasis. Other diseases such as primary hyperparathyroidism, type 1 renal tubular

acidosis (RTA), Crohn's disease, primary hyperoxaluria, and cystinuria are associated with recurrent urolithiasis but account for less than 5% of patients with stone disease. An etiology for urolithiasis can be determined 97% of the time after an appropriate workup. Etiologies of urolithiasis are listed in Table 1. Metabolic abnormalities account for the majority of disease. Sixty percent of calcium stone disease is caused by idiopathic hypercalciuria. Hyperuricosuria, followed by hypocitraturia and hyperoxaluria, is the next most common metabolic abnormality causing disease. Medications that may also play a role in stone disease are listed in the table. High dietary fructose intake is also associated with urolithiasis.

Evaluation

Family physicians must take a thorough history including presenting symptoms, medical history (e.g., gout, bowel disease), medications and supplements, diet, and family history of stone disease or related illnesses. Physical exam of the flank, abdomen, groin, and genitals is most useful, and physicians should use physical exam to rule out other possible diagnoses. Urinalysis with urinary pH and microscopic examination for red blood cells, white blood cells, and crystals should be performed [19]. Hematuria is 67% sensitive and 58% specific for urolithiasis. Presence of white blood cells or crystals can indicate concomitant infection or hyperuricemia. Urine culture should also be obtained to evaluate for infection.

Diagnostic imaging is the next step in evaluation. A prudent and safe first step is to perform an ultrasound of the kidney and collecting system. Patients with a positive ultrasound need not have a CT scan with its attendant radiation. Those with negative ultrasound should progress to unenhanced helical CT – with reported sensitivity of 95–100% and specificity of 94–96% in diagnosing urolithiasis. Advantages of this imaging technique include avoidance of intravenous contrast, short duration (approximately 5 min to perform), ability to visualize all stone types, localization of stone within the ureter, identification of secondary signs of obstruction when a stone has recently passed, and ability to diagnose other abdominal and pelvic pathology when urolithiasis is not present. Additionally, the use of CT scans allows for better quality imaging in obese patients and may be more available compared to ultrasound [19]. Using Hounsfield density helical CT allows one to differentiate uric acid, cystine, and calcium-containing stones from one another and to subtype calcium stones.

Plain radiography is only useful if other conditions are suspected as the cause of pain due to low sensitivity and specificity. Only calcium-containing stones are radiopaque, but this fact is complicated by the fact that calcifications seen on plain radiograph may or may not be associated with the urinary system.

Intravenous urography (IVU) is a less desirable option than ultrasound or CT scan. IVU can usually detect ureteral obstruction based on dilation of the collecting system or ureter, a delayed nephrogram, or delayed excretion of contrast. IVU is limited in that signs of obstruction may not appear acutely, radiolucent stones cannot be visualized, and many other causes of abdominal pain cannot be evaluated. Intravenous contrast is necessary when performing an IVU and can cause postcontrast nephropathy and numerous systemic reactions.

Approach to Management

Urolithiasis complicated by an infected stone and/or urosepsis is an emergency. Emergent urological consultation for either immediate drainage by percutaneous nephrostomy or retrograde ureteral stent insertion is necessary since these patients have a high mortality. Other indications for urgent urological consultation are anuria, bilateral obstruction, obstruction of a sole functioning kidney, hydronephrosis, concomitant pregnancy, and renal failure. Those patients with refractory pain as well as those with potential comorbidities such as arteriopathy or are older than age 60 should also be referred.

In the absence of these conditions, stone size and location determines the next step. Ureteral stones with a width 4 mm or less will spontaneously pass in 80% of patients, while rates fall to 35% at 5 mm and 25% at 7 mm. Patients with stones <5 mm in width should be provided adequate analgesia. Maintaining urine volumes greater than 2.5 L a day is essential [18]. Patients should be instructed to strain their urine and bring in any stones for analysis and should follow up immediately for symptoms of urosepsis. Stone passage may be monitored with plain radiographs and a urological referral made if stones are not passed within 4–6 weeks. At this time, patients with persistent stones are often offered either ureteroscopy to remove stones or extracorporeal shock wave lithotripsy (ESWL) to remove stones.

Antispasmodics

Calcium channel blockers and alpha blockers should be first-line therapy for urolithiasis. These medications not only reduce the pain from renal colic by reducing smooth muscle spasm in the ureter, they also reduce the time of passage of stones <10 mm by 5–7 days. Alpha blockers should be prescribed as follows: doxazosin (Cardura) 4 mg orally per day or tamsulosin (Flomax) 0.4 mg orally per day. If calcium channel blockers are chosen, then nifedipine (Procardia) 30 mg orally per day should be used.

Analgesia

Adequate pain control often requires a combination of nonsteroidal anti-inflammatory drugs (NSAIDs) and narcotics. As a note of caution, patients with reduced renal function should be prescribed NSAIDs only after the risks of further kidney damage are considered and discussed with patients [14]. Any NSAID is acceptable to treat urolithiasis for a short period. Long-term treatment entails more risk, and physicians should consider naproxen (Naprosyn) 500 mg twice daily due to its lower risk of thrombosis. NSAIDs must be held for 3 days prior to ESWL because of antiplatelet effects and risk of bleeding, and aspirin should be held for 7 days prior to ESWL.

Narcotics used for pain control include hydrocodone 5 or 10 mg with acetaminophen 325 mg (Vicodin 10/325) orally every 4–6 h as needed, oxycodone 5 mg with acetaminophen 325 mg (Percocet 5/325) orally every 4–6 h as needed, and codeine 30 mg with acetaminophen 300 mg (Tylenol with codeine No. 3) orally every 4–6 h as needed. An antiemetic such as promethazine (Phenergan) 25 mg orally or ondansetron (Zofran) every 6 h may also be helpful.

Surgical Management

Stone location and size are the primary determinants when choosing which procedure to use for stone removal. ESWL is minimally invasive and is effective for calculi <1 cm in the ureter and <2 cm in the kidney. Basket retrieval through a cystoscope or ureteroscope is indicated for lower ureteral stones not amenable to ESWL [14]. Larger stones may be treated with

percutaneous nephrolithotomy alone or in combination with ESWL [19]. All of these procedures carry minimal surgical risk, and analgesia with either NSAIDs or narcotics is appropriate post procedure. Staghorn renal calculi should always be treated because of their high complication rates. Asymptomatic renal stones do not require treatment but become symptomatic in 50% of patients over 5 years.

Metabolic Evaluation

All patients with stone disease should have a basic workup to identify underlying metabolic or environmental factors causing stone formation. A more in-depth workup should be completed in patients with recurrent urolithiasis.

Minimal evaluation should include urinalysis (including pH) with urine culture, stone analysis when possible, and serum calcium, phosphorus, uric acid, creatinine, and electrolytes. Table 2 shows stone analysis compared with diagnosis.

If no stone is available to analyze, a 24-h urine collection for a stone risk profile while the patient is on their customary diet should be performed. Expert consensus panels recommend this, but there are no trials to determine its effectiveness. The stone risk profile includes urine calcium, oxalate, uric acid, citrate, pH, total volume, sodium, sulfate, phosphorus, magnesium, and urinary saturation of calcium oxalate, brushite, monosodium urate, and uric acid. Once this is completed, dietary modifications to reduce abnormalities in the stone risk profile should be initiated with a

Table 2 Stone composition and diagnosis [14, 15, 17, 18]

Stone composition	Diagnosis
Cystine	Cystinuria
Struvite	Stone due to infection
Uric acid	Hyperuricosuria
	Low pH (gout, diarrhea)
Calcium phosphate	Primary hyperparathyroidism (increased calcium, low phosphorus)
	Renal tubular acidosis (hypokalemia and metabolic acidosis)
	Sodium alkali therapy

Table 3 Dietary changes in response to stone risk profile [14, 17, 18]

	Avoid tea, spinach, dark roughage, chocolate, and nuts
Urinary oxalate >45 mg per day	Take no more than 500 mg of vitamin C daily
Urinary calcium >250 mg per day	Moderate calcium restriction
Uric acid level > 700 mg per day	Restrict protein
Sulfate level > 30 mmol per day	Restrict protein
Low urine pH	Increase intake of potassium-rich citrus fruits
Low urine citrate	Increase intake of potassium-rich citrus fruits
Low urine pH	Increase intake of potassium-rich citrus fruits

concomitant increase in fluid intake to maintain a urine volume of >2.5 L a day. These dietary changes include a sodium restriction of 200 mEq daily for all patients. Other dietary changes are listed in Table 3.

After 1 week, the stone risk profile is repeated and the two completed stone profiles compared. If abnormalities are corrected by dietary modification and increased hydration, then environmental changes are recommended. If abnormalities persist, then appropriate treatment is initiated.

Treatment

In spite of poor evidence, all patients should be told to drink a minimum of 2 L of fluid a day, eat a diet high in potassium-rich citrus fruits, and restrict intake of protein, oxalate, and sodium.

Hyperoxaluria

Non-dietary hyperoxaluria (>45 mg per day) is seen with inflammatory bowel disease, small bowel resection, and intestinal malabsorption of fat. Dietary restriction of oxalate is the main form of treatment. Patients should be counseled to limit intake of oxalate-rich foods and maintain normal calcium consumption [18].

Hypercalciuria

Patients with hypercalciuria (>250 mg per day) associated with hypercalcemia should be evaluated for primary hyperparathyroidism. When hypercalciuria is seen with excess urinary sodium, dietary restriction of sodium 100 mEq per day is recommended. Absorptive hypercalciuria and renal hypercalciuria are the probable causes when the abovementioned conditions are not present. Both can be treated with thiazides such as hydrochlorothiazide 25 mg daily with potassium citrate 20 mEq twice daily. Doses of potassium citrate may be adjusted based on follow-up serum potassium and urinary citrate levels.

Hypocitraturia

High intake of animal proteins is the usual cause of mild to moderate hypocitraturia (100–320 mg per day). It is best treated with potassium citrate 20 mEq twice daily and restriction of animal protein. Chronic diarrhea and renal tubular acidosis (RTA) cause severe hypocitraturia (<100 mg per day). When diarrhea is present, treatment is directed at the diarrhea. Potassium citrate 20–40 mEq twice daily may be given.

Hyperuricosuria

Excess intake of purines causes hyperuricosuria (>700 mg per day) without elevated serum uric acid. Allopurinol (Zyloprim) 300 mg daily and potassium citrate can prevent further stones in combination with dietary restrictions. When hyperuricosuria is found in combination with elevated uric acid and low urinary pH, gout is present. Allopurinol 300 mg daily, along with potassium citrate if urinary pH is low, is recommended. Limitation of non-dairy animal protein may help reduce stone recurrence as well [18].

Prevention of Urolithiasis

There is a poor evidence base for practice patterns to prevent urolithiasis. Regardless, consensus guidelines recommend hydration, dietary therapy, use of potassium citrate, and thiazide diuretics to prevent recurrence in spite of potential adverse effects [15]. Medications used for stone prevention may cause adverse side effects, so periodic monitoring of blood work is recommended [18].

References

1. Crawford P, Crop JA. Evaluation of scrotal masses. Am Fam Physician. 2014;89(9):723–7.

2. Shakiba B, Heidari K, Jamali A, Afshar K. Aspiration and sclerotherapy versus hydrocoelectomy for treating hydrocoeles. Cochrane Database Syst Rev. 2014;11: CD009735.

3. Silay MS, Hoen L, Quadackaers J, et al. Treatment of varicocele in children and adolescents: a systematic review and meta-analysis from the European Association of Urology/European Society for Paediatric Urology Guidelines Panel. Eur Urol. 2019;75 (3):448–61.

4. McConaghy JR, Panchal B. Epididymitis: an overview. Am Fam Physician. 2016;94(9):723–6.

5. Asgari SA, Mokhtari G, Falahatkar S, et al. Diagnostic accuracy of C-reactive protein and erythrocyte sedimentation rate in patients with acute scrotum. Urol J. 2006;3(2):104–8.

6. Centers for Disease Control and Prevention. Sexually transmitted diseases treatment guidelines, 2015.

7. Tracy CR, Steers WD, Costabile R. Diagnosis and management of epididymitis. Urol Clin North Am. 2008;35(1):101–8.

8. Baird DC, Meyers GJ. Testicular cancer: diagnosis and treatment. Am Fam Physician. 2018;97(4):261–8.

9. Hanna NH, Einhorn LH. Testicular cancer–discoveries and updates. N Engl J Med. 2014;371(21):2005–16.

10. Pozza C, Pofi R, Tenuta M, et al. Clinical presentation, management and follow-up of 83 patients with Leydig cell tumors of the testis: a prospective case-cohort study. Hum Reprod. 2019;34(8):1389–403.

11. National Cancer Institute. Testicular cancer screening (PDQ). Health professional version. Bethesda: National Cancer Institute; 2020.

12. DeGeorge KC, Holt HR, Hodges SC. Bladder cancer: diagnosis and treatment. Am Fam Physician. 2017;96 (8):507–14.

13. Preventive Services US. Task Force. Screening for bladder cancer: recommendation statement. Am Fam Physician. 2012;85(4):397–9.

14. Arcangeli G, Arcangeli S, Strigari L. A systematic review and meta-analysis of clinical trials of bladder-sparing trimodality treatment for muscle-invasive bladder cancer (MIBC). Crit Rev Oncol Hematol. 2014; pii: S1040–8428(14)00194–2.

15. Fontenelle L, Sarti T. Kidney stones: treatment and prevention. Am Fam Physician. 2019;99(8):490–6.

16. Guirguis-Blake J. Preventing recurrent nephrolithiasis in adults. Am Fam Physician. 2014;89(6):461–3.

17. Smith-Bindman R, Aubin C, Bailitz J, et al. Ultrasonography versus computed tomography for suspected nephrolithiasis. N Engl J Med. 2014;371(12):1100–10.

18. Pearle MS, Goldfarb DS, Assimos DG, et al. Medical management of kidney stones: AUA guideline. J Urol. 2014;192(2):316–24. https://doi.org/10.1016/j. juro.2014.05.006.

19. Ingimarsson JP, Krambeck AE, Pais VM. Diagnosis and management of nephrolithiasis. Surg Clin N Am. 2016;96(3):517–32. https://doi.org/10.1016/j. suc.2016.02.008.

Part XXI

The Female Reproductive System and Women's Health

Family Planning, Birth Control, and Contraception

Melanie Menning and Peter Schindler

Contents

M. Menning (✉) · P. Schindler
Department of Family Medicine, University of Nebraska
Medical Center, Omaha, NE, USA
e-mail: melanie.menning@unmc.edu;
peter.schindler@unmc.edu

Before discussing family planning, birth control, and contraception, it is crucial to define the terms. Family planning/birth control are contraceptive methods, treatment of infertility, procedures, devices, and behaviors that allow people to obtain their desired number of children and determine the spacing of pregnancies. Contraception is a

© Springer Nature Switzerland AG 2022
P. M. Paulman et al. (eds.), *Family Medicine*,
https://doi.org/10.1007/978-3-030-54441-6_144

subset of family planning/birth control, defined as the intentional use of artificial methods or other practices to prevent pregnancy. The primary forms of contraception are a barrier method, hormonal, nonhormonal IUD, and sterilization.

Contraceptive Use in the United States

As of 2017, there are 72.2 million US women of reproductive age, defined as women aged 15–49, who are using contraception [1]. The most common methods in decreasing order are female sterilization, oral contraception pills, long-acting reversible contraceptives (LARCs), and male condoms [1]. Despite the popularity of modern contraceptive methods, 10% of women of reproductive age are not currently using a contraceptive method to prevent unwanted pregnancy [1]. There are a variety of reasons for not using a contraceptive/ family planning method. Often religion is cited as the principal reason for not using a contraceptive method. Research suggests that many women, regardless of religious affiliation, will use a contraceptive method other than natural family planning in their lifetime [2]. The usage rates are significant because, in general, couples who do not use any method of contraception or birth control have approximately an 85% chance of becoming pregnant over a year [3]. Putting this in perspective, in the United States, the average desired family size is two children [4]. To be able to keep a family size at two or less, a woman must use contraception or birth control/family planning for at least three decades [4].

Women aged 15–19 (18%) have the highest risk of becoming pregnant. The lowest risk group is women aged 40–44 (9%) [2]. Contraceptive use does vary by race and ethnicity. Of women that are of reproductive age, 83% of black women at risk of unintended pregnancy are currently using a contraceptive method. Roughly 90–91% of white, Hispanic, and Asian women are presently using a reliable form of contraception [2]. Another vital aspect to take into consideration is socioeconomic status. About 8% of women living greater than 300% below the poverty line are not currently using a contraceptive method [2]. At a global level, preventing unwanted pregnancies has been a UN Millennium development goal for quite some time. Understanding the basic uptake of contraceptive methods in the USA is essential when considering who is at the greatest risk of unintended pregnancy. In general, understanding local and regional beliefs surrounding contraception and family planning/birth control can aid in providing the most pertinent medical advice and help in dispelling myths and misperceptions of contraceptive methods.

What Are the Most Popular Contraceptive Methods?

In general, the uptake of contraceptive methods is highest among older women and non-Hispanic white women when compared with younger women and non-Hispanic black women [1]. Most (72%) women who use contraception are currently using reversible forms of contraception. Most forms are primarily hormonal methods, such as the pill, implant, patch injectables, vaginal ring, IUDs, and condoms [5]. A minority of women and their partners (28%) rely on permanent methods such as sterilization [5]. Within sterilization, women are more likely than men to have a sterilization procedure performed despite the more invasive nature of the procedure when performed on women. Female sterilization usage is not uniform among subgroups of women. Sterilization is most prevalent among: African Americans and Hispanics, women over the age of 35, women who have birthed more than two children, women living in poverty, women living in rural areas, women who have not attended education at the university level, and women with no health insurance [2].

There are some commonalities among women who most commonly use an IUD or implant. This particular subset of women tends to be 25–34-year-old, born outside of the USA, currently reside in the western region of the USA, and self-described as "other" to a religious group [6]. Women are more likely to choose a long-acting reversible contraceptive method (LARC) if they have had a child or have used a non-LARC hormonal method in the past [6].

Another extremely common contraceptive method is the male condom. Almost six million women list the male condom as the only form of contraception they use. There are known sociodemographic characteristics of individuals who are more likely to use the male condom: Individuals who are between 15 and 19 years of age, uninsured persons, those educated at the university level, and those who have never had a child or are expecting at least one (more) child [5]. While condoms alone are not an effective form of contraception, dual method use (barrier method combined with another form of contraception) offers protection against both pregnancy and STIs. However, only about 8% of women of reproductive age concurrently use multiple contraceptive methods [7].

Teen Contraceptive Use

Preventing unintended pregnancy among teenagers is a way to help avoid the intergenerational perpetuation of poverty [8]. Eighty-two percent of women between the ages of 15 and 19 are using a contraceptive method. Of the 82% of women, 59% were using a highly effective method such as hormonal contraception or IUDs [9]. More specifically, the most common forms of contraception among teenagers are the male condom, combined contraceptive pills, withdrawal technique, injectable hormonal contraception, patch or ring, and the IUD [10, 11]. Most teenagers tend to use a form of contraception when initiating sexual intercourse for the first time [9]. Using some form of contraceptive is especially important as the likelihood of giving birth before age 20 was twice as high for teenage women who had not used a contraceptive method at the time, they initiated sexual intercourse when compared to women who had [9]. Concerning dual methods, the most recent data available show about one fifth of sexually active females aged 15–19 and one-third males the same age report having used both the male condom and a hormonal method the last time they had sex [9].

Provider Tools

CDC- US MEC

There are a wide variety of provider resources available. The most comprehensive tool available is the CDC US Medical Eligibility Criteria (US MEC) for contraceptive use, 2016. The resource provides general recommendations regarding particular contraceptive methods for men and women. The resource is comprehensive and contains recommendations for specific health conditions such as multiple sclerosis and also discusses subpopulations of people such as postpartum or HIV positive individuals on antiretroviral therapy.

WHO Medical Eligibility Criteria for Contraceptive Use

The WHO Medical Eligibility criteria for contraceptive use is another comprehensive guide intended to improve the quality of care in family planning. The document can be found on the WHO website and is downloadable. There is also a free mobile app available. The WHO medical eligibility guide tends to have much of the same types of information as the CDC US medical eligibility guide with additional provider tools such as the "medical eligibility wheel for contraceptive use."

The Family Planning National Training Center (FPNTC)

The goal of the FPNTC is to ensure those who work in the area of family planning have the skills and knowledge necessary to provide comprehensive family planning care. The FPNTC collaborates closely with the National Clinical Training Center for Family Planning (CTCFP) at the University of Missouri-Kansas City, which delivers clinical skills training and resources to health care providers in the Tile X and related public health communities' mainly Planning National Training Center (FPNTC)

Association of State and Territorial Health Officials (ASTHO)1

Per the organization's website, ASTHO is a national not-for-profit organization representing public health agencies across the USA and US territories. The organization exists mainly to track, evaluate, and advise members of public health about health policy. The organization specifically provides guidance and strategies for implementing LARCs at the provider level.

Non-English Resources for Patients

The US National Library of Medicine (MedlinePlus) contains many family planning/contraceptive handouts in multiple languages such as Burmese, Chinese: Mandarin and Cantonese, Dari, Farsi, Hindi, Hmong, Karen, Kinyarwanda, Nepali, Pashto, Portuguese, Russian, Spanish, Tagalong, and Vietnamese. Topics range from Vasectomy care to emergency contraceptive counseling. For those who care for diverse populations with family planning needs, this is considered an essential resource.

Long-Acting Reversible Contraceptives (LARC)

Long-acting reversible contraceptives (LARC) are a variety of contraceptive methods that are effective at preventing pregnancy for a prolonged period without requiring any user maintenance. Types of LARCs include subdermal contraceptive implants, IUDs, and injections. LARCs do not rely on patient compliance; therefore, their typical and actual failure rates are identical (Less than 1%). In general, LARCs have higher efficacy, higher continuation rates, and higher satisfaction rates compared with short-acting contraceptives among adolescents and adults who choose to use them [12–14].

Intrauterine Device (IUD)

Mechanism of action: The IUD is a T-shaped device that is inserted into the uterus. Its main mechanisms of action are to (1) irritate the uterine lining, (2) impairs sperm motility, (3) interfere with fertilization, and (4) inhibit implantation. There are two main types of IUDs available on the US market, progesterone containing (hormone) IUDs and a copper-containing IUD (non-hormonal). Progesterone containing IUDs release low levels of progesterone, which results in thickened cervical mucus, further inhibiting sperm motility. Also, the progestins themselves may impair fertilization. Concerning copper-containing IUDs, the copper ion itself is toxic to human spermatozoa and human ova. The copper IUD also enhances inflammatory responses, which are harmful to spermatocytes and oocytes.

One example of a hormonal IUD is the Levorgestril (LNG) containing Mirena IUD. Levonorgestrel is a potent progestin. It applies a significant effect on human cervical mucus, thickening enough for the mucus to act as a spermicidal barrier. Thick cervical mucus directly inhibits sperm capacitation, which effectively prevents conception. The levonorgestrel also causes atrophy of the endometrium. A sequela of the atrophic endometrium is that leads to a dramatic reduction of menstrual flow.

Availability: There are Five IUDs available in the United States [15]. The copper-containing IUD and four levonorgestrel-releasing IUDs. The LNG containing IUDs range from a total of 13.5 mg to 52 mg levonorgestrel.

Effectiveness: IUDs are incredibly effective; less than 1% of women become pregnant in the first year of having an IUD [3]. IUDs can be used by women of all ages, including adolescents, and by parous and nulliparous women. One crucial educational point for patients is that IUDs do not protect against sexually transmitted infections (STI). IUDs, combined with a barrier method, are an effective combination for preventing pregnancy and STIs.

Contraindications: Pregnancy, puerperal sepsis, immediate placement after septic abortion, distorted uterine cavity, cervical or endometrial cancer (awaiting treatment), gestational trophoblastic disease, breast cancer (progestin IUD only), AIDS not on antiretroviral therapy, pelvic tuberculosis, and unexplained vaginal bleeding

Subdermal Contraceptive Implant

Mechanism of action: The subdermal contraceptive implants are typically a small single etonogestrel-containing rod inserted in the medial aspect of the arm. The implant's main mechanism of action is to inhibit ovulation. A secondary mechanism is an increase in cervical mucus viscosity, which inhibits sperm penetration.

Availability: There is one implant (Nexplanon) currently available in the USA.

Effectiveness: The subdermal implant is highly effective. In some cases, the Nexplanon is more effective than sterilization [12]. Less than 1% of women in the first year of use will become pregnant [3]. Since it is considered a LARC method, the typical and actual use rate is identical. Women of all ages can use the implant. One crucial educational point for patients is that subdermal implants do not protect against STIs. Implants combined with a barrier method are an effective combo for preventing pregnancy and STIs.

Contraindications

Relatively few. There are a few contraindications, such as severe rheumatologic conditions and current pregnancy. Consult provider resources for more in-depth information.

Other Considerations

If a woman desires the implant and it has been greater than 5 days since the initiation of her menstrual period, she must use a backup form of contraception for 7 days or abstain from sexual intercourse for 7 days [16]. After 7 days, if a pregnancy test is negative, then the implant may be placed. If it has less than 5 days since the initiation of the menstrual period, then no additional contraceptive protection is needed.

Injectables

Mechanism of action: Slow-release, medroxyprogesterone acetate (DMPA). One slow-release, 150 mg IM dose of DMPA, is given every 3 months. Contraceptive mechanisms of action for DMPA include ovulation suppression, thickening of the cervical mucus that blocks sperm motility, and endometrial changes that impede/prevent implantation [17].

Availability: One slow-release, 150 mg IM dose of DMPA given every 3 months. DMPA is also available in a micronized formulation for subcutaneous administration every 12 weeks. The subcutaneous preparation delivers a 30% lower total dose (104 mg) than the IM preparation but may suppress ovulation for at least 13 weeks, without being affected by body mass [18].

Effectiveness: DMPA is highly effective and generally well-tolerated contraceptives. For DMPA, cumulative pregnancy rates of 0.1–0.7% have been reported at 1 year [19], 0.4% at 2 years [19].

Other considerations: Bleeding pattern changes occur in between 20% and 40% of DMPA users [20] Approximately 50% of women using DMPA discontinue use by 1 year, primarily because of altered bleeding patterns [20]. Amenorrhea is 21% more likely to occur in women using DPMA [21]. Weight gain of up to 2–3 kg over 1 year has been reported with the use of these contraceptives in clinical trials [22]. Progestogen-only injectable contraceptives are associated with a delay of up to 1 year in the return to fertility after discontinuing use [23].

Data associating a reduction in bone mineral density (BMD) with progestogen-only injectable contraceptives are equivocal. Progestogen-only injectable contraceptives are associated with reduced BMD, but since the "fracture threshold" is not breached, an increased risk for fracture has yet to be demonstrated [24]. BMD normalizes after study drug discontinuation, although a concern in adolescents is that peak bone mass is never reached.

There is a possible etiological association between highly effective contraceptives such as DMPA and the risk of acquiring sexually transmitted infections, including HIV. DMPA does not appear to increase HIV risk among women in the general population, although further investigation is needed to verify this finding [25, 26]. Findings from a recent randomized study suggest an association between exposure to DMPA and the risk of

HIV disease progression, which also urgently requires additional research [26].

Emergency Contraception

Mechanism of action: Emergency contraception is a way to prevent pregnancy after unprotected sex or contraceptive failure; it does not affect an established pregnancy [27]. The majority of dedicated emergency contraceptive products currently on the market are effective when taken within 72 h of unprotected sex (although they are decreasingly effective for up to 5 days after unprotected sex). Nonhormonal copper IUDs inserted up to 5 days after unprotected intercourse can also act as emergency contraception [27].

Availability: There are several products available in the USA, levonorgestrel and ulipristal acetate.

Effectiveness: Levonorgestrel must be taken within 72 h, and ulipristal acetate must be taken within 120 h. The effectiveness of the regimens varies among the method used. Levonorgestrel, for example, about 13 out of 100 women will still become pregnant after taking the pills [3]. On the other hand, ulipristal acetate, about six or out of every 100 women, may become pregnant after taking the pills [3]. The copper IUD is the most effective emergency contraceptive method. One out of 1000 women who use a copper IUD may become pregnant [3].

Combined Hormonal Contraceptives

Mechanism of action: Combined hormonal contraceptives (CHCs) include low-dose estrogen combined oral contraceptives (COCs), the combined hormonal patch, and the combined vaginal ring. The mechanism of action for the combined hormonal contraceptives is generally: ovulation suppression via estrogen and cervical mucus thickening, and endometrial thinning via progestin.

Other considerations: CHCs do not protect against sexually transmitted infections. Certain medications may affect the efficacy of combined hormonal contraceptives. Medications such as rifampin, anticonvulsants, HIV medications, and supplements can lower the efficacy of CHCs.

Vaginal ring: There are two vaginal rings available in the USA currently. The etonogestrel and ethynyl estradiol ring and the segesterone and ethynyl estradiol ring. The rings are very similar in size flexibility and shape but vary in the number of hormones and duration of use. The etonogestrel and ethynyl estradiol ring is a flexible ring that is inserted into the vagina and kept in place for 21 days. Then removed for 7 days for a withdrawal bleed. A new ring is inserted every month. The segesterone and ethynyl estradiol is a ring that is kept in place for 21 days then removed for 7 days. The main difference between the etonogestrel and segesterone ring is that the segesterone ring is not discarded after 21 days. A single Segerterone ring has been approved for 1 year. The contraceptive mechanism of action of the vaginal ring is primarily ovulation suppression [28]. Secondary mechanisms of action are likely cervical mucus thickening and endometrial thinning [28].

Effectiveness: The vaginal ring is not as effective as IUDs and the implant. Failure rates are overall low and very similar to the patch and COCs [29]. With typical use, about nine out of 100 women who use this method may become pregnant [3].

Hormonal patch: There are two formulations of the contraceptive patch available in the USA: The Ethinyl estradiol and norelgestromin patch: releases 25 mcg of EE and 150 norelgestromin and Ethinyl estradiol and levonorgestrel: releases 30 mcg of EE and 125 mcg of LNG per day.

The patch is changed once per week for 3 weeks (21 total days), followed by one patch-free week (7 days) [30, 31]. The patch is most effective if there is no more than a 7-day patch-free interval. The patch should always be changed/applied on the same day of the week (e.g., Sundays for Sunday start).

Effectiveness: The hormonal patch is a highly effective method; about one out of 100 women may become pregnant with perfect use. About nine out of 100 may become pregnant with typical use [3].

Other considerations: There was a theoretical concern regarding body weight and hormonal patch effectiveness. Studies show that BMI does not seem to affect the efficacy of the hormonal patch [32].

Oral contraceptive pill: Mechanism of action is the suppression of ovulation by inhibition of gonadotropin-releasing hormone (GnRH), Luteinizing hormone (LH), and follicle-stimulating hormone (FSH), and the mid-cycle LH surge. Both the progestin and estrogen hormones present in the combined oral contraceptives work together. Estrogen primarily suppresses FSH and subsequently prevents folliculogenesis. The progestin-related mechanisms are responsible for effects on the endometrium, such as thinning of the endometrial lining and thickening of the cervical mucus.

Effectiveness: With typical use, nine out of 100 women may become pregnant. With perfect use, the oral contraceptive pill is over 99% effective [3].

Other considerations: The most common adverse effect of combined oral contraceptive pills is breakthrough bleeding. Occasionally women may experience headaches, abdominal cramping, nausea, breast tenderness, and an increase in vaginal discharge or decreased libido. Most of the side effects can be relieved by switching to a different combined oral contraceptive formulation.

General Guidelines for Combined Hormonal Contraceptives

The combined hormonal contraceptives have some general principles when it comes to selecting candidates. Typically, the general guidelines hold for any form of contraception that uses estrogen and progestin as the two primary hormones. If a woman is over the age of 35 and smokes about a half a pack a day, has risk factors for arterial cardiovascular disease, hypertension (over 160 systolic, history of venous thromboembolism, not on anticoagulation), known ischemic heart disease, history of stroke, complicated valvular heart disease, current

breast cancer, decompensated cirrhosis, hepatocellular adenoma or malignant hepatoma, migraine with aura, and diabetes of over 20-year duration or with complications with the disease such as nephropathy, retinopathy, or neuropathy other forms of contraception should be considered.

Barrier Methods

There are several barrier methods available; the male condom, female condom, diaphragm, cervical cap, spermicide sponge.

Mechanism of action: Prevent sperm from coming into contact with a woman's egg. Some barrier methods also protect against sexually transmitted infections.

Effectiveness: In general, barrier methods are not a very effective way of preventing pregnancy. About 20 women out of 100 may become pregnant when using barrier methods [3].

Condoms: Male and Female

Condoms create a physical barrier that can protect the user from STIs as well as prevent pregnancy. There are two main types of condoms available: male and female condoms. The male condom is a thin sheath worn over the penis during sexual intercourse. The female condom is a thin plastic pouch that lines the vagina. Latex and polyurethane condoms appear to provide the best protection against sexually transmitted infections. All condoms are single-use. 18 out of 100 women may become pregnant over the course of the year with the use of condoms as the primary contraceptive method [3].

Diaphragm and Cervical Cap

The diaphragm is a small, dome-shaped device made of silicone or latex that fits inside the vagina and covers the cervix. It typically is used with a spermicide. The diaphragm must remain in place for 6 h after sex, but not more than 24 h total. The cervical cap is a small plastic dome that fits tightly over the cervix and stays in place by suction. It must also be used with spermicide. Like the diaphragm, the cap must be left in place for at least

6 h after intercourse. About 12% of nonpariuous women and 25% of multiparious women may become pregnant with the diarpham and cervical cap methods [3].

Spermicides

Mechanism of action: Spermicides are chemical compounds that kill sperm on contact. There is only one type of spermicide available in the USA, Nonoxynol-9 (N-9). There are a variety of formulations of N-9 such as a cream, foam, jelly, tablet, suppository, or film. The primary mechanism of action to prevent pregnancy is by stopping and killing sperm before they can reach an egg and fertilize it. Spermicides are typically used in combination with other barrier methods. If used, the spermicide should remain in the vagina at least 6 h after sex.

Effectiveness: Roughly 20–28 out of 100 women each year who use spermicides alone for birth control may become pregnant [3].

Permanent Contraceptive Methods: Tubal Sterilization and Vasectomy

Tubal sterilization and vasectomy for men are highly effective, safe, and permanent methods. The tubal sterilization methods will generally need to be performed in an operating room under anesthesia. Tubal sterilization can be performed postpartum either immediately after a c-section or vaginal delivery or scheduled as an outpatient procedure. The vasectomy can be done as an office procedure under local sedation if necessary. Generally, there are very few contraindications for tubal sterilization and vasectomy. The sterilization methods are intended to be irreversible. Most people who choose sterilization are satisfied with their decision. There is a small proportion of women who regret a tubal sterilization procedure. Among men, there also is a small percentage that does experience regret as well [33]. It is essential that men and women receive appropriate consulting about the permanency of sterilization, including the risks, benefits, and alternatives.

Natural Family Planning

Natural family planning mainly consists of fertility based methods (FAB) to identify the fertile days of the menstrual cycle. This can be done by observing fertility signs such as cervical secretions, and basal body temperature or by monitoring cycle days. The FAB methods can be used alone or in combination with barrier methods.

Effectiveness: It is unclear how effective natural family planning is. The comparative efficacy of fertility awareness-based methods remains unknown [34].

References

1. Daniels K, Abma JC. Current contraceptive status among women aged 15–49: United States, 2015–2017. NCHS data brief, no 327. Hyattsville: National Center for Health Statistics; 2018.
2. Jones RK, Dreweke J. Countering conventional wisdom: new evidence on religion and contraceptive use. New York: Guttmacher Institute; 2011.
3. Hatcher RA et al., eds. Contraceptive technology. 20th revised ed. New York: Ardent Media; 2011.
4. Sonfield A, Hasstedt K, Gold RB. Moving forward: family planning in the era of health reform. New York: Guttmacher Institute; 2014.
5. Kavanaugh ML, Jerman J. Contraceptive method use in the United States: trends and characteristics between 2008 and 2014. Contraception. 2018;97(1):14–21. https://doi.org/10.1016/j.contraception.2017.10.003.
6. Kavanaugh ML, Jerman J, Finer LB. Changes in use of long-acting reversible contraceptive methods among U.S. women, 2009–2012. Obstet Gynecol. 2015;126 (5):917–27.
7. Sonfield A. Why family planning policy and practice must guarantee a true choice of contraceptive methods. Guttmacher Policy Rev. 2017;20:103–7.
8. Meade CS, Kershaw TS, Ickovics JR. The intergenerational cycle of teenage motherhood: an ecological approach. Health Psychol. 2008;27(4):419.
9. Martinez G, Copen CE, Abma JC. Teenagers in the United States: sexual activity, contraceptive use, and childbearing, 2006–2010. Vital Health Stat 23. 2011;31:1–35.
10. Special tabulations of data from Daniels K et al., Current contraceptive use and variation by selected characteristics among women aged 15–44: United States, 2011–2013. Natl Health Stat Report 2015, 86: 1–14.
11. Lindberg L, Santelli J, Desai S. Understanding the decline in adolescent fertility in the United States, 2007–2012. J Adolesc Health. 2016;59(5):577–83. https://doi.org/10.1016/j.jadohealth.2016.06.024.

12. Stoddard A, McNicholas C, Peipert JF. Efficacy and safety of long-acting reversible contraception. Drugs. 2011;71(8):969–80. https://doi.org/10.2165/11591290-000000000-00000.

13. Coles MS, Mays A. Addressing IUD efficacy, eligibility, myths, and satisfaction with adolescents and young adults. In: Optimizing IUD delivery for adolescents and young adults. Cham: Springer; 2019. p. 41–54.

14. Apter D. Contraception options: aspects unique to adolescent and young adult. Best Pract Res Clin Obstet Gynaecol. 2018;48:115–27.

15. Friedman J, Oluronbi RA. Types of IUDs and mechanism of action. In: Optimizing IUD delivery for adolescents and young adults. Cham: Springer; 2019. p. 29–39.

16. Palomba S, Falbo A, Di Cello A, Materazzo C, Zullo F. Nexplanon: the new implant for long-term contraception. A comprehensive descriptive review. Gynecol Endocrinol. 2012;28(9):710–21.

17. Mishell JD. Pharmacokinetics of depot medroxyprogesterone acetate contraception. J Reprod Med. 1996;41(5 Suppl):381–90.

18. Jain J, Dutton C, Nicosia A, Wajszczuk C, Bode FR, Mishell DR Jr. Pharmacokinetics, ovulation suppression and return to ovulation following a lower dose subcutaneous formulation of Depo-Provera®. Contraception. 2004;70(1):11–8.

19. Itriyeva K. Use of long-acting reversible contraception (LARC) and the Depo-Provera shot in adolescents. Curr Probl Pediatr Adolesc Health Care. 2018;48(12):321–32.

20. Zigler RE, McNicholas C. Unscheduled vaginal bleeding with progestin-only contraceptive use. Am J Obstet Gynecol. 2017;216(5):443–50.

21. Draper BH, Morroni C, Hoffman M, Smit J, Beksinska M, Hapgood J, Van der Merwe L. Depot medroxyprogesterone versus norethisterone oenanthate for long-acting progestogenic contraception. Cochrane Database Syst Rev. 2006;3:CD005214.

22. Gallo MF, Lopez LM, Grimes DA, Carayon F, Schulz KF, Helmerhorst FM. Combination contraceptives: effects on weight. Cochrane Database Syst Rev. 2014;1:CD003987.

23. Allen RH, Cwiak C, Kaunitz AM. Progestin injectable contraceptives. In: The handbook of contraception. Cham: Humana Press; 2016. p. 125–38.

24. Lopez LM, Grimes DA, Schulz KF, Curtis KM. Steroidal contraceptives: effect on bone fractures in women. Cochrane Database Syst Rev. 2009;2: CD006033.

25. Morrison CS, Turner AN, Jones LB. Highly effective contraception and acquisition of HIV and other sexually transmitted infections. Best Pract Res Clin Obstet Gynaecol. 2009;23(2):263–84.

26. Stringer EM, Levy J, Sinkala M, Chi BH, Matongo I, Chintu N, Stringer JS. HIV disease progression by hormonal contraceptive method: secondary analysis of a randomized trial. AIDS (London, England). 2009;23(11):1377.

27. Black KI, Hussainy SY. Emergency contraception: oral and intrauterine options. Aust Fam Physician. 2017;46(10):722.

28. Duijkers IJ, Klipping C, Verhoeven CH, Dieben TO. Ovarian function with the contraceptive vaginal ring or an oral contraceptive: a randomized study. Hum Reprod. 2004;19(11):2668–73.

29. Oddsson K, et al. Efficacy and safety of a contraceptive vaginal ring (NuvaRing) compared with a combined oral contraceptive: a 1-year randomized trial. Contraception. 2005;71(3):176–82.

30. Xulane- norelgestromin and ethinyl estradiol patch. US Food and Drug Administration (FDA) approved product information. Revised April, 2017. US National Library of Medicine. http://www.dailymed.nlm.nih.gov. Accessed 27 Feb 2020.

31. TWIRLA (levonorgestrel and ethinyl estradiol) transdermal system. US FDA approved product information. Grand Rapids: Corium International; February 2020. https://www.accessdata.fda.gov/drugsatfda_docs/label/2020/204017s000lbl.pdf. Accessed 30 Mar 2020.

32. Galzote RM, Rafie S, Teal R, Mody SK. Transdermal delivery of combined hormonal contraception: a review of the current literature. Int J Women's Health. 2017;9:315.q.

33. Sharma V, et al. Vasectomy demographics and post-vasectomy desire for future children: results from a contemporary national survey. Fertil Steril. 2013;99(7):1880–5. https://doi.org/10.1016/j.fertnstert.2013.02.032.

34. Grimes DA, Gallo MF, Halpern V, Nanda K, Schulz KF, Lopez LM. Fertility awareness-based methods for contraception. Cochrane Database Syst Rev. 2004;4: CD004860. https://doi.org/10.1002/14651858.CD004860.pub2.

Vulvovaginitis and Cervicitis

107

Charles Fleischer and Shermeeka Hogans-Mathews

Contents

C. Fleischer (✉) · S. Hogans-Mathews
College of Medicine, Florida State University, Tallahassee,
FL, USA
e-mail: Charles.Fleischer@med.fsu.edu;
shermeeka.hogans-mathews@med.fsu.edu

© Springer Nature Switzerland AG 2022
P. M. Paulman et al. (eds.), *Family Medicine*,
https://doi.org/10.1007/978-3-030-54441-6_157

Acute Cervicitis

The appearance of a normal cervix varies widely throughout a woman's lifespan. As estrogen levels rise during puberty, columnar endocervical cells evert onto the squamous ectocervical epithelium at the squamocolumnar junction (metaplasia) and create a transformation zone. This site may be red and friable and can be the source of postcoital and intermenstrual bleeding. During and after menopause, this squamocolumnar junction generally recedes into the endocervical canal and the cervix becomes atrophic with a pale appearance. Subepithelial point hemorrhages may also be seen, and it becomes susceptible to trauma [1]. Cervicitis is inflammation of the uterine cervix that primarily affects the columnar epithelial cells of the endocervical glands but may also affect the squamous epithelial cells of the ectocervix. There are two major diagnostic signs characteristic of cervicitis in which either one or both may be present. These signs include a purulent or mucopurulent endocervical exudate in the endocervical canal or on an endocervical swab and sustained endocervical bleeding induced by gentle palpation or passage of a cotton swab through the cervical os [2].

Cervicitis is usually acute, and well-established etiologies include sexually transmitted infections (STIs), such as *Neisseria gonorrhoeae*, *Chlamydia trachomatis*, *Herpes Simplex Virus* (HSV), *Trichomonas vaginalis*, and *Bacterial vaginosis* (BV). Acute cervicitis may be caused by other infectious agents such as rarer bacteria, viruses, and fungi [1]. Allergens or idiopathic inflammation should also be considered. Cervical infection can ascend (upper-genital-tract infection) and cause endometritis or pelvic inflammatory disease (PID). Therefore, women with cervicitis should be tested for both *Chlamydia trachomatis* and *Neiserria gonorrhoeae* with nucleic acid amplification tests (NAATs) using vaginal, cervical, or urine samples. With cervicitis, BV and Trichomonas should also be tested for and treated if present [2].

Both *Neisseria gonorrhoeae* and *Chlamydia trachomatis* produce varying degrees of an acute inflammatory reaction that affects the glandular epithelium. In a 2018 surveillance report by the Centers for Disease Control and Prevention (CDC), there were 1.8 million cases of Chlamydia, which is the most frequently reported infectious disease, and 583,405 cases of Gonorrhea [3]. Infections can be diagnosed through the assessment of first-catch urine or swab specimens from the endocervix, vagina, or urethra. However, NAATs, which have been cleared by the FDA for provider or self-collected samples from vaginal swabs (equivalent in sensitivity and specificity) [4], have replaced cultures as the gold standard [5]. The sensitivity is usually above 90% and the specificity is around 99%, which contributes to a 20–50% greater detection of *C. trachomatis* infections compared to cultures [4].

As for genital herpes, most recurrent cases are caused by HSV-2 with approximately 50 million persons in the United States infected [6]. Many of these individuals have mild or unrecognized infections but shed the virus intermittently in the anogenital area. Therefore, they can be transmitted by persons who are either unaware that they have the infection or are asymptomatic when transmission occurs [7]. The selected diagnostic test will vary with the overall clinical presentation and can include a viral culture, polymerase chain reaction (PCR), type specific serologic tests, or direct fluorescence antibody [8]. In a patient with active lesions, cell culture and PCR are the preferred tests. The sensitivity of viral culture is low, especially for recurrent lesions, and declines rapidly as lesions begin to heal. NAAT, again, is more sensitive compared to viral cultures, but negative results do not rule out an infection as viral shedding is intermittent [7].

An estimated five million women in the United States are infected annually with Trichomonas [9, 10], and like genital herpes, this may be an underestimate as up to 50–75% of cases are asymptomatic [9, 11] and therefore unreported. *Trichomonas vaginalis* is the cause of approximately 10% of all cases of vaginitis; if left untreated, it may progress to urethritis or cervicitis. Trichomoniasis is also associated with coinfection with other sexually transmitted organisms [9] and is the most common sexually transmitted infection in the world, with 120 million cases reported each year [12]. Microscopy is often the first step in the diagnosis of trichomoniasis due to the convenience and low cost, as well as sensitivity of 60%–70% and specificity of nearly 100% [13, 14]. If trichomonads are visible on microscopy, no further testing is indicated as

Image 1 *Trichomonas vaginalis* parasitic protozoa. This image shows a wet prep microscopy from a vaginal specimen showing trichomonads in a patient presenting with vaginal symptoms. (Obtained from the Centers for Disease Control and Prevention. 1975. Public Health Image Library ID# 17912. https://phil.cdc.gov/Details.aspx?pid= 17912)

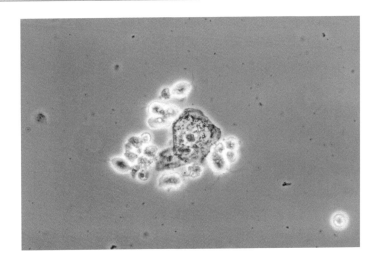

seen on Image 1. However, if microscopy is negative, then the gold standard NAAT with high sensitivity and specificity is performed as opposed to using rapid diagnostic kits, or a culture where results may take up to seven days. For example, the Aptima T. vaginalis assay (Hologic) that has been approved by the US Food and Drug Administration (FDA) has a sensitivity that ranges from 95 to 100 percent and a specificity that ranges from 95 to 100 percent that is superior to other diagnostic tests in all patient populations via vaginal discharge and urine samples [15–18]. It often detects three to five times more *T. vaginalis* infections compared to wet-mount microscopy, which has a sensitivity of 51 to 65 percent. Other NAATs include Amplicor (Roche), AmpliVue (Quidel), BD ProbeTec TV Qx (BD Diagnostics), NuSwab VG (LabCorp), Solana (Quidel), and Xpert TV (Cepheid) assays [19].

Another bacterial cause of cervicitis is *Bacterial vaginosis*, which commonly results in vaginal discharge in women of reproductive age with prevalence ranging from 10% to 50% [20–22]. It is thought to arise when anaerobic vaginal flora overtakes and/or replaces the aerobic vaginal flora, namely, lactobacilli. Typically, *Gardnerella vaginalis* and mycoplasma are increased in number, while lactobacilli comprise a smaller fraction. The exact cause of BV is not clear. However, *G. vaginalis* alone is the most frequent cause and makes up

approximately 40% of BV cases, followed by other anaerobes which include *Mycoplasma hominis, Peptostreptococcus spp.,* and *Mobiluncus spp.* [21–23]. Women with BV are also at a higher risk of acquiring a sexually transmitted disease (STD), such as HIV, gonorrhea, and chlamydia [24, 25]. A diagnosis of BV is established primarily using the Amsel criteria [26], wherein three of the following four criteria have to be met to diagnose BV. The criteria include: Gray, homogeneous discharge; positive amine (fishy) odor or "whiff test" (positive potassium hydroxide (KOH test) – sensitivity 6.58% and specificity 73.6%); vaginal pH > 4.5; >20% clue cells/HPF on microscopy (sensitivity 43.1% and specificity 99.6%) [27]. See Image 2. Cultures are of limited diagnostic value as cultures for *G. vaginalis* in almost all women with symptomatic infections are positive, whereas 50%–60% of healthy asymptomatic women are also positive [12]. The FDA has approved commercial tests that have acceptable performance compared to gram staining, which include a DNA probe-based test for high concentrations of *G. vaginalis* (BD Affirm VPIII), vaginal fluid sialidase activity test (OSOM BVBlue test), and two PCR-based assays that target several BV-associated species (BD Max, Aptima BV).

Lately, *Mycoplasma genitalium* has been increasingly associated with acute cervicitis and an infection can lead to (PID), endometritis,

Image 2 Clue cell. This image shows wet prep microscopy from a vaginal specimen showing a clue cell in a patient presenting with bacterial vaginosis. (Obtained from the Centers for Disease Control and Prevention. 1978. Public Health Image Library ID# 14574. https://phil.cdc.gov/Details.aspx?pid=14574)

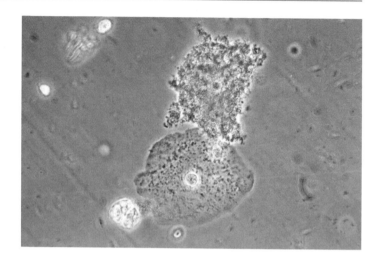

increased risk of HIV transmission, and complications of both pregnancy and childbirth [28, 29]. When a patient's sexual partners are affected, there is also increased economic and emotional burden [1]. *Mycoplasma genitalium* is very difficult to culture, and patients are often asymptomatic [2]. NAAT with PCR or transcription-mediated amplification is therefore used in research facilities and laboratories and may be available for high-risk populations [28, 30]. A prospective multicenter clinical study published in 2019 demonstrated clinical efficacy for the first FDA-cleared transcription-mediated amplification (TMA) NAAT for the detection of *M. genitalium* 16S rRNA [30]. Depending on the specimen, sensitivity and specificity estimates ranged from 77.8% to 98.9% and 97.8% to 99.6%, respectively. However, study limitations include the lack of oropharyngeal or rectal samples and coinfection data for other STIs. Future studies will be needed to further evaluate its role in asymptomatic populations.

A majority of patients with acute cervicitis are asymptomatic and cases are detected incidentally on examination. As intervals for routine gynecologic screening examinations lengthen, cervical infections, especially if asymptomatic, may be missed. Annual wellness examinations and other patient visits outside of routine gynecologic cancer screening visits should, if indicated, include a brief evaluation with a sexual risk assessment and a gynecologic examination. All patients being

evaluated for chlamydia, gonorrhea, or trichomoniasis should also be offered counseling and testing for HIV and syphilis [7].

Chronic Cervicitis

Unlike the more common acute cervicitis, chronic cervicitis is characterized by persistent discharge for at least three months despite the resolution or exclusion of infection [31]. Chronic cervicitis is also usually caused by noninfectious sources, and there is no standard approach to these cases. Noninfectious causes include mechanical or chemical irritation, radiation therapy, systemic inflammatory diseases (such as Behcet syndrome), and malignancy [2]. Chronic cervicitis may remain idiopathic in many women due to unknown or undetectable infectious and non-infectious agents.

Noninfectious causes of both acute and chronic cervicitis include allergens and irritants. Commercial products that can irritate or disrupt the cervicovaginal mucosa include spermicides and contraceptive creams, douching, perfumes, and deodorants. These irritants can disrupt the normal balance of vaginal flora and lead to cervicitis [1]. Irritants also include latex, povidone-iodine, surfactants, topical anesthetics, and cornstarch. Mechanical irritation, caused by trauma from surgical instruments and foreign bodies such as a pessary, diaphragm, tampon, cervical cap, or condom, can also cause cervicitis [2].

Office Evaluation

When approaching a patient with cervicitis, in addition to a focused medical history, visual and olfactory characterization of the discharge, microscopy, pH value of the secretions, and a gynecological examination should be performed. Focused questions should cover vaginal itching or pain, characterization of any discharge (amount, consistency, color, odor), menstrual cycle status, and intermenstrual or postcoital bleeding (Fig. 1). A thorough medication history should focus on antibiotic use, hormones, and any over-the-counter products [31]. Clinicians need to sensitively and appropriately screen for STI risk factors by asking about the patient's symptoms, the partner's symptoms, and a detailed sexual history [1].

Findings present on a cervical examination in a patient with cervicitis may include mucopurulent discharge, cervical friability with sustained easy bleeding when gently palpated or swabbed, vesicular or ulcerative lesions, punctate hemorrhages of the "strawberry" cervix, and cervical motion tenderness (CMT). Diffuse vesicular lesions or ulcerations suggest HSV, while punctate hemorrhages are characteristic of *T. vaginalis*. Condyloma lesions may have a flat, raised, or cauliflower appearance. On bimanual examination, CMT caused by inflammation of the pelvic ligaments is a clear indication of PID which can complicate cervicitis. During the examination, clinicians

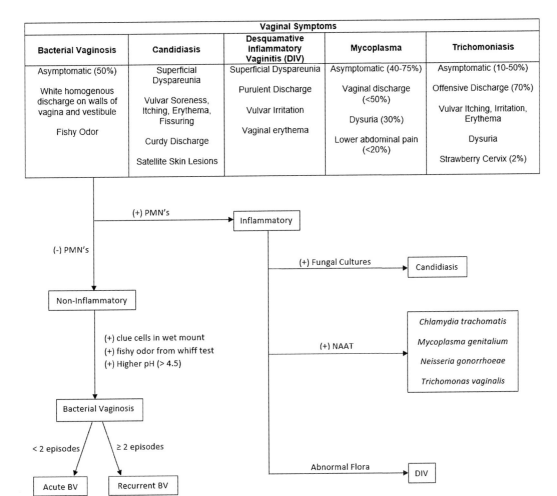

Vaginal Symptoms				
Bacterial Vaginosis	**Candidiasis**	**Desquamative Inflammatory Vaginitis (DIV)**	**Mycoplasma**	**Trichomoniasis**
Asymptomatic (50%)	Superficial Dyspareunia	Superficial Dyspareunia	Asymptomatic (40-75%)	Asymptomatic (10-50%)
White homogenous discharge on walls of vagina and vestibule	Vulvar Soreness, Itching, Erythema, Fissuring	Purulent Discharge	Vaginal discharge (<50%)	Offensive Discharge (70%)
		Vulvar Irritation	Dysuria (30%)	Vulvar Itching, Irritation, Erythema
Fishy Odor	Curdy Discharge	Vaginal erythema	Lower abdominal pain (<20%)	Dysuria
	Satellite Skin Lesions			Strawberry Cervix (2%)

Fig. 1 Approach to the patient with cervicitis

Table 1 Common causes of vaginal discharge with concomitant cervicitis

Bacterial vaginosis	Aerobic vaginitis	Candidiasis	Trichomoniasis
50% asymptomatic	10–20% asymptomatic	60% of women colonized Minority develop symptoms	10–50% asymptomatic 5–15% no abnormal signs
Thin white homogenous discharge, coating walls of vagina and vestibule Offensive fishy odor	Purulent discharge	Vaginal discharge may be curdy	Offensive vaginal discharge in up to 70% Frothy and yellow-green discharge in 10–30%
Absence of vaginitis	Vulval burning or stinging Superficial dyspareunia Vaginal erythema and edema Vaginal ulceration	Vulval soreness, itching, and erythema Vulval fissuring Superficial dyspareunia Satellite skin lesions Vulva edema	Vulva itching/irritation and erythema Dysuria Rarely low abdominal discomfort Vaginitis 2% strawberry cervix visible to naked eye

Obtained from Sherrard J, Wilson J, Donders G, Mendling W, Jensen JS. 2018 European (IUSTI/WHO) International Union against sexually transmitted infections (IUSTI) World Health Organisation (WHO) guideline on the management of vaginal discharge. Int J STD AIDS. 2018;29(13):1258–1272. doi:https://doi.org/10.1177/0956462418785451

should also look for noninfectious causes including abrasions and ecchymosis [1]. When indicated, they should perform smears, cultures, or immunofluorescence assays to confirm or exclude an infection with *N. gonorrhea* or chlamydia [31].

Vaginal discharge concomitant with cervicitis is more commonly caused by infections (up to 90%) such as STIs, with the alteration of vaginal flora resulting in an increase in colonization by different facultative pathogenic microorganisms (i.e., *Gardnerella vaginalis*). These infections include bacterial vaginosis (up to 40%–50% of cases), vulvovaginal candidiasis (20%–25%), and trichomoniasis (15%–20%) (Table 1). If an infectious process is suspected, a sample of the vaginal discharge should be taken from the posterior vaginal vault using a cotton-tipped applicator and smeared on a glass slide, followed by a droplet of 0.9% normal saline. The slide is then evaluated using phase-contrast wet mount microscopy [12]. Compared to real-time PCR, wet mount sensitivity is 40% (95% confidence interval, 19.1% to 63.9%) and specificity is 100% (95% CI, 99.7% to 100%);[19] therefore, if a patient is symptomatic with cervicitis, further testing should be performed using culture or NAAT. A leukocyte-rich urethral or cervical discharge specifically is considered highly suggestive of an infection. With negative detection of trichomonads and greater than 10 white blood cells per high power field seen on microscopy of vaginal fluid, this may indicate a *Chlamydia trachomatis* or *Neiserria gonorrhoeae* infection [2]. A gram stain is also essential as composition of the microbial flora and the purity can be obtained [12].

Treatment

Treatment of cervicitis is directed at etiology and symptomatology. When the etiology is unknown, there is no recommendation for treatment beyond empiric coverage for STIs. Empiric coverage can be provided for women who are found to be at an increased risk for *Chlamydia trachomatis* or *Neiserria gonorrhoeae* infection while considering the feasibility of follow-ups or NAAT [2].

First line empiric treatment is made up of single doses which should be administered upon the visit to increase adherence and is comprised of azithromycin 1 gram orally and ceftriaxone 250 milligrams intramuscularly as this covers for chlamydial, gonorrheal, and mycoplasma infections and is a safe option for pregnant women

[2]. Depending on patient presentation, such as QTc prolongation or hepatotoxicity, azithromycin may be substituted by doxycycline 100 milligrams twice daily for seven days. However, one should be aware that there is a higher prevalence of gonococcal resistance with tetracyclines in the United States. Despite sharing a beta-lactam ring, as the third generation cephalosporins have such a different side chain compared to penicillin, the chances of cross-reactivity are close to 0% [32]. However, if seriously concerned, a clinician may consider using a fluoroquinolone as an alternative to the cephalosporin. Expedited partner therapy should also be provided, and patients should be counseled on abstinence or safe sex practices for seven days after completion of therapy. If cervicitis persists on follow up even after standard treatment of sexually transmitted infections, clinicians would need to consider the cause being *Mycoplasma genitalium*. [1]

As for genital HSV, management should focus on the chronic nature of the disease as well as acute recurrences, which entails the use of antivirals for a minimum of seven to ten days [7]. Valacyclovir may be the preferred antiviral compared to others that require dose administration three to five times a day. Smaller doses of these agents are used for suppressive therapy for those who have experienced more than four to five recurrences per year, and it has successfully reduced recurrence rates by 70%–80%. However, clinicians should periodically assess for discontinuation as recurrences tend to diminish over time.

Treatment of BV in the presence or absence of pregnancy consists of clinically equivalent metronidazole or clindamycin [7]. Although oral and vaginal formulations have similar clinical cure rates of 70–80%, the vaginal preparation is preferred due to less systemic side effects. However, drug and formulation selection should be patient-specific by evaluating drug availability, adverse effects, and previous response to therapies. Metronidazole is available as 500 mg orally twice daily for 7 days, or as a 0.75% vaginal gel with one applicatorful of 5 g (equivalent to 37.5 mg of metronidazole) inserted once daily for a total of 5 days [14]. A one-time administration (orally and

vaginally) is less effective, and therefore not recommended [7]. For clindamycin, a 7-day course of 2% clindamycin cream vaginally (5 g of cream contains 100 mg of clindamycin phosphate) may be used. Alternative regimens include oral clindamycin (300 mg twice daily for seven days), clindamycin ovules (100 mg intravaginally once daily for three days), and single application of clindamycin (Clindesse) as a bioadhesive. These regimens have not been studied extensively and may have lower efficacy for eradicating BV [14]. BV resolves spontaneously in about 30% of pregnant and nonpregnant women, but treatment may reduce the risk of acquiring other STDs. During pregnancy, BV is particularly harmful due to the possibility of a peripartal infection and premature birth. Therefore, regardless of pregnancy status, symptomatic and asymptomatic women should be treated [12]. Recurrent BV treatment is discussed below.

Follow-up

A follow-up visit should be scheduled to allow the provider to determine whether the cervicitis has resolved. Women with a specific diagnosis of chlamydia, gonorrhea, or trichomonas should be offered partner services and instructed to return in three months after treatment for repeat testing because of high rates of reinfection, regardless of whether their sex partners were treated [33]. Test-of-cure to detect therapeutic failure for chlamydia or uncomplicated gonorrhea (i.e., repeat testing 3–4 weeks after completing therapy) is not advised for persons treated with the recommended or alternative regimens, unless therapeutic adherence is in question, symptoms persist, or reinfection is suspected. If symptoms persist or recur, women should be instructed to return for re-evaluation. Retesting is not the same as a test-of-cure (TOC). Retesting for reinfection of chlamydia, gonorrhea, and trichomonas is done routinely. A test-of-cure, however, is performed three to four weeks after treatment and only under the following circumstances: (1) if concern exists regarding persistence of infection despite treatment, (2) if symptoms of infection persist, (3) if lack of adherence to the treatment regimen is suspected, and (4) after treatment of chlamydia during pregnancy [7].

Women with persistent or recurrent cervicitis despite treatment should be reevaluated for possible re-exposure or treatment failure to gonorrhea or chlamydia. If relapse and/or reinfection with a specific STD has been excluded, BV is not present, and sex partners have been evaluated and treated, the management options for persistent cervicitis are undefined; in addition, the utility of repeated or prolonged administration of antibiotic therapy for persistent symptomatic cervicitis remains unknown [7].

The etiology of persistent cervicitis, including the potential role of *M. genitalium,* is unclear. *M. genitalium* might be considered for cases of clinically significant cervicitis that persist after azithromycin or doxycycline therapy in which re-exposure to an infected partner or medical non-adherence is unlikely. In settings with validated assays, women with persistent cervicitis could be tested for *M. genitalium* with the decision to treat with moxifloxacin based on results of diagnostic testing [34]. In treated women with persistent symptoms that are clearly attributable to cervicitis, a referral to a gynecologic specialist can be considered [7].

Special Populations

For cervicitis among special populations, although women with the infection and HIV require the same therapy as those without HIV, treatment is more crucial to reduce cervical HIV shedding and subsequent transmission. The diagnosis and treatment of cervicitis is also the same for pregnant women [7].

Vaginitis

Vaginitis broadly includes conditions that can cause an array of symptoms ranging from discharge, itching, burning, odor, swelling, and more [35]. Vaginitis contributes to many of the gynecological visits to the primary care office. 70% of cases of vaginitis are caused by BV, trichomoniasis, and vulvovaginal candidiasis (VVC) [36]. Vaginitis can be divided into two separate categories: inflammatory versus non-inflammatory (Table 2) [35]. Inflammatory vaginitis involves the presence of vulvar/vaginal edema and erythema or the microscopic presence of polymorphonuclear neutrophils (PMNs). Non-inflammatory vaginitis is the absence of the above characteristics [35].

Inflammatory Vaginitis

Trichomoniasis

As discussed earlier in the cervicitis section of this chapter, *Trichomoniasis* is the most common cause of inflammatory vaginitis [35]. Similar to BV, there is a higher prevalence of *Trichomoniasis* in African-American women (9.6%) compared to non-Hispanic white women (0.8%) [35, 42]. Diagnostic testing was discussed previously; however, it is important to note that Trichomoniasis cannot be diagnosed via Papanicolaou tests (liquid-based or conventional) due to false-positive and false-

Table 2 Classifications of vaginitis

Vaginitis [35]		
Inflammatory	Most common	Least common
	Trichomoniasis Vulvovaginal Candidiasis (VVC)	Atrophic vaginitis or genitourinary syndrome of menopause (GSM) Desquamative inflammatory vaginitis (DIV)) Multimucosal erosive diseases (autoimmune)
Noninflammatory	Most common	Least common
	Bacterial vaginosis (BV)	Vulvovaginal Candidiasis (certain forms) Mixed infections (VVC/BV)

negative results [35]. Retesting at 3 months is recommended by the CDC to due high rates of recurrence but can be performed as early as one month after treatment [35].

Vulvovaginal Candidiasis

In their lifetimes, 70–75% of women are expected to experience at least one episode of VVC [37]. Out of this population, 10–15% are estimated to be asymptomatic colonizers and 5–10% will potentially experience recurrent VVC [37]. The symptoms of VVC including gynecological discomfort, pain, irritation, and hinderances to sexual interactions can cause a great deal of distress including mental anguish and lowered self-esteem [37]. Sequelae of untreated VVC infections include PID, ectopic pregnancy, infertility, spontaneous abortions, changes in menstruation, and increased HIV susceptibility [37].

Factors that contribute to the pathogenicity of Candida can be attributed to its hyphae formation, adhesion, phenotypic switching, extracellular hydrolytic enzyme production, and formation of biofilm [37]. Risk factors for candida infection include uncontrolled diabetes, pregnancy, hormone replacement therapy (HRT), corticosteroid use, and antibiotics are noted to be risk factors related to host [37]. In addition to the risk factors discussed, intrauterine devices, condoms, oral contraceptives, spermicides, clothing habits (i.e., tight-fitting underwear), hygiene, and sexual activity can also contribute to increasing risk of VVC infection [37]. HRT with estrogen and progesterone also seem to play a role in increasing VVC infection. The incidence of VVC in females prior to puberty and after menopause appears to be uncommon [37]. VVC is often seen in pregnancy when the following contributors are present: high carbohydrate diets, immune system suppression, and stress [37]. Receptive oral sexual activity and frequent sexual intercourse have been implicated as proposed risk factors in recurrent VVC [37].

The most common species of VVC include *C. albicans, C. glabrata, Candida krusei, Candida parapsilosis,* and *Candida tropicalis* [37]. There is a concern for resistance as there

has been an increase in C. *glabrata* due to prolonged antifungal treatments and self-medication. C. *glabrata* is more resistant to antifungal medications [37]. Thus, appropriate examination, diagnosis, and treatment of VVC are strongly recommended versus prolonged treatment or recurrent self-treatment. Fortunately, flucytosine and boric acids, which are nonazole antifungals, have been successful at treating *Non-Candida albicans Candida (NCAC)* [37].

VVC can be classified as either uncomplicated or complicated. There are four specific criteria for uncomplicated VVC infection which include the following: nonimmunocompromised status, mild-to-moderate symptoms or findings, *Candida albicans* infection (proven or suspected), and sporadic or infrequent episodes of less than 4 each year [15]. Conversely, classification of *complicated VVC* involves meeting at least one of the following criteria: immunocompromising disease states such as diabetes, severe symptoms, or findings which include fissure formation, extensive erythema of the vulva, and excoriation or recurrent episodes defined as greater than or equal to four episodes in one year, or NCAC (proven or suspected) [15].

Diagnosis of VVC

Abnormal discharge is highly associated with VVC with most patients complaining of a white cottage-cheese-like discharge [40]. Two findings are usually required to diagnose VVC: (1) Aptima test positive for *Candida* or positive fungal vaginal culture or (2) wet-mount microscopy with hyphae, pseudohyphae, or spores present [40]. Unfortunately, the sensitivity of microscopy in identifying VVC is only 50–70% and may not yield the correct diagnosis if the patient has already begun over-the-counter (OTC) treatment with an antifungal prior to vaginal examination [40].

Treatment of VVC

Uncomplicated vulvovaginal candidiasis can be treated with OTC intravaginal medications, prescription intravaginal medications, or prescribed oral agents. Intravaginal treatment options may include application of 5 g of OTC clotrimazole 1% cream once daily for 7–14 days, clotrimazole 2% cream once daily for 3 days, miconazole 2% cream once daily for 7 days, or miconazole 4% cream for 3 days [14, 15]. Other OTC options include miconazole vaginal suppositories in 100 mg (7 day), 200 mg (3 day), and 1200 mg (1 day) dosages or application of tioconazole 6.5% ointment in a 5 g single dosage [14]. Prescribed intravaginal creams and suppositories include butoconazole 2% cream single dose, terconazole creams in 0.4% for 7 days and 0.8% for 3 days in 5 g dosages and an 80 mg vaginal suppository of terconazole for 3 days [14]. Fluconazole is available as a single 150 mg dose oral agent which can be repeated in 72 hours, if needed, and carries the risk of hepatotoxicity [14]. Medication reconciliation and checking for drug-drug interactions is also of paramount importance prior to prescribing fluconazole.

despair and frustration about recurrent infections given the accompanied discharge, odor, and discomfort. Thus, it appears that recurrent BV can certainly take its toll on patients by causing moderate-to-severe impact on overall quality of life and interfering with their sexual functioning and self-esteem [39]. List 1 explores treatment options for recurrent bacterial vaginosis.

List 1 Recurrent Bacterial Vaginosis Treatment

Treatment options for recurrent bacterial vaginosis [35, 39]
Intravaginal metronidazole daily × 10 days, then twice weekly for 4–6 months [35]
Oral tinidazole or metronidazole twice daily × 7 days, then intravaginal boric acid 600 mg daily × 21 days, then intravaginal metronidazole twice weekly for 4–6 months [35]
Secnidazole 2 g single dose [39]

Noninflammatory Vaginitis

Bacterial Vaginosis

Bacterial vaginosis (BV)), which was discussed earlier in the cervicitis section, is a non-inflammatory type of vaginitis and causes up to 30–50% of vaginitis cases [35, 36]. After adjustments are made for poverty, age, and education, ethnic minorities (African-Americans and/or American-Hispanic women) are up to 3 times more likely to have BV than in white non-Hispanic women [35]. Risk factors for recurrence of BV include having a regular sex partner (especially in female to female intercourse) and a history of BV infection [38]. Almost 60% of women will have a recurrence of BV within 12 months after a single treatment. The recurrence may be due to a bacterial biofilm. [35]. Currently, the CDC does not recommend the usage of probiotics in preventing BV infections or recurrences [35]. However, consistent condom use has been shown to decrease BV incidence [35]. Recurrent BV has many psychological, social, and financial implications for patients whom often present in

Atrophic Vaginitis or Genitourinary Syndrome of Menopause (GSM)

Atrophic vaginitis, also known as GSM, affects greater than 50% of postmenopausal women [41]. Patients often present with symptoms that include sexual dysfunction, dyspareunia, vaginal dryness, increased urinary frequency and urgency, vaginal itching and urinary tract infections [41]. Given the fact that primary care physicians may not screen for GSM and that patients may be hesitant to mention symptoms due to embarrassment, this condition often remains untreated and undiagnosed [41]. GSM is a clinical diagnosis that usually presents with the following examination findings: scarce pubic hair, atrophy of labia minora and vaginal canal, pale mucosa, increased vaginal pH, and narrowing of the introitus [41]. Etiologies other than GSM should be considered, such as dermatoses, malignancies, irritants, inflammatory diseases, or infectious vaginitis [41].

Short-term treatment options for GSM include lubricants and moisturizers. Water-based lubricants are recommended compared to silicone, petroleum, and oil-based lubricants. Silicone lubricants have increased risk of genital issues, whereas petroleum and oil-based lubricants can increase the risk of BV and VCC infections [41]. Another option is hyaluronic acid-based vaginal gel which has been shown to improve symptoms of dryness and can be used every 3 days [41]. If prescription therapy is needed, low-dose vaginal estrogen therapy (ET) is recommended, especially due to its efficacy and safety profile compared to systemic estrogen [41]. Low-dose vaginal treatment options include creams, inserts, and vaginal rings. Creams include estradiol-17β (Estrace) and conjugated estrogens (Premarin) both dosed at 0.5–1 g daily for two weeks and progressing to 0.5–1 g one to three times weekly [41]. Vaginal inserts include estradiol hemihydrate (Vagifem, Yuvafem) dosed at 10-μg inserted once daily for two weeks and progressing one insert twice weekly and DHEA (Intrarosa) dosed at 6.5 mg once daily [41]. Vaginal rings include estradiol-17β (Estring) and estradiol acetate (Femring) with instructions to place insert and leave in for 90 days before replacement [41]. Lastly, selective estrogen receptor modulators (SERM), such as Ospemifene (Osphena), are dosed at 60 mg daily and are approved for moderate to severe dyspareunia [41]. Of note, the safety of this medication has not been determined in patients who are at a higher risk for breast cancer as no data has suggested that Osphena stimulates breast tissue [41]. Of note, it may take a few weeks for patients to notice full benefits of therapy. Also, endometrial protection with a progestogen is usually not needed when women are being treated with low-dose vaginal estrogen therapy [41].

Desquamative Inflammatory Vaginitis (DIV)

Often heralded as a diagnosis of exclusion, DIV is a process of chronic inflammation of the vestibule and vagina that is usually seen in white (non-Hispanic) women and perimenopausal women [35]. Etiology of DIV is unclear. However, a lichen planus variant or a vaginal atrophic

bacterial overgrowth may be considered potential sources [36]. Characteristic patients usually present in a hypoestrogenic condition with yellow or brown abnormal discharge, severe dyspareunia, and burning [36]. The clinical hallmark of DIV entails microscopic findings of PMNs, inflammatory cells, and parabasal epithelial cells, in addition to increased vaginal pH and purulent discharge [35]. Upon examination, extraneous vaginal discharge and severe erythema of the vagina and introitus are present [36]. Of note, vaginitis related to estrogen and infectious etiologies must be excluded prior to arriving at the diagnosis of DIV [35]. Trials of clindamycin or intravaginal steroids are treatment options. These include Clindamycin vaginal cream 2% every other night, and hydrocortisone 10% vaginal suppository or hydrocortisone 25 mg suppositories every night [35]. Prolonged therapy for 4–8 weeks is often needed to resolve symptoms [35].

Other Causes of Inflammatory Vaginitis

Other causes of inflammatory vaginitis include lichen planus, pemphigus vulgaris, pemphigoid, and cicatricial pemphigoid. One of the hallmarks of these disorders includes erythematous, shallow, and isolated erosions of the vagina or labia minora [35]. Biopsy is warranted in these cases. For patients with these symptoms, referrals are often necessary to gynecology or dermatology.

Cytolytic vaginosis is caused by Lactobacilli overgrowth which is noted to cause cellular dissolution due to damages of the epithelium of the vagina [38]. This is usually most problematic during the luteal phase of the menstrual cycle [38]. Vulvar dysuria, pruritis, dyspareunia, and erythema with white pasty appearing vaginal walls are hallmark symptoms of cytolytic vaginosis. [39]. Wet prep would reveal lactobacilli and fragmented squamous cells with the absence of leukocytes, yeast, clue cells, and trichomonads [39]. Sodium bicarbonate treats cytolytic vaginosis by raising the pH of the vagina. This can be done as a prepared douche or with a gelatin capsule containing sodium bicarbonate [39].

Approach to the Patient

Obtaining a thorough list of symptoms, sexual history, history of prior vaginal infections as well as hygiene history is important in assisting in workup of vulvovaginitis. Recommendations include obtaining a focused history, performing an adequate gynecological exam (vulva, vestibule, vagina, and cervical inspection) with either testing of vaginal pH, microscopy of vaginal secretions, and amine test or utilizing Aptima test swab for further testing [36]. Patients presenting with concerns for vaginitis may experience an array of adverse emotional and psychological sequelae. Patients may be significantly impacted, leading to sexual dysfunction, decreased self-esteem or negative thoughts of self, frustration, loss of productivity from educational or occupational pursuits, decreased socialization, and effects from pain, discomfort, and inconvenience [38]. For a majority of patients, there can be a host of social issues that arise given the sensitivity involved with gynecological issues. Building rapport with patients and being sensitive, empathetic, and respectful during encounters can help place patients at ease and result in a more productive encounter. Patients with recurrent or abnormal symptoms and issues should be referred to the gynecologist for further evaluation and management.

References

1. Allen, Margaret PA-C, MSL, DFAAPA. Identifying acute cervicitis in an era of less-frequent routine gynecologic examinations. JAAPA. 2018;31(2):50–3.
2. Centers for Disease Control and Prevention. Diseases characterized by urethritis and cervicitis. https://www.cdc.gov/std/tg2015/urethritis-and-cervicitis.htm. Accessed 15 Nov 2020.
3. Centers for Disease Control and Prevention. Sexually transmitted disease surveillance 2018. https://www.cdc.gov/std/stats18/toc.htm. Accessed 15 Nov 2020.
4. Centers for Disease Control and Prevention. Recommendations for the Laboratory-Based Detection of Chlamydia trachomatis and Neisseria gonorrhoeae – 2014. March 14, 2014 / 63(RR02);1–19.
5. Meyer T. Diagnostic procedures to detect chlamydia trachomatis infections. Microorganisms. 2016;4(3):25.
6. Bradley H, Markowitz LE, Gibson T, et al. Seroprevalence of herpes simplex virus types 1 and 2—United States, 1999–2010. J Infect Dis. 2014;209:325–33.
7. Centers for Disease Control and Prevention. Sexually transmitted diseases treatment guidelines, 2015. https://www.cdc.gov/std/tg2015/tg-2015-print.pdf. Accessed 14 Nov 2020.
8. Gupta R, Warren T, Wald A. Genital herpes. Lancet. 2007 Dec 22;370(9605):2127–37.
9. Sobel JD. What's new in bacterial vaginosis and trichomoniasis? Infect Dis Clin N Am. 2005;19:387–406.
10. Huppert JS. Trichomoniasis in teens: an update. Curr Opin Obstet Gynecol. 2009;21:371–8.
11. Klebanoff MA, Carey JC, Hauth JC, et al. Failure of metronidazole to prevent preterm delivery among pregnant women with asymptomatic Trichomonas vaginalis infection. N Engl J Med. 2001;345:487–93.
12. Mylonas I, Bergauer F. Diagnosis of vaginal discharge by wet mount microscopy: a simple and underrated method. Obstet Gynecol Surv. 2011 Jun;66(6):359–68. https://doi.org/10.1097/OGX.0b013e31822bdf31.
13. Cudmore SL, Delgaty KL, Hayward-McClelland SF, Petrin DP, Garber GE. Treatment of infections caused by metronidazole-resistant Trichomonas vaginalis. Clin Microbiol Rev. 2004;17(4):783–93.
14. Committee on Practice Bulletins—Gynecology. Vaginitis in nonpregnant patients: ACOG practice bulletin, number 215. Obstet Gynecol 2020 Jan;135(1):e1-e17.
15. Workowski KA, Bolan GA, Centers for Disease Control and Prevention. Sexually transmitted diseases treatment guidelines, 2015. MMWR Recomm Rep. 2015;64:1.
16. Andrea SB, Chapin KC. Comparison of Aptima Trichomonas vaginalis transcription-mediated amplification assay and BD affirm VPIII for detection of T. vaginalis in symptomatic women: Performance parameters and epidemiological implications. J Clin Microbiol. 2011;49:866.
17. Chapin K, Andrea S. APTIMA® Trichomonas vaginalis, a transcription-mediated amplification assay for detection of Trichomonas vaginalis in urogenital specimens. Expert Rev Mol Diagn. 2011;11:679.
18. Schwebke JR, Hobbs MM, Taylor SN, et al. Molecular testing for Trichomonas vaginalis in women: Results from a prospective U.S. clinical trial. J Clin Microbiol. 2011;49:4106.
19. Miller JM, Binnicker MJ, Campbell S, Carroll KC, Chapin KC, Gilligan PH, Gonzalez MD, Jerris RC, Kehl SC, Patel R, Pritt BS, Richter SS, Robinson-Dunn B, Schwartzman JD, Snyder JW, Telford S 3rd, Theel ES, Thomson RB Jr, Weinstein MP, Yao JD. A guide to utilization of the microbiology laboratory for diagnosis of infectious diseases: 2018 update by the Infectious Diseases Society of America and the American Society for Microbiology. Clin Infect Dis. 2018 Aug 31;67(6):e1–e94.
20. Simoes JA, Giraldo PC, Faundes A. Prevalence of cervicovaginal infections during gestation and accuracy of clinical diagnosis. Infect Dis Obstet Gynecol. 1998;6:129–33.
21. Shanon H. Diagnostic microbiology of bacterial vaginosis. Am J Obstet Gynecol. 1993;165:1240–4.

22. Allsworth JE, Peipert JF. Prevalence of bacterial vaginosis:2001–2004 National Health and Nutrition Examination Survey data. Obstet Gynecol. 2007;109:114–20.

23. Srinivasan U, Misra D, Marazita ML, et al. Vaginal and oral microbes, host genotype and preterm birth. Med Hypotheses. 2009;73:963–75.

24. Myer L, Denny L, Telerant R, et al. Bacterial vaginosis and susceptibility to HIV infection in South African women: a nested case-control study. J Infect Dis. 2005;192:1372–80.

25. Cu-Uvin S, Hogan JW, Caliendo AM, et al. Association between bacterial vaginosis and expression of human immunodeficiency virus type 1 RNA in the female genital tract. Clin Infect Dis. 2001;33:894–6.

26. Amsel R, Totten PA, Spiegel CA, et al. Nonspecific vaginitis. Diagnostic criteria and microbial and epidemiologic associations. Am J Med. 1983;74:14–22.

27. Hillier SL, Krohn MA, Rabe LK, et al. The normal vaginal flora, H2O2-producing lactobacilli, and bacterial vaginosis in pregnant women. Clin Infect Dis. 1993;16(suppl 4):S273–81.

28. Ona S, Molina RL, Diouf K. Mycoplasma genitalium: an overlooked sexually transmitted pathogen in women? Infect Dis Obstet Gynecol. 2016;2016:4513089.

29. Lis R, Rowhani-Rahbar A, Manhart LE. Mycoplasma genitalium infection and female reproductive tract disease: a meta-analysis. Clin Infect Dis. 2015;61(3):418–26.

30. Gaydos CA, Manhart LE, Taylor SN, Lillis RA, Hook EW III, Klausner JD, Remillard CV, Love M, McKinney B, Getman DK, on behalf of the AMES Clinical Study Group. Molecular testing for Mycoplasma genitalium in the United States: results from the AMES prospective multicenter clinical study. J Clin Microbiol. 2019;57:e01125–19.

31. Iqbal U, Wills C. Cervicitis. [Updated 2020 Sep 10]. In: StatPearls. Treasure Island (FL): StatPearls Publishing; 2020 Jan-.

32. Herbert ME, Brewster GS, Lanctot-Herbert M. Medical myth: ten percent of patients who are allergic to penicillin will have serious reactions if exposed to cephalosporins. West J Med. 2000;172(5):341.

33. Hosenfeld CB, Workowski KA, Berman S, et al. Repeat infection with chlamydia and gonorrhea among females: a systematic review of the literature. Sex Transm Dis. 2009;36:478–89.

34. Manhart LE, Broad JM, Golden MR. Mycoplasma genitalium: should we treat and how? Clin Infect Dis. 2011;53(Suppl 3):S129–42.

35. Neal CM, Kus LH, Eckert LO, Peipert JF. Noncandidal vaginitis: a comprehensive approach to diagnosis and management. Am J Obstet Gynecol. 2020;222(2):114–22.

36. Nyirjesy P. Management of persistent vaginitis. Obstet Gynecol. 2014;124(6):1135–46.

37. Gonçalves B, Ferreira C, Alves CT, Henriques M, Azeredo J, Silva S. Vulvovaginal candidiasis: epidemiology, microbiology and risk factors. Crit Rev Microbiol. 2016;42(6):905–27.

38. Mills BB. Vaginitis: beyond the basics. Obstet Gynecol Clin N Am. 2017;44(2):159–77.

39. Faught BM, Reyes S. Characterization and treatment of recurrent bacterial vaginosis. J Womens Health (Larchmt). 2019;28(9):1218–26.

40. Paavonen JA, Brunham RC. Vaginitis in nonpregnant patients: ACOG practice bulletin number 215: ACOG practice bulletin number 215. Obstet Gynecol. 2020;135(5):1229–30.

41. Faubion SS, Sood R, Kapoor E. Genitourinary syndrome of menopause: management strategies for the clinician. Mayo Clin Proc. 2017;92(12):1842–9.

42. Centers for Disease Control and Prevention. Trichomoniasis Statistics. https://www.cdc.gov/std/trichomonas/stats.htm#:~:text=February%2013%2C%202013)-,Prevalence,participated%20in%20NHANES%202013%2D2016. Accessed 06 Jan 2021.

Sabrina Hofmeister and Seth Bodden

Contents

Patients frequently bring forth concerns about disorders of menstruation to primary care providers. These disorders are complex and often have many plausible etiologies. A sound knowledge of anatomy and physiology is necessary to definitively diagnose and manage these conditions. This chapter will outline the etiology, diagnosis, and treatment of some of the most common menstrual disorders which are frequently addressed by family physicians.

Premenstrual Disorders

Premenstrual disorders (PMD) are conditions that occur during the luteal phase and resolve shortly after menstruation. Roughly 80% of menstruating women report symptoms during the luteal phase, and between 2% and 5% of women meet the diagnostic criteria for a premenstrual disorder [1]. The subspecialties of psychiatry and gynecology have developed overlapping but distinct diagnoses that qualify as premenstrual disorders. Premenstrual syndrome (PMS) was defined by

S. Hofmeister (✉)
Family and Community Medicine, Medical College of Wisconsin, Milwaukee, WI, USA
e-mail: shofmeister@mcw.edu

S. Bodden
Medical College of Wisconsin, Milwaukee, WI, USA
e-mail: sbodden@mcw.edu

© Springer Nature Switzerland AG 2022
P. M. Paulman et al. (eds.), *Family Medicine*,
https://doi.org/10.1007/978-3-030-54441-6_145

Table 1 Diagnostic criteria for premenstrual syndrome

Premenstrual syndrome		Premenstrual dysphoric disorder	
Affective symptoms	Somatic symptoms	Column A	Column B
Anger outbursts Anxiety Confusion Depression Irritability Social withdrawal	Abdominal bloating Breast tenderness Breast swelling Headache Joint or muscle pain Extremity swelling Weight gain	Affective lability Irritability or anger Depressed mood Anxiety, tension	Decreased interest in usual activities Difficulty concentrating Lethargy or lack of energy Change in appetite or overeating Sleep changes Feeling overwhelmed Somatic symptoms (see column 2)

the field of OB/GYN and consists of both affective and somatic symptoms. Premenstrual dysphoric disorder (PMDD) was defined by the field of psychiatry and focuses primarily on psychiatric symptoms in its diagnostic criteria.

In order to diagnose a premenstrual disorder, symptoms must occur during the luteal phase and resolve shortly after the onset of menstruation. Other conditions may have symptoms that worsen during the luteal phase, but these can be distinguished from PMD because some symptoms persist throughout the menstrual cycle [1]. When working up a PMD, differential diagnoses should contain conditions that could be worsened in the luteal phase such as depression, anxiety, migraines, endometriosis, and hypothyroidism. A diagnosis of PMS can be made if the patient reports at least one affective and one somatic symptom in the 5 days preceding menses (Table 1). This must have occurred during at least the last three menstrual cycles and symptoms must resolve within 4 days from the onset of menstruation independent of any external pharmacologic therapy. Symptoms must be severe enough to impair functioning in social, academic, or work settings and must occur reproducibly during at least two cycles of reporting [2]. A diagnosis of PMDD may be made if, in the majority of menstrual cycles, at least five symptoms from a combination of both columns (Table 1) are markedly present in the final week before the onset of menses. The symptoms must have been present for the majority of menstrual cycles in the last year and have caused significant distress and alternation in functioning in all relationships and settings. The symptoms must also not be attributable to other medical or psychiatric conditions or pharmacologic treatments and must improve within a few days after

initiation of menses with resolution within a week after menses subside [3].

Because women tend to overestimate the cyclical nature of their symptoms, prospective questionnaires are the most accurate way to diagnose PMS and PMDD [1]. The Daily Record of Severity of Problems (DSRP) seen in Fig. 1 is a valid and reliable tool that can be used to diagnose PMS or PMDD. The DSRP has women rate their symptoms through at least two menstrual cycles. Alternatively, women can administer the DRSP on the first day of their menses if a faster diagnosis is desired.

SSRIs are the first-line treatment for severe symptoms of PMS and PMDD. Sertraline, paroxetine, fluoxetine, citalopram, and escitalopram can be used to treat both the psychiatric symptoms and physical symptoms of PMS and PMDD. A 2013 Cochrane review found that each of the five SSRIs studied had statistically significant benefits on patient-reported symptoms when compared to placebo. Either continuously taking an SSRI or taking it only during the luteal phase has been shown to be beneficial. Higher doses tend to be needed for relief of physical symptoms. Bupropion was not effective for symptom relief of PMS or PMDD. SNRIs such as venlafaxine have been used off-label to treat PMDD [1].

Studies have shown that continuous use of OCPs can provide benefit when treating physical and psychiatric symptoms of PMS and PMDD. It appears that OCPs may be most beneficial in treating the psychiatric symptoms of PMDD; however, there is evidence that OCPs may improve abdominal bloating, mastalgia, headache, weight gain, and swelling of the extremities. Small studies have shown calcium supplementation with calcium

Daily Record of Severity of Problems for Diagnosis of Premenstrual Dysphoric Disorder																																		
Symptoms	Day of menstrual cycle (day 1 is the start of the menstrual period)																																	
	1	2	3	4	5	6	7	8	9	10	11	12	13	14	15	16	17	18	19	20	21	22	23	24	25	26	27	28	29	30	31	32	33	34	35
Felt depressed or sad																																			
Felt hopeless																																			
Felt worthless or guilty																																			
Felt anxious or tense																																			
Had mood swings																																			
Feelings were more easily hurt																																			
Felt angry or irritable																																			
Had conflicts with people																																			
Had less interest in activities																																			
Had trouble concentrating																																			
Felt tired or lacked energy																																			
Had increased appetite																																			
Had food cravings																																			
Slept more or had trouble waking up																																			
Had trouble getting to sleep or staying asleep																																			
Felt overwhelmed																																			
Felt out of control																																			
Had breast tenderness																																			
Had breast swelling or weight gain, or felt bloated																																			
Had headache																																			
Had joint or muscle pain																																			
At least one of the problems noted above caused reduced productivity at work, school, or home																																			
At least one of the problems noted above interfered with hobbies or social activities																																			
At least one of the problems noted above interfered with relationships with others																																			
Menstrual flow: H = heavy, M = medium, L = light or spotting (leave blank for no bleeding)																																			

NOTE: Patients should record the score for each item on each day using the following scale: 1 = not at all, 2 = minimal, 3 = mild, 4 = moderate, 5 = severe, 6 = extreme. If during the mid-follicular phase (days 6 through 10) the patient has an average daily score greater than 3 for any symptom, an alternative diagnosis should be sought. Excused symptoms include appetite for obese patients, insomnia with good reasons, or pain from physical illness. The week before menses, the patient should score at least 4 for at least two days on five symptoms that correlate with premenstrual dysphoric disorder diagnostic criteria (Table 2). The week before menses, the patient should score at least 4 for at least two days on at least one impairment item. The patient must meet these criteria for two consecutive cycles or two out of three cycles. Clinical judgment should correlate with the assessment of daily ratings.

Information from Endicott J, Nee J, Harrison W. Daily Record of Severity of Problems (DRSP): reliability and validity. *Arch Womens Ment Health.* 2006;9(1):41-49.

Fig. 1 Daily Record of Severity of Problems for diagnosis of premenstrual dysphoric disorder

carbonate either 500 mg bid or 1200 mg daily can reduce the symptoms of depression, appetite, and fatigue in women diagnosed with PMS [1]. Cognitive behavioral therapy (CBT) has been shown to improve functioning and depression scores for patients with PMS or PMDD. Lastly, mindfulness-based exercises or acceptance-based CBT may be helpful to reduce symptoms [1].

Amenorrhea and Oligomenorrhea

In order for a woman to have regular menstrual cycles, there must be a complex interaction between the hypothalamic pituitary axis, the ovaries, and the uterine outflow tract. A disruption at one of these sites can result in amenorrhea or oligomenorrhea. The workup for primary amenorrhea and secondary amenorrhea will be discussed separately; however, there is overlap in etiologies of these conditions.

Primary Amenorrhea

Primary amenorrhea is defined as a female who has not achieved menarche by age 16 or has not achieved menarche or developed secondary sex characteristics by age 14 [4]. A thorough history and physical examination should be completed paying particular attention to medications, weight gain or loss, breast and pubic hair development, galactorrhea, headaches, acne, hirsutism, and clitoromegaly.

Given that the most common cause for amenorrhea is pregnancy and lactation, the workup for all amenorrhea should begin with a pregnancy test. If negative, a prolactin, TSH, follicle-stimulating hormone (FSH), and luteinizing hormone (LH) level should be checked. A pelvic ultrasound should also be completed to assess the outflow tract.

Outflow Tract Abnormalities

Outflow tract abnormalities account for roughly 20% of cases of primary amenorrhea [4]. Females with an imperforate hymen will have normal pubertal development but may experience cyclical pain during the onset of puberty. On exam, a bluish bulging mass can be seen at the entrance to the vagina which is called hematocolpos. Referral to a surgeon can reestablish normal menses [4].

Transverse vaginal septum develops in utero, and while location varies, it typically is high in the vaginal cavity [4]. Girls with a transverse vaginal septum have normal pubertal development and may begin to experience cyclical pelvic pain. On exam, a shortened blind vaginal pouch will be seen. Surgery is the definitive treatment for this condition.

Mullerian agenesis is an abnormal development of at least part of the mullerian tract which consists of the fallopian tubes, uterus, cervix, and upper two-thirds of the vagina. It causes 15% of primary amenorrhea and can be diagnosed with pelvic imaging [5]. Mullerian agenesis is associated with other renal and skeletal abnormalities; therefore, patients often require a multidisciplinary team [4].

Androgen insensitivity syndrome is a disorder in which a patient genetically has 46XY chromosomes and has testes that produce male levels of testosterone and anti-mullerian hormone; however, they have a defect in the androgen receptor. Patients develop female external genitalia; however, they do not develop the mullerian tract. Patients may present with inguinal hernias. Androgen insensitivity syndrome can be diagnosed through karyotyping and a testosterone level.

Gonadal Anomalies

Gonadal anomalies account for 30–40% of primary amenorrhea and should be suspected if there is an elevated FSH level [4]. Turner syndrome is classically a 45 XO chromosome genetic abnormality; however, it may also be the result of other X gene abnormalities. It is characterized by women of short stature, webbed neck, low-set ears, widely spaced nipples, short fourth metacarpals, and agenesis of the ovaries. Growth velocity may be slow starting as a toddler and continue into adolescence, and patients tend to have limited secondary sex characteristics. A specialist should manage these patients as replacing recombinant growth hormone, estrogen, and progesterone can help with normal growth and pubertal development. Patients may also have renal, cardiac, or ophthalmologic abnormalities [4]. Gonadal dysgenesis occurs in a woman who has 46XX chromosomes but does not develop functioning ovaries. Imaging will often identify streak gonads. Management should be completed through specialty referral. Swyer syndrome occurs in individuals with 46XY chromosomes who do not develop testes. They do develop normal internal and external female genitalia and require referral to subspecialist to remove testes due to high malignancy risk.

Hypothalamic and Pituitary Causes

Functional hypothalamic amenorrhea, medications, and hyperprolactinemia can cause primary amenorrhea but will be discussed in greater details under secondary amenorrhea. Constitutional delay is a delay in the onset of menarche and typically is found in patients with a family history of delayed puberty. This is a diagnosis of exclusion.

Secondary Amenorrhea

Secondary amenorrhea occurs when women who previously had regular menses cease to have menses for 3 months [5]. Oligomenorrhea is the lack of menstruation for longer than 35 days in adults and 45 days in adolescence [4, 5]. Adolescents may have irregular periods for 3 years following menarche.

For all women with amenorrhea, workup should begin with a b-hCG test to exclude pregnancy. If a thorough history and physical exam does not point to a specific cause, then checking a prolactin, thyroid-stimulating hormone (TSH), estradiol (E2), and follicle-stimulating hormone (FSH) level may provide additional diagnostic insight. Figure 2 outlines the diagnostic workup, and Table 2 outlines medications that can cause amenorrhea [6].

Hypothalamic Pituitary Axis

The hypothalamic pituitary axis plays an important role in controlling the menstrual cycle. When working up amenorrhea, abnormalities in serum prolactin, TSH, or low FSH levels would suggest the etiology is related to the hypothalamic pituitary axis.

Functional hypothalamic amenorrhea (FHA) is the disruption of ovulation caused by stress on the body. FHA can be caused by stressors including undernutrition, excessive exercise, emotional stress, or chronic disease. Classically, this is seen in the female athlete triad in which a woman has low-energy availability, menstrual dysfunction, and low bone mineral density. Labs usually reveal a low FSH and estradiol level. The patient should meet with a nutritionist if undernutrition or an underlying eating disorder is suspected. Menses generally resume when a patient returns to about 90% of ideal body weight [4]. Bone mineral density testing should be conducted in women who have been amenorrheic for 6 months or have a history of a stress fracture [5].

Hyperprolactinemia, diagnosed with an elevated serum prolactin level, often presents with infertility or amenorrhea. Patients may also complain of headaches, bilateral temporal visual field defects, or galactorrhea. Common causes of elevated prolactin levels could include pregnancy, lactation, pituitary adenomas, pituitary stalk disruptions, and medications [6]. Common medications that elevate prolactin include first-generation antipsychotics, methyldopa, and metoclopramide. An MRI of the pituitary is essential to look for masses in the hypothalamic pituitary areas of the brain. Pituitary adenomas >1 cm or adenomas that cause symptoms such as headaches or visual field defects should be referred to a specialist. Dopamine agonists may be used to treat elevated prolactin levels.

There are other disruptions to the hypothalamic-pituitary axis that can cause amenorrhea. Both hyperthyroid and hypothyroid disorders can disrupt menstrual cycles. Sheehan's syndrome, a condition in which the pituitary gland goes through ischemic necrosis due to blood loss, should be suspected in women who experienced a large postpartum hemorrhage. Cushing disease and

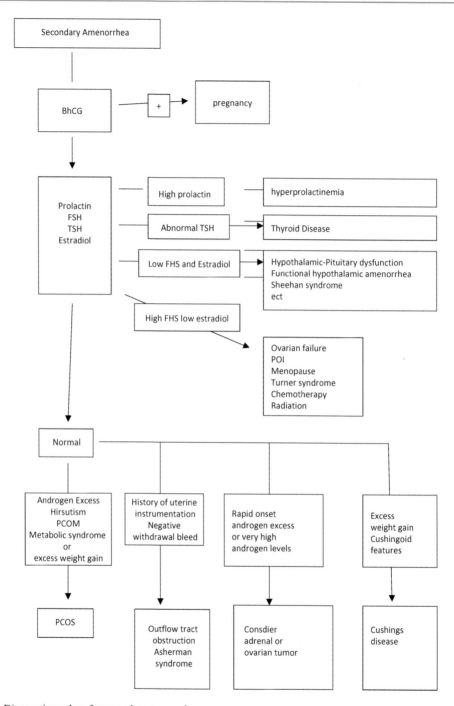

Fig. 2 Diagnostic workup for secondary amenorrhea

congenital adrenal hyperplasia are both rare causes of amenorrhea and should be considered if patients have exam findings concerning for elevated cortisol or elevated androgens [7].

Gonadal dysfunction would be suggested by elevated FSH levels and low estradiol levels. Primary ovarian insufficiency (POI), previously referred to as premature menopause, is the

Table 2 Medications that cause amenorrhea [6]

GnRH suppression	Opioids
Hyperprolactinemia	Glucocorticoids
	Psychotropics
	GI motility agents
	Antihypertensives (verapamil, methyldopa)
Hypophysitis	CTLA-4 antibodies

development of ovarian insufficiency before the age 40. Women experience irregular menses or amenorrhea, hot flashes, and vaginal dryness. Women can be diagnosed with this condition by having two serum FSH levels in the menopausal range, 1 month apart [5]. Estrogen levels will be low but do not necessarily need to be checked. While most causes are idiopathic, Turner syndrome or its variants can cause POI, so karyotyping should be offered to women with POI. Chemotherapy, radiation, or autoimmune disease could also cause POI. Hormone replacement therapy may help with vasomotor symptoms to maintain healthy bone density and should be offered to patients until the natural age of menopause [5].

Outflow tract abnormalities are not a common cause of secondary amenorrhea but should be considered in high-risk populations. Intrauterine adhesions should be considered in women who have had intrauterine or endometrial procedures, particularly uterine curettage. Cervical stenosis should be considered in women who have had cervical procedures, radiation, or even vaginal birth [5]. It may be reasonable to try an estrogen/progestin withdrawal test to evaluate for bleeding. If no bleeding occurs, then an outflow tract abnormality is suggested. Pelvic ultrasound may be helpful in making the diagnosis; however, hysteroscopy may be required in order to diagnose an outflow tract obstruction.

Dysmenorrhea

Dysmenorrhea is defined as cramping abdominal pain occurring with menses [8]. Dysmenorrhea is considered to be primary dysmenorrhea if there is no pelvic pathology found to explain the symptoms. Primary dysmenorrhea often occurs within 6–12 months of menarche when ovulatory cycles are established. It is associated with normal volume menstrual flow and pain subsides after 2–3 days [9]. It is often prostaglandin-mediated. Dysmenorrhea is considered to be secondary dysmenorrhea if underlying pelvic pathology is identified. Often secondary dysmenorrhea occurs in women aged 20–30. Although many women do not find dysmenorrhea to be abnormal and do not seek medical treatment, it is the most common gynecologic condition reported among female adolescents and also affects 60–70% of adult women who menstruate [10, 11].

There are many important questions to ask about when taking a patient history including age of first menstruation, timing of dysmenorrhea onset, relation to menses and menstrual flow severity, description of the pain, sexual history, past medical and family history including chronic pain syndromes, presence of comorbid psychiatric disorders, associated gastrointestinal symptoms, and any previous treatment and response [9]. Patients, especially adolescents, may not be comfortable answering these questions. Upon initial presentation, an abdominal examination should be performed. A pelvic examination is not always necessary if there are not symptoms of a sexually transmitted infection or the patient has not been sexually active [10]. Laboratory evaluation and imaging are generally not helpful for the diagnosis of primary dysmenorrhea but may be helpful in the diagnosis of secondary dysmenorrhea. Table 3 delineates the possible differential diagnoses of dysmenorrhea.

Diagnosis of primary dysmenorrhea can be made from taking a detailed history and limited physical exam [10]. Secondary dysmenorrhea may be diagnosed after the history and physical

Table 3 Differential diagnosis of dysmenorrhea [9, 10]

Primary dysmenorrhea	Secondary dysmenorrhea
	Endometriosis
	Adenomyosis
	Cervical stenosis
	Uterine leiomyomas
	Obstructions of the genital tract:
	Congenital malformations
	Pelvic adhesions
	Uterine polyps
	Pelvic inflammatory disease
	Irritable bowel syndrome or disease
	Ovarian cysts
	Cystitis
	Mood disorders
	Musculoskeletal pain

examination indicate an abnormal cause for the pain or subsequent abnormal laboratory evaluation or imaging or occurs [9].

Treatment of dysmenorrhea must be tailored to the underlying cause. Multiple pharmacologic interventions are effective for the treatment of primary dysmenorrhea in women of all ages. These pharmacologic therapies are targeted at reducing prostaglandin and leukotriene production to reduce overall pain perception. Nonsteroidal anti-inflammatory drugs (NSAIDS) are considered first line [12]. Table 4 is a summary of the frequently used NSAIDS.

Hormonal contraceptives are also considered to be another acceptable first-line option in addition to or in lieu of NSAIDS [10]. These include combined oral contraceptives in pill, patch, or ring form which all work to decrease the thickness of the endometrial lining [12]. Implantable contraceptive progestin rods, intramuscular medroxyprogesterone acetate, or intrauterine devices with levonorgestrel are also effective. Each method has associated risks and other benefits, so the decision to utilize a certain method should be tailored to each patient. Finally, many alternative and complementary therapies can be utilized for treatment of primary dysmenorrhea. These include physical activity which had the largest beneficial effect, acupressure which had a moderate effect, and heat therapy [8, 13]. Many medicinal plants including fennel, chamomile, and *Zataria multiflora* are reported to be effective as well; however, further studies are needed to clearly identify the risks and benefits

Table 4 Recommended NSAIDs and doses for treatment of primary dysmenorrhea [10, 12]

Drug	Loading dose	Maintenance dose
Ibuprofen	800 mg	400–800 mg q 8 h PRN
Naproxen sodium (reduce doses by 50 mg if naproxen)	550 mg	220 mg–550 mg q 12 h PRN
Celecoxib	400 mg	20 mg q 12 h PRN
Mefenamic acid	500 mg	250-500 mg q 6–8 h PRN
Diclofenac potassium	100 mg	50 mg q 6–8 h PRN

of these treatments [14]. If primary dysmenorrhea does not improve within 3–6 months of starting treatment, family physicians should investigate for secondary causes.

If treatment for primary dysmenorrhea has failed or initial history and physical suggests a secondary cause, then imaging or surgical investigation for that cause should be pursued after appropriate referral. Endometriosis is the most common etiology of secondary dysmenorrhea and frequently responds to many of the same treatments utilized for primary dysmenorrhea; however, conservative surgical therapy and suppressive hormonal therapy are sometimes needed [12]. Continual patient education and multidisciplinary support can assist as well with both straightforward and complex cases to improve patient outcomes [10].

Abnormal Uterine Bleeding

Abnormal uterine bleeding (AUB) had many different names prior to 2011 when the International Federation of Gynecology and Obstetrics (FIGO) issued guidance to update and standardize terminology [15]. Terms such as menorrhagia, metrorrhagia, hypo- or hypermenorrhea, polymenorrhea, and dysfunctional uterine bleeding are no longer recommended to be utilized [16]. FIGO recommends the use of the term AUB to describe any change in menstrual volume, frequency, or duration in nonpregnant females [16]. This condition is commonly experienced by approximately 1/3 of reproductive aged women, adds significantly to overall healthcare expenditures, and is well-addressed by family physicians [15]. Table 5 describes some normal features of menstruation.

Diagnosis of AUB can be made if conditions within the acronym PALM-COEIN are present as detailed in Fig. 3 [17]. AUB can be further subcategorized into regularly occurring ovulatory cycles with heavy menstrual bleeding (HMB) or irregularly occurring cycles with likely ovulatory dysfunction (AUB-O) [15].

Evaluation of the patient with AUB should always include a detailed history about menstrual cycle length, variability and volume, sexual history, past medical history of coagulation disorders, and inquiry about fatigue, pain, or mood changes [17]. Physical exam should assess the patient for signs of a bleeding disorder such as bruising or petechiae, sources of extrauterine bleeding such as cervical irritation or endocervical polyps, an enlarged uterus, signs of PCOS such as acne or hirsutism, signs of thyroid disease or galactorrhea, or obesity. Laboratory evaluation is limited but may include a completed blood count (CBC), pregnancy test, thyroid-stimulating level (TSH), prolactin level, sexually transmitted disease testing, cervical cancer screening, assessment for coagulopathy if physical exam is concerning, and possible endometrial sampling. Endometrial sampling is recommended in patients older than 45 or younger if additional risk factors are present such as PCOS, obesity, or failed medical management. Pelvic imaging is often ordered and includes transvaginal ultrasound as the initial test of choice, followed by hysteroscopy or other modality if further evaluation is required [18].

Treatment of AUB depends on the underlying cause. For women who have a structural cause identified, removal of the abnormality can alleviate symptoms. For women with a diagnosed endocrine condition such as hypothyroidism, obesity, or hyperprolactinemia, correction of the endocrine disorder can alter the hypothalamic pituitary axis (HPA) enough to enable the body to resume ovulation and correct the AUB. Correction of coagulopathy or discontinuation of anticoagulants can also alleviate bleeding.

Table 5 Normal menstrual cycle [17]

Frequency	24–38 days
Duration	4–8 days
Volume of blood loss	5–80 ml

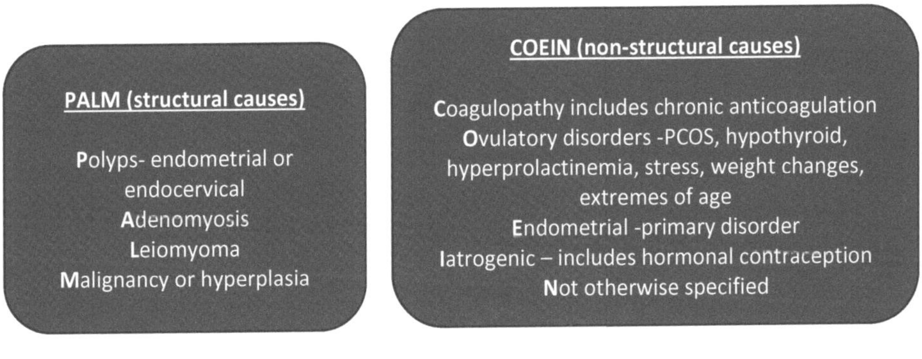

PALM (structural causes)	COEIN (non-structural causes)
Polyps- endometrial or endocervical Adenomyosis Leiomyoma Malignancy or hyperplasia	Coagulopathy includes chronic anticoagulation Ovulatory disorders -PCOS, hypothyroid, hyperprolactinemia, stress, weight changes, extremes of age Endometrial -primary disorder Iatrogenic – includes hormonal contraception Not otherwise specified

Fig. 3 PALM-COEIN

Polycystic Ovarian Syndrome (PCOS)

PCOS is a common condition affecting somewhere between 5 and 20% of women during their reproductive years [19]. The Rotterdam Criteria define PCOS as a condition in which a woman has two of the following three findings: hyperandrogenism – either on clinical exam or found biochemically – oligo-ovulation or anovulation, or polycystic ovarian morphology (PCOM). Androgen excess often presents clinically as hirsutism (terminal hairs in a male-like pattern). Other signs of androgen excess could be acne or alopecia; however, these findings are less specific to androgen excess. While labs are not needed to confirm hyperandrogenism, free and total testosterone along with DHEAS can be checked if the exam is not conclusive [19]. It should be noted that hormonal birth control use in the last 3 months may alter these tests.

Ovarian dysfunction can present in different ways. Oligo-anovulation presents with menstrual cycles lasting longer than 35 days in length or having 10 or less cycles in a year. Women with ovulatory dysfunction may also present with frequent menstrual bleeding or even normal menstrual cycle duration without ovulation [19]. In these patients, a mid-luteal progesterone level or serial ultrasound monitoring can be used to assess ovulation [20]. PCOS may play a role in up to 80% of anovulatory infertility [20].

PCOM is typically found on ultrasound and is defined as having one or more ovary with a volume greater than 10 cm^3 or having an antral follicle count of 12 or greater [21].

Women with PCOS are at increased risk for metabolic dysfunction. Insulin resistance is common with PCOS patients being five to seven times more likely to develop type 2 diabetes mellitus [19]. They are also more likely to develop dyslipidemia. It is therefore recommended to screen for insulin resistance with a 2-h glucose tolerance test and lipid panel every 2–3 years. There are also higher rates of endometrial cancer, anxiety, and depression [19].

Women with PCOS present to their primary care providers with different primary concerns. Treatment should be therefore geared toward the patient's primary concern and treatment goals. In obese patients with PCOS, both calorie restriction and increased exercise are considered first-line treatment for helping with menstrual irregularities, infertility, insulin resistance, and hyperandrogenic symptoms [22].

Infertility is a common presenting symptom for patients with PCOS and accounts for roughly 80% of anovulatory infertility [20]. As stated above, diet and exercise are the first-line treatments for obese patients with infertility. Metformin alone may help establish ovulation in women with anovulatory PCOS and has obvious metabolic benefits. Ovulation induction with clomiphene citrate or letrozole are considered first-line medications for infertility; however, given the risk for multiple gestations, it should be only offered by experienced physicians [20]. If the patient desires to regulate menses but does not desire fertility, OCPs can be considered.

Hyperandrogenism can manifest as hirsutism, acne, and/or alopecia. OCPs have been shown to improve all these symptoms. Hirsutism may also be treated with cosmetic hair removal therapies, androgen receptor blockers, or finasteride [19]. Women suffering from acne can also be treated with topical antimicrobials or topical retinoids. Alopecia can be treated with topical minoxidil.

References

1. Hofmeister S, Bodden S. Premenstrual syndrome and premenstrual dysphoric disorder. Am Fam Physician. 2016;94(3):236–40.
2. American College of Obstetricians and Gynecologists. Guidelines for Women's Health Care: A Resource Manual. Fourth ed. Washington, DC: American College of Obstetricians and Gynecologists; t1:5 2014:608.
3. Diagnostic and Statistical Manual of Mental Disorders. Fifth ed. Washington, DC: American Psychiatric Association; 2013:171–172.
4. Marsh CA, Grimstad FW. Primary amenorrhea: diagnosis and management. Obstet Gynecol Surv. 2014;69 (10):603–12.
5. Klein DA, Paradise SL, Reeder RM. Amenorrhea: a systematic approach to diagnosis and management. Am Fam Physician. 2019;100(1):39–48.
6. Fourman LT, Fazeli PK. Neuroendocrine causes of amenorrhea–an update. J Clin Endocrinol Metab. 2015;100(3):812–24.

7. Pereira K, Brown AJ. Secondary amenorrhea: diagnostic approach and treatment considerations. Nurse Pract. 2017;42(9):34–41.

8. Matthewman G, Lee A, Kaur JG, Daley AJ. Physical activity for primary dysmenorrhea: a systematic review and meta-analysis of randomized controlled trials. Am J Obstet Gynecol. 2018; 219(3):255.e1-.e20.

9. Burnett M, Lemyre M. No. 345-primary dysmenorrhea consensus guideline. J Obstet Gynaecol Can. 2017;39 (7):585–95.

10. ACOG Committee Opinion No. 760. Dysmenorrhea and endometriosis in the adolescent. Obstet Gynecol. 2018;132(6):e249–e58.

11. Bernardi M, Lazzeri L, Perelli F, Reis FM, Petraglia F. Dysmenorrhea and related disorders. F1000Res. 2017; 6:1645.

12. Ryan SA. The treatment of dysmenorrhea. Pediatr Clin N Am. 2017;64(2):331–42.

13. Armour M, Smith CA, Steel KA, Macmillan F. The effectiveness of self-care and lifestyle interventions in primary dysmenorrhea: a systematic review and meta-analysis. BMC Complement Altern Med. 2019; 19(1):22.

14. Sharghi M, Mansurkhani SM, Larky DA, Kooti W, Niksefat M, Firoozbakht M, et al. An update and systematic review on the treatment of primary dysmenorrhea. JBRA Assist Reprod. 2019;23(1):51–7.

15. Kaunitz AM. Abnormal uterine bleeding in reproductive-age women. JAMA. 2019;321(21):2126–7.

16. Elmaoğulları S, Aycan Z. Abnormal uterine bleeding in adolescents. J Clin Res Pediatr Endocrinol. 2018;10 (3):191–7.

17. Cheong Y, Cameron IT, Critchley HOD. Abnormal uterine bleeding. Br Med Bull. 2017;123(1):103–14.

18. Khafaga A, Goldstein SR. Abnormal uterine bleeding. Obstet Gynecol Clin N Am. 2019;46(4):595–605.

19. Azziz R. Polycystic ovary syndrome. Obstet Gynecol. 2018;132(2):321–36.

20. Balen AH, Morley LC, Misso M, Franks S, Legro RS, Wijeyaratne CN, et al. The management of anovulatory infertility in women with polycystic ovary syndrome: an analysis of the evidence to support the development of global WHO guidance. Hum Reprod Update. 2016;22(6):687–708.

21. Bednarska S, Siejka A. The pathogenesis and treatment of polycystic ovary syndrome: What's new? Adv Clin Exp Med. 2017;26(2):359–67.

22. Ring M. Women's health: polycystic ovarian syndrome, menopause, and osteoporosis. Prim Care. 2017;44(2):377–98.

Menopause

Sara M. Pope, Emily Prazak, Steven Elek IV,
Timothy D. Wilcox, and Janelle K. Riley

Contents

S. M. Pope (✉) · E. Prazak
Kaiser Permanente Washington Family Medicine
Residency, Seattle, WA, USA
e-mail: sara.m.pope@kp.org; Emily.R.Prazak@kp.org

S. Elek IV
Navy Medical Center Portsmouth, Portsmouth, VA, USA
e-mail: Steven.Elek@med.navy.mil

T. D. Wilcox
U.S. Naval Hospital Guam, Tutuhan, Guam
e-mail: Timothy.Wilcox@med.navy.mil

J. K. Riley
Naval Branch Health Clinic, Fallon, NV, USA
e-mail: Janelle.Riley@med.navy.mil

© Springer Nature Switzerland AG 2022
P. M. Paulman et al. (eds.), *Family Medicine*,
https://doi.org/10.1007/978-3-030-54441-6_111

Overview

Menopause is a natural occurrence that marks the end of woman's reproductive years. Menopause is often described as an absence of "periods." However, the process is most accurately defined as the permanent cessation of menses. Clinical menopause is recognized after 12 months of amenorrhea [1]. The normal transition period that occurs prior to menopause is known as perimenopause. This transition begins approximately 4 years prior to menopause and is a result of progressive decline in ovarian function. This transition leads to menstrual cycle disruption, with waxing and waning of ovarian function. During perimenopause and menopause, women will experience many symptoms that include hot flashes, vaginal dryness, as well as mood and sleep disturbances [2]. There are several treatment options, both hormonal and nonhormonal, to combat these unwanted symptoms. Since average life span has increased, most women can expect to live at least one third of their life in menopause. The menopausal transition (MT) presents women with unique health concerns related to disease prevention and quality of life.

The Female Reproductive Life Span and the Menopausal Transition

During fetal life, the ovary goes through a series of embryological changes that result in the development of a primordial follicle, which is described as an ovum surrounded by granulosa cells. At the time of birth, a female infant will have approximately two million primordial follicles [4]. By puberty, 400,000 primordial follicles remain. Throughout a woman's reproductive life, only 400–500 of the primordial follicles grow into mature follicles and ovulate. By menopause, few, if any, primordial follicles remain. As the number of primordial follicles approaches zero, the production of estrogen decreases. When production of estrogen falls below a critical value, there is no longer feedback inhibition on the production of follicle-stimulating hormone (FSH) and luteinizing hormone (LH) [4]. Eventually, estrogen production by the ovaries falls to zero and can no longer inhibit the production of FSH and LH. Instead, these gonadotropins are produced in large and continuous quantities. These hormonal changes ultimately lead to cessation of menses [3–5].

Table 1 Stages of menopausal transition

Early perimenopause	Irregular menstrual cycles
	Ovulation may fail to occur
Late perimenopause	>60 days between menstrual cycles
	Skipped menstrual cycles
	Anovulatory cycles
	Episodes of amenorrhea
	Occurs within 1–3 years of FMP
	VMS may begin
Final menstrual period	Defined retrospectively
	Final period before 12 months of amenorrhea
Menopause	Cessation of menses for 12 months
Early postmenopause	2 years following the FMP
	VMS most likely to occur
Late postmenopause	5–8 years after the FMP
	Increased CV risk
	Altered bone metabolism
	Increasing symptoms of urogenital atrophy

FMP final menstrual period, *VMS* vasomotor symptoms

The hallmark of the MT (Table 1) is the change in the menstrual cycles, ultimately leading to cessation of periods. While many women progress through this transition without seeking medical care, a substantial number will have questions about the changes they experience. Women may consult their family physician for advice or reassurance during this time of transition.

Specifically, women may desire to know "what to expect" regarding the timeline of menopause and their menstrual cycles. Such questions can be challenging for the family physician to address, since the MT is characterized by irregularity. Predicting when menopause may occur has historically been difficult; however, in recent years there has been much interest in research directed toward better understanding and anticipating the MT.

The Stages of Reproductive Aging Workshop (STRAW) originally met in 2001 [6] to discuss the existing data on the MT. Since chronological age correlates poorly with menopausal changes, the goal of the workshop was to produce a staging system, analogous to the Tanner system for puberty, which could be used to objectively classify a woman's status in the MT. STRAW divided adult female life into three general phases: reproductive, menopausal transition, and postmenopause. These phases were further divided into seven stages, focused around the final menstrual period (FMP). The reproductive phase was divided into early (Stage 5), peak (Stage 4), and late (Stage 3a, 3b), The menopausal transition was divided into early (Stage 2) and late (Stage 1). Postmenopause, preceded by FMP, was divided into early (Stage +1a, +1b, +1c) and late (Stage +1). The resulting STRAW criteria have been well received and have guided further research in the field. The system was reviewed and updated in 2011 to reflect findings in the subsequent decade [7]. The updated staging system serves as the basis for the following discussion.

Stages of the Menopausal Transition

Late Reproductive Years

Even prior to entering the MT, women may notice changes in the flow or duration of their menses (e.g., "lighter" menses). Declining ovarian function results in decreased fertility. With a decrease in the number of developing follicles, there is a rise in FSH concentration. This is thought to be the result of decreased feedback inhibition of FSH and LH.

Early Menopause Transition

Change in the intermenstrual interval signals the beginning of the perimenopausal period. This change in bleeding patterns is the first symptom noticed by most women. The STRAW + 10 staging system [6, 7] objectively defines this stage as recurrent differences of ≥7 days in the length of consecutive cycles. For example, a woman experiences a cycle of 25 days followed by a cycle of 33 days. To meet the criteria, a similar discrepancy between consecutive cycle lengths should recur within ten cycles [7].

Of course, many women will not present with such detailed records of their periods. The overall concept of cycle length irregularity, however, should be clinically discernible in most instances. The clinical significance of this stage is primarily that it allows physician and patient to be reasonably confident that the menopausal transition has begun. The length of this stage is quite variable.

In late perimenopause, estrogen production falls below a critical level when the number of primordial follicles approaches zero. Women begin to have skipped cycles, episodic amenorrhea, and an increasing frequency of anovulatory cycles. These irregular cycles are the result of dramatic variations in estradiol concentrations.

Late Menopausal Transition

When a woman experiences a gap of greater than 60 days between cycles, she can be said to have entered the "late" phase of MT. This objective landmark is typically easy to discern in the clinical setting and signifies that a woman is likely within 1–3 years of her FMP. This stage has additional clinical significance, as this is the time when many women will begin having menopausal symptoms such as hot flashes.

Final Menstrual Period and Early Postmenopause

The landmark of the FMP is identified in retrospect, when a woman has been amenorrheic for 12 months. The 2 years that follow the FMP are considered the early postmenopausal period and are notable for a high prevalence of vasomotor symptoms.

Late Postmenopause

Late postmenopause describes the phase where menopausal hormone changes have fully stabilized, approximately 5–8 years after the final menstrual period. At this point, many of the symptoms of the menopausal transition will have subsided, but the physiologic implications of the postmenopausal state persist, such as increased cardiovascular risk, altered bone metabolism, and urogenital atrophy [3, 6, 7, 8].

Laboratory Testing

Discerning a woman's status in the menopausal transition should be thought of as a clinical process guided by the menstrual cycle history. Although research efforts are beginning to better characterize the status of several markers (i.e., follicle-stimulating hormone, estradiol, anti-Mullerian hormone) in the various stages of menopause, lab testing is not required for most women entering menopause at an appropriate age. The North American Menopause Society discourages the routine assessment of hormone levels [9]. However, a recent prospective from the Study of Women's Health Across the Nation (SWAN) showed that levels of anti-Mullerian hormone (AMH), along with age, may help estimate when a woman will undergo her FMP [10].

Epidemiology

The average onset of menopause is 51.4 years of age [13]. However, there is considerable variation among women. Approximately 5% of women undergo menopause after age 55, while in another 5%, onset will occur between 40 and 45 [5, 11]. This variation is thought to be due to several factors. Women with family members with early menopause are more likely to also experience early menopause [12]. According to STRAW, smokers both experience an earlier onset and a shorter MT duration. Black women experience a longer MT duration than White women. Lastly, those whose MT onset is earlier experience a longer MT duration [13].

Systemic Effects of Menopause

Menopause reflects a time of significant change for women. All the effects discussed below can have a substantial biopsychosocial impact, and they represent opportunities for the family physician to improve quality of life. The sequelae of menopause are widely underreported, and intentional screening should be considered part of high-quality care for perimenopausal and postmenopausal women.

Vasomotor Symptoms

One of the most common and well-known effects of menopause is the hot flash. Classically, these are "sudden episodes of intense heat that usually begin in the face or chest and spread throughout the body, accompanied by sweating and flushing that typically last 1–5 min" [14]. Physiologically, the symptoms largely result from peripheral vasodilation and inappropriate activation of heat loss mechanisms. Therefore, chills may follow the hot flash, as core body temperature is lowered [15]. Peri- and postmenopausal women are apparently predisposed to these reactions due to a narrowing of the thermoregulatory set zone in the hypothalamus [16]. This has been hypothesized as being related to the hormonal changes of menopause, but the exact mechanism remains unclear.

While estimates vary, a definite majority of women (up to 80%) will experience vasomotor symptoms (VMS) as they pass through menopause [7, 17]. Data on the duration of VMS suggest that the average length of symptoms is 7.4 years. SWAN identified four different subgroups of women in how they experienced VMS over the MT: (1) An early-onset group had VMS early in MT, which persisted after LMP but then declined; (2) later-onset group experienced VMS peaking during the FMP, persisting through and declining into postmenopause; (3) one group with few to none VMS during the MT; and (4) super flashers began VMS before FMP, and it persisted far into postmenopause [13]. It is important for the family physician to realize that both the experience and reporting of VMS will vary greatly between individuals.

On a larger scale, culture and ethnicity have a substantial effect on how women perceive their menopausal symptoms. SWAN showed Black women had the highest rate and longest duration of VMS and were most affected their VMS. Asian women reported the lowest rate of VMS, with Hispanic and White women landing between Black and Asian women. Lower socioeconomic status, less education, smoking, depression and anxiety, and a history of childhood abuse or neglect were associated with increased VMS. Thus, the family physician should make treatment recommendations on an individualized basis, taking the patient's unique experience into account.

Women who seek professional advice for their VMS should be counseled on lifestyle interventions and non-pharmacologic measures that may reduce their symptoms. These include smoking cessation, weight loss, stress reduction, lowering ambient room temperatures, and clothing choices [9, 14]. While supportive evidence for these interventions is limited, most are practical or bring other associated health benefits. The most effective treatment for VMS is hormonal therapy (HT). Other nonhormonal treatments that may reduce symptoms include paroxetine, venlafaxine, clonidine, gabapentin, and pregabalin [14]. Treatment will be discussed in more depth later in this chapter.

Sleep Disturbances

Perhaps one of the most challenging effects of menopause for the family physician to manage is sleep disturbances. In one large study, 38% of peri- and postmenopausal women reported sleep difficulty [18]. The menopausal transition has been shown in multiple studies to be strongly associated with sharp increases in the incidence of sleep disturbance and insomnia and increases over the MT [13]. However, there are numerous potential causes for sleep disruption in peri- and postmenopausal women, and in any given patient, several factors may be at play.

Vasomotor symptoms are a leading and clinically obvious cause for sleep disruption in perimenopause. However, even perimenopausal women without vasomotor symptoms have an increased prevalence of poor sleep [18]. Primary sleep disorders such as sleep-disordered breathing

(SDB), restless leg syndrome, and periodic limb movement disorder all present with increased frequency in menopausal women [19]. Depression, anxiety, and other mood disorders may act as primary or secondary causes of insomnia. The overall health status of the woman must be taken into consideration, as worsening medical conditions can contribute to poor sleep. Medications should be reviewed, and sources of chronic and acute pain should be actively managed.

In summary, the approach to sleep disturbance in perimenopause must be highly individualized and involve careful attention to the patient's specific complaints. Standard sleep hygiene education should be provided. The patient's risk factors for sleep disturbance should be addressed. Several studies have assessed the effect of HT on sleep; however, findings have been mixed and difficult to compare due to the variety of study populations, HT formulations, and tools to evaluate sleep. A recent clinical trial of peri- and post-menopausal women with insomnia symptoms as well as daily hot flashes initially showed the effectiveness of cognitive behavioral therapy (CBT) in women with insomnia during the MT [19].

Urogenital Changes

Nearly all of the tissues of the lower genitourinary tract in females feature estrogen receptors, including the bladder, urethra, and pelvic floor musculature [15]. With the withdrawal of estrogen during menopause, these structures undergo several physiologic changes that can be clinically problematic for women. Previously known as vulvovaginal atrophy, this constellation of findings is now referred to as the *genitourinary syndrome of menopause* (GSM), in order to reflect the broad nature of effects that may be related to this transition.

It is thought that nearly half of women will experience genitourinary symptoms related to menopause [20]. The most commonly reported GSM symptoms are vaginal dryness and dyspareunia. In the SWAN cohort, vaginal dryness increased from 19% to 34% over the MT. The more advanced into the menopausal stage, the more likely vaginal dryness was reported. Women may experience dryness,

irritation, and pain regardless of whether they are sexually active. Those who are sexually active may experience painful intercourse due to lack of lubrication and decreased elasticity of vaginal tissues. Loss of interest in or avoidance of sexual intercourse commonly results [13, 20]. Sexual functioning declines approximately 20 months prior to FMP and slows after FMP [13].

Urinary tract changes, such as urinary frequency, dysuria, and increased susceptibility to urinary tract infections (UTIs), are thought to be at least partially attributable to the hormonal changes of menopause [21]. Urinary incontinence (UI) was reported by 65% of the SWAN cohort at least once over a 9-year period of follow-up. Although UI is frequently reported, this is due to mid-life changes and not necessarily from menopause or decrease in estradiol [13].

The clinical approach includes screening for vaginal symptoms and dyspareunia, which women may be hesitant to voluntarily report. Objective findings on exam may include vaginal pallor and loss of rugae, as well as elevated vaginal pH (>5). It is important for the physician to consider and exclude other causes for the reported symptoms, such as vaginal infection, contact dermatitis, or lichen sclerosus [14, 21].

Once the diagnosis of GSM is established, women should be reassured of the possibility of treatment. Family physicians should be reminded that the symptoms of vulvovaginal atrophy are unlikely to improve without intervention [14]. For women with vaginal symptoms, local estrogen therapy is effective and has very few contraindications. Risk of endometrial stimulation remains a theoretical risk, so the lowest effective dose should be used, and any vaginal bleeding should be investigated [21]. Patients should be appropriately counseled on the unstudied safety profile of long-term use [14]. In women with additional menopausal symptoms, HT can be considered, as it is also effective for the symptoms of GSM.

Cognitive Changes

Many women perceive changes in their cognition during the MT. Memory loss or forgetfulness is one of the most common complaints, but women may also report a decreased ability to concentrate or multitask [9]. Studies investigating this phenomenon have validated some degree of correlation between subjective complaints and objective cognitive performance [31]. It is currently thought that minor declines can be attributable to the menopausal transition period but do not predict level of functioning later in life [9]. However, in any given patient, confounding factors may be in play. For example, subjective cognitive complaints are more common in the presence of mood symptoms and vasomotor symptoms.

Although several trials suggest modest cognitive benefit from HT, conflicting evidence exists [22]. The North American Menopause Society does not recommend HT for cognitive concerns or memory loss. Family physicians should focus efforts on optimizing other aspects of the patient's health by treating depression, reducing VMS, promoting sleep, encouraging physical activity, and avoiding medications that may affect cognition [9].

Mood Changes

The menopausal transition leading up to the final menstrual period appears to be a time of increased risk for symptoms of depression and anxiety. Depressive and anxiety symptoms have been reported more frequently during the late peri- and postmenopause than premenopause [13]. Stressful life events, increased financial strain, lower education, and being Hispanic were greater risks for depressive symptoms than menopausal status [13].

Although women may be more likely to present with non-affective complaints, family physicians should be alert to the possibility that depression and/or anxiety could be contributing to symptoms in the perimenopausal female. General symptoms of depression and anxiety should be carefully distinguished from actual mood disorders. The physician should assess the severity of the symptoms and their effect on functioning. Contributing biopsychosocial factors should be explored. Patients with mild depression or anxiety may benefit from cognitive behavioral therapy, whereas the addition of pharmacotherapy should

be considered in patients with moderate to severe symptoms [9].

Skin and Hair Changes

The hormonal changes of menopause represent one of several factors driving the process of skin aging in postmenopausal women. General systemic aging, along with variables such as sunlight exposure and smoking, also plays a significant role. In general, postmenopausal women may notice thinning of the skin, increased skin laxity and wrinkles, and dryness of the skin [9, 23].

Women may note hair loss or hirsutism. Both changes may be related to a relative increase in androgens in comparison with estrogen in postmenopausal women. Common hair loss disorders include female pattern hair loss and telogen effluvium [9].

Interestingly, estrogen replacement therapy has been shown to improve various characteristics of both the skin and hair in postmenopausal women [9, 23]; however, treatment of skin or hair changes is not considered to be a primary indication for hormonal therapy.

Cardiovascular Disease

Menopause is a time of escalating cardiovascular (CV) risk in women. Over the MT, women will see unfavorable changes in lipid profiles, body fat distribution, metabolic syndrome risk, and vascular health [13]. It is well-known that premenopausal women have, on average, more favorable lipid profiles than men [15]. However, this advantage subsides at menopause, and cardiovascular disease (CVD) remains the number one cause of death in women [9, 15]. As the FMP approaches, the increased LDL levels are associated with a higher risk of plaque presence. While higher levels of HDL may not be protective [13]. The effect of hormonal changes on female lipid profiles led to a large-scale investigation of HT for reduction of CV risk, with the ultimate finding of inadequate benefit and unacceptable risk for routine use of HT in CVD prevention.

Family physicians should be aware of the potential for abrupt changes in lipid profiles in the early postmenopausal period [9]. Aside from this, however, the prevention of cardiovascular disease in peri- and postmenopausal females does not differ substantially from other adult populations. Weight loss, exercise, and smoking cessation should be promoted. Blood pressure and cholesterol levels should be optimized. Diabetes mellitus should be screened for at appropriate intervals.

Osteopenia and Osteoporosis

Bone mineral density loss starts before the FMP, not after menopause. The estrogen deficiency of the MT promotes osteoclast activation, leading to a state in which bone reabsorption exceeds bone formation [24]. Following menopause, risk of fracture grows exponentially with age, and lifetime incidence of osteoporotic fractures is thought to be as high as 40% in Caucasian women [25].

In peri- or postmenopausal women, the evaluation begins with determining risk of fracture. Dual-energy x-ray absorptiometry (DEXA) objectively evaluates bone mineral density and is recommended for average-risk women at age 65. Earlier DEXA screening, however, should be considered in postmenopausal women thought to be at increased risk for osteoporosis [9]. Risk factors to consider include ethnicity (Caucasian and Asian women are at highest risk), low body weight, family history of osteoporosis and fractures, smoking, daily alcohol use, and use of high-risk medications such as systemic glucocorticoids. Some medical conditions can predispose to osteoporosis, such as rheumatoid arthritis or chronic kidney disease [25]. The patient's fall risk should be assessed, and women who have had a prior fragility fracture (fracture with fall from standing) are at particularly high risk for additional fractures. The Fracture Risk Assessment Tool (FRAX) developed by the World Health Organization incorporates many of the above risk factors and can be used to further guide clinical decisions.

Prevention efforts should include educating all women on the importance of adequate calcium and vitamin D intake and weight-bearing exercise. Supplemental calcium and vitamin D should be considered, as the average postmenopausal female receives approximately 500 mg less elemental calcium in her daily diet than recommended levels [25]. Osteoporosis is diagnosed by history of a fragility facture or by a bone mineral density (BMD) T-score < -2.5 at standard sites. In women with osteoporosis, as well as women with osteopenia and an elevated FRAX risk score, treatment should be considered [25]. Available options include bisphosphonates (Fosamax, Actonel, Reclast), selective estrogen receptor modulator (SERM) raloxifene (Evista), recombinant parathyroid hormone (Forteo), and calcitonin (Miacalcin). Estrogen replacement therapy has been shown to decrease fracture risk, but the benefit does not persist beyond discontinuation of therapy [25]. Estrogen replacement therapy is not currently FDA approved for treatment of osteoporosis.

Menopause Treatment

Overview

Most women manage the transition into menopause independently with approximately 10% of women seeking medical care. Symptoms of vaginal dryness, hot flashes, night sweats, and sleep disturbance most commonly prompt women to present to physicians [26]. Hormone therapy (HT) has been the mainstay treatment of menopausal symptoms for over 70 years. While HT is effective treatment for menopausal symptoms, some women may have underlying diseases that preclude use of hormones or wish to avoid risks associated with HT. Thus, there is expanding literature to explore alternative non-hormonal therapies (Table 5).

Hormone Therapy

Hormone therapy may include estrogen therapy alone (ET) or combined estrogen-progesterone therapy (EPT). Estrogen in combination with progesterone or alone is the most effective treatment of menopause-related vasomotor symptoms.

Progesterone alone also reduces vasomotor symptoms but not as effectively as estrogen [27].

Indications

Appropriate indications for HT include vasomotor symptoms such as hot flashes, night sweats, and vaginal dryness. Topical hormone therapy may be sufficient for vaginal symptoms without systemic vasomotor symptoms. Until the publication of the Women's Health Initiative (WHI) in 2002 [28, 29], HT was widely prescribed for the prevention of cardiovascular disease, dementia, and osteoporosis; however, due to the increased health risks discovered by the WHI, prescription of HT for preventative measures ceased. Overall, the physician's decision to offer treatment of vasomotor symptoms may depend on a woman's perception of the severity of symptoms [26].

Effectiveness of Hormone Therapy

Hormone therapy has consistently shown to be effective for treating several menopause symptoms, particularly vasomotor symptoms. A meta-analysis of randomized controlled trials shows incidence of hot flashes with HT reduced by 75% compared to 50% reduction with placebo [26]. Stated another way, estrogen has been shown to reduce the frequency of hot flashes by approximately 2.5–3 hot flashes/day [29]. In addition to decreased risk of fractures, HT may offer a small to moderate improvement in sexual function by improving the vulvovaginal symptoms of vaginal dryness and atrophy [30]. Improvement in sexual function seems to occur via treatment of menopausal symptoms. Improvements in vasomotor symptoms and vaginal dryness can take, on average, 1–2 months after starting therapy [26].

Formulations

Hormone therapy is available in oral tablets, transdermal patches, topical gels and sprays, or intravaginal preparations (Table 2). Estrogen alone may be used in

Table 2 Hormone therapy formulations

Hormone class	Formulation	Medication brand name
Oral estrogen	Estradiol	Estrace
	Esterified estrogen	Menest
	Estropipate	Ortho-Est
	Conjugated equine estrogen (CEE)	Premarin
Oral progestin	Micronized progesterone	Crinone, Endometrin, Prometrium
	Medroxyprogesterone acetate	Provera
Progesterone-release IUD	Levonorgestrel	Mirena, Skyla, Kyleena, Liletta
Oral combination estrogen and progestin	CEE/ medroxyprogesterone	Prempro
	Estradiol/norgestimate	Prefest
	Estradiol/ norethindrone acetate	Activella, Amabelz, Mimvey
	Ethinyl estradiol/ norethindrone	FemHRT, Jevantique Lo, Jinteli
	Estradiol/drospirenone	Angeliq
Estrogen patch	Estradiol	Alora, Minivelle, Vivelle-dot, Climara, Menostar, Dotti
Estrogen-progestin patch	Estradiol/ norethindrone	CombiPatch
	Estradiol/ levonorgestrel	Climara Pro
Topical estrogen	Estradiol gel	Estrogel, Elestrin, Divigel
	Estradiol spray	EvaMist
Intravaginal estrogen ring	Estradiol: Systemic absorption for treatment of vasomotor symptoms	Femring
	Estradiol: Local absorption for treatment of vulvovaginal symptoms only	Estring
Intravaginal estrogen tablet	Estradiol	Vagifem, Yuvafem, Imvexxy
Intravaginal estrogen gel	Estradiol	Estrace
	CEE	Premarin

women without a uterus. However, unopposed estrogen in women with a uterus increases the risk of endometrial hyperplasia [31], so progesterone must be added to estrogen in any woman with a uterus [30]. There is minimal systemic absorption of topical agents, so topical and intravaginal estrogen formulations are safe to use in women with a uterus without the addition of progesterone. Progestin-only formulations are available mainly in oral form; however, off-label use of levonorgestrel-releasing intrauterine devices (IUDs) has been shown to be both safe and effective [32]. Combination formulations are available as well.

Risks of Hormone Therapy

Known side effects of HT include nausea, breast tenderness, and irregular bleeding, especially early in menopause, as ovarian estrogen production fluctuates during this time [26, 27].

The Women's Health Initiative [26, 33, 34] unveiled many previously unknown risks associated with HT. Studies demonstrated that both estrogen therapy (ET) and estrogen-progesterone therapy (EPT) increased risk for stroke, venous thromboembolism (VTE), death by lung cancer, dementia, and gallbladder disease. Treatment with combined EPT also increased the risk of breast cancer and cardiovascular disease (CVD). Treatment with ET alone conversely was found to decrease breast cancer risk and not have an impact on CVD [30, 34].

There are many ways to numerically represent the increased risk posed by ET and EPT. Perhaps the most useful in counseling patients is by using the absolute risk (AR) over a defined time period (see Tables 3 and 4).

When using this data to counsel women on the risks and benefits of HT, there are caveats and nuances to keep in mind. Most data was collected in women with a mean age >60 years with only smaller groups of women in the perimenopausal or younger age group (age 50–59). This poses a major challenge for applying the data to clinical practice, since most women who seek hormone replacement therapy are in this younger age group. Furthermore, later subgroup analyses in the post-stoppage phases

Table 3 Risk of combined hormone therapy in postmenopausal women

Complication	Years of use	Absolute risk (AR)
Coronary event	After 1 year	4/1000
Venous thromboembolism	After 1 year	7/1000
Stroke	After 3 years	18/1000
Breast cancer	After 5.6 years	23/1000
Gallbladder disease	After 7 years	27/1000
Death from lung cancer	After 5.6 years (plus 2.4 years of follow-up)	9/1000
Dementia (>65 years, healthy)	After 4 years	18/1000

Adapted from Marjoribanks et al. [30]

Table 4 Risk of estrogen-only hormone therapy in peri- and postmenopausal women

Complication	Years of use	Absolute risk (AR)
Coronary event	After 1 year	4/1000
Venous thromboembolism	After 1–2 years	5/1000
	After 7 years	21/1000
Stroke	After 7 years	32/1000
Gallbladder disease	After 7 years	45/1000
Breast cancer	No significant increased risk	

Adapted from Marjoribanks et al. [30]

of the WHI-suggested CVD may be slightly reduced, rather than increased when hormone therapy (either ET or EPT) was initiated in women ages 50–59 [34]. However, this same age group also had an increase in breast cancer risk when started on combined HT [35]. Unfortunately, research on hormone replacement in this younger age group continues to be limited, even now 20 years after the WHI. Transdermal preparations may have a somewhat decreased risk of VTE, though further study is needed. Family physicians can expect the literature to continue to evolve in order to address specific factors such as age, proximity to menopause at the time of initiation, duration of HT therapy, and type of hormonal preparation.

Contraindications

Hormone therapy is contraindicated in women with a history of breast cancer, CVD, stroke, dementia, VTE, undiagnosed bleeding, or pregnancy.

Duration

Given the risks associated with HT, it is currently recommended to prescribe HT only in the lowest effective dose for the shortest possible time. Family physicians should regularly discuss with patients the ongoing need for therapy versus discontinuation. Short-term use of systemic HT is also clinically appropriate as hot flashes disappear within a few years of menopause for two thirds of women. Urogenital symptoms on the other hand are not self-limited, and frequently long-term therapy is needed. Topical and intravaginal therapy should be enough for urogenital symptoms [26]. Women with severe symptoms will need to balance the risk and benefits through informed decision-making with their physicians.

Monitoring

Regular review of continued need for HT by a woman and her physician is recommended. No specific interval is currently recommended, though every 3–6 months or at least annually is appropriate.

Intravaginal Hormonal Therapy

For women whose menopause symptoms are primarily vulvovaginal symptoms (e.g., atrophy, dryness, dyspareunia, etc.), the recommended treatment is intravaginal hormone therapy. While systemic hormone therapy will treat these symptoms, intravaginal therapy has significantly decreased risk for breast cancer, VTE, and stroke. Intravaginal HT is available as a cream, ring, or tablet (intravaginal pessary). These delivery systems have been shown to be equally effective at managing the symptoms of vaginal atrophy, with the main adverse side effect being the potential for thickening of the endometrial lining [36]. Caution should therefore be utilized in women with a history of endometrial hyperplasia or estrogen receptor-positive breast cancer. Vaginal moisturizers have similar efficacy to vaginal hormonal therapy and are thus excellent over-the-counter options for women who cannot or prefer not to use intravaginal hormone therapy [36]. Another nonhormonal option is the selective estrogen receptor modulator ospemifene, which is approved by the FDA specifically for moderate to severe vulvovaginal symptoms. As an oral tablet, it is an option for patients who prefer not to use an intravaginal treatment; however, it carries a risk of worsening vasomotor symptoms and an increased risk of VTE [37].

Bio-identical Hormone Therapy

There has been growing popularity of bio-identical hormone therapy (BHT), which technically refers to any hormone therapy that uses the same hormone produced endogenously (specifically 17β-estradiol). However, in lay communities this term is generally used to refer to hormones extracted from plants and modified to be structurally identical to endogenous hormones. These modified hormones are then compounded in variable combinations of estradiol, estrone, progesterone, testosterone, and DHEA by compounding pharmacies. These compounded formulations can take the form of pills, patches, gels, or suppositories. Many women have turned to BHT due to the assumption it is a more "natural" alternative to hormone therapy and thus safer than standardized HT. However; there is significant concern regarding the safety and effectiveness of BHT, as the compounding process is not standardized or regulated and the cost to patients is often quite high. A 2013 Cochrane Review analyzed 23 RCTs comparing efficacy for vasomotor symptoms and adverse events for BHT (unopposed 17 beta-estradiol) vs. placebo vs. conjugated equine estrogens. While there was low to moderate quality evidence that BHT improved vasomotor symptoms when compared to placebo, there was no significant difference in effectiveness when comparing BHT to conjugated equine estrogens. Results comparing the safety profile for BHT vs. HT were mixed, so the claim that BHT is safer than HT remains debatable [38].

Nonhormonal Therapy

Nonhormonal therapy may be an appropriate option for women with contraindications to hormonal therapy or those wishing to avoid risks associated with HT. A variety of treatment modalities have been investigated including antidepressants, clonidine, gabapentin/pregabalin, plant derivatives, acupuncture, hypnosis, and exercise.

Antidepressants

Some selective serotonin reuptake inhibitors (SSRIs) and serotonin-norepinephrine reuptake inhibitors (SNRIs) have been shown to reduce hot flashes, possibly due to the role serotonin plays in mediating hot flashes. Most of the data comes from lower doses of antidepressants (i.e., venlafaxine 37.5–75 mg or paroxetine 12.5–25 mg) for relative short durations (4–12 weeks).

Paroxetine (Paxil): Studies [29] indicate on doses of paroxetine, 12–25 mg daily, women experienced fewer daily hot flashes than women taking placebo (3.2–3.3 versus 1.8 fewer episodes/day). A trial predominantly including women with breast cancer taking tamoxifen on 10–20 mg of paroxetine also had fewer daily hot flashes compared with placebo. Paroxetine was effective at both doses, but not surprisingly, women taking higher doses experienced more adverse effects.

Venlafaxine (Effexor): Additional investigations have shown that women taking venlafaxine at doses from 37.5 to 150 mg/day experienced decrease frequency of hot flashes (30–58% versus 19% compared to placebo). Effects were greater with higher doses, though most evidence is from doses of 37.5–75 mg daily. An RCT with a head-to-head trial comparing venlafaxine to estradiol showed slight superiority of estradiol compared to

venlafaxine 75 mg daily. In this study, where mean hot flashes in the study group were 8/day, venlafaxine resulted in reduction to 5.5 daily episodes compared to 4.4 in the estradiol group [34].

Other SSRIs: Studies comparing fluoxetine (Prozac) and citalopram (Celexa) to placebo have failed to show a significant difference in vasomotor symptoms [29].

Alternative Pharmacological Therapy

Clonidine (Catapres): Meta-analysis shows that clonidine in doses of 0.05–0.15 mg daily may reduce hot flashes compared to placebo. Increased effect was seen at 8 weeks compared to 4 weeks of treatment [29]. Transdermal clonidine at 0.1 mg appears more effective than oral clonidine [26].

Gabapentin (Neurontin) and Pregabalin (Lyrica): A meta-analysis of studies comparing gabapentin and pregabalin compared to placebo showed a mean reduction of 1.62 hot flashes/day after 4 weeks and a mean reduction of 2.77 hot flashes/day after 12 weeks. While HT was still more effective than gabapentin/pregabalin, there was no significant difference between gabapentin/pregabalin and SSRIs [42].

Non-pharmacological Options

Plant and Natural Derivatives: Several naturally derived substances have been studied as an alternative for the treatment of menopause. Phytoestrogens are plant-derived products that have estrogenic activity. Soy isoflavones fit within this category and do show benefit for VMS and vaginal dryness [41] . Meta-analysis of red clover isoflavones, specifically Promensil and Rimostil, also showed possible slight benefit [29, 41]. Black cohosh, although widely utilized, has not been found to be beneficial [43]. Chinese herbal medicines are more challenging to study due to the varying combinations of herbs utilized, but thus far, meta-analyses have not shown a clear benefit. Several other natural products including evening primrose oil, dong quai, and ginseng have shown no benefit [26].

Exercise: Historically there has been much debate regarding the connection between physical activity and menopause symptoms. While physical activity has been anecdotally reported as an acute trigger of VMS, it has also been proposed as a potential treatment for symptoms of menopause. A meta-analysis evaluating exercise as a trigger of hot flashes suggested that daily physical activity may increase the number of self-reported hot flashes (particularly in women with depression

Table 5 Systemic effects and treatment of menopausal symptoms

		Hormonal	Nonhormonal
Vasomotor symptoms (VMS)	Hot flash	ET, EPT (oral, transdermal)	SSRIs: Paroxetine (Paxil)
			SNRIs: Venlafaxine (Effexor)
			Clonidine (Catapres)
			Gabapentin (Neurontin)
			Pregabalin (Lyrica)
			Acupuncture
			Clinical hypnosis
Sleep[a]	Insomnia Poor quality of sleep		Sleep hygiene Cognitive behavioral therapy (CBT) Exercise Acupuncture
Urogenital	Vaginal dryness, irritation, pain Dyspareunia Urinary frequency Dysuria Increased susceptibility to UTIs	ET (transdermal, intravaginal)	Vaginal moisturizers Clomiphene
	Memory loss Forgetfulness Poor concentration Depressive mood Anxiety		Treat depression, offer CBT Reduce VMS Promote sleep Exercise, physical activity Avoiding medications that affect cognition
Skin and hair	Thinning of skin Increased skin laxity, wrinkles Dry skin Hair loss Hirsutism		Reassurance
Cardiovascular	Increased LDL level Decreased HDL level		Weight loss Exercise Smoking cessation Optimize blood pressure, cholesterol level Screen for diabetes mellitus
Bone	Osteopenia Osteoporosis		Calcium, vitamin D Bisphosphonates Selective estrogen receptor modulators Recombinant parathyroid hormone Calcitonin

[a]Consider treating other primary causes: hot flashes, depression, restless leg syndrome, obstructive sleep apnea, or periodic limb movement disorder; *ET* estrogen therapy, *EPT* estrogen-progesterone therapy, *SSRIs* selective serotonin reuptake inhibitors, *SNRIs* serotonin-norepinephrine reuptake inhibitors

or anxiety), but not physiologic hot flashes, meaning women may perceive an increased number of hot flashes with exercise but there is no clear physiologic link for this observation [44]. Conversely, a Cochrane Review evaluating exercise as a treatment modality for vasomotor symptoms failed to show evidence of benefit [45]. Certainly for overall health, exercise remains a component of a healthy lifestyle, but given the current lack of evidence, it is difficult to make specific recommendations to women regarding the role of exercise for VMS.

Acupuncture: Multiple systematic reviews and meta-analyses have demonstrated that acupuncture improves VMS when compared with no treatment; however, there is no significant difference when compared with sham acupuncture [46]. Thus, clinicians may consider recommending acupuncture but should be clear about the limitations with patients.

Clinical Hypnosis: A single RCT compared clinical hypnosis to a control treatment showed a 74% decline in the frequency of hot flashes for the clinical hypnosis group compared to 17% decline for the control group. Similar differences were also noted for hot flash severity [47]. As these results have been demonstrated in only one RCT at this time, additional study will be beneficial to confirm results (Table 5).

Not all women will experience menopausal-related symptoms severe enough to warrant treatment; however, a substantial number will have questions about the changes they are experiencing and ways to maximize their health during the menopausal transition. Future evidence-based research will continue to help guide the family physician to successfully treat each woman in a holistic, individualized manner.

References

1. McKinlay SM. The normal menopause transition: an overview. Maturitas. 1996;23:137.
2. Taffc JR, Dennerstein L. Menstrual patterns leading to the final menstrual period. Menopause. 2002;9:32.
3. Hacker NF, Gambone JC, Hobel CJ. Hacker & Moore's essentials of obstetrics & gynecology [internet]. 6th ed. Philadelphia: Elsevier; 2016. p. 406–13. Available from: https://www.clinicalkey.com/#!/content/book/3-s2.0-B9781455775583000358. Cited 22 Mar 2020
4. White BW, Harrison JR, Mehlmann LM. Endocrine and reproductive physiology [internet]. 5th ed. St. Louis: Elsevier; 2019. p. 170–85. Available from: https://www.clinicalkey.com/#!/content/book/3-s2.0-B9780323595735000088?scrollTo=%23top. Cited 22 Mar 2020
5. Greendale GA, Ishii S, Huang M, Karlamangla AS. Predicting the timeline to the final menstrual period: the study of women's health across the nation. J Clin Endocrinol Metab. 2013;98(4):1483.
6. Soules MR, Sherman S, Parrott E, Rebar R, Santoro N, Utian W, et al. Executive summary: Stages of Reproductive Aging Workshop (STRAW) Park City, Utah, July, 2001. Menopause. 2001;8(6):402–7.
7. Harlow SD. Executive summary of the stages of reproductive aging workshop + 10: addressing the unfinished agenda of staging reproductive aging. J Clin Endocrinol Metab. 2012;97(4):1159–68.
8. Allshouse A, Pavlovic J, Santoro N. Menstrual cycle hormone changes associated with reproductive aging and how they may relate to symptoms. Obstet Gynecol Clin N Am. 2018;45(4):613–28. Available from: https://www.clinicalkey.com/#!/content/playContent/1-s2.0-S0889854518300640?returnurl=https:%2F%2Flinkinghub.elsevier.com%2Fretrieve%2Fpii%2FS0889854518300640%3Fshowall%3Dtrue&referrer=https:%2F%2Fwww.ncbi.nlm.nih.gov%2Fpubmed%2F30401546. Cited 23 Mar 2020
9. Shifren J, Gass M. The North American Menopause Society recommendations for clinical care of midlife women. Menopause. 2014;21(10):1038–62.
10. Finkelstein JS, Lee H, Karlamangla A, Neer RM, Sluss PM, Burnett-Bowie SM, et al. Anti-Mullerian hormone and impending menopause in late reproductive age: the Study of Women's Health Across the Nation. J Clin Endocrinol Metab. 2020;105(4) https://doi.org/10.1210/clinem/dgz283.
11. Gold EB. The timing of the age at which natural menopause occurs. Obstet Gynecol Clin N Am. 2011;38(3):425–40.
12. de Bruin JP, Bovenhuis H, van Noord PA, et al. The role of genetic factors in age at natural menopause. Hum Reprod. 2001;16:2014.
13. El Khoudary SR, Greendale G, Crawford SL, Avis NE, Brooks MM, Thurston RC, et al. The menopause transition and women's health at midlife: a progress report from the Study of Women's Health Across the Nation (SWAN). Menopause. 2019;26(10):1213–27. Available from: https://journals.lww.com/menopausejournal/Fulltext/2019/10000/The_menopause_transition_and_women_s_health_at.20.aspx. Cited 23 Mar 2020
14. Al-Safi Z, Santoro N. Menopausal hormone therapy and menopausal symptoms. Fertil Steril. 2014;101(4):905–15.
15. Hoffman B, Schorge J, Schaffer J, Halvorson L, Bradshaw K, Cunningham F, et al. Chapter 21: Menopausal transition. In: Hoffman BL, Schorge JO, Schaffer JI, Halvorson LM, Bradshaw

KD, Cunningham FG, et al., editors. Williams gynecology. 2nd ed. New York: McGraw-Hill; 2012.

16. Stearns V, Ullmer L, Lopez J, Smith Y, Isaacs C, Hayes D. Hot flushes. Lancet. 2002;360:1851–61.

17. Gold EB, Colvin A, Avis N, Bromberger J, Greendale J, Powell L, et al. Longitudinal analysis of the association between vasomotor symptoms and race/ethnicity across the menopausal transition: Study of Women's Health Across the Nation. Am J Public Health. 2006;97(6):1226–35.

18. Kravitz H, Ganz P, Bromberger J, Powell L, Sutton-Tyrrell K, Meyer P. Sleep difficulty in women at mid-life: a community survey of sleep and the menopausal transition. Menopause. 2003;10(1):19–28.

19. Baker FC, Lampio L, Saaresranta T, Polo-Kantola P. Sleep and sleep disorders in the menopausal transition. Sleep Med Clin. 2018;13(3):443–56. Available from: https://www.ncbi.nlm.nih.gov/pmc/articles/PMC6092036/. Cited 23 Mar 2020

20. Sturdee D, Panay N. Recommendations for the management of postmenopausal vaginal atrophy. Climacteric. 2010;13:509–22.

21. Portman D, Gass M. Genitourinary syndrome of menopause: new terminology for vulvovaginal atrophy from the International Society for the Study of Women's Sexual Health and The North American Menopause Society. Menopause. 2014;21(10):1063–8.

22. Fisher B, Gleason C, Asthana S. Effects of hormone therapy on cognition and mood. Fertil Steril. 2014;101 (4):898–904.

23. Brinkat M, Baron Y, Galea R. Estrogens and the skin. Climacteric. 2005;8(2):110–23.

24. Hofbauer L, Schoppet M. Clinical implications of the osteoprotegerin/RANKL/RANK system for bone and vascular diseases. JAMA. 2004;292(4):490–5.

25. The North American Menopause Society. Management of osteoporosis in postmenopausal women: 2010 position statement of The North American Menopause Society. Menopause. 2010;17(1):25–54.

26. Roberts H. Managing the menopause. BMJ. 2007;334 (7596):736–41.

27. Gass ML, Heights M, Manson JE, Cosman F, Hayes H, Grodstein F, et al. The 2012 hormone therapy position statement of The North American Menopause Society. Menopause. 2012;19(3):257–71.

28. Writing Group for the Women's Health Initiative Investigators. Risks and benefits of estrogen plus progestin in healthy postmenopausal women: principal results from the Women's Health Initiative randomized controlled trial. JAMA. 2002;288(3):321–33. https://doi.org/10.1001/jama.288.3.321. Available from: https://jamanetwork.com/journals/jama/fullarticle/195120. Cited 23 Mar 2020

29. Nelson HD, Vesco KK, Fu R, Nedrow A, Miller J, Nicolaidis C, Walker M, Humphrey L. Nonhormonal therapies for menopausal hot flashes. JAMA. 2006;295 (17):2057–71.

30. Marjoribanks J, Farquhar C, Roberts H, Lethaby A. Long term hormone therapy for perimenopausal and postmenopausal women. Cochrane Database Syst

Rev. 2012;2012(7):CD004143. Available from: https://www.cochranelibrary.com/cdsr/doi/10.1002/146518 58.CD004143.pub4/full. Cited 20 Mar 2020

31. Furness S, Roberts H, Marjoribanks J, Lethaby A. Hormone therapy in postmenopausal women and risk of endometrial hyperplasia. Cochrane Database Syst Rev. 2012;2012(8):CD000402. Available from: https://www.cochranelibrary.com/cdsr/doi/10.1002/14651858.CD000402.pub3/full. Cited 20 Mar 2020

32. Long ME, Faubion SS, MacLaughlin KL, Pruthi S, Casey PM. Contraception and hormonal management in the perimenopause. J Women's Health. 2015;24 (1):3–10. https://doi.org/10.1089/jwh.2013.4544.

33. Anderson GL, Limacher M, Assaf AR, Bassford T, Beresford SA, Black H, et al. Women's Health Initiative Steering Committee. Effects of conjugated equine estrogen in postmenopausal women with hysterectomy: the Women's Health Initiative randomized controlled trial. JAMA. 2004;291(14):1701–12.

34. Mason JE, Chlebowski RT, Stefanick ML, Aragaki AK, Rossouw JE, Prentice RL, et al. Menopausal hormone therapy and health outcomes during the intervention and extended poststopping phases of the Women's Health Initiative randomized trials. JAMA. 2013;310 (13):1353–68. https://doi.org/10.1001/jama.2013.278 040.

35. Rossouw JE, Manson JE, Kaunitz AM, Anderson GL. Lessons learned from the Women's Health Initiative trials of menopausal hormone therapy. Obstet Gynecol. 2013;121(1):172–6.

36. Lethaby A, Ayeleke R, Roberts H. Local oestrogen for vaginal atrophy in postmenopausal women. Cochrane Database Syst Rev. 2016;2016(8):CD001500. Available from: https://www.ncbi.nlm.nih.gov/pmc/articles/PMC7076628/. Cited 20 Mar 2020

37. Mitchell CM, Reed SD, Diem S, Larson JC, Newton KM, Ensrud KE, et al. Efficacy of vaginal estradiol or vaginal moisturizer vs placebo for treating postmenopausal vulvovaginal symptoms: a randomized clinical trial. JAMA. 2018;178(5):681–90. Available from: https://www.ncbi.nlm.nih.gov/pmc/articles/PMC5885 275/. Cited 20 Mar 2020

38. Wurz GT, Kao CJ, DeGregoria MW. Safety and efficacy of ospemifene for the treatment of dyspareunia associated with vulvar and vaginal atrophy due to menopause. Clin Interv Aging. 2014;9:1939–50. https://doi.org/10.2147/CIA.S73753.

39. Gaudard AMIS, Silva de Souza S, Puga MES, Marjoribanks J, da Silva EMK, Torloni MR. Bioidentical hormones for women with vasomotor symptoms. Cochrane Database Syst Rev. 2016;2016(8):CD010407. Available from: https://www.cochranelibrary.com/cdsr/doi/10.1002/14651858.CD010407.pub2/full. Cited 20 Mar 2020

40. Joffe H, Guthrie KA, LaCroix AZ, Reed SD, Ensrud KE, Manson JE, et al. Low-dose estradiol and the serotonin–norepinephrine reuptake inhibitor venlafaxine for vasomotor symptoms: a randomized clinical trial. JAMA Intern Med. 2014;174(7):1058–66.

41. Shan D, Zou L, Liu X, Shen Y, Cai Y, Zhang J. Efficacy and safety of gabapentin and pregabalin in patients with vasomotor symptoms: a systematic review and meta-analysis. Am J Obstet Gynecol. 2019;222(6):564–579.e12. Available from: https://www.clinicalkey.com/#!/content/playContent/1-s2.0-S0002937819327681?returnurl=https:%2F%2Flinkinghub.elsevier.com%2Fretrieve%2Fpii%2FS0002937819327681%3Fshowall%3Dtrue&referrer=https:%2F%2Fwww.ncbi.nlm.nih.gov%2Fpubmed%2F31870736. Cited 20 Mar 2020

42. Lethaby A, Marjoribanks J, Kronenberg F, Roberts H, Eden J, Brown J. Phytoestrogens for menopausal vasomotor symptoms. Cochrane Database Syst Rev. 2013;2013(2):CD001395. https://doi.org/10.1002/14651858.CD001395.pub4.

43. Leach MJ, Moore V. Black cohosh (Cimicifuga spp.) for menopausal symptoms. Cochrane Database of Systematic Reviews 2012, Issue 9. Art. No.: CD007244. https://doi.org/10.1002/14651858.CD007244.pub2.

44. Zhu X, Liew Y, Liu ZL. Chinese herbal medicine for menopausal symptoms. Cochrane Database Syst Rev. 2016;2016(3):CD009023. Available from: https://www.cochranelibrary.com/cdsr/doi/10.1002/14651858.CD009023.pub2/full. Cited 20 Mar 2020

45. Gibson C, Matthews KA, Thurston R. Daily physical activity and hot flashes in the Study of Women's Health Across the Nation (SWAN) Flashes Study. Fertil Steril. 2014;101(4):1110–6.

46. Daley A, Stokes-Lampard H, Thomas A, MacArthur C. Exercise for vasomotor menopausal symptoms. Cochrane Database Syst Rev. 2014;2014(11):CD006108. Available from: https://www.cochranelibrary.com/cdsr/doi/10.1002/14651858.CD006108.pub4/full. Cited 20 Mar 2020

47. Dodin S, Blanchet C, Marc I, Ernst E, Wu T, Vaillancourt C, et al. Acupuncture for menopausal hot flushes. Cochrane Database Syst Rev. 2013;2013(7):CD007410. https://doi.org/10.1002/14651858.CD007410.pub2.

48. Elkins GR, Fisher WI, Johnson AK, Carpenter JS, Keith TZ. Clinical hypnosis in the treatment of postmenopausal hot flashes: a randomized controlled trial. Menopause. 2013;20(3):291–8. Available from: https://www.ncbi.nlm.nih.gov/pmc/articles/PMC3556367/. Cited 20 Mar 2020

Tumors of the Female Reproductive Organs

110

Paul Gordon, Hannah M. Emerson, Faith Dickerson, Surbhi B. Patel, and Genevieve Riebe

Contents

Leiomyoma

General Principles

Definition/Background

Leiomyoma or fibroids arise from monoclonal proliferation or numerous copies of the same or very few cells [1] and are stimulated by estrogen and progesterone. They increase their growth rate during pregnancy and regress after menopause. They vary widely in size from a few millimeters to large masses filling the entire abdomen.

Epidemiology

Leiomyoma is the most common benign neoplasm of the female reproductive tract. It is present in 20–30% of women of reproductive age [2]. However, since many leiomyomata are asymptomatic, the true incidence is unknown. African-American women have a two- to threefold higher incidence than white women [3]. In addition, a systemic review by Stewart et al. [4] describe age, nulliparity, premenopausal state, hypertension, family history, time since parity, food additive, and soybean consumption to have a higher incidence.

P. Gordon (✉) · G. Riebe
Family and Community Medicine, University of Arizona, College of Medicine, Tucson, AZ, USA
e-mail: pgordon@medadmin.arizona.edu

H. M. Emerson · F. Dickerson · S. B. Patel
College of Medicine, University of Arizona, Tucson, AZ, USA
e-mail: hemerson@email.arizona.edu; fdickerson@email.arizona.edu; surbhibpatel@email.arizona.edu

© Springer Nature Switzerland AG 2022
P. M. Paulman et al. (eds.), *Family Medicine*,
https://doi.org/10.1007/978-3-030-54441-6_112

Classification

The easiest classification system is by anatomic location: (1) intramural, entirely within the walls of the uterus; (2) submucous, beneath the uterine lining; (3) subserous, which distorts the outer surface of the uterus; (4) intraligamentous; (5) parasitic, deriving its blood supply from another organ to which is has become attached; (6) pedunculated, attached to the uterus by a stalk; and (7) cervical.

Approach to the Patient

Risk factors have been identified which aid us in our approach to the patient. Fibroids are subject to hormonal stimuli. They arise with menarche and become inactive after menopause.

Diagnosis

History

Nonpregnant women with leiomyoma are often asymptomatic. The most common systems for which they seek treatment are abnormal bleeding and pelvic pain or pressure. If the myoma significantly distorts the uterine cavity, women may be infertile. Additionally, they may experience increased abdominal girth, urinary frequency, low back pain, and dyspareunia. There are also adverse pregnancy outcomes including malpresentation, dysfunctional labor, abnormal placentation, and abruption.

Physical Examination

The bimanual exam is the key physical exam procedure to identify a leiomyoma. A lobular, enlarged structure with a rubbery consistency may be found. Larger lesions can also be felt on abdominal exam.

Laboratory and Imaging

Anemia may be found as a result of abnormal uterine bleeding. Hydronephrosis may also be seen due to ureteral compression from the mass. Pelvic ultrasound remains the test of choice for diagnosis. Sonohysterogram or hysteroscopy can be used to confirm submucous leiomyomata.

Special Testing

MRI should be used sparingly due to its cost and the adequacy of other diagnostic imaging procedure. If there is an atypical lesion and concern for sarcoma is present, MRI would be appropriate. Endometrial biopsy can be performed if there is concern for endometrial cancer (see next section).

Differential Diagnosis

The most important diagnosis to be considered in the differential is leiomyosarcoma. It is rare but aggressive. However, of those rapidly growing leiomyoma (6 cm in 1 year), less than 0.1% of these are malignant. At surgery for women with presumed benign leiomyoma, the FDA estimates the prevalence of 0.277% for any uterine sarcoma and 0.134% for leiomyosarcoma [5]. Other diagnoses include solid ovarian tumors or uterine enlargement due to adenomyosis [1].

Treatment

Behavioral

Women with asymptomatic fibroids require no treatment.

Medications\Immunizations and Chemoprophylaxis

Women with abnormal uterine bleeding will often benefit from a trial of cyclic or continuous oral contraceptives or progestins. Prior to surgery, gonadotropin-releasing hormone (GnRH) agonists can decrease size and stop the bleeding. Long-term use of GnRH agonists has side effects such as osteoporosis. Mifepristone, an antiprogestin, may cause significant decrease in myoma size but may cause endometrial hyperplasia. Repeated intermittent use of ulipristal acetate, a selective P receptor modulator (SPRM), has shown efficacy in decreasing myoma size without causing concerning endometrial hyperplasia [6].

Referrals

For women whose symptoms continue despite treatment with medications, there are several surgical options. However, there are no well-conducted trials with US women comparing expectant management and various surgical procedures [1]. For women who wish to retain their fertility, myomectomy is generally offered. This procedure consists of removing the leiomyoma and then repairing the defect in the uterine wall. Myomectomy can be performed via laparotomy, laparoscopy, or hysteroscopy depending on the size, location, and number of lesions. There are several minimally invasive, uterus-sparing options. Radiofrequency volumetric thermal ablation (RFVTA) uses laparoscopic or transcervical routes using sonography guidance to place needle electrodes that use thermal energy to induce thermal fixation and coagulative necrosis in solid tumors, resulting in fibroid volume reduction and symptomatic relief [7, 8]. For women wishing to avoid surgery and who do not have future child-bearing plans, uterine artery embolization can be used [9]. This procedure using angiography decreases blood flow to the uterus. This procedure has high (80–90%) success rates in decreasing blood flow and size and improving pelvic pressure [1]. However, it has been associated with surgical intervention within 2–5 years post-procedure [9]. For women who have completed childbearing and desire uterus-sparing options, magnetic resonance-guided focused ultrasound (MRgFUS) is also available; however, it is uncertain what the maximum myoma size threshold, candidate profile, and long-term outcomes for this method will be. MRgFUS is an outpatient procedure that involves noninvasive thermoablation that focuses multiple waves of ultrasound energy on a small area of tissue, thereby thermally destroying the tissue, with low short-term morbidity and rapid recovery [10]. Comparison of all three uterus-sparing modalities shows that RFVTA provides more significant fibroid and uterine volume reduction than uterine artery embolization or MRgFUS [10]. Finally, hysterectomy may be offered as a definitive procedure. The Agency for Healthcare Research and Quality (AHRQ) report concludes "The current state of the literature does not permit definitive conclusions about benefit, harm, or relative costs to help guide women's choices" [1].

Counseling

Fibroid tumors can be present in women with recurrent implantation failure, and appropriate counseling regarding their treatment would fall on the family physician [11]. Additionally, there are multiple factors related to successful hysteroscopic endometrial ablation including fibroids that could improve patient counseling.

Prevention

As mentioned above, nulliparity increases the risk of fibroids. Similarly, pregnancy is associated with a reduced risk of fibroids. Mifepristone, an antiprogestin, has been shown to decrease the size of leiomyomata by 50% [12]. Three WNT/beta-catenin pathway inhibitors, i.e., inhibitor of beta-catenin and TCF4 (ICAT), niclosamide, and XAV939, have been shown to block leiomyoma growth and proliferation [13]. Finally, a number of substances have been effective in the chemoprevention of fibroid tumors in quails [14, 15].

Endometrial Carcinoma

General Principles

Definition/Background

Endometrial cancer is the most common gynecological malignancy and the fourth most common cancer in women after breast, lung, and colorectal cancers. Incidence of endometrial carcinoma has increased by 1–2% annually, as has mortality [16]. Various theories to explain this increase included increasing life span and coexisting medical comorbidities in these women.

Epidemiology

The mean age at diagnosis is 60 years [17], and 90% of cases occur in women older than 50 years. 90% of cases occur in women older than 50 years, 20% of women have this diagnosis before menopause, and approximately 5% have disease before age 40 years [18]. Approximately 72% are stage I, 12% are stage II, 13% are stage III, and 3% are stage IV.

Table 1 Classification of endometrial cancer

Type I	Type II	Familial
Low-grade	High-grade	Lynch
Minimal myometrial invasion	Deep myometrial invasion	
Arising in a background of hyperplasia	Serous or clear cell	
Perimenopausal Estrogen-related Younger age Obesity		

Classification

Endometrial cancer is commonly classified into three types (Table 1). The majority of women have Type I. With Type I, a genetic predisposition to obesity can increase one's risk of endometrial cancer. Type II occurs more commonly in older women, is more common in black women, and consists of higher-grade tumors. Genetic disease can represent up to 10% of cases, of which 5% are associated with Lynch syndrome, the hereditary nonpolyposis colorectal cancer syndrome.

Approach to the Patient

Risk factors have been identified, and these should be addressed including the possibility of a hereditary component. These risk factors, which will be discussed below, include obesity, reproductive, and menstrual factors.

Diagnosis

History

Abnormal uterine bleeding including postmenopausal, menorrhagia, or metrorrhagia is the most common presenting symptom for women with endometrial hyperplasia or carcinoma. Atypical glandular cells on cervical cytology should also be evaluated with colposcopy, endocervical curettage, and endometrial biopsy in women older than 35 or those with risk factors for endometrial cancer [19]. Nearly 70% of women with early-stage endometrial cancer are obese. Moreover, the relative risk for death for women with endometrial cancer increases with increasing BMI [20]. Continuous estrogen stimulation, both endogenous and exogenous, can alter the menstrual cycle resulting in anovulation. Anovulation results in continuous unopposed estrogen stimulation since there is no corpus luteum to produce progesterone. Obesity, through the peripheral conversion of androstenedione into estrone, results in increased endogenous estrogen and increases in the relative risk (RR) of endometrial cancer up to three times [21]. Estrogen-producing tumors, cirrhosis, unopposed estrogen therapy, and tamoxifen can also result in increased estrogen stimulation in the uterus. Although tamoxifen is an antiestrogen in breast tissue, it can have estrogenic activity in the endometrium [22]. Unopposed estrogen replacement during menopause increases the RR four to eight times, whereas combined estrogen and progesterone replacement therapy decreases the risk of endometrial cancer. Similarly, progestin-containing oral contraceptives or combined oral contraceptive pill decreases the risk of disease by nearly one-half. This increased risk associated with estrogen therapy continues until 2 or 3 years after cessation of therapy [23]. Nulliparity and diabetes are associated with a two- to threefold increase incidence of disease. Nulliparity is related to infertility rather than intentional prevention of pregnancy. Infertility is related to anovulation as discussed above as opposed to tubal factors. Although the incidence in white women is higher than in black women, stage for stage, black women have a less favorable prognosis. Regarding Type II disease, these patients account for 10% of cases, are not related to estrogen excess, tend to occur at an older age, and are poorly differentiated with serous or clear cell histology.

Physical Examination

In women with abnormal uterine bleeding and risk factors as mentioned above, concern for endometrial cancer must be pursued. Although a physical examination including bimanual may be important, the diagnosis is made based on histology. Endometrial biopsy is an office-based procedure for the family physician [24].

Laboratory and Imaging

There are multiple modalities available to evaluate the endometrium. However, there is no recent ACOG Practice Bulletin to guide the clinician in choosing the modality. Endometrial biopsy (EMB) (with a piston catheter) is a simple procedure with good accuracy [25]. There have been a few retrospective studies comparing its accuracy to dilation and curettage (D&C) [26]. Although D&C was slightly better, it requires a visit to the operating room and anesthesia, whereas office EMB does not. Goldstein and colleagues who "were among the first Americans to publish on the high negative predictive value of thin distinct endometrial echo in postmenopausal patients with bleeding" [27] recommend beginning the evaluation with endovaginal ultrasound (EV-US). If the endometrial stripe is </4 mm in postmenopausal women or </5 mm in premenopausal women, no further diagnostic procedure is necessary (Fig. 1 in Goldstein [28]). Sweet et al. recommend EMB for women <35 years with recurrent anovulation and/or other risks for endometrial cancer. These risks include obese adolescents with 3 years of untreated anovulatory bleeding; women <35 years with chronic anovulation, diabetes, family history of colon cancer, infertility, nulliparity, obesity, or tamoxifen use; for women whose bleeding did not respond to medical therapy [29]. All women >/35 years with suspected anovulatory bleeding should have an EMB performed.

Special Testing

Saline infusion sonohysterography (SIS) can be used to evaluate the endometrial lining if transvaginal ultrasound does not provide adequate visualization. Sterile saline is instilled into the uterine cavity via a small catheter with ultrasound guidance. SIS can provide additional differentiation of focal lesions in addition to diffuse abnormalities such as endometrial hyperplasia. Newer techniques substitute gel for saline, which provides better technical results, and slightly increased sensitivity and specificity of detection of intrauterine lesions, compared to SIS [30]. Patients experience reduced discomfort because gel-instillation sonography uses a smaller amount of gel to distend the uterine cavity [31].

Differential Diagnosis

The differential diagnosis for abnormal uterine bleeding includes both malignancy as discussed above and benign causes. ACOG Practice Bulletin [32] reviews benign causes ▶ Chap. 105, "Selected Disorders of the Genitourinary System". The results of EMB show simple and complex hyperplasia both with and without atypia. The Gynecologic Oncology Group sought to validate the reproducibility of the referring institution's pathologic diagnosis of complex hyperplasia with atypia. They found the level of reproducibility to be poor [33]. Current recommendations are that women with both simple and complex hyperplasia without atypia and those with simple hyperplasia with atypia can be treated with progestins as the risk for endometrial carcinoma is low [21]. Cyclic medroxyprogesterone 10 mg daily for 14 days each month or continuous megestrol acetate 20–40 mg daily are both acceptable as is the placement of a progestin-releasing IUD. However, women with complex hyperplasia with atypia have >40% incidence of coexisting adenocarcinoma, and hysterectomy is the treatment of choice for these women. Alternatively, endometrial intraepithelial neoplasia is a new classification system designed to replace the hyperplasia terminology [34]. If this terminology were to be widely adopted by the pathology community, then this diagnosis may be more useful for clinical decisions than the current hyperplasia classification system.

Treatment

Behavioral

The most important behavioral intervention related to the prevention of endometrial cancer is weight loss, reviewed elsewhere in this text.

Medications\Immunizations and Chemoprophylaxis

As noted above, women with both simple and complex hyperplasia without atypia and those with simple hyperplasia with atypia can be treated with progestins. Cyclic medroxyprogesterone

10 mg daily for 14 days each month or continuous megestrol acetate 20–40 mg daily are both acceptable as is the placement of a progestin-releasing IUD. These women should have a repeat EMB in 3–6 months and referral to a gynecologist if the hyperplasia persists.

Referrals

All women with complex hyperplasia with atypia and those with adenocarcinoma need referral to a gynecologist or gynecologic oncologist, respectively.

Cervical Cancer

General Principles

Definition/Background

Invasive cervical cancer is the third most common gynecologic cancer among women in the United States [35]. There are two histological types of cervical cancer, adenocarcinoma and squamous cell carcinoma. The human papilloma virus (HPV) is detected in 99.7% of all cervical cancer [36], with HPV types 16 and 18 accounting for 70% of those cases [37]. The epidemiology, risk factors, diagnosis, screening, prevention, and treatment of cervical cancer will be reviewed here.

Epidemiology

Worldwide, cervical cancer is the third most common malignancy [37]. There were 13,170 new cases of cervical cancer and 4,250 cervical cancer-related deaths in the United States in 2019. Cervical cancer estimates are higher for particular racial and ethnic groups with incidence and mortality being higher in African-American, American Indian, and Alaskan Native women than white and Asian women in the United States. Estimates are also higher for Hispanic women than non-Hispanic women. The incidence is highest in Hispanics/Latinos at 9.3 per 100,000 and mortality highest in African-Americans with 3.5 deaths per 100,000 cases [38]. There has been an overall decrease of deaths by 30.66% from 1990 to 2007 and a 50% reduction in incidence over 30 years from 1975 to 2006 [39]. From 2007 to 2016, death rates have fallen about 0.7% each year [38].

Risk Factors

Epidemiological risk factors for cervical cancer are well documented. Some are modifiable, which speaks to the importance of patient education and awareness for increased risk. Human papilloma virus (HPV) infection is a well-established risk factor for cervical cancer. Most risk factors are linked with the increased risk of acquiring HPV. These risks include early onset of sexual activity, multiple sexual partners, history of sexually transmitted infections, sexual partner (s) infected with HPV, history of vulvar or vaginal intraepithelial neoplasia or cancer, and immunosuppression [40]. Another major risk factor associated with cervical cancer is smoking [41]. In utero diethylstilbestrol (DES), previous treatment of high-grade precancerous lesions and history of cervical cancer are also risk factors [42]. Although unclear, socioeconomic status, three or more full-term births, young age at first delivery (less than 20 years of age), and oral contraceptive use may also increase risk. Other high-risk groups include refugees and women who have immigrated to the United States from countries where cervical cancer screening is not routinely performed and women without access to health care [43] (Table 2).

Classification

Cervical cancer is classified as squamous cell carcinoma, adenocarcinoma, adenosquamous or mixed carcinomas, and small cell carcinoma. Squamous cell carcinoma accounts for approximately 90% of cervical cancers, adenocarcinoma

Table 2 Risk factors for cervical cancer [44]

Risk factor	Relative risk
Menarche to first coitus <1 year	26.4
Age at first coitus <16 years	16.1
More than three sexual partners before age 20	10.2
Never having a pap smear	8.0
Cigarette smoking >20 years	4.0
History of genital warts	2

comprises the other 10% with adenosquamous, and small cell carcinomas are rare.

Diagnosis

As described in Moore's approach to cancer management, there are four steps involved: (1) Establish the diagnosis. (2) Define the extent of disease. (3) Determine and implement treatment. (4) Follow the patient for evidence of recurrence and/or treatment-related complications [45].

History

Early cervical cancer may be asymptomatic. Common symptoms of cervical cancer include irregular vaginal bleeding, heavy vaginal bleeding, dyspareunia, and postcoital bleeding [40]. Unusual vaginal discharge may be described and can be purulent, malodorous, bloody, watery, or mucinous [46]. Taking a careful history and proper diagnostic testing must be performed as to not mistake these symptoms for cervicitis or vaginitis. Advanced cervical cancer may lead to lower back or pelvic pain and bowel and urinary symptoms. Advanced disease that has invaded nearby structures may lead to vaginal fistula formation (causing vaginal passage of urine or stool), hematuria, or hematochezia. Advanced disease may also present with deep venous thrombosis, ureteral obstruction, and lower leg edema from invasive spread [40].

Physical Examination

When a woman presents with a history or symptoms concerning for cervical cancer, a physical exam should be performed. A pelvic examination including a speculum exam for direct visualization of the cervix is paramount. Palpation of the groin and supraclavicular lymph nodes is part of a complete exam. Visualization of the cervix may demonstrate a normal appearing cervix, visible cervical lesion, or large tumor(s). All lesions that are friable, raised, or appear to be condyloma should be biopsied. Staging examinations also include a pelvic examination with the addition of a rectovaginal exam and calculation of tumor size and parametrial and vaginal involvement.

Laboratory and Imaging

Cervical cytology should be performed for all women when cervical cancer is suspected. HPV co-testing is done in screening but is not used for the diagnosis of cervical cancer when a woman presents with symptoms or has a visible lesion. In the initial evaluation of women with suspected cervical cancer, a cervical biopsy may be performed or may be part of a staging procedure. Imaging (MRI) is typically not used for the diagnosis of cervical cancer, but is useful in staging and evaluation of women with a known malignancy [47].

Differential Diagnosis

The differential diagnosis of cervical cancer includes mimics of the common symptoms of cervical cancer including irregular or heavy vaginal bleeding, postcoital bleeding, and abnormal vaginal discharge. Cervicitis, structural abnormalities, uterine leiomyoma, endometrial polyps, adenomyosis, endometritis, and pelvic inflammatory disease may all cause abnormal uterine bleeding. Visible cervical lesions including nabothian cysts, mesonephric cysts, cervical ectropion, ulcers from STIs, reactive glandular changes, and endometriosis are also on the differential for cervical cancer.

Treatment

Staging

Staging is performed before the proper treatment is chosen. Staging of cervical carcinoma is based on clinical staging as defined by the system set forth by the International Federation of Gynecology [45] and considers the size and invasion of the lesion with stage IV being the most advanced disease [48, 49]. Cervical carcinoma can metastasize hematogenously, lymphatically, or directly to adjacent tissues. A lymph node evaluation must be performed to ascertain involvement as this information could affect treatment options and planning. The most common sites of distant metastasis include the pelvic, aortic, and mediastinal lymph nodes, lungs, liver, and skeleton [50].

Treatment Options

Treatment options depend on staging including localized disease, locally advanced disease, and metastatic or recurrent. Treatment options vary and may include surgery, radiation, brachytherapy, and chemotherapy. The patient's comorbidities, fertility desires, and risk of recurrence should also be considered when determining which treatment is best [50].

Referrals

Patients with diagnosed cervical cancer need referral to a gynecologist oncologist as soon as the diagnosis is made. Referring to other oncology services, such as patient centered support groups, and to a social worker (to help with financial questions or concerns, additional community resources, and support) is helpful for the patient as they are coping with a new diagnosis or recurrent cervical cancer.

Screening

In 2018, the US Preventive Services Task Force (USPSTF) updated the 2012 statement on screening for cervical cancer [51]. These recommendations are similar to the ACS/ASCCP/ASCP and ACOG current guidelines [52].

These recommendations are for women who have a cervix and do not apply to women who have received a diagnosis of a high-grade precancerous cervical lesion, cervical cancer, and exposure to diethylstilbestrol or women who are immunocompromised [42]. These recommendations apply regardless of the patient's sexual history [52]. Screening recommendations from the USPSTF including techniques, initiation, frequency, and management of abnormal screening results will be discussed here.

Techniques

Cervical cytology screening techniques include the more common liquid-based cytology and the conventional Papanicolaou (Pap) smears. Both are considered acceptable forms of screening by the ACOG [43]. These are discussed collectively as cervical cytology. Available HPV DNA tests include HPV high risk, HPV 16 and 18 DNA, and Hybrid Capture 2 HPV DNA. Testing for low-risk HPV types is not useful.

Initiation and Frequency

Cervical cancer screening with a pap smear is recommended to start at age 21 years based on guidelines set forth by the US Preventive Services Task Force in 2018, ACS/ASCCP/ASCP, and ACOG [42, 43, 52]. Annual screening is not recommended for all women. Cytology results from previous pap smears, age, immune status, and previous HPV testing influence recommended screening intervals [51].

The ACS identifies groups that may require more frequent testing including individuals with a history of cervical cancer, history of a high-grade precancerous lesion, HIV, immunosuppression, and in utero exposure to DES [52]. For HIV patients, ACOG recommends a screening pap smear twice in the first year after diagnosis and then annually thereafter [53].

All guidelines mentioned above for cervical cancer screening recommend cytology alone for screening every 3 years for woman ages 21–29 years of age. Screening of women between the ages of 20 and 24 has been shown to have no impact on rates of invasive cancer up to age 30 [54]. For women between the ages of 30 and 65 years, cytology alone can be performed every 3 years according to the USPSTF guidelines [42]. The USPSTF states that in this age group, women who wish to extend screening to every 5 years may do HPV testing alone or cytology with HPV co-testing but that this may lead to additional testing. The ASC/ASCCP/ASCP and ACOG guidelines recommend screening in combination with cytology and HPV testing every 5 years in women ages 30–65 [55].

The USPSTF recommends stopping cervical cancer screening for women older than age 65 with adequate prior screening, not otherwise at risk for cervical cancer [42]. This recommendation defines adequate screening as two consecutive cytology negative pap smears with negative HPV co-testing in the 10 years prior to stopping screening (with the last test within 5 years) or three consecutive negative cytology tests. In addition, women who have had a total hysterectomy and have no history of CIN 1 or 2 or cervical cancer also do not need continued screening. Women who have had a high-grade precancerous lesion should continue testing for 20 years after management of the lesion [52].

The Bethesda system from 2001 is a standardized framework for laboratory reports for cervical cytology. The report attests to specimen adequacy and gives a descriptive diagnosis. There have been three revisions since 1988 [56]. In 2012, experts from national and international health organizations, federal agencies, and professional societies convened to revise the 2006 American Society for Colposcopy and Cervical Pathology Consensus Guidelines. From this meeting arose new evidence-based consensus guidelines for managing women with abnormal cervical cancer screenings tests, CIN, and adenocarcinoma in situ (AIS) [57]. The new longer screening intervals recommended by ASCCP, ACOG, and USPSTF were incorporated into these guidelines. These guidelines are the standard of care for managing abnormal cervical cancer screening tests. They can be found on the ASCCP website (http://www.asccp.org). The 2014 Bethesda System Update is included in the 2015 publication of *The Bethesda System for Reporting Cervical Cytology: Definitions, Criteria, and Explanatory Notes* [56].

Colposcopy

Colposcopy is used to visualize mucosal abnormalities of the cervix that may be suspicious and require biopsy. A colposcope is a low-power magnification device that permits the visualization of abnormalities of the cervix that are consistent with CIN or invasive cancer. During colposcopy, the cervix is washed with a solution of acetic acid which turns areas of the cervix white that have high nucleic acid. Biopsies are then procured and sent for histopathology. Results from colposcopy dictate the next steps in management. The 2015 ASCCP guidelines guide practitioners through the standards of care based on histopathology results. These guidelines can be found on the ASCCP website.

Prevention

Primary Prevention

Behavioral intervention to modify known risk factors for cervical cancer may modify the incidence of cervical cancer. Practitioners can use techniques such as motivational interviewing to help patients decide which risk factors they would like to modify. Primary prevention such as quitting smoking, condom use, using contraception methods other than oral contraceptive pills, and limiting the number of sexual partners can modify an individual's risk.

Medications/Immunizations and Chemoprophylaxis

HPV is associated with development of anogenital cancers including cervical, vaginal, vulvar, and anal. HPV is divided into two classes: non-oncogenic (low-risk) and oncogenic (high-risk). Low-risk HPV genotypes including 6 and 11 are associated with condyloma and mild dysplastic changes that typically do not progress. High-risk HPV types including 16, 18, 31, 33, 35, 45, 52, and 58 are associated with moderate (CIN 2) and severe dysplasia (CIN 3) [37, 50]. As previously noted, the high-risk types are seen in most cervical cancers. Only a small percentage of women with HPV will develop cervical cancer or abnormalities, as HPV alone is usually necessary but not a sufficient precursor for the development of squamous cell carcinoma [43].

Vaccination against the genotypes known to be the etiology of most cervical cancers is given with the intent to reduce the incidence of anogenital cancers. The Food and Drug Administration has approved three vaccines for the prevention of HPV infection. The bivalent three-dose vaccine, Cervarix, is approved for females ages 9–25 years to prevent cervical cancer, CIN1, CIN 2, and adenocarcinoma in situ caused by oncogenic HPV genotypes 16 and 18. The quadrivalent three-dose vaccine is approved for females and males age 9–26 years and protects against HPV genotypes 6, 11, 16, and 18. It is indicated to prevent cancers and intraepithelial neoplasias of the cervix, anus, vulva, vagina, and genital warts associated with the aforementioned genotypes [58]. The newest vaccine, GARDASIL 9, is a nine-valent vaccine against HPV genotypes 6, 11, 16, 18, 31, 33, 45, 52, and 58. It is approved for males and females. There are two recommended vaccine schedules. The first schedule includes two doses, the first dose before age 15 and the second dose 6–12 months after the first dose. The second schedule includes three doses, the first dose after age 15, the second dose 1–2 months after the first dose, and the third dose 6 months after the first dose. The GARDASIL 9 vaccine has the same indications as the quadrivalent vaccine but covers more HPV genotypes [50].

The American Academy of Pediatrics (AAP) and CDC recommend that both boys and girls get routine HPV vaccinations if they are between 11 and 26 years old. Practitioners can administer vaccinations to patients as early as age 9. For those under 15, the two-dose GARDASIL 9 vaccine is recommended. For those over age 15 or with immune deficiencies, the three-dose GARDASIL 9 vaccine is recommended [59]. The CDC recommends that adults between ages 27 and 45 consult their physicians to determine their risk of new HPV infections before getting vaccinated [50].

Long-term effects of HPV vaccination on prevention of cervical cancer and CIN 2 and 3 are unknown; however, studies are currently being done [60]. Since there is no long-term data to help deduce how vaccination may alter the need for screening with cytology or cytology with HPV co-testing and the HPV vaccines do not include all high risk HPV genotypes, women who have been vaccinated against high-risk HPV infection should continue to be screened according to the USPSTF guidelines [42].

Secondary Prevention

The pap smear is a screening tool used to detect changes in cervical cells. In 2015, the American Society for Colposcopy and Cervical Pathology (ASCCP) with partnered organizations revised their 2006 consensus guidelines, recommending management of women with cytological abnormalities. The 2014 Bethesda System terminology [56] is used for cytological classification. Using the algorithms set forth in the ASCCP

2015 guidelines, practitioners are guided through the possible outcomes of cervical cytology from a pap smear based on results, age, and history of previous pap smear results. Within the guidelines, HPV testing only refers to high-risk, oncogenic HPV types only. The 2015 ASCCP guidelines can be accessed at http://www.asccp.org/guidelines.

Ovarian Cancer

General Principles

Definition/Background

Ovarian cancer is the second most common gynecologic malignancy and is the leading cause of death from gynecologic malignancies in the United States [35]. The majority of ovarian malignancies, approximately 90%, are derived from epithelial cells [61]. Epithelial carcinoma of the ovaries, fallopian tubes, and peritoneum are clinically similar, and there are five main subtypes which include high-grade serous carcinoma, endometrioid carcinoma, clear cell carcinoma, mucinous carcinoma, and low-grade serous carcinoma. The other types of ovarian malignancies include germ cell tumors and sex cord-stromal tumors.

Epidemiology

In 2018, there were 22,240 expected cases of ovarian cancer, with an expected 14,070 deaths in the United States [62]. It is the fifth leading cause of death of women in the United States [62]. Based on data from 2014 to 2016, approximately 1.3% of women will be diagnosed with ovarian cancer during their lifetime, and in 2016, the number of women living with ovarian cancer in the United States was 229,875 [63]. Rates for new ovarian cancer in the United States have been falling on average 2.3% for the past 10 years [64]. Only 14.9% of ovarian cancers are diagnosed at stage I, and the 5-year survival rate for ovarian cancer found at stage I is 92.4% [63]. The 5-year survival rate declines with increasing stage, and the overall 5-year survival rate across all stages is 47.6% [64].

Risk Factors

The pathogenic mechanisms for ovarian cancer have yet to be explained. Currently, there are two predominant hypotheses – incessant ovulation and exposure to gonadotropins. The theory of incessant ovulation was born out of data which demonstrated that women with history of pregnancy, lactation, or contraceptive use have a lower incidence of epithelial ovarian cancer. The gonadotropin exposure hypothesis is less supported by data and comes from the observation that experimentally induced ovarian tumors have gonadotropin receptors. Others have suggested that reproductive hormones [65] or chronic inflammation [66] may play a role in ovarian carcinogenesis. Although these separate theories may relate to the heterogeneity of epithelial ovarian cancers, none of them are able to fully explain the pathogenic mechanisms [61].

Family History/Familial Ovarian Cancer Syndromes

The strongest risk factor for ovarian cancer is family history. It is important to differentiate women who have a history of an isolated family member with ovarian cancer and those that may have a rare familial ovarian cancer syndrome from germline mutations including BRCA1 or BRCA2 mutations or Lynch syndrome. Women with Ashkenazi Jewish heritage with a single family member with breast cancer before age 50 or ovarian cancer are also considered to have a high-risk family history.

Reproductive/Hormonal Factors

Overall, the data seems to support the hypothesis of incessant ovulation as a risk for ovarian cancer. Women who are multiparous or who take oral contraceptives have a decreased risk of epithelial ovarian cancer. Women with early menarche and late menopause may be at an increased risk. Women with infertility may also be at an increased risk; however, data is currently inconclusive. The Women's Health Initiative found no increased risk for women on combined estrogen-progestin therapy compared with placebo [67]. Breastfeeding is thought to be protective against epithelial ovarian cancer, but further studies are warranted [68].

Environmental

Environmental risk factors include cigarette smoking and exposure to asbestos, a known carcinogen. Increased risk with perineal use of talcum powder is controversial. The association may be explained by the similar structure between talcum powder and asbestos, and that decades before, some talcum powder was contaminated with asbestos. Smoking increases the risk of mucinous ovarian cancer, with increasing amount of smoking leading to increased risk [69].

Other

Obesity seems to increase the risk of ovarian cancer [70]. Risk also increases with age. Taller individuals are also thought to be at an increased risk of ovarian cancer, with an 8% risk increase per 5 cm height [71].

Diagnosis

History

Ovarian cancer is typically diagnosed at a late stage. However there is evidence demonstrating that women will present with symptoms, even in early stages, that may get overlooked [72, 73]. Ovarian cancer can cause a myriad of symptoms, and distinguishing these symptoms from symptoms that normally occur in women or those that may be caused by a different medical disorder is problematic. Majority of women with epithelial ovarian cancer will present with a pelvic or abdominal symptoms prior to their diagnosis. Abdominal pain or discomfort and abdominal bloating or swelling are the most common symptoms. Patients may note urinary frequency, early satiety, and back pain. What may help distinguish these symptoms from other medical conditions is their more frequent and severe nature in those with ovarian cancer.

Physical Exam

If a pelvic mass is suspected or woman has symptoms suggestive of an epithelial ovarian cancer, a physical exam is warranted and should include an abdominal, pelvic, rectovaginal, and lymph node exam. A lymph node exam should include evaluation of groin and supraclavicular lymph nodes. If a physical exam is suspicious for a mass or other secondary symptoms of ovarian cancer such as ascites are found, further investigation is warranted with labs and imaging.

Laboratory and Imaging

If a physical exam and history is concerning for possible ovarian cancer, a Ca 125 tumor marker and abdominal and transvaginal ultrasound should be obtained. If the physical exam is benign, waiting 2 weeks to see if symptoms resolve prior to ordering pelvic ultrasound is reasonable.

Differential Diagnosis

The differential diagnosis for epithelial ovarian carcinoma and tubal and peritoneal carcinoma is variable depending on the presentation of the patient. Patients can have a myriad of symptoms though typically these will be urologic or gastrointestinal in nature. In women who do not have an adnexal mass on exam and imaging, workup for other causes of their symptoms is warranted and may be done simultaneously.

Staging/Treatment

Referrals

Ovarian, fallopian tube, and peritoneal cancers may require surgery for diagnosis. Primary care providers should refer to a gynecologist oncologist for the staging of these cancers and their surgical management.

Medications/Chemoprophylaxis

After diagnosis, a gynecologist oncologist will make recommendations based on the type and stage of the ovarian cancer. The main treatments for ovarian cancer include surgery, chemotherapy, hormone therapy, radiation, and target therapy. Often, two or more different options will be used to treat ovarian cancer.

Prevention

Routine gynecologic care with a primary care provider is an important component of cancer prevention. As part of an annual wellness exam, providers can help screen for familial cancer syndromes by reviewing the patient's family history and any new health changes. Risk reduction for ovarian cancer can also be discussed including quitting smoking and managing weight to prevent obesity. Those with a known familial cancer syndrome or those at risk should be identified during these routine exams and referred to a gynecologist oncologist and genetic counselor to discuss other options for prevention including chemoprevention, mastectomy, and bilateral salpingo-oophorectomy.

Screening

The yearly well woman exam is an excellent time to evaluate a patient's risk for hereditary breast and ovarian cancer syndromes. Using screening questions to identify those at greater risk is an opportunity to also discuss risk reduction.

The practice bulletin published by ACOG [74] outlines criteria that if met would prompt a clinician to refer a patient for a genetic risk assessment. Genetic risk assessments include a referral to a genetic counselor who will, with the patient's assistance, gather a medical family history and provide education about specific cancers including potential genetic testing and counseling. Women who have a known or suspected ovarian cancer should also be referred to a genetic counselor.

Screening methods for ovarian cancer include measurement of the tumor marker CA 125, serological markers, and ultrasound.

Consensus is that women at average risk should not undergo routine screening for ovarian cancer. The USPSTF gives an evidence level of D for screening asymptomatic women with no known hereditary cancer syndrome [75]. The incidence and prevalence of ovarian cancer makes consideration of a high false-positive rate very important when consider screening. A potential risk of screening is a false-positive result, which may lead to surgery including laparotomy or laparoscopy and other invasive procedures. Benefits include being able to find ovarian cancer at an earlier stage where it may be more curable. A large trial in the United States showed that screening with CA-125 and transvaginal ultrasound compared with usual care did not reduce ovarian cancer mortality and 15% of women who had a false-positive result who underwent surgery had a serious complication [76]. The USPSTF, in their recommendation against routine screening, notes that screening may lead to patient harm, including from invasive procedures such as surgery [75].

Screening with the CA 125 tumor marker and transvaginal ultrasound in women with a familial ovarian cancer syndrome who have not had a prophylactic salpingo-oophorectomy is recommended by the National Comprehensive Cancer Network. However, improved survival rates with this screening combination have not been demonstrated [77, 78]. ACOG recommends bilateral salpingo-oophorectomy at age 35–40 for BRCA1 carriers and at 40–45 for BRCA2 carriers. However, this timing should be individualized based on patient factors, including family history, and desire for future childbearing [79]. Additional screening methodologies may be recommended, and all screening should be directed by a gynecologist or gynecologist oncologist.

References

1. Viswanathan M, Hartmann K, McKoy N, Stuart G, Rankins N, Thieda P, et al. Management of uterine fibroids: an update of the evidence. Evid Rep Technol Assess. 2007;154:1–122.
2. Baird DD, Dunson DB, Hill MC, Cousins D, Schectman JM. High cumulative incidence of uterine leiomyoma in black and white women: ultrasound evidence. Am J Obstet Gynecol. 2003;188(1):100–7.
3. Wise LA, Palmer JR, Spiegelman D, Harlow BL, Stewart EA, Adams-Campbell LL, et al. Influence of body size and body fat distribution on risk of uterine leiomyomata in U.S. black women. Epidemiology. 2005;16(3):346–54.
4. Stewart EA, Cookson CL, Gandolfo RA, Schulze-Rath R. Epidemiology of uterine fibroids: a systematic review. BJOG Int J Obstet Gy. 2017;124(10):1501–12.
5. Food US, Administration D. FDA updated assessment of the use of laparoscopic power morcellators to treat uterine fibroids. FDA safety communication. USFDA: Silver Spring; 2017.
6. Donnez J, Donnez O, Matule D, Ahrendt H, Hudecek R, Zatik J, et al. Long-term medical management of uterine fibroids with ulipristal acetate. Fertil Steril. 2016;105(1):165–173.e4.
7. Brölmann H, Bongers M, Garza-Leal J, Gupta J, Veersema S, Quartero R, et al. The FAST-EU trial: 12-month clinical outcomes of women after intrauterine sonography-guided transcervical radiofrequency ablation of uterine fibroids. Gynecol Surg. 2016;13:27–35.
8. Ghezzi F, Cromi A, Bergamini V, Scarperi S, Bolis P, Franchi M. Midterm outcome of radiofrequency thermal ablation for symptomatic uterine myomas. Surg Endosc. 2007;21(11):2081–5.
9. Gupta JK, Sinha A, Lumsden MA, Hickey M. Uterine artery embolization for symptomatic uterine fibroids. Cochrane Database Syst Rev. 2014;12
10. Taheri M, Galo L, Potts C, Sakhel K, Quinn SD. Nonresective treatments for uterine fibroids: a systematic review of uterine and fibroid volume reductions. Int J Hyperth. 2019;36(1):295–301.
11. Urman B, Yakin K, Balaban B. Recurrent implantation failure in assisted reproduction: how to counsel and manage. A. General considerations and treatment options that may benefit the couple. Reprod Biomed Online. 2005;11(3):371–81.
12. Morales AJ, Kettel LM, Murphy AA. Mifepristone: clinical application in general gynecology. Clin Obstet Gynecol. 1996;39(2):451–60.
13. Ono M, Yin P, Navarro A, Moravek MB, Coon VJS, Druschitz SA, et al. Inhibition of canonical WNT signaling attenuates human leiomyoma cell growth. Fertil Steril. 2014;101(5):1441–9.
14. Ozercan IH, Sahin N, Akdemir F, Onderci M, Seren S, Sahin K, et al. Chemoprevention of fibroid tumors by [−]-epigallocatechin-3-gallate in quail. Nutr Res. 2008;28(2):92–7.
15. Sahin K, Akdemir F, Tuzcu M, Sahin N, Onderci M, Ozercan R, et al. Genistein suppresses spontaneous oviduct tumorigenesis in quail. Nutr Cancer. 2009;61(6):799–806.
16. Siegel R, Ma J, Zou Z, Jemal A. Cancer statistics, 2014. CA Cancer J Clin. 2014;64(1):9–29.
17. Siegel RL, Miller KD, Jemal A. Cancer statistics, 2019. CA A Cancer J Clin. 2019;69(1):7–34.
18. Sorosky JI. Endometrial cancer. Obstet Gynecol. 2008;111(2 Pt 1):436–47.
19. Schnatz PF, Guile M, O'Sullivan DM, Sorosky JI. Clinical significance of atypical glandular cells on cervical cytology. Obstet Gynecol. 2006;107(3):701–8.
20. von Gruenigen VE, Tian C, Frasure H, Waggoner S, Keys H, Barakat RR. Treatment effects, disease recurrence, and survival in obese women with early endometrial carcinoma: a gynecologic oncology group study. Cancer. 2006 15;107(12):2786–91.
21. Sorosky JI. Endometrial cancer. Obstet Gynecol. 2012;120(2 Pt 1):383–97.
22. Fisher B, Costantino JP, Wickerham DL, Redmond CK, Kavanah M, Cronin WM, et al. Tamoxifen for prevention of breast cancer: report of the National Surgical Adjuvant Breast and Bowel Project P-1 Study. J Natl Cancer Inst. 1998;90(18):1371–88.
23. Brinton LA, Hoover RN. Estrogen replacement therapy and endometrial cancer risk: unresolved issues. The endometrial Cancer collaborative group. Obstet Gynecol. 1993;81(2):265–71.

24. Gordon P. Videos in clinical medicine. Endometrial biopsy. N Engl J Med. 2009;361(26):e61.

25. Dijkhuizen FP, Mol BW, Brolmann HA, Heintz AP. The accuracy of endometrial sampling in the diagnosis of patients with endometrial carcinoma and hyperplasia: a meta-analysis. Cancer. 2000;89(8): 1765–72.

26. Leitao MM Jr, Han G, Lee LX, Abu-Rustum NR, Brown CL, Chi DS, et al. Complex atypical hyperplasia of the uterus: characteristics and prediction of underlying carcinoma risk. Am J Obstet Gynecol. 2010;203(4):349.e1–6.

27. Goldstein SR. The role of transvaginal ultrasound or endometrial biopsy in the evaluation of the menopausal endometrium. Obstet Gynecol. 2009;201(1):5–11.

28. Goldstein SR. Modern evaluation of the endometrium. Obstet Gynecol. 2010;116(1):168–76.

29. Sweet MG, Schmidt-Dalton TA, Weiss PM, Madsen KP. Evaluation and management of abnormal uterine bleeding in premenopausal women. Am Fam Physician. 2012;85(1):35–43.

30. Werbrouck E, Veldman J, Luts J, Van Huffel S, Van Schoubroeck D, Timmerman D, et al. Detection of endometrial pathology using saline infusion sonography versus gel instillation sonography: a prospective cohort study. Fertil Steril. 2011;95(1):285–8.

31. Van Den Bosch T, Van Schoubroeck D, Luts J, Bignardi T, Condous G, Epstein E, et al. Effect of gel-instillation sonography on Doppler ultrasound findings in endometrial polyps. Ultrasound Obstet Gynecol. 2011;38(3):355–9.

32. ACOG Committee on Practice, Bulletins – Gynecology, American College of Obstetricians and, Gynecologists. ACOG practice bulletin: management of anovulatory bleeding. Int J Gynaecol Obstet. 2001; 72(3):263–71.

33. Zaino RJ, Kauderer J, Trimble CL, Silverberg SG, Curtin JP, Lim PC, et al. Reproducibility of the diagnosis of atypical endometrial hyperplasia: a gynecologic oncology group study. Cancer. 2006;106(4):804–11.

34. Baak JP, Mutter GL, Robboy S, van Diest PJ, Uyterlinde AM, Orbo A, et al. The molecular genetics and morphometry-based endometrial intraepithelial neoplasia classification system predicts disease progression in endometrial hyperplasia more accurately than the 1994 World Health Organization classification system. Cancer. 2005;103(11):2304–12.

35. Siegel RL, Miller KD, Jemal A. Cancer statistics, 2019. CA Cancer J Clin. 2019;69(1):7–34.

36. Walboomers JM, Jacobs MV, Manos MM, Bosch FX, Kummer JA, Shah KV, et al. Human papillomavirus is a necessary cause of invasive cervical cancer worldwide. J Pathol. 1999;189(1):12–9.

37. Bruni L, Albero G, Serrano B, Mena M, Gómez D, Muñoz J, et al. World: Human papillomavirus and related diseases, summary report 2019. ICO/IARC Information Centre on HPV and Cancer 6/17/19 6/17/19.

38. Howlader N, Noone AM, Krapcho M, Miller D, Brest A, Yu M, et al. Cancer of the Cervix Uteri –

Cancer Stat Facts Available at: https://seer.cancer.gov/statfacts/html/cervix.html. Accessed 13 Nov 2019.

39. Ries L, Melbert D, Krapcho M, Stinchcomb DG, Howlader N, Horner MJ, et al. SEER Cancer Statistics Review, 1975–2005. Bethesda: National Cancer Institute; 2008. Available at: http://seer.cancer.gov/csr/1975_2005/. Accessed 21 Oct 2014

40. Cannistra SA, Niloff JM. Cancer of the uterine cervix. N Engl J Med. 1996;334(16):1030–7.

41. Su B, Qin W, Xue F, Wei X, Guan Q, Jiang W, et al. The relation of passive smoking with cervical cancer: a systematic review and meta-analysis. Medicine. 2018;97 (46):e13061.

42. Moyer VA. U.S, preventive services task F. screening for cervical cancer: U.S. preventive services task force recommendation statement. Ann Intern Med. 2012; 156(12):880–91.

43. ACOG Committee on Practice, Bulletins – Gynecology. ACOG Practice Bulletin no. 109: cervical cytology screening. Obstet Gynecol. 2009;114(6):1409–20.

44. Miller BA, Kolonel LN, Bernstein L. Racial/ethnic patterns of cancer in the United States 1988–1992. Bethesda: NIH Publication; 1996. 96(4101)

45. Moore DH. Cervical cancer. Obstet Gynecol. 2006; 107(5):1152–61.

46. Partridge EE, Abu-Rustum NR, Campos SM, Fahey PJ, Farmer M, Garcia RL, et al. Cervical cancer screening. J Natl Compr Cancer Netw. 2010;8(12):1358–86.

47. Jordan SE, Maliakal C, Schlumbrecht MP, Quintero L, Pearson JM, Wolfson AH, et al. Examining the utility of magnetic resonance imaging compared with physical exam in cervical cancer staging. Gynecol Oncol. 2019;154:119.

48. Bhatla N, Berek JS, Fredes MC, Denny LA, Grenman S, Karunaratne K, et al. Revised FIGO staging for carcinoma of the cervix uteri. Int J Gynecol Obstet. 2019;145(1):129–35.

49. Corrigendum to "Revised FIGO staging for carcinoma of the cervix uteri". Int J Gynecol Obstet. 2019;147(2): 279–80. [Int J Gynecol Obstet 145(2019) 129–135]

50. Stumbar SE, Stevens M, Feld Z. Cervical Cancer and its precursors. Prim Care. 2019;46(1):117–34.

51. Curry SJ, Krist AH, Owens DK, Barry MJ, Caughey AB, Davidson KW, et al. Screening for Cervical Cancer: US Preventive Services Task Force Recommendation Statement. JAMA. 2018;320(7):674–86.

52. Final Recommendation Statement: Cervical Cancer: Screening. U.S. Preventive Services Task Force. 2019. Available at: https://www.uspreventiveservicestaskforce.org/Page/Document/RecommendationStatementFinal/cervical-cancer-screening. Accessed 15 Nov 2019.

53. Practice Bulletin No. 117. Gynecologic care for women with human immunodeficiency virus. Obstet Gynecol. 2010;116(6):1492–509.

54. Sasieni P, Castanon A, Cuzick J. Effectiveness of cervical screening with age: population based case-control study of prospectively recorded data. BMJ. 2009;339:b2968.

55. Saslow D, Solomon D, Lawson HW, Killackey M, Kulasingam SL, Cain J, et al. American Cancer

Society, American Society for Colposcopy and Cervical Pathology, and American Society for Clinical Pathology screening guidelines for the prevention and early detection of cervical cancer. CA Cancer J Clin 2012; 62(3):147–172.

56. Nayar R. The Bethesda system for reporting cervical cytology: definitions, criteria, and explanatory notes. 3rd ed: Cham, Springer International Publishing; 2015, 2015.

57. Massad L, Stewart Einstein MH, Huh WK, Katki HA, Kinney WK, Schiffman M, Solomon D, Wentzensen N, Lawson HW, et al. 2012 Updated consensus guidelines for the management of abnormal cervical cancer screening tests and cancer precursors. J Lower Genital Tract Disease. 2013;17(Supplement 1):S1–S27.

58. Munoz N, Kjaer SK, Sigurdsson K, Iversen OE, Hernandez-Avila M, Wheeler CM, et al. Impact of human papillomavirus (HPV)-6/11/16/18 vaccine on all HPV-associated genital diseases in young women. J Natl Cancer Inst. 2010;102(5):325–39.

59. Committee on Infectious D. HPV vaccine recommendations. Pediatrics. 2012;129(3):602–5.

60. Velentzis LS, Caruana M, Simms KT, Lew J, Shi J, Saville M, et al. How will transitioning from cytology to HPV testing change the balance between the benefits and harms of cervical cancer screening? Estimates of the impact on cervical cancer, treatment rates and adverse obstetric outcomes in Australia, a high vaccination coverage country. Int J Cancer. 2017;141(12):2410–22.

61. Webb PM, Jordan SJ. Epidemiology of epithelial ovarian cancer. Best Pract Res Clin Obstet Gynaecol. 2017;41:3–14.

62 Siegel RL, Miller KD, Jemal A. Cancer statistics, 2018. CA Cancer J Clin. 2018;68(1):7–30.

63. SEER. Cancer statistics. 2014. Available at: http://seer.cancer.gov/statfacts/html/ovary.html. Accessed 22 Nov 2014

64. Cancer Stat Facts: Ovarian Cancer. 2016.; Available at: https://seer.cancer.gov/statfacts/html/ovary.html. Accessed 15 Sept 2019.

65. Risch HA. Hormonal etiology of epithelial ovarian, cancer with a hypothesis concerning the role of androgens and progesterone. J Natl Cancer Inst. 1998;90 (23):1774–86.

66. Ness RB, Cottreau C. Possible role of ovarian epithelial inflammation in ovarian cancer. J Natl Cancer Inst. 1999;91(17):1459–67.

67. Anderson GL, Judd HL, Kaunitz AM, Barad DH, Beresford SA, Pettinger M, et al. Effects of estrogen plus progestin on gynecologic cancers and associated diagnostic procedures: the Women's Health Initiative randomized trial. JAMA. 2003;290(13):1739–48.

68. Luan N, Wu Q, Gong T, Vogtmann E, Wang Y, Lin B. Breastfeeding and ovarian cancer risk: a meta-analysis of epidemiologic studies. Am J Clin Nutr. 2013;98(4):1020–31.

69. Jordan SJ, Whiteman DC, Purdie DM, Green AC, Webb PM. Does smoking increase risk of ovarian cancer? A systematic review. Gynecol Oncol. 2006;103(3):1122–9.

70. Olsen CM, Green AC, Whiteman DC, Sadeghi S, Kolahdooz F, Webb PM. Obesity and the risk of epithelial ovarian cancer: a systematic review and meta-analysis. Eur J Cancer. 2007;43(4):690–709.

71. Dixon-Suen SC, Nagle CM, Thrift AP, Pharoah PDP, Ewing A, Pearce CL, et al. Adult height is associated with increased risk of ovarian cancer: a Mendelian randomisation study. Br J Cancer. 2018;118(8):1123–9.

72. Goff BA, Mandel L, Muntz HG, Melancon CH. Ovarian carcinoma diagnosis. Cancer. 2000;89 (10):2068–75.

73. Yawn BP, Barrette BA, Wollan PC. Ovarian cancer: the neglected diagnosis. Mayo Clin Proc. 2004;79 (10):1277–82.

74. American College of Obstetricians and Gynecologists Committee on Gynecologic, Practice. Committee Opinion No. 477: the role of the obstetrician-gynecologist in the early detection of epithelial ovarian cancer. Obstet Gynecol. 2011;117(3):742–6.

75. Moyer VA. U.S. preventive services task F. screening for ovarian cancer: U.S. preventive services task force reaffirmation recommendation statement. Ann Intern Med. 2012;157(12):900–4.

76. Buys SS, Partridge E, Black A, Johnson CC, Lamerato L, Isaacs C, et al. Effect of screening on ovarian cancer mortality: the prostate, lung, colorectal and ovarian (PLCO) Cancer screening randomized controlled trial. JAMA. 2011;305(22):2295–303.

77. Gaarenstroom KN, van der Hiel B, Tollenaar RA, Vink GR, Jansen FW, van Asperen CJ, et al. Efficacy of screening women at high risk of hereditary ovarian cancer: results of an 11-year cohort study. Int J Gynecol Cancer. 2006;16(Suppl 1):54–9.

78. Olivier RI, Lubsen-Brandsma MA, Verhoef S, van Beurden M. CA125 and transvaginal ultrasound monitoring in high-risk women cannot prevent the diagnosis of advanced ovarian cancer. Gynecol Oncol. 2006;100(1):20–6.

79. American College of Obstetricians and, Gynecologists, ACOG Committee on Practice, Bulletins – Gynecology, ACOG Committee on G, Society of Gynecologic O. ACOG Practice Bulletin No. 103: hereditary breast and ovarian cancer syndrome. Obstet Gynecol. 2009;113(4):957–66.

Benign Breast Conditions and Disease

111

Gabriel Briscoe, Chelsey Villanueva, Jennifer Bepko, John Colucci, and Erin Wendt

Contents

G. Briscoe (✉) · C. Villanueva · J. Bepko · J. Colucci · E. Wendt
David Grant Family Medicine Residency Program, David Grant Medical Center, Fairfield, CA, USA
e-mail: gabriel.w.briscoe.mil@mail.mil; chelsey.villanueva.1@us.af.mil; jennifer.bepko@us.af.mil; john.l.colucci3.mil@mail.mil; erin.d.wendt.mil@mail.mil

© Springer Nature Switzerland AG 2022
P. M. Paulman et al. (eds.), *Family Medicine*,
https://doi.org/10.1007/978-3-030-54441-6_113

Introduction

Benign breast disease is a common occurrence in family medicine. Patients may present with masses, skin lesions, breast pain, breastfeeding complaints, and concerns regarding risk of malignancy. The incidence of benign breast disease rises in a woman's third decade of life and peaks in her fifth and sixth decade of life, whereas the risk of malignancy continues to increase past menopause [1]. Knowledge of basic anatomy and physiology of the breast is important when evaluating breast pain, nipple discharge, breast skin lesions, and breast masses. As with many other conditions, pertinent history taking and physical exam help determine the need for imaging. Many breast conditions may need confirmation with biopsy with those results dictating appropriate follow-up.

Anatomy and Physiology

The breast contains glandular, ductal, fibrous, and fatty tissue. Each breast contains 6–20 lobes made of several lobules within which are 10–100 subsegmental ducts, 20–40 segmental ducts, and 5–10 primary milk ducts that emerge at the areola via 6–10 pinhole openings. More lobes are present in the outer quadrants, especially the upper outer quadrants that are a common location for many breast conditions. Hormonal effects on breast tissue include estrogen on the development and elongation of ductal tissue, progesterone on ductal branching and lobulo-alveolar development, and prolactin on milk protein production [2]. The cyclic nature of estrogen and progesterone during the menstrual cycle increases cell proliferation and can yield changes in breast size and consistency.

History, Physical Exam, and Initial Workup

A patient may present with complaints of pain, nipple discharge, skin lesion, and/or a palpable mass. The initial assessment of breast complaints includes thorough history taking, a clinical breast exam, consideration for imaging, and possibility of biopsy.

Table 1 Elements of history for breast complaint

Symptom characteristics
Onset of symptoms/mass
Change in symptoms/mass over time and relation to the menstrual cycle (if premenopausal)
History of similar symptoms
Discharge: Spontaneous or expressed, location, color, amount, timing with pregnancy/breastfeeding, medications, association with visual changes and/or headaches, presence of recurrent irritation
Pain: Caffeine intake, hormonal therapy, contraception use
Diet and medications: Current medications and history of hormone therapy
Personal and family cancer history: Including breast, ovarian, endometrial, color, prostate cancer, relationship to patient, age of onset
History of breast surgery or biopsies: Document reason and pathology results
Patient information: Reproductive status, reproductive history, lactation status, radiation or chemical exposure, tobacco exposure

Adapted from Andolsek and Copeland [3]

History

A patient with breast complaints should have a thorough history taken to include the duration of symptoms, presence or absence of nipple discharge, pain, skin lesion or palpable mass, change in size of any masses over time, relation of symptoms to menstrual cycle, and systemic symptoms such as fever, malaise, or chills. Potential personal risk factors for benign breast disease would generally depend on the particular lesion as discussed later in the chapter. Potential risk factors for malignant breast disease include female sex, older age, genetic factors, ethnicity, personal or family history of cancer, menstrual and reproductive history, use of hormonal medications, chest radiation exposure, diethylstilbestrol (DES) exposure, and certain benign breast disease. Elements that should be obtained from a thorough history are listed in Table 1.

Breast Self-Examination

While self-identified masses or lesions warrant a clinical exam, there is conflicting current opinion regarding regular self-breast exams. In 2009, the US Preventive Task Force (USPSTF) recommended against teaching breast self-examination (BSE) in all women (Grade D) due to false-positive findings leading to the need for unnecessary imaging and biopsies [4]. However, the USPSTF, American College of Obstetricians and Gynecologists (ACOG), the American Cancer Society (ACS), and the National Comprehensive Cancer Network recommend teaching breast self-awareness by educating patients about the normal feel and appearance of their breasts [4, 5].

Clinical Breast Exam

Similar controversy exists to the utility of the clinical breast exam (CBE) as a screening tool. The USPSTF has concluded that there is insufficient evidence to perform a CBE as a screening tool in women over the age of 40 in countries that provide routine mammography screening again citing the concern of high rates of false-positive results, and subsequent workup may offset potential benefits [6]. The American Academy of Family Physicians concurs that there is insufficient evidence to recommend CBE as a screening tool [7]. Additionally, the ACS no longer recommends the CBE as a screening modality [8]. However, ACOG recommends CBE every 1–3 years from ages 20 to 39 and annually after age 40 [9]. Although debate also exists for the timing and frequency for screening exams, CBE should be performed with any breast-related complaint. CBE has a sensitivity and specificity of 49–69% and 86–99%, respectively [10].

The breast exam includes visual inspection, palpation, and nipple expression. In addition to the breast, the exam should include evaluation of the chest, axillae, and regional lymph nodes. With the patient in the seated position, hand on the waist, conducts a visual inspection for breast asymmetry, size difference, contour changes (dimpling or flattening), skin color, or changes in nipple appearance. Positioning the patient with arms overhead and then on the waist while leaning forward can enhance subtle changes such as skin retractions. Skin changes suggestive of a malignancy include dimpling, puckering, edema, and thickening of the skin (peau d'orange).

Breast palpation should be performed with the patient in both seated and supine positions. While still seated, palpate for cervical, supraclavicular, and axillary lymphadenopathy. In the supine position, the ipsilateral arm to the breast should be placed over the patient's head. The breast tissue is examined using the finger pads and progresses in a systematic fashion (either in a spiral fashion or vertical stripe pattern) without missing any areas, including up to the collarbone and axilla. Palpitation of the nipple includes attempting nipple expression by gently compressing the areola between the thumb and index finger. Consider sending any fluid expressed for evaluation. Clearly document all abnormal findings to include location (by quadrant or in relation to the face of a clock), consistency of any masses (soft, firm), mobility, and margins (well circumscribed, smooth, irregular). Benign lesions are typically without skin changes, smooth, soft to firm texture, mobile, and with well-defined margins, while malignant lesions generally are hard, fixed, immobile, and with poor margins [8, 10].

Imaging

Diagnostic imaging should be performed for any concerning masses. Imaging method is determined by patient's age due to breast density changes over time: women over 30 years of age or younger patients with a higher risk of cancer and palpable breast mass should be initially evaluated with diagnostic mammography with ultrasound [10]. Women under 30 should be evaluated with ultrasound due to increased sensitivity of detecting lesions in dense breast tissue [10]. Breast magnetic resonance imaging (MRI) is not recommended for routine breast cancer screening in women with average risk of developing breast cancer. The ACS recommends MRI screening for women at an increased risk of breast cancer defined as 20–25% or greater lifetime risk of developing breast cancer according to family history risk assessment tools, known BRCA1 or BRCA 2 gene mutations, first-degree relatives with BRCA mutations and without personal genetic testing, a history of chest radiation between the ages of 10 and 30, and genetic syndromes such as Li-Fraumeni, Cowden, or Bannayan-Riley-Ruvalcaba syndrome or an affected first-degree relative [8]. Findings on breast imaging are summarized using the Breast Imaging-Reporting and Data System, or BI-RADS [11]. The most recent update combines all three imaging modalities (ultrasound, mammography, and MRI) to standardize reporting results and provide recommended follow-up imaging and/or biopsy guidelines summarized in Table 2.

Table 2 BI-RADS categories

BI-RADS category	Assessment	Likelihood of malignancy	Follow-up recommended
0	Incomplete	n/a	Additional imaging required, in some states within 30 days
1	Negative	n/a	Routine screening
2	Benign finding(s)	n/a	Routine screening
3	Probably benign	<2%	Short-interval follow-up (repeat mammogram in 6 months) or biopsy
4A	Low suspicion for malignancy	2–10%	Biopsy should be performed
4B	Moderate suspicion for malignancy	10–50%	Biopsy should be performed
4C	High suspicion for malignancy	>50% to <95%	Biopsy should be performed
5	Highly suggestive of malignancy	>95%	Biopsy should be performed and urgent referral to subspecialist
6	Known biopsy-proven malignancy	n/a	Surgical excision when clinically appropriate

Adapted from Salzman et al. [10]

Tissue Sampling

Breast tissue sampling may be indicated for suspicious lesions even with normal mammography, as pathology such as lobular carcinoma may not be visible on imaging. Other indications include breast cysts that recur after aspiration, bloody nipple discharge or bloody cyst fluid, skin changes, asymmetry or thickening on exam, nodularity on exam, inflammatory skin changes that do not respond to antibiotics, suspicious nodes, or microcalcifications on mammography.

Biopsies of suspicious lesions are often performed after diagnostic imaging by a qualified physician. Options for tissue sampling include fine-needle aspiration (FNA), core-needle biopsy (CNB), or excisional biopsy. Localizing modalities include ultrasound, x-ray or stereotactic imaging, and MRI. Considering what type of sampling technique is the clinical discretion of the performing clinician and may also depend on the breast size.

Needle biopsy is performed percutaneously with local anesthesia and is a minimally invasive evaluation of abnormalities. FNA allows for diagnosis and treatment of breast cysts, cytological evaluation of abnormal lymph nodes, or when needle biopsy is not possible. CNB utilizes either a vacuum-assisted or automated biopsy devices. Both FNA and CNB allow for marking the biopsy site with a clip for future follow-up or to guide surgical excision. With adequate sampling, an FNA has 98–99% sensitivity, 99% positive predictive value, and 86–99% negative predictive value in detecting malignancy. However, adequacy is dependent on the physician's training and experience level [12]. Ultrasound-guided CNB has a sensitivity of 99% for palpable lesions and 93% for nonpalpable lesions [12]. However, excisional biopsy should be considered for evaluation and diagnosis of breast masses in addition to providing therapeutic measures. Excisional and incisional biopsies are performed when masses are suspected to be malignant, when less invasive sampling is inconclusive, unavailable, or suggestive of malignancy.

In addition to particular BI-RADS results, certain benign lesions should be considered for biopsy. A complex sclerosing lesion greater than 10 mm should be considered for excisional biopsy. Low-risk lesions including fibroadenomas (simple or complex), hamartomas, fat necrosis, sclerosing adenosis, columnar cell change or hyperplasia, or radial scar less than 10 mm do not necessarily need surgical evaluation unless there is radiographic discordance or it is associated with atypical ductal or lobular hyperplasia. All high-risk lesions that cannot be sampled should be referred for surgical excision [13].

The Triple Test

The triple test includes clinical exam, imaging, and tissue sampling. When performed with concordant results, diagnostic accuracy approaches 100% [12]. Any discordant results may require excisional biopsy. The Triple Test Score (TTS) may aid in interpretation of discordant results. Each component of the test (exam, imaging, tissue sampling) is assigned a score: 1 for benign findings, 2 for suspicious lesions, and 3 for malignant lesions. A score of 3–4 is consistent with benign lesions and may be clinically followed with a repeat exam in 4–6 weeks; >6 indicates possible malignancy that may require surgical intervention. Excisional biopsy is recommended for a TTS of 5 [12]. An approach to management of palpable breast masses is summarized in Fig. 1.

Common Chief Complaints

Breast Pain (Mastodynia/Mastalgia)

Breast pain makes up 66% of breast complaints and can be categorized as cyclical (relating to menses) or noncyclical [10] (Table 3).

Cyclic Versus Noncyclic Breast Pain

Cyclic breast pain correlates to the menstrual cycle typically occurring in the late luteal phase and resolving with menses. It occurs in two-thirds of women, and absence of serious disease can be

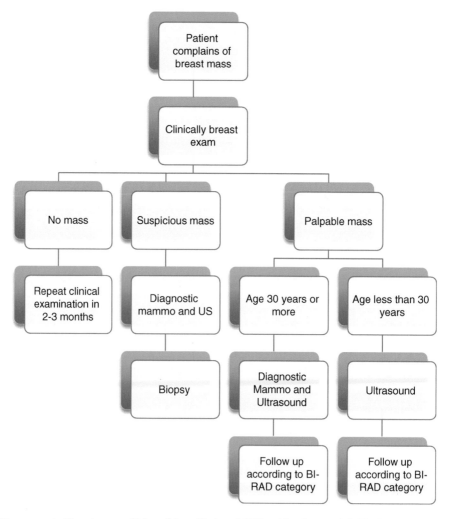

Fig. 1 Management of breast masses (Adapted from Neal et al. [13] and Pearlman and Griffin [14])

offered. Noncyclic breast pain is not correlated with the menstrual cycle and can be due to pregnancy, mastitis, thrombophlebitis, benign or malignant tumors, trauma, hematoma, and cyst rupture or fat necrosis. Though most cases of noncyclic breast pain occur for reasons unknown, they are likely due to anatomic rather than hormonal causes. Noncyclic breast pain can also be attributed to some medications such as hormonal medications, psychiatric medication, cardiac/antihypertensive medications, and antimicrobials [16].

In the initial evaluation of breast pain, it is vital to perform an examination for evaluation of palpable masses which may be contributing to symptoms. If there is a palpable mass associated with

the patient's pain, referral to a breast surgeon for surgical treatment is more likely to be efficacious regardless of the pattern of pain symptoms.

Treatment of Breast Pain

Nonpharmacological Interventions

Many women wear improperly fitted bras; therefore, proper fitting of undergarments, wearing a soft supportive bra during sleep, and wearing of a sports bra during exercise may improve breast pain [16]. Cold or heat compresses and massage may also alleviate symptoms. One clinical trial

Table 3 Summary of management of breast pain

Nonpharmacological interventions
Properly fitting bra, soft supportive bra during sleep, sports bra during exercise
Hot or cold compresses
Massage
Relaxation training
Decreasing dietary fat intake
Methylxanthine/caffeine reduction (coffee, tea, sodas, chocolate)
Vitamin E
Evening primrose oil
Pharmacologic interventions – For patients with severe persistent pain
Nonsteroidal anti-inflammatory drugs (NSAIDs) (oral or topical), acetaminophen
Oral combined contraceptives (low estrogen, high progesterone)
Danazol, low dose or during the luteal phase (FDA approved)
Gestrinone
Tamoxifen, low dose or during the luteal phase (not FDA approved)
Bromocriptine (Parlodel)
Goserelin (Zoladex) and Buserelin

Adapted from Andolsek, Copeland [3] and National Comprehensive Cancer Network [15], and AAFP [10]

demonstrated a reported decreased of symptoms in 61% of women who listened to audiocassettes of progressive muscle relaxation for 4 weeks compared to 25% in women who did not. Dietary changes decreasing dietary fat and methylxanthine/caffeine intake have been suggested; however, to benefit from a lower dietary fat diet, women must decrease their intake to less than 20% of their daily caloric intake, and there is inconsistent evidence to support the reduction or elimination of caffeine in treating breast pain.

Pharmacological Interventions

Vitamin E (alpha-tocopherol) may alter steroidal hormone production and acts as an antioxidant. However, studies have been inconclusive when used for treating fibrocystic breast disease, and it may increase bleeding risk. Evening primrose oil (gamma-linolenic acid), 3000 mg/day in divided doses for 3–6 months, is often recommended for the treatment of breast pain though conflicting data exists regarding its efficacy. Its mechanism includes restoration of the saturated/unsaturated fatty acid balance and decreased steroidal hormone sensitivity since women with cyclic breast pain may have abnormal fatty acid profiles that may cause epithelial hormonal hypersensitivity. Adverse reactions include nausea, bloating, and lowering seizure threshold; thus, it should not be used in patients with a seizure history. Isoflavones, genistein, and daidzein found in soy bind to estrogen receptors and can increase the follicular phase of the menstrual cycle to delay menstruation as well as decrease mid-cycle-luteinizing and follicle-stimulating hormone surges and estradiol levels. Evidence supporting its use is limited. Studies are limited regarding the efficacy of acetaminophen or nonsteroidal anti-inflammatory medications (NSAIDs) for breast pain though oral and topical preparations may be of benefit in those without contraindications though evidence is not consistent for benefit. The best evidence for these preparations is for the topical NSAID diclofenac (Voltaren) which has been shown to be useful in cyclic and non-cyclic breast pain [17].

Hormonally Active Pharmacological Interventions

Hormonally active medications most often used for breast pain are danazol, bromocriptine, or tamoxifen. Possible adverse reactions must be weighed against the potential benefits, and these agents are typically used for 2–6 months then tapered or discontinued. Relapse may occur requiring a second course of the same or different agent.

Danazol is a gonadotropin production and luteinizing hormone surge inhibitor and a weak estrogen antagonist. Currently, it is the only Food and Drug Administration (FDA)-approved medication for breast pain. Initial dosing is 200–600 mg by mouth daily with a maintenance dose of 50–100 mg by mouth daily once symptoms are controlled. This medication is contraindicated for pregnant, lactating patients, as well as those with history of VTE. Common side effects include headache, nausea, emotional lability and depression, fluid retention, vaginal dryness, hirsutism, amenorrhea, weight gain, menstrual irregularities, hot flashes, and acne. Side effects may be lessened with use of 200 mg by mouth daily only during the luteal phase. Treatment can be stopped after 4–6 months with a favorable treatment response lasting for months to years. Clinical trials have shown 59–92% of women reporting relief with danazol therapy with corresponding decreased breast volume and density.

Bromocriptine acts as a prolactin inhibitor/dopamine agonist and can be used for cyclical breast pain. Dosing is 1.25 mg by mouth nightly or 2.5 mg by mouth twice a day. Common side effects include nausea, vomiting, postural hypotension, constipation, and dizziness. Severe symptoms limit its use to women that are unresponsive to other agents or with hyperprolactinemia.

Tamoxifen is a selective estrogen receptor modulator commonly used off-label for breast pain. Dosing is 10–20 mg by mouth daily for 3–4 months or for days 15–25 of the monthly menstrual cycle. Adverse effects include menstrual irregularity, menopausal symptoms, vaginal dryness or discharge, endometrial cancer, and deep vein thrombophlebitis. In controlled trials, tamoxifen demonstrated a reduction in pain in 71–96% of women with cyclic mastalgia and 56% of women with noncyclic mastalgia. Unfortunately there is a high rate of recurrence of symptoms after discontinuation of treatment and the maximum duration of treatment is 6 months.

Gestrinone, a synthetic 19-nortestosterone derivative, has been shown in a double-blind, placebo-controlled study to yield reduction in breast pain at a dose of 2.5 mg by mouth per week. Its action is similar to danazol, and side effects are primarily androgenic.

If oral contraceptives (OCP) and menopausal hormone medications appear causative to breast pain symptoms, the addition of progestational agents (i.e., medroxyprogesterone 5–10 mg 10 days prior to menses, progesterone cream daily the week prior to menses; topical, oral, or parenteral preparations) or switching to a low-estrogen, high-progesterone OCP can relieve cyclic breast pain.

Lastly, gonadotropin-releasing hormone agonists such as goserelin and buserelin (available as subcutaneous implants) induce significant ovarian suppression, and use is limited due to significant menopausal side effect profile. There are some limited data to support the use of goserelin specifically for severe treatment-refractory mastalgia; however treatment duration is limited to 6 months due to effects on bone mineral density [18].

Nipple Pain

The complaint of nipple pain commonly occurs with the onset of breastfeeding. Breastfeeding mothers experiencing pain should have their technique evaluated. Assuring proper positioning and latch as well as releasing the infant's suction prior to removing from the breast are keys to prevention. A certified lactation consultant can be pivotal to the support of the breastfeeding couplet. Topical vitamin E ointment and USP modified lanolin are commonly used but can lead to local skin reactions. Signs of nipple cracking, fissures, blistering, or redness should be examined promptly as well as the infant's mouth. See section on "Mastitis" for further details. If a *Candida* infection is suspected, the nursing mother should receive a course of an oral antifungal, and the infant should be treated as well if topical involvement is present.

Nipple pain in the non-lactating female may be due to local irritation and friction as seen in runners. Small elastic bandages over the nipples and lubricants can be used during activities to reduce the incidence and emollients, or low-dose hydrocortisone creams may decrease symptoms.

Dermatologic conditions can also cause nipple pain. Eczema can manifest as bilateral erythema, scaling and weeping crusts, fissures, vesicles, excoriation, or erosions and can be treated with trigger avoidance and topical steroids. If nipple lesions do not resolve or are accompanied by a mass, then prompt evaluation should be performed. Further evaluation should be undertaken if the lesion is ulcerated or weeping in a middle-aged or older woman as this may suggest Paget's disease of the breast.

Mastitis

Acute mastitis, also known as puerperal or lactation mastitis, commonly occurs within the first 3 months of breastfeeding as a result of cellulitis of the interlobular connective tissue within the mammary gland [1]. Incidence ranges from 7% to 11% of breastfeeding mothers with a higher incidence in first-time mothers. The most common organisms are staphylococcus and streptococcus species. Risk factors for mastitis include improper nursing technique leading to milk stasis, nipple fissuring/cracks allowing entry for bacteria, stress, and sleep deprivation contributing to a weakened immune system and poor milk production [1]. Presentation includes fever, flu-like symptoms, axillary adenopathy, purulent drainage, and leukocytosis. Acute mastitis can develop into abscess formation in approximately 10% of cases and rarely septicemia.

Treatment for mild infection includes warm compresses, oral acetaminophen, and oral antibiotics (i.e., dicloxacillin, a first-generation cephalosporin, or clindamycin for at least 10 days). Feeding techniques should be observed, and improper techniques corrected. Women should continue to nurse or pump frequently unless unable to achieve a good latch. Nursing can continue with intravenous antibiotics and abscess drainage if a good latch is achieved. Cultures of breast milk or purulent material are of little clinical value except when the infection does not respond to conservative management or oral antibiotics. Close follow-up in 48–72 h is warranted, and biopsy should be considered for atypical presentations or persistent/recurrent infections unresponsive to antibiotics.

Recurrent subareolar abscess (Zuska's disease) is a rare bacterial infection of the breast due to squamous metaplasia of one or more lactiferous ducts that obstructs keratin plugs and causes proximal duct dilation. It is characterized by a triad of draining subareolar cutaneous fistulas; chronic thick, pasty nipple discharge; and a history of multiple, recurrent mammary abscess. It is associated with smoking. Treatment includes abscess drainage and excision of the affected duct and sinus tract [1].

Granulomatous mastitis can be due to infection (tuberculosis), foreign material (silicone or paraffin), or systemic autoimmune disease. Microbiologic, immunologic, and histopathologic evaluation is needed for diagnosis. "Idiopathic granulomatous mastitis" describes granulomatous lesions without an identified cause. Recommended treatment includes surgical excision and steroid therapy. Since 50% of cases continue with persistence, recurrence, and complications, long-term follow-up is necessary [1].

Ectopic or Absent Breast Tissue

The most common congenital breast abnormality is supernumerary and aberrant breast tissue. The most common location is near the breast and on the chest wall, vulva, and axilla although documented occurrences have been reported outside of the milk line including the knee, thigh, buttock, face, ear, and neck. Variances in nipple components (polythelia) and glandular tissue (polymastia) occur and usually have a separate duct system from normal breast. Ectopic breast tissue responds to physiological changes similar to normal breast tissue, and malignancies in ectopic breast tissue are rare [1].

Underdeveloped breast tissue can be congenital or acquired. Congenital disorders associated with hypoplasia include ulnar-mammary syndrome, Turner's syndrome, congenital adrenal hyperplasia, and Poland's syndrome that are associated with breast cancer. Acquired hypoplasia is usually a result of trauma or radiotherapy. Amastia, the absence of breast and nipple, and amazia, the presence of nipple but absence of breast tissue, are rare [1].

Nipple Discharge

Nipple discharge occurs in nearly 7% of women referred for breast disorder evaluation with approximately 5% having serious underlying pathology [2]. Pathologic findings include discharge in postmenopausal women or women over 50 years old, persistent discharge, spontaneous discharge, discharge from a single-duct, unilateral discharge, gross or occult bloody discharge, clear or serous discharge, or discharge associated with a mass [10].

Galactorrhea

Galactorrhea is defined as milk production more than 1 year after breastfeeding wean or in nulligravid or postmenopausal women. It is most commonly caused by hyperprolactinemia from pituitary tumor, hypothyroidism, or medications such antipsychotics, metoclopramide, opiates, cocaine, and some antihypertensives [19]. Other causes include renal disease and chest wall inflammation from a thoracotomy, burns, herpes zoster, or topical irritation from clothing. Evaluation involves a thorough history, characteristics of the discharge, and laboratory evaluation including renal function, prolactin, and thyroid-stimulating hormone (TSH) levels. Imaging may be needed. Treatment with dopaminergic agonists can be initiated if prolactin and TSH levels are normal [2].

Non-galactorrheal Discharge

Non-galactorrheal, or non-milky, discharge warrants investigation based on the number of ducts involved. Single-duct etiologies include intraductal papilloma, ductal carcinoma in situ, and Paget's disease, thus warranting further investigation. Multiple duct discharge can be due to fibrocystic changes or ductal ectasia (discussed below) and requires further workup if bloody; otherwise, reassurance can be provided for clear, serous, green-black, or non-bloody discharge that commonly occurs with fibrocystic disease [2]. If the discharge is bloody, galactography can be performed to evaluate for space-occupying lesions. Cytological evaluation of discharge fluid has a 35–47% sensitivity for detecting malignancy and may be of limited diagnostic value.

Mammary Duct Ectasia

Mammary duct ectasia (periductal mastitis or comedomastitis) is a chronic inflammatory reaction resulting in permanent ductal distension. It presents with thick, white or discolored, cheesy nipple discharge; palpable subareolar mass; noncyclic breast pain; or nipple inversion or retraction though it can also be asymptomatic. It can be identified as microcalcifications on mammography. Mammary duct ectasia can mimic invasive carcinoma especially in middle-aged to elderly parous women and may have an association with smoking. Though biopsy may be required to exclude malignancy, mammary duct ectasia should be managed conservatively [1].

Benign Breast Masses

Risk factors for developing benign breast masses include both genetic influences and environmental exposures. On pathologic examination, benign breast lesions are frequently found to have loss of heterozygosity [2]. Population studies have shown that first-degree relatives of patients with breast cancer have a higher rate of benign breast disease [20, 21]. In addition to increased risk of breast cancer, women with BRCA1 or BRCA2 genetic mutations have a high rate of multiple benign lesions [2].

Hormonal factors likely play a large role in the development of breast lesions. Postmenopausal use of estrogen replacement (regardless of concomitant progestin use) may more than double the risk for benign breast lesions [2]. Conversely, tamoxifen use for breast cancer prevention is associated with a 28% decrease in prevalence of benign lesions [2]. OCPs have also shown a decreased risk [21]. Early studies have shown that serum levels of estrogen, insulin, C-reactive protein, and adiponectin are independent risk factors for benign proliferative breast disease although investigation is needed [22]. Some studies have shown that lifestyle modifications such as increased physical activity; increased intake of vegetable oils, nuts, vitamin E, and fiber; and decreased consumption of alcohol, animal fat, and red meat may lower risk of benign breast disease [23].

Benign breast masses are broadly categorized into three histological categories: nonproliferative lesions, proliferative lesions without atypia, and atypical hyperplasia. This grouping correlates to future risk of developing cancer as the degree of cellular proliferation is related to an increased risk of breast cancer in patients with benign breast conditions [24]. Nonproliferative disease carries no increased risk of breast cancer, but proliferative disease without and with atypia has a relative risk of 1.3–1.9 and 4.1–5.3, respectively [14]. Findings on biopsy, age at biopsy, and family history of breast cancer are risk factors for breast cancer for those diagnosed with benign breast masses. Additional risk factors include increased breast density on mammography, high postmenopausal plasma levels of free estradiol and testosterone, and greater than 20 kg (44 lb) weight gain after menopause, early menopause, early menarche, and late childbearing [2].

Statistically, nine out of ten new nodules in premenopausal women are benign [2]. The vast majority of biopsies (approximately 70%) will demonstrate nonproliferative lesions [1]. Current recommendations suggest that all women with a dominant, discrete, palpable lesion should have surgical referral in addition to imaging based on age and risk factors as described above. If nodularity is vague, thickened, or asymmetric, an exam can be repeated at mid-cycle for one or two menstrual cycles in the premenopausal patient. If resolved, reassurance can be provided; otherwise, the patient should be referred to a surgeon with breast imaging.

Nonproliferative Lesions

Nonproliferative lesions are further divided and include fibrocystic changes of cysts and ductal ectasia, mild hyperplasia, nonsclerosing adenosis, periductal fibrosis, simple fibroadenomas, lobular hyperplasia, juvenile hypertrophy, and stromal hyperplasia. Traumatic lesions that include hematomas, fat necrosis, and lesions caused by foreign bodies are also in the category of nonproliferative lesions. Other lesions in the category include benign tumors such as hamartomas, lipomas, phyllodes tumors, solitary papillomas, neurofibromas, giant adenomas, and adenomyoepitheliomas; infections such as granulomas and mastitis; sarcoidosis; squamous and apocrine metaplasia; and diabetic mastopathy.

Cysts

Cysts are fluid-filled, round, or ovoid structures derived from the terminal duct lobular units that occur in one-third of women between 35 and 50 years old. Late menopause, hormone-replacement therapy use, and thin stature are associated with increased prevalence of cysts [2]. Cysts represent approximately 25% of breast lesions [1, 12]. Ultrasonography has the ability to distinguish fluid-filled cysts from solid lesions. Simple cysts as diagnosed on imaging (BI-RADS 2) are almost always benign; therefore, it is not necessary to aspirate these lesions [14]. Complex, complicated, or atypical cysts are characterized by internal echoes, thin septations, thickened/irregular walls, or lack of posterior enhancement on ultrasonography and can be managed with follow-up imaging. An intracystic mass/nodule should be regarded as "suspicious for neoplasm" and consideration for core-needle or surgical biopsy [1]. Non-bloody fluid can be discarded, but if recurrent, a surgical consult should be obtained. Bloody fluid should be sent for pathology, and a surgical consult placed [2] obtained.

Fibrocystic Changes

Fibrocystic changes are the most frequent benign disorder of the breast of premenopausal women between 20 and 50 years of age, encompassing 50% of clinical and 90% of histological presentations [1]. It is commonly described as "lumpy" breasts or nondiscrete, tender, or painful breast nodules in multifocal regions or bilaterally. Symptoms usually begin just prior to menses and diminish once menses start and are rare in postmenopausal women. Both solid lesions including adenosis, epithelial hyperplasia with or without atypia, apocrine metaplasia, radial scar, and papilloma as well as irregular cysts without discrete mass occur. These changes are thought to be a result of estrogen's predominance over progesterone [1]. FNA can provide symptomatic relief and confirm the diagnosis. Aspiration of clear or milky fluid should be followed clinically for at least 3 months to assure that there is no recurrence [1]. Bloody fluid or no fluid aspirated with a palpable mass, residual mass or thickening, or mass recurrence warrants further evaluation and possible excisional biopsy. Mammography and ultrasonography should also be performed prior to further tissue sampling.

Fibroadenomas

Fibroadenoma is the most common benign breast tumor [14]. Typical presentation is a firm, mobile, discrete breast mass, most often unilaterally, though can be multiple and have a bilateral appearance. The peak incidence is 15–35 years of age and is generally discovered by the patient [1]. These lesions tend to grow during pregnancy, in the luteal phase of the menstrual cycle, as well as in the third and fourth decades of life due to an exaggerated hormonal response [2]. If a lesion is clinically and radiographically suspected to be a fibroadenoma, biopsy may be omitted and followed with serial ultrasonography, though some surgeons may recommend that all discrete masses be biopsy proven, especially among BRCA carriers [2]. If performed, biopsy-proven fibroadenomas need not be followed by serial ultrasounds [2]. Fibroadenomas and phyllodes tumors have similar physical and radiographic features, but phyllodes tumors need excision due to risk of malignancy and high rate of recurrence [14].

Fat Necrosis

Fat necrosis of the breast typically presents as a superficial small, ill-defined, painless, or painful inflammatory mass most commonly in the peri-areolar region [1, 24]. Causes include accidental trauma, postoperative changes, or radiation therapy. Affected areas either enlarge, remain unchanged, or resolve spontaneously. If symptoms persist longer than 1 week, biopsy should be performed to rule out malignancy as it can also be associated with carcinoma or any lesion that provokes suppurative or necrotic degradation (i.e., mammary duct ectasia, fibrocystic disease with large cysts) [1]. Areas of fat necrosis present as oil cysts, smooth or microcalcifications, asymmetries, or spiculated masses on mammography. Findings on ultrasonography and MRI are varied and depend on the extent of fibrosis, inflammatory reaction, and amount of liquefied fat. Fat necrosis may clinically and radiographically mimic malignancy but has classic histological characteristics [1]. Needle biopsy may be indicated to further investigate findings though it may be avoided if the MRI is conclusive [25].

Proliferative Lesions Without Atypia

These include usual ductal hyperplasia, complex fibroadenomas, sclerosing adenosis, papilloma or papillomatosis, radial scar, and blunt duct adenosis.

Usual Ductal Hyperplasia

Usual ductal hyperplasia is characterized by proliferation of epithelial cells within the mammary ducts without distorting the architecture of the ducts themselves. Usual ductal hyperplasia does not confer an increase in breast cancer risk, and no additional treatment is needed [1].

Intraductal Papilloma

Intraductal papillomas may present as a breast mass; however, most women will present with serous or serosanguinous nipple discharge [1]. Presentation is during ages of 30 and 50 years [14]. A single, central papilloma is benign and does not confer an increased risk for subsequent breast cancer. However, papillomatosis (at least five separate papillomas in one segment of breast tissue) does increase the risk of malignancy, and therefore, bilateral diagnostic imaging and surgical referral are needed [3]. Up to one-third of women with papillomatosis will have either an existing or subsequent malignancy [14].

Sclerosing Adenosis

Sclerosing adenosis is a benign proliferative disease that can mimic carcinoma on pathology and imaging [1]. It typically presents as a palpable mass or as an incidental finding on screening mammography. No treatment or follow-up is indicated for this lesion.

Radial Scar

Radial scar is often found as an incidental finding on pathology; however, it may mimic carcinoma on imaging [1]. When discovered, patients should be referred to surgery for excisional biopsy to ensure benign diagnosis due to the increased risk for malignancy [14].

Atypical Hyperplasia

Atypical hyperplasia encompasses both atypical ductal hyperplasia (ADH) and atypical lobular hyperplasia (ALH). ADH confers up to fivefold increase in risk for subsequent breast cancer [14]. Premenopausal women with ADH have a significantly higher risk of developing carcinoma compared to postmenopausal women [1]. ADH appears morphologically similar to ductal carcinoma in situ (DCIS); however, architecturally the cells only fill a small portion of the duct [1]. These lesions are often first detected by micro-calcifications on mammography [1]. Due to the increased risk of subsequent cancer, women diagnosed with ADH should be closely monitored with clinical breast examination every 6–12 months, self-breast awareness, and annual mammograms [9, 26]. And for these patients are 30 years old or older, annual MRI can be considered [26]. ALH appears histologically similar to lobular carcinoma in situ (LCIS), the latter being notable for a greater degree of proliferation. ALH is most prevalent in perimenopausal women and typically found as an incidental finding on pathologic examination [1]. Unlike DCIS, ALH is not a precursor lesion to breast cancer and does not need to be excised; however, it is a risk factor for the development of future breast cancer [14].

Breast Disease During Pregnancy

The dynamic changes in estrogen and progesterone levels during pregnancy cause increased breast size, firmness, and nodularity returning to the prepregnancy state within 3 months of breastfeeding cessation. Palpable masses in a pregnant or lactating patient that persists for 2 weeks or longer should be evaluated with ultrasound. Ultrasound-guided biopsy may need to be performed for new solid mass in a pregnant or lactating patient. If biopsy is deferred, then close clinical follow-up and repeat imaging are recommended. Overall, 80% of palpable breast masses present in pregnancy are benign [27].

Fibroadenomas are the most common benign tumor in pregnancy and lactation. Due to growth that may outpace the increase in vascular supply, these tumors may infarct. Lactating adenomas, which occur in the third trimester and during lactation usually, regress after cessation of breastfeeding. Presentation is typically either solitary or multiple, mobile, and discrete lesions less than 3 cm [1]. These lesions may arise in ectopic locations such as the axillae, chest wall, or vulva and often spontaneously resolve. Surgical treatment may be needed for patient comfort, and there is no increased risk of malignancy [1].

Galactoceles are painless, palpable masses that commonly appear after the cessation of breastfeeding. They occur as a consequence of ductal obstruction and milk inspissations. Most do not require aspiration, but ultrasound-guided aspiration may be indicated if the mass is bothersome. Bloody nipple discharge can occur in the third trimester or during lactation due to minimal breast trauma along with epithelial proliferation and new capillary formation. Without a palpable mass, ultrasound can be performed to exclude papilloma or intraductal carcinoma. Ductography or postpartum MRI can be performed if further evaluation is needed. Mastitis has the highest incidence during the first 6 weeks postpartum [27]; see above for further details.

Male Breast Conditions

Gynecomastia

Gynecomastia is the proliferation of glandular breast tissue in men due to disruption of the estrogen to progesterone ratio [28]. It can be categorized as physiologic or nonphysiologic. On exam there is palpable, firm glandular tissue in a concentric mass around the nipple-areolar complex. Physiologic gynecomastia makes up one-fourth of cases, is self-limited, and occurs in newborns, adolescents, and older men. Nonphysiologic gynecomastia covers a wide range of diagnoses, and one-fourth of cases are due to idiopathic or unknown causes. This must be differentiated from pseudogynecomastia that is a proliferation of adipose rather than glandular tissue associated with obesity.

Nonphysiologic conditions include persistent pubertal gynecomastia, medications and substances (10–25%), cirrhosis (8%), primary and secondary hypogonadism (8% and 2%, respectively), hypothyroidism (2%), renal disease (1%), refeeding after starvation, and tumors (3%).

One-half of adolescent males experience gynecomastia typically starting between 13 and 14 years of age or Tanner stage 3 or 4 with resolution in 6 months to 2 years. Persistence beyond 2 years or after 17 years of age warrants further evaluation. If no underlying causes can be found and treatment is desired, testosterone supplementation, estrogen-receptor-modifying agents, or surgical referral are options.

A wide variety of medications are known to cause gynecomastia (see Table 4).

Antipsychotics, antiretroviral, and prostate cancer therapies are common culprits. Lavender, tea tree oil, dong quai, soy consumption of more

Table 4 Agents associated with gynecomastia

Cardiovascular medications
Amiodarone, amlodipine, angiotensin-converting enzyme inhibitors, atorvastatin, diltiazem, fenofibrate, digoxin, nifedipine, rosuvastatin, verapamil, spironolactone
Anti-infectious agents
Antiretroviral agents – didanosine, isoniazid, ketoconazole, penicillamine, metronidazole, minocycline
Hormonal agents
Estrogen agonists, estrogens – *whether taking it himself, or absorbing it from a sexual partner who uses vaginal cream or ring*, testosterone, gonadotropin-releasing hormone agonists, human chorionic gonadotropins, phytoestrogens, clomiphene, bicalutamide, nilutamide, anabolic steroids
Psychiatric medications
Diazepam, fluoxetine, haloperidol, mirtazapine, paroxetine, risperidone, tricyclic antidepressants, venlafaxine
Miscellaneous
Alcohol, amphetamines, alkylating agents, cimetidine, cisplatin, corticosteroids, etomidate, finasteride, flutamide, heroin, hydroxyzine, marijuana, meprobamate, methadone, methotrexate, methyldopa, metoclopramide, minoxidil, omeprazole, phenytoin, ranitidine, reserpine, sulindac, theophylline, vinca alkaloids

Adapted from Andolsek and Copeland [3] and Taboada et al. [25]

than 300 mg per day, and *Tribulus terrestris* in performance-enhancing supplements have also been linked to gynecomastia. Regression occurs with discontinuation of causative agent within 3 months except with the use of anabolic steroids, marijuana, heroin, or amphetamines.

Treatment includes discontinuing any offending agents and treating underlying causes. Tamoxifen has been shown to have modest effect for physiologic, persistent pubertal, or idiopathic gynecomastia. Raloxifene, dihydrotestosterone, danazol, clomiphene, aromatase inhibitors, and surgery are other options.

Approximately 10% of patients with testicular tumors present with gynecomastia alone with Leydig cell tumors having the highest frequency due to estradiol secretion. Adrenal, testicular germ cell, liver, gastric, and bronchogenic tumors can manifest with gynecomastia as well. While obtaining an initial history, care should be taken to explore for constitutional symptoms that may indicate malignancy though male breast cancer accounts for approximately 1% of all breast cancer cases [29].

References

1. Guray M, Sahin AA. Benign breast diseases: classification, diagnosis, and management. Oncologist. 2006;11:435–49.
2. Santen R, Mansel R. Benign breast disorders. N Engl J Med. 2005;353(3):275–85.
3. Andolsek K, Copeland J. Benign breast disease. In: Taylor R, David A, Fields S, Phillips M, Scherger J, editors. Family medicine (Taylor). New York: Springer; 2003.
4. U.S. Preventive Task Force. Screening for breast cancer: U.S. Preventive Service Task Force recommendation statement. Ann Intern Med. 2016. Available from https://annals.org/aim/fullarticle/2480757/screening-breast-cancer-u-s-preventive-services-task-force-recommendation.
5. American College of Obstetricians and Gynecologists. Well-woman visit. ACOG Committee opinion no. 755. Obstet Gynecol. 2018;132:e181–6. Accessed at https://www.acog.org/Clinical-Guidance-and-Publications/Committee-Opinions/Committee-on-Gynecologic-Practice/Well-Woman-Visit?IsMobileSet=false on 23 Nov 2019
6. Nelson H, Tyne K, Naik A, Bougatsos C, Chan B, Humphrey L. Screening for breast cancer: an update for the U.S. preventive services task force. Ann Intern Med. 2009;151(10):727–37.
7. Clinical Preventive Service Recommendation. Breast cancer [Internet]. 2016. Available from https://www.aafp.org/afp/2016/0415/p711.html Accessed 23 Nov 2019.
8. Oeffinger K, et al. Breast cancer screening for women at average risk 2015 guideline update from the American Cancer Society. JAMA. 2015;314(15):1599–614. https://www.cancer.org/cancer/breast-cancer/frequently-asked-questions-about-the-american-cancer-society-new-breast-cancer-screening-guideline.html
9. American College of Obstetricians and Gynecologists. Breast cancer risk assessment and screening in average-risk women. Practice bulletin no. 179. Obstet Gynecol. 2017;130:e1–16.. Reaffirmed in 2019
10. Salzman B, Collins E, Hersh L. Common breast problems. Am Fam Physician. 2019;99(8):505–14. https://www.aafp.org/afp/2019/0415/p505.html
11. Mercado C. BI-RADS update. Radiol Clin N Am. 2014;52:481–7.
12. Klcin S. Evaluation of palpable breast masses. Am Fam Physician. 2005;71:1731–8.
13. Neal L, Tortorelli CL, Nassar A. Clinician's guide to imaging and pathologic findings in benign breast disease. Mayo Clin Proc. 2010;85(3):274–9.
14. Pearlman M, Griffin J. Benign breast disease. Obstet Gynecol. 2010;116:747–58.
15. National Comprehensive Cancer Network. Breast cancer screening and diagnosis. Version 1. 2014 [Internet]. Available from http://www.nccn.org/professionals/physician_gls/f_guidelines.asp
16. Smith R, Pruthi S, Fitzpatrick L. Evaluation and management of breast pain. Mayo Clin Proc. 2004;79:353–72.
17. Goyal A. Breast pain. BMJ Clin Evid. 2014;2014:0812.
18. Mansel RE, Goyal A, Preece P, et al. European randomized, multicenter study of goserelin (Zoladex) in the management of mastalgia. Am J Obstet Gynecol. 2004;191(6):1942–9.
19. Huang W, Molitch M. Evaluation and management of galactorrhea. Am Fam Physician. 2012;85(11):1073–80.
20. Webb P, Byrne C, Schnitt S, Connolly J, Jacobs T, Peiro G, Willett W, Colditz G. Family history of breast cancer, age, and benign breast disease. Int J Cancer. 2002;100:375–87.
21. Bertlesen L, Mellemkjaer L, Balslev E, Olsen J. Benign breast disease among first-degree relatives of young breast cancer patients. Am J Epidemiol. 2008;168:261–7.
22. Catsburg C, Gunter M, Chen C, Cote M, Kabat G, Nassir R, Tinker L, Wactawki-Wende J, Page D, Rohan T. Insulin, estrogen, inflammatory markers, and risk of benign proliferative breast disease. Cancer Res. 2014;74(12):3248–58.
23. Frazier A, Rosenberg S. Preadolescent and adolescent risk factors for benign breast disease. J Adolesc Health Care. 2013;52(5S):S36–40.
24. Hartmann L, Sellers T, Frost M, Lingle W, Degnim A, Ghosh K, et al. Benign breast disease and the risk of breast cancer. N Engl J Med. 2005;353(3):229–37.
25. Taboada J, Stephens T, Krishnamurthy S, Brandt K, Whitman G. The many faces of fat necrosis in the breast. AJR Am J Roentgenol. 2009;192(3):815–25.
26. Practice Bulletin No. 164. Obstet Gynecol. 2016; 127(6). https://www.acog.org/Clinical-Guidance-and-Publications/Practice-Bulletins/Committee-on-Practice-Bulletins-Gynecology/Diagnosis-and-Management-of-Benign-Breast-Disorders
27. Vashi R, Hooley R, Butler R, Geisel J, Philpotts L. Breast imaging of the pregnant and lactating patient: physiologic changes and common benign entities. AJR Am J Roentgenol. 2013;200(2):329–36.
28. Dickson G. Gynecomastia. Am Fam Physician. 2012;85(7):716–22.
29. Weiss JR, Moysich KB, Swede H. Epidemiology of male breast cancer. Cancer Epidemiol Biomark Prev. 2005;14(1):20–6.

Breast Cancer

Birgit Khandalavala and J. Khandalavala

Contents

B. Khandalavala (✉)
Department of Family Medicine, University of Nebraska
Medical Center, Omaha, NE, USA
e-mail: birgit.khandalavala@unmc.edu

J. Khandalavala
Department of Obstetrics and Gynecology, Dignity Health,
Omaha, NE, USA

© Springer Nature Switzerland AG 2022
P. M. Paulman et al. (eds.), *Family Medicine*,
https://doi.org/10.1007/978-3-030-54441-6_152

General Principles

Background

Breast cancer will be diagnosed in one in eight women in the Unites States, making breast cancer the most common cancer in women. The greater likelihood of preclinical detection of the disease, coupled with the emergence of effective treatment regimens, has resulted in declining mortality and a cure rate of over 90% for the majority of women with early disease [1, 2].

Over the past 10–15 years, there has been a paradigm shift in the clinical management of breast cancer, from a previous focus on tumor burden, to a current focus on biology-centered approaches. At the same time, there has been a trend to de-escalate more aggressive therapy and minimize possible negatives of overtreatment [3]. The present breast cancer treatment strategy involves two newer strategies:

1. Limiting targeted therapies to potential responders
2. Promoting more conservative approaches while retaining treatment efficacy

For the primary care provider, the profound ongoing changes, newer terminologies, and treatment complexities will continue to make breast cancer a challenging area [3]. There continues to be national debate and lack of consensus in many areas of breast cancer management, from screening, primary prevention with medications to newer clinical management applications: but the overall goal remains balancing the harms and benefits with input from the patient [4–6].

A patient-centric multispecialty and multimodal approach continues to be the ideal approach for the patient with breast cancer. The primary care provider's involvement is crucial in all aspects of breast cancer care, and it is anticipated that review of revised guidelines and recommendations will be requisite for the practitioner to be able to provide updated personalized care of the patient and to optimize long-term survivorship and cardiovascular health [7–12].

Definition and Classification

Majority of breast cancers (90–95%) arise from the terminal duct lobular units of the collection ducts in the breast. Epithelial cells from the ducts or the lobules begin neoplastic proliferation to produce breast cancer that is of different histological and molecular subtypes. These subtypes determine the type and response to therapy and predict prognosis in conjunction with the anatomic location and spread of the tumor [2, 4–6].

(A) **Histopathological Subtypes**: Tumors arising from the ducts of the breast tissue are known as ductal and from the lobules, as lobular. If the tumor is confined within the duct or lobule, the lesion is referred to as preinvasive, and when it extends outside the duct or lobule, as invasive. Invasive ductal carcinoma accounts for 80–85% of invasive cancers and invasive lobular carcinoma for approximately 10–15% of cases. Invasive ductal carcinoma is now referred to as "no special type" (NST). Preinvasive lesions are known as carcinoma in situ. Ductal carcinoma in situ (DCIS) can progress to invasive cancer which is typically unilateral, while lobular carcinoma in situ can be seen to occur in both breasts. The diagnosis of DCIS has sharply increased as mammography screening rates have increased but ductal carcinoma in situ does not always progress to cancer, and has variable outcomes with 40% of lesions remaining stable, while other precursor lesions can progress to invasive disease. The more recent understanding of DCIS is that the lesions are more of a risk factor, rather than definitive precursors for breast cancer.

(B) **Molecular subtypes**: At the molecular level, breast cancer is considered a "heterogeneous" disease based on gene expression: 4–5 subtypes have been described such as the Luminal A and Luminal B, Basal-like and Human Epidermal growth factor Receptor 2 enriched and Triple negative. To direct therapy, however, subtypes based on surrogate tumor receptor markers are more commonly used and these are categorized by the presence or absence of molecular markers for estrogen and progesterone receptors and epidermal growth factor (*ERBB2*, formerly *HER2 or HER2/neu*). Tumors expressing estrogen and /or progesterone receptors are said to be hormone receptor (HR) positive breast cancers. Approximately 70% of patients with breast cancer have HR+ disease with estrogen receptor (ER) and/or progesterone receptor (PR) expression. HR+ is more common in older women and has a better prognosis with less invasive disease. The cells can also have additional hormone receptors detected in half of the lesions. Epidermal growth factor 2 is amplified or overexpressed in 20% of breast cancers and is associated with poorer prognosis. Systemic therapy for ERBB2-targeted therapy such as Trastuzumab and Tyrosine Kinase Inhibitors has significantly changed the prognosis lately. Triple negative tumors do have hormone receptors or overexpress ERBB2. Approximately 15% of all breast cancers are triple negative and associated with lower survival and a greater likelihood of early metastatic spread. This tumor subtype is more likely to be seen in younger women, African-American or Hispanic race.

Anatomical Subtypes: The eighth edition of the American Joint Committee on Cancer breast cancer staging manual was implemented in 2018. The traditional surgical Tumor/Node/Metastases (TNM) stage of breast cancer was preserved but added into a total of seven items for the complete stage grouping. TNM refers to the size and spread of the primary breast tumor: Stage 1 is local tumors smaller than 2 cm, Stage 2–3 are local larger tumors, and Stage 4 refers to distant metastatic spread. Prognostic biomarkers added to the stage grouping include Tumor Grade, HR status, ERBB2 and Oncotype DX Breast Recurrence Score. Staging for breast cancer is more complex than for any other cancer, with more than 150 combinations of anatomic and prognostic staging groups possible [1, 13].

Pathogenesis

Molecular pathogenesis: The exact mechanism of breast cancer pathogenesis is not known, and the current evidence indicates that there are two pathways, low-grade and high-grade. The low-grade pathway consists of the estrogen receptor phenotype, and estrogen stimulates the growth of cancer cells. The high-grade pathway consists of ERBB2 and triple negative with specific genetic changes and expression of genes involved in cell cycle and cellular proliferation. In the early phases of cancer genesis, the immune system protects against cancer spread; however, once it becomes invasive, this immune microenvironment is altered to promote cancer spread [3].

Epidemiology

Breast Cancer in Females: The majority of the breast cancer diagnosed is in women over 65 years of age, with a median age of 62, and only 5% of all breast cancers occur in women under 40 years old [1, 2]. In the United States in 2018, breast cancer accounted for 30% of cancer cases and 14% of cancer related deaths with an estimated 266,120 new cases of breast cancer, and an estimated 40,920 women deaths from breast cancer [14]. The 5-year survival rate of breast cancer is an estimated 89.7%, ranging from 98.7% when cancer is diagnosed at localized stages to 27% when distant metastases are present. The overall mortality rate from breast cancer has been steadily declining over the past 50 years, for a total decline of 40% through 2017 [1].

In the United States, despite similar incidence, higher mortality is seen in African American women compared to any other ethnic group. Incidence rates have increased among Asian/Pacific Islander, non-Hispanic African American, and Hispanic women [1, 5].

Breast Cancer in Males: Less than 1% of all breast cancers occur in men. Similar to women, male breast cancer risk increases with age. Other risk factors include radiation exposure, *BRCA1/2* gene mutations, family history of breast or ovarian cancer, Klinefelter syndrome, testicular disorders, diabetes, gynecomastia, and obesity [1]. The vast majority of male breast cancers on histology are ductal carcinomas. Overall mortality is higher in males due to older age and more comorbidities [1, 3].

Approach to the Patient

Early Detection

Breast cancer can be diagnosed early in the disease process and is typically found prior to the development of widespread lesions and metastatic spread. Concurrently, effective treatments are widely available in high income countries, making population screening a viable option. As a result of these two important factors, patients at increased breast cancer risk can be identified early with (1) risk factor assessment and (2) screening. This has been the standard of care for the majority of the adult female population in developed countries and correlated with decreased breast cancer mortality [2–4].

Risk Factors and Risk Assessment

The main risk factors for breast cancer are female sex and advancing age. Although other characteristics have been associated with an increased risk of breast cancer, most women in whom invasive breast cancer is diagnosed do not have many other identifiable risk factors. Genetic factors account for 5–10% of increased risk [5, 6].

(A) Genetic factors such as positive family history and deleterious gene sequence from BRCA genes and other account for 5–10% of risk of which the BRCA1 and BRCA2 are the most common. The cumulative risk with age for carriers of the BRCA1 and BRCA2 by age 80 is an average cumulative risk of breast cancer of 72% and 69%, respectively, and at age 70 years, 65% and 45%, respectively.

(B) Lifestyle and other modifiable factors are emerging factors that increase the risk of breast cancer by estimates of 20% or more, and include alcohol, obesity, physical inactivity, and poor nutrition. Physical activity and breast feeding are associated with reduction in risk [3].

Additional risk factors include African American ethnicity for increased cancer mortality, early onset of menarche, nulliparity, and late onset of menopause. Hormonal contraception may increase the risk and remains to be determined conclusively. Local factors such as previous breast biopsy, breast density, prior medical radiation to the chest and previous history of breast cancer are associated with an increased risk of developing breast cancer.

Screening Models for High Risk Assessment

Genetic Risk: The new recommendation from the USPSTF is to conduct routine risk assessment, genetic counseling, and genetic testing for BRCA related cancer screening in high-risk women with personal or family history of breast, ovarian, tubal or peritoneal cancer. One of several brief questionnaires can be used. Routine risk assessment, genetic counseling, or genetic testing is not recommended. Pretesting genetic counseling is preferable. This recommendation was based on evidence that current genetic testing can accurately detect known BRCA1/2 mutations [5, 15].

Overall Risk: In the original Gail model risk factors included age, age at first menstruation, age at first childbirth, family history of breast cancer in first-degree relatives, number of prior breast biopsies, and history of atypical hyperplasia. Newer models include race/ethnicity, prior false-positive mammography results or benign breast disease, body mass index or height, estrogen and progestin use, history of breastfeeding, menopause status or age, smoking, alcohol use, physical activity, education, breast density, and diet. Most models report performance slightly better than age alone as a risk predictor. Additional annual MRI screening may be indicated if risk is greater than 20%.

Radiological Screening: The mammogram has been the mainstay of radiological screening and the standard of care. Breast ultrasound and MRI are additional modalities for screening in certain patients with additional risk factors. Breast self-examination and clinical breast examination are no longer recommended by the majority of guidelines. Shared decision-making regarding breast cancer screening between the provider and the patient is optimal, since many of the choices are highly personal [1–3, 5].

Mammogram Guidelines: For women 50–74 years, there is general agreement regarding the benefits of screening at intervals of 1–2 years, and various guidelines are available. There is lack of consensus regarding age of onset of screening, intervals between screening and optimal imaging for dense breast tissue, as well as stopping rules. Tailored breast cancer screening for above average risk women is yet to be clearly established (Table 1).

The American college of radiology–Breast Imaging and Reporting and Data system (BI-RADS) is a standardized reporting system on mammogram reports. BI-RADS 0 category assessment is that additional imaging evaluation is needed, BI-RADS 1 and 2 indicate negative and benign findings, BI-RADS 3 is probably benign, with follow-up recommended, BI-RADS 4 is suspicious abnormality, and BI-RADS 5 is highly suspicious and tissue sampling with a core biopsy is recommended. BI-RADS 6 is for known biopsy proven malignancy.

Ultrasound is useful for evaluation of localized symptoms and preferred initial imaging in young women. Guided percutaneous biopsy is possible. Breast ultrasonography can also be used to evaluate and biopsy axillary lymph nodes. Ultrasound is often used as the imaging modality following a screening mammogram with BIRADS 2 or BIRADS 3 result.

Magnetic Resonance Imaging provides further information in addition to mammogram of suspicious lesions and can be used for screening in women, with an estimated lifetime risk of breast cancer of greater than 20%. MRI is beneficial in the evaluation of suspicious lesions in women with breast implants and for preoperative assessment of newly diagnosed invasive lobular cancer.

Harms of Screening: The harms of screening include false-positive or overdiagnosis, anxiety, and over treatment. The balance of benefits versus harms of breast cancer screening is controversial. The risk-benefit balance appears to improve with age. A 2013 Cochrane review found that it was unclear if mammographic screening does more harm than good, in that a large proportion of

Table 1 Mammogram recommendations for women based on age

Organization	Age (years)	Recommendations for women
United States Preventative Services Task Force (USPSTF)	40–49 50–74	Individualized Every 2 years for years
American Cancer Society	40–54 >55	Annually Transition to biennial or continue annually Continue screenings with overall good health and 10-year life expectancy
Canadian Guidelines	40–49 50–69	Not recommended Every 2–3 years
European Guidelines	45–74	Every 2–3 years
American College of Obstetricians and Gynecologists (ACOG)	25–39 >40 50 >50–75 >75	May be offered Annually (initiate if patient desires) Initiate no later than Annually or biennially Based on shared decision making
International Agency For Research On Cancer	50–74	Beneficial with risk of overdiagnosis
National Comprehensive Cancer Network	25–39 >40	Every 1–3 years Recommend at age 40 annually

women who test positive turn out not to have the disease [16]. US Preventive Services Task Force found evidence of benefit of screening for breast cancer in women 40 to 70 years of age, to reduce the mortality from advanced breast cancer disease. Much of the controversy stems from the diagnosis of DCIS and treatment of lesions that may not necessarily progress to invasive disease [1, 5, 17].

Diagnosis

Overview

Imaging studies are typically suggestive of malignancy; however, definitive confirmation can only be done with a tissue biopsy. The differential diagnosis of breast cancer consists of mainly benign diseases of the breasts such as fibrocystic disease and rarely, other malignant tumors [2, 4].

History and Clinical Presentation

More than half the breast cancers are diagnosed at an early stage with a mammogram. A palpable lump that can be felt is now seen in only one third of cases, and 90% of cases are early without spread. Majority of the occurrence of breast cancer is seen to be localized at the time of diagnosis, with regional spread to the axilla seen in 31% and distant spread in only 6%. A lump in the axilla, change in breast shape, nipple changes or discharge, and dimpling of the skin changes are uncommon presentations. Metastatic disease may include bone pain, enlarged/palpable lymph nodes, palpable abnormalities in the ribs, spine, or skull.

Diagnostic Workup

Features worrisome on a screening mammogram for malignant tumor include a mass, architectural distortion, asymmetry, and microcalcifications, which require further work-up with a diagnostic mammogram, ultrasound, core needle biopsy, and sometimes breast magnetic resonance imaging. For younger women, or in the presence of increased breast density, an ultrasound may be an additional imaging modality.

Biopsy

A definitive diagnosis requires histopathological confirmation with a biopsy of the concerning tissue. There are standard criteria to establish the diagnosis of preinvasive or invasive ductal or lobular cancer. Surgical reports provide information about the peritumoral vascular invasion and surgical margin status.

Treatment

Overview

Due to the many complexities of breast cancer therapies, a multidisciplinary and individualized plan for each patient needs to be developed with patient preferences and patient reported outcomes to guide the treatment. The modalities of treatment are surgical, radiation, or systemic [1, 2, 4].

Ductal Carcinoma In Situ

The optimal treatment for DCIS continues to be debated as there is no certain way to determine the prognosis of a DCIS lesion. Surgical excision of the lesion with either mastectomy or lumpectomy may be done, often with sentinel node biopsy, and may be combined with adjuvant radiation therapy and /or hormonal therapy However, it is unclear whether surgery or adjuvant radiation therapy for DCIS is always required. In approximately 60% and 75% of DCIS, hormone receptor positive is detected, and endocrine therapy can be administered for 5 years. Several clinical trials are currently underway to determine optimal management and identify prognostic biomarkers [1, 2, 4].

Operable Stage I–III Disease

Loco-Regional Treatment

The surgical resection of the primary tumor is the treatment of choice for curative breast cancer and can consist of lumpectomy or mastectomy, with breast tissue conservation preferred. Sentinel node biopsy or dissection of axillary lymph nodes is done in early breast cancer to evaluate any spread to the axillary lymph nodes or to remove regional tumor spread. The sentinel node biopsy is preferred over the axillary node dissection, since there is less likelihood of lymphedema and other complications. Breast reconstruction can be offered concomitantly with the initial surgery or as a staged procedure. Patients who undergo lumpectomy and those with high-risk disease postmastectomy usually receive adjuvant radiation therapy. This reduces the risk of local recurrence and improves disease free and overall survival for patients with early breast cancer with lymph node involvement by 75% in a dose-effect relationship. Regional nodal irradiation can improve outcomes in select patients and is used as an alternative to Axillary Lymph Node dissection. Strategies to de-escalate the burdens of radiation and newer protocols, including shorter or single intraoperative dose, continue to be developed.

Systemic Therapy

Systemic therapies – endocrine or chemotherapy – have proven to be highly effective and reduce breast cancer mortality in early breast cancer by one third. Therapy is precisely determined by biomarkers, and adverse effects are limited by restricting use to only those patients with a high likelihood of a response. Therapy may be given preoperatively (neoadjuvant), or following definite loco-regional treatment, postoperatively (adjuvant).

Endocrine therapy stops or slows the growth of breast cancer by blocking the interaction of hormones, estrogen and progesterone. Because these therapies tend to be more selective for cancer cells, they usually result in fewer adverse effects. For HR+ tumors, standard adjuvant endocrine therapy after surgery is recommended for all postmenopausal women for 5–10 years with selective estrogen-receptor-modulator such as oral tamoxifen, letrozole, anastrozole, or exemestane. When managing premenopausal patients, Tamoxifen and Zoladex have been used.

The indications for chemotherapy are determined by gene expression panels (such as Oncotype DX, PAM 50, and MammaPrint) for assessment of risk of distant recurrence. The Oncotype Dx 21-Gene Recurrence Score is used most widely in the United States, for patients with early-stage HR+ or ERBB2 + breast cancer. Regimens for chemotherapy include Adriamycin, cyclophosphamide, and Docetaxel, for 12–20 weeks. For triple negative tumors and ERBB2 + breast cancers, neoadjuvant chemotherapy is the standard of care and side effects include cardiac toxicity. Bone modifying agents such as Bisphosphonates and RANK-L antibody Denosumab may serve a dual purpose of improving bone mineral density and improved patient outcomes.

Inoperable Stage IV Metastatic Disease

With rare exception, metastatic breast cancer cannot be cured, and the intent is preserving quality of life with systemic therapies, local palliative resection or radiation therapy for bone, brain, or soft tissue metastases. Trastuzumab has dramatically improved patient outcomes in ERBB2 + metastatic breast cancer. Immunotherapy and "checkpoint" medications are poised to change the dire prognosis.

Surveillance and Follow-up Care

The majority of patients with breast cancer are enjoying long periods of disease-free years, returning to their primary care providers for their long-term care. Surveillance is needed quarterly for the first year, and annual for the next 5 years, with a screening mammography, or breast MRI for high-risk patients. The early onset of menopause may occur with antiestrogen use in younger women. Posttreatment local side effects include lymphedema, reactions at the site of radiation or surgery, acute toxicities such as hair loss, nausea and fatigue, and chronic persistent conditions, such as infertility, premature menopause, cardiotoxicity, neuropathy, cognitive dysfunction, and chronic pain. Between 25% and 60% of women develop chronic pain. Serotonin and norepinephrine reuptake inhibitors may be useful for vasomotor symptoms, chronic pain and fatigue. Financial and psychosocial burdens are additional aspects that may need to be addressed. There is a small but increased risk of other cancers in these patients. Impaired cognition after chemotherapy is common and treatment includes cognitive rehabilitation therapy. Patients with treatment-induced menopause are at risk for bone loss and should be monitored. Primary care clinicians should counsel patients about the importance of maintaining a healthy lifestyle, monitor for posttreatment symptoms that can adversely affect quality of life, and monitor for adherence to endocrine therapy [11].

Evolving Role of Primary Care in Breast Cancer

Chemoprevention

The USPSTF now recommends that clinicians offer to prescribe breast cancer risk-reducing medications, such as Tamoxifen, Raloxifene, or Aromatase Inhibitors, to women who are at increased risk for breast cancer and at low risk for adverse medication effects (recommendation grade B), but not for average risk for breast cancer (recommendation grade D) [6].

Breast Cancer and Cardiovascular Disease

While mortality rate from breast cancer is 1 in 31.5 women, the mortality rate for women with heart disease is 1 in 3.3 women. For older women, cardiovascular disease (CVD) poses a greater mortality threat than breast cancer itself. This is the first scientific statement from the American Heart Association on CVD and breast cancer. The optimal management of cardiac disease in survivors of breast cancer, hence becomes the foremost priority for primary care providers [17].

References

1. American Cancer Society. Breast cancer facts & figures 2019–2020. https://www.cancer.org/content/dam/cancer-org/research/cancer-facts-and-statistics/breast-cancer-facts-and-figures/breast-cancer-facts-and-figures-2019-2020.pdf. Updated 2019. Accessed 26 Oct 2020.
2. Waks AG, Winer EP. Breast cancer treatment: a review. JAMA. 2019;321(3):288–300.
3. Harbeck N, Penault-Llorca F, Cortes J, Gnant M, Houssami N, Poortmans P, Ruddy K, Tsang J, Cardoso F. Breast cancer. Nat Rev Dis Primers. 2019 Sep 23;5 (1):66. https://doi.org/10.1038/s41572-019-0111-2. PMID: 31548545.
4. O'Sullivan CC, Loprinzi CL, Haddad TC. Updates in the evaluation and management of breast cancer. Mayo Clin Proc. 2018;93(6):794–807.
5. Practice Bulletin Number 179: Breast Cancer Risk Assessment and Screening in Average-Risk Women. Obstet Gynecol. 2017 Jul;130(1):e1-e16. https://doi.org/10.1097/AOG.0000000000002158. PMID: 28644335.
6. Pace LE, Keating NL. Medications to reduce breast cancer risk: promise and limitations. JAMA. 2019;322(9):821–3.
7. Hoover LE. Breast cancer screening: ACP releases guidance statements. Am Fam Physician. 2020;101(3):184–5.
8. Nye L. Integrating breast cancer risk management into primary care. Am Fam Physician. 2020;101(6):330–1.
9. Fok RW, Low LL, Quah HMJ, et al. Roles and recommendations from primary care physicians towards managing low-risk breast cancer survivors in a shared-care model with specialists in Singapore – a qualitative study. Fam Pract. 2020.
10. Zoberi K, Tucker J. Primary care of breast cancer survivors. Am Fam Physician. 2019;99(6):370–5.
11. Runowicz CD, Leach CR, Henry NL, et al. American cancer society/American society of clinical oncology breast cancer survivorship care guideline. CA Cancer J Clin. 2016;66(1):43–73.
12. Daly MB, Ross E. Breast cancer chemoprevention – can we make a case for precision medicine? JAMA Oncol. 2019;5(11):1542–4.
13. Giuliano AE, Connolly JL, Edge SB, et al. Breast cancer – major changes in the American joint committee on cancer eighth edition cancer staging manual. CA Cancer J Clin. 2017;67(4):290–303.
14. National Cancer Institute. Surveillance, Epidemiology, and End Results Program. Cancer Stat Facts: Female Breast Cancer. Statistics at a Glance. Accessed 13 April 2021 from https://seer.cancer.gov/statfacts/html/breast.html

15. Mills J, Fakolade A. Risk assessment, genetic counseling, and genetic testing for BRCA-related cancer. Am Fam Physician. 2020;101(4):239–40.

16. Gøtzsche PC, Jørgensen KJ. Screening for breast cancer with mammography. Cochrane Database Syst Rev. 2013 Jun 4;2013(6);1–73:CD001877. https://doi.org/10.1002/14651858.CD001877.pub5. PMID: 23737396; PMCID: PMC6464778.

17. Screening for breast cancer: recommendation statement. Am Fam Physician. 2016; 93(8). https://www.aafp.org/afp/2016/0415/afp20160415p711.pdf

Selected Disorders of the Female Reproductive System

113

Ashley Wilk, Ashley Falk, and Niyomi DeSilva

Contents

A. Wilk (✉) · A. Falk · N. DeSilva
Florida State University College of Medicine Family
Medicine Residency at BayCare Health System, Winter
Haven, FL, USA
e-mail: ashley.wilk@baycare.org;
Niyomi.DeSilva@baycare.org

P. M. Paulman et al. (eds.), *Family Medicine*,
https://doi.org/10.1007/978-3-030-54441-6_155

Acute Pelvic Pain in Women

Background

Pelvic pain is a common presentation in primary care. Although studies are lacking, estimates are that 1 in 7 women has acute or chronic pelvic pain in their lifetime. Causes of acute pelvic pain include reproductive, genitourinary, gastrointestinal, and musculoskeletal etiologies [1]. Various definitions for acute pelvic pain exist, but most agree chronic pelvic pain is present for at least 6 months [2]. This section will focus on acute pelvic pain and an evidence-based approach using clinical history and physical examination skills.

History

An accurate and thorough history is key to the evaluation of acute pelvic pain. First, it is important to classify patients by those of reproductive age versus those who are postmenopausal. The patient should be asked about the quality, intensity, location, timing, duration, and radiation of the pain as well as the exacerbating and alleviating factors. Inquiry should also be made into associated symptoms (urinary, gastrointestinal, and musculoskeletal). Past medical and surgical histories should be obtained, with special attention to gynecologic or abdominal pathology. Sexual history should be taken with emphasis on last menstrual period, sexual partners, and history of sexually transmitted infections [3].

Physical Exam

The physical exam should first assess the immediacy of the patient's condition. Attention to vital signs and abdominal exam may reveal fever, hypotension, tachycardia, guarding, or rebound on abdominal exam. These findings prompt immediate surgical referral as they could indicate ruptured ectopic pregnancy, hemorrhagic ovarian cyst, or ruptured appendicitis.

The clinician must then determine if the woman's symptoms are from an abdominal or pelvic source, which can be done through physical exam. It is critical to first assess for evidence of peritoneal irritation. Signs of peritoneal irritation include involuntary guarding, rebound tenderness, and increased pain with an increase in intra-abdominal pressure, such as with movement or cough [4]. Following the abdominal exam, a pelvic exam should be performed for further assessment of the patient's symptoms. The examination should begin by visual inspection of the external genitalia. Speculum examination is necessary to visualize the cervix and vagina. Abnormal vaginal or cervical discharge should be noted and sample obtained for further evaluation. Gonorrhea and chlamydia testing should be performed at this time. Bimanual exam should be performed next. One should take note of the position of the uterus and any masses or tenderness. Cervical motion tenderness commonly represents peritonitis of the reproductive tract but may also reflect irritation of adjacent structures. There are definite limitations to pelvic examination including experience of the examiner, patient anxiety, and body habitus [5].

Labs

All premenopausal patients should receive a urine pregnancy test as part of the evaluation. Urine b-hCG tests are sensitive to 25 mIU per mL and positive 3–4 days after implantation [6]. A vaginal wet mount should be obtained and ideally interpreted with microscopy to assess for presence of *T. vaginalis*. White blood cells on wet mount would support a diagnosis of pelvic inflammatory disease (PID). Gonorrhea and chlamydia testing should be performed. Studies have found that vulvovaginal samples are more sensitive than endocervical samples for detecting chlamydia in both symptomatic and asymptomatic women [7]. Vulvovaginal samples were also found to have the highest sensitivity for detecting gonorrheal infection in a similar study [8]. Other laboratory studies are ordered based on physical exam and history findings. Leukocytosis may be seen in PID, appendicitis, and pyelonephritis, and thus if suspected, a CBC should be obtained. Studies have found that only 60% of women with PID have leukocytosis [9]. Blood type and cross-matching should be performed if there has been substantial hemorrhage. In the pregnant patient, Rh testing is performed if there is concern for threatened abortion [4]. Blood cultures are performed if there is concern for disseminated infection. Urinalysis and culture are performed when a patient has urinary-related complaints.

Imaging

Imaging modalities such as ultrasonography, computerized tomography (CT), and magnetic resonance imaging (MRI) are excellent choices in the evaluation of acute pelvic pain due to their high accuracies [10]. The American College of Radiology (ACR) recommends transvaginal and transabdominal ultrasound in the evaluation of acute pelvic pain in both pregnant and non-pregnant patients in the reproductive age group. An MRI is second line in this population if ultrasound is inconclusive or nondiagnostic. CT abdomen and pelvis with contrast should be used only in nonpregnant, reproductive age patients if MRI is not available, as radiation dosage should be taken into consideration. CT, however, demonstrates the improved diagnostic performance in identifying gastrointestinal and urinary etiology of pelvic pain. CT scan is 95–100% sensitive in diagnosing appendicitis, whereas transabdominal ultrasound is approximately 67% sensitive. IV contrast is required for optimum accuracy in diagnosing pyelonephritis, pelvic venous thrombosis, and most bowel pathologies [11].

Diagnosis/Management

To determine the etiology in a woman presenting with acute pelvic pain, the clinician must utilize the diagnostic tools discussed above. Top priority is to rule out life-threatening conditions, such as ectopic pregnancy, ruptured tubo-ovarian abscess, and appendicitis [3].

The Pregnant Patient

Ectopic pregnancy should be considered in all pregnant women presenting with abdominal or pelvic pain. Women with history of previous ectopic, tubal surgery, and tubal pathology or who have an intrauterine contraceptive device in place are at an increased risk of ectopic pregnancy. Transvaginal ultrasound is the imaging modality of choice. Early referral is recommended given surgery is the principal treatment option [12].

The most common cause of abdominal or pelvic pain in the pregnant patient is spontaneous abortion. These women often present with dull or cramping pain that may be either constant or intermittent. Vaginal bleeding may be an accompanying symptom. The cervical os should be visualized on speculum exam, which can then be used for classification of the abortion. Pelvic ultrasound is instrumental in the diagnosis. These findings will guide the management either medically or surgically [13].

Infectious Gynecologic Causes of Pelvic Pain

Endometritis

Endometritis, an infection of the lining of the uterus, may occur postpartum or as part of an ascending infection. Women with recent instrumentation of the endometrial cavity such as hysteroscopy or dilation and curettage are at increased risk of endometritis as are women with a previous episode of PID preceded by confirmed infection with chlamydia or gonorrhea. Symptoms of endometritis typically include pelvic pain, general malaise, abnormal vaginal discharge, and bleeding. Postpartum endometritis is associated with fundal tenderness and foul-smelling vaginal discharge. Fever may be present. Antibiotics, both parenteral and oral, are the mainstay of treatment. Due to the polymicrobial nature of endometritis, a combination of broad-spectrum antibiotics with both gram- positive and gram-negative coverage is recommended. Providers should also consider adding metronidazole, given as a reported association between bacterial vaginosis and endometritis [14].

Pelvic Inflammatory Disease (PID) and Tubo-Ovarian Abscess (TOA)

PID is most common in women aged 20–29. Clinically, the diagnosis has been made based on abdominal tenderness with or without adnexal or cervical motion tenderness on bimanual examination, with supporting laboratory findings. Studies have found that clinical symptoms are not as sensitive or specific as laparoscopy [15]. The CDC recommends empiric treatment for PID in sexually active women if they are experiencing pelvic or lower abdominal pain if no cause is identified for illness other than PID in a patient with cervical motion tenderness, uterine tenderness, or adnexal tenderness. To further enhance the specificity of the minimum criteria and support a diagnosis of PID, the patient should also have either an elevated temperature (>101 F), abnormal cervical or vaginal discharge, increased numbers of WBCs on wet prep, elevated ESR, elevated CRP, or documentation of infection with *N. gonorrheae* or *C. trachomatis*. The recommended outpatient treatment is 250 mg of IM ceftriaxone in a single dose plus 100 mg of doxycycline twice daily for 14 days with or without 500 mg metronidazole twice daily for 14 days. An alternative to doxycycline is 1 gm of azithromycin once a week for 2 weeks [14].

Tubo-ovarian abscess is a complication of untreated PID; however, women over age 40 and those with IUDs in place are also at risk. If abscess rupture is suspected, prompt surgical evaluation is necessary. Clinical signs include hypotension, tachycardia, tachypnea, peritoneal signs, or acidosis. In the absence of evidence of rupture, surgical exploration and treatment are generally advised in women with signs of sepsis. Premenopausal women without signs of hemodynamic instability and an abscess less than 9 cm in diameter are candidates for antibiotic therapy alone [16]. Antibiotic therapy should include coverage for sexually transmitted pathogens (*N. gonorrheae* and *C. trachomatis*) as well as anaerobes. The CDC recommends a minimum of 2 weeks of antibiotic treatment and close follow-up if outpatient treatment is being considered [14].

Infectious Gynecologic Causes of Acute Pelvic Pain

See Table 1.

Noninfectious Gynecologic Causes of Acute Pelvic

Dysmenorrhea

Dysmenorrhea is a common cause of pelvic pain and is defined as painful cramps that occur with menstruation. Onset is typically 6–10 months after onset of menses. Primary dysmenorrhea refers to menstrual pain in the absence of pelvic pathology. Pelvic examination is necessary only in those individuals that are sexually active. The treatment options for primary dysmenorrhea

Table 1 Infectious causes of acute pelvic pain

Diagnosis	Risk factors	Clinical signs	Treatment
Pelvic inflammatory disease	Sexually active IUD *N. gonorrhea/C. trachomatis* infection	Fever >101 F Abdominal pain Vaginal discharge +/− CMT on bimanual exam	One time dose of 250 mg IM Ceftriaxone +100 mg of doxycycline BID for 14 days +/− metronidazole Alternate to doxycycline is 1 gm of azithromycin q week for 2 weeks
Tubo- ovarian abscess	Typically a complication of PID, thus presentation per above.	Signs of rupture Hypotension Tachycardia Tachypnea Peritoneal signs Acidosis	If hemodynamically unstable, surgical consultation is advised If abscess less than 9 cm give 250 mg ceftriaxone x 1 dose, 100 mg doxycycline BID for 14 days and metronidazole 500 mg BID for 14 days
Endometritis	Postpartum Postoperative (D&C, hysteroscopy) Previous gonorrhea/ Chlamydia infection	Fundal tenderness Foul-smelling vaginal Discharge +/− fever	Hospital admission with broad spectrum antibiotic (gram positive and gram negative) +/− metronidazole

include nonsteroidal anti-inflammatory drugs and hormonal contraceptives. Secondary dysmenorrhea should be suspected when additional symptoms such as abnormal uterine bleeding, dyspareunia, and noncyclic pain are present and when pelvic examination is abnormal, thereby suggesting an underlying pathology. Further evaluation of secondary dysmenorrhea should start with transvaginal ultrasound once infectious etiologies, such as gonorrhea and chlamydia, have been ruled out.

Endometriosis is the most common cause of secondary dysmenorrhea. Pelvic exam may reveal retroversion, decreased uterine mobility, adnexal masses, or uterosacral nodularity. The pain of endometriosis is typically cyclical and may be associated with dyspareunia, dysuria, and dyschezia. Adenomyosis is associated with menorrhagia with possible intermenstrual bleeding. Bimanual exam is likely to reveal an enlarged, tender, boggy uterus in adenomyosis. Leiomyomata presents with cyclic pelvic pain with menorrhagia, and fibroids may be appreciated on pelvic examination. The treatment of dysmenorrhea associated with endometriosis is combined oral estrogen-progesterone; however, depot medroxyprogesterone, the etonogesterel implant (Nexplanon), and the levonorgestrel-releasing intrauterine device (Mirena) have also been proven effective [17].

Ovarian Cysts

Functional ovarian cysts are relatively common in women of reproductive age; they tend to be asymptomatic and resolve over the course of 4–8 weeks with expectant management. The rupture of a follicular cyst causes a release of fluid, which may cause acute pain due to irritation of the peritoneum. The pain may be severe initially; however, it resolves without treatment. Corpus luteum cysts, being more vascular, can lead to severe hemorrhage and pain similar to a ruptured ectopic. Stable patients were previously evaluated through surgical laparoscopy if the diagnosis was not certain; however, CT scan can replace the diagnostic laparoscopy. Hemodynamic compromise, uncertainty of torsion, symptoms unrelenting for over 48 h, increasing hemoperitoneum on ultrasound, or decreasing hemoglobin are indications for surgical intervention [18].

Adnexal Torsion

Adnexal torsion is an uncommon gynecologic emergency that occurs when the ovary, fallopian tube, or both twist on the utero-ovarian ligament. Prompt diagnosis is necessary to ensure surgical restoration of the blood supply in order to salvage the ovary and tube. This is often difficult as it presents similarly to other pelvic and abdominal conditions and the imaging features associated with torsion may be non-specific. The patient typically presents with acute onset abdominal pain. Other clinical features are leukocytosis, nausea/vomiting, palpable abdominal mass, and fever. Doppler studies should be performed in addition to ultrasonography if torsion is suspected, as lack of arterial or venous flow to/from the involved adnexa is often seen. A normal Doppler study does not necessarily rule out adnexal torsion. Ultrasonography with Doppler has been shown to be more accurate in diagnosing adnexal torsion compared with CT scan in some studies [19].

Nongynecologic Causes of Acute Abdominal Pain

Gastrointestinal

Appendicitis is the most common nongynecologic cause of acute pelvic pain. Patients generally present with right lower quadrant abdominal pain with migration of pain from the periumbilical area. Fever, psoas sign, rebound tenderness, and rigidity may also be found on physical examination. If the diagnosis remains unclear, imaging studies with either ultrasonography or CT are useful in making the diagnosis.

Diverticulitis should be suspected in the adult patient with left lower quadrant abdominal pain, fever, and leukocytosis. Patients with suspected diverticulitis are often evaluated with CT scan, which is useful if the differential also includes appendicitis [1].

Urinary Tract Disorders

Pyelonephritis, lower urinary tract infection, and nephrolithiasis can lead to acute pelvic pain. Lower urinary tract infections usually present with dysuria, urgency, frequency, and suprapubic tenderness. Urinalysis and culture can confirm the diagnosis, and the patient can be treated with appropriate oral antibiotics. Similar symptoms are often seen in pyelonephritis with the addition of fevers, chills, and costovertebral angle and flank tenderness. If uncomplicated, outpatient management with appropriate antibiotics is warranted.

Nephrolithiasis often presents with severe, colicky pain which radiates from the flank into the pelvis. Associated nausea and emesis may be seen. Urinalysis is positive for blood, and imaging studies reveal the stone and a dilated ureter or kidney. Expectant management with pain control and IV or oral hydration is the mainstay of treatment [15].

Conclusion

In the evaluation of acute pelvic pain, the clinician must first rule out the emergent, life-threatening conditions. Given the broad differential, a complete and thorough history, physical examination, and urine pregnancy test are indicated in every patient presenting with pelvic pain. Ordering the appropriate labs and imaging as discussed above will often lead to the correct diagnosis and treatment.

Toxic Shock Syndrome

Menstrual toxic shock syndrome (TSS) emerged as a public health threat to women of reproductive age in 1979–1980. While sporadic cases have been documented since the 1920s, the dramatic increase in the number of cases in the 1980s prompted research that determined an association with high-adsorbency tampons. The incidence of TSS has declined after some of the brands of tampons were discontinued [20]. TSS is caused by a specific strain of S. aureus that produces toxin TSST-1 and enterotoxins A–E. The toxins act as superantigens stimulating a release of cytokines, prostaglandins, and leukotrienes. CDC reports TSS to include symptoms of fever (temperature greater than 102), diffuse macular erythroderma, desquamation (1–2 weeks after the onset of rash), hypotension, and involvement of three or more organ systems [21]. Nonmenstrual TSS is most often a result of postsurgical, postpartum, postabortion, or nonsurgical cutaneous infections (Table 2).

Table 2 Diagnosis of toxic shock is based on the presence of two major criteria, or one major criteria and one minor criteria

TSS major criteria (all must be present)	Minor criteria (three or more)
Fever (temp >102 F) Rash Erythroderma followed by desquamation of mucous membranes: oral, vaginal and conjunctival Hypotension (systolic BP < 90)	CNS: Altered mental status w/o focal deficit Cardiovascular: Distributive shock, arrhythmia, nonspecific ST wave EKG changes, and heart failure Pulmonary: Pulmonary edema, respiratory distress syndrome Gastrointestinal: Nausea, vomiting, and diarrhea hepatic Elevated liver-associated enzymes renal: Elevated blood urea nitrogen Hematologic: Thrombocytopenia, anemia, leukopenia musculoskeletal: Creatinine kinase greater than twice the upper limit of normal Metabolic: Hypocalcemia, hypophosphatemia

Chronic Pelvic Pain

Background

Chronic pelvic pain (CPP) is defined as a non-menstrual, noncyclical pelvic pain that has been present for at least 6 months. Further, it is defined as not being related to malignancy. CPP must be severe enough to interfere with daily activities and may often require medical or surgical treatment [22–29]. Reported prevalence rates range from 3.8% to 24% in women aged 15–73 years [29], roughly 15% of the female population [30]. Pelvic pain is the single most common indication for referral to gynecology [31]. The economic impact, including both direct and indirect health care costs, exceeds 2 billion dollars a year in the USA [29, 31]. CPP is often associated with negative behavioral, cognitive, sexual, and emotional consequences [32], as well as increased drug and alcohol use [24, 29]. Patients with CPP are more likely to have a history of spontaneous abortion, military service, c-section delivery, sexually transmitted disease, nongynecologic surgery, non-pelvic somatic complaints, multiple sexual partners, and psychosexual trauma and abuse [23, 25–27, 30, 33].

The pathophysiology of CPP is poorly understood and is often multifactorial. CPP is rarely found to be due to a single cause [31]. An underlying diagnosis is not found in up to 60% of patients with CPP [29, 30]. Symptoms are often suggestive of urinary tract, gastrointestinal, pelvic floor, or gynecological sources [34]. This complex interaction of organ systems, along with the psychological burden associated with chronic pain, has led to the recommendation to treat pelvic pain with a multidisciplinary approach [23, 25–27, 33].

History

A thorough history is critical in evaluating a patient with CPP. A full review of systems is indicated [30], as is a full history of previous workup for the pain, including all surgical and nonsurgical diagnostic approaches [23, 30]. It is important also to discuss with the patient how CPP affects her daily activities and sexual function and satisfaction. Treatments tried in the past, both those that provided relief and those that did not, are helpful in teasing out the next steps in both diagnosis and management [23].

One should have a discussion with the patient regarding her pain, in terms of character, quality, intensity, radiation, and causative and alleviating factors [30]. It is important for the provider to differentiate between visceral, somatic, and neuropathic pain when taking a history. Visceral pain is typically reported as dull, crampy, and poorly localized. It can be associated with nausea, vomiting, and sweating due to autonomic feedback [30]. Somatic pain, because it originates from muscles, bones, and joints, will be reported as sharp or dull and is localized. Neuropathic pain is reported as burning or paresthesia [30].

Physical Exam

The physical exam for a patient with chronic pelvic pain is similar to that for a patient presenting acutely and should be performed gently [23], and chaperones should always be present, with at least one person of the medical team being female [30]. The exam should begin with a gait analysis, paying attention to her movement and her sitting pose. Heart and lung exam, as well as appropriate HEENT exam, should also be part of this comprehensive evaluation. The abdomen should be inspected for scars, masses, and tenderness, as well as rebound or fluid shifting.

A pelvic exam should be performed last and should be performed after the patient voids [29]. Inspection of the tissues of the external genitalia is key to note discoloration, scarring, or signs of dermatologic or infectious processes [30]. A moist cotton swab can be used to determine any point tenderness of the external structures [23]. A gentle digital exam can help determine if there is pelvic floor weakness, spasms, or tenderness. A speculum exam is necessary to inspect the internal vaginal vault, and samples can be obtained for Pap smear (as appropriate), wet prep, and cultures for sexually transmitted infection testing. It is important to note the appearance of the cervix and if there is discharge present. Use of one half of the speculum with pressure placed posteriorly or anteriorly in the vaginal vault can help assess for pelvic organ prolapse. The pelvic exam is completed with a bimanual exam, noting any cervical motion tenderness and tenderness with palpation of the posterior portion of the bladder or of the ovaries and uterus themselves.

A rectal examination is also warranted in the evaluation of CPP. It should include anoscopy to evaluate for lesions, internal hemorrhoids, inflammation, fissures, fistulas, or abscesses. Colonoscopy may be warranted if the patient has a report of hematochezia or is greater than age 50. Psychological assessment should be included as part of the complete evaluation of a patient with CPP and should be performed by a health psychologist or psychiatrist who is familiar with CPP [26,

27]. Factors to be considered with this assessment include the patient's understanding and meaning of her pain; impact on her functional roles; emotional functioning; coping mechanisms; knowledge of what can exacerbate her pain; quality of her relationships with her family, friends, and care team; and social support [26, 27].

Labs and Imaging

Due to the multifactorial etiology and pathophysiology of the source of pelvic pain, a six-point system has been developed to assist the physician in guiding the workup. Named "UPOINT," it consists of recommendations for *u*rinary, *p*sychological, *o*rgan specific, *i*nfectious, *n*eurological, and *t*ender musculature causes [34]:

- *Urological*: assess urine flow and voiding diary; consider cystoscopy, ultrasound, and flowmetry
- *Psychological*: assess for depression, history of abuse, pregnancy losses, coping mechanisms (catastrophizing), and feelings of hopelessness or helplessness
- *Organ Specific*: assess genital and urinary structures and anorectal exam and asks questions regarding sexual dysfunction and stooling patterns
- *Infectious*: take samples for urine and genital infections, consider stool cultures
- *Neurological*: assess complaints of paresthesias and dysesthesias, perform neurologic testing as part of examination to include sensory reflexes, and muscular function testing
- *Tender Musculature*: assess by palpating pelvic floor muscles, abdominal muscles, and gluteal muscles

Labs that are indicated in the evaluation of CPP include b-hCG; Pap smear (as indicated by age and history of past pathology on Pap smears); gonorrhea and chlamydia testing; wet prep evaluation for yeast, bacterial vaginosis, and trichomoniasis; hemoccult testing; urinalysis; and urine culture. Other testing to consider includes ESR and CRP to evaluate for chronic inflammatory processes, such as inflammatory bowel disease or antitissue transglutaminase antibody tests for celiac disease [23].

Imaging commonly performed includes a pelvic ultrasound to evaluate the bladder, uterus, and ovarian structures. Transvaginal ultrasound is more sensitive to evaluate for pelvic masses and adenomyosis than transabdominal scanning [26, 27]. In other cases, an MRI may be indicated, as this was found in one study to determine the cause of CPP in up to 39% of cases [30]. MRI is useful for characterizing pelvic masses and is the imaging modality of choice for diagnosing adenomyosis [26, 27]. Laparoscopy, cystoscopy, and hysteroscopy allow direct visualization of the involved structures and can also be useful for the evaluation of CPP.

Diagnosis and Management

The four most common causes of CPP include endometriosis, adhesions (intra-abdominal/intrapelvic), interstitial cystitis, and irritable bowel syndrome [30]. Several organs and organ systems have been implicated in the cause of CPP:

- Bladder pain syndrome
- Urethral pain
- Vulvar pain syndrome
  - Generalized
  - Local
- Vestibular pain
- Clitoral pain
- Dysmenorrhea
- Pelvic floor muscle pain
- Coccyx pain
- Irritable bowel syndrome
- Chronic anal pain
- Pelvic bone stress fracture

The most common cause of chronic pelvic pain is endometriosis [30], defined as the presence of endometrial tissue outside of the endometrial cavity. Incidence is 1–7% and affects primarily nulliparous women in their 20s and 30s. Unfortunately, diagnostic laparoscopy to determine the presence of endometriosis is negative in half of the cases. Adenomyosis is defined histologically as the presence of endometrial glands and stroma deep within the stroma of the uterus. It is a condition in which the uterus is often enlarged and boggy and is associated with pain, dysmenorrhea, and menorrhagia. Adenomyosis is diagnosed with use of US or MRI and has an incidence in up to 70% of cases of CPP, occurring in the fourth and fifth decades of life [26, 27]. Adhesions can arise from chronic pelvic inflammatory disease, prior surgery, endometriosis, or unknown factors [26, 27]. Somewhat controversial as a cause of CPP, adhesions are found in up to 50% of patients undergoing laparoscopic evaluation for CPP. Up to 33% of women who suffer from CPP have a history of pelvic inflammatory disease, thought to be related to adhesions that resulted from the infection [26, 27]. Uterine fibroids are associated with pain, dysmenorrhea, pressure, and menorrhagia.

Interstitial cystitis is a nongynecological source of CPP that is manifested by bladder pain, urinary frequency, urgency, or nocturia. Pain is often suprapubic. Bladder pain syndrome is thought to be caused by a defect in the permeability of the urothelial glycosaminoglycan layer leading to mast cell activation, histamine release, neurogenic inflammation, and upregulation of afferent nerve signals. Childbirth, surgery, bacterial infections, instrumentation, or autoimmune processes are considered possible insults contributing to bladder pain syndrome. After initial evaluation to rule out infection, voiding diaries can help with diagnosis and to monitor treatment. Cystoscopy to perform intravesical potassium sensitivity has a specificity of 83% and sensitivity of 73% [23].

Irritable bowel syndrome is the presence of abdominal pain three or more days a month and is associated with changes in stool frequency or form (loose vs. solid). IBS is a diagnosis of exclusion, and other causes such as Crohn's, celiac disease, lactose intolerance, and milk/food allergies must be ruled out. Up to 79% of patients with CPP have IBS, and 60% will have associated dysmenorrhea [30].

Treatment

Medications implicated in the treatment of CPP are primarily analgesics, such as NSAIDs. Naproxen is the preferred NSAID due to long half-life. Medications such as gabapentin and carbamazepine, phenytoin, and clonazepam have also been found to be useful as they inhibit the excessive stimulation of accessory neurons. Tricyclic antidepressants such as amitriptyline have been found to assist with CPP as well, restoring sleep and improving pain tolerance. The use of opioids in the treatment of CPP is controversial, although it may allow return of normal function of the patient if pain is controlled. Due to risk of addiction and the comorbid psychological diagnoses often associated with CPP, it is recommended that opioid use for treatment of CPP be a last resort [23] and in a tertiary center equipped and experienced for management of chronic pain [33]. Selective serotonin reuptake inhibitors (SSRIs) and tricyclic antidepressants (TCAs) have level III evidence in the treatment of refractory pain [23].

CPP associated with endometriosis is often managed with hormonal treatment, such as estrogen-progestin combinations, progestins alone, danazol, or GnRH agonist, with or without NSAID therapy. The theory is CPP that varies with menstrual cycling will respond to the suppression of the hypothalamic-pituitary-gonadal axis.

NSAIDs are considered first line therapy for interstitial cystitis, although studies have not found NSAIDs or opioids to be routinely effective. Pentosan polysulfate sodium (PPS) is approved by the FDA for the treatment of interstitial cystitis and is thought to mimic the normal glycosaminoglycan layer that protects the urothelium that is dysfunctional. Treatment may require up to 6 months to be effective but is effective in up to 32% of patients. Dietary modifications have also been suggested in the treatment of interstitial cystitis, such as elimination of foods suspected to aggravate the urothelium including caffeine, alcohol, spicy and acidic foods, artificial sweeteners, and carbonated beverages [23].

IBS can be treated with dietary modifications. Diarrhea-predominant IBS may respond to loperamide, cholestyramine, and rifampin. Constipation-predominant IBS is treated with supplemental fiber, stool softeners, and cathartics such as lactulose and polyethylene glycol. TCAs, muscle relaxants, and SSRIs have also been helpful in treating IBS [30].

It should not be overlooked that women who suffer from CPP also may suffer from concomitant psychosocial problems as related to past history of abuse, both sexual and emotional, as well as anxiety and depression. Treatment of these comorbid conditions is key in treating the whole patient and necessary for success.

Surgical Interventions and Approach to Management of CPP

Denervating procedures, such as presacral neurectomy and uterosacral ligament resection, have been studied as treatment modalities for CPP. The results in the randomized controlled trial (RCT) are inconsistent and cannot be recommended [33].

Hysterectomy may be indicated in the treatment of CPP, and up to 18% of hysterectomies are performed for CPP [33]. Hysterectomy is an acceptable treatment for endometriosis, adenomyosis, and uterine fibroids.

Adhesion lysis was not found to be beneficial except in the setting of severe adhesions. Hydrodistention of the bladder by urogynecologists with intravesical instillations with dimethyl sulfoxide or bacille Calmette-Guérin has been shown to decrease pain.

Conclusion

Chronic pelvic pain is a multifactorial process, can involve more than one organ system, and should be treated with a multidisciplinary approach to include physical therapy for pelvic floor muscle dysfunction and psychiatry or behavioral health specialists. Successful treatment requires a positive patient-provider relationship. First-line medications indicated for the treatment of CPP include NSAIDs and hormone therapy for appropriate indications (i.e., endometriosis). Narcotics are not indicated in the treatment of chronic pelvic pain, except in the most extreme of cases and with the assistance of a pain management treatment facility.

Infertility

Introduction and Background

Primary care offices are often where patients with concern for infertility initially seek care. Infertility is defined as failure to achieve pregnancy within 12 months of unprotected sexual intercourse or therapeutic donor insemination in women younger than 35 years old [35]. In women over age 35, it is defined by failure to achieve pregnancy within 6 months. Several studies indicate that approximately 80–90% of couples without significant comorbidities conceive within 1 year of attempting conception, 95% after 2 years [35]. Fecundability is a term used to describe the probability of achieving pregnancy in one menstrual cycle. Fecundability has been shown to decrease after 3 months of attempted conception and decreases with the advancing age of the female partner.

Infertility affects up to 15% of opposite-sex couples in the USA [36]. Appropriate workup should be offered to patients who meet the definition of infertility or are otherwise at high risk of infertility based on additional medial conditions. Women over the age of 35 should undergo prompt workup and intervention after 6 months of failure to conceive. Women over the age of 40 and those with medical conditions known to cause infertility warrant immediate evaluation and treatment. Relevant medical conditions include amenorrhea; oligomenorrhea; uterine, tubal, or peritoneal disease; endometriosis stage III or IV; and either known or suspected male infertility [36].

Female Factor Infertility

According to the World Health Organization (WHO), female factor infertility is the etiology in 37% of cases in developed countries. Initial workup of female infertility includes review of patient's past medical and surgical history, thorough physical exam, and laboratory workup. Historical elements that should be reviewed include menstrual history (age of menarche, cycle lengths and characteristics, and signs of ovulation), previous methods of contraception, timing of sexual intercourse in relation to ovulatory cycle, sexual dysfunction, prior pregnancy history, previous surgical procedures and hospitalization, and gynecologic history (including sexually transmitted infections, pelvic inflammatory disease, abnormal Pap smears and associated treatments, endometriosis, or uterine fibroids), as well as any previous infertility workup or treatment that has been performed [36]. Endocrine history including thyroid disease, hirsutism, and galactorrhea should be addressed as well as family history of birth defects or premature menopause. Current medications and dietary supplements should be reviewed. Social history should be taken with attention to use of nicotine-containing products, alcohol, and/or illicit drugs. Physical exam should include full assessment with special attention to patient's vitals, thyroid, breasts, and pelvis. Note should be made of thyroid enlargement or nodules, signs of excessive androgens, breast secretions, and Tanner stage of sexual development. Pelvic examination should assess for vaginal or cervical abnormalities, secretions, or discharge, excessive tenderness of the pelvis, presence of masses, uterine shape, position, and mobility.

Female infertility workup evaluates structural abnormalities, ovulatory function, and ovarian reserve. Ovarian reserve is the term used to describe reproductive potential of the ovaries based on the number of oocytes available for potential fertilization [37]. Ovarian reserve can be evaluated through serum tests of a woman's level of anti-mullerian hormone (AMH) or basal follicle-stimulating hormone (FSH) plus estradiol. Transvaginal ultrasound with antral follicle count can also assist in this evaluation. Ovarian preserve correlates with expected response of future ovarian stimulation treatments. Ovarian reserve is considered to be diminished when AMH is less than 1 ng/mL, antral follicle count is less than 5–7, FSH is over 10 IU/L, or if there is history of fewer than 4 oocytes at the time of egg retrieval following in vitro fertilization stimulation [37]. AMH is produced by antral follicles and remains stable throughout the menstrual cycle. This allows AMH to be assessed at any point during the menstrual cycle. Diminished AMH correlates with diminished ovarian reserve. Antral follicle count can be assessed using transvaginal ultrasound to evaluate the number of follicles in both ovaries measuring 2-10 mm in size. Fewer than 5–7 follicles is considered to be a low antral follicle count. A low count is associated with a diminished response to ovarian stimulation. Antral follicle count can be low in hypothalamic amenorrhea or with hormonal contraceptives. It is elevated in the setting of polycystic ovarian syndrome (PCOS). FSH and estradiol levels should be measured between cycle days 2–5. FSH values over 10 IU/L are associated with less response to ovarian stimulation treatment. Estradiol levels assist in analyzing FSH results. Elevated estradiol levels over 60–80 pg/mL may suppress FSH levels and indicate decreased ovarian reserve [37]. Women with elevated FSH level prior to age 40 or with unexplained ovarian insufficiency should be screened to determine if they are fragile X carriers.

Ovulatory function is typically assessed with a woman's menstrual history and/or serum progesterone measurement [38]. Progesterone values greater than 3 ng/mL in the mid-luteal cycle suggest ovulation but do fluctuate over the course of a few hours. Furthermore, ovulatory dysfunction is defined as repeated levels of luteal progesterone less than 3 ng/mL, history of oligiomenorrhea/amenorrhea, or both. Up to 33% of women with regular menstrual cycles every 25–35 days are anovulatory, so ovulation must be confirmed with further evaluation. This can be performed in a variety of ways including progesterone measurement in mid-luteal cycle, positive luteinizing hormone (LH) testing, cervical mucus changes, or basal body temperatures. Possible etiology of anovulation include obesity, hypothalamic dysfunction, pituitary dysfunction, or, most commonly, PCOS. Hyperprolactinemia and thyroid disease may also cause ovulatory dysfunction including inadequate luteal phase or amenorrhea. As such, serum thyrotropin and prolactin levels should be checked during workup [38].

Gynecologic imaging can assist in evaluating fallopian tube patency, pelvic pathology, and ovarian reserve. Tubal factors are evaluated with hysterosalpingography (HSG) and hysterosalpingo-contrast sonography while uterine factors are evaluated with HSG, transvaginal ultrasound, sonohysterography, and hysteroscopy. HSG is a procedure performed to view the uterus and fallopian tubes, evaluating tubal patency. Radiopaque contrast is injected through the cervix while fluoroscopy imaging is performed. The negative predictive value of HSG to evaluate tubal patency is much higher than the positive predictive value [35].

Male Factor Infertility

Male factor infertility, according to the WHO, was reported to be the causal factor in about 10% of cases of infertility in developed countries. Overall, male factor may be contributory in up to 40% of cases in addition to the female factor. As such, evaluation for male infertility including medical history, physical exam, and lab workup including semen analysis is recommended when initiating infertility workups. Those with male infertility often are found to have no sperm or low sperm count in ejaculate, termed azoospermia and oligozoospermia, respectively. Poor sperm motility, otherwise known as asthenozoospermia, is found in nearly 80% of infertile men. Teratozoospermia, or abnormal sperm morphology, is another factor that may contribute to male infertility [39].

Etiology of male infertility can be divided into four main categories. Endocrine and systemic medical disorders account for 2–5% of male infertility cases, mostly frequently related to secondary hypogonadotropic hypogonadism. Primary testicular defects in sperm production are identified in

65–80% of male infertility cases while sperm transport disorders account for 5%. 10–20% are without specific identifiable cause and normal sperm analysis and are termed idiopathic male infertility [39].

Workup of male fertility should focus on evaluating for potentially reversible or treatable causes. Subsequently, workup should aim to identify those who may benefit from assistive reproductive technology. Evaluation should include thorough history, physical examination, and semen analysis. It may also include endocrine testing, genetic testing, and imaging of glands and ducts [39].

Semen sample should be collected following 2–7 days of abstinence from ejaculation to allow for accurate sperm count. Since sperm concentration in semen samples can be variable, submission of two samples obtained at least 1 week apart is recommended [39].

Unexplained Infertility

Up to 30% of couples show evidence of female ovulation as well as tubal patency and normal semen analysis; this is termed "unexplained infertility." For these couples, emphasis should be placed on optimizing the overall health of both partners and timing intercourse based on ovulation. Possible treatment avenues may include stimulated ovulation with clomiphene and/or intrauterine insemination. In vitro fertilization has not been shown to be of significant benefit in couples with unexplained infertility [40].

Endometriosis

The presence of endometrial tissue outside of the uterus is known as endometriosis. It was first described over 150 years ago, and yet no unified theory of its origin exists [41]. Endometrial tissue has been found in several locations outside the uterus, including on the ovaries, fallopian tubes, posterior cul-de-sac, inside the peritoneal cavity, and on the bowel. In rare cases, it has been found within the lungs, brain, bone, and even on the skin [41–45].

Epidemiology

Endometriosis is seen in approximately 15% of all women within the reproductive age. It is the most common cause of chronic pelvic pain and 40% of infertility [43, 44]. Approximately 50% of all women with endometriosis experience infertility [46].

Risk factors include early menarche, late menopause, low BMI, Muellerian anomalies, nulliparity, prolonged menses, shorter lactation intervals, and first-degree relatives with endometriosis.

Pathophysiology

Since no single theory has been proven, the pathogenesis of endometriosis is considered multifactorial. The most widely accepted one is retrograde menstruation, proposed by Sampson in the 1920s [43]. It proposes that endometrial tissue is retrogradely transported up through the fallopian tubes and eventually into the peritoneal cavity. From there, it has the ability to implant essentially anywhere throughout the body. This was proven evident in a study where 90% of women evaluated during their menstrual cycle were found to have menstrual blood within their peritoneal fluid [44]. Coelomic metaplasia is another concept that was brought forth in the 1960s. It was theorized that the peritoneum contains undifferentiated cells which are transformed into endometrial tissue as they are influenced by endogenous hormonal or immunological factors that promote this differentiation [44, 45]. Benign metastasis is another theory that suggestion spread of endometrial cells through lymphatic or hematological distribution. Endometrial implants found in the brain, bone, and lungs are evidence of such mechanism.

Implantation of endometrial tissue in ectopic sites is not the only factor that affects endometriosis. The foreign cells need the correct environment in order to proliferate and survive. Several processes have been suggested. Impaired cell-mediated immunity prevents the clearance of ectopic endometrial cells and fragments

[43]. Leukocytes are unable to recognize the cells as abnormal for its location and are resistant to natural killer cells [44]. The endometrial cells are further potentiated by the immune system. The increased numbers of leukocytes in the peritoneal fluid leads to increased inflammation and capillary formation which result in increased vascularization, thereby providing increased blood flow to the implanted endometrial cells. Upregulation of TNF alpha, IL-8, and cytokines helps the neovascularization and proliferation, further stabilizing the implanted tissue. VEGF has been shown to directly correlate to the stage of disease. Elevated levels of macrophages cause further inflammation due to being bound to a portion unique to endometriosis. This limits the phagocytic ability and increases the production of IL-6, leading to increased inflammation. Increased levels of prostaglandins have also been noted in peritoneal fluid, contributing to increased pain.

Infertility in endometriosis is thought to be directly linked to increased inflammation. Impaired ovulation and inappropriate oocyte formation are thought to be a result of the inflammatory state. The luteal phase is also disrupted, most likely secondary to dysregulation of progesterone receptors. Inflammation can also negatively affect sperm motility, embryo formation, and implantation.

Treatment

Treatment options for endometriosis are fairly limited and are not always effective, especially long-term. Many have side effects, leading to limited use of the treatment and subsequently immediate return of symptoms. NSAIDs and OCPs are considered first line therapy for endometriosis [46]. Pain is best controlled with NSAIDs, although there is inconclusive evidence of efficacy. They work by inhibition of COX-1 and COX-2 activity, downregulating prostaglandin production, thereby inducing endometrial cell apoptosis [46, 47]. Side effects of NSAIDs include peptic ulcers, increased bleeding risk, and anovulation [48]. OCPs inhibit gonadal estrogen which suppresses ovarian activity. The result

is a reduced production of prostaglandins, thereby decreasing inflammation. Continuous use or shorter days off OCPs produce the best results as it limits the recovery phase of estrogen synthesis. Drawbacks of OCP use include increased risk of thromboembolic events in tobacco smokers over the age of 35. OCP use is limited in women who desire fertility in the near future. Unfortunately, cessation of OCPs results in an almost immediate return of symptoms.

Various other hormonal treatments have also been investigated. Progestins block mechanisms at the central and peripheral levels, leading to a decrease in estrogen-induced proliferation. The atrophic endometrium thereby enters a pseudo-pregnancy state, decreasing pain. Nexplanon, which is depomedroxyprogesterone, produces similar results. Side effects include possible weight gain, breast tenderness, and menstrual irregularities. Hormonal IUDs such as levonorgestrel-releasing can improve dysmenorrhea, pelvic pain, dyspareunia, and the size of the ectopic endometrial tissue. Synthetic androgen derivatives were first explored several decades ago, as they induce a hypoestrogenic-hyperandrogenic state. While they limit endometrial tissue growth, the side effects of elevated levels of androgen make this a less desirable option [46, 49].

Second-line treatment options include GnRH analogues which suppress the receptors of the pituitary. This leads to hypoestrogenism which manifests as amenorrhea and atrophy of the endometrial tissue. While up to 50% of patients experience symptom reduction, the use of GnRH analogues is limited as it can mimic menopause with hot flashes, depression, urogenital atrophy decreased libido, loss of bone density, and worsening of lipid profiles. Aromatase inhibitors decrease the levels of estrogen by downregulating the conversion of steroidal precursors. With the decrease in estrogen, endometrial tissue growth is inhibited and COX-2 mediated inflammation is reduced. Reversible side effects include headaches, nausea, diarrhea, flushing, joint pain, and stiffness, along with bone density loss. Adding HRT or bisphosphonates can help reduce the severity of the side effects. Melatonin can also be used as a natural antioxidant and to combat free radicals that are related to endometriosis. It has been shown to decrease the size of endometrial tissue and increase antioxidant activity. VEGF has been directly correlated to the severity of the disease. By inhibiting VEGF, angiogenesis is halted, depriving the endometrial implants of blood supply that is necessary for implantation and proliferation. Although animal studies have been conducted, no human trials have been established at this time [46, 49].

References

1. Karnath BM, Breitkopf DM. Acute and chronic pelvic pain in women. Hosp Physician. 2007;43:41–8.
2. Curry RW Jr, George P, Samrag N. Acute pelvic pain: evaluation and management. Compr Ther. 2004;30:173–84.
3. Kruszka PS, Krusszka SJ. Evaluation of pelvic pain in women. Am Fam Physician. 2010;82:142–6.
4. Yudin MH, Wiesenfeld HC. Acute pelvic pain. In: Zenilman JM, editor. Sexually transmitted infections: diagnosis, management, and treatment. Sudbury: Jones & Bartlett Learning; 2012. p. 145–53.
5. Padilla LA, Radosevich DM, Milad MP. Accuracy of pelvic examination in detecting adnexal masses. Obstet Gynecol. 2000;46:593–8.
6. Chard T. Pregnancy tests: a review. Hum Reprod. 1992;7:701–10.
7. Schoeman SA, Stewart CM, Booth RA, Smith SD, Wilcox MH, Wilson JD. Assessment of best single sample for finding chlamydia in women with and with- out symptoms: a diagnostic test study. BMJ. 2012;345:e8103.
8. Stewart CM, Schoeman SA, Booth RA, Smith SD, Wilcox MH, Wilson JD. Assessment of selftaken swabs versus clinician taken swab cultures for diagnosing gonorrhoea in women: single centre, diagnostic accuracy study. BMJ. 2012;345:e8107. https://doi.org/10.1136/bmj.e8107.
9. Jaiyeoba O, Soper DE. A practical approach to the diagnosis of pelvic inflammatory disease. Infect Dis Obstet Gynecol. 2011;2011:753037. https://doi.org/10.1155/2011/753037.. Epub 2011 Jul 26
10. Cicchiello LA, Hamper UM, Scoutt LM. Ultrasound evaluation of gynecologic causes of pelvic pain. Obstet Gynecol. 2011;38:85–114.
11. American College of Radiology. ACR appropriateness criteria. Acute pelvic pain in the reproductive age group. Ultrasound Q. 2011;27:205.
12. Jurkovic D, Wilkinson H. Diagnosis and management of ectopic pregnancy. BMJ. 2011;342.d3397.
13. Dighe M, Cuevas C, Moshiri M. Sonography in first trimester bleeding. J Clin Ultrasound. 2008;36:352.
14. Centers for Disease Control and Prevention. Sexually transmitted diseases treatment guidelines, 2010. MMWR. 2010;59:63–7.
15. Bartlett EC, Levison WB, Munday PE. Pelvic Inflammatory disease. BMJ. 2013;346:f3189.
16. Lareau SM, Beigi RH. Pelvic inflammatory disease and tubo-ovarian abscess. Infect Dis Clin N Am. 2008;22:693.
17. Osayande AS, Mehulic S. Diagnosis and initial management of dysmenorrhea. Am Fam Physician. 2014;89:341–6.
18. Kim JH, Lee SM, Lee JH, et al. Successful conservative management of ruptured ovarian cysts with hemoperitoneum in healthy women. PLoS One. 2014;9:e91171.
19. Chiou SY, Lev-Toaff AS, Masuda E, et al. Adnexal torsion: new clinical and imaging observations by sonography, computed tomography, and magnetic resonance imaging. J Ultrasound Med. 2007;26:1289–301.
20. Reingold A, Harget NT, Shands KN, et al. Toxic shock syndrome surveillance in the United States, 1980–1981. Ann Intern Med. 1982;96:875.
21. CDC. Toxic shock syndrome. 2011 case definition. CSTE position statement. http://wwwn.cdc.gov/nndss/ conditions/toxic-shock-syndrome-other-than-streptococ cal/case-definition/2011
22. Alappattu MJ, Bishop MD. Psychological factors in chronic pelvic pain in women: relevance and application of the fear-avoidance model of pain. Phys Ther. 2011;91(10):1542–50. https://doi.org/10.2522/ptj.20100368. Epub 11 Aug 2011. Review. PubMed PMID: 21835893; PubMed Central PMCID: PMC3185223
23. Bordman R, Jackson B. Below the belt: approach to chronic pelvic pain. Can Fam Physician. 2006;52 (12):1556–62. PubMed PMID: 17279236; PubMed Central PMCID: PMC1783755
24. Daniels JP, Khan KS. Chronic pelvic pain in women. BMJ. 2010;341:c4834. https://doi.org/10.1136/bmj.c4834.
25. de Bernardes NO, Marques A, Ganunny C, Bahamondes L. Use of intravaginal electrical stimulation for the treatment of chronic pelvic pain: a randomized, double-blind, crossover clinical trial. J Reprod Med. 2010;55(1–2):19–24.
26. Jarrell JF, Vilos GA, Allaire C, Burgess S, Fortin C, Gerwin R, Lapensée L, Lea RH, Leyland NA, Martyn P, Shenassa H, Taenzer P, Abu-Rafea B, Chronic Pelvic Pain Working Group, Society of Obste- tricians and Gynaecologists of Canada. Consensus guidelines for the management of chronic pelvic pain. J Obstet Gynaecol Can. 2005;27(9):869–910. English, French
27. Jarrell JF, Vilos GA, Allaire C, Burgess S, Fortin C, Gerwin R, Lapensée L, Lea RH, Leyland NA, Martyn P, Shenassa H, Taenzer P, Abu-Rafea B, Chronic Pelvic Pain Working Group, SOGC. Consensus guidelines for the management of chronic pelvic

pain. J Obstet Gynaecol Can. 2005;27(8):781–826. English, French

28. Montenegro ML, Gomide LB, Mateus-Vasconcelos EL, Rosa-e-Silva JC, Candido-dos-Reis FJ, Nogueira AA, Poli-Neto OB. Abdominal myofascial pain syndrome must be considered in the differential diagnosis of chronic pelvic pain. Eur J Obstet Gynecol Reprod Biol. 2009;147(1):21–4. https://doi.org/10.1016/j.ejogrb.2009.06.025. Epub 22 Jul 2009. Review

29. Montenegro ML, Vasconcelos EC, Candido Dos Reis FJ, Nogueira AA, Poli-Neto OB. Physical therapy in the management of women with chronic pelvic pain. Int J Clin Pract. 2008;62(2):263–9. Epub 7 Dec 2007. Review

30. Stein SL. Chronic pelvic pain. Gastroenterol Clin N Am. 2013;42(4):785–800. https://doi.org/10.1016/j.gtc.2013.08.005. Epub 23 Oct 2013. Review

31. Latthe P, Mignini L, Gray R, Hills R, Khan K. Factors predisposing women to chronic pelvic pain: systematic review. BMJ. 2006;332(7544):749–55. Epub 16 Feb 2006. Review. PubMed PMID: 16484239; PubMed Central PMCID: PMC1420707

32. Morrissey D, Ginzburg N, Whitmore K. Current advancements in the diagnosis and treatment of chronic pelvic pain. Curr Opin Urol. 2014;24(4):336–44. https://doi.org/10.1097/MOU.0000000000000062. Review

33. Vercellini P, Viganò P, Somigliana E, Abbiati A, Barbara G, Fedele L. Medical, surgical and alternative treatments for chronic pelvic pain in women: a descriptive review. Gynecol Endocrinol. 2009;25(4):208–21. https://doi.org/10.1080/09513590802530940.. Review

34. Latthe P, Latthe M, Say L, Gülmezoglu M, Khan KS. WHO systematic review of prevalence of chronic pelvic pain: a neglected reproductive health morbidity. BMC Public Health. 2006;6:177. Review. PubMed PMID: 16824213; PubMed Central PMCID: PMC1550236

35. Infertility workup for the women's health specialist. ACOG Committee Opinion No. 781. American College of Obstetricians and Gynecologists. Obstet Gynecol. 2019;133:e377–84.

36. Practice Committee of the American Society for Reproductive Medicine. Diagnostic evaluation of the infertile female: a committee opinion. Fertil Steril. 2015;103(6):e44–50.

37. Practice Committee of the American Society for Reproductive Medicine. Testing and interpreting measures of ovarian reserve. Fertil Steril. 2015;103: e9–e17.

38. Lindsay TJ, Vitrikas KR. Evaluation and treatment of infertility. Am Fam Physician. 2015;91(5):308–14.

39. Winters BR, Walsh TJ. The epidemiology of male infertility. Urol Clin North Am. 2014;41:195.

40. Jose-Miller AB, Boyden JW, Frey KA. Infertility. Am Fam Physician. 2007;75(6):849–56.

41. Stilley JA, Birt JA, Sharpe-Timms KL. Cellular and molecular basis for endometriosis-associated infertility. Cell Tissue Res. 2012;349(3):849–62.. (44)

42. Vercellini P, Viganò P, Somigliana E, Fedele L. Endometriosis: pathogenesis and treatment. Nat Rev Endocrinol. 2014;10:261.

43. Macer ML, Taylor HS. Endometriosis and infertility: a review of the pathogenesis and treatment of endometriosis-associated infertility. Obstet Gynecol Clin N Am. 2012;39(4):535–49. https://doi.org/10.1016/j.ogc.2012.10.002.

44. Burney RO, Giudice LC. Pathogenesis and pathophysiology of endometriosis. Fertil Steril. 2012;98(3):511–9. https://doi.org/10.1016/j.fertnstert.2012.06.029.. Epub 20 Jul 2012

45. Prefumo F, Todeschini F, Fulcheri E, Venturini PL. Epithelial abnormalities in cystic ovarian endometriosis. Gynecol Oncol. 2002;84:280.

46. Zito G, Luppi S, Giolo E, Martinelli M, Venturin I, Di Lorenzo G, Ricci G. Medical treatments for endometriosis-associated pelvic pain. Biomed Res Int. 2014;2014:191967. https://doi.org/10.1155/2014/191967.. Epub 07 Aug 2014

47. Pall M, Fridén BE, Brännström M. Induction of delayed follicular rupture in the human by the selective COX-2 inhibitor rofecoxib: a randomized double-blind study. Hum Reprod. 2001;16:1323.

48. Brown J, Crawford TJ, Allen C, et al. Nonsteroidal anti-inflammatory drugs for pain in women with endometriosis. Cochrane Database Syst Rev. 2017;1: CD004753.

49. Practice Committee of the American Society for Reproductive Medicine. Treatment of pelvic pain associated with endometriosis: a committee opinion. Fertil Steril. 2014;101:927.

Disorders of the Neck and Back

James Winger

Contents

Disorders of the Back

Low Back Pain (LBP)

General Principles

Definition/Background

Low back pain (LBP) is a heterogeneous condition with high prevalence, high morbidity, and large economic burden. According to the 2010 Global Burden of Disease Study, low back pain ranked highest among 291 studied disorders in terms of years lived with disability (YLDs), with a global point prevalence estimated to be 9.4% (95% CI 9.0–9.8) [1]. In 2005, direct expenditures for spine problems in the United States were estimated at $85.9 billion, which represented 9% of the total national healthcare expenditures, similar to costs associated with arthritis, cancer, and diabetes, and only exceeded significantly by those for heart disease and stroke [2]. In the United States between 2004 and 2008, it is estimated that over two million episodes of back pain resulting in presentation for emergency care occurred, yielding an incidence rate of 1.39/ 1,000 person-years [3]. In workers 40–65 years of age, back pain costs employers an estimated $7.4 billion/year in lost productive time [4]. Commonly, disorders of the neck and back are self-limiting conditions, which require only judicial use of imaging and rarely more invasive treatments. Many national and international groups have produced high-quality, evidence-based recommendations to aid in the diagnosis and treatment of low back pain (Table 1) [5].

J. Winger (✉)
Department of Family Medicine, Loyola University Chicago Stritch School of Medicine, Maywood, IL, USA
e-mail: jwinger@lumc.edu

© Springer Nature Switzerland AG 2022
P. M. Paulman et al. (eds.), *Family Medicine*,
https://doi.org/10.1007/978-3-030-54441-6_116

Table 1 2007 recommendations on the diagnosis and treatment of low back pain from the American College of Physicians and the American Pain Society

1. Patients should be classified at initial presentation into the following groups: Nonspecific low back pain, back pain potentially associated with radiculopathy or spinal stenosis, or back pain potentially associated with another specific spinal cause. The history should include assessment of psychosocial risk factors that predict the risk for chronic disabling back pain
2. Clinicians should not routinely order imaging or other diagnostic testing in patients with nonspecific back pain
3. Diagnostic imaging and testing should be pursued when severe or progressive neurological deficits are present or when severe underlying conditions are suspected
4. Patients suspected to have either radiculopathy or spinal stenosis should be evaluated with MRI or CT only if potential candidates for surgery or epidural steroid injection
5. Clinicians should provide patients' educational materials regarding the course and prognosis of back pain, advice to remain active, and self-care options
6. For most patients, the first-line medication options are acetaminophen or nonsteroidal anti-inflammatory drugs
7. Clinicians should consider the addition of nonpharmacologic therapy with proven benefits in those not initially improving. For acute low back pain, spinal manipulation; for chronic or subacute low back pain, intensive interdisciplinary rehabilitation, exercise therapy, yoga, acupuncture, massage therapy, spinal manipulation, cognitive-behavioral therapy, or progressive relaxation

Epidemiology

A 2002 survey in the United States indicated that low back pain, defined as posterior trunk pain between the costal margins and inferior gluteal folds, was present for at least 1 day in the last 3 months in 26.4% of respondents, with men and women exhibiting similar responses. Prevalence rates were reported highest among Native Americans and lowest among Asian Americans. Increasing income and higher education levels had moderating effects on reported back pain [6]. Throughout the adult life cycle, prevalence rates increase until the 60–65 year age group and then again decline, with the peak incidence of LBP in the third decade of life [7]. Commonly reported factors associated with LBP include anxiety, depression, job dissatisfaction, low levels of social support, low educational status, poor coping skills, ongoing litigation, smoking, and obesity [8]. While the incidence of LBP is increasing, as are its associated medical costs, no commensurate improvements are seen in health status [2].

Progression to chronic LBP that lasts more than 6 weeks is a costly complication, both in terms of medical expenditures and work absences. In those experiencing activity-limiting pain, most will experience recurrent episodes [7], and up to 40% of those with initial back pain episodes will experience pain chronically [9]. Psychosocial factors (depression, anxiety, coping mechanisms, attitudes, stress, and job satisfaction) better

predict the transition from acute to chronic back pain than do patient-specific anatomic factors [8].

The majority of the societal morbidity associated with LBP is accounted for by disability. Disability 1 year after initial lumbosacral injury has been shown to be predicted by injury severity, specialty of the first healthcare provider seen after injury, worker-reported physical disability, number of pain sites, "very hectic" job, no offer of accommodation, and previous injury involving a month or more off of work. These factors produce a model predicting disability with a 0.88 (95% CI 0.86–0.90) area under the receiver operating characteristic (ROC) curve [10].

Natural History

LBP is frequently described as a self-limiting condition in that initial episodes resolve in 90% of individuals within 3 months of onset [9]. Pooled data analysis indicates that the greatest improvement occurs in the first 6 weeks following initial injury with slower improvement through 52 weeks. However, LBP has a high propensity for recurrence and persistence, and levels of pain, disability, and work absence remain mostly constant after 90 days. A 2008 study indicated that in a cohort of nearly 1,000 patients, more than half of those initially absent from work had returned by 14 days and 83% by 3 months; nearly 30% had persistent pain at 12 months' time [9]. Many patients experience at least one recurrence in the first 12 months following a low back pain episode with a prior episode of LBP being the only strong predictor of future recurrence [11].

Anatomic sites of acute lumbosacral pain vary and may include paraspinal musculature, collagenous structures (tendon and ligament), intervertebral disk, annulus fibrosus, facet joints, central canal stenosis, spinal nerve roots, and the vasculature.

Clinical Presentation

The experience of many individuals with LBP is that of pain and dysfunction that gradually resolve over several days and allow return to the usual activities of daily living [9]. Most individuals with an episode of LBP will not present to medical attention.

History

Focused history in a patient presenting with LBP will include onset of symptoms, location of pain, timing of pain, interventions that provide palliation or provocation, and any associated symptoms. Assessment for signs suggesting neurological involvement, such as radiation of pain, weakness, numbness, sensory changes, or bowel and bladder dysfunction, is likewise important. Description of any previous episodes of back pain should be elicited during the interview, as well as any current or pertinent past medical history. Interview of a patient presenting with low back pain should pay particular attention to established risk factors for back pain such as known trauma, previous low back pain, missed work, occupational mechanism, and preexisting mood disorder [12].

In addition to standard interviewing approaches, certain additional queries in individuals with low back pain are aimed at identifying neurosurgical emergency, vertebral fracture, or malignancy. A retrospective study of 206 patients with spinal cord or cauda equina compression noted that the presence of bowel and bladder dysfunction as well as saddle sensory disturbance yielded a specificity of 0.92 and a likelihood ratio of 3.46 of such compression [13]. Interestingly, this same study noted that these symptoms showed stronger association with MRI diagnosis

than did physical examination of the lower extremities, even while only marginally raising the clinical suspicion of neurological compression. A 2013 study evaluating the benefit of screening questions addressing the presence of malignancy indicated that only a prior history of malignancy is informative [14]. The same study also found that prolonged corticosteroid use, older age, and trauma increased the pretest probability of spinal fracture by 15–43% when present individually and greater when present in combination. Thus, there is relatively little evidence favoring reliance on the so-called "red flag" symptoms to trigger changes in management.

Physical Exam

Examination of the patient with back pain is attentive to the presence and extent of signs indicating neurological involvement. Observation of the patient's gait, stance, and posture (absence or alteration of normal lordosis or kyphosis) may provide diagnostic clues. Inspection while attending to patient modesty should include the entire back and posterior pelvis but also the upper and lower extremities. The sequelae of trauma may present as disfigurement, edema, or ecchymosis. Asymmetry and muscle wasting may indicate chronic motor neuropathy. Palpation of bony and other landmarks may assist in the localization of a primary pain source. The spinal range of motion in coronal, sagittal, and axial planes may be useful as an indicator of which movement types trigger a patient's pain; however, this specific assessment is noted to be highly examiner dependent.

A neurologic exam is performed on all patients and should include both upper and lower extremities (Table 2). Manual muscle testing should focus on nerve root myotome testing rather than on specific individual muscles, and strength should be scored with the standard 0–5 scale. Testing of nerve root strength may be assessed as follows: single-leg rising from a chair without the use of hands (quadriceps/L4), heel walking (tibialis anterior/L5), and toe walking (gastrocnemius/S1). The examiner must be aware that deficits in balance or preexisting weakness may affect motor strength testing results. Assessment of pinprick and light touch sensation should be

Table 2 Strength, sensation, and deep tendon reflexes associated with the commonly impinged nerve roots

Nerve root	Strength testing	Sensory innervation	Deep tendon reflexes
C5	Shoulder abduction	Lateral arm	Biceps (C5, C6)
C6	Elbow flexion, wrist extension	Lateral forearm	Brachioradialis
C7	Elbow extension, wrist flexion	Middle of the hand dorsum	Triceps
C8	Finger flexion	Medial forearm	–
T1	Finger abduction	Medial arm	–
L3	Hip flexion	Distal upper leg	–
L4	Knee extension	Anterior knee	Knee jerk (patellar)
L5	Ankle dorsiflexion (heel walking)	Dorsum of the foot	Hamstring reflex (L5, S1)
S1	Ankle plantar flexion (toe walking)	Lateral foot	Ankle jerk (Achilles)

compared to the unaffected contralateral side. Numbness should be specified by dermatomal distribution and may include examination of the perineum and sacral distributions. Evaluation of vibration and position sense may be useful if central processes are included in the differential diagnosis. Signs of upper motor neuron (UMN) dysfunction, such as Hoffmann's reflex, a positive Babinski's sign, or hyperreflexia, may suggest etiology for lower motor neuron dysfunction. Pertinent reflexes include the knee jerk (L4), hamstring reflex (L5, S1), and ankle jerk (S1), as graded on the standard 0–4 scale. Depending on the extent of neurological manifestations, assessment of perineal sensation and anal sphincter tone may be appropriate.

Nerve tension tests such as the straight-leg raise (SLR) and seated slump test (SST) may suggest neural impingement but are positive in most symptomatic individuals with and thus have a poor positive predictive value when applied to all patients with low back pain. In the SST, the patient is seated on the edge of the examination table. With the hands clasped behind the back and neck flexed with the upper body "slumped" forward, the examiner passively extends the knee. A positive finding is reproduction and radiation of the patient's pain beyond the knee. Having the patient extend his or her neck, thus relieving neural tension and lessening or relieving the pain, may provide confirmation of this finding. The SLR is performed with the patient supine and the ipsilateral hip flexed to 90° while the examiner passively extends the ipsilateral knee. A positive test is reproduction and radiation of the patient's pain prior to 60° of knee

extension and further relief of such pain with knee flexion. This maneuver may be modified by Lasègue's sign: dorsiflexion of the ipsilateral ankle increasing neural tension and thus worsening the pain response. The femoral stretch test (FST) for upper (L2, L3, L4) lumbar nerve root impingement is performed with the patient prone as the examiner passively and slowly flexes the ipsilateral knee. Reproduction of the patient's typical lower extremity pain constitutes a positive test. The crossed SLR (cSLR) and crossed FST (cFST) are performed on the lower extremity contralateral to a patient's typical radiating pain.

The cSLR and cFST are poorly sensitive but highly (>90%) specific [15]. Thus, neural tension tests may be better applied only to those with presenting symptoms already suggestive of radiculopathy.

In 2011, Suri et al. evaluated the accuracy of physical exam maneuvers for the diagnosis of midlumbar (L2, L3, L4) and low lumbar (L5, S1) nerve root impingement. The study compared standardized, expert-level examinations to MRI findings in patients presenting to a physiatry spine practice with acute or subacute symptoms suggestive of nerve root impingement. Exam maneuvers testing positive that either increased the likelihood ratio >4.0 or exhibited 100% specificity for midlumbar nerve root impingement were FST, cFST, sit-to-stand test, medial ankle sensation, and patellar reflex assessment. Achilles reflex testing was the only exam maneuver in which a positive test either increased the likelihood ratio >5.0 (+LR 7.1) [15].

Further examination should include the hips and sacroiliac joints. Range of motion of the femoroacetabular joints should be assessed along with the response to the loading of the acetabular labra. The acronymically named FABER test, also known as Patrick's test, stresses the SI joint by flexing, abducting, and externally rotating the contralateral hip while applying posterior pressure to the ipsilateral anterior pelvis and contralateral knee. A positive response is reproduced pain in the contralateral SI joint.

Given the contribution of psychosocial issues to acute and chronic low back pain, assessment of biopsychosocial stressors should be performed. Minimally, screening for common mood disorders such as anxiety and depression should be done. The presence of nonorganic signs or nonanatomic pain distributions does not exclude orthopedic pain generators but may indicate a need for further psychiatric workup.

It is estimated that a brief physical examination and neurological examination of the L4, L5, and S1 dermatomes, myotomes, and deep tendon reflexes should be sufficient to identify 99% of potentially serious spinal pathology [16].

Radiographic and Laboratory Diagnosis

There has been much studied and written about the utilization of imaging strategies as applied to back pain. Published recommendations discourage imaging in the first 4 weeks after presentation [17, 18]. In a 2007 clinical guideline paper, the American College of Physicians and the American Pain Society wrote: "Clinicians should not routinely obtain imaging or other diagnostic tests in patients with nonspecific low back pain [5]." Supporting these recommendations, a 2009 random effects meta-analysis of 1,806 patients evaluated the effect of immediate lumbar imaging on clinical outcomes at 3 and 6 months' time when compared to usual care without imaging; no differences were found with regard to pain or function levels at the specified time points [18]. Risks of unnecessary imaging include radiation exposure (CT, roentgenography), identification of abnormal tissues with unknown relation to a patient's pain source, diminished self-perceived health, and unnecessary healthcare utilization [17].

Plain-film radiography is best used as an initial evaluation only when vertebral compression fracture is of utmost concern, such as those with osteoporosis or with chronic steroid use. When appropriate, plain-film radiography of the spine should include standing anteroposterior and lateral view of the lumbar spine. In adolescent athletes in whom spondylolisthesis is considered, oblique views of the lumbosacral spine should be obtained. European guidelines actively discourage the use of plain-film radiography and MRI for nonspecific back pain unless in the context of referral for a second opinion [19].

Advanced imaging may play an important role in the evaluation of a patient when severe (urinary retention, saddle anesthesia) or progressive neurologic deficits are present (Fig. 1) or when high-morbidity conditions such as metastatic cancer, vertebral infection, or the cauda equina syndrome are suspected [5]. Magnetic resonance imaging is generally preferred over CT due to the lack of ionizing radiation and better visualization of soft tissues and the spinal canal. In patients with signs and symptoms suggestive of nerve root compression or spinal stenosis, evaluation with MRI or CT should only be done in individuals who are potential candidates for surgery or image-guided epidural steroid injection [5].

Radiographic abnormalities are common in the spine and show poor correlation with patients' presenting pains [20]. A 2000 study of 408 patients demonstrated no significant associations between segmental distribution of symptoms and the presence of anatomic impairment, while only severe nerve compression and disk extrusion were shown to be strongly predictive (OR 2.72 and 3.34) of pain present below the knee [21].

Differential Diagnosis

Nonspecific Low Back Pain

It is theorized that the majority of acute low back pain has paraspinal anatomic structures as a pain generator. Paraspinal musculature, spinal ligaments, and annulus fibrosis of the intervertebral disk are all poorly imaged and may be sites of

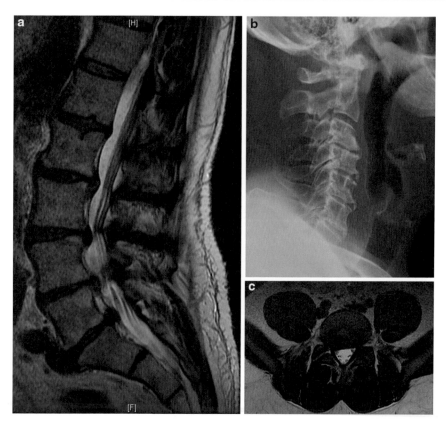

Fig. 1 Imaging of the pathologic spine. (**a**) T2-weighted sagittal MRI image of the lumbar spine of a 64-year-old man reveals multilevel spondylosis with disk pathology including protrusion and extrusion with migration at levels L3–L4, L4–L5, and L5–S1. (**b**) Plain-film x-ray image of lateral cervical spine in an 84-year-old woman shows extensive and widespread spondylosis and osteoarthritis with anterior bridging osteophytes and ossification of the anterior longitudinal ligament and moderate to severe disk degeneration. (**c**) T2-weighted axial MRI image of the lumbar spine of a 22-year-old man at the L5–S1 level demonstrates right foraminal disk protrusion and disk bulge, causing mild central canal stenosis, severe right-sided neuroforaminal narrowing, and moderate left-sided neuroforaminal narrowing with mild bilateral facet hypertrophy

injury that account for the most common types of low back pain [17].

Osteoarthritis

Degenerative osteoarthritis of the axial spine is estimated to be present in 40–85% of individuals [21], and arthritis in general is a leading cause of disability and decreased quality of life. Spondylosis (lumbar spine degeneration) has been defined as intervertebral disk degeneration and same vertebral-level osteophytosis. As in other joints, spinal arthritis is characterized by changes to the articular cartilage and subchondral bone, inflammatory response of the synovium, and inappropriate bone and cartilage overgrowth.

Radiographic features of spondylosis include vertebral osteophytosis, disk space narrowing, and facet joint osteoarthritis. Recent longitudinal studies with a large number of patients have highlighted the discordance between radiographic findings and patient symptoms [21].

Intervertebral Disk Herniation

Progressive failure of the successive layers of the annulus fibrosus is responsible for the ultimate failure of the structure of the intervertebral disk. Gradual desiccation of nuclear material results in a centrifugal disorganization of collagenous layers in the inner and outer annuli. This disorganized tissue cracks and fissures, eventually resulting in channels that permit herniation of the nuclear material through the annulus.

Disk herniation occurs typically in a posterior (paramedian) or posterolateral direction, these being the weakest areas of the disk. Depending on the anatomic location of the disk disfigurement, resultant symptoms may border on radiculopathy (posterolateral) to frank myelopathy or neurogenic claudication (paramedian). Disk disfigurement may range from disk bulge to herniation, protrusion, and extrusion [22].

The hallmark of disk herniation presentation is radiating pain. While the outer layer of the annulus fibrosus is poorly innervated, like other chronically degenerative collagenous tissues, the pathologic outer annuli exhibit neoinnervation that show positive staining for substance P, which has been associated with pain generation [22]. Paresthesias and numbness may be present and with prolonged symptoms weakness may occur in the distal musculature from lower motor neuron compromise.

Diagnosis is commonly clinical, based on a combination of reported radicular pain in a dermatomal distribution, neuropathic signs, and positive nerve-tension testing findings. As up to 30% of asymptomatic individuals have radiographic evidence of lumbar disk pathology, radiographic study is not commonly indicated without severe or rapidly progressive neuropathic symptoms [23].

Spinal Stenosis

Degenerative lumbar spinal stenosis describes the effects of degenerative changes in the spinal canal on the vascular and neural elements of the lumbar spine [24]. Symptoms vary and may include gluteal or lower extremity pain that may occur with or without back pain, especially when seen in older patients. Walking and upright exercise typically worsen symptoms, and patients may relieve symptoms with forward flexion or recumbent posture. As in other syndromes mediated by degeneration, symptoms are slowly progressive. While not supported by extant literature, certain exam findings may be associated with the diagnosis of spinal stenosis: the Romberg test, thigh pain exacerbated by extension, sensorimotor deficits, leg cramps, and abnormal Achilles tendon reflexes

all may be present. Prognosis may only be favorable in up to one half of patients, with few treatments significantly altering the course of the disease. If needed for diagnostic or interventional purposes, MRI or CT myelogram are the preferred imaging modalities.

Osteoporosis

Osteoporosis is estimated to affect up to 30% of all women over the age of 65. Associated fractures occur in up to 50% of all affected individuals, leading to profound morbidity and healthcare resource utilization. The United States Preventive Services Task Force currently recommends screening via dual-energy x-ray absorptiometry (DEXA) in women with increased fracture risk aged 60–64 and all women aged greater than 65 [25]. In addition to age and sex, risk factors include low BMI, personal history of fracture, Caucasian or Asian race, > two alcoholic drinks daily, caffeine and tobacco use, history of falls, low level of physical activity, low calcium and vitamin D intake, and use of certain predisposing medications. Initial treatment includes fall prevention education, intake of calcium >1,200 mg/ day, intake of vitamin D >800 IU/day, and treatment with bisphosphonate osteoclast inhibitor medication. Compression fractures of the vertebra are the most common type of osteoporotic fracture and may be painful; symptoms usually resolve over the course of 3–4 months. Up to 4% of patients presenting to primary care offices with back pain will have a vertebral compression fracture [14]. Patients with vertebral compression fractures usually do not present with pain radiation, as there typically is no neural compromise. Plain-film radiography may indicate a loss of vertebral height associated with compression fracture, and diagnosis of low-impact fractures in susceptible individuals should prompt further investigation. Currently, there are no serum biochemical markers used to aid in diagnosis [25].

Neoplasia

Fewer than 1% of individuals presenting to primary care offices with back pain will be diagnosed with a malignancy [14], and the spine is a more common site of metastasis than primary tumor.

Risk factors for spinal malignancy include age >50 years, history of malignancy, and recent unintended weight loss. Symptoms include unrelenting pain that is not improved with rest and may be worse at night. Initial evaluation may include plain-film radiography enhanced by the erythrocyte sedimentation rate.

Symptomatic secondary metastases are estimated to occur in approximately 10% of all cancer patients, and cadaveric studies find 30–90% prevalence of spinal metastases [26]. Spinal metastases are most likely to originate from the breast, lung, prostate, or hematopoietic system and may arise via hematogenous spread, local extension via lymphatics, or perineurium or extension through the intervertebral foramina.

Primary spinal tumors are rare, affecting 2.5–8.5/100,000 patients yearly [27]. Multiple myeloma is a malignant clonal proliferation of plasma cells characterized by the presence of these cells in the bone marrow and monoclonal immunoglobulins in the serum and/or urine. Rarely, a solitary plasmacytoma may be the only manifestation of disease and may be present in the vertebral column. These tumors commonly present with spinal cord compression; thus, serum and urine protein electrophoresis should be performed in all patients with pathological vertebral fractures in which primary malignancy is not evident. Lymphomas may arise in the bones or compress the spinal cord via invasion of the epidural space.

Facet Syndrome

The lumbar zygapophyseal joint is a commonly cited source of spinal pain; dysfunction may be associated with unilateral or bilateral pain radiating to one or both buttocks, groin, and thighs but not proceeding below the knee. Pathological degeneration of the synovial joint may be noted on CT evaluation, and thus intra-articular anesthetic injection has long been a treatment for this condition. However, as with many other areas of degeneration within the axial skeleton, there is incomplete correlation between radiographic findings and patients' reports of pain [28]. Thus, today diagnostic anesthetic block of the small nerve fibers innervating the facet joints (medial branch block or MBB) is considered a gold standard for lumbar facet joint syndrome diagnosis. Due to the fleeting response to MBB seen in treated patients, a longer-lived treatment is now utilized: lumbar medial branch neurotomy (LMBN). Thermal coagulation at temperatures in excess of 80 °C denature intracellular proteins and produce results that last on average, longer than those achieved with MBB [28]. A 10-year clinical audit noted that among 174 patients treated with LMBN, 68% exhibited good or excellent results.

Ankylosing Spondylitis

Characteristic of the spondyloarthropathies is ankylosing spondylitis (AS). It is an inflammatory arthritis that commonly affects the axial spine with possible extension to peripheral joints, eyes, and bowel. AS exhibits symptoms onset in the late teens, but the delay between the symptom presentation of lumbosacral pain and stiffness and eventual diagnosis averages 8 years [29], primarily due to the difference in distinguishing the symptoms of AS from nonspecific mechanical low back pain in the young active population. While there is limited diagnostic utility in plain-film radiology, MRI has permitted the identification of the inflammatory sequelae of this disease, aided by serum markers of inflammation such as ESR and CRP.

Visceral Diseases

Uncommonly, back pain may be the only presenting concern in a patient with organ system-based disease. Typically, visceral pain referred from intra-abdominal and retroperitoneal organs differs in quality from musculoskeletal pain; however, this difference may be subtle and overlooked.

Dissecting thoracic or abdominal aortic aneurysm is described as "tearing" pain that is acute and severe. This condition is found in up to 4% of those patients over 50 with increased prevalence in smokers and those with diagnosed hypertension and hyperlipidemia. Some patients will have a pulsatile abdominal mass, and presentation may include diaphoresis and signs of impending circulatory failure such as hypotension and tachycardia [30].

Myocardial infarction may present as mid-thoracic pain that radiates to the left arm or axilla. It is most common in those older than 45, with risk factors including family history, hyperlipidemia, hypertension, obesity, and others. Presenting symptom constellation may include diaphoresis, dyspnea, anterior chest heaviness or pain, nausea, vomiting, and a sense of impending doom.

Acute low back pain associated with abdominal pain in a woman of childbearing age may indicate ectopic pregnancy. Back pain is described as part of a classic symptom triad including amenorrhea and vaginal bleeding. Hypovolemic shock may be present in up to 20% of cases, and associated back pain may be located in the L1 and L2 dermatomes of the pelvic organs.

Acute pancreatitis commonly presents with "boring" thoracolumbar pain when the pancreatic duct is obstructed. Patients with acute pancreatitis may have a history of gallstones or binge drinking, and diagnosis is usually achieved with assessment of serum lipase and amylase as well as CT demonstration of glandular inflammation.

Vague back pain that occurs with increasing gastric acidity levels may represent a duodenal ulcer. Inflammation, injury, and ulceration of the mucosal lining of the digestive tract are associated with *H. pylori* infection, smoking, and alcohol ingestion.

Urological conditions such as nephrolithiasis and urinary tract infection commonly present with varying back pain. Ascending urinary tract infections may exhibit low lumbar pain or perinephric pain from ribs 9–11 on either side of the low thoracic spine if pyelonephritis has developed. Unilateral thoracolumbar pain radiating to the ipsilateral flank and toward the groin may indicate a ureteral stone [30].

Management

Stratified Primary Care Management

Multiple international management recommendations for low back pain recommend stratification of patients into groups based on risk for morbid pathology and risk of progression to chronic back pain. A 2011 study known as STarT Back evaluated this model on the basis of economic and patient-centered metrics when compared to usual care in English general practices [31]. This study included greater than 850 adult patients and evaluated changes in the Roland Morris Disability Questionnaire (RMDQ) at 12 months' time as well as quality-adjusted life years (QALY) and healthcare costs between stratified and non-stratified groups. Individuals were stratified into one of three groups: "low-risk" patients had one visit and were educated as to the good prognosis and that further treatment was not necessary nor beneficial; the medium-risk group was referred for further physiotherapy; and the high-risk group was referred for "psychologically informed physiotherapy" [31]. The stratified (interventional) group had significantly improved RMDQ scores at 4 and 12 months and 0.039 additional QALYs and cost savings compared to the nonstratified control group. The low-risk group intervention was found to be noninferior to usual care, indicating that the minimum intervention did not lead to worse outcomes than the current best practices. Differences were present between matched risk groups at 4 and 12 months but lost statistical superiority at the latter time point [31].

Another study of stratification in family medicine practice demonstrated similar results. In 2014, Foster published results showing modest improvements in patient overall outcomes, improved use of healthcare resources, and reduced sick certification without increased healthcare costs. Direct patient benefits of stratification intervention included improvements to physical function, fear avoidance beliefs, satisfaction, and work absenteeism. Changes to physician behaviors included decreased NSAID prescription, increased appropriate referral to physical therapy, and fewer sickness certifications [32].

A subsequent 2018 study of 1,700 patients was unable to reproduce these positive findings and demonstrated no improvement in patient function or healthcare utilization with stratified care [33].

Thus, stratified care for low back pain may demonstrate clinical and economic benefits and can be implemented successfully into a family medicine practice. Further research may reveal if certain populations show improved outcomes from stratified care.

Activity

For most patients, especially those with nonspecific low back pain, rapid return to normal activities, including work, are recommended. However, these patients should initially avoid heavy lifting, twisting, and bodily vibration [5].

Bed Rest

The harmful physiological adaptations to organismal inaction are dramatic and well established. The complications of bed rest are myriad. Muscle mass loss may approach 2% daily in the first 3 weeks of enforced rest; this is primarily due to catabolism of muscle proteins by enzymes activated by inactivity. Joint stiffness and loss of capsular compliance begin soon after immobilization. The risk of thromboembolic event, pulmonary atelectasis, and pressure ulcers rises along with inactivity.

When bed rest is prescribed for acute lumbosacral injury, the aforementioned complications are risked. Bed rest in acute low back pain is not associated with either quicker resolution of pain or return to regular activity. Regular activity as tolerated maximizes the return to function and decreases patient pain score report.

Pharmacological

Nonopiate Analgesics

For most patients with low back pain, acetaminophen and nonsteroidal anti-inflammatory drugs (NSAIDs) are the first-line pharmacological treatment. Acetaminophen is recommended by the American Pain Society and American College of Physicians as the initial pharmacological treatment of nonspecific back pain due to its record of safety in other settings of musculoskeletal pain. Acetaminophen carries a low risk of harm; it is not associated with the risk of either gastrointestinal bleeding or myocardial infarction and is relatively well tolerated [34]. Hepatotoxicity may be seen at doses approaching the recommended maximum daily allowance (3 g/day), and so caution must be taken in those patients with preexisting liver conditions or heavy alcohol use.

NSAIDs exert their anti-inflammatory, analgesic, and antipyretic effects via the inhibition of the cyclooxygenase (COX)-2 enzyme. Nonselective NSAIDs (celecoxib) also inhibit COX-1, which is responsible for gastric mucosal protection via prostaglandin production. A review of different NSAID formulations indicates similar efficacy when compared to placebo in acute and chronic back pain and similar intrafamily efficacy. Thus, treatment decisions may rely on side effect profile, prior response to NSAIDs, cost, and dosing schedule. Each member of the class is associated with gastrointestinal and renal adverse effects, including gastrointestinal ulcers, hemorrhage, and perforation, as well as decreased glomerular filtration. A 2006 meta-analysis of 138 individual studies revealed an approximate twofold classwide risk elevation in myocardial infarction when compared to placebo, except naproxen, which showed no such increased risk. Cardiovascular, gastrointestinal, and renal risks should be taken into account prior to prescribing or recommending NSAIDs for nonspecific low back pain. The long-term use of NSAIDs may be combined with misoprostol, a prostaglandin that decreases the risk of gastrointestinal ulceration, or a proton pump inhibitor [34].

Opiate Receptor Agonists

There exists significant controversy regarding the use of opiate receptor agonist medication in low back pain. Opiate receptors are widely distributed throughout the brain, spinal cord, and intestinal tract and are activated by morphine and its derivatives and homologues. While considered the strongest class of pain relievers, they carry significant potential for dependence and abuse due to their effects on the dopaminergic reward system of the brain. In 2009, the American Pain Society and the American Academy of Pain Medicine published joint guidelines on the use of opioids for chronic noncancer pain to aid practitioners in decisions regarding this class of medication [35]. Primary among these recommendations include time-limited rather than symptom-limited course of medication. Common adverse effects include constipation, nausea, somnolence, and pruritus.

Tramadol is a synthetic agent with weak affinity for the α-opiate receptor. Clinically, it has greater efficacy than NSAIDs and is relatively comparable to weak opiates [35]. Tramadol has similar adverse effect tolerability to acetaminophen-opioid combinations; however, it has been linked to the serotonin syndrome when used in combination with serotonin receptor antagonists.

Skeletal Muscle Relaxants

Medicines known as "skeletal muscle relaxants" are related neither pharmacologically nor structurally. Those commonly used for the relief of musculoskeletal spasticity are baclofen, carisoprodol, cyclobenzaprine, metaxalone, methocarbamol, tizanidine, and orphenadrine. It is unclear if these medications work to relax muscles or if their effects stem mostly from sedation [34]. Medications in this grouping have been shown to demonstrate short-term pain relief for acute low back pain, but no agent has been shown to be more effective than others [36]. These medications carry a high rate of adverse side effects, and sedation commonly limits their use. Several studies have indicated the equivalence of benzodiazepines when compared to skeletal muscle relaxants for acute low back pain, suggesting similar benefit. All medications here referenced may be more effective when combined with an NSAID or acetaminophen [36].

Antidepressants

Certain antidepressants with noradrenergic antagonist activity may have pain-modulating properties independent from their effects on mood disorders. Tricyclic antidepressants (TCAs) such as amitriptyline have long been used in chronic pain conditions, and, in recent years, serotonin and norepinephrine reuptake inhibitors (SNRIs) such as duloxetine, venlafaxine, desvenlafaxine, and others carry similar indications. TCAs show small benefit over placebo for chronic nonspecific pain in some meta-analyses, while SNRIs have shown benefits for certain types of chronic pain. High rates of adverse effects limit the use of these medications and prevent their use as a first-line treatment [36].

Systemic Corticosteroids

While it has been suggested that the inflammatory response associated with extruded intervertebral disk nuclear material may be stemmed with oral corticosteroids, several studies in the setting of lumbar radicular pain have demonstrated no improvement versus placebo. Similarly, despite the euphoric effect achieved by some patients, these medications are also without effect in non-specific acute low back pain [34].

Disease-Modifying Antirheumatic Drugs (DMARDs)

There is no role for antitumor necrosis factor (TNF)-α biologic therapy in the treatment of non-specific low back pain [34].

Exercise

Whether done in the home setting or under the guidance of a physical therapist, stretching, and strengthening activities are commonly prescribed for acute nonspecific back pain. A meta-analysis of 11 studies utilizing the McKenzie (directional preference) method indicated significant improvement in pain and disability after 1 week of therapy [37], resulting in a recommendation for usage [strength of recommendation taxonomy (SORT) B]. Evidence suggests that there is a mild benefit for exercise protocols in chronic nonspecific back pain and little to no improvement when compared to other treatments in acute back pain [38].

Back School

Education is commonly utilized in the treatment of low back pain; it is apparent, however, that there is little to no standardization on what constitutes back school curriculum, and thus, these approaches vary widely. A 2016 review analyzed 273 trials that studied the effects of back schools on nonspecific low back pain; four were deemed to be rigorous enough to meet inclusion criteria. Given the paucity of high-quality evidence available, the authors were unable to comment on the efficacy of back schools for acute and subacute nonspecific LBP [39].

Psychological Intervention

Cognitive-behavioral therapy (CBT) is a method of psychotherapy that attempts changing cognitive processes to affect changes in behavior, thought, and emotional responses. CBT has been applied to chronic pain settings with varying results. In the setting of chronic pain, CBT has improved pain experience, positive coping, and social role function when compared to placebo or other treatments [40].

Spinal Manipulation

A 2004 Cochrane meta-analysis concluded that spinal manipulation was superior only to sham treatments and inert interventions. It demonstrated no advantage over "usual care," analgesic medication, physical therapy, exercise, or back school. Chronic pain applications were found to yield similar results. These results were unaffected by the presence of pain radiation, study quality, manipulator, nor therapy combinations [41].

Acupuncture

A Cochrane review of studies investigating the use of acupuncture in the treatment of low back pain found acupuncture to be effective for pain relief and equivalent to other complementary or conventional treatments. For short-term relief of chronic pain, acupuncture was more effective than sham procedure and placebo. Data regarding the effects on short-term low back pain were inconclusive [42].

Epidural Steroid Injection

The use of epidural steroid injections in the treatment of pain for lumbar radiculopathies as well as spinal stenosis is increasing. A meta-analysis of 38 placebo-controlled trials evaluating the effect of epidural steroid injection in lumbar radiculopathy and spinal stenosis showed brief and nonsustained effects of injection in lumbar radiculopathy that were below predefined set points for clinical significance. There were no effects in spinal stenosis. Neither patient characteristics nor technical factors had an effect on these results [43].

Surgery

Evidence is very clear that there are limited roles for surgery of the spine outside the conditions of sciatica, pseudoclaudication, or spondylolisthesis [44]. Prolonged or worsening neurological symptoms in the setting of diagnosed disk disease unresponsive to or inappropriate for ESI should stimulate referral for surgical evaluation.

Lumbar diskectomy is the most common operation in the United States for reasons related to disk herniation, but there remains poor evidence supporting its use when compared to conservative treatments. Newer treatments in minimally invasive spine surgery (MISS) offer lower perioperative morbidity to patients.

The largest and longest-term comparison between nonsurgical and surgical approaches was published as the 10-year follow-up to the Maine lumbar spine study ($n = 400$) [44]. Ten years after initial presentation, postsurgical patients were more likely to be satisfied with their current condition when compared to the medically managed patients (71% vs. 56%, $P = 0.002$), whereas there was insignificant difference between the two groups with regard to improvement in the initial presenting symptom and work and disability status [44].

Chronic Low Back Pain

Low back pain of greater than 6 months duration develops in a small percentage of patients. These conditions carry a very low likelihood of a specific diagnosis, and symptomatic cure is unlikely. Treatment should be supportive, with efforts aimed at improving pain and function. While the mechanisms of initial injury and chronic pain propagation are unclear, it is proposed that these disorders are primarily mechanically induced, and then maladaptive physical and cognitive compensations produce a mechanism for an ongoing pain.

A recent systematic review demonstrated predictors favoring persistent disabling back pain: maladaptive coping behaviors, nonorganic signs, functional impairment, significant comorbidities, and psychiatric comorbidities. Factors such as low level of fear avoidance and functional impairment predict recovery at 1-year time [45].

The transition from acute to subacute to chronic pain appears to be one strongly mediated by psychosocial factors rather than anatomic or disease-based factors. Therefore, interventions attempting to prevent chronicity transformation have utilized psychological approaches.

Disorders of the Neck

Cervical Radiculopathy

General Principles

A common cause of neck pain is impingement of the cervical nerve roots exiting the spine. This is frequently caused by disk pathology, facet joint osteophytes, or degenerative disk disease, further affected by intraneural edema or inflammatory mediators such as substance P. The annual incidence of cervical radiculopathy has been found to be 83 in 100,000 persons [22].

The nomenclature of the cervical nerve roots differs from that elsewhere in the spine. The presence of an eighth cervical nerve root determines that most cervical nerve roots exit the spinal canal superior to their correspondingly named vertebra; the C7 nerve root exits at the level of the C6–C7 intervertebral disk. The exception to this rule is the eighth cervical nerve root, which exits between the C7 and T1 vertebral levels. The most commonly affected nerve root is the C7 root, which is impinged at the level of the C6–C7 intervertebral disk.

Presentation

When compared to chronic spondylosis of the cervical spine, pain associated with radiculopathy is more commonly unilateral [46]. The most common mechanism of acute cervical radiculopathy is that of annular failure of the intervertebral disk resulting in disk deformation or frank extrusion of nuclear material. Chronic radicular symptoms, which may persist in up to two thirds of patients, are more commonly associated with chronic spondylosis, usually characterized by facet joint osteophytosis or disk degeneration [22].

As with lumbar radiculopathy, the clinical presentation is highly dependent on the exact impinged nerve root or roots; however, clinical and symptom overlap does occur. Pain in proximal nerve root distribution is accompanied by distal distribution neuropathy (paresthesias or other sensory dysfunction). Commonly, referred pain from unilateral cervical radiculopathy is vaguely localized to the ipsilateral neck, shoulder, or medial scapular border [46], whereas radicular pain may follow a dermatomal distribution.

On physical examination, pain is usually exacerbated by neck extension as well as neck rotation toward a patient's symptomatic side, which narrows the neural foramen (Spurling's sign). Conversely, a patient may find mild relief with neck flexion, shoulder abduction, and scapular retraction. Altered deep tendon reflexes corresponding to the affected nerve root may be present. Upper motor neuron findings such as hyperreflexia, clonus, and Hoffman's sign should be absent: their presence should stimulate search for myelopathic conditions.

Diagnosis

The differential diagnosis of cervical radiculopathy encompasses pathologies of the neck, shoulder, viscera, and extremities. Thus, trauma, myelopathy, degenerative spondylosis, rotator cuff pathology, myocardial ischemia, zoster, and other conditions should be considered at differential diagnosis [46]. As noted with lumbar radiculopathy, plain-film x-ray is of limited use, given the poor correlation between findings and the patient's report of symptoms. Similarly, in the absence of certain findings suggesting cancer, myelopathy, or acute pathologies, it is recommended that practitioners delay advanced imaging until after a suitable period of conservative treatment has failed [47]. MRI or CT are best utilized as a confirmatory test of nerve root compromise, in anticipation of referral to spine subspecialist and possible interventional treatment, with limited evidence available to recommend for or against the use of electromyography (EMG) [47].

Management

The prognosis of cervical radiculopathy is optimistic and well described [26, 46]. The majority of patients will improve over time, with 75–90% having no or minimal further sequelae. Management decisions must be made with reference to this high rate of recovery.

The following interventions have insufficient evidence to recommend or discourage their use: medication, physical therapy, traction, cervical manipulation, and cervical collar. Several of these have demonstrated improvement in patients' symptoms in uncontrolled trials. Cervical manipulation has been rarely associated with emergent vascular and nonvascular complications then requiring definitive surgical treatment [47]. Similar consideration should be used when applying pharmacological treatments to cervical radiculopathy as were discussed with regard to lumbar radiculopathy.

Injection of an anti-inflammatory steroid and anesthetic mixture into the epidural space may provide symptom relief for up to 60% of patients and delay or negate the need for surgery in an additional 25% [47]. Rare but potential complications such as spinal cord damage and death may be considered when developing an interventional treatment plan for those patients with cervical radiculopathy.

Surgical referral is appropriate in individuals who have documented cervical radicular symptoms that are intolerable and resistant to a prolonged (6 weeks) course of conservative treatment.

Acute Cervical Strain

General Principles

The acute cervical strain caused by acceleration-deceleration and subsequent energy transfer to the neck is known as whiplash. It commonly occurs during motor vehicle accidents, but also during sporting activities. It may result in a variety of bony and soft tissue injuries, manifest by myriad symptoms. This constellation is known as whiplash-associated disorders (WAD) [48]. These conditions generally have a positive prognosis, with 87% and 97% cited as having recovered from their injuries at 6 and 12 months; however, this optimism is debated [48].

Presentation

Common symptoms after motor vehicle accident (MVA) are neck pain (88–100%) and headache (54–66%), but also commonly seen are neck stiffness, shoulder pain, arm pain or numbness, and others [48]. As in other injuries of the axial spine, issues surrounding the compensation for injury and work delay clinical improvement. In 2001, Côté reviewed a Canadian study investigating the association between insurance systems and claim-closure and compensation times after WAD. In the no-fault province of Quebec, the median claim-closure time was 30 days and 4.1% of claimants were still compensated at 1 year. In Saskatchewan under the tort system, the median claim-closure time was 433 days and 57% were still compensated at 1 year, implying extra-physiological influences to recovery [49].

Diagnosis

An acute cervical injury in the setting of an appropriate mechanism of injury is suitable for the diagnosis of whiplash-associated disorders. Care must be taken not to overlook other conditions that can be present with cervical and cranial trauma, such as fracture, intracranial hemorrhage, mild traumatic brain injury (mTBI), and others. Typically, diagnostic testing and imaging are only utilized to exclude these other conditions.

Management

Management of whiplash should be multimodal and include an assessment of psychological wellness in accordance with the biopsychosocial model. Patients' beliefs, coping strategies, locus of control, and disability should also be measured [48]. It has been suggested that active interventions may be more effective in those with WAD. These have been shown to be beneficially long term on pain, global perceived effort, or participation in daily activities [48]. Patients should be educated and reassured regarding the positive prognosis. Active therapy for comorbid mood disorders should be addressed immediately.

Return-to-clinic and emergency room visit criteria should be discussed. If applicable, continuing care of mTBI should be provided.

Prognosis

The prognosis of acute whiplash is favorable for most individuals. Age, gender, baseline neck pain, baseline headache, and radicular complaints all have independent influence on recovery. It is well recognized that nonmedical factors may also strongly affect recovery. The above Canadian study further noted that when Saskatchewan changed its insurance systems from tort to no-fault, it achieved a 54% reduction in median time to claim closure [49]. The influence of jurisdiction on recovery is further highlighted by chronic whiplash, which is low in historically no-fault provinces (Québec), less litigious countries (Greece), and where whiplash is not compensated (Lithuania) [49].

Cervical Myelopathy

General Principles

Chronic atraumatic compression of the cervical spinal cord due to spondylosis is the most common cause of spinal cord compression in the world [50]. It is understood that 40–60% of untreated cervical spondylotic myelopathy (CSM) cases will progress with worsening neuropathy, neuroinflammation, and apoptosis. Radiographic evidence of cervical stenosis is insufficient to produce the syndrome, as some patients with significant stenosis never develop myelopathy for reasons that are unclear.

Presentation

The clinical presentation in CSM varies greatly, depending on the site and type of lesion and whether it produces motor or sensory and upper motor neuron or lower motor neuron signs in the upper or lower limbs [50]. Onset is typically between ages 50 and 70, of insidious onset and progressive and unremitting. These characteristics may help distinguish it from other neuropathic syndromes, such as peripheral compression or multiple sclerosis.

Symptoms may include neck and/or upper limb pain, weakness, numbness or loss of sensation in the upper or lower extremities, and bladder symptoms such as incontinence or urinary frequency.

Physical exam may reveal signs consistent with upper motor neuron dysfunction: hyperreflexia and/or clonus, Hoffman's sign, Babinski's reflex, multilevel nerve root weakness, sensory loss, or signs of spasticity in the lower limbs [50].

Diagnosis

Plain-film x-ray is commonly obtained in individuals with CSM. With the advent of cross-sectional imaging, however, MRI and intrathecal enhanced CT (CT myelography) have become the studies of choice to evaluate this condition [50], as they are able to aid in the calculation of intracanalar dimensions. The role of EMG is to evaluate for the presence of other conditions that may mimic the findings of CSM, such as peripheral compressive lesions. Cerebrospinal fluid and blood analysis may be used to similarly exclude other neurological conditions [50].

Management

Myelopathy is a progressive disorder and little evidence exists that nonoperative treatment halts or reverses its progress. Thus, nonoperative treatment (intermittent bed rest, the use of collar, anti-inflammatory medication, and discouragement of high-risk activities) is reserved only for asymptomatic patients or those with mild symptoms [50]. Referral or comanagement with a neurologist or neurosurgeon is recommended. For individuals with moderate to severe or rapidly progressive myelopathic symptoms, immediate surgical referral is warranted.

References

1. Hoy D, March L, Brooks P, Blyth F, Woolf A, Bain C, et al. The global burden of low back pain: estimates from the global burden of disease 2010 study. Ann Rheum Dis. 2014;73(6):968–74.
2. Martin BI, Deyo RA, Mirza SK, Turner JA, Comstock BA, Hollingworth W, Sullivan SD. Expenditures and health status among adults with back and neck problems. JAMA. 2008;299(6):656–64.

3. Waterman BR, Belmont PJ, Schoenfeld AJ. Low back pain in the United States: incidence and risk factors for presentation in the emergency setting. Spine J. 2012;12 (1):63–70.

4. Ricci JA, Stewart WF, Chee E, Leotta C, Foley K, Hochberg MC. Back pain exacerbations and lost productive time costs in United States workers. Spine (Phila Pa 1976). 2006;31(26):3052–60.

5. Chou R, Qaseem A, Snow V, Casey D, Cross JT, Shekelle P, Owens DK. Diagnosis and treatment of low back pain: a joint clinical practice guideline from the American College of Physicians and the American Pain Society. Ann Intern Med. 2007;147(7):478–91.

6. Deyo RA, Mirza SK, Martin BI. Back pain prevalence and visit rates: estimates from U.S. national surveys, 2002. Spine (Phila Pa 1976). 2006;31(23):2724–7.

7. Hoy D, Brooks P, Blyth F, Buchbinder R. The epidemiology of low back pain. Best Pract Res Clin Rheumatol. 2010;24(6):769–81.

8. Cohen SP, Argoff CE, Carragee EJ. Management of low back pain. BMJ. 2008;337:a2718.

9. Henschke N, Maher CG, Refshauge KM, Herbert RD, Cumming RG, Bleasel J, et al. Prognosis in patients with recent onset low back pain in Australian primary care: inception cohort study. BMJ. 2008;337:a171.

10. Turner JA, Franklin G, Fulton-Kehoe D, Sheppard L, Stover B, Wu R, et al. ISSLS prize winner: early predictors of chronic work disability: a prospective, population-based study of workers with back injuries. Spine (Phila Pa 1976). 2008;33(25):2809–18.

11. Stanton TR, Henschke N, Maher CG, Refshauge KM, Latimer J, McAuley JH. After an episode of acute low back pain, recurrence is unpredictable and not as common as previously thought. Spine (Phila Pa 1976). 2008;33(26):2923–8.

12. Patrick N, Emanski E, Knaub MA. Acute and chronic low back pain. Med Clin North Am. 2014;98(4):777–89, xii

13. Raison NTJ, Alwan W, Abbot A, Farook M, Khaleel A. The reliability of red flags in spinal cord compression. Arch Trauma Res. 2014;3(1):e17850.

14. Downie A, Williams CM, Henschke N, Hancock MJ, Ostelo RWJG, de Vet HCW, et al. Red flags to screen for malignancy and fracture in patients with low back pain: systematic review. BMJ. 2013;347:f7095.

15. Suri P, Rainville J, Katz JN, Jouve C, Hartigan C, Limke J, et al. The accuracy of the physical examination for the diagnosis of midlumbar and low lumbar nerve root impingement. Spine (Phila Pa 1976). 2011;36(1):63–73.

16. Airaksinen O, Brox JI, Cedraschi C, Hildebrandt J, Klaber-Moffett J, Kovacs F, et al. Chapter 4: European guidelines for the management of chronic nonspecific low back pain. Eur Spine J. 2006;15(Suppl 2):S192–300.

17. Deyo RA, Jarvik JG, Chou R. Low back pain in primary care. BMJ. 2014;349:g4266.

18. Chou R, Fu R, Carrino JA, Deyo RA. Imaging strategies for low-back pain: systematic review and meta-analysis. Lancet. 2009;373(9662):463–72.

19. Savigny P, Watson P, Underwood M. Guideline development group. Early management of persistent non-specific low back pain: summary of NICE guidance. BMJ. 2009;338:b1805.

20. Beattie PF, Meyers SP, Stratford P, Millard RW, Hollenberg GM. Associations between patient report of symptoms and anatomic impairment visible on lumbar magnetic resonance imaging. Spine (Phila Pa 1976). 2000;25(7):819–28.

21. Goode AP, Carey TS, Jordan JM. Low back pain and lumbar spine osteoarthritis: how are they related? Curr Rheumatol Rep. 2013;15(2):305.

22. Roh JS, Teng AL, Yoo JU, Davis J, Furey C, Bohlman HH. Degenerative disorders of the lumbar and cervical spine. Orthop Clin N Am. 2005;36(3):255–62.

23. Jegede KA, Ndu A, Grauer JN. Contemporary management of symptomatic lumbar disc herniations. Orthop Clin North Am. 2010;41(2):217–24.

24. Kreiner DS, Shaffer WO, Baisden JL, Gilbert TJ, Summers JT, Toton JF, et al. An evidence-based clinical guideline for the diagnosis and treatment of degenerative lumbar spinal stenosis (update). Spine J. 2013;13(7):734–43.

25. Sweet MG, Sweet JM, Jeremiah MP, Galazka SS. Diagnosis and treatment of osteoporosis. Am Fam Physician. 2009;79(3):193–200.

26. Sciubba DM, Gokaslan ZL. Diagnosis and management of metastatic spine disease. Surg Oncol. 2006;15(3):141–51.

27. Sundaresan N, Boriani S, Rothman A, Holtzman R. Tumors of the osseous spine. J Neuro-Oncol. 2004;69 (1–3):273–90.

28. Varlotta GP, Lefkowitz TR, Schweitzer M, Errico TJ, Spivak J, Bendo JA, Rybak L. The lumbar facet joint: a review of current knowledge: part II: diagnosis and management. Skelet Radiol. 2011;40(2):149–57.

29. Sengupta R, Stone MA. The assessment of ankylosing spondylitis in clinical practice. Nat Clin Pract Rheumatol. 2007;3(9):496–503.

30. Klineberg E, Mazanec D, Orr D, Demicco R, Bell G, McLain R. Masquerade: medical causes of back pain. Cleve Clin J Med. 2007;74(12):905–13.

31. Hill JC, Whitehurst DG, Lewis M, Bryan S, Dunn KM, Foster NE, et al. Comparison of stratified primary care management for low back pain with current best practice (start back): a randomised controlled trial. Lancet. 2011;378(9802):1560–71.

32. Foster NE, Mullis R, Hill JC, Lewis M, Whitehurst DGT, Doyle C, et al. Effect of stratified care for low back pain in family practice (impact back): a prospective population-based sequential comparison. Ann Fam Med. 2014;12(2):102–11.

33. Cherkin D, Balderson B, Wellman R, Hsu C, Sherman KJ, Evers SC, et al. Effect of low Back pain risk-stratification strategy on patient outcomes and care processes: the MATCH randomized trial in primary care. J Gen Intern Med 2018; 33(8):1324–1336. https://doi.org/10.1007/s11606-018 -4468-9. Epub 2018 May 22.

34. Chou R. Pharmacological management of low back pain. Drugs. 2010;70(4):387–402.

35. Chou R, Fanciullo GJ, Fine PG, Adler JA, Ballantyne JC, Davies P, et al. Clinical guidelines for the use of chronic opioid therapy in chronic noncancer pain. J Pain. 2009;10(2):113–30.

36. Chou R, Huffman LH. Medications for acute and chronic low back pain: a review of the evidence for an American pain society/American college of physicians clinical practice guideline. Ann Intern Med. 2007;147(7):505–14.

37. Guild DG. Mechanical therapy for low back pain. Prim Care. 2012;39(3):511–6.

38. Hayden JA, Van Tulder MW, Malmivaara AV, Koes BW. Meta-analysis: exercise therapy for non-specific low back pain. Ann Intern Med. 2005;142(9):765–75.

39. Poquet N, Lin CW, Heymans MW, van Tulder MW, Esmail R, Koes BW, Maher CG. Back schools for acute and subacute non-specific low-back pain. Cochrane Database Syst Rev. 2016;4:CD008325.

40. Vibe Fersum K, O'Sullivan P, Skouen JS, et al. Efficacy of classification-based cognitive functional therapy in patients with non specific chronic low back pain: a randomized trial. Eur J Pain. 2013;17(6):916–28.

41. Assendelft WJ, Morton SC, Yu EI, Suttorp MJ, Shekelle PG. Spinal manipulative therapy for low back pain. Cochrane Database Syst Rev. 2004;1(1):CD000447.

42. Furlan AD, van Tulder M, Cherkin D, Tsukayama H, Lao L, Koes B, Berman B. Acupuncture and dry-needling for low back pain: an updated systematic review within the framework of the cochrane collaboration. Spine (Phila Pa 1976). 2005;30(8):944–63.

43. Chou R, Hashimoto R, Friedly J, et al. Epidural Corticosteroid Injections for Radiculopathy and Spinal Stenosis: a systematic review and meta-analysis. Ann Intern Med. 2015;163:373–81. https://doi.org/10.7326/M15-0934.

44. Atlas SJ, Keller RB, Wu YA, Deyo RA, Singer DE. Long-term outcomes of surgical and nonsurgical management of sciatica secondary to a lumbar disc herniation: 10 year results from the Maine lumbar spine study. Spine (Phila Pa 1976). 2005;30(8):927–35.

45. Chou R, Shekelle P. Will this patient develop persistent disabling low back pain? JAMA. 2010;303(13):1295–302.

46. Eubanks JD. Cervical radiculopathy: nonoperative management of neck pain and radicular symptoms. Am Fam Physician. 2010;81(1):33–40.

47. Bono CM, Ghiselli G, Gilbert TJ, Kreiner DS, Reitman C, Summers JT, et al. An evidence-based clinical guideline for the diagnosis and treatment of cervical radiculopathy from degenerative disorders. Spine J. 2011;11(1):64–72.

48. Peeters GG, Verhagen AP, de Bie RA, Oostendorp RA. The efficacy of conservative treatment in patients with whiplash injury: a systematic review of clinical trials. Spine (Phila Pa 1976). 2001;26(4):E64–73.

49. Côté P, Cassidy JD, Carroll L, Frank JW, Bombardier C. A systematic review of the prognosis of acute whiplash and a new conceptual framework to synthesize the literature. Spine (Phila Pa 1976). 2001;26(19):E445–58.

50. Toledano M, Bartleson JD. Cervical spondylotic myelopathy. Neurol Clin. 2013;31(1):287–305.

Christopher Jensen

Contents

Hand and Wrist

Infectious and Inflammatory

Paronychia

Paronychia refers to an inflammatory process of the tissues of the lateral nail fold, frequently following minor trauma. This response is subdivided into acute (<6 weeks) and chronic (>6 weeks).

C. Jensen (✉)
Department of Family Medicine, University of Nebraska Medical Center, Omaha, NE, USA
e-mail: cjensenj@unmc.edu

© Springer Nature Switzerland AG 2022
P. M. Paulman et al. (eds.), *Family Medicine*,
https://doi.org/10.1007/978-3-030-54441-6_146

Typical presentation consists of erythema, swelling, and tenderness of the affected area. As with most soft tissue infectious, treatment must follow evaluation to exclude abscess formation. In the absence of an abscess, treatment consists of soaking in warm water or antiseptic with application of topical antibiotic; severe cases or cases which fail to respond to this may require systemic antibiotic therapy. If oral antibiotics are considered, risk factors for MRSA (incarceration, hospitalization, or known colonization) should dictate therapy. If there is known exposure to oral flora as in patients prone to nail chewing or dental work, Augmentin is ideal.

In the event of abscess formation, incision and drainage (I&D) should be performed. Digital block can provide excellent anesthesia for the procedure after which an 11 blade may be run parallel to the nail on the affected side to allow for drainage of purulent material. Warm soaks should be maintained after I&D to facilitate ongoing drainage, and in most cases, antibiotic therapy is not needed following the procedure [13].

Felon

Infection of the soft tissue (pulp) of the fingertip is referred to as a felon and commonly arises from either a puncture wound of the fingertip or spread of infection from an untreated paronychial infection. This typically presents as a painful red swollen fingertip, but importantly this should not extend proximal to the distal interphalangeal (DIP) joint as the septated compartments of the digital pulp confine the spread of the infection. Evaluation for the presence of abscess is critical in determining the necessary course of treatment and is most easily done through soft tissue ultrasound of the area. The presence of abscess mandates incision and drainage and in many cases operative intervention. Regardless of the presence of abscess, patients should undergo antibiotic therapy including staphylococcal and streptococcal coverage which can be further guided by culture obtained during I&D.

Herpetic Whitlow

Herpetic whitlow is a viral infection of the distal finger which can be caused by human herpes virus 1 or 2. This commonly presents as one or more vesicular lesions, but importantly the pulp space is not directly involved, and therefore on examination the fingertip should not be tense. Distinction of this from a felon is important as drainage of the lesions of whitlow should be avoided if possible; incision and drainage may result in spread of the virus and increase the chance of secondary bacterial infection. If the diagnosis is in doubt, confirmation can be obtained through viral culture, Tzanck smear, or antigen testing of fluid from a lesion. The condition is self-limited with typical resolution within 2–3 weeks though recurrence is common, present in between 20% and 50% of patients. Treatment primarily consists of symptomatic management with anti-inflammatories and elevation of the affected region. Limited evidence suggests chronic acyclovir may reduce the rates of recurrence [17].

Tenosynovitis

Infectious tenosynovitis represents an inflammatory response within the tendon and its surrounding synovial sheath. This is most commonly the result of local penetrating trauma but can, in rare cases, be the result of hematogenous seeding. While this can occur in any tendon sheath and associated synovium, the most common site is in the hand and wrist and is subdivided into flexor and extensor disease. Flexor tenosynovitis presents with four key features (Table 1), while extensor disease can present much more subtly than its flexor counterpart. Typical presentation consists of local redness and tenderness, most often of the wrist. A high degree of suspicion should therefore be maintained in dorsal wrist cellulitis, especially if the patient's response to antibiotic therapy is poor [3].

Treatment of the infection is guided by the severity of presentation. Hospital admission with intravenous antibiotic therapy is advised with specific coverage tailored to the mechanism of exposure. Bite wounds should be treated based on the oral flora of the offending creature; water exposure should cause consideration of pseudomonal coverage. Early evaluation by an orthopedic surgeon is advisable as irrigation, open washout, and serial debridement can be required to clear the infection.

Table 1 Knavel's signs – in combination, these have been shown to have sensitivity of greater than 90% for pyogenic tenosynovitis. Specificity is significantly lower (approximately 50%). Other considerations should include palmar abscess or (in patients who are anticoagulated) hemorrhage [10]

Sign	Sensitivity	Specificity
The affected finger is held in slight flexion	91.4%	51.3
The affected tendon displays fusiform swelling	94.3	51.3
The affected tendon is tender to palpation	91.4	69.2
Passively extending the involved digit produces pain	97.1	53.8

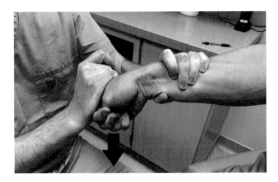

Fig. 1 The Finklestein test is performed by having the patient grasp their thumb within their other digits. The examiner then applies ulnar force to the hand. A positive test consists of significant pain at the radial styloid

De Quervain's Tenosynovitis

Atraumatic radial wrist pain can indicate inflammatory change in the extensor pollicis brevis or abductor pollicis longus tendons, commonly called De Quervain's tendinopathy. This is thought to be an overuse injury though etiology is not fully understood. Diagnosis is suggested by a positive Finkelstein's test (see Fig. 1). In mild cases, immobilization with a thumb spica splint can be performed. In severe cases or when a patient is suffering disability, treatment may be attempted with glucocorticoid injection between the two tendons. In the event a patient's symptoms are refractory to both, surgical evaluation may be considered.

Intersection Syndrome

Commonly mistaken for De Quervain's tendonitis, intersection syndrome presents similarly with pain in the dorsal and thenar wrist but can be distinguished by pain located more proximally and dorsally as opposed to over the radial styloid as seen in De Quervain's. Treatment consists of activity modification through reduction use of wrist extensors. If that fails local steroid injection where the first and second dorsal compartments cross can be considered, ideally under ultrasound guidance.

Traumatic

Mallet Finger

This injury consists of a tear of the extensor tendon at the DIP joint, most often due to sudden forced flexion of the extended joint against resistance. The result is a tendon which may be abnormally stretched, torn, or avulsed from the distal phalanx. Patients present with a DIP joint which can be passively extended but is unable to be extended actively. In rare cases patients may have limitation in passive extension which, if present, should raise the concern for debris from the injury trapped in the joint space. If found this merits further evaluation and possible surgical intervention. In its absence, treatment consists of rigid adherence to splinting of the DIP joint in full extension for 6 weeks. Extension must be maintained during this time, and the patient should be advised that the digit should be held in extension manually during any periods when the splint is removed or exchanged.

Jersey Finger

Forced extension of the DIP joint against resistance can result in damage to the flexor digitorum profundus tendon. This will typically present with volar DIP pain and a finger which is held in extension at rest. There may or may not be a palpable volar mass along the normal course of the tendon representing the torn and retracted tendon. The examiner will commonly find a DIP joint in which active flexion is weak (partial tear) or absent (complete tear) when the metacarpophalangeal (MCP) and proximal interphalangeal (PIP) joint are held in extension. Management of jersey finger is surgical, and prompt referral to an orthopedic hand surgeon is warranted in all cases to limit disability. In the interim, the DIP joint should be splinted in partial flexion.

Central Slip Extensor Tendon Injury

Forced flexion of the PIP joint from an extended position can result in a tear of the central slip of the extensor tendon. This allows the lateral bands to displace around the joint in the volar direction. The characteristic deformity which develops consists of a PIP joint which is flexed with concurrent hyperextension of the DIP joint, referred to as a boutonnière deformity though this can develop gradually and will frequently be absent on initial presentation. Treatment for the injury is extension splinting of the PIP joint continuously for 6 weeks.

Scaphoid Fracture

The scaphoid is both the largest carpal bone and the most likely to sustain fracture, most often with forced wrist extension or axial compression such as sustained in a fall onto an outstretched hand. Patients generally present with radial wrist pain, immediately proximal to the first metacarpal, frequently accompanied by reduced grip strength. Classically tenderness is expected in the anatomic snuffbox but may also be present distal to Lister's tubercle or along the dorsal wrist crease. Plain films of the wrist are the initial radiographic study and should include a dedicated scaphoid view. The physician should however be aware that acute fractures have a false-negative rate reported as at least 20%. If suspicion remains high, following a negative radiograph, acute MRI, or, if not available, CT can clarify the diagnosis. In the event, advanced imaging is delayed in a patient with suspicious presentation; the patient should be placed in a thumb spica splint.

If a scaphoid fracture is found, surgical evaluation is mandated if there is any evidence of instability. This includes fractures of the proximal pole, displacement of more than 1 mm, comminuted fractures, or unstable fractures of any other carpal bones. As the potential for disability in cases of non-union is high, referral may be considered even in the absence of these signs or if the patient's circumstances would benefit from a more rapid return to work or sport.

Hamate Fracture

Much like a scaphoid fracture, hamate fractures will commonly result from a fall on an outstretched hand but are also common with a direct impact injury to the palm of the hand from a bat, club or racquet in sports. The area of maximum tenderness is generally the hypothenar eminence but can be more diffuse. The hook of hamate pull test can help confirm the diagnosis (see Fig. 2). Initial imaging is by plain film, but sensitivity of this is low and if negative advanced imaging with CT should be considered. In the event of a fracture, there can be concurrent injury to both the ulnar nerve and artery, so assessment for sensory loss and Allen's test for arterial patency should be performed. If neurovascular compromise is present, the patient should undergo urgent surgical evaluation. If no surgical intervention is required, the patient should be placed in a short-arm cast. If swelling is significant at time of

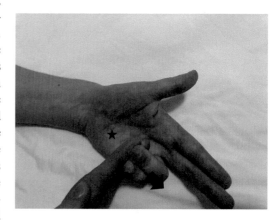

Fig. 2 The hook of hamate pull test is performed with the patient flexing the last two digits with the wrist in ulnar deviation The examiner then attempts to extend the fingers against resistance. A positive test consists of pain in the region of the hamate (*)

presentation, a volar splint may be used as initial therapy.

Elbow

Radial Head Subluxation

Classically referred to as nursemaid's elbow, this is a common injury in children under 5 in which the annular ligament slips over the head of the radius. This is commonly caused by traction on the forearm, typically with the hand pronated. Most often parents report a recent history of non-use of the affected extremity, and the patient typically does not have significant discomfort so long as the arm is not manipulated. X-ray may be used if the diagnosis is in doubt but should not be relied on as positioning for the film can cause reduction of the displacement. Multiple maneuvers have been suggested to reduce the subluxation with the highest rate of success found on hyperpronation of the affected extremity. The physician should hold the affected elbow in one hand, applying pressure medially to the radial head. The other hand can then be used to hyperpronate the hand. If the patient is not using the arm within 30 min of reduction, further evaluation for additional injury to the elbow including radiographic exam should be considered.

Olecranon Bursitis

Bursitis can develop as the result of prolonged pressure, injury, infection, or other inflammatory insult. In the olecranon this acutely presents as warm painful swelling of the elbow. Of note, unlike an effusion or infection of the elbow joint itself, extension should not exacerbate pain in bursitis. The diagnosis can be made clinically; however if the physician suspects infection or crystalline etiology, the bursa may be aspirated. If this is done, following the procedure the area should be compressed as it will, in the majority of cases, reaccumulate. Treatment of non-infectious bursitis consists of protecting the bursa from ongoing trauma and compression to prevent fluid reaccumulation. If allowed to persist chronically, the bursal sac may thicken and require surgical intervention to correct.

Lateral Epicondylitis

Classically referred to as tennis elbow, this is an overuse injury causing degenerative change in the extensor carpi radialis brevis (ECRB) tendon as it inserts into the lateral epicondyle. Typical presentation is pain just distal to the lateral epicondyle, which on exam can be aggravated by extension of the wrist against resistance [8]. Multiple therapies have been advocated to treat the condition including counter-force bracing, eccentric exercise programs, and injections of steroids or prolotherapy using injections of glucose or platelet-rich plasma, but evidence for clear efficacy of any of the techniques is lacking [2].

Medial Epicondylitis

Similar in both mechanism and presentation to lateral epicondylitis, this condition is a degenerative injury of the flexor mechanism of the wrist as it inserts into the medial epicondyle. Pain is typically present at and just distal to the medial epicondyle and is exacerbated by flexion of the wrist against resistance. As with lateral epicondylitis, multiple therapies are recommended, and evidence for their efficacy is not compelling.

Arm

Humeral Fractures

Supracondylar Fracture

Supracondylar fractures are the most common elbow fracture in pediatric populations and are significant both due to the technique used in proper imaging and the potential for neurovascular compromise. Patients typically present with elbow pain, swelling, and significantly reduced ROM at the elbow following a fall onto an outstretched hand. Adequate analgesia should be given immediately to facilitate a high-quality neurovascular examination. In cases with visible deformity, splinting should be considered prior to radiographic examination as repositioning of the extremity may cause further neurovascular injury. Orthopedic consultation is warranted in most cases though a posterior splint and sling may be considered if the fracture is nondisplaced and the patient is neurovascularly intact [4].

Mid-Shaft Humeral Fracture

Mid-shaft fractures will most frequently occur from a direct impact of the humerus but should also be considered in cases of pain after rapid contraction of the musculature of the arm such as with throwing or arm wrestling. Patients typically present with local tenderness, frequently with associated bruising. The examiner should take care to perform a thorough neurovascular examination including ulnar, radial, and median nerve as radial nerve runs adjacent to the bone in this area. If any neurovascular compromise is found, emergent evaluation by an orthopedic specialist is indicated. Most other cases are treated non-operatively, but as functional bracing is frequently required for optimal outcomes, orthopedic evaluation is generally warranted.

Proximal Humeral Fracture

Proximal injuries of the humerus typically require high-energy collisions in the young population (sports or motor vehicle crashes) but can occur with low-energy falls in the over 50 population. Evidence supports that non-displaced fractures can be treated non-operatively with a sling [6] and there is increasing evidence [12] that injuries with a single displaced fragment may be as well, however at this time the majority of cases with any displaced fragments warrant orthopedic evaluation.

Bicep Tears

Acute Tear of the Long Head of the Proximal Bicep

Injury to the long head of the biceps tendon will most frequently present following an acute injury with patients frequently reporting an audible pop associated with onset of pain. The pain itself is generally described as radiating distally from the anterior shoulder and is exacerbated by flexion or supination of the forearm. This may be accompanied by a visible deformity in which the shortening of the muscle belly causes a localized bulge along the humerus though this can be subtle in patients with obesity [19]. The examiner will frequently note localized tenderness in the bicipital groove and, if the patient presents acutely, swelling and bruising of the proximal arm. Therapy is generally conservative as rupture of the long head is associated with only mild to moderate loss of strength but in patients who rely on physical strength or find the cosmetic result of the tear unacceptable surgical intervention is reasonable.

Acute Tear of the Distal Bicep

Distal bicep tears will typically present with acute pain in the anticubital fossa following injury. Bruising may be present acutely but visible muscular deformity is rare. Patients are expected to have increased pain and weakness with resisted flexion or supination at the elbow. The diagnosis can be further suggested by the squeeze test, a lack of forearm motion with compression of the bicep, or the hook test (see Fig. 3). The diagnosis is confirmed through the use of musculoskeletal ultrasound or MRI. All patients with a distal tear should undergo orthopedic evaluation as delayed intervention is associated with worsened functional outcomes

Shoulder

Glenohumeral Dislocation

Anterior Glenohumeral Dislocation

The vast majority (>95%) of shoulder dislocations occur anteriorly. Patients will typically present following an impact to an abducted externally rotated arm which forces the head of the humerus to move anteriorly but can uncommonly occur as the result of a fall onto the arm or direct impact from behind. Patients will typically present with decreased and painful range of motion in the

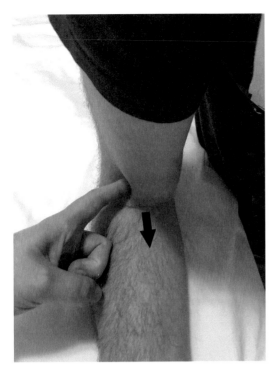

Fig. 3 The hook test is performed with the patient's hand in supination. The examiner slides his finger behind and then pulls forward on lateral aspect of the distal bicep tendon. Inability to grasp the tendon suggests a complete distal bicep tear

shoulder and will frequently have a visible or palpable deformity of the joint. In comparison with the patient's other shoulder, the examiner may note a more flattened appearance as the humeral head shifts anteriorly and inferiorly. This shift can cause injury to the axillary nerve or rotator cuff. The former is most easily assessed through sensory evaluation of the proximal third of the affected arm, while the latter is discussed later. Assessment of distal pulses allows for evaluation of axillary arterial damage. Multiple techniques are described to reduce an anterior dislocation, and most are beyond the scope of this text, but the Stimson technique bears mentioning as it has a high rate of success and can be performed without a skilled assistant. To perform this, the patient is positioned prone on a gurney with the dislocated shoulder dangling. 20–30 lb of weight are suspended from the affected arm, and the shoulder is allowed to passively relocate. The patient is sedated and allowed to rest in this position; >90% of dislocations reduce within 30 min [11].

Posterior Glenohumeral Dislocation

Posterior dislocation are a rare injury which can occur following direct impact to the anterior shoulder but should also be considered in cases where the patient has undergone violent muscle contractions as in cases of seizure or electrical shock. Patients generally present with inability to externally rotate a painful arm and may demonstrate a visibly flattened anterior shoulder with visible or palpable posterior displacement of the humeral head. Reduction is performed with the arm held in adduction with elbow bent. A sheet is hooked over the forearm and used to apply axial traction downward. Success rates vary but are reduced with duration and extent of dislocation

Inferior Glenohumeral Dislocation

Inferior dislocations most commonly occur following an impulse applied to a maximally abducted arm as in a patient who grasps an overhead object while falling. Patients present with an arm which is held in maximal abduction and cannot be adducted. Despite its rarity this injury merits discussion as it is associated with high rates of injury to adjacent structures making a thorough neurovascular evaluation critical. Reduction is performed through traction directed axially along the humerus. An assistant is frequently required to hold the patient in place as traction is applied

Imaging. In patients with suspected glenohumeral dislocation, pre- and post-reduction radiographs allow for confirmation of the diagnosis, successful reduction, and assessment for any associated bony injuries. These should include the traditional AP and axillary view but also a scapular "Y" view. If plain films are inconclusive but posterior dislocation is strongly suspected, subsequent CT scan may improve sensitivity of the evaluation. If imaging demonstrates that the reduction has failed, orthopedic intervention and open reduction may be required.

Aftercare. Following reduction, neurovascular evaluation should be repeated to assess for any damage done in the course of reduction. Patients are then immobilized using a sling, traditionally for 3 weeks though there is evidence for reduced loss of range of motion with only 1 week of immobilization in patients over 30. Regardless of age patients should be instructed to maintain passive range of motion in the affected arm through pendulum swings during the period of immobility. Following this physical therapy may be useful in regaining lost range of motion and preventing redislocation.

Rotator Cuff Injuries

Presentation. The presentation of patients with rotator cuff tears is variable but generally includes pain which is exacerbated with overhead motion. Onset typically follows trauma or repetitive strain in young populations but as patients age may be subtle and atraumatic. A number of exam maneuvers have been proposed to aid in diagnosis of tears, but evidence that the location of pain on physical examination can localize the injury is poor [7]. Injury of the cuff as a whole is suggested by inability to smoothly adduct the arm from overhead to the side or by evidence of shoulder impingement. This can be demonstrated by the Hawkins-Kennedy or Neer's tests (Figs. 4 and 5, respectively)

Imaging. Imaging studies can be used for confirmation of cuff injury. Plain film has limited value but does suggest the diagnosis if the humeral head is found to be displaced [9]. In the hands of a skilled operator, ultrasound has been demonstrated to be accurate in the diagnosis of tears, but MRI appears to be more accurate in gauging the extent of a tear and degree of tendon retraction [16].

Treatment. It is classically believed that the majority of patients are able to be treated conservatively with physical therapy, but key exceptions which are worth noting include patients who have had an acute or acute on chronic full thickness tears which result in significant loss of function. Within that population patient outcomes following acute surgical intervention have been shown to be improved. Of note, recent data does suggest that even patients exhibiting small tears may have

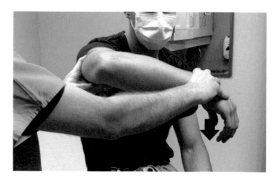

Fig. 4 To perform the Hawkins-Kennedy test, the patient flexes the elbow and shoulder to 90 degrees. The examiner then applies downward force to the hand while stabilizing the upper extremity proximal to the elbow. Pain in the shoulder region suggests shoulder impingement

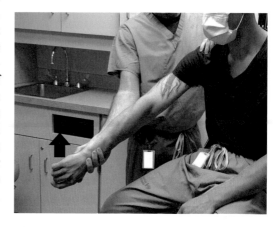

Fig. 5 Neer's maneuver is performed by passively flexing the shoulder while using the other hand to prevent the patient from shrugging. Pain suggests shoulder impingement

improved functional outcomes following surgical intervention [14].

Subacromial Bursitis

The subacromial bursa lies between the rotator cuff and the acromion and is frequently inflamed by any of the processes above but can also arise from systemic inflammatory disease. Typical patients will present pain of the proximal third of the lateral arm of the affected side. Unlike a rotator cuff tear which can present with very similar pain, bursitis should, in theory, not cause a lack of strength; however guarding on the part of the patient may make this distinction difficult in practice. Steroid injection into the bursa can be useful both diagnostically and therapeutically as a full return to baseline following injection makes other shoulder pathology unlikely. Even with full pain relief, physical therapy can be an important adjunctive therapy to prevent recurrence.

Frozen Shoulder

Frozen shoulder or adhesive capsulitis is a poorly understood condition which manifests as gradual and progressive limitation in active and passive range of motion. It typically presents in the 50s and 60s with onset more common in patients with comorbidities, most prominently diabetes. Examination is expected to show reduction in active and passive range of motion, frequently with associated pain. In contrast to subacromial bursitis, steroid injection is not expected to relieve this discomfort. The utility of imaging is mostly in exclusion of alternative diagnoses, with X-ray findings limited to at most osteopenia. MRI may be considered but will generally be expected to demonstrate only capsular thickening. Treatment is controversial and poorly supported by evidence but will frequently include range of motion exercises and potentially glucocorticoid injection. If the patient fails to demonstrate improvement, orthopedic consultation may be helpful [5].

Clavicular Fracture

A fracture of the clavicle can commonly occur following a fall on an outstretched arm or direct trauma to the bone. Patients typically present with localized point tenderness, often with associated visible deformity which can result from bony displacement or hematoma formation.

Mid-Shaft Clavicle Fracture

The vast majority of clavicle injuries (70–80%) occur mid-shaft and shortening, and displacement is common. Evaluation should include neurovascular exam of the extremity and assessment for underlying injury to the lung and pleura. X-ray is generally sufficient to confirm the diagnosis. Indications for orthopedic evaluation of mid-shaft fractures include evidence of neurovascular or lung injury, skin tenting over the site, and open fracture or concurrent glenoid fracture (as this leaves the upper extremity without bony attachment to the thorax). There is controversy regarding the degree of displacement which should mandate operative intervention, but data [20] supports the non-operative management of fractures with less than 2 cm displacement.

Distal Clavicle Fracture

Distal fractures are subdivided into categories (Table 2) based on the location and characteristics of the injury. Types 1, 3, and 4 may be able to be managed non-operatively. Management of type 2 fractures is controversial. Non-operative management has very high rates of non-union without operative intervention [15], but some evidence suggests this may not significantly impact patients' functional outcomes. In all cases non-operative management consists of sling immobilization with physical therapy for range of motion and strengthening once tenderness has resolved [1].

Proximal Clavicle Fracture

While quite rare, accounting for less than 3% of clavicle fractures, those involving the proximal third of the bone are significant for several points. First, due to the bony overlap and often minimal displacement, X-ray lacks sensitivity for proximal fractures, and if negative, CT should be considered [18]. Second, due to the much higher forces typically required to cause a proximal clavicle fracture, there is a very high (>80%) rate of clinically significant neck, head, or intrathoracic injury in traumatic fractures, mandating operative intervention in most cases. In patients who present with atraumatic (stress) fractures, management is with sling immobilization as in distal fractures.

Table 2 Classification and management of distal clavicular fractures

Fracture category	Definition	Management
Type 1	Fracture lateral to coracoclavicular ligament Ligaments remain intact on both fragments preventing displacement	Non-operative
Type IIA	Fracture medial to coracoclavicular ligament Ligaments remain intact but only insert on distal fragment allowing superior displacement	Operative
Type IIB	Coracoclavicular ligament injury allowing displacement of medial fragment	Operative
Type III	Intra-articular fracture involving AC joint	Non-operative
Type IV	Physeal fracture in children Ligaments intact	Non-operative
Type V	Comminuted fracture	Operative

References

1. Anderson K. Evaluation and treatment of distal clavicle fractures. Clin Sports Med. 2003;22(2):319–26.
2. Bisset L. A systematic review and meta-analysis of clinical trials on physical interventions for lateral epicondylalgia * commentary. Br J Sports Med. 2005;39 (7):411–22.
3. Clark DC. Common acute hand infections. Am Fam Physician. 2003;68(11):2167–76.
4. Cuomo AV, Howard A, Hsueh S, Boutis K. Gartland type I supracondylar humerus fractures in children. Pediatr Emerg Care. 2012;28(11):1150–3.
5. Ewald A. Adhesive capsulitis: a review. Am Fam Physician. 2011;83(4):417–22.
6. Gaebler C, Mcqueen M, Court-Brown C. Minimally displaced proximal humeral fractures epidemiology and outcome in 507 cases. Acta Orthop Scand. 2003;74(5):580–5.
7. Itoi E, Minagawa H, Yamamoto N, Seki N, Abe H. Are pain location and physical examinations useful in locating a tear site of the rotator cuff? Am J Sports Med. 2006;34(2):256–64.
8. Johnson GW, Cadwallader K, Scheffel SB, Epperly TD. Treatment of lateral epicondylitis. Am Fam Physician. 2007;76(6):843–8.
9. Keener JD, Wei AS, Kim HM, Steger-May K, Yamaguchi K. Proximal humeral migration in shoulders with symptomatic and asymptomatic rotator cuff tears. J Bone Joint Surg Am. 2009;91(6):1405–13.
10. Kennedy CD, Lauder AS, Pribaz JR, Kennedy SA. Differentiation between pyogenic flexor tenosynovitis and other finger infections. Hand. 2017;12(6):585.
11. Kothari RU, Dronen SC. Prospective evaluation of the scapular manipulation technique in reducing anterior shoulder dislocations. Ann Emerg Med. 1992;21 (11):1349–52.
12. Launonen AP, Sumrein BO, Reito A, Lepola V, Paloneva J, Jonsson KB, et al. Operative versus non-operative treatment for 2-part proximal humerus fracture: a multicenter randomized controlled trial. PLoS Med. 2019;16(7):e1002855.
13. Leggit J. Acute and chronic paronychia. Am Fam Physician. 2017;96(1):44–51.
14. Moosmayer S, Lund G, Seljom US, Haldorsen B, Svege IC, Hennig T, et al. At a 10-year follow-up, tendon repair is superior to physiotherapy in the treatment of small and medium-sized rotator cuff tears. J Bone Joint Surg. 2019;101(12):1050–60.
15. Oh JH, Kim SH, Lee JH, Shin SH, Gong HS. Treatment of distal clavicle fracture: a systematic review of treatment modalities in 425 fractures. Arch Orthop Trauma Surg. 2010;131(4):525–33.
16. Okoroha KR, Fidai MS, Tramer JS, Davis KD, Kolowich PA. Diagnostic accuracy of ultrasound for rotator cuff tears. Ultrasonography. 2019;38(3): 215–20.
17. Rubright JH, Shafritz AB. The herpetic whitlow. J Hand Surg Am. 2011;36(2):340–2.
18. Throckmorton T, Kuhn JE. Fractures of the medial end of the clavicle. J Shoulder Elb Surg. 2007;16 (1):49–54.
19. Virk MS, Cole BJ. Proximal biceps tendon and rotator cuff tears. Clin Sports Med. 2016;35(1):153–61.
20. Waldmann S, Benninger E, Meier C. Nonoperative treatment of midshaft clavicle fractures in adults. Open Orthop J. 2018;12(1):1–6.

Disorders of the Lower Extremity

116

Jeff Leggit, Ryan Mark, Chad Hulsopple, Patrick M. Carey, and Jason B. Alisangco

Contents

J. Leggit (✉) · R. Mark · C. Hulsopple · P. M. Carey
Department of Family Medicine, Uniformed Services
University of the Health Sciences, Bethesda, MD, USA
e-mail: jeff.leggit@usuhs.edu; chad.hulsopple@usuhs.
edu; patrick.m.carey.mil@mail.mil

J. B. Alisangco
Fort Belvoir Family Medicine Department, Fort Belvoir
Community Hospital, Fort Belvoir, VA, USA

© Springer Nature Switzerland AG 2022
P. M. Paulman et al. (eds.), *Family Medicine*,
https://doi.org/10.1007/978-3-030-54441-6_118

The lower extremities provide the stable platform for locomotion and all movements while upright. They are subject to much higher force loads than the upper extremities. Walking has an impact force of 1.2–3 times a patient's body weight (BW), and running can increase the impact force anywhere from 7–10 times BW. Compounded over a lifetime, the lower extremities are subject to tremendous loads. Multiple intrinsic and extrinsic factors increase the risk for lower extremity injuries. These include but are not limited to musculoskeletal abnormalities (e.g., pes cavus), obesity, advancing age, chronic illness (e.g., diabetes, COPD), training errors, certain medication use, and previous trauma.

This chapter will discuss in detail those conditions most commonly seen and managed by the family physician in an ambulatory setting as well as those less common entities that have high morbidity if not properly recognized.

Hip Injuries

Hip Fracture

General Principles
General principles worldwide there are approximately 1.66 million hip fractures per year, with 95% occurring in adults age 60 or greater. Mortality rates associated with hip fracture approach 14% in the first 30 days following the fracture and 17–37% within the first year. Aging is associated with several impairments including osteoporosis, muscle weakness, imbalance, hearing loss, and presbyopia. These age-related factors combined with comorbid medical disorders and polypharmacy place seniors at high risk for falls and subsequent hip fractures. With the aging population, it is estimated there will be more than six million hip fractures per year by 2050 [1].

Diagnosis
Classically, patients will present with sudden onset of hip pain and inability to walk after a fall. However, it is important to remember those with minimal displacement or impaction fractures may be able to ambulate. Insufficiency fractures

(normal stress to abnormal bone causing a fracture) may occur in the absence of overt trauma. Additional presenting complaints concerning for hip fracture include pain in the groin, thigh, buttock, or knee. Physical exam will show localized tenderness in the hip and groin with limited range of motion.

Initial assessment of the patient with a hip fracture should focus on a complete history and physical exam as there may be coexisting injuries (e.g., traumatic brain injury). Radiographic examination should include anterior/posterior (AP) pelvis and cross-table lateral hip views with careful avoidance of frog leg positioning due to risk of fracture displacement. Computed tomography (CT) scanning is useful when plain films are inconclusive. Any elderly or at-risk patient (i.e., chronic steroid use or known osteoporosis) with hip pain and a history of a fall requires a thorough radiographic assessment. The differential diagnosis includes dislocation, ligamentous sprain, muscle injury, and chondral or labral pathology. (Note that many of these conditions may coexist with any fracture.) See Table 1 for a list of differential diagnosis for hip-related pain.

Treatment
Immediate treatment of an isolated hip fracture (except avulsion fractures) consists primarily of providing adequate analgesia and urgent orthopedic surgery consultation. Most fractures should be repaired surgically within 48 h. However, nonoperative management is appropriate when surgical risk is too great or when life expectancy is limited.

The family physician may be asked to assist with pre- and perioperative management to include cardiac risk evaluation. The most current American Heart Association and American College of Cardiology guidelines should be consulted for the latest recommendations, but in general if there are no active cardiac conditions and the patient had been able to walk a flight of stairs, surgery can proceed [2].

Antithrombotic agents should be used for at least 10–14 days and up to 35 days postoperatively per the American Academy of Chest

Table 1 Differential diagnosis of hip pain disorders of the lower extremity

Very common	Common	Infrequent	Referred
Osteoarthritis Tendinopathy[a] Muscle strains[a] Bursitis[b] Iliotibial band syndrome (proximal) Sacroiliac disorders	Synovitis (femoral acetabular) Inguinal hernia Labral tear Femoral acetabular impingement Nerve entrapment[c] Stress fracture Traction apophysitis[d] Acute fractures Chondral lesions Snapping hip [e] Tensor fascia lata syndrome Bony contusion (iliac crest) Coccyx injury	Hip dislocation and subluxation Sportsman's groin (sports hernia, athletic pubalgia) Pubic symphysis dysfunction (osteitis pubis) Osteonecrosis (avascular necrosis) Ligamentum teres rupture Inflammatory or crystalline arthropathy Slipped capital femoral epiphysis Legg-Calve-Perthes disease – Os acetabuli (extra ossification at superior surface of acetabulum) Malalignments	Lumbar/sacral disk/nerve pathology Septic arthritis Claudication, aorta/iliac insufficiency (Leriche's syndrome) Herpes zoster Pelvic/abdominal pathology Tumor Complex regional pain syndrome

[a]Gluteal, iliopsoas, adductor, quadriceps, hamstring, piriformis
[b]Greater trochanteric, iliopsoas, ischial
[c]Lateral femoral cutaneous (meralgia paresthetica), iliohypogastric, ilioinguinal, genitofemoral, femoral, saphenous, obturator
[d]Ischial tuberosity (origin of the hamstrings); anterior inferior iliac spin (origin of the rectus femoris); anterior superior iliac spine (the origin of the sartorius); pubic symphysis (origin of the adductor brevis and longus/gracilis)
[e]Internal due to iliopsoas or labral pathology and external due to iliotibial band

Physicians. While there is no consensus to the exact regiment or optimal duration, it is agreed up that antithrombotic prophylaxis with a combination of pharmacologic and mechanical device should be used. Aspirin is not recommended as a single pharmacologic agent for prophylaxis following surgery for hip fracture [3].

The family physician has a major role in primary and secondary fracture prevention which are very similar and include risk factor reduction through smoking cessation, moderation of alcohol use, osteoporosis management (prevention, detection, and treatment), and fall prevention (to include home assessment). Reducing polypharmacy and medication reconciliation should also be addressed. High-risk medications include sedatives, hypnotics, behavioral health medicines, antihypertensives, and anticoagulants. Although the best strategy for restoring mobility and function after a fracture has not been determined, a combination of weight-bearing exercise, proprioception/balance training, and muscle strengthening is

advocated. Prophylaxis with bisphosphonates should be offered regardless of osteoporosis status to those patients with hip fractures receiving a prosthetic. The use of bisphosphonates has been shown to increase prosthetic survival [2]. Bisphosphonates should be administered along with appropriate doses of calcium and vitamin D unless contraindications exist. A recent review of cushioned hip protectors showed that they have little effect on hip fractures and compliance is poor at best [4].

Stress Fractures

General Principals

Lower extremity stress fractures account for 80–90% of all stress fractures and up to 20% of sports related injuries [5]. Table 2 lists intrinsic and extrinsic risk factors which must be addressed for prevention as well as recurrence avoidance. Around the hip, femoral neck stress fractures

Table 2 Intrinsic and extrinsic risk factors for stress fractures and overuse injuries of the lower extremity

Intrinsic risk factors		Extrinsic risk factors	
Hormonal factors Leg length abnormality Foot abnormality	(E.g., estrogen deficiency) Functional* vs. true** Pes cavus/planus Rearfoot varus Hypermobile first ray Short first ray or long second ray	Training regimen*	Volume Intensity Duration Inadequate recovery time New activity Poor technique
Hip	Excessive hip external rotation Femoral ante/retroversion		
Knee	Genu valgum/varum Patella alta Tibia vara/torsion		
↓ Muscle endurance ↓ Bone mass ↓ Lower body muscle mass		Medications	
		Improper nutritional habits	♀ athlete triad
		Running surface	Hard Soft Canted
Muscle imbalance Genetic factors Metabolic factors		Smoking	
		Environmental factors	Hot Cold Humid
		Improper equipment	Shoe**
*Functional leg length abnormality is measured by relative heights of iliac crests standing and or umbilicus to medial malleolus. Difference of ≥1 cm is considered significant and prompts evaluation for true leg length abnormality vs. functional due to pelvic obliquity. Treat with shoe inserts in shorter side or manipulation of obliquity **True leg length abnormality is measured from a fixed point to a fixed point – anterior superior iliac spine to medial malleolus. Difference of >1 cm is considered significant and should prompt evaluation (scanogram) and treatment (foot insert or surgical correction)		*Stress fractures (as well as overuse conditions) are preceded by 4–12 weeks of an increase in physical demand without adequate recovery time interposed Recommendation is to only increase one parameter at time and not more than 10% a week **Minimalist vs. shock absorber or pronator vs. supinator (evidence-based recommendations cannot be made and sound training practices are more prudent than shoe type in preventing injuries) Loss of structural support from worn shoes (q 6 months or 500 miles)	

(FNS) are associated with high morbidity if not promptly diagnosed and appropriately managed. Female athletes and those unaccustomed to running or impact forces (e.g. basic military recruit) are the most common patient populations. Pain can be focal or diffuse and even radiate to the knee.

Diagnosis

There is a paucity of physical exam findings related to bone stress injury, and a high index of suspicion is required for proper identification. It would be prudent to have patients be non-weight-bearing while awaiting a definitive diagnosis. Definitive diagnosis requires radiographic confirmation. Plain radiography should be ordered but radiographic findings often lag or are very

difficult to appreciate. Bone scans lack specificity and remain positive for months to years even after a patient has fully recovered and therefore are not recommended. Magnetic resonance imaging (MRI) is the modality of choice for diagnosis.

Consider bone mineral density testing if history of multiple low-risk stress fractures or a single high-risk stress fracture.

Treatment

Stress fractures can be segregated into low and high risk depending on their location and ability to heal. See Table 3 for a list of each type of fracture and treatment recommendations based on type. If confirmed, all patients with FNS should be referred for definitive management and immediately be placed on non-weight-

Table 3 Low- and high-risk stress fractures of the lower extremity

Low risk	High risk
Generally occurs to cortical bone	*Generally occurs to cancellous (spongy) bone*
Femoral shaft	Femoral neck
Medial tibia	Patella
First to fourth metatarsal	Anterior tibial diaphysis
Treatment recommendations	Talus
Must off-load (can use crutches, cast, walking boot, or rigid shoe depending on site). Gradually resume weight-bearing as symptoms allow while restoring strength and flexibility	Tarsal navicular
	Fifth metatarsal
Correct risk factors	**Treatment recommendations**
	Refer to musculoskeletal specialist due to high morbidity
	Correct risk factors

bearing status of the involved lower extremity [6]. Treatment of FNS consists of internal fixation vs. strict non-weight-bearing. Stress fractures of the tension side, superior aspect of the femoral neck, should be considered urgent and referred to an orthopedic surgeon. Stress fractures of the compression side, inferior aspect of the femoral neck, may be treated with non-weight-bearing status dependent on the severity of the fracture. Treatment, in the primary care setting, should focus on the identification and modification of risk factors. The majority of low-risk stress fractures will heal with conservative management between 8 and 14 weeks. Management of high-risk stress fractures should include a strong consideration for referral.

Avulsion Fractures

The hip contains a number of apophyseal sites which are subject to injuries ranging from apophysitis to fractures (avulsions or stress). See Fig. 1 for hip and upper leg anatomy. Avulsion injuries are rare and are more commonly seen in the adolescent population secondary to muscle contraction against an open growth plate. Unless an avulsed fragment is displaced >2 cm, nonoperative management is recommended and consists of partial weight-bearing in conjunction with decreased activity for a 3–6 week period. This is followed by gradual resumption of activity as pain allows. Correction of any modifiable risk factors (Table 2) is required to prevent recurrence.

Hip Dislocation

General Principles
The focus of this section is simple dislocations of the femoral head outside of the acetabulum. Complex dislocations have an associated fracture, and after the dislocation is reduced, fracture management dictates therapy. Dislocations are not subtle injuries and require immediate referral to an orthopedic surgeon. The most common mechanism of injury is a high-energy motor vehicle accident which carries the risk of other major traumatic injuries. Other mechanisms include a fall from a height, automobile-pedestrian accidents, and athletic injuries [7]. Posterior dislocations are most common and present as a flexed, adducted, and internally rotated leg. Anterior dislocations are rare and more likely to occur during sporting events. These patients will present with the lower extremity in external rotation with slight flexion and abduction.

Diagnosis
Because of the high-energy mechanism of injury, a thorough clinical examination should be performed beginning with airway, breathing, and circulation following standard Advanced Trauma Life Support® protocols. Additionally it is important to assess for neurologic or vascular injury. An AP pelvis radiograph is usually adequate for the diagnosis of a hip dislocation. A posteriorly dislocated femoral head appears smaller than the contralateral side and will be outside of the acetabulum, while an anteriorly dislocated femoral head appears larger. A cross-

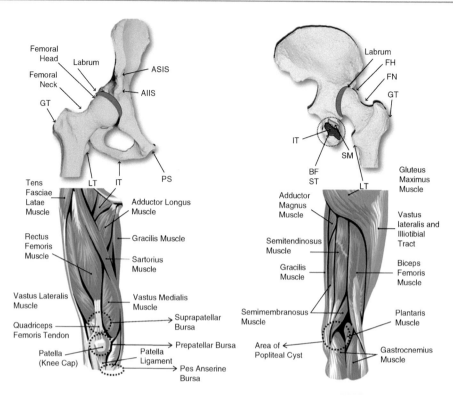

Fig. 1 Hip and upper leg anatomy. AIIS anterior inferior iliac spine (rectus femoris origin), ASIS anterior superior iliac spine (sartorius origin), PS pubic symphysis (adductor brevis/longus and gracilis origin), IT ischial tuberosity (hamstring origin (BF biceps femoris/ST semitendinosus/ SM semimembranosus)), GT greater tuberosity (gluteus medius/minimus insertion), LT lesser tuberosity (iliopsoas insertion), FH femoral head, FN femoral neck (Muscle figures adapted and used by permission from fpnotebook.com)

table lateral film provides a second view of the relationship of the femoral head to the acetabulum. Unless there is suspicion of an occult femoral neck fracture, a CT is not needed prior to emergent reduction. The differential diagnosis is the same as for fractures but includes subluxations.

Treatment

Hip dislocation is a severe injury that requires prompt attention. Emergent reduction reduces the period of avascularity to the femoral head and should be accomplished as atraumatically as possible and ideally within 6 h. If neurovascular compromise is not present, a fracture should be ruled out prior to any attempts at reduction. If there is no associated fracture on postreduction films and proper joint alignment is achieved, the leg should be extended and externally rotated, and a knee immobilizer should be placed to prevent inadvertent flexion at the hip. All patients with hip dislocation must be referred to an orthopedic surgeon who will guide rehabilitation. Patients are at risk for avascular necrosis and subsequent osteoarthritis (OA). They should be encouraged to maintain an ideal body weight as well as core and hip strength to mitigate morbidity.

Femoroacetabular Impingement (FAI) Syndrome

General Principles

Femoroacetabular impingement (FAI) syndrome comprises a constellation of bony overgrowth conditions secondary to adaptation or malformation in and around the hip joint. There can be involvement of the acetabulum, the femoral head, or a combination of the two

[8]. The impingement deformities include acetabular overgrowth or acetabular retroversion (abnormal position changing the way the femur articulates with the acetabulum) producing a pincer (pinching) lesion and femoral neck bony buildup producing a cam or "pistol-grip" deformity (abutting up against a normal acetabulum). However, the most common is a mixed type with features of both (see Fig. 2). The condition is most commonly seen in the athlete population, with an increased prevalence identified in the young, the female, and the Caucasian populations. Long-standing FAI may lead to acetabular labral injury, damage to the articular cartilage and osteoarthritis.

Diagnosis

Pain related to FAI is insidious in onset, and patients will commonly complain of groin pain but can also experience pain in the buttock, lateral or anterior thigh, and low back. There is often a reduced range of motion and/or pain in internal rotation and flexion. Patients may state that they need to frequently change positions while sitting to alleviate pain. Diagnosis is usually delayed because of the vague nature of the complaints and the lagging radiographic changes.

Young athletic males more commonly are affected by cam lesions. Cam-type deformities can lead to chondral damage, labral tears, and

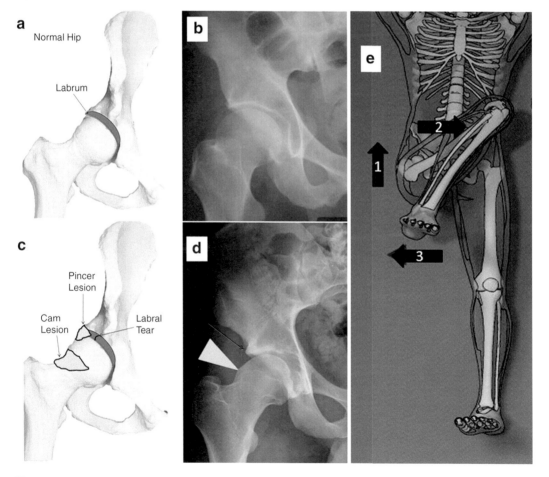

Fig. 2 Femoroacetabular impingement and FADIR test. (**a**) Normal hip anatomic model. (**b**) Normal hip AP radiography. (**c**) Hip anatomic model with cam and pincer lesion and labral tear. (**d**) AP radiography with cam lesion (*yellow arrowhead*) and pincer lesion (*red arrowhead*). (**e**) FADIR test: flexion (*arrow #1*), adduction (*arrow #2*), internally rotate (*arrow #3*) (FADIR image adapted with permission from fpnotebook.com)

early OA due to abnormal abutment forces on the acetabular labrum. Middle-aged active women are more likely to present with pincer lesions. Their pain results from the over-coverage of the femoral head or acetabular retroversion which appears on plain films as an anterior osteophyte from the superior lateral acetabulum. As mentioned earlier, a mixed cam and pincer deformity is the most common presentation (see Fig. 2). Patients with concomitant labral tears may present with mechanical symptoms of clicking and catching.

Evaluation should include a complete lumbar and lower extremity physical exam specifically assessing for obvious anatomic malalignments (leg length discrepancy, lower limb valgus/varus position, pes cavus/planus), decreased range of motion, and hip weakness. The tests most consistent with FAI include a painful supine impingement test or FADIR test (hip flexion to 90°, **ad**duction, and **i**nternal **r**otation; see Fig. 2) along with a painful resisted straight leg raise. (The pattern of inspection, palpation, range of motion, motor strength, and special tests constitutes the essential elements of all musculoskeletal physical examinations and will be repeated throughout the chapter.)

If FAI is suspected, radiographs should be obtained, including at minimum a standing pelvis AP and a lateral view. Additional images such as frog leg and possibly a Dunn view (AP pelvis with the hip at 20° abduction and either 45° or 90° flexion) may further help to evaluate femoral head/neck morphology. Plain MRI has little role in FAI evaluation; however MR arthrogram can serve two purposes: first the contrast material can help identify chondral and labral lesions which have important treatment implications, and secondly the intra-articular anesthesia injected for the procedure can serve a diagnostic role in identifying the hip joint as the primary source of pain. CT is utilized for defining the three-dimensional bony abnormalities but is reserved for the treating surgeon for surgical planning. The differential diagnosis includes tendinopathies and chondral or labral pathologies (see Table 1).

Treatment

Recent evidence suggests that conservative management with a physical therapy-based treatment plan results in improvement of functional status and pain reduction for patients with FAI. Additional pain control, either orally or via intra-articular injections, may be used to augment physical therapy. Exercises directed at strengthening the hip abductors, pelvic stabilizers, and abdominal core muscles as well as correcting any contractures of the hamstrings, iliopsoas, quadriceps, or iliotibial band are recommended regardless whether nonsurgical or surgical options are pursued [9]. (This reference contains examples of home exercise handouts for a variety of conditions and is suggested for prescribing home rehabilitation therapy.) Arthroscopic surgery is the definitive treatment for FAI. The mainstay of surgery is the removal of any mechanical obstructions. One of the benefits of surgical intervention is the ability to correct underlying soft tissue injury, such as labral tears, as well as removal of the mechanical obstruction.

Acetabular Labral Tear (ALT)

General Principles

The acetabular labrum is a fibrocartilaginous structure lining the acetabular socket (see Fig. 1). It is vascularized only in the outer third and pain-sensing nerve fibers parallel the blood supply. The lack of robust blood supply explains why the labrum has a poor potential to heal; a similar concept will be discussed in the knee meniscus. The hip labrum serves to aid in stability and force disbursement. Acetabular labral tear (ALT) is both common and frequently asymptomatic. A cadaveric study found that 93–96% of hips demonstrated a tear of the acetabular labrum [10].

An ALT can result from an acute injury or abnormal force pattern stemming from femoral acetabular incongruities (e.g., FAI). Symptomatic ALTs can present suddenly after a traumatic event, but much more often present with an insidious onset of groin, lateral, anterior, and posterior hip pain. Acetabular labral tears are undiagnosed for an average of 2 years owing to their vague pain pattern and lack of distinct physical exam techniques.

Diagnosis

ALT often presents as anterior groin pain that worsens with loading of the joint. This can include prolonged periods of standing, sitting, or walking. Sharp pain often accompanied by mechanical symptoms such as clicking or catching is frequently described. When patients are asked to identify the painful area, they will cup the hip with their forefinger and thumb ("C" sign). As with all disorders of the hip, physical examination must include a visual inspection for lower extremity malalignments, points of tenderness, range of motion, motor strength, and special tests. The FADIR test, described earlier (see Fig. 2), has the most substantiating evidence for intra-articular pathology and therefore can guide one in the direction of diagnosis. Other tests have been described but lack quality supporting evidence.

Imaging of the painful hip should begin with radiographs, including at a minimum a weight-bearing AP (whenever possible radiographs should be weight-bearing for any lower extremity conditions). In patients with a suspected ALT, radiographs should be analyzed for abnormal morphology of the acetabulum and femoral head, including anatomy predisposing to FAI (see Fig. 2). MRI with contrast (MR arthrogram) is the imaging modality of choice and can demonstrate a displaced labral flap or irregular labral morphology. A paralabral cyst is a small collection of fluid communicating with the labrum or the cartilage-labral junction, when noted is pathognomonic of a labral tear. Intra-articular anesthetic hip injection can also be helpful in the diagnosis of intra-articular pathology. This injection can be done at the time of MR arthrogram or separately via ultrasound-guided injection or fluoroscopy. Just as in FAI, if intra-articular anesthesia alleviates the pain, the hip joint can be assumed to be the source of the pain. Arthroscopy remains the gold standard for the diagnosis of ALT. No single patient history or clinical examination findings are "stand alone" in their ability to diagnose ALT. An emphasis on the summative patient history, clinical examination findings, imaging modalities,

and intra-articular anesthetic injection response is needed to diagnose a symptomatic ALT. The differential diagnosis (Table 1) includes tendinopathies, FAI, and chondral lesions.

Treatment

A trial of conservative management, including relative rest and oral analgesic medications, combined with a focused physical therapy protocol is recommended. Therapy should focus on strengthening the hip, pelvis, and abdominal core musculature in addition to addressing flexibility deficits (see Ref. [9] for home exercises). A trial of intra-articular injection with steroid under imaging guidance can be offered; however one must keep in mind that repeated injections with corticosteroid may damage chondral surfaces and are not recommended. Additional intra-articular injectable therapies are available but lack high-quality supporting evidence at this time. When conservative measures do not control the patient's symptoms or when functional limitations remain unsatisfactory, a referral for orthopedic surgery is appropriate.

Greater Trochanteric Pain Syndrome (GTPS) or Trochanteric Bursitis

General Principles

GTPS is a common overuse syndrome involving one or a combination of greater trochanteric bursae, iliotibial (IT) band and gluteus medius and gluteus minimus muscle and/or tendon (see Fig. 1). The primary action of these muscles is hip abduction. There may be up to 3–4 bursae in this region. A bursa is a small synovial-lined structure that helps tissues glide over one another, as when a tendon slides over another tendon or bone. Greater trochanteric bursitis previously was theorized to be caused by repetitive trauma from friction which leads to bursitis or inflammation in the region. More recent evidence from imaging studies have shown most patients with the diagnosis of bursitis have little or no bursal inflammation and more commonly tendinopathy (disease of the tendon) of the hip abductors [11].

Diagnosis

GTPS is characterized by pain and tenderness over the bony prominence of the posterior lateral thigh. Pain may start after a specific trauma or have an insidious onset. Patients may complain of pain in the lower buttocks and the lateral aspect of the thigh when lying on the hip, walking, running, climbing stairs, or when standing on the affected leg. Pain may radiate down the lateral aspect of the leg along the pathway of the IT band.

Evaluation of a patient with GTPS should include a full history and physical exam of the back, pelvis, and lower extremities. The presence of weakness, contractures, asymmetry, and pain in other areas such as the lower back, groin, knees, ankles, and feet can contribute to the syndrome. The family physician should assess for malalignments of the lower extremity, gluteus medius weakness, and tightness of the IT band. Pain on direct palpation is the most sensitive and specific finding. Often the culprit is a gluteal insertional tendinopathy. Active abduction, engaging of the gluteus medius/minimus muscles,

and passive adduction, stretching of the involved muscle, are painful and can exacerbate this lateral hip pain. Reproduction of index pain with a 30 s single-leg stance test is highly suggestive of a gluteal tendinopathy and is also used to detect a positive Trendelenburg sign. A positive or abnormal Trendelenburg sign is when the patient demonstrates an abnormal lateral pelvic tilt while assuming a single-legged stance on the affected side in an effort to overcome hip weakness on the painful limb (see Fig. 3).

GTPS is a clinical diagnosis. Imaging is pursued when the diagnosis remains unclear or the patient is not responding to appropriate therapy. Plain film radiography may show trochanteric exostoses or osteophytes suggesting calcific tendinopathy or bursopathy in long-standing cases of GTPS. MRI may show degenerative changes to the gluteus medius and minimus tendons. Ultrasonography has emerged as an effective imaging modality for identification of normal vs. pathologic appearance of the structures involved. An added benefit of ultrasonography is

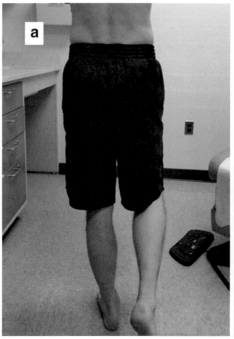
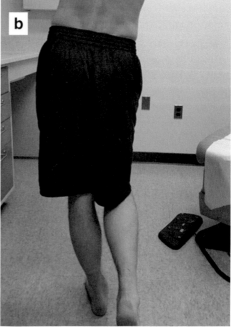

Fig. 3 Trendelenburg sign – patient stands on affected leg and lifts the unaffected leg from floor. (**a**) Normal response – ability to maintain pelvis in neutral position. (**b**) A positive or abnormal sign manifested by inability to maintain neutral posture when standing on the affected leg (non-weight-bearing hip will drop below the weight-bearing hip)

the ability to perform a dynamic exam for reproduction of patient reported symptoms.

Treatment

GTPS typically responds to conservative measures, such as activity modification, physical therapy (PT) aimed at strengthening the hip (specifically the gluteal muscles – see Ref. [9] for home exercises), and correction of any contractures. Weight loss is appropriate if indicated and can dramatically improve pain. Interventions to relieve pain are required if pain precludes daily activities, sleep, and/or participation in rehabilitative exercises. (These principals hold true for all lower extremity conditions.) Ice massage may suffice, but the short-term use of acetaminophen or NSAIDs may be warranted. If these modalities do not provide adequate symptomatic relief, corticosteroid injection into the associated bursa can be entertained. Long-term studies have shown steroid injections alone to be inferior to PT, and they should not be used as sole treatment. (This concept also holds true for most overuse conditions.) While studies on the effectiveness of regenerative (platelet-rich plasma – PRP) and proliferative (prolotherapy) injection therapies have lacked consistency, their use in treating various tendinopathies is growing in popularity and use [12]. They should be considered when pain and dysfunction persist despite appropriate rehabilitation. These treatments should be performed in conjunction with strengthening and stretching. Extracorporeal shock wave therapy has shown potential benefit and may be an option. Surgical treatment is reserved for patients who have completed a minimum of 6–12 months of conservative management but remain symptomatic.

Quadriceps and Hamstring Injuries

General Principles

Injuries to the anterior and posterior thigh are extremely common and can be a source of long-term morbidity especially for the high-level athlete. Thigh injuries can account for up to 13.5% of all sports injuries [13]. The quadriceps muscles, comprised of the rectus femoris and vastus lateralis/intermedius/medialis, are the primary knee extensors. The hamstring muscles are the primary knee flexors and consist of the bicep femoris, semimembranosus, and semitendinosus. The quadriceps have different origins but a common insertion point (superior pole of the patella), while the hamstrings are the opposite (see Fig. 1). Both muscle groups are prone to acute injuries (avulsions, tendon tears/strains, muscle contusions/tears) and chronic tendinopathies. It is important to remember that the hamstring muscles (with the exception of the short head of the biceps femoris) and the rectus femoris of the quadriceps are biarticular muscles (span two joints) and thus are more prone to injury.

Diagnosis

When attempting to identify the etiology of thigh pain, there are two important factors to consider, the location and the mechanism of injury. Contusions will be focal and the result of a direct blow or fall, while tears/strains usually occur with bursts of speed/kicking/stretching, both can have significant bruising and swelling. A chronic poorly localized pain pattern should raise suspicion of a stress fracture or referred pain (see Table 1). Pain at the bony origin raises the suspicion of an avulsion injury. While strains more commonly occur at the myotendinous junction.

Range of motion should be gently assessed. Strength testing can be challenging in the acute setting as loss of strength can be secondary to pain as well as injury. The degree of pain and weakness is a predictor of injury severity and thus recovery time. Special tests for referred pain (i.e., radiculopathy or sacroiliac dysfunction) are reserved for those cases that are not straightforward or are not responding to appropriate treatment. Imaging with ultrasound or MRI is largely reserved for refractory cases or when the diagnosis is in question, with the exception of suspected stress fracture as discussed earlier in this chapter.

Treatment

The first 24 h is the most critical time for quadriceps contusions. The goal is to maintain maximal flexion and minimize bleeding. This is accomplished by having the patient flex the knee as much as possible and maintaining this position for 24 h with the use of an elastic bandage and the almost continuous use of ice over the tender area. Soft tissue therapy (i.e., massages) is contraindicated acutely for risk of rebleeding. After the first 24 h, patients can begin a gentle stretching program to tolerance and progress as symptoms dictate. Local control of pain can be accomplished with oral (acetaminophen, NSAIDs) and topical (lidocaine, NSAIDS) analgesics or ice. NSAID use has not been found to decrease the incidence of complications, specifically myositis ossificans. Once full range of motion is achieved, then strengthening should commence (see Ref. [9] for home exercises). Symptom-based progression is discussed in greater detail under the treatment section of calf injuries. Symptom-based progression serves as a template for rehabilitation principles for quadriceps and hamstring injuries as well. Treatment of quadriceps strains is largely the same as to treatment of quadriceps contusions, keeping in mind that patients may take a longer amount of time for full recovery from strain as compared to contusion.

Large contusions can lead to the development of myositis ossificans (MO), a calcification of a hematoma. MO present as a hardening mass. Currently, there is no adequate therapy to treat once present. If there is no history of trauma to explain the calcified mass, a workup for a tumor should be undertaken.

Hamstring tears can be divided into types 1 and 2. Type 1 occurs at the proximal portion of the long head of the bicep femoris and is the result of an explosive burst, i.e., sprinting. Type 2 occurs at the ischial tuberosity at the origin of the semi-membranosus and is related to excessive stretch (i.e., full knee extension combined with hip flexion) [14]. (see Fig. 1). The rehabilitation is similar, though type 1 injuries have a tendency to recover quicker compared with type 2 injuries, and patients should be advised as such. Rehabilitation begins with restoring full range of motion followed by a focus on regaining strength and culminates in activity- or sport-specific drills (see Ref. [9] for home exercises). The use of a thigh compression sleeve is recommended in the acute, chronic, and rehabilitative setting. These injuries have a high rate of recurrence, with prior hamstring injury being identified as a leading risk factor for future injury. Because of this the high-level athlete may be best served with a referral to a specialist for rehabilitation recommendations. Chronic hamstring and quadriceps tendinopathies are treated similar to GTPS and are also discussed in ▶ Chap. 55, "Athletic Injuries." They require addressing risk factors, biomechanical assessment, and strengthening of the involved muscle groups as well as the core muscles (see Table 2).

Knee Injuries

Meniscal Injuries

General Principles

The medial and lateral menisci are semicircular fibrocartilage structures with perfect congruity between the femur and tibia (see Fig. 4). This perfect congruity allows the menisci to dissipate force and provide joint stability as well as lubrication. Similar to the acetabular labrum, the adult menisci are only vascularized on the periphery, which leads to the concept of red and white zones (red zone with blood supply and white zone without blood supply). In general, red zone injuries have the potential to heal, while white zone injuries cannot heal. This is an important concept in treatment recommendations. Pain fibers parallel the vascularity and thus are located around the periphery as well. Loss of function leads to abnormal joint forces and accelerates cartilage damage and ultimately osteoarthritis.

Meniscus tears are categorized by type and location. Horizontal, radial, vertical (which includes bucket-handle tears), root tears, ramp lesions, and complex (which are a combination of the previous types) are frequently described. Horizontal and complex tears are most common and typically exist on the osteoarthritis spectrum. Radial and vertical tears are common in acute injuries, whereas root tears and ramp lesions are typically higher-energy injuries associated with ACL tears. In a study of patients aged 50–90 years, the prevalence of meniscus tear

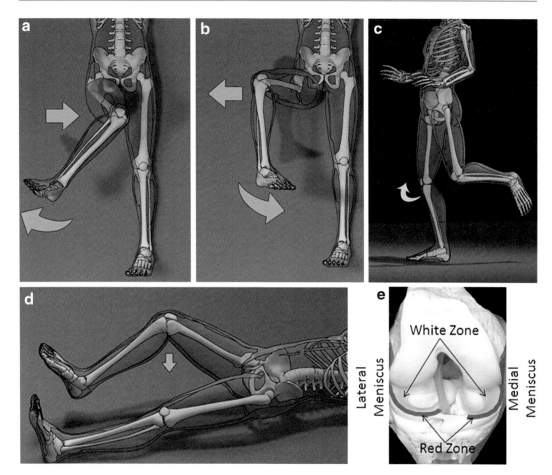

Fig. 4 Meniscal signs and anatomy. (**a**) McMurray test for medial meniscus – with fingers on medial and lateral joint line, flex the hip and knee maximally. Apply a valgus force (in direction of *straight arrow*) to the knee while externally rotating the foot (in direction of *curved arrow*) and passively extending the knee. A positive test is pain (with or without an associated click/snap) located on a respective joint line during movement (sensitivity ~65%; specificity ~65%). (**b**) McMurray test for lateral meniscus – with fingers on medial and lateral joint line, flex the hip and knee maximally. Apply a varus stress (in direction of *straight arrow*) during internal rotation of the foot (in direction of *curved arrow*) and passive extension of the knee. A positive test is pain (with or without an associated click/snap) located on a respective joint line during movement (sensitivity ~65%; specificity ~65%). (**c**) Thessaly test – hold patient's outstretched hands while he or she stands flat-footed on the floor, internally and externally rotating three times with the knee flexed 20°. A positive test is pain in respective joint compartment with movement (sensitivity ~85%; specificity ~90%). (**d**) Bounce home test – flex knee to 45 degrees and allow knee to fully passively extend (direction of *arrow*). A positive test is pain with passive extension (sensitivity ~45%; specificity ~75%). (**e**) Anatomic model of lateral and medical meniscus of right knee showing *red zone* (vascularized) and *white zone* (nonvascularized) (Figures **a**, **b**, **c**, **d** adapted with permission from fpnotebook.com)

was 31% [15]. Meniscal tear treatment has traditionally been with an arthroscopic partial meniscectomy (APM). While APM use has decreased over the last 15 years, it is still the most common orthopedic surgical procedure in the United States with 700,000 arthroscopic partial meniscectomies every year [16]. Recently the utility of this traditional practice has been called into question.

Diagnosis

Acute meniscal injuries present after a traumatic event. This can be a sudden noncontact twisting event (the most common mechanism) or through contact as in a football tackle. The presence of an acute effusion varies; an effusion generally denotes an injury to the vascularized red zone. Pain is the predominant feature. Other important historical elements are catching or locking, defined as a mechanical symptom of "something" inside the joint not allowing full pain-free range of motion. Physical examination findings can include a variable amount of intra-articular swelling (it is important to differentiate between soft tissue and intra-articular swelling), pain to palpation along the relevant joint line (anterior and posterior medial, anterior and posterior lateral), and pain with one or more of the meniscal tests (see Fig. 4). A thorough assessment for other ligamentous injuries (cruciate, collateral, patellar) is required as their injury has an impact on treatment recommendations.

Plain films consisting of an AP, lateral, and patellar view should generally be ordered if one is considering an acute meniscal tear in order to rule out a fracture, but other than showing an effusion, they are not diagnostic. Despite being able to adequately diagnose an isolated meniscal injury with history and physical exam in >90% of patients, an MRI is almost always ordered to confirm an acute meniscal tear. In addition to confirming the clinical suspicion, MRI is invaluable at detecting concomitant ligamentous injury and the presence of osteoarthritis or cartilage damage which have treatment recommendation implications. Unfortunately the MRI sensitivity of ramp lesions is only 48% [16].

Chronic (usually degenerative) injuries present with pain along the relevant joint line, intermittent swelling, and possible mechanical symptoms of locking and catching but lack the acute history of a traumatic event (although a careful history may reveal an antecedent event years previous that may have initially damaged the meniscus). Physical examination is similar as in the evaluation for acute injuries (see Fig. 4). The decision to image depends on the patient's symptoms and treatment preferences. A weight-bearing AP and lateral radiograph should be ordered as well as a patellar view (sunrise or merchant) to evaluate the presence and degree of OA which may affect treatment options. If the patient complains of true locking

(a mechanical block to range of motion), then an MRI is warranted to confirm the diagnosis. Caution must be taken in interpreting meniscal tears on MRI though as they are present in approximately 20% of people without knee symptoms <40 years of age and up to 70% >65 years of age [17]. The differential diagnosis includes OA, chondral lesions, and patellofemoral pain syndrome (see Table 4).

Treatment

In general, patients under 40 and those without significant OA or cartilage damage are ideal candidates for meniscal repair. Acute meniscal tears warrant referral and should be repaired within 8 weeks of the injury. In chronic, degenerative tears, unless the patient has true mechanical symptoms (locking or catching), a discussion of treatment outcomes and joint decision-making is warranted. Since repair is generally not possible and once meniscal tissue is removed its function is lost permanently, symptom management becomes the treatment goals. Several randomized clinical trials have showed no significant differences in terms of knee pain relief, improved knee function, or patient satisfaction between APM and lower extremity strengthening exercises over 2–5 years of follow-up [18].

Baker's Cyst (Popliteal Cyst)

General Principles

Named after Dr. William Baker who first described the condition in 1877, a Baker's cyst is more properly termed a popliteal cyst. It is a fluid-filled mass generally resulting from the distention of a preexisting bursa in the popliteal fossa, most commonly the medial gastrocnemius-semimembranosus bursa (see Fig. 1). Unlike other bursa, this one is connected via a valvular opening in the joint capsule posterior to the medial femoral condyle and is present in up to 40–54% of healthy adult knee [19].

Diagnosis

Patients generally complain of fullness behind the knee. A mass can usually be seen and

Table 4 Differential diagnosis of knee and calf disorders of the lower extremity

Very common	Common	Infrequent	Referred
Knee			
• Ligamentous injury (ACL, PCL, MCL, LCL) • Patellofemoral syndrome • Bursitis [a] • Patellar tendinopathy • Osteoarthritis • Chondral lesions • Iliotibial band syndrome (distal) • Meniscal injury	• Osteochondrosis (Sinding-Larsen-Johansson and Osgood-Schlatter) • Less common tendinopathy (quadriceps, proximal hamstring, popliteus) • Patellar instability (can be all directions) • Popliteal cyst	• Plica syndrome • Fat-pad syndrome (Hoffa syndrome) • Osteochondritis dissecans • Crystal-induced arthropathy • Stress fracture • Nerve entrapments (common peroneal, saphenous)	• Pigmented villonodular synovitis • Popliteal artery entrapment syndrome • Fabella syndrome
Calf			
• Gastrocnemius [b] • Stress fracture • Medial tibial stress syndrome [c] • Achilles tendinopathy	• Soleus [b] • Plantaris [b] • Fracture • Anterior tibial stress syndrome [d]	• Compartment syndrome (exertional and acute) • Nerve entrapment [e] • Achilles tendon rupture	• Infection • Tumor • Deep vein thrombosis
Differential diagnosis for acute hemarthrosis			
• Ligamentous injury • Meniscal injury • Patella injury • Extensor mechanism injury • Osteochondral injury • Fracture • Avulsion			

[a]Suprapatellar, prepatellar, deep infrapatellar, gastrocnemius, semimembranosus, sartorius, pes anserine, MCL bursa, distal iliotibial band, fibular collateral ligament, popliteus tendon
[b]Includes muscle strain/tears and tendinopathies
[c]Pain along posterior medial aspect of tibia believe to be periostitis of posterior tibial muscle, flexor digitorium longus and/or the soleus attachment on tibia
[d]Pain along the anterior aspect of tibia believe to be periostitis of anterior tibial muscle attachment on tibia
[e]Peroneal, sural, tibial

palpated in the prone patient with the knee fully extended. With knee flexion to around 45°, the cyst usually disappears or decreases in size. Confirmation can be obtained via ultrasound or MRI and should be performed if any doubt exists about the masses' etiology. A ruptured popliteal cyst can present with acute pain and signs of inflammation. An evaluation for a deep vein thrombosis (DVT) should be considered in this setting. The differential diagnosis includes tumors both benign and malignant as well as meniscal cysts and DVTs (see Table 4). Although popliteal cysts are most commonly found between the medial head of the gastrocnemius and semimembranosus, they have been reported in other areas. If a posterolateral cyst is discovered, further evaluation should be performed to rule out a meniscal cyst or soft tissue tumor as lateral presentation of popliteal cysts is unusual.

Treatment

Management is not dictated by the cyst but rather by the pathology that causes the cyst. OA with or without concomitant meniscal injury is usually the underlying cause in the majority of patients.

In those patients having mechanical symptoms due to a large cyst, ultrasound-guided aspiration can provide temporary relief, but the cyst will invariably return if the underlying pathology is not remedied.

Knee Bursitis

General Principles

There are multiple bursas around the knee that can become symptomatic (see Fig. 1 and Table 4). Irritation of any of these bursas can cause knee pain. Definitive treatment lies in treating the underlying cause of the bursa irritation and not the irritation itself (see discussion on victims and culprits under GTPS). Local control of pain can be accomplished with oral (acetaminophen, NSAIDs) and topical (lidocaine, NSAIDs) analgesics or ice massages. Injections can be performed with steroids or other agents such as dextrose or platelet-rich plasma. Due to the great variability in bursa location, ultrasound-guided injections are recommended. It must be emphasized though that these are temporary measures and the underlying cause must be elucidated and corrected. Pes anserine bursitis will be discussed as it is prototypical and extremely common. Prepatellar bursitis will be mentioned as it has some unique features that must be taken into account.

Pes Anserine Bursitis

The diagnosis is easily made by tenderness at the pes anserine area and an appropriate history. The pes anserine bursa is generally located on the proximal medial portion of the tibia just superficial to the distal tibial insertion of the superficial medial collateral ligament (MCL) of the knee (see Fig. 1). This is the site for the common insertion point for the conjoined tendons of the sartorius, gracilis, and semitendinosus muscles. There is great individual variability in its exact location with most bursas lying between the three conjoined tendons and the tibia, less frequently between the MCL and the tendons, or between the tendons themselves. Because of the close approximation to the distal portion of the MCL, any history of a twisting injury or contact preceding the pain would warrant valgus loading of the knee in 0° and 30° to ensure the MCL is not sprained. In addition, medial meniscal tears can

sometimes be confused or coexist with pes anserine bursitis (see Table 4). Treatment of pes anserine bursitis pain should include the local therapies mentioned in the "General Principles" section of knee bursitis and most importantly a search for and correction of the contributing factors:

- OA of the knee – as many as 75% of patients with OA have symptoms of pes anserine bursitis; knee and hip strengthening are the mainstays for OA treatment.
- Obesity – even a modest weight loss of ~5% may alleviate the pain.
- Valgus knee deformity, alone or in combination with collateral instability – bracing may be beneficial.
- Pes planus (i.e., flat foot) – consider foot orthoses.
- Diabetes mellitus (DM) – common comorbidity in a variety of bursitis. It is unclear if it is the obesity that accompanies DM or if it is the DM itself which causes the bursitis and it is also unclear if good glycemic control will minimize musculoskeletal complaints.
- Medial meniscal tear – loss of stability increases the forces over the pes anserine; see discussion on meniscal injuries for treatment recommendations.
- Saphenous nerve injury (from surgery, trauma, or mass effect) – needs a high index of suspicion for diagnosis and then must treat the cause.

Prepatellar Bursitis

Special note should be made concerning prepatellar bursitis, as an infectious etiology can be the cause. The following in declining order can be responsible for prepatellar bursitis [20]:

- Direct trauma (e.g., a fall on the patella or direct blow to the knee)
- Recurrent minor injuries associated with overuse (e.g., repeated kneeling)
- Septic or pyogenic process
- Crystal deposition (e.g., gout, pseudogout)

If there is any concern for an infection (erythema, warmth, fluctuance), then at a minimum, an aspiration is required to analyze fluid content (white blood cells, protein, lactate, glucose, crystals, Gram stain, culture). Ultrasound greatly facilitates both confirmation of an enlarged bursa sac and is invaluable if an aspiration is considered. Fortunately, even if the bursa is infected, conservative treatment is warranted with aspiration of as much material as possible, and oral antibiotics that are narrowed once laboratory results are known (always consider methicillin-resistant *Staphylococcus aureus* and local antibiotic resistance patterns). Incision and drainage or bursectomy is reserved for patients with severe, refractory, or chronic/recurrent disease.

Fractures and Dislocations of the Knee

General Principles

Acute fractures of the knee are the result of trauma and are associated with an acute hemarthrosis. The differential diagnosis for an acute traumatic hemarthrosis in order of precedent is ligamentous injury (ACL being #1), peripheral meniscal injury, or a fracture (see Table 4). Quadriceps and patellar tendon tears are extra-articular structures but are associated with a large amount of soft tissue swelling. Their diagnoses are generally not difficult to make. Patients are unable to extend the knee and, because of their immediate loss of function, almost always present to the emergency room.

An acute fracture will present with focal tenderness over the involved bony area. Range of motion is usually limited by pain and unless there is a concomitant ligamentous/meniscal injury, special tests for the knee are normal. Plain radiography, at a minimum AP and lateral, is usually adequate to confirm the diagnosis, but if negative and clinical suspicion is high, an MRI would be warranted. Although CT is the imaging modality of choice for bony abnormalities, MRI will be able to diagnose the fracture as well as any other soft tissue abnormality that might be missed on CT. All fractures of the knee, which invariably are intra-articular, should be managed in conjunction with an orthopedist or a sports medicine physician in a timely fashion. (i.e., 48 h) In the interim depending on the degree of swelling, a compression wrap or hinged knee brace can be applied. Knee immobilizers are particularly painful and uncomfortable for patients and should never be left on for an extended period of time. If an in-person consultation cannot be achieved in an adequate timeframe, a telephone consultation to a specialist for treatment recommendations is warranted. Adequate pain control can generally be achieved with acetaminophen and/or NSAIDs.

Osteochondral defects and stress fractures can present more subtly and subacutely; therefore, a high index of suspicion is required. Osteochondral defects are focal areas of articular injury with damage to both the cartilage and the adjacent subchondral bone. Trauma is the leading cause of a focal osteochondral defect in a previously normal bone in the skeletally mature. The term osteochondral defect encompasses the entity known as osteochondritis dissecans (OCD). The acronym OCD is sometimes applied both to osteochondral defects and osteochondritis dissecans but technically should be reserved for the latter and will be the case in this chapter. The cause of OCD remains unknown but may include one or all of the following factors: genetic predisposition, defective skeletal development, vascular insult, and trauma. OCD usually begins in adolescents although its sequelae, premature OA may not become apparent until adulthood. Knee OCD frequency is reported to be 20/100,000 in 10–20-year-olds. Symptoms of any osteochondral defect include activity-related pain, catching or locking of the affected joint, and/or a transient effusion. OCD is often misdiagnosed as patellofemoral syndrome. Plain radiography includes AP view, lateral view, sunrise or merchant view, and a notched view, but an MRI is often required for diagnosis and is essential for staging. Adult osteochondral defects may present as an acute fracture or insidious as in an OCD.

When discovered, osteochondral defects should be at a minimum co-managed with an orthopedist or a sports medicine provider. Prognosis and treatment is dependent primarily on the stability of the lesion and the age of the patient.

Adolescents with stable lesions can heal, but the skeletally mature are very unlikely to heal on their own [21].

Stress fractures of the knee are not common and require a high index of suspicion. Plain radiography can be suggestive, but generally an MRI is needed to confirm diagnosis. Management involves decreasing force loads and correcting any mitigating factors (see previous discussion on stress fractures).

Patella dislocations occur almost always laterally with the medial patellofemoral ligament tearing. As in other ligamentous injuries, it can occur due to direct trauma or from sudden change in direction or muscular contractions. It is not unusual for the patella to spontaneously relocate. After radiographs are obtained to document fractures and if the patella remains dislocated, administering an adequate amount of intra-articular anesthesia and gently elevating the patella while providing a medially direct force accomplish the reduction. Postreduction radiographs are recommended. There is invariably an injury to the lateral femoral condyle and the accompanying facet of the patella as the patella dislocates over the lateral femoral condyle. After knee bracing with a patellofemoral brace, all patients should be referred to orthopedics for management as primary repair is recommended for some patient populations.

A complete knee dislocation is a major traumatic event that should be managed in an emergency room/hospital setting similar to a hip dislocation. In addition to the ligamentous and potential osteochondral abnormalities associated with the injury, the integrity of the popliteal artery must be evaluated in all cases.

Lower Leg/Ankle/Foot Injuries

Calf Injuries

General Principles

Injuries to the posterior lower leg (calf) are common, with a higher prevalence of calf injuries in athletes greater than 40 years old [22]. The muscles of the superficial posterior compartment of

the lower leg are the gastrocnemius, soleus, and the plantaris. The gastrocnemius and soleus muscles are known as the triceps surae (some anatomists believe they are one muscle with three heads combining at the Achilles tendon to insert on the posterior calcaneus) (see Fig. 5). Together these muscles function as the primary plantar flexor of the ankle. Most injuries to these muscles occur with sudden explosive movements or prolonged impact activities. The gastrocnemius is a biarticular muscle of the lower extremity and is composed of a medial and lateral head originating on their respective femoral condyles. The soleus has a broad origin on the proximal tibia and fibula. Over 90% of injuries in the calf involve only the gastrocnemius muscle, with 86% of those injuries in the medial head, and 14% in the lateral head [23]. The plantaris muscle has significant anatomic variability of its presence and location. When present, it originates just medial to the lateral head of the gastrocnemius and traverses proximally between the gastrocnemius and popliteus muscles and distally between the gastrocnemius and soleus muscles. The function of the plantaris is debated; injury to its muscle or tendon must remain in the differential of calf pain. The popliteus muscle originates from the lateral condyle as a component of the posterolateral corner of the knee and inserts on the posterior aspect of the proximal tibia. Although not a traditional calf muscle, it is included for discussion as it can be a source of pathology in the proximal calf area either due to a tendinopathy or compression of the neurovascular bundle that lies in close approximation to the muscle tendon.

Diagnosis

Gastrocnemius injuries are commonly acute in origin, occurring with explosive or dynamic eccentric loading of the calf with activities such as sprinting or jumping. As an example, a tennis leg is a common injury to the medial head of the gastrocnemius that occurs with knee extension and sudden ankle dorsiflexion. The associated pain of this acute injury is described as a tearing or stabbing sensation, and most patients have difficulty bearing full weight on the injured leg. There may be a variable amount of swelling or

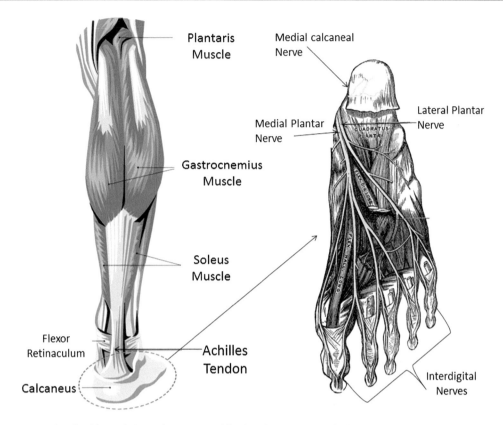

Fig. 5 Posterior distal leg and plantar foot anatomy (distal leg image adapted with permission from fpnotebook.com). Plantar foot adapted from *Gray's Anatomy* 20th edition from 1918 (Lewis) in the public domain following expiration of its patent. Available online at http://bartleby.com/107/)

bruising, depending on the degree of muscle injury. Active plantar flexion of the ankle with the knee extended, and passive or active dorsiflexion of the ankle can reproduce the patient's pain. An isolated or concomitant Achilles tendon tear must be ruled out. Both diagnoses have similar mechanisms of injury but are differentiated by physical exam and imaging. Achilles tendon integrity is assessed with careful palpation to identify a defect despite the considerable swelling around the tear. Also, perform the Thompson squeeze test by placing the patient in the prone position and squeezing the proximal calf musculature. The nomenclature of the Thompson squeeze test can be confusing; a negative squeeze test is when plantar flexion is present, indicating an intact muscle-tendon complex, and a positive test is when plantar flexion is not present, indicating a disruption of the muscle-tendon complex. It is less misleading to describe the motion observed when squeezing the posterior calf as opposed to saying a negative or positive test. Some passive plantar flexion may be present in up to 10% of complete Achilles tendon ruptures from an intact plantaris muscle or activation of the deep posterior compartment muscles of the leg. Likewise, the lack of passive plantar flexion does not indicate a complete tear. Two case reports demonstrate a positive calf squeeze, and upon surgical evaluation, only a tear of the gastrocnemius was identified in the triceps surae [24]. Pursue further imaging with ultrasound or MRI if clinical suspicion remains high for an Achilles tendon injury despite a normal or equivocal physical exam. An ultrasound is the least expensive and rapidly obtained. However it is operator dependent and an intact plantaris can be mistaken for an intact

Achilles tendon, and a large hematoma can obscure the tear.

Plantaris injuries are commonly acute in origin with the same mechanism of injury as gastrocnemius injuries. Symptoms are similar but not as severe. Swelling and bruising are not always apparent because the plantaris muscle and tendon lie deep to the gastrocnemius. These injuries are usually located in the mid-calf and are more distal to the injuries of the medial head of the gastrocnemius. As the plantaris usually does not contribute to the Achilles tendon, the calf squeeze test will be negative, resulting in passive ankle plantar flexion. An exception to this would be if the Achilles tendon was involved in the acute injury.

Contrary to gastrocnemius and plantaris muscle injuries, soleus muscle injuries characteristically are of a chronic nature. The chronicity of these injuries may occur because the soleus contains predominantly slow-twitch muscle fibers, whereas the gastrocnemius is comprised of both fast- and slow-twitch muscle fibers. Distance runners and those who engage in hill running are more vulnerable to soleus injuries. Palpation of the calf reveals deep muscle soreness and minimal to no swelling or contusion. A functional exam of the soleus muscle can help elucidate the diagnosis by the patient performing active plantar flexion with heel raises on a step with the knee flexed to 20–30°. The gastrocnemius is tested by repeating the functional exam with the knee in full extension. If the patient's pain is exacerbated while the knee is flexed, but reduced or absent with knee extended, this finding is highly suggestive of a soleus muscle injury.

As mentioned earlier in GTPS, a complete physical examination should include the entire kinetic chain looking for leg length discrepancies, pes cavus or pes planus, flexibility deficits, and strength deficits such as hip weakness with the Trendelenburg test (see Fig. 3). Table 4 provides a differential diagnosis for lower leg complaints.

Treatment

Treat these injuries in a phased approach. A detailed description is provided and serves as a model for other muscle or tendon injuries (e.-g., groin, quadriceps, and hamstring injuries). The initial phase protects an acute injury from further damage while restoring the range of motion. Calf compression is helpful for posterior calf injuries and accomplished with commercial compression sleeves or elastic bandages; the latter is more prudent to treat an acute injury avoiding neurovascular compression by adjusting the amount of compression. Ice is recommended for acute injuries and utilizes pain medication (i.e., acetaminophen or NSAIDs) as needed. Occasionally severe injuries require modification of weight-bearing with crutches and immobilization, either with a posterior splint or a commercial walking boot. Revisit the need for immobilization and the patient's weight-bearing status every 3–5 days as restoring normal range of motion and their ability to weight bear is essential. Heel lifts can assist in pain relief by shortening the muscle-tendon unit. If a heel lift is used for acute pain management, it should be removed as soon as pain allows, usually 3–5 days, avoiding a permanently contracted muscle-tendon unit.

Once the patient can walk without a limp, test their ability to do a heel lift. If they have minimal pain, the patient may begin the next phase of recovery with active rehabilitation that consists of strengthening the gastrocnemius-soleus complex with repetitive heel raises and progressive loading (see Ref. [9] for home exercises). Plyometric exercises and activity-specific training can begin after the patient can tolerate progressively loading without recurrence of pain or dysfunction. Every patient's injury recovery time is variable. Functional assessments should guide treatment advances to include the ability to walk without a limp, ability to do heel lifts without significant pain, progressive loading, and pain-free functional activity.

The continued use of a calf compression sleeve is an option and patient dependent. To prevent a recurrence, patients should maintain a strengthening program of the lower extremity. The use of foot orthosis can be considered for leg length abnormalities or pes cavus or planus.

Achilles Tendon Rupture

General Principles

The Achilles tendon has poor vascularity 2–6 cm proximal to its insertion on the calcaneus (see Fig. 5). This watershed area is at risk for tendinopathies and rupture. Men are approximately four times more likely to have an Achilles tendon rupture. The age-adjusted incidence, regardless of gender, peaked at 41 years old with a mean incidence of about 69/100,000/person-year [25]. The mechanism of injury is the same as for acute calf injuries described above, which is a vigorous contraction of the calf muscle with explosive or dynamic movements, while the ankle is in a dorsiflexed position. The exact pathophysiology of an Achilles tendon rupture is unknown, but underlying tendinopathy and impaired blood flow appear to be correlated to this injury. All fluoroquinolones demonstrate an increased risk of Achilles tendinopathy. Ofloxacin and norfloxacin are the only two fluoroquinolones that demonstrate a significant risk of Achilles tendon rupture, and the concomitant use of corticosteroids did not have a significant increase in that risk. After 30 days from the initial exposure to the medication, the risk of Achilles tendon rupture returns to the patient's baseline. The highest risk of Achilles tendinopathy and rupture was seen in those patients 60 years of age and older [26].

Diagnosis

An oft-heard complaint is "someone kicked me in the back of the leg." An audible snap is common, with an antalgic gait and minimal power with push-off, but the patient is otherwise able to compensate with the muscles of the deep posterior compartment and the plantaris muscle. Most complain of intense pain, but a case series demonstrated that up to one-third of patients had no pain with an acute rupture [27]. It is speculated that these patients had chronic tendinopathy, and the rupture relieved the discomfort from tendinopathy. Acutely significant swelling and ecchymosis are usually present. Careful palpation of the tendon will reveal a gap but can be obscured due to the inflammation or a hematoma. As above, the entire calf musculature should be examined to identify gastrocnemius, soleus, or plantaris injuries (see Table 4).

Strength testing demonstrates markedly decreased plantar flexion. The calf squeeze test described above usually demonstrates a positive test with no passive plantar flexion of the ankle. As mentioned earlier, with a complete rupture, plantar flexion may be present, and conversely loss of plantar flexion is not 100% sensitive or specific for a complete rupture. Ruptures are missed in up to 25% of patients due to multiple variables to include a confounding exam. These estimates were made before the widespread availability of ultrasound and MRI. If a tendon rupture is suspected despite a negative or equivocal exam, obtain advanced imaging studies to avoid the high morbidity of a missed rupture.

Treatment

Traditionally, the treatment of Achilles tendon ruptures was surgical for the active population and nonoperative for the elderly or those with significant comorbidities. Recent studies demonstrate that nonoperative treatments are a viable option for active populations when coupled with modern rehabilitation techniques. Nonoperative treatment includes physical therapy combined with progression from non-weight-bearing in a cast or a walking boot to a walking boot with incremental reductions in the height of heel wedges guided by a clinical and radiographic assessment of the tendon integrity. The re-rupture rates are low, and the risk difference between the operative and nonoperative groups is small at 1.6%. The operative group has a 3.3% higher-risk difference of complications (i.e., infection, DVT, wound adhesion) [28]. Early functional rehabilitation within the first 2 weeks of surgery with weight-bearing and various exercise-based interventions is inconclusive because of the high variability and lack of standardization of exercises. However, higher patient satisfaction is demonstrated with the transition from a rigid cast to functional bracing within 2 weeks of surgery [29]. A referral is recommended to an orthopedic surgeon unless the physician has considerable experience in managing Achilles tendon ruptures, including casting and splinting. Informed and shared decision-making is paramount to determine the most appropriate treatment course.

Plantar Fasciopathy (PF)

General Principles

Plantar fasciopathy (PF), also known as plantar fasciitis, is the most common cause of heel pain in adults, affecting more than 2 million annually in the United States. The peak incidence is between 40 and 60 years old [30]. Higher-risk populations include runners and occupations with prolonged standing. Physical factors that predispose patients to PF include limited ankle dorsiflexion and obesity.

A complicated fibrous network richly invested with small nerves connects the plantar fascia to the structures of the foot. The plantar fascia consists of medial, central, and lateral bands originating on the plantar aspect of the calcaneus. PF occurs most frequently in the central band, which extends distally dividing into five bands that insert on the metatarsophalangeal joints. Its primary function is to provide both static and dynamic support of the longitudinal arch.

Biomechanical dysfunction leading to microtears at its calcaneal attachment is thought to be the etiology. Plantar fasciitis is a misnomer in most patients because the histopathology of PF reveals degenerative tissue with a lack of traditional inflammatory cells, which directly impacts the treatment options [31]. However enthesopathic conditions such as seronegative spondyloarthropathies can present with pain and inflammation of the plantar fascia due to an autoimmune inflammatory process.

Diagnosis

The classic patient presentation is increased pain upon the first steps after sleeping or prolonged sitting that improves or diminishes in severity after a few minutes of ambulation. Radicular pain is atypical and should alert the physician to an alternative diagnosis such as nerve compression. Perform an inspection of the lower extremity to identify comorbidities or kinetic chain dysfunction to include true or functional leg length abnormalities and foot abnormalities such as pes cavus or planus (see Table 2). Usually swelling or bruising is absent in PF and if present raises the concern for an alternate diagnosis. Physical exam findings include sharp pain and tenderness over the medial plantar calcaneal region which is accentuated with great toe extension and ankle dorsiflexion. Ankle dorsiflexion can be limited due to PF pain and posterior calf tightness. Both of these factors need to be considered as a part of the rehabilitation program. Palpation and percussion of the posterior tibial nerve, especially the medial calcaneal and lateral plantar branches, should be performed to ensure they are not the source of the pain (see Fig. 5).

PF is a clinical diagnosis. Imaging is reserved to rule out other conditions. Plantar calcaneal spurs are present in patients with and without symptoms of PF. The formation of heel spurs is hypothesized to be an adaption to bony stress at the plantar fascia origin on the calcaneus. The most common mimickers of PF are heel fat-pad syndrome and neuropathies, but it is possible to have multiple concurrent pathologies, and one may beget the other [32] (see Table 5 for differential diagnosis).

Treatment

The natural history of PF is a self-limited resolution in about 90% of patients, but this may take up to 12 months. There are a myriad of treatments with limited evidence as well as conflicting and mixed results. Therefore a conservative, least invasive, cost-effective approach is prudent. Obesity is an extrinsic risk factor for musculoskeletal conditions and should be addressed. If training errors are revealed, these should be corrected. If biomechanical dysfunction is discovered, this should be corrected (e.g., lower extremity and core weakness, flexibility deficits, leg length abnormality, pes cavus, or planus) (see Table 2). Initial treatment is aimed at controlling pain to allow normal activities of daily living (ADLs) and then progressing to meet the patient's desired activity goals. In the acute setting, pain relief is the primary goal and can be accomplished with ice massage, oral, topical, or injectable pain

Table 5 Differential diagnosis of ankle and food disorders of the lower extremity

Very common	Common	Infrequent	Referred
Ankle sprain	Achilles tendon rupture	First MTP joint sprain (turf toe)	Radiculopathy
Plantar	Fractures	Calcaneal abnormalities (retrocalcaneal,	Chronic regional pain
fasciopathy	Metatarsalgia (multiple	Haglund)	syndrome
Tendinopathy [a]	causes)	Enthesopathies of autoimmune	Septic arthritis
Stress fracture	Toe abnormality [b]	conditions	Neoplasm
Osteoarthritis	Hallux valgus	Fat-pad atrophy	Vascular disorders
	Interdigital nerve	Nerve compression [c]	
	entrapment	Osteochondrosis [d]	
	Corns/calluses	Hallux rigidus	
	Sesamoid disorders	Lisfranc injury	
		Plantar fascia rupture	
		Cuboid subluxation	
		Plantar fibromatosis	
		Sinus tarsi syndrome	
		Tarsal coalition	

[a]Achilles, posterior tibialis, peroneal (fibularis), flexor hallucis
[b]Hammer, mallet, claw, curly
[c]Posterior tibial-tarsal tunnel, lateral plantar, medial calcaneal, peroneal (superficial, deep)
[d]Calcaneal (Sever), navicular (Köhler), metatarsal head (Freiberg)

medications. No difference was found in pain or functional outcomes in patients with plantar heel pain, whether they were placed in custom or pre-fabricated foot orthoses [33]. As tolerated, proceed with the stretching and strengthening of the foot and lower extremity. In addition to plantar fascia stretching, the triceps surae should be stretched (see Ref. [9] for home exercises). Standing with just the toes on a step or placing a towel under the toes while performing heel raises with the eccentric lowering of the heel into dorsiflexion stretches both the Achilles tendon and plantar fascia and is a form of eccentric loading and strengthening. Eccentric strengthening occurs when the muscles are lengthened while contracting to control the dorsiflexion of the ankle and has shown to have superior outcomes to corticosteroid injections into the plantar fascia [34]. No evidence-based recommendations can be made for orthoses such as counterforce braces, socklike sleeves, or dorsiflexion splints, but some patients demonstrate anecdotal improvement with their use. These orthoses should not be used in isolation but as part of a comprehensive treatment regimen that includes stretching, strengthening, and the correction of extrinsic risk factors.

Consider injection therapies for refractory cases of chronic PF. Corticosteroids combined with an anesthetic can provide immediate short-term relief after the injection and can help to confirm the source of pathology. Their repeated use is discouraged for the risk of fat-pad atrophy or plantar fascia rupture. In general, utilize this treatment for severe pain that limits ADLs or restricts rehabilitation. Injection therapies with prolotherapy, PRP, and botulinum toxin are options for recalcitrant cases with varying levels of evidence. Low-frequency shock wave therapy treatments may have a role in the treatment of PF when other conservative measures fail, but patient outcomes are mixed in the literature. Surgery is a last resort, and the diagnosis must be revisited if the patient is not responding to other treatments.

Metatarsalgia

General Principles

Metatarsalgia is pain at the metatarsals, which is a nonspecific term for any painful condition around the forefoot, generally at the metatarsal heads. It is a symptom rather than a condition, and the treatment is determined by identifying the underlying cause (i.e., the victims and culprits concept discussed in GTPS). The first digit absorbs 40% of impact forces of the foot. Any condition that alters this force distribution can contribute to metatarsalgia. The second metatarsal head is affected more often due to its relative inflexibility when compared to the other digits, its proximity to the main force absorber (i.e., the first digit), and a common anatomical variant of a shortened first metatarsal [35]. The following section will discuss common causes of metatarsalgia in greater detail with a more extensive list in Table 5.

Diagnosis

Metatarsalgia has a gradual onset of pain without trauma. Obtaining an occupational history can identify modifiable risk factors. Inquiring about recent exercise patterns is paramount because a delayed diagnosis of a stress fracture can result in significant morbidity (see Table 2 for risk factors). Inspect the entire kinetic chain for apparent abnormalities. Local tenderness is present with palpation of the plantar metatarsal heads. Weight-bearing plain radiographs may be ordered to assess for additional bony pathology. Utilize advanced imaging with ultrasound and MRI to evaluate for other pathologies (e.g., stress fractures, neuralgia, and sesamoiditis). Salient findings for the specific diagnosis will be discussed under their respective sections.

Treatment

Successful long-term treatment resides with identifying the cause of the patient's symptoms. For generalized metatarsalgia without a specific etiology, a metatarsal pad or bar can be used to off-load the metatarsal heads. If the patient has noticeable anatomic changes, consider a custom foot orthotic.

Interdigital Nerve Compression

A variety of conditions cause compression and swelling of the interdigital nerves of the toes (see Fig. 5). A Morton's neuroma, which is actually a neuritis and not a true nerve tumor, occurs most commonly between the third and fourth digit. Paresthesias can be present and amplified with direct palpation along the nerve's distribution. Compression of the metatarsal heads by squeezing both sides of the forefoot can cause the affected interdigital nerve to have a painful click or snap between the two opposing bones (i.e., Mulder's sign).

Symptomatic relief with an anesthetic block can be diagnostic and if combined with a corticosteroid, therapeutic. A dorsal approach is highly recommended to avoid complications. Ultrasound guidance is advocated to ensure precise delivery under direct visualization. Recurrence can be treated with either chemical or surgical nerve ablation techniques, but successful long-term management includes correction of the biomechanical causes of nerve compression.

Sesamoiditis

Sesamoiditis is a generic term for pain located around the sesamoid complex of the foot. The sesamoid complex absorbs the most force for the first ray. There are two sesamoid bones embedded, respectively, in the lateral and medial heads of the flexor hallucis brevis at the first MTP joint. They function to improve the power of flexion at the MTP joint and to absorb the majority of forces along the medial aspect of the foot. Either sesamoid can be bipartite, and patients with pes cavus have a higher risk for sesamoid injuries [36].

Patients present with pain upon palpation of the affected sesamoid and with great toe dorsiflexion. Treatments include correcting biomechanical dysfunction and redistributing impact forces at the sesamoids with various types of padding (e.g., dancer's pads) and foot orthoses. Imaging is not required unless the diagnosis is uncertain or the patient is not responding to conservative treatments. If required plain films, including an axial sesamoid view, can be challenging to interpret. An MRI is more definitive as it will reveal the presence of stress fractures, soft tissue swelling, or other concomitant pathology. The differential diagnosis for the athletic population includes first MTP joint sprain or turf toe. Turf toe is an acute injury that can be recalcitrant to healing, as it is difficult to unload this area entirely. It is frequently treated with rest and custom orthoses.

Distal Tibia/Fibula/Ankle/Foot Fractures

Acute fractures of the ankle are common but usually present with the same mechanism as an ankle sprain which is discussed in ▶ Chap. 55, "Athletic Injuries." The foot and leg are the most common locations for stress fractures because of the high, repetitive force loads imparted. As mentioned earlier, they are preceded by new mechanical stresses for which the body has not had time to accommodate. See Table 3 for low- and high-risk stress fractures and management.

References

1. Chen DX, Yang L, Ding L, Li SY, Qi YN, Li Q. Perioperative outcomes in geriatric patients undergoing hip fracture surgery with different anesthesia techniques: a systematic review and meta-analysis. Medicine (Baltimore). 2019;98(49):e18220.
2. Rodriguez CR, Parrish DO, Kumar A. Common fractures. FP Essent. 2013;405:1–6, 9-46; quiz 7-8, 7-51
3. Flevas DA, Megaloikonomos PD, Dimopoulos L, Mitsiokapa E, Koulouvaris P, Mavrogenis AF. Thromboembolism prophylaxis in orthopaedics: an update. EFORT Open Rev. 2018;3(4):136–48.
4. Santesso N, Carrasco-Labra A, Brignardello-Petersen R. Hip protectors for preventing hip fractures in older people. Cochrane Database Syst Rev. 2014;3
5. Kahanov L, Eberman LE, Games KE, Wasik M. Diagnosis, treatment, and rehabilitation of stress fractures in the lower extremity in runners. Open Access J Sports Med. 2015;6:87–95.
6. McCormick F, Nwachukwu BU, Provencher MT. Stress fractures in runners. Clin Sports Med. 2012;31(2):291–306.
7. Foulk DM, Mullis BH. Hip dislocation: evaluation and management. J Am Acad Orthop Surg. 2010;18(4): 199–209.
8. Mallets E, Turner A, Durbin J, Bader A, Murray L. Short-term outcomes of conservative treatment for femoroacetabular impingement: a systematic review and meta-analysis. Int J Sports Phys Ther. 2019;14(4):514–24.
9. Safran MR, Zachazewski JE, Stone DA. Instructions for sports medicine patients. 2nd ed. Philadelphia, PA: Elsevier/Saunders; 2012.. xv, 1311 p.
10. Groh MM, Herrera J. A comprehensive review of hip labral tears. Curr Rev Musculoskelet Med. 2009;2(2): 105–17.
11. Redmond JM, Chen AW, Domb BG. Greater trochanteric pain syndrome. J Am Acad Orthop Surg. 2016;24(4):231–40.
12. Ellis J, Schneider JR, Cloney M, Winfree CJ. Lateral femoral cutaneous nerve decompression guided by preoperative ultrasound mapping. Curcus. 2018;10(11): e3652.
13. Machotka Z. Anterior thigh pain. In: Bruckner & Khan's clinical sports medicine. 5th ed. Sydney: McGraw-Hill; 2017. p. 659–78.
14. Askling C, Schache A. Posterior thigh pain. In: Bruckner & Khan's clinical sports medicine. 5th ed. Sydney: McGraw-Hill; 2017. p. 679–712.
15. Gee SM, Tennent DJ, Cameron KL, Posner MA. The burden of meniscus injury in young and physically active populations. Clin Sports Med. 2020;39(1):13–27. https://doi.org/10.1016/j.csm.2019.08.008.
16. Mordecai SC, Al-Hadithy N, Ware HE, Gupte CM. Treatment of meniscal tears: an evidence based approach. World J Orthop. 2014;5(3):233–41. http://www.wjgnet.com/2218-5836/full/v5/i3/233.htm. https://doi.org/10.5312/wjo.v5.i3.233.
17. Mezhov V, Teichtahl AJ, Strasser R, Wluka AE, Cicuttini FM. Meniscal pathology-the evidence for treatment. Arthritis Res Ther. 2014;16:206.. open access http://arthritis-research.com/content/16/2/206
18. Sihvonen R, Paavola M, Malmivaara A. Finnish degenerative meniscal lesion study (FIDELITY) group, et al. arthroscopic partial meniscectomy versus sham surgery for a degenerative meniscal tear. N Engl J Med. 2013;369:2515–24.
19. Herman AM, Marzo JM. Popliteal cysts: a current review. Orthopedics. 2014;37(8):e678–84.
20. Baumbach SF, Lobo CM, Badyine I, et al. Prepatellar and olecranon bursitis: literature review and development of a treatment algorithm. Arch Orthop Trauma Surg. 2014;134(3):359–70.
21. Nakamura N, Rodeo SA, Alini M, Maher S, Madry H, Erggelet C. Physiology and pathophysiology of musculoskeletal tissues. In: Miller MD, Thompson SR, editors. Delee & Drez's orthopaedic sports medicine: principles and practice. 4th ed. Philadelphia: Elsevier; 2015. p. 3–19.
22. Mckean KA, et al. Musculoskeletal injury in the masters runners. Clin J Sport Med. 2006;16(2):149–54. https://doi.org/10.1097/00042752-200603000-00011.
23. Weishaupt D, Schweitzer ME, Morrison WB. Injuries to the distal gastrocnemius muscle: MR findings. J Comput Assist Tomogr. 2001;25:677–82. https://doi.org/10.1097/00004728-200109000-00003.
24. Douglas J, Kelly M, Blachut P. Clarification of the Simmonds–Thompson test for rupture of an Achilles tendon. Can J Surg. 2009;52(3):E40–1.
25. Ganestam A, Kallemose T, Troelsen A, Barfod KW. Increasing incidence of acute Achilles tendon rupture and a noticeable decline in surgical treatment from 1994 to 2013. A nationwide registry study of 33,160 patients. Knee Surg Sports Traumatol Arthrosc. 2015;24 (12):3730–7. https://doi.org/10.1007/s00167-015-3544-5.
26. Alves C, Mendes D, Marques FB. Fluoroquinolones and the risk of tendon injury: a systematic review and meta-

analysis. Eur J Clin Pharmacol. 2019;75(10):1431–43. https://doi.org/10.1007/s00228-019-02713-1.

27. Gravlee JR, Hatch RL, Galea AM. Achilles tendon rupture: a challenging diagnosis. J Am Board Fam Pract. 2000;13:371–3.

28. Ochen Y, Beks RB, Heijl MV, Hietbrink F, Leenen LPH, Velde DVD, et al. Operative treatment versus nonoperative treatment of Achilles tendon ruptures: systematic review and meta-analysis. BMJ. 2019;364: k5120. https://www.bmj.com/content/364/bmj.k5120.

29. Zellers JA, Christensen M, Kjær IL, Rathleff MS, Silbernagel KG. Defining components of early functional rehabilitation for acute achilles tendon rupture: a systematic review. Orthop J Sports Med. 2019;7(11):23259671 1988407. https://doi.org/10.1177/2325967119884071.

30. Lareau CR, Sawyer GA, Wang JH, DiGiovanni CW. Plantar and medial heel pain: diagnosis and management. J Am Acad Orthop Surg. 2014;22(6):372–80.

31. Monteagudo M, Albornoz PMD, Gutierrez B, Tabuenca J, Álvarez I. Plantar fasciopathy: a current concepts review. EFORT Open Rev. 2018;3(8):485–93. https://doi.org/10.1302/2058-5241.3.170080.

32. Neufeld SK, Cerrato R. Plantar fasciitis: evaluation and treatment. J Am Acad Orthop Surg. 2008;16(6):338–46.

33. Rasenberg N, Riel H, Rathleff MS, et al. Efficacy of foot orthoses for the treatment of plantar heel pain: a systematic review and meta-analysis. Br J Sports Med. 2018;52:1040–6.

34. Rathleff MS, Thorborg K. 'Load me up, Scotty': mechanotherapy for plantar fasciopathy (formerly known as plantar fasciitis). Br J Sports Med. 2015;49: 638–9.

35. Espinosa N, Brodsky JW, Maceira E. Metatarsalgia. J Am Acad Orthop Surg. 2010;18(8):474–85.

36. Dedmond BT, Cory JW, McBryde A Jr. The hallucal sesamoid complex. J Am Acad Orthop Surg. 2006;14(13):745–53.

Osteoarthritis

Natasha J. Pyzocha and Douglas M. Maurer

Contents

N. J. Pyzocha (✉)
98point6, Seattle, WA, USA

D. M. Maurer
Office of the Surgeon General Defense Health
Headquarters, Falls Church, VA, USA
e-mail: douglas.maurer4.mil@mail.mil

© Springer Nature Switzerland AG 2022
P. M. Paulman et al. (eds.), *Family Medicine*,
https://doi.org/10.1007/978-3-030-54441-6_119

General Principles

Definition/Background

Osteoarthritis (OA) is a degenerative joint disease characterized by cartilage deterioration and hypertrophy of bone. OA can present in almost any joint in the body, but the knee is the most common location to develop this condition [1]. Other common locations include the fingers, hips, and spine. OA develops when degeneration exceeds chondrocyte remodeling leading to cyst formation, further cartilage loss, and decreased joint use that further decreases the physiologic stimulation of chondrocyte activity. OA threatens patients' ability to participate in healthy physical activity, thereby predisposing them to increased cardiovascular disease, weight gain, diabetes, and potential loss of independence [2].

Epidemiology

OA is one of the most common chronic medical conditions and the most common type of arthritis [1]. In 2020, the Centers for Disease Control reported that OA affects over 32.5 million US adults [3]. Estimated costs from hospital expenditures due to joint replacement surgery in 2013 accounted for $16.5 billion, or 4.3% of the combined costs for all hospitalizations in 2013 [3]. For privately insured patients, OA was the most expensive hospitalized condition amounting to over $6.2 billion in hospital costs [3]. Risk factors include genetics, acute or recurrent trauma, advancing age, female gender, and obesity [4].

Classification

In 1981, the American College of Rheumatology (ACR) organized a subcommittee to develop criteria to better define OA [5]. The committee developed two methods of classification: traditional inclusion criteria and classification trees. A superior approach according to the ACR is using the tree model in which the appropriate tree is utilized based on patient data. Although clinical data is sufficient to diagnose OA, laboratory and radiographic data may improve sensitivities and specificities. The three joints evaluated were the knee, hip, and hands. There are several classification schemes for OA but the ACR is the most widely used.

Osteoarthritis of the Knee

Traditional inclusion criteria of the knee developed in 1989 include knee pain plus at least three of the following six clinical characteristics: greater than 50 years of age, morning stiffness for less than 30 min, crepitus on active motion of the knee, bony tenderness, bony enlargement, or no palpable warmth. Using these criteria, there is a sensitivity of 95% and specificity of 69% in diagnosing OA [5].

Knee osteoarthritis classical clinical criteria [5]

- Knee pain
- Plus at least three of the following
  - Greater than 50 years old
  - Morning stiffness for less than 30 min
  - Crepitus on active motion of the knee
  - Bony tenderness
  - Bony enlargement
  - No palpable warmth

Using the classification and regression tree technique (CART), three trees were formed for knee OA. The first tree was based on clinical features alone, clinical features with laboratory findings, and combined clinical, laboratory, and radiographic features. Sensitivities for these trees were 89%, 88%, and 94%, respectively, and specificities were 88%, 93%, and 88%, respectively [5].

Osteoarthritis of the Hip

The traditional inclusion criteria for diagnosing OA of the hip developed in 1991 include hip pain plus at least two of the following features: erythrocyte sedimentation rate (ESR) of less than 20 mm/h, radiographic osteophytes (femoral or acetabular), or joint space narrowing on radiography (superior, axial, or medial). These criteria accurately diagnose OA with a sensitivity of 89% and specificity of 91% [6].

Hip osteoarthritis classical clinical criteria [6]

- Hip pain
- Plus at least two of the following
  - Erythrocyte sedimentation rate of less than 20 mm/h
  - Radiographic osteophytes (femoral or acetabular)
  - Joint space narrowing on radiography (superior, axial, or medial)

Two classification trees were developed for the hip. The trees were made with and without radiographs. The tree that did not incorporate radiographic features included internal rotation of less than 15°, pain on internal rotation, morning stiffness, age, ESR, and flexion of less than 115°. This tree had a sensitivity and specificity of 86% and 75%, respectively. With the addition of radiographs assessing for radiographic osteophytes and axial space narrowing, the sensitivity and specificity improved to 91% and 89%, respectively [6].

Osteoarthritis of the Hands

Traditional inclusion criteria for OA of the hands developed in 1990 include hand pain (including hand aching or stiffness) plus at least three of the following: hard tissue enlargement of two or more of ten selected joints (second and third distal interphalangeal (DIP) joints, the second and third proximal interphalangeal (PIP) joints, and the first carpometacarpal (CMC) joint of both hands), enlargement of two or more DIP joints, fewer than three swollen metacarpalphalangeal (MCP) joints, and deformity of at least one of the ten selected

joints. These traditional inclusion criteria yielded a sensitivity of 94% and specificity of 87% [7].

Hand osteoarthritis classical clinical criteria [7]

- Hand pain (including hand aching or stiffness)
- Plus at least three of the following
  - Hard tissue enlargement of two or more of ten selected joints (second and third distal interphalangeal joints, second and third proximal interphalangeal joints, first carpometacarpal of both hands)
  - Hard enlargement of two or more distal interphalangeal joints
  - Fewer than three swollen metacarpophalangeal joints
  - Deformity of at least one of the ten selected joints

Classification trees with and without radiographic features were created and found to be identical in that there was no statistical difference in the inclusion criteria. The sensitivity and specificity of the two trees were 92% and 98%, respectively. As a result, hand OA is often classified by only clinical features [7].

Approach to the Patient

OA is most likely seen in the older patient with insidious onset of pain, swelling, and morning stiffness in the affected joints. History and physical exam can guide a primary care provider's suspicion for OA. Consider an alternate diagnosis in the presence of acute pain, swelling, erythema, fever, or rash. Radiologic and laboratory studies may also be necessary if an alternate diagnosis is suspected.

Diagnosis

History

OA is often diagnosed by an overall clinical picture using the patient's age, history, physical examination, and radiographic findings. No single clinical feature is absolutely sensitive or specific in making the diagnosis. Patients initially present

Table 1 X-rays for osteoarthritis [11]

Knee	Anteroposterior weight bearing, lateral, oblique
Hip/pelvis	Anteroposterior weight bearing
Spine	Anteroposterior, lateral
Hand	Anteroposterior, lateral, oblique, magnified view
Foot	Anteroposterior, lateral, oblique, magnified view

with symptoms to include pain, limited morning stiffness, and reduced function [8].

Physical Examination

Some common signs include crepitus, joint swelling, restricted movement, and bony enlargement [8]. In later stages, joint deformity may be present [8]. Erythema, fever, severe local inflammation, and progressive pain may suggest another diagnosis [8]. In the presence of an effusion, consider aspiration and fluid analysis.

Laboratory and Imaging

According to the European League for Rheumatism, three symptoms (persistent knee pain, limited morning stiffness, and reduced function) and three signs (crepitus, restricted movement, and bony enlargement) in a patient with risk factors for OA can make the diagnosis, and imaging may not be necessary. With all six of these factors present, the probability of seeing OA on a radiograph is 99% [8]. Laboratory tests and radiographs are not needed to accurately diagnose OA, but testing may rule out the likelihood of another process occurring. Radiographic findings may be misleading and disproportionately severe when compared to pain or the clinical examination.

Laboratory tests are typically normal for uncomplicated osteoarthritis. White blood cell count derived from synovial fluid would be expected to be less than 2,000 per mm^3 (2.0×10^9 per L) [9].

Radiologic abnormalities that are often present include joint space narrowing, osteophytes, and subchondral sclerosis [10]. For the evaluation of knee OA, a weight-bearing anteroposterior, lateral, and oblique views should be ordered. For

the evaluation of hip/pelvis OA, an anteroposterior weight-bearing film should be ordered. For the evaluation of spine OA, an anteroposterior and lateral film should be ordered. For the evaluation of hand OA, an anteroposterior, lateral, and oblique film should be ordered. A magnified view of the specific joint may also be beneficial. For the evaluation of foot OA, an anteroposterior, lateral, and oblique film should be ordered. A magnified view of the specific joint may also be beneficial (Table 1) [11].

Differential Diagnosis

The differential diagnosis for OA includes crystal-induced arthritis, gout, pseudogout, rheumatoid arthritis, ankylosing spondylitis, psoriatic arthritis, septic joint, osteoporosis, metastatic cancer, multiple myeloma, scleroderma, Reiter's syndrome, systemic lupus erythematosus, and Lyme disease.

Treatment

The treatment of OA is directed towards reduction of symptoms and preventing disability. To manage the symptoms of OA, patients and healthcare providers often consider multiple approaches [1]. Although there are no pharmacologic therapies that prevent the progression of joint damage due to OA, many medications may help alleviate the symptoms. The goal of therapy is to control pain and swelling, minimize disability, and improve quality of life.

Lifestyle Modifications

Nonpharmacologic treatment of OA should be the cornerstone to management and should be tried first, followed by pharmacologic augmentation to relieve pain when necessary. Symptoms of OA are typically relieved with rest; however, resting the affected joint may lead to muscle atrophy and decreased joint mobility. Rest is only recommended for a short period of time (typically 12–24 h for acute pain) after which active and passive joint motion and exercises should resume.

Alternatively, high and low intensity aerobic exercises are beneficial for improvements in functional status, pain, gait, and aerobic capacity [12]. Exercising also decreases the incidence of obesity which is strongly associated with the development of OA. The relative risk of developing knee OA in patients with a high BMI (no specific BMI) was 1.5 for men and 2.1 for women [13]. In a follow-up study using the same population, the risk of developing OA was reduced following weight loss. A 10 lb. weight loss over 10 years reduced the probability of developing knee OA by 50% [14]. Given these implications, weight loss is recommended to help treat and prevent worsening of OA.

Medications

Topical Medications

Topical NSAIDs or capsaicin can be used as treatment in patients with mild disease, who cannot tolerate oral agents, have contraindications to oral agents, or those that may have an increased risk of adverse side effects. Topical NSAIDs can sometimes provide only modest or short-lived benefit and capsaicin may cause local irritation. There are no trials that directly compare topical therapies. Topical NSAIDs may be helpful for the treatment of OA of the hand or knee [15]. Capsaicin has shown mild to moderate efficacy in randomized trials in hand and knee OA in comparison with placebo [16].

Acetaminophen and Anti-Inflammatories

Oral medications are often the mainstay treatment used to treat OA [1]. Acetaminophen is no longer considered first line for OA as evidence has shown that nonsteroidal anti-inflammatory drugs (NSAIDs) are superior for improving knee and hip OA (15). There are certain subsets of patients where acetaminophen may be considered over NSAIDs to include patients older than 65 years and those with an increased bleeding risk. Acetaminophen, if chosen, should be started initially on an as-needed basis, but in patients with persistent symptoms, regular use may be initiated at doses up to 4 g/day [17]. Acetaminophen is generally safe but hepatotoxicity can occur at high doses, especially in patients who concurrently are at risk for hepatic function impairment due to lifestyle choices, polypharmacy, or underlying pathophysiology. In patients who take acetaminophen on a chronic daily basis, consider laboratory testing to assess for hepatotoxicity.

Nonsteroidal anti-inflammatory drugs work by preventing inflammation and controlling pain by blocking cyclooxygenase (COX-1 and COX-2 enzymes) [1]. The side effect profile of NSAIDs is not always favorable, and each year, more than 100,000 patients are hospitalized for gastrointestinal complications resulting from NSAID use with 15% of these patients dying from these complications [1]. NSAIDs should be avoided in patients with prior gastrointestinal ulcers or bleeding and in patients who are taking anticoagulants [18]. Inhibition of the COX-1 enzyme is responsible for the associated gastrointestinal toxicity [18]. In addition, NSAIDs are limited in patients with cardiovascular and renal complications. The choice of an NSAID is based upon a variety of factors, and there is no convincing evidence that any of the available NSAIDs are more effective than any other for OA of the knee or hip [19]. A short to medium acting NSAID is generally used on an episodic basis in patients with non-inflammatory OA. In inflammatory OA, longer therapy at a higher dosage may be required to control symptoms. If one NSAID is not effective after 2–4 weeks on a maximal dosage, then consider the use of a different NSAID. Aim to use NSAIDs on an as needed basis at the lowest dose required to control the patient's symptoms. COX-2 inhibitors were developed to provide relief of pain without associated gastrointestinal complications; however, COX-2 inhibitors have a similar risk of serious adverse gastrointestinal effects as other NSAIDs in long-term users [18]. Chronic use of COX-2 inhibitors has also been associated with an increased cardiovascular risk [18]. Consider treating gastrointestinal symptoms associated with NSAID use with antacids, H2 blockers, or preferably proton pump inhibitors. In patients being treated chronically with daily NSAIDs, consider obtaining a complete blood count, blood urea nitrogen, creatinine, and aspartate aminotransferase.

Intra-Articular Injections

Intra-articular injections are common treatments for OA patients with moderate to severe pain that is not adequately controlled by oral medications. Clinical evidence suggests that the benefit is short lived, and usually patients report symptoms returning after 1–4 weeks [20]. Corticosteroids are proven to be effective at reducing pain in knee OA, although duration and efficacy of these treatments is controversial [2]. Corticosteroids decrease pain by roughly one third, but provide that benefit for only approximately 1 week [2, 20]. A dose equivalent to 50 mg of prednisone may be required to show benefit at 16–24 weeks [20]. The ACR suggests that a dose of 40 mg triamcinolone be used for injections to provide adequate pain relief [20]. Triamcinolone appears to be more efficacious than either methylprednisolone or betamethasone [2]. There is concern that long-term treatment could promote joint destruction and tissue atrophy; however, studies tend to suggest that changes are more likely due to the underlying disease than the steroid injection [20]. It is recommended that the same joint not be treated more than four times a year. Intra-articular glucocorticoid injections are generally well-tolerated and septic arthritis is rare.

Hyaluronic acid is a secondary medication option for intra-articular injections. In long-term studies of patients with symptomatic hip degenerative joint disease, however, intra-articular injection of hyaluronic acid was no better than placebo [21]. In a Cochrane review, hyaluronic acid and hylan products were found to be superior to placebo in efficacy; however, the sample size was small and many different types of viscosupplementation were used. The study found beneficial effects on pain, function, and patient global assessment especially at the 5- and 13-week postinjection period. In some analyses, viscosupplements were comparable in efficacy to systemic forms of treatment but with more local reactions and fewer systemic side effects [22]. The use of these medications remains controversial.

Opioids

In patients with significant OA symptoms not adequately treated with acetaminophen, NSAIDs, or joint injections, a low potency opioid analgesic may be considered. Tramadol is a weak opioid that does not produce gastrointestinal bleeding or renal problems. A Cochrane review showed that tramadol or tramadol/paracetamol decreased pain intensity, produced symptom relief, and improved function, but these benefits were small [23]. Adverse events were not shown to be life threatening, and the drug may have had some synergistic effect with acetaminophen [23]. It is recommended not to use nontramadol opiates due to the increased risk for adverse events [24].

Other Pharmacologic Options

In patients with OA in multiple joints, who may not be able to tolerate NSAIDs, or who have not responded satisfactorily to other interventions, duloxetine can be considered. Duloxetine works on desensitizing central nociceptive processing through selective inhibition of serotonin and norepinephrine uptake. At doses of 60 to 120 mg daily, duloxetine was found to have a relative risk of 30 and 50% improvement in pain intensity of 1.49 (95% CI 1.31–1.70) and 1.69 (95% CI 1.27–2.25), respectively, for knee OA compared to placebo after 10 to 13 weeks of treatment [25]. Medication side effects included constipation, diarrhea, dizziness, dry mouth, fatigue, and somnolence. Gabapentin at a dose of 600 mg daily similarly was shown to reduce pain and improve functional status in patients with knee OA but this medication took longer than traditional therapy to work, around 3 months [26]. It had similar side effects to the duloxetine.

In patients with moderate to severe OA of the hip or knee and inadequate response to standard therapy, tanezumab was shown to significantly reduce pain and improve function in comparison to placebo but there was also an increase in total joint replacements following treatment [27]. As a monoclonal antibody which inhibits nerve growth factor binding and reduces pain hypersensitivity, further research is needed to determine the clinical significance of its efficacy and adverse effect profile.

Referrals

Consider referring patients for assistive devices or braces if patients have restrictions of their activities of daily living. Occupational therapy may be helpful for hand-related or specific work issues. Physical therapy may be helpful for all other patients with the exception of hip osteoarthritis. A recent study in 2014 showed that physical therapy was no more effective than sham therapy in reducing pain and improving function in adults with hip osteoarthritis [28].

Complementary and Alternative Therapy

Controversy exists about the effectiveness of glucosamine, chondritin, vitamin D, diacerein, avocado soybean unsaponifiables, and fish oil. In some studies, glucosamine was found to reduce the pain of moderate to severe OA of the knee to improve function and slow the progression of joint space narrowing with an onset of benefit at 4 weeks [29, 30]. A Cochrane review found that some formulations of glucosamine (as a Rotta brand pharmaceutical preparation) were effective in improving OA symptoms but non-Rotta preparations were shown to be ineffective [29]. Due to clear lack of evidence, this should not be routinely recommended.

Other complementary therapies such as curcumin, *Boswellia serrata,* ultrasound therapy, acupuncture, magnet therapy, ginger, leaches, laser light therapy, platelet-rich plasma, dextrose prolotherapy, tai chi, balneotherapy, autologous chondrocyte implantation, and ice massage may be helpful in treating OA but there is limited evidence [31–43].

Surgical Options

Surgical options are often last-line therapy for OA. Joint replacement should be considered for patients with restriction of joint mobility, weekly exertion-induced pain that restricts exercising, or severe OA; however, the final treatment decision should be made individually [44]. Arthroscopy with arthroscopic debridement and lavage is not an effective treatment for OA of the knee [45]. In one randomized control trial (RCT), arthroscopic surgery plus medical and physical therapy was no more effective than medical and physical therapy alone [46]. Obese patients with BMI >30 are no longer considered as great a risk of hardware failure after total joint replacement as previously thought [44].

Special consideration and optimization of medical therapy should be considered prior to surgical options. Refer to an orthopedic surgeon if pain persists despite continued medical management.

Patient Education and Activation

Patients should be educated on this chronic condition that worsens over time. They should know common symptoms of OA and those symptoms that may lead to a different etiology. Patients should try to control pain primarily with oral medications and may need to escalate care depending on the severity of their symptoms. They should be given references on where to obtain more information.

Prognosis

Further degeneration of the joint is likely to progress with aging. Obesity and weight gain will lead to further stress and destruction of the joint. Progression is most strongly associated with age, joint space width, femoral head migration, femoral osteophytes, bony sclerosis, Kellgren/Lawrence hip grade 3 (x-rays with moderate multiple osteophytes, definite narrowing of joint space, some sclerosis, and possible deformity of the bone contour), baseline hip pain, and Lequesne index score ≥ 10 (a scoring system developed to assess severity of OA, ≥ 10 is considered severe) [47].

References

1. Najm WI, Reinsch S, Hoehler F, Tobis JS, Harvey PW. S-adenosyl methionine (SAMe) versus celecoxib for the treatment of osteoarthritis symptoms: a double-blind cross-over trial. BMC Musculoskelet Disord. 2004;5:6.
2. Hepper CT, Halvorson JJ, Duncan ST, et al. The efficacy and duration of intra-articular corticosteroid injection for knee osteoarthritis: a systematic review of level I studies. J Am Acad Orthop Surg. 2009;17:638–46.
3. Osteoarthritis. Atlanta (GA): Centers for Disease Control and Prevention; 2014. http://www.cdc.gov/arthritis/data_statistics/cost.htm. Accessed 17 Mar 2020.
4. Evangelou E, Chapman K, Meulenbelt I, et al. Large-scale analysis of association between GDF5 and FRZB variants and osteoarthritis of the hip, knee, and hand. Arthritis Rheum. 2009;60:1710–21.
5. Altman R, Asch E, Bloch D, Bole G, Borenstein D, Brandt K, Christy W, Cooke TD, Greenwald R, Hochberg M. Development of criteria for the classification and reporting of osteoarthritis. Arthritis Rheum. 1986;29(8):1039.
6. Altman R, Alarcón G, Appelrouth D, Bloch D, Borenstein D, Brandt K, Brown C, Cooke TD, Daniel W, Feldman D. The American College of Rheumatology criteria for the classification and reporting of osteoarthritis of the hip. Arthritis Rheum. 1991;34(5):505.
7. Altman R, Alarcón G, Appelrouth D, Bloch D, Borenstein D, Brandt K, Brown C, Cooke TD, Daniel W, Gray R. The American College of Rheumatology criteria for the classification and reporting of osteoarthritis of the hand. Arthritis Rheum. 1990;33(11):1601.
8. Zhang W, Doherty M, Peat G, et al. EULAR evidence-based recommendations for the diagnosis of knee osteoarthritis. Ann Rheum Dis. 2010;69:483–9.
9. Manek NJ, Lane NE. Osteoarthritis: current concepts in diagnosis and management. Am Fam Physician. 2000;61(6):1795–804.
10. McAlindon T, LaValley M, Schneider E, et al. Effect of vitamin D supplementation on progression of knee pain and cartilage volume loss in patients with symptomatic osteoarthritis: a randomized controlled trial. JAMA. 2013;309:155–62.
11. Swagerty DL, Hellinger D. Radiographic assessment of osteoarthritis. Am Fam Physician. 2001;64(2):279–87.
12. Bosomworth NJ. Exercise and knee osteoarthritis: benefit or hazard? Can Fam Physician. 2009;55:871–8.
13. Felson DT, Anderson JJ, Naimark A, Wlaker AM, Meenan RF. Obesity and knee osteoarthritis. The Framingham study. Ann Intern Med. 1988;109(1):18.
14. Felson DT, Zhang Y, Anthony JM, Naimark A, Anderson JJ. Weight loss reduces the risk for symptomatic knee osteoarthritis in women. The Framingham study. Ann Intern Med. 1992;116(7):535.
15. Derry S, Moore RA, Rabbie R. Topical NSAIDs for chronic musculoskeletal pain in adults. Cochrane Database Syst Rev. 2012;9:CD007400. https://doi.org/10.1002/14651858. CD007400.pub2
16. Deal CL, Schnitzer TJ, Lipstein E, Seibold JR, Stevens RM, Levy MD, Albert D, Renold F. Treatment of arthritis with topical capsaicin: a double-blind trail. Clin Ther. 1991;13(3):383.
17. Brandt KD, Bradley JD. Should the initial drug be used to treat osteoarthritis pain be a nonsteroidal anti-inflammatory drug? J Rheumatol. 2001;28:467–73.
18. Deeks JJ, Smith LA, Bradley MD. Efficacy, tolerability, and upper gastrointestinal safety of celecoxib for treatment of osteoarthritis and rheumatoid arthritis: systematic review of randomised controlled trials. BMJ. 2002;325:619–23.
19. Watson MC. Non-aspirin, non-steroidal anti-inflammatory drugs for osteoarthritis of the knee. Cochrane Database Syst Rev. 2000;1:CD000142. https://doi.org/10.1002/14651858. CD000142.pub2
20. Arroll B, Goodyear-Smith F. Corticosteroid injections for osteoarthritis of the knee: meta-analysis. BMJ. 2004;328:869–70.
21. Richette P, Ravaud P, Conrozier T, et al. Effect of hyaluronic acid in symptomatic hip osteoarthritis: a multicenter, randomized, placebo-controlled trial. Arthritis Rheum. 2009;60:824–30.
22. Bellamy N, Campbell J, Welch V, Gee TL, Bourne R, Wells GA. Viscosupplementation for the treatment of osteoarthritis of the knee. Cochrane Database Syst Rev. 2006;2:CD005321. https://doi.org/10.1002/14651858. CD005321.pub2
23. Cepeda MS, Camargo F, Zea C, Valencia L. Tramadol for osteoarthritis. Cochrane Database Syst Rev. 2007;1:CD005522. https://doi.org/10.1002/14651858. CD005522.pub2
24. Nuesch E, Rutjes AWS, Husni E, Welch V, Juni P, Nuesch E. Oral or transdermal opioids for osteoarthritis of the knee or hip. Cochrane Database Syst Rev. 2010;1:CD003115. https://doi.org/10.1002/14651858. CD003115.pub4

25. Wang ZY, SHI S, Li SJ, Chen F, Chen H, Lin HZ, Lin JM. Efficacy and safety of duloxetine on osteoarthritis knee pain: a meta-analysis of randomized controlled trials. Pain Med. 2015;16(7):1373.

26. Enteshari-Moghaddam A, Azami A, Isazadehfar K, Mohebbi H, Habibzadeh A, Jahanpanah P. Efficacy of duloxetine and gabapentin in pain reduction in patients with knee osteoarthritis. Clin Rheumatol. 2019;38 (10):2873–80.

27. Schnitzer TJ, Easton R, Pang S. Effect of Tanezumab on joint pain, physical function, and patient global assessment of osteoarthritis among patients with osteoarthritis of the hip or knee. JAMA. 2019;322 (1):37–48.

28. Bennell KL, Egerton T, Martin J, et al. Effect of physical therapy on pain and function in patients with hip osteoarthritis. A randomized clinical trial. JAMA. 2014;311(19):1987–97.

29. Towheed TE, Maxwell L, Anastassiades TP, et al. Glucosamine therapy for treating osteoarthritis. Cochrane Database Syst Rev. 2007;4:CD002926. https://doi.org/10.1002/14651858. CD002946.pub2

30. Pavelka K, Gatterova J, Olejarova M, Machacek S, Giacovelli G, Rovati LC. Glucosamine sulfate use and delay of progression of knee osteoarthritis: a 3-year, randomized, placebo-controlled, double-blind study. Arch Intern Med. 2002;162:2113–23.

31. McAlindon TE, LaValley MP, Gulin JP, Felson DT. Glucosamine and chondroitin for treatment of osteoarthritis: a systematic quality assessment and meta-analysis. JAMA. 2000;283:1469–75.

32. Rutjes AWS, Nuesch E, Sterchi R, Juni P. Therapeutic ultrasound for osteoarthritis of the knee or hip. Cochrane Database Syst Rev. 2010;1:CD003132. https://doi.org/10.1002/14651858. CD003132.pub2

33. Berman BM, Lao L, Langenberg P, Lee WL, Gilpin AM, Hochberg MC. Effectiveness of acupuncture as adjunctive therapy in osteoarthritis of the knee: a randomized, controlled trial. Ann Intern Med. 2004;141:901–10.

34. Wolsko PM, Eisenberg DM, Simon LS, et al. Double-blind placebo-controlled trial of static magnets for the treatment of osteoarthritis of the knee: results of a pilot study. Altern Ther Health Med. 2004;10:36–43.

35. Altman RD, Marcussen KC. Effects of a ginger extract on knee pain in patients with osteoarthritis. Arthritis Rheum. 2001;44:2531–8.

36. Bandolier. Avocado/soybean unsaponifiables for OA. 2004. Available from http://www.jr2.ox.ac.uk.offcampus.lib.washington.edu/bandolier/band122/b122-3.html

37. Andereya S, Stanzel S, Maus U, et al. Assessment of leech therapy for knee osteoarthritis: a randomized study. Acta Orthop. 2008;79:235–43.

38. Brosseau L, Welch V, Wells GA, de Bie R, Gam A, Harman K, Morin M, Shea B, Tugwell P. Low level laser therapy (classes III) for treating osteoarthritis. Cochrane Database Syst Rev. 2007;1:CD002056. https://doi.org/10.1002/14651858. CD002046.pub3

39. Khoshbin A, Leroux T, Wasserstein D, Marks P, Theodoropoulos J, Ogilvie-Harris D, Gandhi R, Takhar K, Lum G, Chahal J. The efficacy of platelet-rich plasma in the treatment of symptomatic knee osteoarthritis: a systematic review with quantitative synthesis. Arthroscopy. 2013;29: 2037–48.

40. Rabago D, Patterson JJ, Mundt M, Kijowski R, Grettie J, Segal NA, Zgierska A. Dextrose prolotherapy for knee osteoarthritis: a randomized controlled trial. Ann Fam Med. 2013;11:229–37.

41. Song R, Lee EO, Lam P, Bae SC. Effects of tai chi exercise on pain, balance, muscle strength, and perceived difficulties in physical functioning in older women with osteoarthritis: a randomized clinical trial. J Rheumatol. 2003;30:2039–44.

42. Verhagen AP, Bierma-Zeinstra SMA, Boers M, Cardoso JR, Lambeck J, de Bie R, de Vet HCW. Balneotherapy for osteoarthritis. Cochrane Database Syst Rev. 2009;2:CD006864. https://doi.org/10.1002/14651858. CD00684.pub4

43. Brosseau L, Yonge KA, Robinson V, Marchand S, Judd M, Wells G, Tugwell P. Thermotherapy for treatment of osteoarthritis. Cochrane Database Syst Rev. 2007;1:CD004522. https://doi.org/10.1002/14651858. CD004522.pub4

44. Brouwer RW, Jakma TSC, Verhagen AP, Verhaar JAN, Bierma-Zeinstra SMA. Braces and orthoses for treating osteoarthritis of the knee. Cochrane Database Syst Rev. 2007;1:CD004020. https://doi.org/10.1002/14651858. CD004020.pub2

45. Moseley JB, O'Malley K, Petersen NJ, et al. A controlled trial of arthroscopic surgery for osteoarthritis of the knee. N Engl J Med. 2002;347:81–8.

46. Kirkley A, Birmingham TB, Litchfield RB, et al. A randomized trial of arthroscopic surgery for osteoarthritis of the knee. N Engl J Med. 2008;359: 1097–107.

47. Wright AA, Cook C, Abbott JH. Variables associated with the progression of hip osteoarthritis: a systematic review. Arthritis Rheum. 2009;61:925–36.

Scott G. Garland and Nathan P. Falk

Contents

S. G. Garland (✉) · N. P. Falk (✉)
Florida State University College of Medicine Family
Medicine Residency at BayCare Health System, Winter
Haven, FL, USA
e-mail: scott.garland@baycarc.org;
nathan.falk@med.fsu.edu

© Springer Nature Switzerland AG 2022
P. M. Paulman et al. (eds.), *Family Medicine*,
https://doi.org/10.1007/978-3-030-54441-6_120

Joint pain is a common complaint in primary care. Pain can be considered acute (days), subacute (weeks), or chronic (generally lasting more than 3 months). Accurately diagnosing the cause of joint pain, encouraging continuity of care, and working with multidisciplinary teams using the right blend of therapeutic modalities give patients the best chance for good long-term outcomes. This chapter will focus, in particular, on diseases that commonly present with joint pain.

Differential Diagnosis of Joint Pain

Step 1: A Thorough Medical History

The key step in diagnosing any of the arthritides is a careful history. By definition, arthritis is acute or chronic inflammation of a joint often accompanied by swelling, erythema, and warmth within any individual joint. Most commonly, arthritis presents with some degree of joint pain. A careful medical history allows for determination of inflammatory and mechanical (degenerative) joint disease.

The history should pinpoint the exact location of the pain. Is the problem limited to one joint (monoarticular), several joints (oligoarticular), or many joints (polyarticular)? Is the problem limited to small joints, large joints, or both? Is the pain truly within the joint? If the pain surrounds the joint (periarticular), this leads to suspicion for soft tissue inflammatory conditions (tendinopathy, bursopathy, enthesopathy). If the pain is more diffuse, systemic disorders come to mind. Is the pain symmetric? Rheumatoid arthritis, systemic lupus erythematosus, polymyositis, Sjögren's syndrome, and scleroderma are commonly polyarticular and symmetric. Other conditions that tend to be polyarticular and asymmetric include psoriatic arthritis, ankylosing spondylitis, and other spondyloarthropathies. Joint stiffness, reduced joint range of motion, swelling, constitutional symptoms (fever, chills, sweats, weight loss), local or generalized weakness, a history of trauma or injury, and the presence of fatigue are other important elements of the medical history. It is important to also define exacerbating and alleviating factors as well as the extent, timing, and waxing/waning nature of symptoms.

The history will help determine to what degree joint complaints are associated with rest and physical activity. Symptoms that are exacerbated by physical activity suggest a mechanical component (particularly when combined with locking or a "give-way" sensation). Morning stiffness describes joint stiffness after a period of generalized inactivity (e.g., overnight sleep). While many individuals can be "slow to get going" in the morning, stiffness lasting for more than an hour is not normal and suggests a systemic inflammatory disease. Patients with degenerative disease, such as osteoarthritis, will more commonly complain of stiffness as the day progresses. Non-inflammatory joint pain typically increases with physical activity. Other historical features supporting an inflammatory component to the joint pain include midday fatigue and joint swelling. A sleep history is important as many patients describe significant interruptions to their sleep habits associated with many of the arthritides. Assessing activities of daily living provides good insight into functional limitations. Asking about tasks such as standing from a chair without assistance, showering, washing, or combing hair and the ability to climb stairs is helpful. Determining how the pain has limited the patient's overall ability to function helps to establish a baseline and determine realistic treatment goals. A thorough past medical, surgical, travel, and occupational history provides additional clues into the source and etiology of the joint pain.

Step 2: Physical Examination

Everyone presenting with joint pain should have a thorough physical examination that focuses on the musculoskeletal system while looking for systemic clues in all major organ systems such as the skin. The vital signs should be reviewed. A general physical exam can provide clues to systemic illness. Skin lesions, organomegaly, lymphadenopathy, pulmonary or cardiac auscultatory changes, and neurological findings all point to different etiologies of joint pain. Observe the patient's gait. Look for obvious deformities or muscular atrophy. Palpate individual joints for synovial thickening, fluctuance, or laxity. Note passive and active ranges of motion, particularly of the affected joints. Passive range of motion (ROM) is often greater than active ROM in arthritic joints. Test strength and sensation. An accurate documentation of the physical examination, particularly the musculoskeletal exam, is time-consuming but is important to assess changes over time. Utilize any electronic medical record system embedded templates if available. Formal dynamometry can be used to track changes in strength over time (e.g., grip strength).

A thorough history and physical examination should lead (in most cases) to a short list of diagnostic possibilities. Based on the history and examination, laboratory and radiographic studies help pinpoint the final diagnosis and guide appropriate treatment.

Rheumatoid Arthritis (RA)

Background and Pathophysiology

Rheumatoid arthritis (RA) is a chronic, systemic, inflammatory disease that affects synovial joints in a symmetric distribution. In most patients without proper therapy, RA is chronic and progressive. Early diagnosis and treatment is important to improve long-term outcomes and potential remission. Early treatment, optimally within 12 weeks of symptom onset, with disease-modifying antirheumatic drugs (DMARDs) gives the best

chance of achieving remission [1]. RA occurs in all racial and ethnic groups and is seen more commonly in women (3:1) [2]. Prevalence estimates suggest 1.5 million US adults are affected by RA [3]. First-degree relatives have a twofold to threefold higher risk for developing RA. The disease occurs in all age groups but is more common with increasing age and peaks between the fourth and sixth decades of life. The leading cause of death in RA is cardiovascular disease, and overall mortality is 2.5 times higher in patients with RA as compared to the general population [4].

The definitive cause of RA is unknown. In susceptible individuals, an external trigger, such as infection or trauma, triggers an autoimmune cascade that results in joint inflammation, synovial hypertrophy, joint destruction, and potentially other extra-articular manifestations. A history of parental substance abuse is associated with an increased risk for developing RA in adulthood [5]. Sixty percent of patients with RA in the United States share an epitope on the HLA-DR4 cluster, suggesting some element of genetic risk [6]. Several other genes have weaker associations with RA but may contribute. Following an environmental insult, synovial cell hyperplasia and endothelial activation lead to progressive inflammation with articular damage and bony destruction. Abnormal cytokine and inflammatory mediator production along with activation of both T-cell and B-cell lineages contribute to the pathophysiology of RA. The proliferation of synovial cells and subsynovial vessels leads to synovial proliferation, pannus formation, and articular destruction.

Clinical Presentation

The hallmark presentation of RA involves a persistent, symmetric small joint polyarthritis of the hands, wrists, and feet. In decreasing frequency, the knee, shoulder, ankle, cervical spine, hip, and elbow can also be involved (as can, theoretically, any synovial joint). Most patients have an insidious onset over weeks to months. Morning stiffness is common, and patients report increasing difficulty with routine activities of daily living such as personal hygiene, dressing, and combing their hair. Constitutional symptoms (low-grade fever, malaise, fatigue) are common as well. Large joints often become symptomatic later in the course of the disease. The small joints of the hands and feet should be carefully examined for swelling, warmth, tenderness, and changes in range of motion (ROM). Interosseous muscular atrophy is a common early finding. With progressive joint destruction, characteristic joint deformities (such as boutonniere, swan neck, ulnar deviation, or hammertoe) develop. Rheumatoid nodules can develop particularly along the extensor surface of the ulna. Knee effusions are relatively common in RA and may contribute to progressive muscular atrophy of the quadriceps with resulting instability. The hips and cervical spine are also commonly involved in RA. Atlantoaxial instability is more common in patients with early and severe arthritis of the hands and in those on high doses of corticosteroids.

Because RA is a systemic inflammatory process, most patients will exhibit extra-articular manifestations of the disease. Malaise and fatigue are the most common systemic symptoms. Rheumatoid nodules occur in 25% of RA patients. Cardiovascular disease is more prevalent in RA patients. RA is also associated with pericardial effusions, pericarditis, myocarditis, and coronary arteritis. Hematologic malignancies such as non--Hodgkin's lymphoma are more common in patients with RA. Pulmonary complications include pleural effusions, pulmonary fibrosis, nodular lung disease, and bronchiolitis obliterans. RA is also associated with secondary Sjögren's syndrome.

Diagnosis

The diagnosis of RA is based upon the combination of clinical, laboratory, and radiographic findings. In 2010, the American College of Rheumatology (ACR)/European League Against Rheumatism (EULAR) developed classification criteria to assist in the early detection of RA [7]. This classification represents an update to the 1987 ACR classification criteria as an attempt to better identify patients early in the course of the

Table 1 2010 ACR-EULAR classification criteria for rheumatoid arthritis [7]

	Score
A summative score of 6/10 from elements A through D is consistent with RA	
(A) Joint involvement	
1 large joint	0
2–10 large joints	1
1–3 small joints (with or without involvement of large joints)	2
4–10 small joints (with or without involvement of large joints)	3
>10 joints (at least 1 small joint)	5
(B) Serology (at least 1 test result is needed for classification)	
Negative RF and negative ACPA	0
Low-positive RF or low-positive ACPA	2
High-positive RF or high-positive ACPA	3
(C) Acute phase reactants (at least 1 test result is needed for classification)	
Normal CRP and normal ESR	0
Abnormal CRP or abnormal ESR	1
(D) Duration of symptoms	
<6 weeks	0
6 weeks	1

disease and initiate effective treatment. According to the ACR/EULAR guidelines, patients who have one joint with definitive synovitis that is not explained by another disease process should be tested for RA (Table 1).

Laboratory and Imaging Studies

Selected laboratory tests, undertaken after a careful history and physical examination, can help confirm the diagnosis of RA. The erythrocyte sedimentation rate (ESR) and C-reactive protein (CRP) levels are markers of inflammation. Both are typically elevated in RA. CRP also corresponds over time to radiographic progression of RA. Common complete blood count (CBC) findings associated with RA include an anemia of chronic disease (normochromic, normocytic) and thrombocytosis. Autoantibodies, including rheumatoid factor (RF), antinuclear antibody (ANA), and anticitrullinated protein antibodies (ACPA; tested commonly as anti-CCP), are normally the most helpful laboratory tests to aid in the diagnosis of RA. Anti-CCP antibodies have a sensitivity and specificity equal to (or better than) RF for the diagnosis of RA [8]. Patients without RA but who have elevated anti-CCP levels may be at risk of progression to RA [9]. The presence of both anti-CCP and RF is highly specific for the diagnosis of rheumatoid arthritis. As with RF, the presence of anti-CCP antibodies indicates a worse disease prognosis.

Plain radiographs are the preferred initial images in RA. Plain films can show erosions and can be followed serially to mark disease progression. Magnetic resonance imaging (MRI) provides more accuracy and allows for earlier detection of joint changes. MRI is much more costly and is typically used to assess abnormalities of the cervical spine. While ultrasonography is rapidly growing in use for musculoskeletal imaging, its role in RA is evolving. Ultrasound can identify joint effusions in deep joints such as the hip or shoulder and can identify synovial vascularization. As an office-based technology, ultrasonography offers promise in the evolving care for RA patients [10].

Treatment

Successful treatment of RA includes a multidisciplinary, interprofessional team employing a variety of modalities including diet, exercise, stress management, physical therapy, behavioral health, medications, and (potentially) surgery. Patient-centered care focusing on specific treatment goals, patient and family education, and long-term expectations facilitates success.

Nonpharmacologic Treatment

Multiple nonpharmacologic modalities are available to help relieve pain, improve function, and maintain (or enhance) strength and range of motion in patients with RA. The application of heat is effective to relieve pain and stiffness. Hot packs, paraffin baths, ultrasonography, and other modalities may provide relief and also help to prepare affected joints for range of motion and strengthening exercises. Orthotic devices and splints also play an important

role in managing patients with RA. These devices can reduce pain, enhance function, reduce deformity, and provide proper mechanical joint alignment. Since most RA patients complain of fatigue and reduced cardiorespiratory endurance, a program of therapeutic exercise is important to maintain aerobic capacity and muscular strength. Involving occupational therapists, physical therapists, and exercise scientists can help provide individualized programs of splinting and exercise prescription to optimize physical function while mitigating the risk of injury.

Pharmacologic Therapy

Multiple medication options exist for the treatment of RA. These options include nonsteroidal anti-inflammatory drugs (NSAIDs) and disease-modifying antirheumatic drugs (DMARDs) including biologics, corticosteroids, and non-biologic agents. Selecting the right therapy for the right patient to optimize outcome while minimizing toxicity can be challenging. Therapy with DMARDs should utilize a treat-to-target approach with a goal to reduce disease activity by 50% within 3 months and achieve remission or low disease activity within 6 months [6]. If initial DMARD therapy has not reached target, then alternative therapy should be considered.

NSAIDs and Corticosteroids

NSAIDs and corticosteroids are typically used to provide pain relief and reduce inflammation as a "bridge" for the 3–6 months before DMARD therapy takes effect [11]. NSAIDs do not alter or slow joint destruction and are insufficient monotherapy for RA.

DMARDs

Once the diagnosis of RA has been made, the goal is to control the disease activity, slow joint damage, provide symptomatic relief, and improve overall patient function. The DMARDs and biologic agents are most effective in accomplishing these goals. Vaccination requirements should be administered for patients who are being considered for therapy with DMARD or biologic therapy. The recommendations vary slightly depending on the drug being considered. It should be noted that while patients on prednisone and other immunosuppressive agents can and should receive inactivated vaccines, their protective antibody response might be blunted. Every patient should be screened for hepatitis B and hepatitis C infections or latent tuberculosis before starting DMARD or biologic therapy as the therapies may reactivate the disease.

DMARDs can be classified as biologic and nonbiologic agents. Common nonbiologic DMARDS include hydroxychloroquine (HCQ), sulfasalazine (SSA), azathioprine (AZA), methotrexate (MTX), and leflunomide. For treating RA, MTX and SSZ are generally recognized to be the most active with the best risk-benefit ratios. MTX is typically used alone, or in combination with other medications, for moderate to severe RA and can be administered either orally or subcutaneously. The biologic DMARDS include five tumor necrosis factor alpha (TNF-α) inhibitors: etanercept, infliximab, golimumab, certolizumab, and adalimumab. Biologic DMARDs are typically reserved for use when nonbiologic DMARD (e.g., MTX) has not induced a remission or as initial therapy if a patient has many poor prognostic indicators to include erosive disease, positive serological markers, and extra-articular manifestations. Patients on anti-TNF-α therapy should avoid live viral vaccines.

Other non-TNF biologic DMARDs are available. These include rituximab (most often used in combination with MTX), anakinra, abatacept, tofacitinib, baricitinib, and tocilizumab. Recent guidelines have been published to guide changes in medication doses, combinations, and switching agents [11] (Table 2).

Surgery

Surgery can provide pain relief, correct deformities, and improve function. Joint fusions, joint replacement, myofascial release, and other techniques are based on patient age, joint(s) involved, functional disability, and disease stage. Patients with cervical spine instability and refractory pain or neurological compromise are candidates for surgical intervention as well.

Clinical Course and Disease Activity

2011 ACR/EULAR guidelines provide separate definitions of remission of RA for use in clinical trials and clinical practice [12]. Disease activity can be measured in clinical practice with a Boolean-based method or with the Simplified Disease Activity Index (SDAI). Remission with the Boolean-based method requires patients to meet all of the following: (a) tender joint count ≤1; (b) swollen joint count ≤1; (c) CRP ≤1 mg/dL; and (d) patient global assessment ≤1 (based on a 0–10 scale survey). Remission categorized by SDAI requires patients to have a score of ≤3.3 which includes the following: simple sum of the tender joint count (using 28 joints), swollen joint count (using 28 joints), patient global assessment (0–10 scale), physician global assessment (0–10 scale), and low CRP levels. To assess progression, patients are generally categorized into four stages: I (early RA), II (moderate progression), III (severe progression), and IV (terminal progression). Similar scales are available to quantify patients' functional capacity: Class I, able to perform activities of daily living; Class II, able to perform self-care and vocational activities, limited in other activities; Class III, able to perform self-care but limited in vocational activities; and Class IV, limited in ability to perform self-care. Using established scales and scoring criteria allows for clear communication between patients and multiple members of the healthcare team to determine the best treatment strategies for each individual patient.

Differentiating Rheumatoid Arthritis from Osteoarthritis

RA and OA are both relatively common clinical conditions. Since the treatment is different, early recognition and differentiation of the two conditions are clinically important. Patients with RA typically complain of morning stiffness, whereas the pain associated with OA increases through the

Table 2 Indications for initiating and switching DMARDs [11]

Disease activity	Recommendation
Early RA (<6 months)	Provide DMARD combination therapy in patients with moderate or high disease activity and poor prognostic features (functional limitation, extra-articular disease, positive RF or anti-CCP antibodies, bony erosions on X-ray)
	Use anti-TNF agent MTX in those with high disease activity and poor prognostic features – except for infliximab, which is used in combination with MTX only (i.e., do not use infliximab as monotherapy)
Established RA if prognosis is not mentioned, use or switch to a nonbiologic or biologic DMARD regardless of prognostic features	Initiating and switching among nonbiologic DMARDs In patients who deteriorate after 3 months of DMARD monotherapy from low to moderate/high disease activity, add MTX, hydroxychloroquine, or leflunomide if no poor prognostic features For patients with persistent moderate/high disease activity after 3 months of MTX or MTX-DMARD combination therapy, add or switch to a different non-MTX DMARD
	Switching from nonbiologic to biologic DMARDs In patients with persistent moderate/high disease activity after 3 months of MTX monotherapy or MTX-DMARD combination therapy, add or switch to an anti-TNF biologic agent, abatacept, or rituximab In patients with persistent moderate/high disease activity after 3 months of intensified DMARD combination therapy or after a second DMARD, add or switch to an anti-TNF biologic agent
	Switching among biologic agents because of lack or loss of benefit In patients with persistent moderate/high disease activity not benefitting after 3 months of anti-TNF biologic therapy, switch to another anti-TNF biologic agent or a non-TNF biologic agent In patients with persistent moderate/high disease activity not benefitting after 6 months of non-TNF biologic therapy, switch to another non-TNF biologic agent or an anti-TNF biologic agent
	Switching biologic agents due to adverse effects In patients with high disease activity and serious event associated with anti-TNF biologic therapy, switch to a non-TNF biologic agent In patients with moderate or high disease activity after failure of non-TNF biologic therapy because of either a serious or a non-serious adverse event, switch to another non-TNF biologic agent or an anti-TNF biologic agent

ACR American College of Rheumatology, *CCP* cyclic citrullinated peptide, *DMARD* disease-modifying antirheumatic drug, *MTX* methotrexate, *RA* rheumatoid arthritis, *RF* rheumatoid factor, *TNF* tumor necrosis factor

day and with use. The small joints of the hands and feet are symmetrically involved in RA and the distal interphalangeal joints rarely involved. OA often is less symmetric and typically impacts larger weight-bearing joints (hips, knees). However, distal and proximal interphalangeal joints of the hands are commonly symmetrically involved in OA. Soft tissue swelling and warmth are more common in RA. Plain films in RA show periarticular osteopenia and marginal erosions.

OA patients often have bony osteophytes on physical examination or radiography. Laboratory findings in OA are normal, whereas RA shows elevations of ESR and CRP along with elevations in RF, anti-CCP, and characteristic CBC changes (anemia, thrombocytosis).

Juvenile Idiopathic Arthritis

Juvenile idiopathic arthritis (JIA) has a wide range of presentations in children. JIA was formerly known as juvenile rheumatoid arthritis (JRA) and is one of the most common chronic inflammatory diseases of childhood. The etiology is unknown, and multiple subtypes exist. Evidence suggests that antibiotic exposure in childhood potentially increases individual risk for JIA [13].

The diagnosis of JIA is based on history and physical examination. Arthritis must be present for at least 6 weeks before the diagnosis of JIA can be considered definitive. Onset occurs before the age of 16. The primary complaint is joint pain (which may manifest as a limp). Children often complain of pain less than adults, however, and in such cases, there is typically cessation of normal joint use such as refusing to stand in a toddler or infant. Onset can be either insidious or abrupt. Morning stiffness is common as is the "gelling phenomenon" (stiffness after periods of rest). An evanescent rash or psoriasis is the most common dermatologic findings. Physical examination is characterized by the presence of arthritis manifested by swelling, warmth, and erythema. Synovitis is common, and children will often hold joints in a position of maximal comfort (e.g., hip in flexion, abduction, and external rotation or knee in partial flexion). Range of motion is limited depending on the degree of pain and swelling. Complications resulting from any of the subtypes of JIA include joint contractures, muscular atrophy, uveitis, and leg length discrepancies.

Clinically, the International League of Associations for Rheumatology has subdivided JIA into multiple categories [14]. These categories include systemic-onset JIA, oligoarticular JIA, polyarticular JIA, psoriatic arthritis, enthesitis-related JIA, and undifferentiated arthritis. In systemic-onset JIA, children appear systemically ill and often complain of myalgias and arthralgias. An evanescent rash of the trunk and extremities is common. Organomegaly and lymphadenopathy may occur. Complaints of chest pain or shortness of breath should raise concern for serositis and a careful examination for rubs, rales, or gallop rhythms. Complications include hemolytic anemia, pericarditis, and (rarely) macrophage activation syndrome.

In oligoarticular JIA, fewer than four (and often only one) joints are involved. Oligoarticular JIA typically impacts weight-bearing joints (knees and ankles). Affected children do not look systemically ill and often walk without a limp despite obvious joint swelling. Anterior uveitis is present in up to 20% of children with oligoarticular (and polyarticular arthritis), and slit-lamp screening is important in these subtypes to exclude ocular disease [14]. Children with polyarticular JIA have five or more joints affected. Small and large joints can be affected, and rheumatoid nodules can be seen in active disease. Children with rheumatoid nodules generally are positive for rheumatoid factor.

Psoriatic arthritis in children is typically milder in children than in adults. It is monoarticular and involves the distal interphalangeal joints in 50% of cases. Nail pitting is present in over two-thirds of cases. Enthesis-related arthritis involves inflammation of the insertion of tendons and ligaments into bone. Pain and tenderness of periarticular structures are common. Additional diagnostic criteria include sacroiliac tenderness, positive HLA-B27 antigen screening, male gender, age over 6 years, the presence of anterior uveitis, and a first-degree relative with related spondyloarthropathies. Rare complications of enthesitis-related JIA additionally include restrictive lung disease and aortic insufficiency. Children with undifferentiated arthritis often have manifestations in multiple JIA categories.

The diagnosis of JIA is clinical. There are no diagnostic laboratory studies. Laboratories are helpful to rule out other disorders, help classify the type of arthritis, and determine the presence of any extra-articular manifestations of disease. Laboratory markers are also used to follow renal or hepatic function in children on various JIA treatment regimens.

The goal of treatment in patients with JIA is to control pain, maximize function, and minimize disability [15]. Current treatment regimens are available based on the following criteria: (a) history of arthritis in four joints, (b) arthritis in five joints, (c) active sacroiliac arthritis, (d) systemic arthritis (inactive), and (e) systemic arthritis (active). The first group (four joints) generally includes patients with psoriatic arthritis, enthesitis-related arthritis, and undifferentiated arthritis. In this group, nonsteroidal anti-inflammatory drugs (NSAIDs) are often useful for monoarticular disease. Intra-articular steroids and methotrexate are the next-line agents followed by treatment with TNF-α inhibitors. For patients with disease in five joints (RF-negative/RF-positive polyarthritis, psoriatic arthritis, enthesitis-related arthritis, and undifferentiated arthritis), NSAIDs have less of a role. Methotrexate and intra-articular steroids are used more commonly. Leflunomide and IL-6 inhibitors (tocilizumab) are alternatives to methotrexate. TNF-α inhibitors are next-line therapy as is abatacept or rituximab. Patients with active sacroiliac arthritis frequently respond to TNF-α inhibitors if they fail to respond to NSAIDs and/or methotrexate.

Patients with active systemic arthritis are treated with corticosteroids after a brief (2-week) NSAID trial. For patients with systemic JIA, anakinra is effective. Tocilizumab has recently been approved for use in systemic JIA as well. Patients who have active arthritis, but no signs of active systemic disease, are treated with NSAIDs, intra-articular injections, and methotrexate. Anakinra or TNF-α is typically used as second-line therapy.

Successful management of children with JIA is best served with an interprofessional and multidisciplinary approach. In addition to rheumatology, patients often benefit from consultation with physical therapy, occupational therapy, behavioral health, and social services to help manage this complex disease.

Reactive Arthritis (Reiter's Syndrome)

Reactive arthritis (formerly known as Reiter's syndrome) is an autoimmune response to infection associated with multiple gastrointestinal (GI) and genitourinary (GU) species [16]. *Shigella* sp., *Salmonella*, *Campylobacter*, and *Chlamydia trachomatis* have been most commonly implicated, but many others have also been associated with this syndrome. Clinically, reactive arthritis typically presents with uveitis/conjunctivitis ("can't see"), noninfectious urethritis ("can't pee"), and arthritis ("can't bend my knee").

Other symptoms include malaise, fatigue, and fever. Physical findings include an asymmetric oligoarthritis that typically involves the weight-bearing joints of the lower extremity and the fingers or toes, so-called sausage digits. While conjunctivitis is the most common eye disease associated with Reiter's syndrome, more worrisome eye diseases such as scleritis, uveitis, episcleritis, and corneal ulceration may be found on ocular exam. Urethral discharge, vulvovaginitis, balanitis circinata, and cervicitis are common genitourinary findings. Although uncommon, keratoderma blennorragicum, a psoriasiform rash, may be seen on the palms and soles. Other skin and nail findings include erythema nodosum and onychodystrophy.

Reactive arthritis typically follows 2–4 weeks after an antecedent GU/GI infection. Reactive arthritis is most common in young men [17]. The frequency of reactive arthritis relates to population rates of HLA-B27. The diagnosis of reactive arthritis is based on history and physical examination. There are no specific laboratory tests. CBC, ESR, CRP, HLA-B27, HIV, tuberculin skin testing, urinalysis, and serologies/cultures (particularly for sexually transmitted infections) can rule out associated disease. There is no curative therapy for reactive arthritis. Treatment is symptomatic or targeted toward the underlying disease [18]. While NSAIDs are frequently used as initial therapy, sulfasalazine, methotrexate, and anti-TNF agents are useful second-line agents for patients with persistent symptoms and no relief from NSAIDs. Any underlying disease that is identified should be treated accordingly.

Systemic Lupus Erythematosus

Background and Pathophysiology

Systemic lupus erythematosus (SLE) is a chronic inflammatory disorder affecting multiple organ systems. SLE can impact any organ system but most commonly involves the skin, musculoskeletal system, renal system, cardiovascular system, hematopoietic system, and nervous system. While the exact cause is unknown, SLE is an autoimmune disorder that is characterized by autoantibody formation and inflammation. T cells have traditionally been implicated as playing a central role in SLE pathogenesis, but other inflammatory cells clearly are implicated. Circulating immune complexes interact with native tissues and activate complement and the inflammatory cascade. Genetic defects in lymphocyte signaling, apoptosis, and the clearance of immune complexes have been identified. Interferon regulatory factor 5 (IRF-5) genetic polymorphisms associated with SLE have been identified in different ethnic populations.

The annual incidence of SLE is roughly 5 cases per 100,000 individuals. Higher rates of SLE are reported in blacks and Hispanics. Most cases (90%) occur in women, particularly after reaching childbearing age. Male cases are described in individuals with Klinefelter syndrome (XXY), suggesting a hormonal contribution to the pathogenesis of SLE. Survival rates for SLE patients have improved markedly over the past several decades. Ten-year survival rates currently exceed 90%.

Clinical Presentation

One of the characteristic manifestations of SLE is a malar rash that spares the nasolabial folds. Other common features include other mucocutaneous abnormalities, joint pain, fever, neurological events (seizures or stroke), proteinuria/cellular casts in urine sediment/renal insufficiency, lymphadenopathy, sicca symptoms, and pleuritis. Abnormalities in hematologic indices are common as well. Clinically, the mnemonic "SOAP BRAIN MD" has been applied to the 11 ACR classification criteria for SLE (Table 3): S (serositis) O (oral ulcers) A (arthritis) P (photosensitivity) B (blood disorders) R (renal involvement) A (antinuclear antibodies) I (immunologic data dsDNA) N (neurologic findings) M (malar rash) D (discoid rash). EULAR has further defined SLE to require elevated ANA levels as an entry point for disease identification. After ANA levels are confirmed, then the diagnosis is based on a weighted score system which includes constitutional, hematologic, neuropsychiatric, mucocutaneous, serosal, musculoskeletal, renal, and immunology domains. The updated criteria have a sensitivity of 96.1% and a specificity of 93.4% for the diagnosis of SLE [19].

Fever, fatigue, and weight loss are the most common constitutional complaints in patients with SLE (new-onset or with flare of active disease). Joint pain is the most common musculoskeletal complaint, followed by myalgias and arthritis. The arthritis is typically symmetrical, and pain may be out of proportion to the degree of joint swelling. Avascular necrosis is more common in patients with SLE, especially those taking corticosteroids. Malar rash, discoid rash, and photosensitivity are the most common cutaneous features. Other associated cutaneous findings include Raynaud's phenomenon, telangiectasia, livedo reticularis, alopecia, discoid lesions, and urticarial.

CNS involvement is common in SLE. The most common are seizures, stroke, and mental status changes (psychosis). The ACR has developed case definitions for multiple neuropsychiatric syndromes associated with SLE including delirium, psychosis, or seizures [20]. Pulmonary findings associated with SLE include pleurisy, pneumonitis, interstitial lung disease, pulmonary hypertension, and an exudative pleural effusion. Corresponding physical findings would include pulmonary rubs, rales, and dullness to percussion. Complaints of chest pain in patients with SLE should not be ignored. Pericarditis is the most common cardiovascular complication of SLE. Patients with pericarditis typically complain of chest pain that is relieved by leaning forward. Pulmonary hypertension can present with progressive dyspnea.

Table 3 2019 European League Against Rheumatism/American College of Rheumatology (EULAR/ACR) classification criteria for systemic lupus erythematosus (SLE) [19]

Entry criteria				
Antinuclear antibodies (ANA) at a titer of $\geq$1:80 on HEp-2 cells or an equivalent positive test				
Additive criteria				
Clinical domain and criteria	**Weight**	**Clinical domain and criteria**		**Weight**
Constitutional		**Renal**		
Fever	2	Proteinuria >0.5 g/24 h		4
Hematologic		Renal biopsy class II or V lupus nephritis		8
Leukopenia	3	Renal biopsy class III or IV lupus nephritis		10
Thrombocytopenia	4	**Serosal**		
Autoimmune hemolysis	4	Pleural or pericardial effusion		5
Neuropsychiatric		Acute pericarditis		6
Delirium	2	**Immunology domain and criteria**		**Weight**
Psychosis	3	**Antiphospholipid antibodies**		
Seizure	5	Anti-cardiolipin antibodies OR		
Mucocutaneous		Anti-β_2GP1 antibodies OR		
Non-scarring alopecia	2	Lupus anticoagulant		2
Oral ulcers	2	**Complement proteins**		
Subacute cutaneous OR discoid lupus	4	Low C3 OR low C4		3
Acute cutaneous lupus	6	Low C3 AND low C4		4
Musculoskeletal		**SLE-specific antibodies**		
Join involvement	6	Anti-dsDNA antibody* OR		
		Anti-Smith antibody		6

To classify systemic lupus erythematous (SLE), patients must first meet the entry criteria of elevated ANA titer. Additive criteria are then added but only the highest weighted criterion per domain is counted toward the total score. SLE classification requires at least one clinical criterion and $\geq$ 10 points. Occurrence of a criterion on at least one occasion is sufficient to be counted. Criteria do not need to occur simultaneously

Anti-β_2GP1 anti- β_2-glycoprotein 1, *anti-dsDNA* anti-double-stranded DNA

Laboratory Findings

Patients with suspected SLE should have a complete blood count (with differential), basic metabolic profile (creatinine and glomerular filtration rate), and formal urinalysis (microscopy). The CBC may reveal leukopenia, anemia, lymphopenia, and/or thrombocytopenia. Abnormalities in urine sediment may include proteinuria or casts. The metabolic profile examines renal function (changes in glomerular filtration rate), looking for signs of lupus nephritis. Erythrocyte sedimentation rates and C-reactive protein levels are often elevated in SLE. Complement protein levels (C3, C4, and CH50) are commonly depressed consumption in active lupus nephritis.

There are multiple autoantibody tests available to aid in the diagnosis of SLE. Antinuclear antibody (ANA) testing is 95% sensitive for SLE but is not specific. However, based on EULAR/ACR criteria, the diagnosis of SLE requires a positive ANA test or equivalent (Table 3). Anti-dsDNA is highly specific but has a lower sensitivity. Levels vary with disease activity. Anti-Sm is the most specific antibody test for SLE but has a very low sensitivity.

Anti-cardiolipin antibodies, anti-β2GP1 antibodies, and lupus anticoagulant testing are laboratory tests that can identify antiphospholipid antibodies that may be associated with the antiphospholipid antibody syndrome. All patients with a diagnosis of SLE should be tested for concurrent antiphospholipid antibody syndrome.

Treatment

The updated European League Against Rheumatism (EULAR) recommendations provide sound guidance for the treatment of SLE [21]. For patients who do not have major organ involvement, corticosteroids and antimalarials are helpful. Traditionally, hydroxychloroquine has been the cornerstone therapy for SLE to prevent flares and reduce disease mortality. NSAIDs can be used for short periods as well if there is not risk of exacerbating underlying organ disorder, particularly renal disease. For cases refractory to steroids and antimalarials, immunosuppressive agents such as azathioprine, methotrexate, and mycophenolate are also useful for certain manifestations and control of systemic disease. Cyclophosphamide can be used in severe life-threatening situations for patients not responding to immunosuppressive therapy. The monoclonal antibody belimumab can be used in patients with frequent relapses. Rituximab should be reserved for organ-threatening disease. Additional guidelines for the management of lupus nephritis were published by the ACR in 2012 [22].

As with many of the rheumatic diseases, an interprofessional, multidisciplinary team is helpful to maximize clinical outcomes for patients with SLE. Consultations with multiple specialties including rheumatology, neurology, nephrology, pulmonology, cardiology, dermatology, hematology, and maternal fetal medicine may be necessary. Patient education is also important. Patients should avoid any known triggers for SLE flares. Patients should wear sunscreen and minimize ultraviolet light exposure to reduce photosensitivity reactions. Patients with SLE often require vitamin D supplementation. Exercise is important to maximize functional capacity, avoid muscular atrophy, and maximize bone mineralization. Patients with SLE should not smoke or use tobacco products.

Raynaud's Disease (Primary Raynaud's Phenomenon)

Primary Raynaud's phenomenon, or Raynaud's disease, is a reactive vasospasm of the fingers and toes typically in response to stress or cold exposure. Primary Raynaud's phenomenon is not associated with any other systemic illness. Secondary Raynaud's phenomenon is associated with

some other form of clinical illness typically autoimmune in nature with scleroderma, SLE, and mixed-connective tissue disorder being the most common. The cause of Raynaud's disease remains unknown. The disease is slightly more common in women and has no racial predilection unless it is associated with an autoimmune disorder. It most commonly occurs in the second and third decades of life. Raynaud's disease is characterized clinically by pallor (white), followed by cyanosis (blue), and erythema (red) on rewarming. The fingers are most commonly affected followed by the toes and ears [24].

When evaluating patients for Raynaud's disease, a careful history is important. This should particularly include a prior history of frostbite and prior repetitive use of vibrating tools, which predispose to vasospasm. Occupational exposures to organic solvents have also been associated with Raynaud's disease. Secondary Raynaud's phenomenon has been associated with autoimmune diseases (scleroderma, SLE), infectious syndromes (hepatitis B and C), neoplastic syndromes (leukemia, lymphoma), environmental exposures, medications (beta-blockers, methylphenidate, oral contraceptives), and hematologic (polycythemia) and metabolic syndromes (diabetes, pheochromocytoma). Historically, the color demarcation between affected and unaffected areas of skin is remarkable. The digits should be examined for sclerodactyly, ulceration, and capillary blush. Nail fold microscopy can reveal abnormalities in capillary loops. Immersing the patient's affected extremity in ice water can often reproduce the symptoms but is typically not necessary for diagnosis. Laboratory testing is helpful in ruling out potential causes of secondary Raynaud's phenomenon, in particular antinuclear antibodies. Diagnostic criteria for primary Raynaud's phenomenon have been established [23] and include trigger by exposure to cold/ stress, bilateral (symmetric) involvement, no necrosis, no underlying systemic cause, normal capillary findings on microscopy, and no laboratory evidence of inflammation or antinuclear factors.

The mainstay of treatment for Raynaud's disease centers on patient education and lifestyle change. Patients should be instructed to wear warm socks, gloves, or mittens and avoid unnecessary cold exposure. Tobacco cessation is important (nicotine is a potent vasoconstrictor). If conservative strategies fail, calcium channel blockers are the traditional pharmacological treatment [23]. Nifedipine (30–120 mg of extended release) is typically the agent of choice. Topical nitroglycerin (1%) and the prostaglandin analogue (iloprost) have shown promise in limited numbers of studies, but extended use data is lacking.

Systemic Sclerosis

Systemic sclerosis (SSc; scleroderma) is a systemic autoimmune disorder, which results in abnormal collagen deposition in the skin and internal organs resulting in progressive fibrosis of the skin, lungs, heart, gastrointestinal tract, and kidneys. Systemic sclerosis represents a broad spectrum of disease with multiple clinical forms. CREST syndrome (calcinosis, Raynaud's phenomenon, esophageal dysmotility, sclerodactyly, and telangiectasias) is a form of scleroderma characterized by cutaneous systemic sclerosis typically involving regions distal to the elbows and knees. Diffuse cutaneous systemic sclerosis is more severe and often involves the internal organs to some degree. Diffuse systemic sclerosis has a more fulminant course with organ involvement and rapid progression. The ACR/EULAR criteria for classification of systemic sclerosis were revised in 2013 [24] (Table 4).

Three important processes are involved in the pathophysiology of SSc: (1) alterations in cellular and humoral immunity, (2) excessive collagen deposition, and (3) fibroproliferative disease of small arteries/arterioles. The resulting vasculopathy and tissue fibrosis result in organ dysfunction and clinical disease. While the exact etiology is not known, exposure to silica, solvents, and/or radiation in genetically susceptible individuals has all been hypothesized to trigger the disease [25]. Viruses (herpesvirus, cytomegalovirus, parvovirus) have also been proposed to accelerate the disease in genetically susceptible individuals. SSc is more common in women. There appears to be a higher incidence rate in blacks as compared to whites. In the United States, the highest

Table 4 ACR/EULAR revised systemic sclerosis classification criteria [24]

Item	Sub-item(s)	Score[a]
Skin thickening of the fingers of both hands extending proximally to the metacarpophalangeal joints (presence of this criterion is sufficient criterion for SSc classification)	None	9
Skin thickening of the fingers (count the higher score only)	Puffy fingers	2
	Sclerodactyly (distal to the metacarpophalangeal joints but proximal to the proximal interphalangeal joints)	4
Fingertip lesions (count the higher score only)	Digital tip ulcers	2
	Fingertip pitting scars	3
Telangiectasia	None	2
Abnormal nail fold capillaries	None	2
Pulmonary arterial hypertension and/or interstitial lung disease (maximum score is 2)	Pulmonary arterial hypertension	2
	Interstitial lung disease	2
Raynaud's phenomenon	None	3
Systemic sclerosis-related autoantibodies (maximum score is 3)	Anti-centromere	3
	Anti-topoisomerase I	3
	Anti-RNA polymerase III	3

[a]The total score is determined by adding the maximum score in each category. Patients with a total score equal to or greater than 9 are classified as having definite systemic sclerosis

prevalence of SSc is in the Choctaw Indian tribe. The peak incidence is 30–50 years of age.

Patients with SSc present with signs and symptoms involving many different organ systems. Skin complaints include tightness and induration (edema), sclerodactyly, pruritus, and pigmentary change. Vascular phenomena typically present as secondary Raynaud's phenomenon. Telangiectasias are also common. Gastrointestinal complaints include reflux, dyspepsia, and altered bowel habits (constipation, diarrhea, incontinence). Respiratory manifestations include dyspnea and cough. Musculoskeletal complaints include myalgias, arthralgias, weakness, and decreased joint range of motion. Common physical findings include sclerodactyly, microstomia, telangiectasia, rales, and an accentuated P2 (pulmonary hypertension).

The diagnosis of SSc is based on history and physical examination. Baseline laboratory studies (CBC, CPK, ESR, B-NP, autoantibody profiles) can help exclude other causes and follow disease progression. Endoscopy, echocardiography, and pulmonary function tests can provide further insight to track target organ function.

There is no cure for scleroderma. Treatment is designed to optimize function of involved organ systems, prevent complications, and provide symptomatic relief. Patients should routinely be encouraged to stop smoking [26]. Investigational therapies are under way to treat skin fibrosis. Pruritus is best managed with moisturizers and antihistamines. Raynaud's phenomenon can be managed with lifestyle changes and calcium channel blockers. Treatment of pulmonary hypertension includes either bosentan, ambrisentan, or sildenafil [25]. Severe SSc-related pulmonary hypertension can be treated with epoprostenol infusions. Antacids, histamine blockers (H2), and proton pump inhibitors can treat common reflux symptoms associated with SSc. Cyclophosphamide is used to treat pulmonary fibrosis in patients with SSc, and nintedanib can be used to slow the rate of pulmonary function decline.

As with other conditions, the broad spectrum of SSc may require input and guidance from a range of consultants. Coordinating care and communication in patients with extensive disease can be a challenge. Rheumatology, pulmonology, cardiology, gastroenterology, surgery, nephrology, physical therapy, occupational therapy, and other services may need to be involved. Developing a robust patient-centered team with clear lines of communication is important to reduce morbidity and improve outcomes.

Sjögren's Syndrome

Sjögren's syndrome is a chronic inflammatory autoimmune disorder. It involves lymphocytic infiltrates within exocrine organs and is characterized by the combination of keratoconjunctivitis sicca or xerophthalmia (dry eyes), xerostomia (dry mouth), and parotid enlargement. Extraglandular features include arthralgias, myalgias, arthritis, lymphadenopathy, neuropathy, and Raynaud's phenomenon. The EULAR/ACR classification for Sjögren's syndrome includes a weighted score based on five categories: (a) labial salivary gland with focal lymphocytic sialadenitis and focus score of ≥ 1 foci/4 mm^2 (3 points); (b) positive anti-SSA or anti-Ro antibodies (3 points); (c) ocular staining score ≥ 5 (or van Bijsterveld score ≥ 4) in at least one eye (1 point); (d) Schirmer's test ≤ 5 mm/5 min in at least one eye (1 point); and (e) unstimulated whole saliva flow rate ≤ 0.1 mL/min (1 point). If a patient has four or more points and does not have an excluding criteria (i.e., history of head or neck radiation, active hepatitis C infection, AIDS, sarcoidosis, amyloidosis, graft versus host disease, IgG4-related disease), then they meet the criteria for Sjögren's syndrome diagnosis [27].

Sjögren's syndrome is more common in patients with HLA-DR52 and affects women nine times more often than men [28]. Sjögren's syndrome is more common in older adults, with an average age of onset in the fourth and fifth decade of life. It is hypothesized that Sjögren's syndrome is triggered by viral disease, though proof remains inconclusive. Many medications (antidepressants, antihistamines, anticholinergics, diuretics, beta-blockers) can also cause xerostomia but should not be confused with Sjögren's syndrome. Outside of sicca symptoms (dry eyes and dry mouth), patients most commonly present with parotitis and cutaneous complaints such as dry skin and pruritis. Dryness of the aerodigestive tract can result in a chronic cough, dysphagia, and a globus sensation. Common physical findings relate to ocular and oral dryness. Angular cheilitis; dental caries; a dry, erythematous, smooth tongue; and chapped lips are common. Parotid gland enlargement occurs in 20–60% of Sjögren's syndrome patients.

The diagnosis of Sjögren's syndrome is based on clinical history (sicca symptoms) and physical examination. Laboratory testing to quantify salivary (sialometry) and lacrimal (Schirmer's test) function is supportive of the diagnosis. Autoantibodies are common in Sjögren's syndrome with anti-SSA and anti-SSB being the most common. Treatment options for Sjögren's syndrome patients are limited and primarily focus on symptom relief. Liberal use of ocular lubricants, skin lubricants, and vaginal lubricants can help mitigate dryness. Humidifiers and frequent sips of water can help alleviate dry mouth. Pilocarpine, artificial saliva, and cevimeline have been used for more severe cases of xerostomia [29]. If major organs are involved, the use of immunosuppressive therapy (cyclophosphamide), rituximab, or systemic corticosteroids is appropriate. Such cases are best managed in the context of a multidisciplinary team including rheumatology, pulmonology, and nephrology depending on the extent of extraglandular disease. Sjögren's syndrome patients should have appropriate eye health and oral health professionals as part of this team.

Polymyalgia Rheumatica (PMR)

Polymyalgia rheumatica (PMR) is a chronic inflammatory disorder that typically affects individuals over the age of 50. The cause of PMR is not known. The pathology of PMR is similar to giant cell arteritis or temporal arteritis. The disease appears to be polygenic in origin, perhaps triggered by an environmental factor (likely a virus) that results in cytokine production due to macrophage and T-cell activation. Polymyalgia rheumatica has an annual incidence of approximately 53 cases per 100,000 persons over age 50 annually in the United States. PMR is more common in white patients (rare in blacks) and more common in women [30]. The median age at the time of diagnosis is 72 years. One in three patients with polymyalgia rheumatica also has temporal arteritis.

The predominant clinical features of PMR are pain or weakness of the hips, shoulders, and neck that are usually associated with morning stiffness. Patients may also complain of constitutional symptoms including fatigue, weight loss, and low-grade fever. In 2012, EULAR/ACR published scoring criteria for patients with PMR: (a) morning stiffness >45 min (2 points), (b) hip pain and limited ROM (1 point), (c) rheumatoid factor (RF) and anticitrullinated protein antibody (CCP) negative (2 points), and (d) no peripheral joint pain (1 point) [31]. Patients with four or more points are likely to have PMR (compared to other spondyloarthropathies or inflammatory arthritides). On physical examination, patients may have a low-grade temperature. They often appear fatigued. Patients have normal muscle strength and no atrophy. There is tenderness to palpation, particularly of the hip and shoulder girdles, but many investigators feel that this is due to synovitis. ROM is often reduced due to the pain. Imaging is not routinely used for diagnosis. The erythrocyte sedimentation rate is the most sensitive (but not specific) laboratory test for PMR. ESR is almost always >40 mm/h and characteristically exceeds 100 mm/h. Creatine phosphokinase levels are normal as are ANA, complement, RF, and anti-CCP levels.

Corticosteroids are generally the cornerstone of treatment for patients with PMR. Patients generally respond well to a prednisone dose of 12.5 to 25 mg/day. If a patient does not respond quickly (within 2–4 weeks) to corticosteroids, other diagnoses should be considered. Patients often require steroids for a prolonged period (1–2 years). Patients on chronic steroid therapy should receive calcium and vitamin D supplementation and regular DEXA scans to assess bone health [32]. When attempts are made to wean a patient off prednisone, the dose is decreased by only 1 mg/month. Methotrexate and TNF-α inhibitors have also been used as steroid-sparing treatments for PMR.

Giant Cell Arteritis (Temporal Arteritis)

Giant cell arteritis (GCA; temporal arteritis) is a cell-mediated inflammatory systemic vasculitis. GCA is the most common systemic vasculitis in adults. Pathophysiology of GCA is characterized by inflammation of the vascular wall of affected arteries (e.g., the temporal artery) which results in endothelial injury, luminal narrowing, and distal ischemia. Like polymyalgia rheumatica, GCA typically presents in patients over 50 years of age [33]. The disease incidence peaks in the eighth decade of life. GCA is more common in women (3:1) and in whites of Northern European descent.

The onset of GCA is variable. Some patients have an insidious onset, while for others it is abrupt. Often there is a constitutional prodrome with patients complaining of anorexia, malaise, myalgias, night sweats, and weight loss in the preceding days to weeks. Headache is the most common symptom associated with GCA (present in three quarters of patients) [34]. The headache is most commonly temporal-occipital in location and described as "throbbing" and "continuous." Many patients are tender to palpation over the temporal artery. Jaw claudication and shoulder and/or hip/pelvic girdle pain are often present as well (as in PMR). Some patients with GCA report visual symptoms. Symptoms are often transient, but sudden loss of vision is a poor sign and can be permanent without immediate treatment. The most common visual symptoms included blurring, visual loss, diplopia, hemianopia, or amaurosis fugax.

Patients with GCA (as in PMR) typically have an elevated ESR (50 mm/h to over 100 mm/h). Definitive diagnosis requires a temporal artery biopsy (TAB). Treatment should not be withheld pending biopsy results, and specimens are more likely to be positive if obtained within 24 h of beginning treatment. Recently, the use of color duplex ultrasonography has shown promise as a diagnostic complement to TAB. High-resolution MRI has been used for a similar purpose. The ACR [35] and others [36] have developed diagnostic criteria for GCA including (a) age over 50, (b) new-onset localized headache, (c) temporal artery tenderness to palpation (or decreased pulsation), (d) ESR 50 mm/h, and (e) positive TAB (vasculitis with mononuclear infiltration). High-dose corticosteroid therapy is the cornerstone of therapy for GCA [37]. Patients with visual symptoms have a markedly increased chance of visual improvement if steroid therapy is initiated within 24 h. Oral prednisone (40–60 mg/day; some sources suggest 80–100 mg/day in patients with visual or neurological symptoms consistent with GCA) should be started immediately while arranging for TAB. Intravenous methylprednisolone (250–1000 mg/day for 3 days) is an alternative to oral prednisone. Once symptoms have improved, steroids should be tapered to the lowest dose necessary to suppress symptoms. Patients often require prolonged treatment with corticosteroids. Symptoms and measurement of acute phase reactants serve as a guide to tapering the dose of corticosteroids. Methotrexate, tocilizumab (an interleukin-6 receptor monoclonal antibody), and TNF-α antagonists have been used as steroid-sparing agents in patients requiring higher doses of prednisone (5–10 mg/day) for prolonged periods of time. GCA is best managed in consultation with a rheumatologist in the context of high-dose steroids and surgery consultation required to assist with TAB. Ophthalmology consultation in the context of visual changes should be entertained if the diagnosis is uncertain.

Ankylosing Spondylitis

Ankylosing spondylitis (AS) is a chronic inflammatory seronegative spondyloarthropathy primarily involving the spine (sacroiliac joint and axial skeleton). The disease is more common in men (3:1) and typically presents during adulthood. More than half of the patients with ankylosing spondylitis present complaining of low-back pain. Features distinguishing AS from mechanical low-back pain include morning stiffness, pain that is unrelieved with rest, and pain that awakens patients from sleep [38]. The pain associated with AS often radiates to the buttocks but rarely below the knee (as seen with sciatica). The onset of pain is often insidious and tends to improve with exercise. Fatigue is reported in 65% of patients. Extra-articular manifestations of AS include uveitis, pulmonary, cardiovascular, renal, gastrointestinal, and metabolic bone diseases. Patients may also have peripheral joint involvement (large joints are more commonly involved than small joints) or complain of other sites of enthesopathic pain (e.g., Achilles tendon, plantar fascia) [38, 39]. Onset after the age of 40 is unusual. Over 90% of Caucasian patients with AS are HLA-B27 positive. However, only 1–2% of patients who are positive for HLA-B27 develop ankylosing spondylitis, suggesting a role of other factors in the onset of disease [40].

Early diagnosis of AS is important to maximize functional outcomes. The diagnosis of AS is based on a combination of clinical and radiographic findings [41, 42] (Table 5). The insidious onset of low-back pain that is worse in the morning, relieved with activity, lasting for more than 3 months in patients under the age of 40 should raise the suspicion for AS [43].

Physical examination should include documentation of lumbar range of motion in particular. The two most commonly used tests to assess spinal flexion are Schober's test and Moll's flexion test. Schober's test is performed with the patient standing. Identify the top of the sacrum,

and mark a spot on the spine 10 cm above and 5 cm below. In normal individuals, this distance increases by at least 5 cm with forward flexion. The Moll's lateral flexion test is performed by marking a point 20 cm above the iliac crest at the midaxillary line. This distance increases by at least 3 cm with lateral flexion in normal individuals. Uveitis (typically unilateral) is the most common extra-articular manifestation of AS [44], but the cardiopulmonary, renal, gastrointestinal, and neurovascular systems can all be involved.

Radiographic studies help to confirm the diagnosis of AS [45]. Involvement of the sacroiliac joint is required to diagnose AS. Radiographic signs of AS include vertebral "squaring" (erosions of the margins of the vertebral bodies) and sclerosis of the vertebral margins (Romanus lesion). Sacroiliac disease is usually bilateral in AS. If the disease has progressed, patients develop a characteristic "bamboo spine" appearance on X-ray. Power Doppler ultrasonography, MRI, and CT also reveal characteristic signs of sacroiliitis. The ESR is elevated. It is easy to measure the flexibility of the spine, which is decreased in most patients.

The goals of treatment of ankylosing spondylitis are to decrease pain and maintain functional status [46]. No specific disease-modifying treatment currently exists for patients with AS. NSAIDs are the initial drugs of choice to control inflammation and decrease pain. Sulfasalazine is helpful in patients who are

Table 5 New York and Rome criteria for diagnosis of ankylosing spondylitis [33, 34]

New York criteria	Rome criteria
Low-back pain with inflammatory characteristics Limitation of lumbar spine motion in sagittal and frontal planes Decreased chest expansion Bilateral sacroiliitis grade 2 or higher∗ Unilateral sacroiliitis grade 3 or higher∗	Low-back pain and stiffness that is not relieved by rest for >3 months Thoracic pain and stiffness Limited motion in the lumbar spine Limited chest expansion History of uveitis

∗Diagnose ankylosing spondylitis if patient presents with any clinical criteria	Diagnosis ankylosing spondylitis when any clinical criteria present with bilateral sacroiliitis grade 2 or higher radiographic sacroiliac (SI) grades
	    Grade 0 – Normal
	    Grade 1 – Suspicious
	    Grade 2 – Minimal sacroiliitis
	    Grade 3 – Moderate sacroiliitis
	    Grade 4 – Ankylosis

unresponsive to NSAIDs. TNF-α antagonists are effective in the treatment of AS. Infliximab, adalimumab, golimumab, certolizumab pegol, and etanercept have all been approved by the FDA as therapy for AS when NSAID therapy has failed. Ixekizumab, an interleukin-17 inhibitor, can be considered as a second-line initial therapy or when NSAIDs and TNF-α antagonists have failed. Patients should be screened for hepatitis B, HIV, and latent tuberculosis before initiating TNF-α antagonist therapy. Complex cases are best managed in the context of a multidisciplinary team including rheumatology, pulmonology, ophthalmology, cardiology, physical therapy, and orthopedic surgery depending on the extent of disease [46, 47].

Psoriatic Arthritis

Psoriatic arthritis is a seronegative inflammatory arthritis that is variable and occurs in about 7–42% of patients with psoriasis (▶ Chap. 120, "Common Dermatoses"). Psoriasis typically precedes the appearance of arthritis by several years. The onset is typically insidious with patients primarily complaining of stiffness and pain. Psoriatic arthritis is also associated with enthesopathy (inflammation at the insertion of ligament/tendon into bone). The Achilles tendon and plantar fascia are commonly involved. One-third of patients will exhibit dactylitis or sausage digit. Skin findings are consistent with psoriasis and include scaly erythematous plaques, guttate lesions, and erythroderma. Psoriatic nail changes (pitting, hyperkeratosis, Beau's lines, transverse ridging) are common. With the exception of skin disease, extra-articular findings are less common in psoriatic arthritis patients than in other inflammatory arthritides. Guidelines for diagnosis [48] include the Classification Criteria for Psoriatic Arthritis (CASPAR) scoring system (3 points total from the following):

- Active psoriasis (2 points)
- History of psoriasis – no active psoriasis (1 point)
- Family history of psoriasis – no active psoriasis (1 point)

- Dactylitis (1 point)
- Juxta-articular new bone formation (1 point)
- Serum RF negative (1 point)
- Nail dystrophy (1 point)

There are no diagnostic laboratory tests for psoriatic arthritis. ESR and CRP are often elevated. X-rays often show joint space narrowing of the interphalangeal joints with periostitis and may show the characteristic "pencil-in-cup" deformity. NSAIDs are the initial treatment of choice, and several DMARDs have been approved for the treatment of psoriatic arthritis including methotrexate, sulfasalazine, cyclosporine, leflunomide, and TNF-α antagonists [49]. If patients have an inadequate response to nonbiologic DMARDs, biologic therapy can be helpful. Biologic options include TNF-α antagonists (adalimumab, certolizumab, etanercept, golimumab, infliximab), interleukin-17 inhibitors (ixekizumab, secukinumab), interleukin-12/23 inhibitors (ustekinumab), CD80/86 receptor antagonists (abatacept), and Janus kinase inhibitors (tofacitinib). Apremilast (a phosphodiesterase-4 inhibitor) is a nonbiologic approved by the FDA for treatment of psoriatic arthritis in adults.

References

1. Nell VPK, Machold KP, Eberl G, et al. Benefit of very early referral and very early therapy with disease modifying anti-rheumatic drugs in patients with early rheumatoid arthritis. Rheumatology. 2004;43(7):906–14.
2. Ahlmén M, Svensson B, Albertsson K, et al. Influence of gender on assessments of disease activity and function in early rheumatoid arthritis in relation to radiographic joint damage. Ann Rheum Dis. 2010;69(1): 230–3.
3. Myasoedova E, Crowson CS, Kremers HM, et al. Is the incidence of rheumatoid arthritis rising? Results from Olmsted County, Minnesota, 1995–2007. Arthritis Rheum. 2010;62(6):1576–82.
4. Sparks JA, Chang SC, Liao KP, et al. Rheumatoid arthritis and mortality among women during 36 years of prospective follow-up: results from the Nurses' Health Study. Arthritis Care Res. 2016;68(6):753–62.
5. Fuller-Thomson E, Liddycoat JP, Stefanyk M. The association between a history of parental addictions and arthritis in adulthood: findings from a representative community survey. Int J Popul Res. 2014;2014: 1–10. https://doi.org/10.1155/2014/582508.

6. Aletaha D, Smolen JS. Diagnosis and management of rheumatoid arthritis: a review. JAMA. 2018;320(13): 1360–72.

7. Aletaha D, Neogi T, Silman AJ, et al. 2010 Rheumatoid arthritis classification criteria: an American College of Rheumatology/European League Against Rheumatism collaborative initiative. Arthritis Rheum. 2010;62(9): 2569–81.

8. Niewold TB, Harrison MJ, Paget SA. Anti-CCP antibody testing as a diagnostic and prognostic tool in rheumatoid arthritis. Q J Med. 2007;100:193–201.

9. Ford JA, Liu X, Marshall AA, et al. Impact of cyclic citrullinated peptide antibody level on progression to rheumatoid arthritis in clinically tested cyclic citrullinated peptide antibody–positive patients without rheumatoid arthritis. Arthritis Care Res. 2019; 71(12):1583–92.

10. Rizzo C, Ceccarelli F, Gattamelata A, et al. Ultrasound in rheumatoid arthritis. Med Ultrason. 2013;15(3): 199–208.

11. Singh JA, Saag KG, Bridges SL Jr, et al. 2015 American College of Rheumatology guideline for the treatment of rheumatoid arthritis. Arthritis Rheumatol. 2016;68(1):1–26.

12. Felson DT, Smolen JS, Wells G, et al. American College of Rheumatology/European League Against Rheumatism provisional definition of remission in rheumatoid arthritis for clinical trials. Arthritis Rheum. 2011;63(3):573–86.

13. Arvonen M, Virta LJ, Pokka T, et al. Repeated exposure to antibiotics in infancy: a predisposing factor for juvenile idiopathic arthritis or a sign of this groups' greater susceptibility to infections? J Rheumatol. 2015;42(3):521–6.

14. Petty RE, Southwood TR, Manners P, International League of Associations for Rheumatology, et al. International League of Associations for Rheumatology classification of juvenile idiopathic arthritis: second revision, Edmonton, 2001. J Rheumatol. 2004;31:390–2.

15. Cassidy J, Kivlin J, Lindsley C, Nocton J. Ophthalmologic examinations in children with juvenile rheumatoid arthritis. Pediatrics. 2006;117(5):1843–5.

16. Beukelman T, Patkar NM, Saag KG, et al. 2011 American College of Rheumatology recommendations for the treatment of juvenile idiopathic arthritis: initiation and safety monitoring of therapeutic agents for the treatment of arthritis and systemic features. Arthritis Care Res. 2011;63(4):465–82.

17. Carter JD, Hudson AP. Reactive arthritis: clinical aspects and medical management. Rheum Dis Clin N Am. 2009;35(1):21–44.

18. Kim PS, Klausmeier TL, Orr DP. Reactive arthritis: a review. J Adolesc Health. 2009;44(4):309–15.

19. Aringer M, Costenbader K, Daikh D, et al. 2019 European League Against Rheumatism/American College of Rheumatology classification criteria for systemic lupus erythematosus. Arthritis Rheumatol. 2019;71 (9):1400–12.

20. Hochberg MC. Updating the American College of Rheumatology revised criteria for the classification of systemic lupus erythematosus. Arthritis Rheum. 1997;40(9):1725.

21. Fanouriakis A, Kostopoulou M, Alunno A, et al. 2019 update of the EULAR recommendations for the management of systemic lupus erythematosus. Ann Rheum Dis. 2019;78(6):736–45.

22. Bertsias G, Ioannidis JP, Boletis J, et al. EULAR recommendations for the management of systemic lupus erythematosus. Report of a task force of the EULAR standing committee for international clinical studies including therapeutics. Ann Rheum Dis. 2008;67(2): 195–205.

23. Hughes M, Herrick AL. Raynaud's phenomenon. Best Pract Res Clin Rheumatol. 2016;30(1):112–32.

24. van den Hoogen F, Khanna D, Fransen J, et al. 2013 Classification criteria for systemic sclerosis: an American College of Rheumatology/European League Against Rheumatism collaborative initiative. Arthritis Rheum. 2013;65(11):2737–47.

25. Allanore Y, Simms R, Distler O, et al. Systemic sclerosis. Nat Rev Dis Primers. 2015;1(1):1–21.

26. Hissaria P, Roberts-Thomson PJ, Lester S, et al. Cigarette smoking in patients with systemic sclerosis – reduces overall survival. Arthritis Rheum. 2011;63 (6):1758–9.

27. Shiboski CH, Shiboski SC, Seror R, et al. 2016 American College of Rheumatology/European League Against Rheumatism classification criteria for primary Sjögren's syndrome: a consensus and data-driven methodology involving three international patient cohorts. Arthritis Rheumatol. 2017;69(1):35–45.

28. Gálvez J, Sáiz E, López P, et al. Diagnostic evaluation and classification criteria in Sjögren's syndrome. Joint Bone Spine. 2008;76(1):44–9.

29. Price EJ, Rauz S, Tappuni AR, et al. The British Society for Rheumatology guideline for the management of adults with primary Sjögren's syndrome. Rheumatology. 2017;56(10):e24–48.

30. Caylor TL, Perkins A. Recognition and management of polymyalgia rheumatica and giant cell arteritis. Am Fam Physician. 2013;88(10):676–84.

31. Dasgupta B, Cimmino MA, Maradit-Kremers H, et al. 2012 provisional classification criteria for polymyalgia rheumatic: a European League Against Rheumatism/ American College of Rheumatology collaborative initiative. Ann Rheum Dis. 2012;71(4):484–92.

32. Dejaco C, Singh YP, Perel P, et al. 2015 Recommendations for the management of polymyalgia rheumatica: a European League Against Rheumatism/ American College of Rheumatology collaborative initiative. Arthritis Rheumatol. 2015;67(10):2569–80.

33. Cantini F, Niccoli L, Storri L, et al. Are polymyalgia rheumatica and giant cell arteritis the same disease? Semin Arthritis Rheum. 2004;33(5):294–301.

34. Waldman CW, Waldman SD, Waldman RA. Giant cell arteritis. Med Clin North Am. 2013;97(2):329–35.

35. Hunder GG, Bloch DA, Michel BA, et al. The American College of Rheumatology 1990 criteria for the classification of giant cell arteritis. Arthritis Rheum. 1990;33:1122–8.

36. Giant DB, Cell Arteritis Development Group. Concise guidance: diagnosis and management of giant cell arteritis. Clin Med. 2010;10(4):381–6.
37. Hoffman GS. Giant cell arteritis. Ann Intern Med. 2016;165(9):ITC65–80.
38. van der Linden S, van der Heijde D. Ankylosing spondylitis. Clinical features. Rheum Dis Clin N Am. 1998;24(4):663–76.
39. Eriksson JK, Jacobsson L, Bengtsson K, Askling J. Is ankylosing spondylitis a risk factor for cardiovascular disease, and how do these risks compare with those in rheumatoid arthritis? Ann Rheum Dis. 2017;76(2): 364–70.
40. Reveille JD, Ball EJ, Khan MA. HLA-B27 and genetic predisposing factors in spondyloarthropathies. Curr Opin Rheumatol. 2001;13(4):265–72.
41. Moll JM, Wright V. New York clinical criteria for ankylosing spondylitis. A statistical evaluation. Ann Rheum Dis. 1973;32(4):354–63.
42. Goie HS, Steven MM, van der Linden SM, et al. Evaluation of diagnostic criteria for ankylosing spondylitis: a comparison of Rome, New York and modified New York criteria in patients with a positive clinical screening test for ankylosing spondylitis. Br J Rheumatol. 1985;24(3):242–9.
43. Braun J, Sieper J. Ankylosing spondylitis. Lancet. 2007;369(9570):1379–90.
44. Stolwijk C, van Tubergen A, Castillo-Ortiz JD, Boonen A. Prevalence of extra-articular manifestations in patients with ankylosing spondylitis: a systematic review and meta-analysis. Ann Rheum Dis. 2015; 74(1):65–73.
45. van der Heijde D, Landewé R. Imaging in spondylitis. Curr Opin Rheumatol. 2005;17(4):413–7.
46. Ward MM, Deodhar A, Gensler LS, et al. 2019 update of the American College of Rheumatology/Spondylitis Association of America/Spondyloarthritis Research and Treatment Network recommendations for the treatment of ankylosing spondylitis and nonradiographic axial spondyloarthritis. Arthritis Care Res. 2019; 71(10):1285–99.
47. Dagfinrud H, Kvien TK, Hagen KB. Physiotherapy interventions for ankylosing spondylitis. Cochrane Database Syst Rev. 2008;1:CD002822.
48. Taylor W, Gladman D, Helliwell P, et al. Classification criteria for psoriatic arthritis: development of new criteria from a large international study. Arthritis Rheum. 2006;54(8):2665–73.
49. Singh JA, Guyatt G, Ogdie A, et al. 2018 American College of Rheumatology/National Psoriasis Foundation guideline for the treatment of psoriatic arthritis. Arthritis Rheumatol. 2019;71(1):5–32.

Selected Disorders of the Musculoskeletal System

Patrick Anderl

Contents

P. Anderl (✉)
Family Medicine, Univeristy of Nebraska Medical Center,
Omaha, NE, USA
e-mail: patrick.anderl@unmc.edu

© Springer Nature Switzerland AG 2022
P. M. Paulman et al. (eds.), *Family Medicine*,
https://doi.org/10.1007/978-3-030-54441-6_148

Fibromyalgia

General Principles

Definition/Background

Fibromyalgia is a chronic, idiopathic, non-articular disorder of pain regulation. Its etiology is unknown, and pathophysiology is uncertain [1]. Though initially called fibrositis, there is no evidence of inflammation in any of the affected tissues [2]. There are no diagnostic laboratory tests for fibromyalgia. Diagnosis is symptom based and often requires a clinician familiar with these chronic widespread pain conditions for confirmation of the diagnosis [3].

Like many other chronic pain syndromes, fibromyalgia can be a controversial diagnosis and at times has been considered psychogenic or psychosomatic. More recently, however, it has been classified as a form of central nervous system sensitization [4].

Epidemiology

Fibromyalgia is the most common cause of chronic widespread musculoskeletal pain [1, 2]. It has been observed in all ages and is more common in women than in men. Prevalence increases with age and peaks between 60 and 79 years, where it is estimated to affect >7% of women [5]. Prevalence in the general population is estimated to be between 1% and 6% depending based on which diagnostic criteria is used, but overall fibromyalgia is likely under recognized in clinical practice [6].

Diagnosis

Fibromyalgia should be suspected in anyone complaining of pain of at least 3 months duration. Several classification criteria have been proposed, but the gold standard continues to be symptom based diagnosis [3]. There are no confirmatory tests or biomarkers.

History

The cardinal symptoms of fibromyalgia are widespread musculoskeletal (also termed multisite) pain, fatigue, and sleep disturbances, but other cognitive, neurologic, and somatic complaints are common [7]. Most patients complain of myalgias, arthralgias, and swollen joints, though synovitis is not present on exam. Fatigue and unrefreshing sleep can be triggered by even minor physical activity, although prolonged inactivity also exacerbates symptoms. Cognitive disturbances, poor attention, and difficulty completing tasks are often described and referred to as "fibro fog" [8]. Depression and anxiety are common coexisting disorders [9]. Other somatic complaints include headache, paresthesias, nondescript abdominal or chest pain, IBS symptoms, pelvic pain, and bladder symptoms. Autonomic complaints include dry eye, Raynaud phenomenon, hypotension, and tachycardia. Patients may also complain of weather-related exacerbations and other environmental hypersensitivities.

Physical Examination

The usual findings include mild to severe tenderness on palpation of various soft tissue sites. There should be no soft tissue or joint swelling or redness. Common tender points include, but are not limited to, the occiput, low cervical spine, trapezius, supraspinatus, second rib, lateral epicondyle, buttock, greater trochanter, and knee [10].

Neurologic testing may reveal subtle findings suggesting peripheral neuropathy or minor sensory and motor abnormalities [11]. Fibromyalgia does not cause any focal neurological deficits. The remainder of physical exam and testing is usually unremarkable.

Classification

There have been several published classification criteria for fibromyalgia. Most were developed and used for clinical research and epidemiologic studies but have not been validated for patient diagnosis [3]. The older 1990 American College of Rheumatology (ACR) classification criteria have been used in most clinical and therapeutic trials.

A different classification system is used in clinical settings. In 2010 the Analgesic, Anesthetic, and Addiction Clinical Trial Translocations Innovations Opportunities and Networks (ACTTION) and American Pain Society (APS) formulated the ACTTION-APS pain taxonomy (AAPT) in order to help differentiate FM from other chronic pain disorders [12].

The 1990 ACR criteria requires symptoms of widespread pain occurring both above and below the waist affecting both sides of the body as well as identification of at least 11 of 18 specifically defined tender points [10]. The inability to standardize the tender point examination was the main impetus in moving away from these criteria.

The 2010 ACR preliminary diagnostic criteria uses a subjective symptom survey called the widespread pain index (WPI) and a symptom severity scale (SSS) rating to assist in diagnosis [13]. It does not require a tender point exam. See Table 1 for the WPI score criteria. See Table 2 for the SSS score criteria.

Fibromyalgia is diagnosed if all of the following are met:

- WPI > 7 and SSS > 5 OR WPI 3–6 and SSS > 9
- Symptoms have been present for at least 3 months
- There is no other more likely alternative diagnosis

The AAPT diagnostic criteria listed in Table 3 are much more subjective and, as a result, easier to use clinically. Diagnosis requires multisite pain (MSP) and sleep problems or fatigue present for greater than 3 months.

Differential Diagnosis

Appropriate diagnosis of fibromyalgia requires the exclusion of other causative conditions. Alternative diagnoses to consider include systemic rheumatic diseases, myopathies, endocrinopathies, myofascial pain syndrome, and neurologic disorders. It is also

Table 1 Widespread pain index score

Widespread pain index (final score will be 0–19)			
How many areas has the patient had pain in the last week?			
Shoulder girdle, left	Shoulder girdle, right	Hip, left (buttock or trochanter)	Hip, right (buttock or trochanter)
Upper arm, left	Upper arm, right	Lower arm, left	Lower arm, right
Upper leg, left	Upper leg, right	Lower leg, left	Lower leg, right
Jaw, left	Jaw, right	Neck	Chest
Upper back	Lower back	Abdomen	

Adapted from Wolfe et al. [13]

Table 2 Symptom severity scale score

Symptom severity scale score (final score will be 0–12)			
Indicate the level of severity of each symptom listed below over the last week, where: 0 = no problem 1 = slight of mild problems, mild or intermittent 2 = moderate, considerable problems, often present 3 = severe, pervasive, continuous			
Fatigue	0	1	2	3
Waking unrefreshed	0	1	2	3
Cognitive symptoms	0	1	2	3
Somatic symptoms[a]	0 None	1 Few	2 Moderate	3 Many
Final score will be 0–12				

Adapted from Wolfe et al. [13]

[a]Somatic symptoms can include muscle pain, irritable bowel syndrome, fatigue/tiredness, memory problem, muscle weakness, headache, abdominal cramping, numbness/tingling, dizziness, insomnia, depression, constipation, abdominal pain, nausea, nervousness, chest pain, blurry vision, fever, diarrhea, dry mouth, itching, wheezing, Raynaud's phenomenon, hives, tinnitus, vomiting, heartburn, oral ulcer, change in taste, seizures, dry eye, shortness of breath, loss of appetite, rash, sun sensitivity, hearing difficulties, easy bruising, hair loss, frequent urination, bladder spasms

Table 3 AAPT diagnostic criteria

The following symptoms present for 3 or more months		
Pain in six or more of the following nine sites		
Head	Left arm	Right arm
Chest	Abdomen	Upper back
Lower back	Left leg	Right leg
Moderate to severe sleep problems OR fatigue		

Adapted from Arnold et al. [12]

helpful to consider overlapping disorders such as functional somatic syndromes, chronic fatigue syndrome, and psychiatric disorders.

Laboratory and Imaging

Lab studies should focus on ruling out other alternative diagnoses being considered. This often includes CBC, thyroid function tests, inflammatory markers, and basic metabolic chemistries.

Routine imaging is not recommended.

Polysomnography may be warranted if the patient has symptoms of obstructive sleep apnea.

Approach to the Patient

Fibromyalgia is a difficult and controversial diagnosis for many primary care providers. Patients are commonly referred to rheumatology specialists for management, though most rheumatologists do not provide primary care for fibromyalgia [14]. Published treatment guidelines recommend that management of patients with fibromyalgia should be carried out in the primary care setting [15].

Treatment

Treatment should be viewed through the biopsychosocial model of illness and directed at the cardinal symptoms of fibromyalgia. Hallmarks of treatment include patient education, exercise, management of coexisting conditions, and pharmacologic therapy. Patients respond best to multidisciplinary, individualized treatment programs such as those implemented in a patient-centered medical home management framework [14–16]. Self-efficiency should be a goal of treatment. Unfortunately, most patients with fibromyalgia continue to have some level of chronic pain and fatigue despite treatment but can continue to live normal and active lives.

Patient Education

Patient education and shared decision-making has been shown to have a beneficial effect on pain scores and decrease in overall resource use and healthcare costs [17]. Patients should be reassured that despite the uncertain pathogenesis, fibromyagia is a real disease process. They should be educated regarding the nature of centralized pain dysregulation and assured that fibromyalgia is a benign disease. Comorbid stress, mood, and sleep disorders should be acknowledged, and education about maladaptive chronic illness behavior should be considered.

Exercise

Exercise is strongly recommended as a treatment for fibromyalgia and has been shown to decrease pain and improve physical function and health-related quality of life [17, 18]. Patients should be counseled that they will likely experience a temporary increase in pain upon initiating an exercise regimen, but this can be mitigated by individualizing treatment programs based on patient preference and comorbidities. Cardiovascular fitness training and low-impact aerobic activities such as brisk walking, biking, swimming, and water aerobics are usually well tolerated. Exercise should be initiated at whatever intensity and duration is possible and gradually increased to a target of 30 min three times per week. Even if patients cannot achieve this goal, they should be encouraged to continue exercising at whatever level is tolerated. Specific written exercise "prescriptions" can be helpful, as adherence is generally poor without persistent health care coaching [1].

Behavioral and Coexisting Disorders

In patients with fibromyalgia, the lifetime prevalence of anxiety is 60%, and depression is 74% [1]. Chronic overlapping pain conditions are common and include functional somatic syndromes such as irritable bowel syndrome, chronic fatigue syndrome, headaches, bladder and pelvic pain syndromes, and temporomandibular disorders [19]. Inadequate management of these conditions can worsen pain directly or indirectly and adversely affect fibromyalgia severity. In addition to disease appropriate treatment of these comorbidities, cognitive behavioral therapy, mind-body therapies, and stress reduction techniques can be helpful.

Medications

Pharmacologic therapy should be started at low dose and titrated up slowly. In the case of inadequate response or intolerable side effects, alternative agents should be preferentially selected based on a patient's most prominent symptoms. Clinically significant improvement occurs in 25–45% of patients treated with medications [20]. Off-label use of medications is common.

The tricyclic antidepressant (TCA) amitriptyline is considered first-line therapy [21]. Other medication class options include tricyclic muscle relaxants, serotonin-norepinephrine reuptake inhibitors (SNRI), and anticonvulsants. Amitriptyline (Elavil) is started at 10 mg at bedtime and may be increased by 5 mg every few weeks. The common effective range is 20–30 mg with a maximum dose of 75 mg. Cyclobenzaprine (Flexeril) is started at 5–10 mg at bedtime and titrated up to 30–40 mg divided daily.

Pregabalin (Lyrica), duloxetine (Cymbalta), and milnacipran (Savella) are the only drugs approved by the US Food and Drug Administration for treatment of fibromyalgia [1]. Pregabalin and gabapentin (Neurontin) are used to help patients with more severe sleep disturbances. Duloxetine and milnacipran can treat concomitant depression, fatigue, and pain symptoms.

Medications should be trialed for at least 3 months at the recommended dose before switching agents. Patients who respond to medication should be maintained on the lowest effective dose for at least 12 months. The decision to wean off medication should be individualized; many patients remain on medication indefinitely.

There is no evidence that acetaminophen (Tylenol), nonsteroidal anti-inflammatory drugs (NSAIDs), or opioid analgesics are effective in fibromyalgia. On the contrary, treatment with opioids results in poorer outcomes [22].

Myofascial Pain Syndrome

General Principles

Definition/Background
Myofascial pain syndrome (MPS) is a soft tissue pain disorder with symptoms similar to fibromyalgia. Both are characterized by painful trigger points; however MPS differs in that the trigger points are located in just one anatomic region rather than generalized, and the course is self-limited rather than chronic. MPS is not associated with fatigue or sleep disturbances.

Classification
MPS can be viewed as a spectrum of regional pain disorders. Myofasical trigger points can be caused by acute injury, repetitive microtrauma related to work or every day activities, or chronic strain of sedentary habits. Examples include whiplash injuries, occupational repetitive or overuse syndrome,

non-specific low back and cervical strain, tension headaches, and temporomandibular joint syndrome [23].

Approach to the Patient

Diagnosis

History and Physical Examination
There are no universally accepted diagnostic criteria for MPS [23].

Patients typically complain of deep aching pain located in one localized area, centered around a specific trigger point. Myofascial trigger points can be palpated, usually within a tight band of muscle of fascia. Etiology of the pain should be investigated with a thorough patient history.

Treatment
MPS is treated similarly to fibromyalgia; however prognosis is better, and patients usually respond well to local treatments. The expected clinical course and prognosis should be described to the patient as early as possible. Heat and cold modalities, topical pain relief creams, and passive stretch are common first-line therapies with few adverse reactions. For refractory cases, trigger point injections with a local anesthetic or corticosteroid, dry needling, and prolotherapy have been shown to be effective [23].

As with fibromyalgia, if patients develop chronic symptoms, treatment should focus on patient validation, education, and self-efficiency.

Complex Regional Pain Syndrome

General Principles

Background/Classification
Complex regional pain syndrome (CRPS) is a chronic pain disorder characterized by regional soft tissue changes and disproportionately severe pain arising from a previous injury.

Symptoms can include pain, swelling, decrease range of motion, sensory and vasomotor skin changes, and bone demineralization. This condition has also been referred to as reflex sympathetic dystrophy, causalgia, and transient osteoporosis [24].

The exact cause of CRPS is unknown but, like fibromyalgia, is suspected to be related to underlying central nervous system sensitization [25]. Common inciting events include fracture, soft tissue crush injuries, sprains, and surgery.

There are two recognized subtypes: type I and type II. In type I cases, there is no evidence of underlying nerve injury. This represents 90% of CRPS patients [24]. Type II refers to cases in which peripheral nerve injury is present. There are also "warm" and "cold" subtypes, referring to associated vasomotor skin symptoms, but these are not universally accepted.

Epidemiology

CRPS is more common in women than men, with an incidence of around 5–20 per 100,000 per year [25].

Approach to the Patient

Diagnosis

History and Physical Examination

The main symptoms of CRPS typically present within 4–6 weeks of an identifiable inciting event or injury. The most common complaint is pain. It is usually described as a continuous deep burning or tearing pain. Pain is usually associated with functional motor impairments including loss of strength or decreased range of motion. Patients may also complain of sensory or autonomic changes including differences in skin temperature, color, or edema. Trophic changes such as decreased hair growth, joint contraction, and skin atrophy may develop later in the course of disease [25].

Physical exam will typically reveal evidence of the inciting injury; however, the extent of symptoms should no longer be fully explained by the initial trauma. Findings will extend beyond the original region involved and cross through different nerve root distributions. Symptoms usually extend to the distal limb.

Laboratory and Imaging

There is no gold standard test to diagnose CRPS [24]. Plain radiographs or bone scintigraphy of the affected and contralateral limbs can be helpful to distinguish subtle bone changes.

Diagnostic Criteria

The Budapest Consensus Criteria aids in clinical diagnosis [26]. This includes:

- Continuing pain disproportionate to the inciting event
- Reports of one symptom in each of following categories:
  - Sensory: Hyperaesthesia or allodynia
  - Vasomotor: Temperature asymmetry, skin color changes, skin color asymmetry
  - Sudomotor: Edema, sweating changes, or asymmetry
  - Motor/trophic: Decreased range of motion, motor dysfunction (weakness, tremor, dystonia), or hair/skin/nail changes
- Findings of one sign in two or more of the following categories:
  - Sensory: Hyperalgesia to pinprick or allodynia to light touch, temperature, deep somatic pressure, or joint movement
  - Vasomotor: Greater than one degree Celsius skin temperature asymmetry or skin color change or asymmetry
  - Sudomotor: Edema, sweating changes, or sweating asymmetry
  - Motor/Trophic: Decreased range of motion, motor dysfunction (weakness, tremor, dystonia), or hair/skin/nail changes.
- And having no other diagnosis that that better explains the signs and symptoms.

Differential Diagnosis

The variety of signs and symptoms of CRPS makes for a broad differential diagnosis. Common alternative causes include compartment syndrome, peripheral vascular disease, DVT, peripheral neuropathy, rheumatoid arthritis, erythromelalgia, conversion, and facticious disorders.

Prognosis and Treatment

The prognosis for CRPS is uncertain. Spontaneous resolution of symptoms has been described, but most patients have some degree of permanent disability. Spontaneous recurrence is also possible and can occur in a different limb than the original episode [25].

Due to the unpredictable course of the disease, goals of treatment focus on restoration of function, management of pain and disability, and improvement in quality of life.

A multidisciplinary approach including physical therapy (PT), occupational therapy (OT), psychosocial support, and pain management is recommended [24].

Referrals

PT and OT should be initiated as quickly as possible after diagnosis as treatment is more effective when begun early [24]. Patients should be instructed that the symptoms they experience are neutrally mediated and do not indicate tissue damage. It is important to note that most therapies utilized to rehabilitate the affected limb will likely result in some level of pain.

Referral to a pain management specialist is recommended in patients with progressive symptoms who have an unsatisfactory response to initial conservative measures. Trigger point injections can be effective and are safer than other interventional options. There is limited and conflicting evidence for sympathetic nerve blocks for treatment of CRPS. Spinal cord stimulators have not been shown to improve functional outcomes or improve pain scores [24].

Comorbid behavioral health disorders can interfere with rehab goals and should be addressed appropriately.

Medications

Pain medications should be used to the extent that it allows for active participation in the rehab process. Common first-line medication includes NSAIDs. Adjuvant medications such as gabapentin or pregabalin are used for neuropathic pain. Bisphosophonates can be effective in patients with evidence of abnormal bone scans. Calcitonin, glucocorticoids, and opioids have been prescribed but have a less favorable risk to benefit ratio [24].

Neuroma

General Principles

Definition/Background

Neuromas are painful benign nervous system tumors that develop as a result of nerve injury. When injured, nerve endings regenerate in an unregulated fashion, resulting in neuroinflammation and disorganized growth, forming a neuroma. Most are asymptomatic which makes incidence difficult to estimate, but studies have placed incidence after amputation between 1% and 7.8% [27]. They have potential to develop anywhere in the body, but several common locations have been described and named. Injury prevention and repair of intraoperative nerve injury are key strategies for management.

Classification

There are three categories of neuromas: neoplasms, traumatic neuromas, and neuromas as a part of a syndrome.

Examples of true neoplastic neuromas include vestibular or acoustic neuroma, nerve sheath myxoma, and others. Acoustic neuromas develop on the vestibular portion of the eighth cranial nerve and cause hearing loss, tinnitus, and sometimes vertigo. They are diagnosed with neuroimaging and can be treated by surgery and radiation [27].

Traumatic neuromas can develop from a sharp, blunt, or traction injury. They are common after elective hand or knee surgery. Stump neuromas can also develop after amputation. A Morton's neuroma is a specific traumatic interdigital neuroma of the foot. It causes burning pain in the intermetatarsal space, most commonly between the third and fourth metatarsals. They are diagnosed with ultrasound and are treated conservatively with metatarsal support devices, shoe inserts, and, if severe, intralesional steroid injection. Surgery is only required in refractory cases [27].

Neuromas can also occur as part of a syndrome. Neurofibromatosis is a genetic syndrome that results in the growth of multiple central and peripheral nervous system neuromas. Multiple endocrine neoplasia 2B involves the trio of mucosal neuromas, thyroid carcinoma, and pheochromocytoma.

Approach to the Patient

Diagnosis

History and Physical Examination
History will reveal some sort of trauma or recent surgery to the affected region. Patient complaints include burning, tingling, numbness, or sharp pain. A hard lump is usually felt and can reproduce an electric shock sensation on palpation.

Imaging
Diagnosis is mainly reliant on history and physical exam. Plain radiographs are done to rule out underlying bone injury. Ultrasound (US), computed tomography (CT), and magnetic resonance imaging (MRI) are rarely necessary.

Treatment and Prevention
Prevention is essential to management. Many neuromas form as a result of surgery, so surgeons should reconnect severed nerve endings intraoperatively wherever possible to prevent neuroma formation. Surgical repair should not be under tension. If the two ends cannot be rejoined, as in the case with amputation, it is common to bury the nerve into nearby muscle tissue for targeted muscle reinnervation.

In the case of already formed neuromas, there is no consensus on best treatment practice which can vary based on neuroma location and etiology. Ice packs and relative rest can alleviate symptoms. Pain is resistant to most pharmacologic therapy, yet prescriptions for NSAIDs and local anesthetic creams are common. Intralesional steroids are reserved for refractory cases. Surgical excision is an option but recurrence rates range from 15% to 50% [27].

Dupuytren's Contracture

General Principles

Background
Dupuytren's disease, also called Dupuytren's contracture, is a fibroproliferative disorder that results in shortening and thickening of the palmar fascia, leading to progressive and symptomatic flexion contracture of the fingers.

Epidemiology
Dupuytren's disease is most common in whites of Northern European descent. It is more common in men than women, and average age at onset is 60 years old. Studies have suggested an autosomal dominant with incomplete penetrance genetic inheritance pattern [24].

It is more prevalent in patients with diabetes and has been associated with smoking, increased alcohol intake, manual labor or exposure to vibrations, low body mass index, and some anticonvulsant drugs [28].

Approach to the Patient

Diagnosis

Physical Examination
Dupuytren's disease begins as a palpable palmar nodule and progresses to a thickened peritendinous band of tissue resulting in a flexion contracture of the fingers. It is most common in the fourth and fifth digits. Skin tethering, puckering, and pitting, dimpling, and tenderness of the skin are common.

The Hueston's tabletop test is a simple procedure that can assist in diagnosis. It is positive if the patient is unable to lay their fingers, palm down, flat on a table [28].

Imaging is not usually warranted, and the diagnosis can be made clinically.

Treatment

Treatment is indicated as the contracture shows signs of progression and begins to impair function. For mild cases, the nodule can be injected with steroids to slow progression. One study showed that intermittent triamcinolone acetonide (Kenalog) injections every 4–6 weeks for 4–5 months led to significant regression [29]. Enzymatic collagenase injections and percutaneous needle aponeurotomy are alternatives to surgery that are also being investigated.

Referrals

Surgical referral is warranted if the metacarpal phalangeal joint contracture is greater than 30° or if there is any contracture of the proximal interphalangeal joint. Surgery is usually successful but the recurrent rate is high [30].

Ganglion Cyst

General Principles

A ganglion cyst is a benign fluid-filled mass overlying a joint or tendon sheath. They can occur anywhere on the body but are most common in the hand and wrist. Seventy percent are found on the dorsal wrist, 20% on the volar wrist, and the remaining 10% at other body sites [31]. They are commonly diagnosed in the second to fourth decades of life with a female predominance.

Approach to the Patient

Diagnosis

Physical Examination

Ganglion cysts present as an obvious palpable firm, round, smooth mass overlying a joint line. If they are large enough to exert mass effect on surrounding structures, patients may complain of joint tenderness, decreased range of motion, sensory, or motor loss.

Differential Diagnosis, Imaging, and Special Testing

Transillumination is an easy technique that can be done in an office setting to help ganglion cysts from other soft tissue nodular lesions. Ganglion cysts will transilluminate, while epidermoid cysts, lipomas, rheumatoid nodules, and tenosynovial giant cell tumors will not [31].

Consider gouty tophi in patients with a history of gout.

Infectious tenosynovitis can present as periarticular swelling but is accompanied by redness and swelling and preceded by a puncture or bite wound.

Ultrasound and MRI can also be useful but are usually reserved for pre-surgical planning.

Treatment

Treatment includes surgical and nonsurgical options. Around 50% of ganglion cysts will resolve spontaneously with observation [31].

For symptomatic patients, simple in-office aspiration can be attempted; however, recurrence rates are over 50% at 1 year [31]. If the cyst recurs within 1 month after aspiration, repeat attempts are unlikely to be successful. If symptoms are controlled for a longer period of time, repeat aspiration can be considered.

Surgical referral is warranted in patients with persistent symptoms despite conservative therapy. Surgical resection is more effective than aspiration with a less than 10% recurrence rate [31].

Closed rupture of ganglion cyst or "bashing it with a bible" is not recommended.

Selected Disorders of Bone

Benign Tumors

General Principles

Nonmalignant bone tumors are often discovered incidentally during evaluation for a different condition. When symptomatic, patients may complain of pain or swelling which can easily be confused for other musculoskeletal ailments which contribute to a delay in diagnosis.

Age of presentation, pain characteristics, and radiographic appearance can help assist in diagnosis. Treatment of these benign tumors ranges from observation to surgical removal.

Osteoid Osteoma

Background

Osteoid osteoma is a bone-forming tumor characterized by a small nidus of reactive bone identified on XR. It accounts for 12% of all benign bone tumors and is most common in the second decade of life. It is 2–3 times more common in males than females [32]. It is typically found in the long bones: femur, tibia, and humerus. Less commonly it presents in the posterior element of the spine.

History and Physical

Osteoid osteoma has a classic presentation of nocturnal bone pain dramatically improved with aspirin or NSAID medications [33]. Depending on the site, patients may also present with limp, leg-length discrepancy, localized swelling, and tenderness.

Imaging

Radiographs will show a small, less than 2 cm (0.75 in.), round osteolytic nidus surrounded by bone sclerosis. This is classically found in the cortex. About 25% of cases will present with a "target pattern" of central ring-like calcification [32].

Treatment and Prognosis

Treatment depends on symptoms. If pain can be managed with NSAID medication, observation with serial radiographs every 4–6 months is reasonable. Treatment for symptomatic lesions includes surgical resection or percutaneous radio-frequency ablation of the nidus. Untreated osteoid osteomas will spontaneously resolve over the course of months to years [34].

Osteochondroma

Background

Osteochondroma is a cartilage-capped bony over-growth arising from the surface of a bone. It is the most common primary bone tumor, accounting for 30% of benign bone tumors. It is most common in the second decade of life and is 1.5 times more common in males [35]. It has a predilection for the distal femur, proximal humerus, and proximal tibia.

History and Physical

Osteochondromas typically present as a painless palpable mass on the axial skeleton. They may cause pain and swelling if fractured. They may rarely grow large enough to compression of local neurovascular structures.

Imaging

Radiographs are sufficient for diagnosis. The bony protuberance can be pedunculated or sessile, typically growing away from the epiphysis and toward the diaphysis. The cartilage cap is thicker in childhood and progressively narrows into adulthood [35].

Treatment and Prognosis

Most osteochondromas do not need treatment. They continue to grow through adolescence and stop growing as the growth plate closes. There is a small lifetime risk of malignant transformation to chondrosarcoma, especially if the cartilage cap is greater than 2 cm (0.75 in.) thick or if it is increasing in size after skeletal maturity [33]. In these cases, treatment is surgical excision of the entire cartilage cap.

Enchondroma

Background

Enchondroma is a cartilage-forming neoplasm found in the marrow cavity. It is more common in women and can be found any time from the second to sixth decades of life with a peak in the in the 30s and 40s. They usually occur in the long bones with a predominance for the hands [36].

History and Physical

The majority of enchondromas are asymptomatic and are found incidentally. Pathologic fractures are more common with lesions in the hands and feet [36].

Imaging

Enchondromas are sharply defined and oval shaped. Endosteal scalloping and calcifications are common [33].

Treatment and Prognosis

Enchondromas are usually self-limited. If they require excision, simple curettage is sufficient. Recurrence is rare.

Non-ossifying Fibroma

Background

Non-ossifying fibroma is a developmental cortical defect, or "bone scar," in which normally ossified areas are instead filled with a fibrous connective tissue. They present in the second decade of life with no gender predominance. They are most common in the tibia and fibula [36].

History and Physical

These lesions are asymptomatic and are usually discovered during workup for unassociated trauma.

Imaging

Non-ossifying fibromas are small, irregular lytic lesions with sclerotic scalloped borders. They may have a more atypical appearance as they fill in with normal bone and resolve.

Treatment and Prognosis

They do not require any further treatment of follow-up. They fill in during adolescence and rarely recur.

Malignant Tumors

General Principles

Malignant bone cancers account for less than 1% of diagnosed cancers each year. Delay in diagnosis is common due to their rarity and the frequency of other musculoskeletal complaints. Lesions are often discovered during workup for suspected fracture rather than bone malignancy. Plain XR imaging is the first diagnostic step and is often sufficient for diagnosis. Due to the significant morbidity and mortality involved, prompt referral to orthopedic cancer specialists is recommended [37].

Approach to the Patient

History and Physical

The primary presenting symptom of a malignant bone cancer is pain, tenderness, and decreased range of motion. Unexplained relapsing and remitting fevers may also be present. Nighttime pain is commonly cited but is only present in 20–30% of patients with a primary malignant bone tumor [38].

Diagnosis

Plain radiograph is the preferred primary imaging study for malignant bone tumors. Any XRs which show potential malignancy should prompt advanced imaging. MRI is superior to CT for evaluating local metastasis. Bone scans and chest CT are helpful for identifying systemic metastasis.

Early referral to a comprehensive cancer center can maximize survival and quality of life [39]. Biopsy confirms the diagnosis, establishes tumor grade, and helps direct treatment.

Primary Osteosarcoma

Background

Osteosarcoma originates from malignant mesenchymal stem cells that differentiate into osteoblasts, the normal bone-forming cells. It is the most common bone cancer and the third most common childhood malignancy. Lesions classically develop in the metaphyses of long bones at the growth plate and thus tend to occur at the age of maximum bone growth. Median incidence is from 12 to 16 years old. Tumors can metastasize regionally or systemically and most often metastasizes to the lungs or to the bones of another extremity [40].

Osteosarcoma is associated with a few specific risk factors. The genetic syndromes Li-Fraumeni syndrome and retinoblastoma have higher incidence of osteosarcoma. History of radiation, previous implanted metal orthopedic prostheses, and Paget disease all have increased risk [39].

Imaging

Osteosarcoma is characterized radiographically by dense sclerosis of the metaphysis. Most tumors extend into the soft tissue and have radiating calcification in a "sunburst" pattern. Both osteosclerotic and lytic lesions can be present [39].

Treatment and Prognosis

Current treatment for osteosarcoma includes preoperative chemotherapy, surgical resection, and postoperative chemotherapy. This approach has helped 90–95% of patients with osteosarcoma avoid limb amputation [37]. Neoadjuvant chemotherapy can decrease the size of the primary tumor size and any pulmonary metastases, while adjuvant chemotherapy helps decrease risk of postsurgical metastasis. Radiation therapy is rarely used.

Five-year survival rate is more than 70% in people with non-metastatic disease but less than 30% if metastases are present. Unfortunately, nearly 20% of patients initially present with lung metastases [41]. Metastatic lesions that remain after chemotherapy are often surgical resected.

Ewing's Sarcoma

Background

Ewing's sarcoma is the second most common type of bone cancer. Its cell origin is unknown, but it is classified in a group of tumors known as small blue round cell tumors.

Like osteosarcoma, this cancer primarily affects children and adolescents during the period of peak bone growth. Unlike osteosarcoma, it typically affects the pelvis, diaphysis of long bones, ribs, and scapula. Common sites of metastasis include the lungs and other bones. There are few known risk factors for Ewing's sarcoma, though it has been associated with some specific genetic translocations [40].

Imaging

Radiographic appearance of Ewing's sarcoma is characterized by bone destruction. Radiating calcification "sunburst" pattern and lamellated "onion skin" periosteal reaction can be seen but are not pathognomonic [39].

Treatment and Prognosis

Like osteosarcoma, treatment for Ewing's sarcoma is neoadjuvant chemotherapy, surgical resection, and adjuvant chemotherapy. However, the use of radiation therapy is effective as an alternative therapy for lesions not amenable to surgical resection.

Metastasis at the time of diagnosis is the most significant negative prognostic factor for Ewing's sarcoma. Survival rates are comparable to osteosarcoma [41].

Chondrosarcoma

Background

Chondrosarcoma is malignant cartilage-producing tumor. It is the least common bone cancer. It usually manifests in people in their fifth to eighth decades of life and affects the central skeleton: pelvis, vertebrae, and proximal long bones. It can develop through malignant transformation of other benign cartilage tumors such as enchondromas [39].

Imaging

Plain radiographs may suggest the presence of a chondrosarcoma based on location and lesion appearance, but CT scan is optimal for evaluating tumor size and local extension. Typical XR appearance is an eccentric calcified osteolytic lesion, and CT can differentiate between mineralized and unmineralized cartilage matrix [29].

Treatment and Prognosis

Chondrosarcoma is generally resistant to chemotherapy. Surgical resection is the primary treatment. Radiation is reserved for lesions where surgical margins cannot be achieved. Tumor grade is the major prognostic indicator in chondrosarcoma. The vast majority of these tumors are low grade and survival rates after surgical resection are favorable [40].

References

1. Clauw DJ. Fibromyalgia: a clinical review. JAMA. 2014;311:1547.
2. Goldenberg DL. Fibromyalgia syndrome. An emerging but controversial condition. JAMA. 1987;257:2782.
3. Goldenberg DL. Diagnosing fibromyalgia as a disease, an illness, a state, or a trait? Arthritis Care Res (Hoboken). 2019;71:334.
4. Pomares FB, Funck T, Feier NA, et al. Histological underpinnings of grey matter changes in fibromyalgia investigated using multimodal brain imaging. J Neurosci. 2017;37:1090.
5. Wolfe F, Ross K, Anderson J, et al. The prevalence and characteristics of fibromyalgia in the general population. Arthritis Rheum. 1995;38:19.
6. Jones GT, Atzeni F, Beasley M, et al. The prevalence of fibromyalgia in the general population: a comparison of the American College of Rheumatology 1990, 2010, and modified 2010 classification criteria. Arthritis Rheumatol. 2015;67:568.
7. Wolfe F, Clauw DJ, Fitzcharles MA, et al. Fibromyalgia criteria and severity scales for clinical and epidemiological studies: a modification of the ACTR Preliminary Diagnostic Criteria for Fibromyalgia. J Rheumatol. 2011;38:1113.
8. Walitt B, Ceko M, Khatiwada M, et al. Characterizing "fibrofog": subjective appraisal, objective performance, and task-related brain activity during a working memory task. Neuroimage Clin. 2016;11:173.
9. Loge-Hagen JS, Saele A, Juhl C, et al. Prevalence of depressive disorder among patients with fibromyalgia: systematic review and meta-analysis. J Affect Disord. 2019;245:1098.
10. Wolfe F, Smythe HA, Yunus MB, et al. The American College of Rheumatology 1990 criteria for the classification of fibromyalgia. Report of the multicenter criteria committee. Arthritis Rheum. 1990;33:160.
11. Lodahl M, Treister R, Oaklander AL. Specific symptoms may discriminate between fibromyalgia patients with vs without objective test evidence of small-fiber polyneuropathy. Pain Rep. 2018;3:e633.
12. Arnold LM, Bennett RM, Crofford LJ, et al. AAPT diagnostic criteria for fibromyalgia. J Pain. 2019;20:611.
13. Wolfe F, Clauw DJ, Fitzcharles MA, et al. The American College of Rheumatology preliminary diagnostic criteria for fibromyalgia and measurement of symptom severity. Arthritis Care Res (Hoboken). 2010;62:600.

14. Hadker N, Garg S, Chandran AB, et al. Efficient practices associated with diagnosis, treatment and management of fibromyalgia among primary care physicians. Pain Res Manag. 2011;16:440.

15. Fitzcharles MA, Ste-Marie PA, Goldenberg DL, et al. Canadian Pain Society and Canadian Rheumatology Association recommendations for rational care of persons with fibromyalgia: a summary report. J Rheumatol. 2013;40:1388.

16. Arnold LM, Gebke KB, Choy EH. Fibromyalgia: management strategies for primary care providers. Int J Clin Pract. 2016;70:99.

17. Macfarlane GJ, Kronisch C, Dean LE, et al. EULAR revised recommendations for the management of fibromyalgia. Ann Rheum Dis. 2017;76:318.

18. Bidonde J, Busch AJ, Schachter CL, et al. Aerobic exercise training for adults with fibromyalgia. Cochrane Database Syst Rev. 2017;(6):CD012700.

19. Maixner W, Fillingim RB, Williams DA, et al. Overlapping chronic pain conditions: implications for diagnosis and classification. J Pain. 2016;17:T93.

20. O'Malley PG, Balden E, Tomkins G, et al. Treatment of fibromyalgia with antidepressants: a meta-analysis. J Gen Intern Med. 2000;15:659.

21. Rico-Villademoros F, Slim M, Clandre EP. Amitriptyline for the treatment of fibromyalgia: a comprehensive review. Expert Rev Neurother. 2015;15:1123.

22. Goldenberg DL, Clauw DJ, Palmer RE, Clair AG. Opioid use in fibromyalgia: a cautionary tale. Mayo Clin Proc. 2016;91:640.

23. Borg-Stein J. Treatment of fibromyalgia, myofascial pain, and related disorders. Phys Med Rehabil Clin N Am. 2006;17:491.

24. Harden RN, Oaklander AL, Burton AW, et al. Complex regional pain syndrome: practical diagnostic and treatment guidelines, 4th ed. Pain Med. 2013; 14:180.

25. Borchers AT, Gershwin ME. Complex regional pain syndrome: a comprehensive and critical review. Autoimmun Rev. 2014;13:242.

26. Harden RN, Bruehl S, Stanton-Hicks M, Wilson PR. Proposed new diagnostic criteria for complex regional pain syndrome. Pain Med. 2007;8:326.

27. Zabaglo M, Dreyer MA. Neuroma. [Updated 2019 Nov 15]. In: StatPearls [Internet]. Treasure Island: StatPearls Publishing; 2020. https://www.ncbi.nlm.nih.gov/books/NBK549838/

28. Shih B, Bayat A. Scientific understanding and clinical management of Dupuytren disease. Nat Rev Rheumatol. 2010;6:715.

29. Ketchum LD, Donahue TK. The injection of nodules of Dupuytren's disease with triamcinolone acetonide. J Hand Surg. 2000;25:1157–62.

30. Trojian TH, Chu SM. Dupuytren's disease: diagnosis and treatment. Am Fam Physician. 2007;76:86–9.

31. Suen M, Fung B, Lung CP. Treatment of ganglion cysts. ISRN Orthop. 2013;2013:940615.

32. Olvi LG, Lembo GM, Santini-Araujo E. Osteoid osteoma. In: Santini-Araujo E, Kalil R, Bertoni F, Park YK, editors. Tumors and tumor-like lesions of bone. London: Springer; 2015. p. 127–49.

33. Arkader A, Gebhardt MC, Dormans JP. Bone and soft-tissue tumors. In: Weinstein SL, Fllynn JM, editors. Lovell and Winter's pediatric orthopaedics. 7th ed. Philadelphia: Wolters Kluwer Health; 2014.

34. Aboulafia AJ, Kennon RE, Jelinek JS. Benign bone tumors of childhood. J Am Acad Orthop Surg. 1999;7:377.

35. Park YK. Osteochondroma. In: Santini-Araujo E, Kalil R, Bertoni F, Park YK, editors. Tumors and tumor-like lesions of bone. London: Springer; 2015. p. 265–71.

36. Biermann JS. Common benign lesions of bone in children and adolescents. J Pediatr Orthop. 2002;22:268.

37. Ferguson JL, Turner SP. Bone cancer: diagnosis and treatment principles. Am Fam Physician. 2018;98 (4):205–13.

38. Widhe B, Widhe T. Initial symptoms and clinical features in osteosarcoma and Ewing sarcoma. J Bone Joint Surg Am. 2000;82(5):667–74.

39. Marina N. Malignant bone tumors. In: Lanzkowsky P, editor. Manual of pediatric hematology and oncology. 5th ed. London: Academic; 2010. p. 739–57.

40. Lieberman JR. Malignant bone tumors. In: AAOS comprehensive orthopaedic review. Rosemont: American Academy of Orthopaedic Surgeons; 2009. p. 417–42.

41. Anderson ME. Update on survival in osteosarcoma. Orthop Clin North Am. 2016;47(1):283–92.

Part XXIII

The Skin and Subcutaneous Tissues

Wanda Cruz-Knight

Contents

General Principles

According to a study conducted by the American Academy of Dermatology, one in every four people who present to a primary care physician (PCP) will have a skin-related problem; roughly 85 million Americans have skin disorders [1]. Therefore, skin conditions are a common cause of patient visits in the primary care setting. While most presentations are minor or easily identifiable, PCPs must be able to promptly recognize these conditions to determine appropriate management.

Diseases of the integumentary system include everything related to the surface of the body. Table 1 outlines the most common skin disease categories and their types based on the International Classification of Diseases, Ninth Revision (ICD-9) and billing data from 2013 [1].

The dermatoses are divided into conditions affecting the skin, nails, and hair. This chapter will focus on the most common dermatoses. While common dermatoses may be accompanied by inflammation, the term dermatitis refers to inflammation of the skin and is not synonymous with dermatoses [2]. Causes of dermatosis may be multifactorial or unknown; most commonly dermatoses are categorized into autoimmune disorders, bacterial, fungal, viral, and genetic. The most common autoimmune disorders are vitiligo, lupus, and alopecia areata. *Staphylococcus aureus* and *Streptococcus pyogenes* are the most common bacterial. Tinea can cause skin infections such as athlete's foot. Ashy dermatosis is

W. Cruz-Knight (✉)
Family Medicine, University of South Florida Morsani School of Medicine, Clearwater, FL, USA

GME BayCare Medical Group, Tampa, FL, USA

USF-MPM Family Medicine, Clearwater, FL, USA
e-mail: Wanda.Cruz-Knight@baycare.org

© Springer Nature Switzerland AG 2022
P. M. Paulman et al. (eds.), *Family Medicine*,
https://doi.org/10.1007/978-3-030-54441-6_153

Table 1 Common skin disease categories and their types based on the International Classification of Diseases, Ninth Revision (ICD-9) and billing data from 2013

Disease category	Disease type
Acne	Acne
Atopic dermatitis/eczema	Atopic dermatitis; eczema; dyshidrosis
Actinic damage	Actinic keratosis; solar dermatitis; sunburn; actinic dermatitis
Bullous diseases	Dermatitis herpetiformis; pemphigus; pemphigoid; other bullous dermatoses; erythema multiforme
Congenital abnormalities	Various hereditary and congenital conditions and anomalies, including ichthyosis congenita, vascular hamartomas, and congenital ectodermal dysplasia
Connective tissue disorders	Lupus; dermatomyositis; scleroderma; diffuse connective tissue disease
Contact dermatitis	Contact dermatitis; diaper rash; nonspecified dermatitis
Cutaneous infections	Bacterial skin infections, including tuberculosis and leprosy; cellulitis; carbuncles; impetigo; onychia
Cutaneous lymphoma	Mycosis fungoides/Sezary syndrome; parapsoriasis
Drug eruptions	Drug dermatitis; Stevens-Johnson syndrome
Hair and nail disorders	Alopecia; telogen effluvium; hirsutism; hair and nail anomalies
HPV/warts/molluscum	Warts, including genital warts; molluscum contagiosum
Melanoma	Malignant melanoma
Nonmelanoma skin cancer	Basal cell carcinoma; squamous cell carcinoma; Kaposi sarcoma; carcinoma in situ
Noncancerous skin growths (benign neoplasms/keloids/scars/cysts)	Lipomas; benign neoplasms; hemangiomas; chalazions; cysts, including pilonidal, Pilar, and sebaceous; corns, calluses, and keratoderma; keloids; scars and fibrosis
Pruritus	Pruritus not otherwise specified; psychogenic skin disease; lichenification
Psoriasis	Psoriasis
Rosacea	Rosacea
Seborrheic dermatitis	Seborrheic dermatitis
Seborrhea	Seborrheic dermatitis; blepharitis
Ulcers	Ulcers, all stages and causes; pyoderma gangrenosum
Urticaria	Psoriasis
Viral	Fungal diseases herpes simplex; herpes zoster; viral exanthemata; dermatophytosis; dermatomycosis; candidiasis
Vitiligo	Vitiligo
Wounds and burns	Burns, all degrees; lacerations; wounds; abrasions; bites; foreign bodies, e.g., splinters

commonly caused by HIV. Finally, genetic susceptibility can predispose people to dermatoses.

There are many skin-related disorders. This chapter will focus on common conditions that most primary care providers will encounter and manage.

Acne

Acne vulgaris is the most common skin condition in the United States, affecting 20% of young people [3]. The severity of acne correlates with puberty, although acne may persist into the 20s and 30s in 64% and 43% of individuals, respectively [3]. Acne can affect the skin in varying degrees from mild involvement to severe presentations leading to facial disfigurement, scarring, and hyperpigmentation. Adolescents and young adults with acne often struggle with the psychosocial effects of acne and may have a higher rate of depression [4].

The pathogenesis of acne vulgaris is complex. Originating within the pilosebaceous follicles, there are four main processes involved in the production of comedones or microcomedones that lead to pimples, papules, or skin scarring, sebum overproduction in the follicles, abnormal shedding of follicular epithelium, follicular colonization by *Cutibacterium acnes*, and inflammation [5]. Excessive androgen hormones or hypersensitivity of sebaceous glands to normal levels of androgen is believed to be the cause of sebum overproduction, with activation of the inflammatory pathway at all stages of acne progression [6]. Genetic factors, diet, psychological stress, tobacco smoke, and damage to the skin integrity may also be involved in the development or progression of acne.

Clinical manifestations of acne vary dependent on type. Table 2 describes the different types of acne lesions; the extent and severity of skin lesions vary widely depending on inflammatory nature and body's response to follicular irritation

Table 2 Clinical manifestation: acne vulgaris occurs in areas of the body with hormonally responsive sebaceous glands such as the face, neck, chest, upper back, and upper arms

Types of acne lesions	Description	Image	Examples
Non-inflammatory acne			
Closed comedones	<5 mm; dome-shaped; smooth; skin-colored, whitish, or grayish papules		Whiteheads
Open comedones	<5 mm papules with a central, dilated, follicular orifice containing gray, brown, or black, keratotic material	https://dermnetnz.org/topics/comedonal-acne/	Blackheads
Giant comedones	>5 mm papules, sebaceous material in pores usually black/brown		Large blackhead-appearing lesions
Solar comedones	Small skin-colored papule from sun damage and usually form in older adults, primarily on the cheeks	https://dermnetnz.org/topics/comedonal-acne/	Mixed white and black sebaceous material
Inflammatory acne			
Papulopustular acne	<5 mm inflamed, relatively superficial papules and pustules		Pus-filled pustules
Nodular acne	>0.5 mm pustules or >1 cm nodules that are deep-seated, inflamed, often tender		Nodular acne

Table 3 Differential diagnosis of acne vulgaris

Inflammatory facial lesions	Non-inflammatory facial lesions	Trunk and extremities	Acneiform eruptions
Rosacea	Sebaceous hyperplasia/seborrheic dermatitis	Folliculitis	Drug-induced acne
Periorificial dermatitis	Nevus comedonicus	Keratosis pilaris	Neonatal cephalic pustulosis
Pseudofolliculitis barbae	Adnexal tumors	Hidradenitis suppurativa	Acne cosmetica
Facial angiofibromas in tuberous sclerosis	Favre-Racouchot syndrome	Steatocystoma multiplex	Acne mechanica
Acne fulminans	Miliaria	Acne fulminans	Occupational acne and chloracne

and activation of inflammatory pathways. Treatment options are based on individual presentation and extent and severity of skin involvement.

Approach to the Patient

Diagnosis of acne vulgaris is dependent on history and physical examination. While there are no laboratory tests to confirm a diagnosis of acne, testing may be warranted when there is suggestion of underlying hyperandrogenism, abscess formation, or other conditions needing additional testing. Patient history is an important element of identifying risk factors that may promote/exacerbate acne formation or guide treatment options.

Patients should be asked information regarding:

- Onset of acne.
- Current medications (there are medications that can exacerbate acne).
- Menstrual history (females) and association with menstrual cycle [7].
- Family history of acne (there is a familial predisposition to acne).
- Systemic symptoms, joint pains, myalgias in patients with severe acne.
- Questions regarding virilization.
- Medical history to include history of prior acne treatment and response.
- Skin care regiment.
- Psychosocial impact.

On physical examination, attention to lesion type and distribution, signs of hyperandrogenism in young children and females, and the presence of skin scarring and post-inflammatory hyperpigmentation are important factors in determining extent/severity of acne, ruling out other skin conditions that may mimic acne, and guiding treatment options. The differential diagnosis of acne can be approached based on location of lesions, onset and duration, and inflammatory versus non-inflammatory nature; Table 3 will outline some of these conditions.

Treatment Options

Treatment of acne vulgaris is based on severity of lesions, location on the skin, and hormonal and dietary history. The decision to use a topical versus an oral therapeutic approach is also dependent on presentation and individual history. Topical treatment options may be available over the counter and by prescription dependent on the formulation and strength needed when individualizing the therapeutic plan [8]. Topical agents are divided into bacteriostatic and bactericidal and are widely available in different formulations and strengths [9, 10]. It is recommended that topical antibiotics not be used as monotherapy due to increased risk of resistance to *C. acnes*. The treatment is aimed at counteracting follicular hyper-proliferation and sebum production, decreasing the levels of

C. acnes on the skin surface, and attacking the inflammatory pathways. Topical retinoids, benzoyl peroxide, azelaic acid, and salicylic acid are effective against comedone formation, with retinoids being preferred as first-line therapy [11]. For patients with mild to moderate inflammatory acne, a topical antibiotic should be added to benzoyl peroxide therapy, as the treatment has been shown to be more effective [9]. For patients with moderate to severe inflammatory acne, an oral antibiotic is recommended along with the use of a topical retinoid and benzoyl peroxide [11].

Oral isotretinoin is reserved for patients with severe, recalcitrant, nodular acne. While women with signs of hyperandrogenism once evaluated for other conditions may benefit from use of oral contraceptives. It is recommended that oral antibiotics be used for limited therapeutic courses, up to 3–4 months. Topical retinoids may be used for acne prevention. A skin care regiment is also an important component of treatment. Use of gentle cleansers and selection of noncomedogenic skin care products and cosmetics are recommended. Facial peels and other cosmetic treatments target hyperpigmentation and scarring and help to improve the psychosocial impact of acne. Referral to a dermatologist is recommended for recalcitrant acne or failed treatment with appropriate management.

Atopic Dermatitis

Atopic dermatitis also known as eczema is an inflammatory skin disease that includes skin dryness, erythema, oozing, and crusting that can lead to lichenification of the skin [12]. While the causes of eczema are not clear, it is believed to be due to genetic predisposition to environmental allergens with skin destruction from pruritus causing much of the disease burden of patients and family. Atopic dermatitis affects up to 25% of children and 2–3% of adults [13]. One out of ten people will develop eczema in their lifetime, with 60% of those predisposed becoming symptomatic in their first year of life and 90% before the age of 5 [14].

Approach to the Patient

History, onset, and clinical presentation are key diagnostic tools. While pruritus is the hallmark for diagnosis, eczema, age of onset, and location of dry skin in skin folds are other criteria [15]. Identifying triggers improves burden of disease. There are no specific labs to aid in diagnosing eczema, although skin biopsy for atypical presentations. Allergy testing can aid with treatment options.

Treatment

Treatment of atopic dermatitis is dependent on severity, skin involvement, causative agents if identified, and medical history. The goal of treatment is reduction of symptoms and prevention. Reducing inflammatory response with topical anti-inflammatory preparations and protecting skin with barriers that prevent cracking and dry skin are important. Patients with severe or refractory eczema may require autoimmune modulators, phototherapy, or systemic treatment [16].

Other common dermatoses are listed in Table 4.

Family and Community Implication of Common Dermatoses

The overall burden of diseases that make up the dermatoses is significant. Yearly over $80 billion healthcare dollars are spent on management of these diseases [20, 21]. Likewise, many of the dermatoses cause skin scarring and deformities that have psychological implications. The chronic condition of some of the dermatoses discussed also affects quality of life and increases burden of suffering. Treatment options continue to improve as research and development continue to address the need for improved management of diseases that make up common dermatoses.

Table 4 Other common dermatoses

Common dermatosis	Epidemiology	Approach to the patient	Diagnosis	Treatment
Androgenetic alopecia, also referred to as hereditary thinning or balding	Affects about 50 million men and 30 million women [17]	Clinical and family history counseling and management of psychosocial implications	Family history Diffuse hair thinning over the central scalp, while the frontal hairline is usually retained in women Gradual recession of the frontal hairline, gradual thinning in the temporal areas, producing a reshaping of the anterior part of the hairline in men Labs: Dehydroepiandrosterone (DHEA) sulfate and testosterone analysis	Identifying and treating other causes of hair loss, i.e., fungal, damage from hair products, thyroid disorders, or iron deficiency Minoxidil: Androgen-independent hair growth stimulator Finasteride: 5-alpha reductase type 2 inhibitors Hair transplant/plugs Hormones to correct imbalance
Psoriasis	Over seven million Americans affected [18] Occurs in all age groups but has the highest prevalence among ages 45 and 64	Clinical and family history – a complex immune-mediated disease in which T lymphocytes, dendritic cells, and cytokines (interleukin [IL]-23, IL-17, and tumor necrosis factor [TNF]) play a central role	Clinical presentation of erythematous papules and plaques with silver scale, may also be accompanied by joint pain and other systemic symptoms No available labs except to exclude other differential diagnosis Skin biopsy if history and physical exam is inconclusive Differential diagnosis may include seborrheic dermatitis, atopic dermatitis, lichen chronicus, fungal infections	Address psychosocial aspect Mild to moderate disease responds to topical corticosteroid therapy, retinoid therapy, or phototherapy; topical tacrolimus or pimecrolimus may be used as alternatives or as corticosteroid-sparing agents for facial involvement Severe psoriasis requires phototherapy or systemic therapies such as retinoids, methotrexate, cyclosporine, apremilast, or biologic immune-modifying agents
Rosacea	Over 16 million Americans affected [19] Common among white people of all ages and races with these groups more commonly affected: Ages 30 and 60 Faired skin, blond hair, and blue-eyed individuals Menopausal women Family history of rosacea	Family history, history of onset and exacerbating factors, psychosocial implications	Diagnosis is based on clinical presentation and history Persistent centrofacial redness, phymatous skin changes (e.g., rhinophyma), papules, pustules, flushing, telangiectases, burning or stinging sensations, edema, and skin dryness Ocular involvement may include lid margin telangiectases, conjunctival injection, ocular irritation, or other signs and symptoms	Psychosocial Mild to moderate disease treated with topical metronidazole, azelaic acid, and topical ivermectin Oral antibiotic therapy, tetracycline, doxycycline, and minocycline are indicated for severe rosacea

References

1. Lim W, Collins SAB, Resneck JS Jr, Bolognia JL, Hodge JA, Rohrer TA, Van Beek MJ, Margolis DJ, Sober AJ, Weinstock MA, Nerenz DR, Begolka WS, Moyano JV. The burden of skin disease in the United States Henry. J Am Acad Dermatol. 2017;76:958–72.
2. Coulson IH, Benton EC, Ogden S. Diagnosis of skin disease. In: Griffiths C, Barker J, Bleiker T, et al., editors. Rook's textbook of dermatology. 9th ed. Oxford: Wiley-Blackwell; 2016. Part 2: Chap. 4:1–26.
3. Bhate K, Williams HC. Epidemiology of acne vulgaris. Br J Dermatol. 2013;168:474–85. https://doi.org/10.1111/bjd.12149.
4. Horne J, Health Psychologist, Middlemore Hospital, Auckland, New Zealand. Chief Editor: Dr. Amanda Oakley, Dermatologist. Psychosocial factors in dermatology. Hamilton; DermNet NZ. April 2015.
5. Toyoda M, Morohashi M. Pathogenesis of acne. Med Electron Microsc. 2001;34(1):29–40.
6. O'Neill AM, Gallo RL. Host-microbiome interactions and recent progress into understanding the biology of acne vulgaris. Microbiome. 2018;6:177.
7. Stoll S, Shalita AR, Webster GF, et al. The effect of the menstrual cycle on acne. J Am Acad Dermatol. 2001;45:957.
8. Gamble R, Dunn J, Dawson A, et al. Topical antimicrobial treatment of acne vulgaris. Am J Clin Dermatol. 2012;13(3):141–52.
9. Tan HH. Topical antibacterial treatments for acne vulgaris: comparative review and guide to selection. Am J Clin Dermatol. 2004;5(2):79–84.
10. Haider A, Shaw JC. Treatment of acne vulgaris. JAMA. 2004;292:726.
11. Bienenfeld A, Nagler AR, Orlow SJ. Oral antibacterial therapy for acne vulgaris: an evidence-based review. Am J Clin Dermatol. 2017;18(4):469–90.
12. Weidinger S, Novak N. Atopic dermatitis. Lancet. 2016;387:1109.
13. Eichenfield LF, Tom WL, Chamlin SL, Feldman SR, Hanifin JM, Simpson EL, et al. Guidelines of care for the management of atopic dermatitis: section 1. Diagnosis and assessment of atopic dermatitis. J Am Acad Dermatol. 2014;70(2):338–51.
14. Beltrani VS, Boguneiwicz M. Atopic dermatitis. Dermatol Online J. 2003;9(2):1.
15. LeBovidge JS, Elverson W, Timmons KG, et al. Multidisciplinary interventions in the management of atopic dermatitis. J Allergy Clin Immunol. 2016;138(2):325–34.
16. Eichenfield LF, Tom WL, Berger TG, et al. Guidelines of care for the management of atopic dermatitis: section 2. Management and treatment of atopic dermatitis with topical therapies. J Am Acad Dermatol. 2014;71:116.
17. Genetics Home Reference. National Institutes of Health U.S. Library of Medicine. https://ghr.nlm.nih.gov/condition/androgenetic-alopecia#statistics. Accessed 30 May 2020.
18. Menter A, Gottlieb A, Feldman SR, Van Voorhees AS, et al. Guidelines of care for the management of psoriasis and psoriatic arthritis: Section 1. Overview of psoriasis and guidelines of care for the treatment of psoriasis with biologics. J Am Acad Dermatol. 2008;58(5):826–50.
19. Okhovat J-P, Armstrong AW. Updates in rosacea: epidemiology, risk factors, and management strategies. Curr Dermatol Rep. 2014;3:23–8.
20. American Academy of Dermatology/Milliman. Burden of skin disease. 2017. www.aad.org/BSD
21. Guy GP, Machlin SR, Ekwueme DU, Yabroff KR. Prevalence and costs of skin cancer treatment in the US, 2002–2006 and 2007–2011. Am J Prev Med. 2015;48:183–7.

Micah Pippin

Contents

M. Pippin (✉)
Family Medicine, LSUHS Shreveport Family Medicine
Residency, Alexandria, LA, USA
e-mail: mpipp2@lsuhsc.edu

© Springer Nature Switzerland AG 2022
P. M. Paulman et al. (eds.), *Family Medicine*,
https://doi.org/10.1007/978-3-030-54441-6_147

Bacterial Infections of the Skin

Impetigo

General Principles
Impetigo is a common bacterial infection affecting the superficial epidermis resulting in bullous and non-bullous skin eruptions.

Epidemiology
While children ages 2–5 are the most frequently affected, impetigo can manifest in persons of any age. *Staphylococcus aureus* and group A beta-hemolytic *Streptococcus pyogenes* are responsible for most cases; however, anaerobic bacteria are also implicated in disease development. The non-bullous subtype comprises a majority of cases, while bullous impetigo has a lower incidence and is caused exclusively by *Staphylococcus* and its epidermolytic toxins [1]. Certain medical comorbidities, such as diabetes mellitus, may predispose patients to impetigo.

Diagnosis

History and Physical Examination
The non-bullous form can be further categorized into primary, affecting intact, healthy skin, and secondary, infecting a previously disrupted epidermis. Diagnosis is clinical and based on a typical presentation and skin manifestation. An initial maculopapular lesion gives way to thin-walled vesicles that rupture and produce the characteristic honey-colored crusts. The typical distribution includes the nares and perioral area, with the extremities also being affected. Bullous impetigo is more often seen on the trunk, axilla, and intertriginous locations. Large, fluid-filled blisters collapse into flaccid bullae with a resulting thin, brown crust. Both bullous and non-bullous lesions are usually self-limited and resolve without scarring.

Treatment
Topical antibiotics, such as mupirocin, have demonstrated increased effectiveness versus placebo in the management of impetigo. Diffuse or severe infections and outbreaks may require systemic

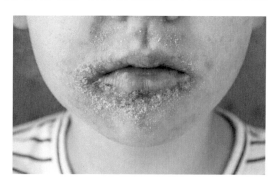

Fig. 1 Impetigo of the face

treatment; however, adverse effects and emerging antimicrobial resistance to oral antibiotics make topical therapies preferable. Specifically, oral penicillin and macrolides are no longer indicated due to resistance. There is currently insufficient evidence to recommend topical disinfectants or popular herbal treatments for impetigo [1]. The most serious complication is acute post-streptococcal glomerulonephritis; however, there is no data to support antibiotics as effective prevention of impetigo's nephritogenic potential [1, 2] (Fig. 1).

Erysipelas

General Principles
Erysipelas, historically known as "St. Anthony's Fire," is a bacterial skin infection of the dermis and lymphatics, often affecting the lower extremities and face and presenting similarly to cellulitis.

Epidemiology
Group A Streptococci is the most common causative organism entering through breaks in the skin and disseminating through the lymphatic system. Risk factors for erysipelas include obesity, diabetes mellitus, venous insufficiency, lymphedema, and any disruption of the cutaneous protective barrier [2, 3].

Diagnosis

History and Physical Examination
Fevers, chills, and malaise often precede the characteristic painful rash featuring an area of

well-demarcated erythema with raised edges. The lower extremities are predominantly affected, while facial erysipelas also occurs and may develop secondary to nasopharyngeal streptococcal infection [2, 3]. Linear streaks of erythema may represent progression through the lymphatic system. The rashes' sharp margins help distinguish erysipelas from the deeper and less confined cellulitis infection.

Treatment

Antibiotics with coverage for streptococci should be administered with penicillin being first-line treatment. Most patients can be managed outpatient with oral preparations; however, severe infections may require intravenous antibiotics and hospitalization (Fig. 2).

Cellulitis

General Principles

Similar to erysipelas, cellulitis is an acute bacterial infection affecting the dermis; however, it also invades deeper into the skin's subcutaneous tissues.

Epidemiology

The majority of cellulitis presentations are attributed to the Gram-positive cocci *Streptococcus* and *Staphylococcus aureus*. In the case of animal bites, Gram-negative bacteria have been isolated. Methicillin-resistant *Staphylococcus aureus*

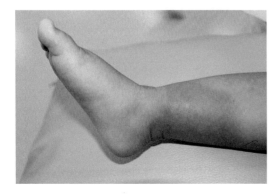

Fig. 2 Erysipelas of the lower extremity

(MRSA) is continuing to grow as a cellulitis pathogen.

Any event or condition that compromises the integrity of the skin such as trauma, venous insufficiency, lymphedema, tinea pedis, diabetes, or obesity may increase susceptibility to acquiring cellulitis.

Diagnosis

History and Physical Examination

Typical findings suggestive of cellulitis include an area of erythema, pain, edema, and heat, most often occurring in a lower extremity. The findings are more diffuse than erysipelas and lack the sharply demarcated border. Purulence suggests *Staphylococcus aureus* as the etiologic organism. Systemic symptoms such as fever and malaise may accompany the cutaneous manifestations.

Evaluation

In general, clinical evaluation is sufficient for diagnosis; however, laboratory analysis and blood cultures should be pursued if sepsis is suspected. Inspection for the presence of an abscess is a vital component of the physical examination and can be difficult. In recent years, ultrasound has emerged as an effective technique in discovering abscess formation [4, 5].

Treatment

In cases of mild, uncomplicated cellulitis, oral antibiotics with coverage for *Streptococcus* and methicillin-sensitive *Staphylococcus aureus* (MSSA), such as cephalexin, should be initiated. If purulence is noted, or risk factors for MRSA are present, coverage for resistant *Staphylococcus* is needed and can be achieved with the addition of oral trimethoprim/sulfamethoxazole or clindamycin. Orbital cellulitis, a variant affecting the tissue surrounding the eye, mandates inpatient treatment and consultation with ophthalmology [2]. Severe cellulitis infections and patients with signs of sepsis or shock should also be treated inpatient with broad-spectrum intravenous antibiotics. Individual patient history and local

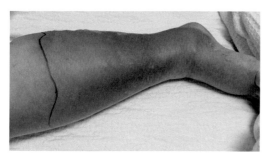

Fig. 3 Cellulitis of the lower extremity

resistance patterns should direct treatment choices and augment standard guidelines (Fig. 3).

Folliculitis

General Principles
Folliculitis is a superficial inflammation of the hair follicles caused by infection and less frequently chemicals or trauma.

Epidemiology
Bacterial pathogens are most often responsible for folliculitis, and, of these, *Staphylococcus aureus* is the most prevalent. *Pseudomonas aeruginosa* may be encountered after exposure to unsanitary bathing reservoirs, and the resulting infection is frequently referred to as "hot tub folliculitis." There are significantly fewer folliculitis cases of fungal etiology, most of which are reported in patients with travel history or immunodeficiency. There may be a male gender preference for folliculitis secondary to frequent shaving.

Diagnosis

History and Physical Examination
A folliculitis diagnosis is clinically attained by observation of perifollicular papules and pustules with a surrounding ring of erythema. The lesions may be asymptomatic to painful depending on the degree of inflammation and can occur anywhere hair follicles are present.

Evaluation
Cultures may be obtained in recalcitrant cases; however, they are rarely required.

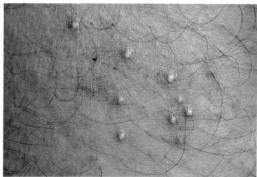

Fig. 4 Folliculitis

Treatment
Topical mupirocin and fusidic acid are first-line therapies for uncomplicated cases. Diffuse, resistant, or recurrent infections should be treated with oral antibiotics such as cephalexin or dicloxacillin. If MRSA infection is suspected or confirmed by culture, trimethoprim/sulfamethoxazole, clindamycin, or doxycycline may be administered systemically [2]. *Pseudomonas* folliculitis is generally self-limited, and antibiotic treatment is not warranted (Fig. 4).

Furuncles and Carbuncles

General Principles
Furuncles and carbuncles, also known as boils, can be viewed as an intermediate in the continuum of skin infections from folliculitis to abscess. While folliculitis affects the superficial tissue around hair follicles, furuncles invade deeper into the subcutaneous tissue and may develop an accumulation of purulent material. Carbuncle refers to an aggregation of individual furuncles resulting in a more diffuse eruption.

Epidemiology
Staphylococcus aureus, often inhabiting healthy skin and the nares, is the most common causative organism and is seeded in the hair follicle through disruptions of the protective cutaneous barrier. Conditions that compromise skin integrity, such as eczema, diabetes, obesity, and poor hygiene, predispose patients to infection [2, 6]. Young

adults and males exhibit an increased predilection for furuncle and carbuncle formation.

Diagnosis

History and Physical Examination
Furuncles present as a tender, erythematous, fluctuant, nodule with superficial pustule formation. Carbuncles are clustered furuncles affecting a larger area and with multiple, purulent drainage sites. Any region of skin occupied by hair follicles can host these infections; however, the neck, face, axilla, groin, back, and buttocks are the most favorable sites of outbreak. Associated lymphadenopathy may manifest and systemic, constitutional symptoms such as fever and malaise can accompany localized inflammation.

Evaluation
The diagnosis can be made based on history and physical examination; however, cultures of expressed purulent material are often obtained to guide management strategies.

Treatment
The mainstay of treatment is incision and drainage of the lesion or lesions and may require subsequent initiation of empiric oral antibiotics. The same categories of antibiotics implemented for folliculitis are utilized, such as cephalosporins or dicloxacillin. If an MRSA etiology is suspected or cultured, antibiotic coverage should be selected to target this organism. Adjunctive topical antibiotics may be offered (Fig. 5).

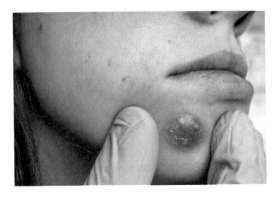

Fig. 5 Carbuncle of the face

Hidradenitis Suppurativa

General Principles
Hidradenitis suppurativa is a chronic and progressive inflammatory condition of the follicular pilosebaceous units located in intertriginous areas. Along with the extensive somatic complaints associated with hidradenitis suppurativa, significant psychologic impact is observed, resulting in an increased adverse impact on quality of life compared to other dermatologic conditions [7].

Epidemiology
Hidradenitis suppurativa has a female predominance and occurs more frequently in blacks and patients with a personal family history. Disease onset is common to young adulthood, and there is an increased incidence in cigarette smokers and the obese. Associated conditions include diabetes mellitus, metabolic syndrome, polycystic ovarian syndrome, and Crohn disease [7].

Diagnosis

History and Physical Examination
Localized painful nodules are present in the mild form of hidradenitis suppurativa and may progress to abscess formation and a broadened distribution in moderate disease. The axillae are the most commonly involved sites, with the gluteal folds, groin, perianal area, perineum, and inframammary regions also affected. Diffuse and recurrent sinus tracts, scarring, and contractures occur in the severe manifestation of the condition. The Hurley classification system is implemented to clinically stage the severity of hidradenitis suppurativa and direct treatment strategies [7].

Treatment
Lifestyle modification, including weight loss and smoking cessation, are the primary non-pharmacologic treatments for hidradenitis suppurativa. Topical clindamycin is the first-line management for mild disease and may be combined with oral tetracycline for moderate presentations. Biologics, specifically adalimumab, are indicated for severe or recalcitrant disease, at

which point, dermatology referral would be warranted [7]. Surgical measures, including punch debridement and incision and drainage, may be performed for acute relief; however, wide excision is the definitive treatment. Combinations of these treatment modalities may be implemented and are often indicated.

Screening for depression should be performed, and resources for the patient's psychological well-being should be made available [7] (Fig. 6).

Abscess of Skin

General Principles

A skin abscess is an accumulation of purulent material within the skin and subcutaneous tissues resulting in a painful and inflammatory focus of infection.

Epidemiology

Staphylococcus aureus, whether MSSA or MRSA, are the predominant bacteria responsible for cutaneous abscesses. Risk factors for abscess

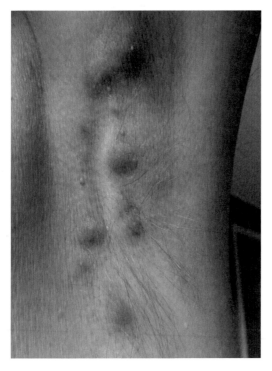

Fig. 6 Axillary hidradenitis suppurativa

formation are similar to cellulitis, furuncles, and carbuncles and include breaks in the skin, venous insufficiency, immunosuppression, diabetes mellitus, and obesity. Abscesses can affect any demographic.

Diagnosis

History and Physical Examination
Classic findings of erythema, tenderness, induration, and fluctuance are generally sufficient to make the diagnosis. Common locations for abscess formation include the extremities, axillae, groin, and buttocks [8].

Evaluation
If the physical examination is ambiguous, and the diagnosis is in question, ultrasound evaluation has demonstrated efficacy in distinguishing an abscess from cellulitis [8, 9]. Laboratory analysis is merited if signs of sepsis are present such as fever and tachycardia.

Treatment
Incision and drainage are required for successful treatment of cutaneous abscesses. Guidelines have stated that antibiotic use is unnecessary following successful surgical debridement of uncomplicated abscesses; however, new evidence suggests that the addition of oral antibiotics improves infection resolution rates and decreases recurrence risk. Also, in the case of complicated abscesses, of concurrent cellulitis, or when systemic symptoms manifest, antibiotic initiation is encouraged. If antimicrobials are implemented, coverage of MRSA with trimethoprim/sulfamethoxazole or clindamycin is recommended. Cephalosporins have not demonstrated effectiveness and are not suggested [8]. After incision and drainage of a typical abscess, packing is no longer advised as it has been shown to increase discomfort and has no effect on recurrence.

Prevention of bacterial skin infections such as folliculitis, furuncles, carbuncles, and abscesses through decolonization with intranasal mupirocin and topical chlorhexidine washes has been suggested; however, the efficacy of these measures has not been substantiated by statistically significant evidence (Fig. 7).

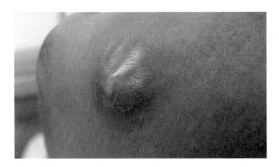

Fig. 7 Abscess of the back

Necrotizing Fasciitis

General Principles
Necrotizing fasciitis is a rare, limb- and life-threatening, rapidly invasive infection of the subcutaneous tissue and fascia.

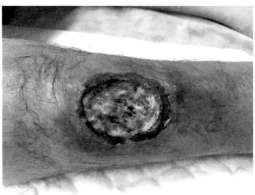

Fig. 8 Necrotizing fasciitis of the lower extremity

Epidemiology
Most cases are secondary to a polymicrobial bacterial infection; however, different subtypes of necrotizing fasciitis are monomicrobial and have even been attributed to fungal elements. Risk factors include obesity, diabetes mellitus, hypertension, chronic kidney disease, venous insufficiency, immunodeficiency, and alcohol and drug abuse [10]. Diabetes mellitus is the most significant comorbidity and is associated with increased rates of limb amputations [10]. One subset of necrotizing fasciitis seen mostly in people with diabetes is Fournier's gangrene, a life-threatening infection of the male genitalia.

Diagnosis

History and Physical Examination
The initial presentation resembles cellulitis and demonstrates localized erythema, edema, and pain. As the infection progresses, vesicles, bullae, necrosis, and crepitus may develop. Distinguishing necrotizing fasciitis from cellulitis may be difficult; however, disproportionate pain on examination and pain outside the margin of erythema may indicate a more extensive infection. Systemic manifestations such as fever, confusion, septic shock, and multiple organ failure result in a high mortality rate and necessitate urgency with evaluation and intervention.

Evaluation
While laboratory and radiographic investigation may assist in making the diagnosis, surgical exploration should not be delayed when clinical suspicion is high.

Treatment
Early surgical debridement and fasciotomy are critical and should be accompanied by empiric broad-spectrum intravenous antibiotic administration. Repeat surgical debridement is often necessary (Fig. 8).

Erythrasma

General Principles
Erythrasma is a bacterial rash of the skin's stratum corneum commonly affecting interdigital and intertriginous locations and often confused with fungal infections.

Epidemiology
Corynebacterium minutissimum is the causative organism [11]. Healthy adults, especially African Americans, are predominantly affected while patients who live in hot, humid climates, are obese, or have diabetes mellitus are more susceptible to infection.

Diagnosis

History and Physical Examination
The eruption is characterized by a well-demarcated, hyperpigmented, and erythematous, macular patch with variable degrees of pruritus. Wood lamp examination exhibits a coral-red fluorescence and may aid in diagnosis.

Treatment
Topical therapy with clindamycin or erythromycin is effective in managing localized infections, while oral erythromycin or clarithromycin may be necessary for extensive disease. Recurrence is common, but the risk may be curtailed by the implementation of proper hygiene and weight loss lifestyle modification.

Viral Diseases of the Skin

Herpes Simplex

General Principles
Herpes simplex is a lifelong neurocutaneous disorder occurring secondary to viral pathogens that lay dormant in neurons until they episodically recur and manifest as mucocutaneous eruptions.

Epidemiology
Herpes simplex virus type 1 (HSV-1) is predominantly responsible for non-genital infections, although herpes simplex virus type 2 (HSV-2) can cause herpes labialis and other variations. The virus is acquired through direct contact and fomite transmission and is most often encountered through nonsexual contact in childhood. Adolescents and adults are often infected through kissing and sharing utensils and straws. There is a gender preference for females, and risk factors for infection include early sexual experiences, frequent and multiple sexual partners, history of a partner with oral lesions, and personal history of non-HSV sexually transmitted infections [12].

Diagnosis

History and Physical Examination
Oral HSV-1 is the most likely presentation to be encountered in the primary care setting. As with other herpetic infections, a prodrome of fever and malaise may precede the mucocutaneous eruption. Primary HSV-1 infection, also known as herpetic gingivostomatitis, is characterized by multiple vesicles on swollen erythematous bases distributed throughout the oral mucosa and lips and subsequently ulcerating into severely painful lesions. Regional lymphadenopathy is often observed. The course of this disease, through the complete resolution of all symptoms, may take up to 2 weeks.

Recurrent labial herpes is often heralded by sensations of paresthesias, itching, and burning at the location of the future eruption and is stimulated by illness, stress, trauma, and UV light exposure [12]. Clusters of painful vesicles appear on the lip's vermillion border, which then ulcerate and crust over followed by resolution in about 1 week. Recurrence rates differ between patients, with some never experiencing a herpetic flare. With subsequent manifestations, the symptoms are often less severe, and the clinical course is abbreviated.

Herpetic keratitis results from an ocular viral infection and must be treated urgently to avoid chronic scarring of the cornea and blindness [12]. Herpetic whitlow affects the hands and digits and is frequently acquired by children who suck their thumbs and bite their nails and healthcare workers who examine patients without proper personal protective equipment. Wrestlers may encounter herpes gladiatorum, which commonly appears on the torso after skin-to-skin contact. In patients with eczema, an HSV outbreak may superimpose itself over atopic areas resulting in a dermatologic emergency known as eczema herpeticum [12].

Evaluation
The diagnosis of herpes simplex can usually be made through a careful history and physical examination. In atypical presentations, or when the diagnosis is in question, viral cultures, PCR,

serology, antibody testing, and Tzanck smears can be implemented to confirm suspected infection.

Treatment

Children with acute, primary herpetic gingivostomatitis can be managed effectively with oral acyclovir suspension. Systemic treatment with nucleoside analogs, such as acyclovir and valacyclovir, is indicated for recurrent herpes labialis outbreaks. Topical therapies can be applied; however, they are not as effective as oral preparations. In patients with numerous recurrences, prophylactic antivirals can be administered (Fig. 9).

Genital Herpes

General Principles

Genital herpes is a prevalent sexually transmitted infection characterized by recurrent, vesicular eruptions of the groin secondary to a lifelong, acquired viral infection.

Epidemiology

Genital herpes may be caused by HSV-1 and HSV-2 infections. Historically, groin outbreaks were predominantly attributed to HSV-2; however, changes in sexual practices have increased HSV-1 prevalence to half of all new cases acquired [13]. Risk factors for viral acquisition include black race, female sex, numerous and unsafe sex encounters, and the presence of other sexually transmitted infections. Also, individuals with HSV-2 have an increased risk of acquiring HIV.

Diagnosis

History and Physical Examination

Outbreaks of genital herpes include single and clustered vesicles that ulcerate, causing pain, itching, and burning. Areas affected include the genitals, perineum, perianal areas, buttocks, and upper thighs, and associated lymphadenopathy may be present. Primary infections may be accompanied by malaise and fever, while subsequent outbreaks are generally less severe and are sometimes preceded by a prodrome. HSV-1 eruptions are often milder, and recurrences are less frequent than HSV-2 infection. Concurrent HIV-positive status increases the severity of HSV-2 flare-ups. Some patients remain asymptomatic carriers, and viral shedding may occur without active expression of the disease.

Evaluation

In patients with clinical disease, type-specific confirmatory testing is recommended to guide management and counseling. Active lesions should be analyzed by PCR, while asymptomatic patients with a history of outbreaks should be evaluated with serologic testing. Partners of HSV-infected patients should also receive type-specific serologic testing to assess their risk of HSV acquisition.

Treatment

Management of genital herpes may be episodic for acute eruptions, or suppressive to prevent recurrence or transmission. Nucleoside analogs such as acyclovir are all equally effective at decreasing the duration and severity of symptoms. Suppressive therapy can reduce the risk of HSV transmission to at-risk partners; however, in patients with HSV-2 and concurrent HIV, suppressive treatment is ineffective at reducing the spread of genital herpes [13].

In pregnant patients with genital herpes, suppressive therapy should be initiated from 36 weeks to term, and laboring women with active lesions should be offered elective cesarean delivery.

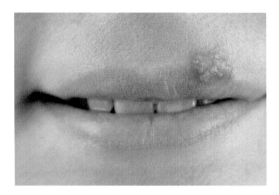

Fig. 9 Herpes labialis on the lip's vermillion border

Herpes Zoster

General Principles
Herpes zoster, or shingles, is the cutaneous manifestation of the reactivation of the dormant varicella virus inhabiting neurons of infected individuals. Zoster represents a pervasive syndrome, and its sequelae can result in chronic debilitation.

Epidemiology
Shingles occur secondary to varicella zoster, the same virus responsible for chickenpox and to which most American adults have been exposed. Reactivation of the dormant pathogen results in the characteristic eruption associated with zoster. With age, the risk of manifesting the disease increases significantly as the immune system naturally weakens, while immunosuppressive disorders such as HIV also confer susceptibility.

Diagnosis

History and Physical Examination
The classic shingles rash is often preceded by a prodrome of symptoms, including fever, malaise, and abnormal skin sensations such as itching and burning. The typical outbreak consists of maculopapular lesions confined to a single, unilateral dermatome which develop into clear, then cloudy, vesicles. Crusting eventually occurs, followed by rash resolution in 2–4 weeks. Scarring and pigmentation changes may develop, and nerve injury secondary to inflammation can result in a chronic pain syndrome known as postherpetic neuralgia. Most rashes are distributed along the dermatomes between T1 and L2; however, viral reactivation in the fifth cranial nerve can result in a condition known as zoster ophthalmicus [14].

Evaluation
In most cases, the diagnosis can be made clinically; however, PCR analysis of vesicular fluid can be utilized for atypical presentations or when the diagnosis is in question.

Treatment
Acyclovir, famciclovir, and valacyclovir decrease the duration of symptoms and pain severity,

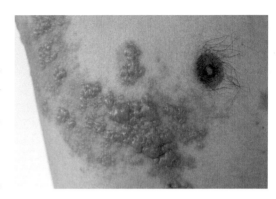

Fig. 10 Herpes zoster of the trunk

especially if initiated within 72 h of the eruption. Adjunctive glucocorticoids may help with discomfort and inflammation; however, they do not decrease the incidence of postherpetic neuralgia, as previously recorded. Acetaminophen and nonsteroidal anti-inflammatories are recommended for the management of mild to moderate symptoms. Postherpetic neuralgia may be treated topically with lidocaine patches or capsaicin cream and systemically utilizing anticonvulsants, tricyclic antidepressants, and, in severe cases, opioids [14].

For herpes zoster prevention, the Advisory Committee on Immunization Practices recommends the use of the recombinant zoster vaccine known as Shingrix beginning at age 50. Two doses of Shingrix are delivered 2–6 months apart and are encouraged even if its predecessor, Zostavax, was previously administered [15] (Figs. 10 and 11).

Viral Warts

General Principles
Warts are benign neoplasms resulting from a viral infection of the skin's epidermal layer.

Epidemiology
Viral warts arise secondary to human papillomavirus. Many different subtypes of this virus exist and manifest with unique presentation and at different locations of the body. In general, cutaneous

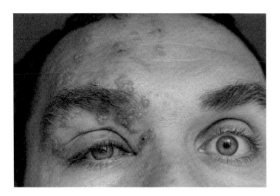

Fig. 11 Zoster ophthalmicus

warts occur most commonly in childhood, while mucosal and genital warts arise in sexually active adolescents and adults, most often in women. Risk factors for epidermal warts include immunosuppression, contact with infected individuals, nail-biting, and walking barefoot.

Diagnosis

History and Physical Examination

Warts present as hyperkeratotic papules and plaques with pathognomonic thrombosed capillaries appearing as small, black dots. Verruca vulgaris appear most commonly on the hands with periungual variations developing adjacent to nails. Plantar warts sprout near pressure points on the soles of the feet and may exhibit discomfort. Planar warts, occurring most often on the face, can be more challenging to diagnose due to their flat appearance and lack of characteristic thrombosed vessels [16]. Sexually transmitted, condylomatous warts erupt on the skin and mucous membranes of the genitalia and anus and, if left untreated, may develop into large, cauliflower-like vegetations known as condyloma acuminatum.

Treatment

Most warts will resolve spontaneously; however, they can cause discomfort and cosmetic concern, and some cases are recurrent or recalcitrant to therapy. Several different treatment modalities exist, none of which has good evidence for consistent effectiveness or superiority to one another.

Topical application of salicylic acid and cryotherapy are management options often implemented in primary care settings. Imiquimod is frequently utilized for condylomatous warts and may be used as second-line therapy for recalcitrant cutaneous warts. Laser ablation, photodynamic therapy, immunomodulation with injected candida antigen, and surgical removal are all emerging treatment options that may be available in secondary care settings [16] (Figs. 12 and 13).

Molluscum Contagiosum

General Principles

Molluscum contagiosum is a highly transmissible viral infection of the skin's keratinocytes spread by direct patient contact, indirect fomite exposure, or autoinoculation through scratching.

Epidemiology

The poxvirus molluscum contagiosum virus is responsible for the epidermal lesions. Children are most commonly infected; however, sexually active adults and immunocompromised individuals may also develop symptoms. The characteristic rash generally appears 2–6 weeks after viral exposure and may persist for months to years.

Diagnosis

History and Physical Examination

Flesh and pink-colored, pearly, dome-shaped papules with central umbilication appear and range in size from 1 mm to 1 cm in diameter. Common eruption locations include the face, trunk, limbs, and axilla and spare only the palms and soles. The anogenital region, abdomen, and thighs are more frequently subject to an outbreak in sexually transmitted infections. Erythema and inflammation may develop as part of the normal immune response or may indicate a secondary bacterial infection.

Treatment

Because the lesions resolve spontaneously, the treatment of non-irritating molluscum is unnecessary. Removing children from school or daycare is

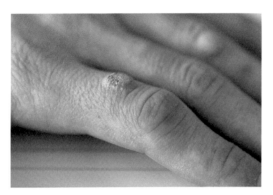

Fig. 12 Viral wart of the index finger

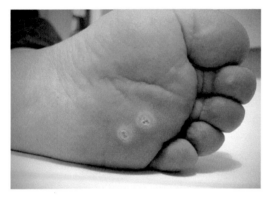

Fig. 13 Plantar warts

also not warranted [17]. If treatment is desired for cosmetic or other reasons, several in-office modalities exist. Topical cantharidin application, curettage, and liquid nitrogen cryotherapy are all appropriate management options. Scratching avoidance, proper hygiene practices, and safe sex in adults may all prevent molluscum transmission (Fig. 14).

Fungal Infections of the Skin

Dermatophytoses

General Principles

Tinea disorders are a group of cutaneous infections caused by dermatophytes, fungal organisms that affect keratinized structures such as the skins' stratum corneum, hair, and nails.

Epidemiology

Trichophyton rubrum is the most common causative fungal species in humans; however, several different dermatophytes can result in infection. Tinea corporis and tinea capitis, which occur on the body and scalp, respectively, mainly occur in prepubescent children. Tinea cruris results in a groin outbreak and almost exclusively develops in males. Tinea pedis, an interdigital foot manifestation, is commonly known as "athlete's foot" and occurs in patients who walk barefoot in communal areas and have persistently sweaty feet. Both tinea cruris and tinea pedis are most frequently found in adolescents and young adults and often occur concurrently. Tinea manuum, an eruption on the hand, can be secondary to autoinfection from scratching an affected foot and is commonly referred to as two feet-one hand syndrome. Dermatophytes may also affect facial hair in adult males, a diagnosis known as tinea barbae. In wrestlers, a version called tinea gladiatorum occurs. Tinea conditions are more common in warmer climates, and individuals with excessive perspiration, diabetes mellitus, and immunocompromise and who wear occlusive garments are predisposed to infection.

Diagnosis

History and Physical Examination

Tinea, in all its forms, generally appears as a pruritic, erythematous, scaling, annular rash with central clearing and an advancing border. The lesions may be isolated or may confluence into a more diffuse eruption. Tinea capitis is associated with localized alopecia. If left untreated, scalp infections may progress to a boggy and indurated inflammatory condition known as a kerion. Tinea cruris infects the skin of the thighs opposite the scrotum but spares the actual genitalia. This feature, as well as a lack of satellite lesions, can help differentiate tinea cruris from candida intertrigo. Tinea pedis classically affects the toe webs; however, it can spread to the plantar and lateral aspects of the foot, commonly referred to as a "moccasin pattern" [18].

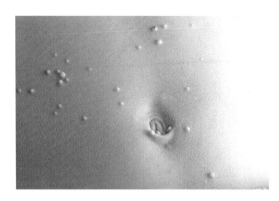

Fig. 14 Molluscum contagiosum of the abdomen

Evaluation

The diagnosis of tinea can often be made clinically by observing the characteristic rash; however, microscopy using potassium hydroxide (KOH) preparations can aid when the diagnosis is in question. While Wood lamp examination can demonstrate fluorescence with some dermatophyte infections, its uses are limited and false negatives may occur if the area viewed has recently been washed. Knowledge of erythrasma's coral-red fluorescence by Wood lamp can help exclude this bacterial infection from the differential when investigating possible dermatophyte rashes. Histology using periodic acid-Schiff (PAS) stains can be performed but is rarely indicated.

Treatment

For localized infection, topical azoles, such as ketoconazole, or allylamines, such as terbinafine, are effective. For severe, diffuse, or recalcitrant cases, oral preparations of antifungals such as terbinafine or itraconazole can be implemented. Oral ketoconazole is no longer recommended due to hepatotoxicity. Tinea capitis must be managed with systemic antifungals with griseofulvin commonly used in children and azoles and allylamines used in adults. Sporicidal shampoos may be used as adjunctive management of tinea capitis. Nystatin is used for candida infections and is not effective against dermatophytes. Topical steroids are currently categorized as a mistreatment for tinea

infections. They may initially help with pruritus and inflammation; however, the rash will recur, or its characteristic appearance will be obscured in a condition known as tinea incognito.

Prevention can be achieved by improved hygiene, non-occlusive clothing, and removal of moist garments after perspiration (Figs. 15 and 16).

Onychomycosis

General Principles
Onychomycosis is a prevalent fungal infection affecting the nails of the hands and, more commonly, the feet.

Epidemiology
Trichophyton rubrum and other dermatophytes cause a majority of onychomycosis cases; however, non-dermatophyte molds and yeast are increasingly implicated in nail infections. Old age, obesity, and tinea pedis increase the risk for onychomycosis, while conditions such as diabetes mellitus and psoriasis predispose patients to infection [19].

Diagnosis

History and Physical Examination
Discoloration and thickening of the nail plate are the classic findings on physical examination and can progress to nail distortion and discomfort in advanced disease.

Evaluation
Microscopy using KOH, fungal cultures, histologic evaluation with PAS staining, and PCR are all available to confirm the diagnosis.

Treatment
Multiple treatment modalities are implemented in the management of onychomycosis. Protracted courses of oral antifungals such as terbinafine are often prescribed, and newer topical preparations such as efinaconazole are demonstrating

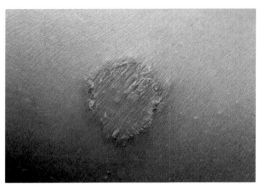

Fig. 15 Tinea corporis

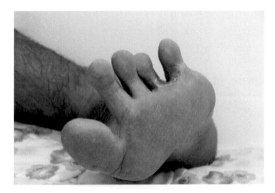

Fig. 16 Tinea pedis

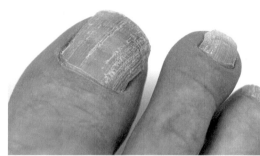

Fig. 17 Onychomycosis of the toenails

Yeast

General Principles
Candidiasis, or yeast infections, represent a group of non-dermatophyte fungal eruptions that affect the epithelium of cutaneous and mucosal surfaces.

Epidemiology
Yeast infections are overwhelmingly caused by *Candida albicans* with other candida species also causing pathology. Candida intertrigo is the most common cutaneous manifestation and affects the moist and friction-laden skin of intertriginous locations. A variation known as candida diaper dermatitis affects the groin and buttocks of newborns and infants. Thrush is an oral, mucocutaneous disorder affecting newborns and at-risk adult hosts. Candidal vulvovaginitis and candida balanitis are yeast infections of the female and male sexual organs, respectively. Obesity, excessive perspiration, diabetes mellitus, frequent steroid or antibiotic use, and any condition that compromises immune functioning place patients at increased risk for yeast infections [21].

Diagnosis

History and Physical Examination
The cutaneous candida rash is characterized by a pruritic, erythematous, finely scaling eruption with associated satellite lesions that occur in

improved efficacy. Traditionally, due to the cost and adverse events associated with systemic treatments, confirmatory testing has been recommended before initiation of oral treatments. New studies suggest that empiric therapy with terbinafine, without organism verification by KOH, may be preferred as the cost of terbinafine is minimal, and hepatotoxicity is less significant than previously speculated [20]. Some guidelines still suggest confirmatory testing. Also, following baseline liver function tests before initiating terbinafine, subsequent laboratory monitoring may not be necessary unless symptoms arise or a history of liver dysfunction is present. Due to the high cost of newer topical therapeutics, the diagnosis should be confirmed with PAS histology before their initiation. Nail debridement may also be implemented to improve cure rates (Fig. 17).

intertriginous areas such as the axillae, groin, inframammary and sub-pannus regions. Infants commonly present with a diaper dermatitis variant of this condition, which may feature maceration and fissures. Thrush is defined by white plaques adherent to the tongue and oral mucosa, which, when removed, reveal erythematous epithelium. In females, itching, burning, and dysuria are accompanied by a white, curdy discharge and erythematous, tender vaginal mucosa in the vulvovaginal manifestation of candida infections. Uncircumcised men are at increased risk for balanitis, which causes tender, erythematous inflammation of the glans and shaft of the penis [2].

Evaluation

Diagnosis is mainly clinical; however, KOH-aided microscopy of the skin and tongue and vaginal wet preps can be implemented if other conditions cannot be excluded by the history and physical examination alone. Budding yeast and septate hyphae are positive findings visualized on microscopy.

Treatment

Management of most cutaneous yeast infections can be accomplished with the application of a topical antifungal such as nystatin or one of the topical azole preparations. Thrush can be eradicated by nystatin oral suspension, and some adults may require systemic treatment with fluconazole. Uncomplicated vulvovaginal candidiasis can be treated with a single dose of oral fluconazole or a number of azole intravaginal creams. Severe, recurrent, and recalcitrant cases of vaginal yeast infections may require multiple doses of fluconazole over an established treatment duration. Therapies for balanitis are similar to those for vulvovaginal disease [2]. Steroid creams and ointments may help initially with discomfort and inflammation; however, they should not be utilized as they can prolong the course of infection.

Medication review, as well as lifestyle modification, including weight loss, avoidance of excessive perspiration and occlusive garments, and

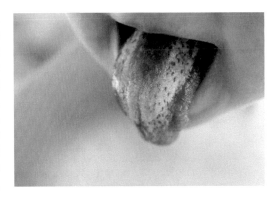

Fig. 18 Oral candidiasis (thrush)

frequent diaper changes, may prevent future candida outbreaks (Fig. 18).

Tinea Versicolor

General Principles

Tinea versicolor, or pityriasis versicolor, is a common fungal infection of the torso and proximal extremities, which is named for the variable pigmentation presentations that appear based on the patient's complexion and skin tone.

Epidemiology

Tinea versicolor is caused by *Malassezia*, a fungal component of healthy skin flora, which becomes pathogenic in patients who live in hot and humid conditions, have oily skin, are immunodeficient, or who have a genetic predisposition. Adolescents and young adults are primarily affected due to the hospitable environment provided by their skin's increased sebum production. Pityriasis versicolor has no gender or racial predominance [22].

Diagnosis

History and Physical Examination

As the name implies, tinea versicolor is characterized by numerous, scaling ovals of varied pigmentation. The typical distribution involves the neck, trunk, and extremities with single well-defined lesions that confluence into larger patches and plaques. The eruption may be erythematous to hyperpigmented in lighter complexions and hypopigmented in darker-skinned patients. Light pruritus may occur, but most presentations are asymptomatic.

Evaluation

The diagnosis can be made clinically; however, Wood lamp fluorescence and KOH preparations may be utilized when the diagnosis is unclear. The spores and hyphae visualized on microscopy have been traditionally described as "spaghetti and meatballs."

Treatment

Topical antifungals such as ketoconazole are the preferred first-line treatments, and other over-the-counter preparations such as selenium sulfide may also be implemented topically. Oral antifungals can be used as second-line agents in severe, recurrent, and recalcitrant cases; however, systemic ketoconazole is no longer recommended due to hepatotoxicity (Figs. 19 and 20).

Infestations

Lice/Pediculosis

General Principles

Pediculosis is an obligate blood ectoparasite infestation resulting in symptoms of intense pruritus. This misunderstood condition provokes anxiety for patients, parents, and school healthcare personnel, leading to an often undue burden for those involved.

Epidemiology

Pediculus humanus capitis, *Pediculus humanus corporis*, and *Pthirus pubis* affect the scalp, body, and pubic region, respectively. Transmission is less pervasive than is commonly perceived and requires direct, close contact due to the louse's inability to jump or fly. Pediculosis capitis is often observed in school-aged children, while pediculosis corporis should be suspected in individuals with poor hygiene or who live in crowded conditions. Pediculosis pubis is found in sexually active adolescents and adults.

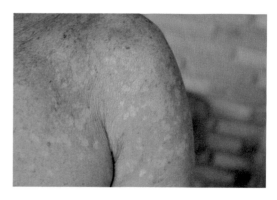

Fig. 19 Tinea versicolor of the trunk and upper extremities

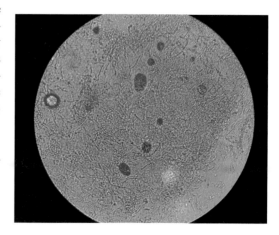

Fig. 20 Spores and hyphae visualized on microscopy of tinea versicolor skin scrapings "spaghetti and meatballs"

Diagnosis

History and Physical Examination

The diagnosis of pediculosis requires direct visualization of at least one live louse and can be aided by a lighted magnifying lens and a fine-toothed nit comb. Observation of nits alone does not indicate an active infestation and does not warrant intervention. Body lice are often found in the seams of clothing upon examination [23]. Family members should be examined if the diagnosis is confirmed.

Treatment

The insecticidal agent permethrin is the preferred first-line agent for the management of pediculosis. As with other non-ovicidal treatment options, permethrin should be administered on two occasions

7–10 days apart. Non-insecticidal preparations are available such as benzyl alcohol 5% lotion and dimethicone solution and may be used as second-line therapeutics in some populations [23]. Ovicidal agents such as malathion, spinosad, and ivermectin may be used in refractory cases or in areas where resistance to permethrin is documented [23]. Malathion is restricted in children under 6 years of age, and lindane should no longer be used due to neurotoxicity in humans.

Wet combing is a nonpharmacologic management option often implemented by patients wanting to avoid adverse events from chemical exposure. This intervention is time-consuming and has variable success rates.

Pediculosis pubis should be managed with permethrin 1%, with malathion 0.5% lotion, or oral ivermectin as second-line therapies [23]. Patients with pubic lice should be screened for sexually transmitted infections, and sex partners from the last month should be treated [23]. Recommendations for pediculosis corporis include hot-water washing clothing and bedding and an increased emphasis on personal hygiene.

A "no-nit" policy for schools and daycares is not recommended as only live lice indicate an active infestation. Because the likelihood of transmission is low, children should not be removed from school during treatment, even when an active infestation is present (Figs. 21 and 22).

Scabies

General Principles

Scabies is a common mite infestation transmitted to patients via skin-to-skin or fomite contact. The resulting dermatitis is intensely pruritic and follows a characteristic body distribution. Because scabies is often misdiagnosed, careful attention to history, physical examination, and diagnostic methods must be considered for prompt and accurate identification.

Epidemiology

The fertilized female *Sarcoptes scabiei* mite burrows through the stratum corneum, releasing eggs and fecal material. The larvae hatch and emerge to

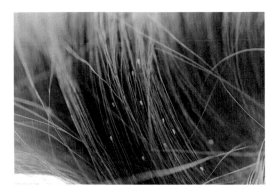

Fig. 21 Nits attached to the hairs of a patient with pediculosis humanus capitis

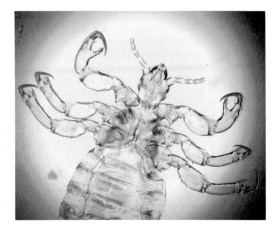

Fig. 22 Louse visualized on microscopy

the skin's surface to mate and repeat the cycle. The typical severely pruritic eruption is preceded by mild symptoms while the body develops a hypersensitivity reaction to the mite products. This initial delay can take up to 6 weeks and may confuse an already tricky diagnosis [23]. Individuals living in overcrowded conditions, and those with poor hygiene or nutritional status, are at increased risk for infestation.

Diagnosis

History and Physical Examination

Erythematous papules, pustules, vesicles, and nodules occur most commonly on the hands, wrists, axilla, waistline, buttocks, and genitalia. The face and neck are spared in adults; however, infants may present with lesions on these areas as

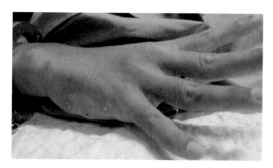

Fig. 23 Hand with scabies dermatitis

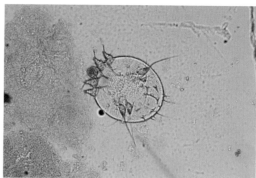

Fig. 24 *Sarcoptes scabiei* mite visualized on microscopy

well as the palms and soles. The pathognomonic burrows of webs and creases are not always apparent.

Evaluation

Microscopy of skin scrapings is used to identify mites, eggs, and fecal particles diagnostic for scabies infestation. Dermoscopy is increasingly being utilized in the evaluation of scabies [23].

Treatment

Topical permethrin cream is the first-line therapy and should be applied from the neck down. The application should remain overnight or at least 8 h and should be repeated in 1 week. Oral Ivermectin is another treatment option; however, it should only be prescribed for patients who have failed an appropriate course of topical permethrin. Patient education is critical in the management of scabies. Bedding and clothing should be washed at a temperature of at least 122°F (50°C) and hot, machine dried [23]. Close contacts should be identified, and recent sex partners should be treated. Individuals should be informed that symptoms may persist up to 2 weeks after successful treatment (Figs. 23 and 24).

Chiggers

General Principles

Trombiculosis or "chiggers" is the infestation of human skin by the Trombiculidae mite larva resulting in a pruritic rash of the groin and ankles [24].

Epidemiology

The *Trombicula* mites, also known as the harvest mites, progress to their larval stage on blades of grass where they attach to human skin and migrate to areas where they are hindered by constrictive clothing such as the ankles and waistline. In the northern United States, chiggers occur in the spring and summer months, while the warmer climate of the south sponsors the harvest mite year-round [24].

Diagnosis

History and Physical Examination

A pruritic eruption of clustered papules and pustules occurs in the typical distribution of the ankles, legs, and waistline. Symptoms are self-limited and resolve within 72 h; however, a hypersensitivity reaction may lead to prolonged edema and urticaria [24].

Treatment

Prevention with DEET-containing insect repellants applied to the skin and garments is effective. Symptomatic treatment of pruritus can be achieved with antihistamines and topical steroids.

Bedbugs

General Principles

The downward trend in bedbug incidence in the twentieth century has reversed over the last two decades with a resurgence in infestations secondary to pesticide resistance, frequent travel, lack of public education, and ineffective pest control programs [25]. Contrary to general perceptions, these obligate blood parasites are responsible for a significant burden on patients, including substantial psychological distress and financial strain.

Epidemiology

The light-aversive insects belonging to the family Cimicidae remain hidden within the proximity of its host's sleeping area. They are drawn to the warmth and carbon dioxide produced by humans, inconspicuously feeding, thanks to the anesthetic properties of their saliva [25]. The components of this saliva are responsible for the host reaction and subsequent dermatitis. Increased population density and high resident turnover rates increase the risk of infestation. The false assertion that poor hygiene contributes to patient susceptibility bolsters the stigma associated with bedbugs [25].

Diagnosis

History and Physical Examination

The cutaneous manifestations of a bedbug infestation are varied, which can lead to diagnostic difficulty and a broad differential. A pruritic, erythematous, maculopapular rash affecting unclothed areas is typical; however, patients may also present with papules, vesicles, and wheals. Linear rows of bites referred to as "breakfast, lunch, and dinner" have been classically associated with bedbug dermatitis. Secondary bacterial infections can occur from the excoriation of the intensely pruritic bites.

Treatment

The cutaneous reaction to bedbugs is self-limited and usually resolves within 1–2 weeks. No intervention has demonstrated efficacy at altering the natural history of bedbug eruptions; however, topical steroids and antihistamines can manage pruritus, while topical antibiotics can treat secondary bacterial infections.

The Environmental Protection Agency (EPA) and the Centers for Disease Control and Prevention (CDC) endorse a comprehensive, integrated

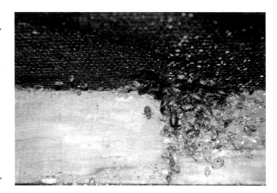

Fig. 25 Bedbug infestation of a bed frame

pest management strategy for addressing site infestation [25]. Multiple pest eradication modalities should be implemented under the supervision of professional exterminators. Due to bedbugs' resistance to temperature extremes, non-washable items should be treated at 120 °F (48.9 °C) or hotter for at least 2 h or 23 °F (−5 °C) or colder for 5 days [25] (Fig. 25).

References

1. Hartman-Adams H, Banvard C, Impetigo JG. Diagnosis and treatment. Am Fam Physician. 2014;90(4):229–35.
2. Clebak KT, Malone MA. Skin infections. Prim Care. 2018;45(3):433–54.
3. Michael Y, Shaukat NM. Erysipelas. StatPearls [internet]. Treasure Island (FL): StatPearls Publishing; 2020.
4. Maxwell-Scott H, Kandil H. Diagnosis and Management of Cellulitis and Erysipelas. Br J Hosp Med (Lond). 2015;76(8):C114–7.
5. Sullivan T, de Barra E. Diagnosis and Management of Cellulitis. Clin Med (Lond). 2018;18(2):160–3.
6. Ramakrishnan K, Salinas RC, Agudelo Higuita NI. Skin and soft tissue infections. Am Fam Physician. 2015;92(6):474–83.
7. Wipperman J, Bragg DA, Litzner B. Hidradenitis Suppurativa: rapid evidence review. Am Fam Physician. 2019;100(9):562–9.
8. Pastorino A, Tavarez MM. Incision and drainage. StatPearls [internet]. Treasure Island (FL): StatPearls Publishing; 2020.
9. Subramaniam S, Bober J, Chao J, Zehtabchi S. Point-of-care ultrasound for diagnosis of abscess in skin and soft tissue infections. Acad Emerg Med. 2016;23 (11):1298–306.
10. Leiblein M, Marzi I, Sander AL, Barker JH, Ebert F, Frank J. Necrotizing fasciitis: treatment concepts and

clinical results. Eur J Trauma Emerg Surg. 2018;44 (2):279–90.

11. Groves JB, Freeman AM. Erythrasma. StatPearls [internet]. Treasure Island (FL): StatPearls Publishing; 2020.

12. Usatine RP, Tinitigan R. Nongenital herpes simplex virus. Am Fam Physician. 2010 1;82(9):1075–82.

13. Groves MJ. Genital herpes: a review. Am Fam Physician. 2016;93(11):928–34.

14. Saguil A, Kane S, Mercado M, Lauters R. Herpes zoster and Postherpetic neuralgia: prevention and management. Am Fam Physician. 2017;96(10):656–63.

15. Maltz F, Shingrix FB. A new herpes zoster vaccine. P T. 2019;44(7):406–33.

16. Lynch MD, Cliffe J, Morris-Jones R. Management of Cutaneous Viral Warts. BMJ. 2014;27, 348

17. Badri T, Gandhi GR. Molluscum Contagiosum. StatPearls [internet]. Treasure Island (FL): StatPearls Publishing; 2020.

18. Ely JW, Rosenfeld S, Seabury Stone M. Diagnosis and Management of Tinea Infections. Am Fam Physician. 2014;90(10):702–10.

19. Gupta AK, Versteeg SG, Shear NH. Onychomycosis in the 21st century: an update on diagnosis, epidemiology, and treatment. J Cutan Med Surg. 2017;21 (6):525–39.

20. Mikailov A, Cohen J, Joyce C, Mostaghimi A. Cost-effectiveness of confirmatory testing before treatment of Onychomycosis. JAMA Dermatol. 2016;152 (3):276–81.

21. Martins N, Ferreira IC, Barros L, Silva S, Henriques M. Candidiasis: predisposing factors, prevention, diagnosis, and alternative treatment. Mycopathologia. 2014;177(5–6):223–40.

22. Renati S, Cukras A, Bigby M. Pityriasis Versicolor. BMJ. 2015;350:h1394.

23. Gunning K, Kiraly B, Pippitt K. Lice and scabies: treatment update. Am Fam Physician. 2019;99(10):635–42.

24. Alexander L, Buckley CJ. Chigger bites. StatPearls [internet]. Treasure Island (FL): StatPearls Publishing; 2020.

25. Studdiford JS, Conniff KM, Trayes KP, Tully AS. Bedbug infestation. Am Fam Physician. 2012;86 (7):653–8.

Skin Tumors

122

Elisabeth L. Backer

Contents

E. L. Backer (✉)
Department of Family Medicine, University of Nebraska
Medical Center, Omaha, NE, USA
e-mail: ebacker@unmc.edu

© Springer Nature Switzerland AG 2022
P. M. Paulman et al. (eds.), *Family Medicine*,
https://doi.org/10.1007/978-3-030-54441-6_149

General Principles

While the current US Preventive Services Task guidelines [1] may not promote routine screening, children, adolescents, and young adults who have fair skin should be counseled about limiting their exposure to ultraviolet (UV) radiation in order to reduce the development of skin cancer. Attention should be paid to examining the skin during regular physical examinations, in addition to evaluating lesions that are concerning to patients or have undergone changes of any kind.

Risk factors for skin cancer include light skin, sunny or high-altitude climates, prior sunburns, atypical nevi, prior history of skin cancer, and a family history of skin cancer as well as exposure to radiation. Those older than 65 years of age are at greater risk for cancerous skin tumors such as squamous cell carcinoma (SCC), basal cell carcinoma (BCC), and melanoma.

Approach to the Patient

History

It is important to ascertain the duration of the onset of a skin tumor, as well as its associated symptoms such as pain, pruritus, and possibly paresthesias. While some skin growths can be linked to acute illnesses, others may have a connection to chronic symptoms including fatigue, weight loss, and malaise – thus a review of systems would be helpful. Other associated factors that may need to be explored include the patient's vocation and hobbies, travel history, sun exposure, prior skin cancers, and prior skin treatments.

Physical Examination

Once the patient's overall condition and general health have been assessed, the skin tumor itself can be evaluated based on type of growth (such as nodule, cyst, papule, or scar), the color of the lesion (such as red in erythroplakia, or black in melanoma), the shape of the tumor (such as dome shaped in keratoacanthoma, or irregular in melanoma), and the texture of the growth itself (such as soft in lipoma and rough in actinic keratosis). Vascular characteristics should also be noted, often heralding neovascularization of cancerous growths. Sun damage and scarring should also be assessed. Dermoscopy aids in magnification of lesions – and by distinguishing between benign and suspicious lesions, can decrease unnecessary biopsies.

The final diagnosis of a skin lesion is frequently determined by biopsy and the resulting histopathology. A referral to a dermatologist may be in order for lesions that are not clearly benign, those that are suspicious of malignancy or those requiring specific treatment or cosmetic outcomes.

Keratosis

Seborrheic Keratosis (SK)

See (Fig. 1).

General Principles

Definition
SKs are very common pigmented benign skin tumors, occurring mainly on the torso and face, consisting of mature keratinocytes. They form as epidermal cells and undergo localized proliferation – and generally occur after age 30–50. Certain cases are linked to a genetic predisposition. When SKs arise more numerously and more rapidly, it can be a sign of underlying disease, such as a GI tract malignancy or lung cancer (Leser-Trelat sign).

Epidemiology
SKs can be somewhat more common and more plentiful in men. The incidence tends to increase with advancing age.

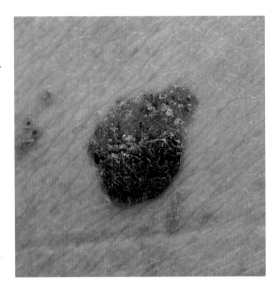

Fig. 1 Seborrheic keratosis. (Image provided by Dept of Dermatology, UNMC)

Classification
Common SKs – also known as basal cell papilloma or solid seborrheic keratosis

Reticulated SKs – also known as adenoid seborrheic keratosis

Inflamed SKs – associated redness and irritation

Diagnosis

History
Patients will usually describe a discolored, slow growing skin lesion (expanding over months to years) that is not associated with any pruritis or tenderness. Some patients attempt to remove the lesion through scratching. When exposed to friction, these lesions can become inflamed or irritated – and can show signs of bleeding [2].

Physical Examination
SKs are round to oval and can vary in size from a few millimeters to several centimeters in diameter. Their typical appearance is that of a "stuck on" lesion, which feels waxy or rough to touch. Color variations range from tan, to light brown, to dark brown and almost black. When inflammation is present, SKs look reddish in color. Under magnification of a dermoscope, the surface shows keratin cysts and comedo-like openings.

Special Testing

When SKs appear atypical or inflamed, a biopsy or removal of the lesion may be warranted.

Differential Diagnosis

SKs need to be differentiated from pigmented BCCs, malignant melanoma, SCCs, solar lentigos, acrochordons, verrucae vulgaris, nevi, and actinic keratoses.

Treatment

No specific treatment is needed for most SKs. Cryotherapy, light electrocautery, or shave biopsy can be utilized if lesions are to be removed [3]. Most patients prefer cryotherapy as no specific wound care is required.

Referrals

Patients with extensive lesions may benefit from a dermatology referral.

Counseling

Treatment of SKs may result in scarring and post-inflammatory hyper- or hypopigmentation.

Patient Education

Patients can be reassured regarding the benign nature of SKs; they do however tend to increase in number with age and can be a cosmetic concern.

Actinic Keratosis (AK) or Solar Keratosis

General Principles

Definition

AKs present as single or multiple scaly lesions on sun-exposed areas of fair-skinned individuals. They occur on a continuum with SCC, and while most AKs do not progress to SCC, 60% of SCC arise out of preexisting AKs. AKs are linked to chronic ultraviolet (UV) radiation exposure and are made up of atypical keratinocytes.

Epidemiology

AKs represent the most common reason for dermatology visits. They usually occur in middle-aged men and are often found in older adults. In areas of high sun concentration such as the Southwestern US or Australia, they may occur at a younger age. Certain skin types are especially susceptible, as are outdoor workers and outdoor enthusiasts. Immunosuppressed patients and those with organ transplants are at a heightened risk for AKs and SCC.

Approach to Patient

Diagnosis

History

Patients will report having noticed an erythematous, scaly lesion over months to years. At times AKs can feel sensitive to touch or be slightly pruritic.

Physical Examination

AKs are typically diagnosed by inspection as well as touch. The lesions can appear reddish, yellow-brown, or skin-colored, while their surface feels rough or sandpapery. Their size varies between 3 and 10 mm. They can occur as isolated or scattered lesions and are commonly located on the face, ears, neck (thinner lesions) and on the forearms, hands, and legs (thicker lesions). Clinical variations include classic, hypertrophic, atrophic, and pigmented AKs, as well as actinic cheilitis and those with a horn.

Special Testing

A deep shave or punch biopsy is advised when SCC is suspected or when lesions appear atypical, including those that have grown rapidly, are tender or ulcerated, or those that fail to respond to treatment

Differential Diagnosis

AKs need to be differentiated from SCC, BCC, inflamed seborrheic keratosis, eczema, and discoid lupus erythematosus and porokeratosis.

Treatment

Since AKs can lead to the development of SCC, treatment is usually recommended. When multiple lesions are present, topical medication may be preferred. Cryotherapy is effective for the majority of lesions: thinner lesions can be treated for 5–10 s, whereas thicker lesions may need >10 s or repeat applications. Two freeze-thaw cycles are typically used.

Medications

Local twice daily application of 5% 5-fluorouracil for days to even weeks can be effective, but can cause skin irritation. Topical imiquimod 5% cream can also be considered, but may be less effective. Chemical peels as well as photodynamic therapy are very effective. The latter is used in conjunction with a skin sensitizing agent.

Referrals

In patients with extensive or atypical lesions, a dermatology referral may be appropriate.

Counseling

Patients should be warned that topical agents such as 5-FU or imiquimod can lead to significant skin irritation. Cryotherapy can result in areas of hypopigmentation and scarring.

Patient Education/Prevention

Skin monitoring for new or recurring lesions is advised. Sun protection and broad-spectrum sunscreen is advised. Patients should avoid the sun during the peak hours in the spring and summer [4].

Pigmented Lesions

Nevus (Mole)

General Principles

Definition

Melanocytic nevi are pigmented macules or papules. They consist of groups of melanocytes which can be found in the epidermis, dermis, or subcutaneous tissue. Nevi can be classified by history as acquired [5] or congenital melanocytic nevi. Acquired melanocytic nevi can be divided by histopathology as junctional, dermal, and compound nevi. Other variants include atypical, blue, halo, or Spitz nevi. Dermoscopy [6] allows for further detailed categorization based on the amount and distribution of pigmentation.

Epidemiology

Nevi are commonly seen in Caucasians. They are acquired during childhood into adulthood, with most adults having about 20 nevi. Nevi that arise de novo in older adulthood may need to be evaluated.

Types of Nevi

Junctional Nevus

This nevus presents as tan to dark brown macule with smooth, round borders – and is found at the dermo-epidermal junction.

Dermal Nevus

This nevus is situated exclusively in the dermis, does not produce melanin, and is therefore usually skin colored.

Compound Nevus

This nevus has elements of both a junctional and a dermal nevus, is tan to dark brown in color, and presents as pigmented papule with a smooth or papillomatous surface.

Atypical Nevus

This nevus has atypical and irregular features to it, given the uneven distribution of melanocytes, thereby having some clinical similarity to melanoma [7]. Atypical nevi have also been called dysplastic nevi. The prevalence of atypical nevi is 2–8% in Caucasians. FAMM is a familial syndrome marked by multiple and atypical moles and the presence of melanoma in first- or second-degree relatives. This syndrome increases the risk of developing melanoma.

Blue Nevus

This nevus presents as a firm, blue to gray-black papule to nodule, and arises out of melanin-producing dermal melanocytes. It occurs in late adolescence.

Halo Nevus

Also known as Sutton's nevus, this nevus has an area of hypopigmentation surrounding the nevus itself. The decrease in melanin which gives rise to the halo is termed "leukoderma" and is based on an inflammatory response. Halo nevi are found on the chest, abdomen, and back, occurring in 1–5% of Caucasian children. Spontaneous regression of the nevus is seen over time.

Spitz Nevus

This nevus is typically found in childhood and presents as a red, hairless papule, usually <1 cm in size. When found in adulthood, melanoma may need to be excluded.

Congenital Nevus

Unlike acquired nevi, this nevus can be sizable and is present at birth; it has an increased risk of developing into melanoma especially when it is large or irregular.

Approach to Patient

Diagnosis

History

Patients may report noticing a new mole or changes within an existing mole. It is vital to obtain a personal history with respect to sun exposure and a family history regarding melanoma.

Most lesions occur during the younger years into adulthood, and are asymptomatic. Those that are pruritic or tender may point to underlying malignant changes. Involution of lesions can occur by age 60.

Physical Examination

Nevi can present as flesh-colored, tan, pink, brown, blue, or gray-black lesions. A complete skin exam is key to identifying new or changing nevi, or those that have unusual characteristics (the "ugly duckling" sign [8]). Melanocytic nevi with atypical features [7] need to be differentiated from melanoma. The ABCDE description is commonly utilized [9]:

A: Asymmetry
B: Border irregularity
C: Color variation
D: Diameter greater than 5 mm.
E: Evolution (changes in shape, color or size of lesion)

Dermoscopy [6] aids the further evaluation of nevi through magnification and assists with distinguishing nevi from melanomas. Whereas nevi are symmetrical in appearance with a regular pigment network, melanomatous lesions are often asymmetrical, have blue or white coloring and an irregular pigment network when seen through a dermoscope. Two or more of the latter three features should prompt a biopsy.

Special Testing

Any atypical or suspicious or symptomatic nevus may need to be biopsied. An excisional full thickness biopsy is advised when melanoma needs to be excluded.

Differential Diagnosis

BCC, dermatofibroma, seborrheic keratosis, traumatic tattoo, and solar lentigo.

Treatment

Most benign appearing nevi can be observed over time. If a mole becomes symptomatic, it may need to be removed. Thin or protruding dermal nevi can be removed via shave biopsy. A punch biopsy is useful for smaller lesions that are less than 5 mm in diameter.

Behavioral

Medications

No specific medication is indicated for nevi.

Referrals

Large, very atypical, or multiple dysplastic appearing nevi may warrant a dermatology referral.

Counseling

Removal of lesions may lead to scarring, keloid formation, or hypopigmentation.

Patient Education

As described below, patients should be counseled to report any changes to their moles. Symptomatic lesions or those that bleed, and should be further evaluated as well.

Prevention

As a general guideline, sun protections should be advised. Patients with multiple acquired melanocytic nevi should pursue periodic total body skin examinations.

Solar Lentigo or Actinic Lentigo

See (Fig. 2).

General Principles

Definition

Solar lentigos, commonly known as "liver spots" or "old age spots," are 1–3 cm pigmented epidermal macules, arising out of proliferation of normal melanocytes and keratocytes from chronic sun exposure [10]. The face, neck, back, shoulders, and extremities are usually affected. While these are benign lesions, they can undergo malignant transformation to form lentigo maligna melanoma.

Epidemiology

These lesions usually occur equally in men and women. They most often present in middle-aged Caucasians or Asians, but can occur at an earlier age in sunny climates.

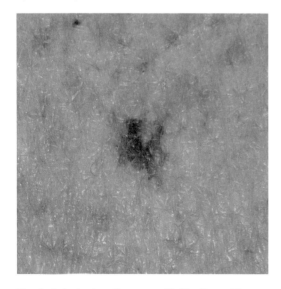

Fig. 2   Solar lentigo. (Image provided by Dept of Dermatology, UNMC)

Classification

Solar lentigo: Most common lentigo, appearing brown and flat. Lesions can enlarge to 3–4 cm.

Pigmented solar lentigo: Also called spreading actinic keratosis, this solar lentigo looks like a seborrheic keratosis.

Lentigo maligna: This lentigo is also flat, but has distinct color variations including black flecks, and heralds transformation into a superficial spreading melanoma or melanoma in situ.

Peutz-Jeghers Syndrome: Multiple lentigos are seen on mucus membranes. This syndrome also features intestinal polyps.

Approach to Patient

Diagnosis

History

Patients report brown spots or macules on sun-exposed areas. These lesions multiply with age and turn darker in the summer and lighter in the winter months.

Physical Examination

Solar lentigos present as tan to brown/black flat macules. They can range from a few mm to 2–4 cm in size. The forehead, cheeks, nose, lips, hands, and forearms are most often affected, as they represent sun-exposed areas, but these lesions can also be seen on the back and chest. When dermoscopy is used, abnormal pigment distribution may herald a developing malignancy.

Special Testing

When a lesion is suspicious, a wide elliptical excision may be best. A punch biopsy can be useful when the lesion develops an area of rapid change.

Differential Diagnosis

Seborrheic keratosis, nevi, lentigo maligna melanoma, pigmented actinic keratosis.

Treatment

Observation may suffice. Smaller unsightly lesions can be treated with cryotherapy for as little as 5 s. If lentigo maligna is suspected, these lesions should be biopsied.

Medications

If lightening of these lesions is desired, hydroquinone 4% cream can be applied bid for several weeks. A triple combination cream made up of fluocinolone 0.01%, hydroquinone 4%, and tretinoin 0.05% is also available. Chemical peels or use of azelaic acid 20% cream bid for 2–4 weeks has been effective. Pigmented solar lentigos also respond to topical fluorouracil application for up to 10 days.

Referrals

Larger lesions or those appearing very atypical or undergoing rapid changes would benefit from a dermatology consult.

Counseling

Treatments can lead to hypopigmentation, localized irritation, and at times uneven bleaching.

Patient Education/Prevention

Any changing or symptomatic lesions should be further evaluated. Sun protection is advised to limit the formation of solar lentigos.

Malignant Skin Tumors

Melanoma

See (Fig. 3).

General Principles

Definition

Melanomas represent the most serious type of skin cancer. They are characterized by the irregular growth and expansion of abnormal melanocytes, spreading locally through lymphatic and systemically by hematogenous routes. Most melanomas are confined to the epidermis; infiltration of the dermis can lead to metastases. Whereas they can arise out of existing nevi, the majority (70%) of melanomas arise de novo.

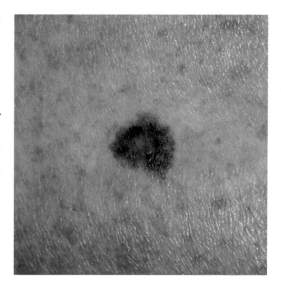

Fig. 3 Melanoma. (Image provided by Dept of Dermatology, UNMC)

Epidemiology

Melanomas account for the most skin cancer deaths, yet make up only 1% of all skin cancer types [11]. While older men are most often affected, melanomas are one of the most common cancers found in the younger population. Superficial spreading and lentigo maligna melanomas occur slightly more often in females. In the United States, about 100,000 cases of melanoma are diagnosed a year and approximately 7000 deaths are attributed to melanoma. Earlier diagnosis has led to a rise in the 5-year survival rate. Affected areas include the torso, head and neck in males, and the extremities in females.

Classification

The four major subtypes are: superficial spreading, nodular, lentigo maligna, and acral melanoma.

Superficial Spreading Melanoma

This subtype represents 70% of melanomas. It commonly arises from an existing nevus, has multiple color variations, and spreads gradually in a horizontal fashion. It is found on backs and lower extremities.

Nodular Melanoma

Representing 15–30% of cases, this second most common subtype of melanoma appears as a uniformly dark, raised lesion, with possible associated ulceration or hemorrhage. Nodular melanomas can have a depth of greater than 2 mm at the time of diagnosis.

Lentigo Maligna Melanoma
Occurring in 10–15% of cases, this less common subtype of melanoma arises from a lentigo and spreads horizontally; it is seen in older patients in sun-exposed areas on the face and forearms.

Acral Melanoma
This subtype makes up less than 5% of melanomas, but is common in darker-skinned individuals. It presents as a dark macule or patch with raised areas and if often seen on soles or palms. It can also show signs of bleeding or ulceration.

Less common melanoma subtypes include **amelanotic melanoma** and **subungual melanoma**. In amelanotic melanoma, the lesion is pink in color and expands over time. In subungual melanoma one can see a darkly pigmented band within the nail, arising out of the nail matrix. It can also present as a mass below the nail plate.

Approach to Patient

Diagnosis

History
Patients usually present with a new or changing skin lesion. Melanomas can be symptomatic (pruritic or tender) and associated with bleeding and scabbing. When reviewing the patients' history, several risk should be explored. These include a family history of melanoma, atypical or larger nevi, sun exposure vocationally or recreationally, sunburns at a young age, fair complexion, tanning-bed exposure, immunosuppression, or advanced age.

Physical Examination
Most melanomas present with discoloration and uneven pigmentation. Variations in color include brown, black, pink, pale, or gray tones. The margins of these lesions are irregular and the surfaces uneven. The clinical diagnosis can be challenging

[12]. When dermoscopy is utilized, it improves the sensitivity and specificity and assists in differentiating between an atypical nevus and a melanoma. Beyond the lesion itself, examining the surrounding lymph nodes is advised.

Laboratory and Imaging
A definitive diagnosis is made through histopathology. When metastases are suspected, imaging of the chest and CT imaging may be useful in staging. Testing of liver enzymes should also be considered.

Special Testing
Lesions suspicious for melanoma should be biopsied. A complete full-thickness excisional biopsy with additional 1–3 mm margin is preferred. A punch biopsy can be useful for diagnostic purposes; it is also useful when a lesion is located on a sensitive area such as the face or a distal extremity. When a partial incisional biopsy is undertaken, it should be aimed at the most atypical section of the lesion. A very thin lesion that is less suspicious can be removed via a deep shave biopsy. A nail biopsy should entail the nail matrix. The final pathology report is key to the further work-up and ultimate treatment plan. Staging is based on the depth of the lesion (Breslow tumor thickness reflects the depth of malignant cell invasion of the dermis), the presence or absence of ulceration, and the mitotic rate. The Clark level of anatomic invasion is also taken into account. In melanomas that exceed a depth of 1 mm, a sentinel node biopsy is done to determine the further prognosis.

Differential Diagnosis
Pyogenic granuloma, pigmented BCC, common or atypical melanocytic nevus, traumatized nevus, blue nevus, solar lentigo, hemangioma, inflamed SK, and dermatofibroma.

Treatment
Tumor thickness is used in guiding further skin excision and is the most important prognostic factor. Survival diminishes with increased thickness. At 1 mm or less, the 10-year survival is 92%; at >4 mm, the rate drops to 50% [13].

The re-excision margin varies depending on the Breslow depth. A margin of 0.5 cm is needed for melanoma in situ, 1 cm in melanomas of <1.0 mm depth, 1–2 cm in those with depth of 1.01–2.0 mm, and 2 cm in melanomas deeper than 2.0 mm.

Medications
Off label use of topical imiquimod (Aldara) has been explored. Vaccines may also play a role in adjuvant therapy.

Referrals
Whenever changes in an existing mole are observed, or a new growing lesion is detected, referral to a dermatologist should be considered. A plastic surgery referral may also be indicated, especially when lesions are areas that are difficult to biopsy.

Counseling
Biopsies can lead to scarring. Healing can be slow and compromised on the extremities. Incomplete lesion removal may lead to further surgery.

Patient Education
Early detection saves lives. Vigilance as to new or changing skin lesions should be encouraged. Smart phone applications for melanoma detection have been developed [14].

Prevention
Limiting sun exposure and following strict sun protective measures is advised. Regular follow-up and detailed skin exams are encouraged.

Basal Cell Carcinoma (BCC)

See (Fig. 4).

General Principles

Definition
This is the most common form of skin cancer, arising out of the basal layer of the epidermis

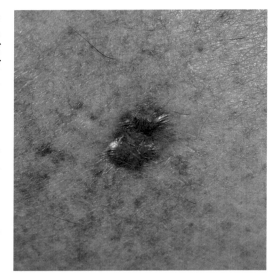

Fig. 4 Basal cell carcinoma. (Image provided by Dept of Dermatology, UNMC)

and its appendages. While it is readily treatable by a variety of methods, it can be locally invasive and destructive, or very seldom, metastasize.

Epidemiology
BCCs make up 8 out of 10 nonmelanoma skin cancers, affecting mainly Caucasian patients over age 40 with a history of extended sun exposure. The incidence increases with age. Men are more often affected than women. States closer to the equator such as Hawaii and California have a higher incidence of BCC. Overall risk factors include UV radiation, tanning beds, phototherapy, and ionized radiation. Certain phenotypes with light hair and eye color and those with a personal history of BCC are also at greater risk.

Classification Based on Histopathology

Nodular BCC
As the most common BCC lesions, these can be pigmented or nonpigmented, and often have an irregular surface or ulceration at the center.

Superficial BCC
These BCC lesions are flat, scaly, and plaque-like in presentation. A reticular infiltration can be seen.

Sclerotic/Morphea-Form BCC

These lesions are accompanied by fibrous stroma, are whitish and have ill-defined margins.

Approach to Patient

Diagnosis

History

Patients will describe a nodule, scabbing, or ulcerating lesion, which appears to be expanding slowly over time.

Physical Examination

The majority of BCCs are located on the face (70%), with 15% found on the trunk. BCCs most often present as a singular firm nodule or papule (nodular BCC), 3–10 mm in size, which can appear pearly in nature. When ulcerated, the border can be described as rolled. BCCs can also appear flat and scaly (superficial BCC) or whitish/fibrous (morphea-form BCCs). Multiple lesions can occur. Dermoscopy is helpful in establishing the diagnosis and can show branching vessels.

Special Testing

Shave or excisional biopsy can establish the diagnosis, but a wider excision with 1–3 mm margins may be needed to sufficiently remove the BCC. Shave biopsy is preferred in areas of skin preservation.

Differential Diagnosis

Dermal nevi, epidermal inclusion cysts, sebaceous hyperplasia, and SCC can mimic nodular BCC, whereas nummular eczema, benign lichenoid keratoses, and amelanotic melanoma can look like superficial BCC. Scleroderma must be distinguished from morphea-form BCC.

Treatment

The treatment depends on the site and extent of the lesion. Cryotherapy is best used for thin, superficial BCC lesions. Mohs surgery is indicated for cosmetically sensitive regions of the face. This form of surgery involves microscopic, incremental removal of layers of the tumor, until the area is tumor free. When complete surgical excision of a BCC lesion can be undertaken, no further treatment is needed. Electrodessication and curettage can be utilized for incompletely removed lesions. Surveillance for local recurrence is advised. When BCC lesions are very large or located in difficult to treat areas, or when palliative treatment is appropriate, radiation therapy can be helpful. Light therapy is another treatment option and involves application of photosensitizing agents to the BCC.

Medications

5FU elicits an inflammatory response that causes destruction of superficial BCC lesions. Imiquimod (Aldara) 5% cream, which is typically applied daily for 6 weeks, has a similar yet more severe effect.

Counseling

Scarring can follow removal of lesions. Local recurrences can occur.

Patient Education/Prevention

Sun avoidance or sun protection through wearing of hats, sun screen, and UV-obstructing clothing is recommended, best done before age 18.

Squamous Cell Carcinoma (SCC)

See (Fig. 5).

General Principles

Definition

SCC is a malignant tumor arising from epithelial keratinocytes as a result of sun exposure or other carcinogens such as ionized radiation. It rarely metastasizes (in 2–6% of cases), and can be effectively treated when diagnosed at an early stage.

Epidemiology

SCC is generally seen in the Caucasian population, occurring more often in men over 55 years of

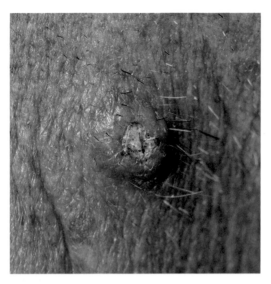

Fig. 5 Squamous cell carcinoma. (Image provided by Dept of Dermatology, UNMC)

age on sun exposed areas. These men often work outdoors, but industrial workers exposed to chemicals can also be affected. Darker skinned individuals can develop SCC from other etiologies. Transplant patients on immunosuppressants are at risk for SCC. Actinic keratosis is a precursor to SCC. SCC can occur in skin damaged by sun, radiation, scars, or burns.

Classification

Bowen's Disease: This is classified as SCC in situ, and presents as a scaly, hyperkeratotic macule or plaque.

Keratoacanthoma: This is a variant of SCC, arising rapidly and presenting with a central keratotic core.

Oral SCC: This is usually a more aggressive form of SCC.

Erythroplasia of Querat (Penile SCC): Also known as Bowen's disease of the penis, this presents with an erythematous plaque on the glans and foreskin and has been linked to HPV.

Vulvar SCC: This form of SCC is also linked to HPV and can be seen in immunocompromised women.

Approach to Patient

Diagnosis

History
Most patients will notice a nodule or non-healing, often scaly scab, which arises over several weeks to months.

Physical Examination
Depending on the form of SCC, patients can present with a thick keratotic scale, an indurated papule or plaques, or an ulcerated nodule. SCC in situ often appears red and scaly. Surrounding areas should also be evaluated for lymph node involvement and other signs of sun damage. Dermoscopy can be helpful [6].

Laboratory and Imaging
If the diagnosis is in question, a biopsy can be performed. CT imaging is useful for staging purposes.

Special Testing
Shave, punch, or excisional biopsies are used for diagnostic purposes and should extend into the dermis. Excising the lesion with a 4 mm margin most often allows for removal of the tumor. Mohs surgery is needed in cases with microscopic invasion.

Differential Diagnosis
The differential diagnosis for SCC includes actinic keratosis, BCC, psoriasis, and Lichen planus. SCC in situ can present similar to nummular eczema.

Treatment
The choice of treatment is often determined in conjunction with a specialist referral to dermatology and/or plastic surgery. Many factors influence the decision including the site, size, shape, and nature of the lesion.

Localized SCC can be considered completely removed if the excisional biopsy denotes negative margins; otherwise a repeat excision must be performed.

High-risk SCCs, and those arising on the face, are best suited for Mohs surgery. Assessment for invasion of the surrounding tissue is important.

Low-risk, small SCC (less than 1 cm in diameter) can be treated with electrodessication and curettage.

Radiation may also be indicated for certain cases, especially when the lesion is not readily accessible surgically. It can decrease the tumor size, but may lead to scarring and also telangiectasia.

Medications
Superficial SCC can be treated with 5 FU.

Referrals
Consultation with dermatology and/or plastic surgery is advised in patients with larger or high-risk lesions, and when Mohs surgery is indicated.

Counseling
Patients should be counseled about the possibility of metastases, even though it is rare. Scarring may result from treatment.

Patient Education
Sun avoidance and sun protection is advised. Since SCC may recur, clinical follow-up is considered important.

Keratoacanthoma (KA)

General Principles

Definition
This nonaggressive form of skin cancer presents as a dome-shaped nodule arising from the epithelium, and is made up of a central keratin-filled crater. It is thought to be a variant of SCC and can develop and expand rapidly.

Epidemiology
KAs occur predominantly in men over age 50 who are of Caucasian descent and have a history of sun exposure. Other risk factors include skin color, trauma, genetics, and chemical carcinogens. Most often a solitary lesion is seen on the neck, face, ears, and hands.

Approach to the Patient

Diagnosis

History
Patients present with a dome-shaped nodule marked by rapid growth over several weeks.

Physical Examination
These lesions are usually singular, 5 mm to 2.5 cm in size, skin-colored or red, nodular in shape, and firm to touch. The dome shape and central keratotic plug distinguishes these lesions. Dermoscopy cannot reliably distinguish between KAs and SCCs.

Special Testing
The diagnosis is made through both clinical and histopathological assessment. An excisional biopsy extending into the subcutaneous fat is advised. It is important to differentiate this lesion from an SCC.

Differential Diagnosis
SCC, nodular BCC, sebaceous cyst, molluscum contagiosum, Kaposi sarcoma, and dermatofiroma.

Treatment
While lesions can undergo spontaneous regression over time, this can lead to a disfiguring scar. An excisional biopsy is usually advised, especially when an SCC is suspected. When a shave biopsy is undertaken, it may need to be followed by electrodesiccation and curettage.

Referrals
A dermatology referral may be necessary if the lesion is large or in an area of cosmetic concern.

Counseling
Patients should be counseled about possible scarring. In the case of incomplete removal, a follow-up procedure may be required.

Patient Education/Prevention
Avoidance of sun exposure and wearing of sun protective clothing is advised.

Kaposi Sarcoma

General Principles

Definition

Kaposi sarcoma (KS) is an angio-proliferative disorder associated with Human Herpes Virus 8 (HHV-8), marked by violaceous nodules. Lesions occur on the skin, but can also be found in other sites such as the oral cavity, GI tract, lymph nodes, and respiratory tract.

Epidemiology

In the United States these lesions occur predominantly in male patients and HIV patients, but also in immunocompromised individuals. Other variants of KS are noted in patients of European or African descent [2].

Classification of KS

Endemic or Classical KS: This type of KS is found in elderly males of European, especially Mediterranean descent.

African KS: This type of KS involves lymph nodes; it is seen in young men and children living in equatorial Africa.

Iatrogenic KS: This type of KS is associated with immunosuppressant therapy and organ transplants.

Epidemic KS: This type is associated with AIDS.

Approach to Patient

Diagnosis

History

Most often patients initially notice a painless ecchymotic macule or nodule. Occasionally ulceration and bleeding can occur, and larger lesions on the extremities can be of functional hindrance, especially if swelling and fibrosis accompany the lesions.

Physical Examination

Lesions typically are oval in shape, have a red or purplish hue, feel firm to touch, and can present as macules, papules, plaques, or nodules. Usually the lesions are situated in the dermis, but can erode the overlying epidermis, forming an ulcer. Lesions can become confluent and associated lymphedema can occur in extremities. In the mouth lesions commonly occur on the hard palate, but can be seen on the uvula and gingiva.

Laboratory and Imaging

On biopsy one finds an intradermal nodule with atypical endothelial cells lining the vascular channels. Pulmonary nodules and pleural effusions can be seen on chest xray (CXR). HIV testing is advised.

Special Testing

The diagnosis is made by skin biopsy.

Differential Diagnosis

Malignant melanoma, pyogenic granuloma, dermatofibroma, hemangioma, ecchymosis, and bacillary angiomatosis.

Treatment

Individual lesions can be removed by excision. Other local interventions include radiotherapy, cryosurgery, or laser surgery.

Medications

More aggressive treatment options may be necessary for complex cases and include intralesional or systemic chemotherapeutic agents. HIV treatment should be addressed in cases associated with HIV disease. In patients on immunosuppressants such as prednisone or methotrexate, consideration should be given to holding such if possible.

Referrals

Consultations may include referrals to dermatology and to oncology.

Counseling

Scarring may occur as a result of local treatments and skin biopsies. Mortality rates increase with GI or pulmonary involvement.

Patient Education

The disease can recur and careful vigilance for such is advised.

Vascular Lesions

Hemangioma

General Principles

Definition
Hemangiomas are known as benign blood vessel growths. When they occur in early infancy, they are known to expand rapidly within the first year of life and then disappear spontaneously by age 5 years [15].

Epidemiology
Hemangiomas occur slightly more often in females.

Classification
Capillary hemangiomas of infancy: These are also known as strawberry nevi and are soft, red to purple nodules or plaques, occurring at or just after birth.

Cavernous hemangiomas: These are somewhat darker vascular malformations associated with swelling of the deeper tissues. They are often larger and can contain arteriovenous shunts. Varicosities can be seen at the skin surface.

Cherry angiomas: Also called senile angiomas or Campbell de Morgan spots, these are common, benign, red, dome-shaped vascular lesions with capillary proliferation, which increase with age.

Approach to the Patient

Diagnosis

History
Patients will notice a red or purplish skin lesion that typically appears to be enlarging over time. Adults may express concern over the cosmetic appearance of cherry angiomas.

Physical Exam
Capillary hemangiomas are often soft red to purple nodules, which do not blanch completely. They occur on the face, trunk, legs, and mucosal membranes. Cavernous hemangiomas present as soft swellings, often multinodular and blue in color, which are easily compressed. Cherry angiomas are small, red, soft papules that occur mainly on the trunk and proximal extremities; they typically blanch with pressure.

Laboratory and Imaging
The diagnosis of hemangiomas is made clinically. Deeper or larger lesions may require imaging to evaluate the full extent of the lesion. Specialist referral is recommended when hemangiomas are found overlying the midline of the spine, as underlying neural tube defects can be associated with such.

Differential Diagnosis
Pyogenic granuloma, melanoma, and bacillary angiomatosis.

Treatment
Most hemangiomas involute spontaneously by age 5 years. Deeper lesion may not recede completely, especially when mucous membranes are involved. Pulse-dye laser treatment can be used for lesions that are larger or impair function. No treatment is needed for cherry angiomas, unless cosmesis is a concern. Pulsed-dye laser, cryotherapy, and electrocautery can be utilized.

Behavioral
Most hemangiomas are asymptomatic but can present cosmetic concerns. Those that are larger and exposed can become ulcerated and may need to be protected.

Medication
Both prednisone and propranolol have been successful in the treatment of hemangiomas.

Referrals
Pediatric surgery or pediatric dermatology consultations should be considered in larger hemangiomas, or those prone to bleeding, ulceration, or scarring.

Counseling
Guidance to parents is important, especially when awaiting spontaneous resolution of hemangiomas

over time. Medical and surgical treatments are accompanied by possible side effects such as scarring or depigmentation. Adults with cherry angiomas can be reassured.

Patient Education
Expectant management may suffice in hemangiomas. Cherry angiomas will likely become more numerous with age.

Angiokeratoma

General Principles

Definition
Angiokeratomas are vascular lesions, likely formed by increased venous pressure within dilated superficial dermal blood vessels, with hyperkeratosis of the overlying epidermis. Most commonly these lesions occur on the genitalia as red-to-purple papules.

Epidemiology
The onset of these lesions is typically between 20 and 50 years of age.

Classification
Angiokeratoma of Fordyce: Multiple angiomas are seen on the scrotum or vulva.
Solitary Angiokeratomas: A single lesion can be present.
Fabry-Anderson Syndrome: This syndrome is marked by numerous cutaneous angiokeratomas forming around puberty and is associated with an X-linked inborn error.

Other Vascular Malformations
These include Angiokeratomas of Mibelli, occurring on the dorsal aspects of digits.

Approach to the Patient

Diagnosis

History
Patients typically report the onset of red, purple, or black papules that can bleed with trauma.

Physical Exam
These discolored papules are usually 2–3 mm in size and most often occur on the scrotum and vulva. Vascular lacunae can be seen with dermoscopy.

Special Testing
No specific testing is required. Dilated blood vessels can be seen if a biopsy is performed.

Differential Diagnosis
Melanoma, hemangioma, Kaposi sarcoma, and pyogenic granuloma.

Treatment
Lesions can be removed by excision, electrodessication, and curettage or laser therapy. This is usually only done for cosmetic purposes.

Referrals
When Fabry-Anderson Syndrome is suspected, referral for treatment of the underlying disease is indicated. A dermatology consult is helpful when considering laser therapy.

Counseling
Patients should be cautioned that scarring can result from treatment of these lesions.

Patient Education
Since these lesions often occur on the genitalia, patients may need to be reassured that these findings are not associated with sexual transmission.

Venous Lake

General Principles

Definition
These lesions arise out of dilated venous capillaries, are usually dark-blue to purple in color, and are most often seen on the lips, face, and ears of older patients.

Epidemiology
Venous lakes occur in men/women after age 50 years, mainly on areas of sun-damaged skin.

Approach to the Patient

Diagnosis

History
Venous lakes usually appear without symptoms, but can bleed if traumatized or become tender when thrombosed.

Physical Exam
Venous lakes are dark-blue to purple, round or oval papules to nodules. They are usually compressible (unlike blue nevi) and soft and can appear grapelike in structure on detailed examination [2].

Special Testing
None needed, as the diagnosis is made clinically.

Differential Diagnosis
Nodular melanoma, pyogenic granuloma, and Kaposi sarcoma.

Treatment
Lesions do not usually regress spontaneously. If cosmetic treatment is desired, or the lesion is traumatized and bleeds often, vascular laser treatment or electrocoagulation can be pursued.

Referrals
If the lesion undergoes change or seems atypical, a dermatology referral may be indicated.

Counseling
Lesions tend to stabilize over time. If treatment is pursued, scarring could result.

Patient Education
Sun protection is advised, and further sun exposure should be avoided.

Pyogenic Granuloma

General Principles

Definition
This is a fast growing, red or dark colored vascular nodule, seen on the skin or mucosa, often arising in response to localized trauma. It is made up out of rapidly proliferating endothelial cells and fibroblasts.

Epidemiology
Pyogenic granulomas occur most often in the second and third decade of life and during pregnancy. Both men and women are equally affected.

Approach to Patient

Diagnosis

History
Patients will present with a new nodule, which has often only been present for a few days or weeks. At times there is a preceding history of trauma to the skin – and while tenderness may be reported, recurrent bleeding from the sight can be common.

Physical Examination
Pyogenic granulomata present as red to purple, small, pedunculated single papules or nodules. Their surface is usually smooth, and can be covered by a yellow discharge. They appear friable, can have erosions, and bleed rather easily. These lesions most often occur on fingers and toes, or on the torso [2].

Special Testing
Pathological evaluation can differentiate lesions from amelanotic malignant melanoma.

Differential Diagnosis
Bacillary angiomatosis, angiosarcoma, melanoma, and Kaposi sarcoma.

Treatment
Surgical removal via shave biopsy is advised, followed by electrodessication or curettage of the base of the lesion. Since there can be a fair amount of bleeding involved, silver nitrate or aluminum chloride may need to be applied topically for hemostasis. Recurrence is possible following incomplete removal of the lesion.

Referrals
In atypical presentations, or if lesion recur or are numerous, a dermatology referral is advised.

Counseling
Surgical removal may lead to scar formation.

Patient Education
Follow-up is advised if the lesion recurs or if the healing seems incomplete.

Nonpigmented Nonvascular Lesions

Dermatofibroma

See (Fig. 6).

General Principles

Definition
Dermatofibromas are common, benign, dermal fibrous lesions made up of histiocyte cells. They occur on the lower extremities, and often arise as a result of minor trauma such as a local insect bite. Synonyms include solitary histiocytoma.

Epidemiology
These lesions occur most often in adults – more frequently in women.

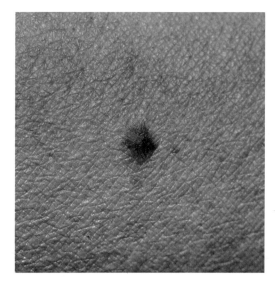

Fig. 6 Dermatofibroma. (Image provided by Dept of Dermatology, UNMC)

Approach to Patient

Diagnosis

History
Dermatofibromas appear over months to years; patients might recall minor trauma to the skin, or notice mild tenderness or itching associated with the lesion. Most lesions remain stable, but can regress spontaneously.

Physical Examination
Dermatofibromas present as solitary firm nodules or papules on the legs and arms. They are <1 cm in size and are typically pink or brown in color. By applying lateral compression, one can elicit the tell-tale "dimpling sign." The center of the lesion can show post-inflammatory hypo- or hyperpigmentation.

Special Testing
Dermoscopy shows a central scar-like lesion with peripheral hyperpigmentation. If the lesion is removed for cosmetic reason, or because of uncertainty of the diagnosis, Spindle cells can be recognized on dermatopathology. Uncommon histological variants of dermatofibromas exist.

Differential Diagnosis
Lesions that mimic dermatofibromas include dermatofibrosarcoma protuberance, malignant melanoma, hypertrophic scar formation, BCC, melanotic nevi, keratoacanthoma, and pilar cysts.

Treatment
No treatment is required, but if the diagnosis is uncertain, the lesion becomes symptomatic or undergoes changes, or if the patient desires removal for cosmetic purposes, this is best done by a punch or elliptical excision. Cryotherapy can treat protruding lesions that become irritated.

Medications
No topical agents are indicated.

Referrals
If the diagnosis seems uncertain, a dermatology referral may be in order.

Counseling
Removal of the lesion may result in a scar.

Patient Education
Most dermatofibroma can be observed; re-evaluation is advised for changing lesions.

Acrochordon or Skin Tag

General Principles

Definition
Acrochordons are outgrows of normal skin, appearing as pedunculated lesions on stalks.

Epidemiology
Acrochordons increase in number with age, obesity, and pregnancy. They are also associated with diabetes.

Approach to Patient

Diagnosis

History
Patients notice skin tags in areas of increased friction around the neckline, axilla, inguinal, or inframammary regions. They often report snagging of the skin tags on jewelry or clothing.

Physical Examination
Whereas most skin tags are flesh-colored pedunculated lesions, they can turn red or black when becoming irritated or undergoing torsion.

Special Testing
Acrochordons are diagnosed clinically.

Differential Diagnosis
Neurofibroma and nevus.

Treatment
No specific treatment is required. If removal is desired, fine-grade scissor removal, cryotherapy, or electrodesiccation are effective. Larger lesions may require local anesthesia with 1% lidocaine with epinephrine. Hemostasis can be accomplished through use of aluminum chloride or silver nitrate.

Medication
No medication is routinely advised.

Referrals
No referrals are usually needed.

Counseling
Use of silver nitrate can lead to skin pigmentation.

Patient Education
Lesions do not typically recur.

Keloids

General Principles

Definition
Hypertrophic scars and keloids arise from an excessive fibroproliferative tissue response following injury to the skin. While hypertrophic scars are limited to margins of the original wound and can regress, keloids extend beyond the injury site into the surrounding skin and do not diminish over time.

Epidemiology
Keloids often occur in the third decade, affect men and women equally, and are most prevalent in patients with darkly pigmented skin. They are often seen on the trunk, earlobes, shoulders, and upper back. While they can arise spontaneously, especially on the sternal region, they usually follow an injury to the skin such as with vaccination, acne, an abrasion, a piercing, cryosurgery, or an excision.

Approach to Patient

Diagnosis

History
Most often patients report an injury to their skin. While the lesion is usually asymptomatic, some keloids can be tender or pruritic.

Physical Examination

Lesions can be skin-colored, but often seem red in appearance. They have a firm, hard texture and are often linear in configuration. Keloids extend beyond the borders of the original injury.

Special Testing

This is usually a clinical diagnosis and does not require specialized testing.

Differential Diagnosis

Dermatofibrosarcoma protuberans, sarcoidosis, desmoid tumor, and foreign body granuloma.

Treatment

Lesions that are excised can recur, unless adjunctive therapy is targeted at limiting reformation, and is best undertaken by a plastic surgeon or very experienced surgeon. Vascular scars may respond to laser treatment.

Medications

Intralesional triamcinolone (0.1–0.5 ml of the 10–40 mg/ml strength) may reduce the size and volume of the lesion – reduce the tenderness or pruritus – and potentially flatten it. This can be repeated monthly if needed. Combination therapy with FU has also been used. Imiquimod may also show some efficacy.

Referrals

Patients with larger or more symptomatic keloids may benefit from a referral to a plastic surgeon or dermatologist.

Counseling

Hypertrophic scars may regress, but keloids can continue to expand over time. Removal of these lesions may lead to further scarring or skin damage.

Patient Education

These lesions are considered to be benign, but can be associated with emotional distress in patients. If any changes or enlargement of these lesions occurs, re-evaluation may be necessary. Patient may want to avoid elective cosmetic surgery if they have a tendency to form keloids or hypertrophic scar tissue.

Lipoma

General Principles

Definition

A lipoma is a small soft tissue growth located in the subcutaneous tissue, consisting of mature fat cells (adipocytes) within a fibrous capsule. Lipomas are the most common benign soft tissue neoplasms.

Epidemiology

These lesions typically are seen in adults with increased adipose tissue.

Classification

Hereditary Multiple Lipomatosis: This is an autosomal dominant condition, occurring predominantly in men.

Pleomorphic Lipomas: These lipomas consist of both adipocytes and giant cells.

Angiolipomas: These lipomas are marked by capillary vessels in addition to adipocytes.

Spindle Cell Lipomas: These lipomas contain spindle cells.

Approach to Patient

Diagnosis

History

Patients will typically report a soft, non-painful lump underneath their skin.

Physical Examination

Palpation reveals a soft, round to oval, non-tender subcutaneous mass, ranging from 1 to 10 cm in size. It can be multilobulated. Patients can have several lipomas. Certain cases are linked to a genetic condition called familial multiple lipomatosis.

Special Testing

Most lipomas are diagnosed clinically. Ultrasound examination can confirm the diagnosis if needed. Rapidly expanding lipomas can be suspicious of liposarcomas – and can be further assessed through MRI studies.

Differential Diagnosis

Epidermal cysts, liposarcomas, and ganglion cysts.

Treatment

Most lipomas do not require any treatment. Large or tender lipomas, or those that are of cosmetic concern, can be surgically excised. Various techniques can be utilized, including elliptical excision of the skin with subsequent dissection of the lipoma from the surrounding tissues, followed by skin closure. Smaller incisions may also suffice, with extrusion of the lipomatous tissue through the incisional opening. If the lipoma is of a significant size, liposuction can be utilized.

Medications

In order to shrink lipomas over time, triamcinolone 10 mg/ml can be injected monthly over several months.

Referrals

Large lipomas, or those situated in anatomically intricate regions, may be best referred to a dermatologist or surgeon.

Counseling

Potential scarring can result from treatment. Recurrences are uncommon.

Patient Education

While these lesions are usually benign, and reassurance suffices, those that expand rapidly or become painful should be reevaluated.

Epidermal Cyst

See (Fig. 7).

General Principles

Mucocutaneous cysts are made up of a closed sac, filled with semisolid material arising from the epithelium that lines the sac. Pseudocysts are made up of mucin from underlying joint space

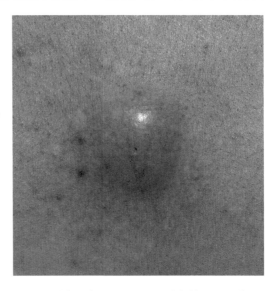

Fig. 7 Epidermal cyst. (Image provided by Dept of Dermatology, UNMC)

(digital mucinous cyst) or occur with rupture of minor salivary gland (mucocele).

Definition

Epidermal cysts are formed within the epithelium of a hair follicle; they contain keratin, not sebum.

Classification

Milia: Milia are 1–2 mm superficial, firm keratin-containing subepidermal cysts occurring on the face. They are common in newborns.

Epidermal inclusion cysts: These improperly called "sebaceous cysts" are keratin containing cysts that occur secondary to traumatic implantation of epidermis within the dermis.

Ruptured epidermal cysts: These cysts are marked by rupture of their thin wall and associated severe local inflammatory responses.

Epidemiology

Epidermal cysts occur in young to middle aged individuals and are more frequently seen in men.

Milia occur in infants to adults, occurring equally in men and women.

Approach to Patient

Diagnosis

History
Patients describe a small bump with a central punctum, often presenting insidiously. These lesions can become painful when inflamed or infected.

Physical Exam
On exam one finds a dermal/subcutaneous nodule (0.5–5 cm in size), with an overlying skin pore, and pasty, malodorous keratin contents – occurring on either the face, neck, trunk, or scrotum. This nodule can appear inflamed, especially when rupturing spontaneously. Infected cysts are usually large and fluctuant.

Laboratory Testing
Culture is not advised.

Special Testing
Pathology is to be pursued if there is an unusual presentation.

Differential Diagnosis
Keratoacanthoma, lipoma, abscess, pilar cyst, ganglion cyst, and dermoid cyst.

Treatment
While observation is encouraged in small, asymptomatic cysts, surgical excision is advised in larger, symptomatic cysts. Incision and drainage of a fluctuant cyst is indicated, with complete removal advised only after the inflammation has resolved.

Excision can be done through 3–4 mm incision or punch biopsy, first removing the cyst contents and then pulling out the cyst itself through the incisional opening [16]– or via a larger incision.

Behavioral

Medications
No antibiotics are advised for ruptured cysts, except when surrounding cellulitis is present.

Referrals
Patients can be referred to a dermatologist or plastic surgeon if cosmetic concerns exist.

Counseling
Cyst recurrences are possible, especially when incompletely removed. Local scarring may occur.

Patient Education
Patient should be counseled about possible cyst enlargement or rupture.

Oral Lesions

General Principles

Oral lesions that cannot be rubbed off and that remain visible even after irritation has resolved, are suspicious of being premalignant, especially if they are located on the ventral surface of the tongue or the floor of the mouth.

Definition

The terms "leukoplakia" and "erythroplakia" refer to white and red mucosal, intra-oral lesions, respectively. Whereas certain lesions may represent hyperkeratosis or be caused by local irritation, at least 25% (or up to 80% in erythroplakia) may eventually progress to oral cancer.

Epidemiology

Leukoplakia typically occurs between age 40 and 70 years, and is more common in men. Risk factors include exposure to HPV, tobacco, and alcohol.

Classification

Leukoplakia: White, distinctly defined or raised mucosal area

Erythroplakia: Localized, red area often arising within plaque of leukoplakia

Oral Hairy Leukoplakia : Variant of leukoplakia, associated with EBV, in patients with
HPV

Approach to the Patient

History
Patients often do not report any symptoms, and
these lesions may go undetected for an extended
period of time, with only occasional discomfort or
episodes of bleeding.

Physical Exam
White plaque-like or verrucous lesions (with or
without ulceration) or red velvety areas are seen
within the mouth, affecting the lower lip, tongue,
sublingual region, or buccal mucosa. Lymph
nodes may be enlarged.

Laboratory Testing and Imaging
Biopsy of these lesions is advised to exclude
dysplasia or carcinoma, especially in tobacco
users. Referral to specialist such as an oral surgeon may be indicated.

Differential Diagnosis
Condylomata accuminata, lichen planus, oral candidiasis, SCC, and bite callus or hyperkeratosis.

Treatment
Surgical excision of lesion advised; CO_2 laser or
cryotherapy may also be used. Close follow-up is
important.

Behavioral
Avoidance of tobacco use or other irritants such as
alcohol is advised. HPV vaccinations may reduce
incidence of oral cancers.

Referrals
Oral surgery or ENT referral indicated for removal
of lesions or further consultation.

Patient Education
Patients should be counseled regarding close
observation for recurrences and any new intra-
oral lesions, as well as avoidance of any possible
triggers.

Surgical Techniques
The decision as to which surgical technique to
employ hinges on various factors, including
whether the nature of the lesion is malignant or
benign. It is also important to consider the location of the lesion (slower healing anticipated for
lower extremity lesions/wounds), the skin type of
the individual (e.g., with regard to keloid formation) and the possible complications such as scar
formation.

The least invasive technique may be best for
good cosmetic results, but if malignancy is presumed, care should be taken to remove the entire
lesion carefully – with an adequate margin, such
as through an elliptical excision. A punch biopsy
is also suitable for the complete removal of a
smaller lesion.

Cryotherapy
This can be used for a variety of lesions, including
actinic keratosis, thin BCC, verrucae, and seborrheic keratosis. Shorter freezing cycles lasting 5–
15 s are sufficient for thin lesions or areas with
delicate skin. Longer freezing cycles of 30 s are
often required for thicker lesions such as seborrheic keratosis or BCCs. Side effects include
hypopigmented scar formation and potential
incomplete eradication of lesion.

Punch Biopsy
This technique is helpful for removal of small skin
lesions such as atypical nevi as well as for determination of the underlying pathology of a lesion.
After cleaning of the skin, local anesthetic is
injected, after which a punch is used to remove
the lesion via gentle pressure and rotation of the
punch, until the dermis is penetrated and the subdermal fat is reached. The specimen is then sent to
the pathology lab. The wound should be approximated with 1–2 sutures if a larger punch (4–6 mm
or greater) is used. Smaller wounds can heal
through secondary intention.

Shave Biopsy
This method can be used to remove benign lesions
such as skin tags, and dermal nevi, as well as pyogenic granulomata. It is also suitable for removal of
superficial BCC and for diagnostic purposes, except
for lesions potentially representing melanoma, as full

thickness depth is vital for staging. A Dermablade, razor blade, or scalpel can be used after the lesion has been marked, cleaned, and local anesthetic has been injected. Thickness up to the mid-dermis can be achieved; the specimen is then sent to pathology. If hemostasis is needed aluminum chloride (Drysol), silver nitrate or pressure can be applied. Silver nitrate may leave a stain.

Excisional Biopsy

This technique is best suited for removal of sebaceous cysts, lipomata, BCC, or SCC, and suspected melanomatous lesions. After marking and cleaning the skin area, local anesthetic is injected and the lesion removed with a margin of approximately 3 mm. An elliptical excision along the skin lines may provide the best cosmetic effect. The specimen is sent to pathology. Interrupted sutures are used to approximate the wound margins.

Curettage and Electrodessication

This technique can be used to treat an incompletely removed small or superficial SCC or BCC, a pyogenic granuloma, or as part of the destruction of the base of a keratoacanthoma. It is also useful to destroy small benign skin lesions. After cleaning of the skin and injection of the local anesthetic, the curette is used to remove abnormal tissue, until the firm base of normal skin tissue is reached. Electrocautery is applied at the base and the cycle of curettage and cauterization is repeated two more times. Hemostasis is accomplished through the cauterization itself. This technique may leave a scar.

Sun Exposure Protection

Basic Principles

It is best to avoid sun exposure between mid-morning and mid-afternoon (10 am and 2 pm). Sun burns occur quicker at higher altitudes and especially in those with fairer complexions.

UVA and UVB rays are transmitted through the atmosphere; some of the UVB rays are absorbed by the earth's ozone layer. UVA rays are thought to be more damaging, can penetrate glass, and reach the deeper skin layers such as the dermis. UVA rays can be found in tanning beds and causes wrinkling, photo-aging, and skin cancer. UVB rays are stronger mid-day and during the summer months, causing sunburns, cataracts, and skin cancer.

Sun screens can be divided into those with a physical ingredient or a chemical ingredient. Those with a physical ingredient contain zinc oxide or titanium oxide block or reflect sun rays and scatter them before they penetrate the skin. Those with a chemical ingredient such as avobenzone, PABA, or octisalate absorb the UV rays before they damage the skin.

Broad-spectrum sunscreens provide protection against both UVA and UVB rays. Higher sun protection factor (SPF) indicates better UVB protection, with SPF of 15 blocking approximately 94% of such rays, SPF of 30 blocking 97%, and SPF of 45–50 blocking 98% of rays. A minimum of SPF 30 is recommended for sun protection, as such can reduce not only sunburn, but also actinic keratosis, SCC, and melanoma.

Sun screen should be applied in adequate amounts 30 min prior to sun exposure in order to bind to the skin. Reapplication of sunscreen is important, especially after sweating or water activity, at least every 2 h. Even on cloudy days, up to 80% of UV rays reach the earth.

References

1. USPSTF. Skin cancer: screening recommendations. https://www.uspreventiveservicetaskforce.org
2. Fitzpatrick T, et al. Color atlas and synopsis of clinical dermatology. 2nd ed. New York: McGraw-Hill; 1992.
3. Wood L, et al. Effectiveness of cryosurgery vs curettage in the treatment of seborrheic keratoses. JAMA Dermatol. 2013;149:108.
4. Thompson S, et al. Reduction of solar keratoses by regular sunscreen use. N Engl J Med. 1993;329:1147.
5. Hunt R, et al. Acquired melanocytic nevi (moles). http://www.uptodate.com, Oct 2018.
6. Kittler H, et al. Diagnostic accuracy of dermoscopy. Lancet Oncol. 2002;3:159.
7. Tucker M, et al. Clinically recognized dysplastic nevi. A central risk factor for cutaneous melanoma. JAMA. 1997;277:1439.

8. Scope A, et al. The "ugly duckling" sign: agreement between observers. Arch Dermatol. 2008;144:58.

9. Tsao H, et al. Early detection of melanoma: reviewing the ABCDEs. J Am Acad Dermatol. 2015;72:717.

10. Schaffer J, et al. Benign pigmented skin lesions other than melanocytic nevi. http://www.uptodate.com, May 2018.

11. Siegel R, et al. Cancer statistics, 2019. CA Cancer J Clin. 2019;69:7.

12. Swetter S, et al. Melanoma: clinical features and diagnosis. http://www.uptodate.com, Dec 2019.

13. Breslow A. Thickness, cross-sectional areas and depth of invasion in the prognosis of cutaneous melanoma. Ann Surg. 1970;172:902.

14. Kassianos A, et al. Smartphone applications for melanoma detection by community, patient and generalist clinician users: a review. Br J Dermatol. 2015;172:1507.

15. Habif T, et al. Clinical dermatology. 3rd ed. Oxford: Oxford University Press; 1996.

16. Zuber T. Minimal excision technique for epidermoid (sebaceous) cysts. Am Fam Physician. 2002;65:1409.

Selected Disorders of the Skin

123

Carlton J. Covey, Stephen D. Cagle Jr, and
Brett C. Johnson

Contents

C. J. Covey (✉) · B. C. Johnson
Travis Family Medicine Residency Program, Travis Air
Force Base, Fairfield, CA, USA
e-mail: brett.johnson.23@us.af.mil

S. D. Cagle Jr
Scott Family Medicine Residency Program, Scott Air
Force Base, O'Fallon, IL, USA

© Springer Nature Switzerland AG 2022
P. M. Paulman et al. (eds.), *Family Medicine*,
https://doi.org/10.1007/978-3-030-54441-6_125

Disorders of Hypopigmentation

Vitiligo

Vitiligo is an acquired loss of pigmentation characterized by the absence of epidermal melanocytes. The destruction of melanocytes is thought to be autoimmune in nature, but the pathogenesis is not understood. It is the most frequent cause of depigmentation; approximately 1–2% of the population is affected with no propensity for gender or race. There is a positive family history in 30% of cases, lending to a relatively strong genetic component, and half of all cases of vitiligo occur prior to the age of 20 but can occur at any age [1]. Vitiligo is further classified as type A or type B. Type A is three times more common, more generalized, and more associated with immunologic diseases. Type B is less common, more rapidly progressive, but less generalized in appearance and follows a dermatomal appearance [2]. Lesions are milk-white hypopigmented macules and patches with discrete margins, which are symmetrically distributed [3]. Commonly affected areas for both types include the face, backs of hands, axillae, and genitalia. The scalp, lips, and mucous membranes may also be affected. Vitiligo can also occur at sites of trauma, such as the elbows or knees, and in previously sun-damaged skin [2]. Vitiligo is associated with thyroid disorders in up to 30% of cases, and there are also reported associations with alopecia areata, psoriasis, adrenal insufficiency, pernicious anemia, and type I diabetes [2]. Laboratory examination to exclude these associated systemic disorders should include thyroid studies, basic chemistry labs, fasting glucose, and a complete blood count. The diagnosis of vitiligo is made by physical exam revealing well-demarcated, uniformly white macules without signs of inflammation. A Wood's lamp can be used in fair-skinned individuals to accentuate hypopigmented areas. Skin biopsy and histologic examination reveal the absence of epidermal melanocytes.

Available literature does not show a higher predilection in dark-skinned individuals, but easier recognition of skin manifestations may increase perceived disfigurement and social stigmata in these patients. Although a benign condition, it can have a major impact on feelings of stress, self-consciousness, and sexual relationships leading to low self-esteem and depression.

Management

The goal of treatment is to restore melanocytes to the skin, which requires activation and migration of melanocytes located in the hair follicles. Therefore, skin with little hair, such as the hands or feet, responds poorly to treatment. Modalities should be chosen on the basis of disease severity, cost and accessibility, and treatment response. Treatment usually takes 6–12 months and should be started early in the course of disease. Combination therapies, such as phototherapy plus topical or oral steroids, are more effective than either alone at producing repigmentation [4]. Moderate- to high-potency topical steroids, or topical calcineurin inhibitors (tacrolimus [Protopic] and pimecrolimus [Elidel]), for 6–9 months are preferred for localized vitiligo [2]. Whereas narrowband ultraviolet B phototherapy (NB-UVB) is added as the disease spreads. In patients with extensive generalized depigmentation who do not respond to phototherapy, depigmentation of the surrounding skin should be considered. All patients with vitiligo should minimize sun exposure and apply broad-spectrum sunscreens to help minimize the contrast between tanned skin and hypopigmented skin.

Pityriasis Alba

Pityriasis is a common hypopigmentation skin disorder in prepubescent children with a history of atopic dermatitis. The most common sites affected are the face, neck, and arms [5]. The lesions begin as a nonspecific erythema but gradually become scaly and hypopigmented with pruritus occasionally present. It is often confused with vitiligo, but vitiligo lesions do not scale. Potassium hydroxide preparation is negative in pityriasis, distinguishing it from tinea infections. The condition is benign and improves after puberty, which can help reassure patients and their families. No treatment is necessary; however, low-potency topical steroids (applied twice daily) and sunscreens are first-line treatments [3]. High-potency topical steroids can be used on erythematous inflammatory lesions, but the depigmentation is not affected by any treatment. Pimecrolimus (Elidel) cream 1% and tacrolimus (Protopic) ointment (0.03% or 0.1%), applied twice daily, are nonsteroidal alternatives for treatment.

Tuberous Sclerosis

Tuberous sclerosis (TS) is the second most common neurocutaneous syndrome, affecting 1 in 6000 newborns, and is marked by childhood seizures and mental retardation but can affect several organ systems [6]. Congenital hypopigmented macules are generally oval or ash leaf shaped located on the arms, legs, and trunk. However, adenoma sebaceum is the most common cutaneous manifestation of TS. The lesions are small (1–5 mm), smooth, firm, yellow-pink papules with telangiectasia [7]. Skin manifestations may be the earliest sign of TS and occur in 80% of patients by 1 year of age [8]. Skin biopsy shows normal melanocytes which excludes vitiligo as the diagnosis. TS is an autosomal dominant disease, and genetic counseling should be offered in persons with a family history of TS. There is no treatment for the skin manifestations, but they offer an early window for diagnosis and referral, for the management of other clinical manifestations of TS.

Disorders of Hyperpigmentation

Pityriasis Versicolor (Tinea Versicolor)

Tinea versicolor is a common superficial fungal infection caused by *Malassezia* sp. It occurs most commonly in tropical climates and commonly affects adolescents and young adults [9]. The skin lesions (macules, patches) are generally hypopigmented, but can be hyperpigmented or erythematous, often with a fine scale which can be scraped for microscopy. It is most commonly found on the upper trunk and upper extremities in adults, but facial involvement is common in children [10]. Tinea versicolor shares common clinical findings with other skin disorders and therefore confirmation of the diagnosis with potassium hydroxide (KOH) is recommended. In one-third of individuals, a Wood's lamp will reveal yellow to yellow-green fluorescence [11]. First-line therapies include topical azole antifungals such as ketoconazole or topical adapalene (Differin) gel [12]. Topical selenium sulfide 2.5% applied for 10 min daily for 7 days and 2% ketoconazole shampoo applied to affected areas for 5 min prior to showering for three consecutive days are effective regimens [13]. Oral ketoconazole and itraconazole, both at doses of 200 mg/day for 5 days, are also effective and appropriate for patients with a large surface area burden for topical treatment [14]. Oral terbinafine (Lamisil) and griseofulvin are not effective in treating tinea versicolor. Hypo- or hyper-pigmentation can be present even after successful treatment. The presence of scale and positive KOH preparation confirms treatment failure.

Photosensitivity Dermatitis

Phototoxic reactions are nonallergic and induced by the use of systemic or topical medications or by contact with certain plants and foods in combination with sun exposure. Skin manifestations are generally confined to sun-exposed areas and result in erythema within minutes to hours of sun exposure [15]. Reactions can range from imperceptible erythema followed by prolonged hyperpigmentation to a sunburn-like reaction, edema with vesicles, and bullae [16]. Common medications associated with photosensitivity include antibiotics (fluoroquinolones, sulfonamides, and tetracyclines), diuretics (furosemide, hydrochlorothiazide), diltiazem, nonsteroidal anti-inflammatory drugs (NSAIDs), aspirin, and topical retinoids. Common foods include lemons, limes, celery, dill, and carrot juice [15]. Treatment is removal of the offending agent. When this occurs, the eruption generally resolves spontaneously. Oral steroids may be needed for severe cases with a significant inflammatory response. Avoidance of the offending agent (medication or food), direct sunlight, and tanning facilities is paramount. The use of clothing with ultraviolet filters and sunscreen can minimize the risk of a photosensitivity reaction.

Lichen Planus

Lichen planus (LP) is an inflammatory skin and mucous membrane reaction of unknown etiology. Mean age of onset for men and women is in the fifth decade of life, and it is rare in children younger than 5 years of age. A positive family history is found in 10% of patients. In the past, it has been thought that liver disease is a risk factor for cutaneous LP, specifically hepatitis C infection [17]. However, this association is based on studies showing weak associations and prevalence rates that range from 0% to 63%. Therefore, screening for hepatitis C in patients with diagnosed lichen planus is also controversial. Medications such as ACE-inhibitors, beta-blockers, and thiazide diuretics have been implicated in LP eruptions.

Clinical Presentation

Clinical features are characteristic and follow the six P's of lichen planus: pruritic, planar, polyangular, purple, plaques, or papules. The planar surface reveals a lacy, reticular pattern of crisscrossing whitish lines (Wickham's striae). Patterns can include annular, diffusely papular, or linear and most commonly affect ankles, volar surfaces of the wrists, forearms, and legs [18]. The clinical course is unpredictable as spontaneous remission can occur in a few months, but most commonly, LP lasts for approximately 4 years. Mucosal LP can occur with or without cutaneous eruptions; oral lichen planus is associated with concomitant vulvovaginal lesions 25% of the time [18]. Cutaneous manifestations can be erosive or nonerosive and can arise on the tongue, lips, buccal mucosa, glans penis, and anus. While a skin biopsy is the gold standard for diagnosis, the diagnosis usually can be made clinically by history and characteristics on physical exam.

Treatment

High-potency topical steroids (clobetasol, fluocinonide) are used as initial treatment for cutaneous and oral LP. Intralesional (triamcinolone acetonide 5–10 mg/ml every 3–4 weeks) and oral steroids (4 week course and taper of prednisone) can also be used for hypertrophic and generalized severely pruritic LP, respectively [17]. Azathioprine can be used as an alternative to steroids. Phototherapy with narrowband UVB or PUVA can also be used for generalized disease. Cyclosporine (6 mg/kg/day) is reserved for patients with severe disease. Calcineurin inhibitors, such as topical tacrolimus (Protopic) and pimecrolimus (Elidel), and aloe vera gel have all been shown to be effective in treating mucous membrane LP if topical steroids are not tolerated [17]. Antihistamines can be used as adjunctive therapy for intense pruritus.

Cutaneous Lupus Erythematosus

Systemic lupus erythematosus (SLE) is a chronic multisystem inflammatory disorder that is potentially fatal. The disease has no single diagnostic marker and is diagnosed using a combination of clinical and laboratory criteria [19]. Diagnosis and treatment can prevent significant morbidity and mortality. The prevalence of the disease is higher in African American females and persons of Hispanic and Asian descent.

Clinical Presentation

Patients with SLE will present with myriad of symptoms; however, cutaneous manifestations are the most common sign. General symptoms such as fatigue and fever (in the absence of infection) are also common. There are three subsets of cutaneous SLE: chronic (discoid), subacute, and acute lupus erythematosus [20]. Chronic type lesions are sharply demarcated erythematous raised lesions that can be round (discoid) and may have a scale. Lesions are normally found distributed asymmetrically on the face and scalp and can last for months. Rheumatologic lab tests such as antinuclear antibody (ANA), anti-double-stranded (ds) DNA, and erythrocyte sedimentation rate (ESR) are usually normal. Subacute lesions can be induced by medications such as hydrochlorothiazide and calcium channel blockers. They can be papulosquamous or annular-polycyclic and occur on the trunk, sparing the knuckles, axillae, and lateral part of the trunk. Subacute lesions are rarely noted below the waist;

ANA, ds-DNA, and ESR are usually positive, and lesions are likely to recur [20]. Classically, acute lesions present as a superficial, non-pruritic, erythematous plaques on sun-exposed areas of the body. The face (butterfly rash), chest, shoulders, extensor surfaces of the arms, and dorsal aspect of the hands are the most common areas. Acute lesions are almost always associated with SLE, whereas other types are less strongly associated. Cutaneous SLE is a clinical diagnosis but confirmatory skin biopsy may be needed when diagnostic uncertainty is present. Both non-scarring and scarring alopecia occur in more than 20% of cases of SLE [20].

Treatment

Photosensitivity is present in all types of cutaneous SLE, and ultraviolet rays from the sun can both induce or exacerbate cutaneous symptoms. Patients should avoid exposure to direct sunlight and use a daily broad-spectrum sunscreen with a sun protection factor (SPF) of 15 or higher [20]. Topical corticosteroids are first line for the treatment of all forms of cutaneous SLE and are used up to three times a day if needed, even on the face. It is common to start with a low- to medium-potency steroid and advance to high potency in those who do not respond. An alternative to corticosteroids is topical calcineurin inhibitors. If either of these treatments fail, antimalarial medications such as hydroxychloroquine or chloroquine are indicated [20]. Dapsone can be used when antimalarials fail or are not tolerated. Third-line therapies include azathioprine, methotrexate, and isotretinoin. Oral corticosteroids should be reserved for patients that fail topical steroid treatment or have a large burden of disease and fail antimalarial treatment.

Corns and Calluses

Corns and calluses result from hyperkeratosis associated with stimulation of the epidermis secondary to chronic pressure or friction on the skin [21]. Risk factors include poorly fitting shoes and anatomical pathology (bunions, hammer toes, claw toes, elevated metatarsals, and varus or valgus inverted hind foot) leading to abnormal pressure points on the foot. Hyperkeratosis is a normal protective physiologic response; however, it becomes pathologic when the corn or callus becomes large enough to cause symptoms.

Clinical Presentation

Because structural abnormalities are an important risk factor, a thorough examination of the foot and ankle is paramount in the evaluation of corns and calluses. Corns are distinguished from calluses often by location as well as the presence of a central conical core of keratin. They are usually located over non-weight-bearing surfaces and are painful when direct pressure is applied. Two subtypes of corns exist: the hard corn and the soft corn. Hard corns are typically located on the dorsolateral aspect of the fifth phalanx or the dorsum of the interphalangeal joint of the lesser toes [21]. The absorption of an extreme amount of moisture from perspiration between the toes leads to soft corns. They most commonly occur between the fourth and fifth web space and are caused by wearing a shoe that is too tight across the toes. Calluses typically form at sites of friction, pressure, and irritation such as the heel or under metatarsal heads. In contrast to corns, calluses do not possess a conical core and have undefined margins [21]. Both entities can be painful and interfere with daily activities.

Corns and calluses are of particular concern for individuals with peripheral arterial disease or diabetes. These patients classically have significantly reduced sensation and pain perception in the distal extremities leading to an increased risk of tissue breakdown, ulceration, and infection.

Management

Removal or redistribution of pressure is the first-line treatment for corns and calluses. Orthotic devices, inserts, or changing footwear can be helpful in patients with foot abnormalities, but the devices vary greatly and preclude recommendations. Donut pads and metatarsal bars can help redistribute pressure. Symptomatic relief of a hard corn can often be achieved through debridement of the lesions and removal of the keratin plug [21]. Patients with a soft corn should be advised to wear shoes with a roomy toe box, low heels, and soft upper portion. Keratinolytic medications (40% salicylic acid plaster) should be used to remove the excessive keratin. Paring down the lesion with a sharp blade is also an option. Appropriate patients (nondiabetics) can be instructed to use a pumice stone or emery board, after soaking the foot in warm water, to help reduce the size of the lesion.

If conservative treatments do not achieve symptomatic relief, corrective surgery may be necessary. A number of procedures exist to correct the underlying cause rather than simply excise the hyperkeratotic area.

Nail Abnormalities

Physical examination of the nails is often overlooked by family physicians, but may reveal localized abnormalities that should be treated or offer a window to an underlying systemic disease requiring further workup. The three most common conditions of the nails the family physician encounters are onychomycosis, ingrown toenails, and subungual hematomas.

Tinea Unguium (Onychomycosis)

Although occurring in 10% of the general population, onychomycosis is much more common in the older adult occurring in 20% of those older than 60 years and 50% of those older than 70 years [22]. Toenails are affected more often than fingernails and are most often caused by dermatophytes of the *Trichophyton* genus. There are five classes of onychomycosis based on morphologic appearance [23]. Distal onychomycosis is the most common and, as its name implies, affects the distal aspect of the nail. Proximal subungual infections invade the nail plate from below and cause the nail to separate. This pattern is the most common form in patients with human immunodeficiency virus infection (HIV). Superficial infection pattern appears to have powder-like patches of transverse striae on the surface of the nail. The nail plate is not thickened as is seen in other infection patterns. Psoriatic nail changes and trauma-related dystrophy can mimic onychomycosis [24]. Histologic examination of distal nail clippings with periodic acid-Schiff (PAS) staining is the best way to diagnose onychomycosis and differentiate it from dystrophic changes resulting from psoriasis. In contrast, potassium hydroxide (KOH) testing, or nail culture procedures, yields many more false negative results (poor sensitivity). If KOH or culture methods are used, it is important to collect distal nail particles as well as subungual debris with a curette. Confirmatory testing, prior to treatment, is controversial. Immediate treatment, with terbinafine, is more cost effective than performing KOH or PAS testing first, with little impact on patient safety [25]. Fingernail infections are generally caused by the *Candida albicans* species and are associated with chronic mucocutaneous candidiasis.

Management

Onychomycosis can negatively affect patient's lives via social stigma and disruption of daily activities or prevention of leisure activities. Treatment is often difficult with a 5-year recurrence rate of approximately 30–50% [26]. Some common poor prognostic factors include >50% areas of nail involvement, significant lateral nail disease, subungual hyperkeratosis, white/yellow/brown streaks in the nail, and patients with poor peripheral circulation or immunosuppression. Oral antifungals are the treatment of choice. Terbinafine (Lamisil) is the first-line treatment with a higher cure rate, lower relapse rate, and fewer side effects than itraconazole. Continuous dosing (terbinafine 250 mg/day for 12 weeks) has been shown to be superior to intermittent treatment, but pulse dosing of itraconazole (200 mg twice a day for 1 week per month × 3 months) is an alternative to continuous dosing

[23]. Routine interval laboratory testing of liver function, in persons without a history of hepatic disease, is unnecessary [27]. Complete resolution takes time (12–18 months to replace a diseased nail), and the nail surface is likely to still look infected after the 12-week treatment course. The use of oral antifungals is discouraged in patients with liver, renal, or heart disease. Superficial dermatophyte infections respond to topical antifungals and can be offered as an option. Cicloopirox nail lacquer has a low cure rate but can be offered to those who desire a trial of topical antifungal prior to initiating systemic therapy [24]. Although topical antifungals are not used to treat active onychomycosis, they can be used to help prevent recurrence. A twice-weekly application of terbinafine cream in the nail area, and between the toes, has been suggested for prevention [26]. Painful or extremely infected nails can be surgically removed.

Ingrown Toenails

Ingrown toenails are common and most commonly affect the large toe. Ingrown toenails occur when the periungual skin is penetrated by the nail, entering the dermis and causing a foreign body reaction which results in a painful toe [28]. Risk factors include tightly fitted shoes, trauma, hyperhidrosis, poor foot hygiene, or excessive trimming of the lateral nail plate. Characteristic signs and symptoms include pain, edema, exudate, and excessive granulation tissue. Indications for treatment include significant pain or infection or recurrent paronychia. Conservative therapy can be used when there is minimal inflammation and pain without purulent drainage. Frequent warm water soaking for 10–20 min, followed by application of a topical antibiotic or topical steroid several times daily, can be tried initially [29]. Other conservative methods include placing wisps of cotton, dental floss, or a gutter splint under the lateral nail edge. There is no evidence to suggest that any of these methods increases the risk of infection. Pre-procedure antibiotics are not indicated and do not reduce healing time or morbidity [30]. The most common surgical procedure to treat an ingrown toenail is partial avulsion of the lateral edge of the nail followed by matricectomy using 80–88% phenol. Phenolization after partial avulsion is more effective at preventing recurrence than partial avulsion alone, although there is an increase in postoperative infections [29]. The regular use of post-procedure antibiotics is not indicated.

Subungual Hematoma

Trauma to the nail and bleeding of the underlying nail bed cause immediate pain secondary to increasing pressure and separation of the nail plate. Puncturing the nail with an electrocautery device, or a red-hot paperclip, is the quickest and most effective method of draining the blood [31]. It is important to avoid the lunula (white crescent part of the nail), and its underlying nail matrix, during the procedure. No anesthesia is required for this procedure. It is important to tell patients that nail discoloration may persist until the nail has completely grown out.

Alopecia

Alopecia is defined as the absence of hair where it is supposed to be present. Growing hairs are termed anagen hairs and make up approximately 85% of all hair. They are securely anchored to the scalp and generally remain in this phase for 3 years. The resting or telogen phase lasts about 100 days and makes up the other 15% of all hair (with some in a catagen or transition phase). Normal shedding of hair occurs daily; however, abnormal hair loss can be pathologic or physiologic. Use of a wig may be recommended for management of both pathologic and physiologic hair loss regardless of cause.

Pathologic Hair Loss

There are four main types of pathologic hair loss. They are categorized according to the degree of scalp involvement (focal or diffuse), as well as the presence of or absence of scarring. Physical exam

and a thorough history will yield the correct categorization of hair loss for the majority of patients. Early recognition and diagnosis are important to aid in timely treatment, which may help to prevent further hair loss.

Telogen Effluvium

Telogen effluvium is the most common form of pathologic hair loss and typically follows a major life stressor such as a serious illness or injury, childbirth, or excessive dieting/rapid weight loss. Physiological causes include anemia, thyroid disorders, and several medication classes (beta-blockers, anticoagulants, oral contraceptives). Laboratory studies may be indicated if an underlying systemic disorder is suspected [32]. Whatever the etiology, the hair follicle enters into the resting phase (telogen phase) and causes diffuse, non-scarring hair loss, without causing complete baldness. The hair follicle, in essence, resets its biological clock and undergoes a normal involutional process [33]. This process takes approximately 100 days, so hair loss is typically seen 2–3 months after the inciting event. Conversely, when the precipitating event is removed, hair loss corrects itself in about 100 days, but may last longer than 4–6 months, fluctuating with times of normal and abnormal hair loss, depending on the inciting event [33, 34]. Physical examination typically reveals generalized hair loss as well as a positive hair pull test (place 40–60 hairs between the thumb and forefinger and pull slowly to the end of the hairs) [32]. The test is considered positive if greater than 10% of the hairs are removed. Treatment consists of stress reduction or identifying and treating the medical cause [32, 33]. Although difficult at times, patients should be reassured that no medication is needed for treatment. As stress wanes, the hair follicles regain normal physiologic activity, hair loss subsides, and regrowth occurs naturally.

Anagen Effluvium

Anagen effluvium is a sudden loss of hair follicles in their growing phase and can cause 80–90% hair loss. Chemotherapy, radiation, or toxic chemicals typically cause this, though inflammatory diseases such as alopecia areata and pemphigus are also culprits [35]. Anagen effluvium can manifest as either patchy or diffuse hair loss. Hair shedding typically begins 1–3 weeks after starting chemotherapy and is usually complete after 1–2 months. Hairs of the scalp are the most largely effected, though there can be hair loss of the eyebrows, eyelashes, pubic hair, and axillary hair as well [36]. Hair follicle stem cells are spared from destruction; therefore, the hair loss from anagen effluvium is not permanent [37]. Scalp cooling has been shown to reduce the risk of chemotherapy-induced hair loss by 55% [38]. No medication has been shown to prevent anagen effluvium.

Alopecia Areata

Alopecia areata is characterized by rapid hair loss in a sharply defined area. Its incidence is about 0.1–0.2% of the population of the United States. The etiology is unknown, but genetic factors may play a role. The association of alopecia areata with thyroid disorders and vitiligo suggests an autoimmune etiology; however, the significance of this association is unknown. Alopecia areata manifests as a non-scarring form of focal hair loss that can occur in a single patch or multiple patches. The affected skin shows smooth, circular, discrete areas of complete hair loss. The periphery of the circular areas may have short stubs of hair that remain (exclamation point hair). The hair loss can occur at any age, but it is more common in children and young adults, with up to 66% of people affected being less than 30 years of age [32]. The onset of the hair loss is typically rapid (a few weeks) and can potentially affect the entire body (alopecia universalis) but the scalp remains the most commonly affected. Overall, as many as 50% of patients with alopecia areata will recover within 1 year; for those with 1–2 patches of focal hair loss, recovery is as high as 80% [39]. Factors associated with a high likelihood prolonged hair loss or relapse are onset in childhood, severe disease affecting scalp and the body, duration of more than a year, associated nail disease (pitting

of the nail plate), or a family history of alopecia areata [40]. Unfortunately, there are currently no curative treatments for alopecia areata. Treatments help to control but do not cure or prevent the spread of alopecia areata. Intralesional injection of corticosteroids is the first-line treatment in patients with less than 50% of the scalp affected. Injection of triamcinolone acetonide (5–10 mg per ml) into the hairless patch every 2–6 weeks stimulated hair growth in 60–67% of cases. The use of high-potency topical corticosteroids has been controversial in the past; however, clobetasol propionate, 0.05%, applied to the area in a thin layer for 6 weeks and then off 6 weeks has been found to be both highly effective and safe in children [41]. Topical minoxidil (Rogaine) 5% concentration can also be used in individuals with greater than 50% of the scalp affected. It is best used in combination with other treatments, such as topical corticosteroids or anthralin. Other treatments include topical immunotherapy such as dinitrochlorobenzene, and tars, which induce an irritant or allergic contact dermatitis that promotes hair growth during healing [33].

Cicatricial (Scarring) Alopecia

Cicatricial alopecia causes permanent hair loss due to the destruction of hair follicles by inflammatory, autoimmune, or non-follicular process. It can be widespread or localized and can be classified as primary or secondary. In primary scarring alopecia, the follicle is the target of inflammation and common causes include discoid lupus, folliculitis decalvans, lichen planopilaris, acne keloid, and dissecting cellulitis of the scalp. In secondary scarring alopecia, the follicles are destroyed by a non-follicular process such as neoplasm, radiation, infection, surgery, and physical or chemical burns [40]. A biopsy is recommended to help support the diagnosis and determine the etiology. Scarring alopecia is an indication for dermatologic referral. Treatment depends upon the level of activity of the disease causing the scarring. Certain causes such as discoid lupus and lichen planopilaris may respond to topical, intralesional, or systemic steroids. Folliculitis decalvans will often respond to long-term antibiotic treatment with doxycycline, minocycline, erythromycin, Bactrim, or rifampin. If scarring is severe, surgical treatments including scalp stretching (removal of bald area and stretching the adjacent scalp over the removed area) or hair transplantation will be needed for treatment.

Traumatic Alopecia

Traumatic alopecia results from hair being forcefully extracted from the head or the breaking of hair shafts by friction, traction, pressure, or other physical trauma. Typical causes include cosmetic practices, trichotillomania, and pressure on the head as occurs on the occiput of infants who lie on their back. Common cosmetic practices that can cause traumatic alopecia (trichorrhexis nodes) include tight braiding, use of hair extensions, frequent brushing with nylon bristles, as well as most hair-straightening practices. Traction alopecia from braids or hair weaves can be detected along the frontal and temporal hairlines. Longstanding traction can lead to cicatricial alopecia and permanent hair loss. If no clear etiology, laboratory evaluation to include a complete blood count, iron studies, copper level, liver function tests, thyroid stimulating hormone level, and serum and urine amino acid levels is reasonable [32]. Treatment includes behavior modification to curtail hair trauma practices and/or managing underlying systemic illness that leads to increased hair fragility.

Trichotillomania is consciously or habitually plucking, cutting, or pulling hair in a bizarre manner and is a self-induced form of traumatic alopecia. Although it can be normal in children, it is closely related to obsessive-compulsive disorder in some children and adults. The mainstay of treatment is helping the patient find a different way to express their emotional needs. Psychiatric referral may be necessary.

Fungal Infection (Tinea Capitis)

Fungal infections can lead to scarring and non-scarring alopecia. Black dot tinea capitis is the most common form in the United States and preferentially affects African American children between 3 and 9 years of age [24]. Similar manifestations in adults should lead one to consider other diagnoses or consider a concomitant immunocompromised condition. Hair, within the scaly patches of hair loss, break off flush with the scalp and appear as a black dot. Diagnosis of tinea capitis can be confirmed with a Wood's lamp, fungal culture, or 10% KOH examination, but most physicians treat tinea capitis if the presentation is typical. First-line treatment of tinea capitis in children has traditionally been with 6–12 weeks of griseofulvin. Newer studies have shown that terbinafine (Lamisil) and fluconazole (Diflucan) have equal effectiveness and safety and shorter treatment courses. Terbinafine has similar efficacy in tinea capitis caused by Microsporum species but requires similar duration of treatment (6–12 weeks) as griseofulvin. Fluconazole has similar effectiveness with only 3–6 weeks of treatment [42]. Topical antifungals are not effective as they do not penetrate the hair shaft. However, concomitant treatment with 1% or 2.5% selenium sulfide shampoo or 2% ketoconazole shampoo should be used in the first 2 weeks of treatment to help decrease the risk of transmission [24]. There should be consideration of treating all close contacts with one of the aforementioned shampoo regimens for 2–4 weeks.

Physiologic Hair Loss

Androgenic alopecia (male pattern baldness) affects greater than 50% of men by 50 years of age and 40–50% of women by 60 years of age. It manifests as bitemporal hair thinning followed by loss of hair over the crown. Symptoms for women are not as severe as in men. Rapid hair loss or hair loss accompanied by pruritus, burning, or tenderness should lead one to consider other diagnoses. An association between male pattern baldness with cardiovascular disease and prostate cancer has been reported; however, the strength of the associations, if any, needs to be clarified. Treatment of androgenic alopecia includes both surgical and nonsurgical options. Medical options include topical minoxidil

(Rogaine) and oral finasteride (Propecia). Topical minoxidil prolongs the anagen phase of hair follicles and pushes resting hair follicles into the growing phase. Minoxidil, at 5% concentration, has been found effective for both hair preservation and regrowth in both men and women but is much more effective in the preservation of existing hair. It should be applied twice daily and benefits may take up to a year to be noticed [43]. Discontinuation of the medication results in continued hair loss and use should be indefinite. There are minimal side effects associated with topical minoxidil. Finasteride is an oral type II 5a-reductase inhibitor that blocks the conversion of testosterone to DHT. At treatment dosing (1 mg per day), it has been found to decrease circulating DHT by two-thirds. When used for 2 years, the medication was able to prevent further hair loss in 83% of men between the ages of 18 and 41 [43]. As with minoxidil, treatment should continue for 12 months to assess the drug's efficacy and must be continued indefinitely to maintain that efficacy. Finasteride can cause decreased libido, erectile dysfunction, and ejaculatory dysfunction and is a pregnancy category X medication. Finasteride can also significantly decrease serum levels of prostate-specific antigen. There is weak evidence showing that combination of finasteride and minoxidil works better than either alone, and this may be an option. Platelet-rich plasma (PRP) scalp injections are a novel treatment option, but more data is needed in order to recommend this modality. Possible surgical approaches for androgenic alopecia include follicle transplant, scalp reduction, and a transition flap.

References

1. Plensdorf S, Martinez J. Common pigmentation disorders. Am Fam Physician. 2009;79(2):109–16.
2. Habif TP. Clinical dermatology: a color guide to diagnosis and therapy. 6th ed. St. Louis: Elsevier; 2016. p. 770–5.
3. Nicolaidou E, Katsambas AD. Pigmentation disorders: hyperpigmentation and hypopigmentation. Clin Dermatol. 2014;32(1):66–72.
4. Ezzedine K, Whitton M, Pinart M. Interventions for vitiligo. JAMA. 2016;316(16):1708.
5. Habif TP. Clinical dermatology: a color guide to diagnosis and therapy. 6th ed. St. Louis: Elsevier; 2016. p. 777.
6. Kohrman MH. Emerging treatments in the management of tuberous sclerosis complex. Pediatr Neurol. 2012;46(5):267–75.
7. Habif TP. Clinical dermatology: a color guide to diagnosis and therapy. 6th ed. St. Louis: Elsevier; 2016. p. 999–1002.
8. Hemady N, Noble C. An infant with a hypopigmented macule. Am Fam Physician. 2007;75(7):1053–4.
9. Gupta AK, Bluhm R, Summerbell R. Pityriasis versicolor. J Eur Acad Dermatol Venereol. 2002;16(1):19.
10. Bouassida S, Boudaya S, Ghorbel R, et al. Pityriasis versicolor in children: a retrospective study of 164 cases. Ann Dermatol Venereol. 1998;125(9):581.
11. Schwartz RA. Superficial fungal infections. Lancet. 2004;364(9449):1173.
12. Shi TW, Ren XK, Yu HX, et al. Roles of adapalene in the treatment of pityriasis versicolor. Dermatology. 2012;224(2):184–8.
13. Kallini JR, Riaz F, Khachemoune A. Tinea versicolor in dark-skinned individuals. Int J Dermatol. 2014;53(2):137–41.
14. Stulberg DL, Clark N, Tovey D. Common hyperpigmentation disorders in adults: part II. Am Fam Physician. 2003;68:1963–8.
15. Habif TP. Clinical dermatology: a color guide to diagnosis and therapy. 6th ed. St. Louis: Elsevier; 2016. p. 576, 769.
16. Kutlubay Z, Aysegul S, Burhan E, et al. Photodermatoses, including phototoxic and photoallergic reactions (internal and external). Clin Dermatol. 2014;32:73–9.
17. Habif TP. Clinical dermatology: a color guide to diagnosis and therapy. 6th ed. St. Louis: Elsevier; 2016. p. 310–20.
18. Usatine RP, Tinitgan M. Diagnosis and treatment of lichen planus. Am Fam Physician. 2011;84(1):53–60.
19. Hochberg MC. Updating the American College of Rheumatology revised criteria for the classification of systemic lupus erythematosus. Arthritis Rheum. 1997;40(9):1725.
20. Habif TP. Clinical dermatology: a color guide to diagnosis and therapy. 6th ed. St. Louis: Elsevier; 2016. p. 680–94.
21. Freeman DB. Corns and calluses resulting from mechanical hyperkeratosis. Am Fam Physician. 2002;65(11):2277–80.
22. Thomas J, Jacobson GA, Narkowicz CK, et al. Toenail onychomycosis: an important global disease burden. J Clin Pharm Ther. 2010;35(5):497–519.
23. Westerberg DP, Voyack MJ. Onychomycosis: current trends in diagnosis and treatment. Am Fam Physician. 2013;88(11):762–70.
24. Ely JW, Rosenfeld S, Stone MS. Diagnosis and management of tinea infections. Am Fam Physician. 2014;90(10):702–10.
25. Mikailov A, Cohen J, Joyce C, et al. Cost-effectiveness of confirmatory testing before treatment of onychomycosis. JAMA Dermatol. 2016;152(3):276–81.

26. Habif TP. Clinical dermatology: a color guide to diagnosis and therapy. 6th ed. St. Louis: Elsevier; 2016. p. 969–74.

27. Stolmeier DA, Stratman HB, McIntee TJ, et al. Utility of laboratory test result monitoring in patients taking oral terbinafine or griseofulvin for dermatophyte infections. JAMA Dermatol. 2018;154(12):1409–16.

28. Habif TP. Clinical dermatology: a color guide to diagnosis and therapy. 6th ed. St. Louis: Elsevier; 2016. p. 976.

29. Heidelbaugh JJ, Hobart L. Management of ingrown toenail. Am Fam Physician. 2009;79(4):303–8. 4

30. Reyzelman AM, Trombello KA, Vayser DJ, et al. Are antibiotics necessary in the treatment of locally infected ingrown toenails? Arch Fam Med. 2000;9 (9):930–2.

31. Tully AS, Trayes KP, Studdiford JS. Evaluation of nail abnormalities. Am Fam Physician. 2012;85(8):779–87.

32. Phillips TG, Slomiany P, Allison R. Hair loss: common causes and treatment. Am Fam Physician. 2017;96 (6):371–8.

33. Habif TP. Clinical dermatology: a color guide to diagnosis and therapy. 6th ed. St. Louis: Elsevier; 2016. p. 923–7.

34. Whiting DA. Chronic telogen effluvium: increased scalp hair shedding in middle-aged women. J Am Acad Dermatol. 1996;35(6):889.

35. Kanwar AJ, Narang T. Anagen effluvium. Indian J Dermatol Venereol Leprol. 2013;79(5):604–12.

36. Patel M, Harrison S, Sinclair R. Drugs and hair loss. Dermatol Clin. 2013;31(1):67–73.

37. Paller A, Moncini A, Hurwitz S. Non-scarring alopecias with hair shaft abnormalities, chapter 8. In: Hurwitz's clinical pediatric dermatology: a textbook of skin disorders of childhood and adolescence. 4th ed. Edinburgh: Elsevier; 2011.

38. Hyoseung S, Jo SJ, Kim DH, et al. Efficacy of interventions for prevention of chemotherapy-induced alopecia: a systematic review and meta-analysis. Int J Cancer. 2015;136(5):E442–54.

39. Gilhar A, Etzioni A, Paus R. Alopecia areata. N Engl J Med. 2012;366(16):1515–25.

40. Alkhalifah A. Alopecia areata update. Dermatol Clin. 2013;31(1):93–108.

41. Lenane P, Macarthur C, Parkin PC. Clobetasol propionate, 0.05%, vs hydrocortisone 1%, for alopecia areata in children: a randomized clinical trial. JAMA Dermatol. 2014;150(1):47–50.

42. Chen X, Jiang X, Yang M, et al. Systematic antifungal therapy for tinea capitis in children. Cochrane Database Syst Rev. 2016;5:CD004685.

43. Varothsi S, Bergfeld WF. Androgenetic alopecia: an evidence based treatment update. Am J Clin Dermatol. 2014;15(3):217–30.

Part XXIV

The Endocrine and Metabolic System

Dyslipidemias

Cezary Wójcik

Contents

General Principles

Definition of Dyslipidemias

Dyslipidemias refer to abnormal function and/or levels of plasma lipoproteins. In routine clinical practice, they are detected by altered plasma lipid levels, which can be elevated (hyperlipidemia) or decreased (hypolipidemia). Normal lipid levels

C. Wójcik (✉)
Oregon Health Sciences University, Portland, OR, USA
e-mail: wojcikc@ohsu.edu

© Springer Nature Switzerland AG 2022
P. M. Paulman et al. (eds.), *Family Medicine*,
https://doi.org/10.1007/978-3-030-54441-6_126

are not synonymous to desirable (optimal or physiological). Hyperlipidemias are of extreme clinical importance due to being the root cause of atherosclerosis leading to atherosclerotic cardiovascular disease (ASCVD). The normal level of low-density lipoprotein cholesterol (LDL-C) is <100 mg/dL, while the non-HDL-C desirable level is <130 mg/dL. High-density lipoprotein cholesterol (HDL-C) is considered low when <40 mg/dL in men and <50 mg/dL in women. Triglycerides (TGs) are elevated when >175 mg/dL [1].

Lipids and Lipoproteins

Lipoproteins are particles composed of lipids (C, cholesterol; TGs, triglycerides; phospholipids) and proteins (apolipoproteins, Apo). The standard lipid panel (LP) measures total TG and cholesterol content in a particle (-C), but not particle count (-P), which can be measured directly by NMR technique or by surrogate markers (e.g., ApoB or ApoA1 levels). Chylomicrons are synthesized in the intestinal epithelium (TG:C ratio 10:1) and hydrolyzed at endothelial surface of capillaries by lipoprotein lipase (LPL) to chylomicron remnants (ChR), removed by the liver. The liver synthesizes very low-density lipoprotein VLDL-P (TG:C ratio 5:1), hydrolyzed by the same LPL to intermediate-density lipoprotein (IDL-P) and then low-density lipoprotein (LDL-P), which is poor in TG and rich in C. LDL-P and other ApoB-containing lipoproteins (e.g., ChR, VLDL-P, and IDL-P) may penetrate the arterial intima, promoting the development of atherosclerotic plaques. High-density lipoprotein (HDL-P, measured by surrogate markers HDL-C or ApoA1) participates in reverse cholesterol transport from plaques to the liver. However, HDL-C levels >100 mg/dL are pro-atherogenic. LDL-P are bound to LDL receptors (LDLr) on hepatocytes. This complex is endocytosed: LDL-P is degraded, while LDLr is recycled to bind more LDL-Ps. However, PCSK9 (proprotein convertase subtilisin/kexin type 9), a protein secreted by hepatocytes, binds to LDL-P/LDLr complex leading to LDLr degradation. Cholesteryl ester transfer protein (CETP)

exchanges cholesteryl esters from LDL-P and HDL-P for TG from VLDL-P. In patients with metabolic syndrome and type 2 DM, VLDL-P is overloaded with TG, and CETP activity is increased. This leads to the formation of small, dense, cholesterol-poor LDL-Ps, which remain longer in the circulation. It also leads to the formation of small, unstable, cholesterol-poor HDL-P. ApoA1 is lost in the urine leading to decreased HDL-C [2, 3].

Epidemiology

Western lifestyle increases the prevalence of dyslipidemia worldwide. In the USA, mean LDL-C levels decreased from 126.2 mg/dL (1999–2000) to 111.3 mg/dL (2013–2014). The age-adjusted prevalence of high LDL-C (≥130 mg/dL) decreased from 42.9% (1999–2000) to 28.5% (2013–2014). Approximately 17% of adults (~25% of males and <10% of females) have low HDL-C. Approximately 25% of adults had high triglyceride levels (≥150 mg/dL) [4].

Screening for Dyslipidemias in Adults

The US Preventive Services Task Force (USPSTF) has abandoned previous recommendations of screening for dyslipidemia, replacing them with recommendations about statin use for the primary prevention of cardiovascular disease [5]. The 2018 ACC/AHA/Multisociety cholesterol guideline recommends lipid screening every 4–6 years with a fasting or nonfasting lipid panel. However, if abnormalities are identified and interventions are implemented, including lifestyle or drug therapy, lipid testing is endorsed every 4–12 weeks after each change and between 3 and 12 months once desired lipid levels are achieved [1].

Screening for Dyslipidemias in Children

USPSTF found insufficient evidence to recommend for or against routine screening for dyslipidemias in infants, children, and adolescents 20 years or younger [6]. The 2018 ACC/AHA/Multisociety cholesterol guideline states that in children and adolescents without cardiovascular risk factors or family history of early CVD, it may be reasonable to measure a fasting lipid profile or nonfasting non-HDL-C once between the ages of 9 and 11 years and again between the ages of 17 and 21 years [1]. Moreover, in children and adolescents with a family history of either early CVD or significant hypercholesterolemia, the same guideline states that it is reasonable to measure a fasting or nonfasting lipoprotein profile as early as age 2 years to detect familial hypercholesterolemia or rare forms of hypercholesterolemia [1].

Classification

Dyslipidemias can be divided into primary (genetic) and secondary.

Classic Fredrickson's classification distinguishes the following:

- *Type I (familial hyperchylomicronemia syndrome, FCS)*: TG to TC ratio ~10:1, TG >1,000 mg/dL; presentation often in children with abdominal pain (recurrent pancreatitis) and eruptive xanthomas. No elevated atherosclerotic cardiovascular disease (ASCVD) risk. Prevalence ~1:1,000,000. FCS phenotype is most often caused by homozygosity of the gene encoding LPL or several associated factors regulating its activity.
- *Type IIa (familial hypercholesterolemia, FH)*: LDL-C usually ≥190 mg/dL, in homozygous FH (HoFH) often up to 400 mg/dL and above. Subjects with mild mutations and heterozygous FH (HeFH) may have LDL-C <190 mg/dL. Early ASCVD, sometimes in children and adolescents. Tendon xanthomas and corneal arcus at age <45 are frequent findings. FH phenotype is classically caused by LDL receptor mutations but can be seen with mutations of ApoB, PCSK9 (gain of function), or LDLRAP1 (recessive). Prevalence HoFH 1:250,000, HeFH 1:250.

- *Type IIb (familial combined hyperlipidemia, FCH)*: LDL-C, TG elevated, low HDL-C, TG to TC ratio ~5:1, atherogenic, frequent with metabolic syndrome. Prevalence ~1:100–1:200. Polygenic inheritance.
- *Type III (dysbetalipoproteinemia)*: IDL-P and ChR elevated, TC ~300 mg/dL, TG ~300 mg/dL, tuberoeruptive xanthomas, orange palmar xanthomas, atherogenic. Caused by ApoE2/E2 genotype or rare ApoE mutations, often silent, unmasked by environmental factors in <20% of ApoE2/E2 homozygotes. Prevalence ~1:200.
- *Type IV (hypertriglyceridemia)*: TC ~250 mg/dL, TG 400–1,000 mg/dL, low atherogenicity, exacerbated by alcohol and poor diet. Prevalence ~1:100–1:200. Polygenic inheritance.
- *Type V (mixed hyperlipidemia)*: TC ~250 mg/dL, TG >1,000 mg/dL, both chylomicrons and VLDL-P elevated, can present in childhood similar to type I or later in life with type 2 DM, gout, and metabolic syndrome. Prevalence ~1:100–1:200. Polygenic inheritance.

Dyslipidemias not included in the Fredrickson classification:

- *Elevated lipoprotein (a)*: Lp(a) is a prothrombotic and atherogenic lipoprotein, with a specific Apo(a) covalently bound to ApoB, often found in families with early ASCVD. Twenty percent of US population has elevated Lp(a) >50 mg/dL, considered a risk-enhancing factor for ASCVD. The higher Lp(a) level, the higher the risk. Patients with high Lp(a) often develop aortic valvular disease in addition to CAD.
- *Inherited low HDL-C*: hypoalphalipoproteinemia is usually associated with increased ASCVD. Includes rare Tangier's disease and lecithin-cholesterol acyltransferase (LCAT) deficiency, which in its heterozygous form is known as fish-eye disease. Very rare forms of low HDL-C (ApoA1 Milano) are cardioprotective.
- *Inherited high HDL-C*: very high HDL-C levels (>100 mg/dL) are not cardioprotective,

as they often reflect deficient function of HDL-P and are associated with atherosclerosis.

- *Inherited low LDL-C*: hypobetalipoproteinemia, autosomal dominant, ApoB deficiency, heterozygote patients have LDL-C <20 mg/dL, decreased ASCVD risk. Homozygote ApoB deficiency can present similarly to abetalipoproteinemia, which is autosomal recessive, microsomal transfer protein (MTP) deficiency presents in childhood (homozygotes only) with symptoms of deficiency of fat-soluble vitamins; LDL-C and VLDL-C are undetectable.
- *PCSK9 loss-of-function mutations*: loss-of-function PCSK9 mutations lead to moderate (heterozygous) LDL-C decrease (40–60 mg/dL) or more pronounced LDL-C (homozygous) decrease (~20 mg/dL) and are associated with decreased ASCVD risk, without any adverse effects.
- *Familial combined hypolipidemia*: autosomal recessive, ANGPTL3 mutations; all lipid levels are very low, including HDL-C; decreased ASCVD risk.
- *Sitosterolemia*: autosomal recessive, ABCG5/8 mutations, with or without elevated LDL-C, caused by accumulation of toxic plant stanols and sterols, normally not absorbed into systemic circulation, increased risk of ASCVD, tendon xanthomas. Prevalence ~1:1,000,000.
- *Cerebrotendinous xanthomatosis (CTX)*: rare, autosomal recessive, caused by CYP27A1 mutations, normal LDL-C levels, resulting from accumulation of cholestanol, increased ASCVD risk, mimics HoFH plus cataracts and neurological abnormalities. Prevalence ~1:50,000.
- *Cholesteryl ester storage disease, LAL (lysosomal acid lipase) deficiency*: high LDL-C and TG, very low HDL-C, elevated LFTs, unexplained hepatosplenomegaly and hepatosteatosis. *Wolman's disease* is caused by complete LAL absence, fatal ~1 year of age, due to anemia, liver failure, and cachexia. Prevalence ~1:50,000.

Secondary dyslipidemias can be subdivided by causative condition into lifestyle induced (high-cholesterol/high-fat diet, sedentary lifestyle, alcohol), endocrine (metabolic syndrome/DM, hypothyroidism, Cushing, polycystic ovarian syndrome), drug induced (cyclosporine, progestins, thiazides, betablockers, retinoids, estrogens, steroids, atypical antipsychotics, protease inhibitors), pregnancy, renal (chronic renal disease, nephrotic syndrome), infectious (HIV, hepatitis), hepatic (obstructive liver disease, cholestasis leading to buildup of lipoprotein X), storage disease (Gaucher's), and others (anorexia nervosa, cancer, transplant patients). Atherogenic dyslipidemia associated with metabolic syndrome, obesity, and/or type 2 DM is characterized by high TG, low HDL-C, and normal or only slightly elevated LDL-C. However, there is a significant increase in LDL-P, which can be measured directly by NMR or increased ApoB, which correlates better with increased ASCVD risk than LDL-C [1–3].

Diagnosis of Dyslipidemias

History

Patients with dyslipidemia often have signs and symptoms of atherosclerosis in different locations; therefore, it is important to inquire about exertional chest pain, history of abnormal EKG, stress test, intermittent claudication, erectile dysfunction, diagnosed CAD, or stroke/TIA. High TG level may cause recurrent pancreatitis in adults and children. History of intermittent abdominal pain and skin eruptions characterizes patients with FCS. Infants with hypo- and abetalipoproteinemia present with failure to thrive, steatorrhea, and developmental delay. Recurrent Achilles tendonitis in a child or adolescent may indicate FH. Family history should focus on premature ASCVD, early death, unusual skin/tendon lesions, pancreatitis, or known lipid disorders. It is important to review dietary habits, smoking history, alcohol use, exercise, and use of any medications or dietary supplements.

Physical Examination

Many physical findings are present in patients with dyslipidemias. Excess cholesterol and/or TG form deposits in different tissues. *Xanthelasmas* are flat, demarcated cholesterol deposits in subcutaneous tissue usually in or close to eyelids. Xanthelasmas are common and nonspecific, often a familial trait unrelated to dyslipidemia, never related to TG elevation. Larger and more tuberous cholesterol deposits are called xanthomas. *Tendon xanthomas*, specifically Achilles tendon xanthomas, are found in FH, CTX, and sitosterolemia patients, often at an early age. *Tuberoeruptive xanthomas* on elbows and knees as well as *palmar xanthomas* are found in dysbetalipoproteinemia. *Arcus senilis* is a grayish/white C/phospholipid deposit in the corneal margin. When found at <45 years of age, it is associated with dyslipidemia; later in life is a nonspecific finding. Clouding of the entire cornea is a characteristic of fish-eye disease. *Eruptive xanthomas* are TG accumulations in the form of small papules often with an inflammatory base, found in hyperchylomicronemia. Fundoscopic eye exam in children suspected to have HoFH may reveal ischemic optic neuropathy. *Lipemia retinalis* is a creamy white appearance of retinal vessels associated with high TG levels. *Orange tonsils* are characteristic of Tangier's disease. Hepatosplenomegaly can be found in patients with type I or type V dyslipidemia, as well as with LAL deficiency. A systolic ejection murmur at the right upper sternal border can be auscultated in patients with HoFH or very high Lp(a) levels, reflecting aortic stenosis (AS) resulting from xanthomatous infiltration of aortic valves (valvular AS) and root (supravalvular AS). Patients with CTX show cataracts and various neurological symptoms: ataxia, dysarthria, dementia, and seizures [2, 7].

Laboratory and Imaging

It is important to distinguish measured C levels within lipoprotein particles (-C) from the actual levels of particles themselves (-P). LP provides information about TC, LDL-C, HDL-C, VLDL-C, as well as TG. Non-HDL-C is calculated by subtracting HDL-C from TC. When LP is collected, nonfasting TG levels can be 20–40% higher than fasting. When LDL-C is calculated by the Friedewald formula [LDL-C = TC−(HDL-C + TG/5)], it becomes inaccurate with TG >200 mg/dL and unreliable with >400 mg/dL. It is also inaccurate at low LDL-C (<70 mg/dl) and TG (≥150 mg/dL) levels. Therefore, in such cases calculation using the new Martin formula is preferred, or a direct LDL-C measurement should be obtained. Nonfasting samples can be used for risk assessment in primary prevention and for assessment of baseline LDL-C levels before the initiation of statin therapy in primary and secondary prevention. Checking TSH and UA for proteinuria will rule out two common secondary causes of dyslipidemia. Extent of preclinical atherosclerosis can be measured by three noninvasive methods: carotid intima-media thickness (CIMT), obtained by US; coronary calcium score (CACS), obtained by a limited CT scan; and screening coronary CT angiogram (CCTA) requiring iv contrast prior to CT. CIMT is no longer endorsed by major guidelines, but it is useful in younger populations. CACS has received full endorsement as a definite tool to demonstrate the presence of subclinical disease. CACS of zero allows reclassification of patients to low risk and withholding of statin therapy except in smokers and patients with diabetes and strong family history of heart disease [1].

Special Testing

Advanced lipid tests include combinations of measurements, obtained by different proprietary techniques. Caution is advised when using those tests, as many of them lack high-level evidence for their use, especially in the general population. An exception is ApoB and LDL-P level testing. LDL-C and LDL-P can be discordant in up to 30% of individuals, especially those with metabolic syndrome. LDL-P or ApoB is a better predictor of CV risk than LDL-C. ApoB ≥130 mg/dL corresponds to LDL-C ≥160 mg/dL and is considered a risk-enhancing factor. High-sensitivity HS-CRP evaluates for potential intra-vascular inflammation, considered as a risk-enhancing factor favoring statin therapy. Elevated Lp(a) levels $\geq$50 mg/dL or $\geq$125 nmol/L are considered another risk-enhancing factor. Relative indications for its measurement are family history of premature ASCVD or personal history of ASCVD not explained by major risk factors. Lp(a) increases ASCVD risk especially at higher levels. Evidence is lacking to use HDL and LDL subfractions as well as more comprehensive inflammatory panels. Genotyping ApoE helps diagnose dysbetalipoproteinemia (Apo E2/E2), and it can also disclose increased risk of Alzheimer's disease (ApoE4/E4). Cholestanol and sitosterol measurements evaluate the proportion of cholesterol from intestinal absorption vs. synthesis in order to potentially guide therapeutic decisions [1–3].

Differential Diagnosis

Treatable, secondary causes of dyslipidemia need to be ruled out before concluding that it is a primary, i.e., genetic, problem. Most cases of dyslipidemia reflect a combination of genetic and environmental factors.

Treatment

Mild dyslipidemias are often amenable to therapeutic lifestyle modifications (TLMs) which are the baseline of therapy for primary and secondary ASCVD prevention. However, pharmacologic therapy is often required. The 2018 ACC/AHA/Multisociety guideline algorithm for initiation of lipid-lowering therapy in secondary prevention is presented in Fig. 1. While statins remain the first-line therapeutic agents, an LDL-C threshold of $\geq$70 mg/dL is introduced to add ezetimibe and PCSK9 inhibitors. The primary prevention algorithm is presented in Fig. 2. Lipid-lowering therapy should be initiated without calculating risk in patients with LDL-C $\geq$190 mg/dL and patients aged 40–75 with DM and LDL-C 70–189 mg/dL.

For patients with DM younger than 40, initiation of statin therapy is favored when they have one or more of the following risk enhancers: 1) long duration of DM ($\geq$10 years for type 2 and $\geq$20 years for type 1); 2) albuminuria $\geq$30 mcg/mg creatinine; 3) eGFR $<$60 mL/min/1.73 m; 4) retinopathy; 5) neuropathy; and 6) ABI $<$0.9. For patients aged 40–75 and LDL-C 70–189 mg/dL, 10-year ASCVD should be calculated using pooled cohort equations [8]. For patients in low-risk category ($<$5%), no treatment is needed. For patients in the intermediate-risk category ($\geq$7.5%– 20%) and selected patients in the borderline-risk category (5%–7.5%), initiation of moderate-intensity statin therapy is advised, especially if the presence of risk-enhancing factors (Fig. 2) favors initiation of statin therapy. In cases of doubt, obtaining CACS helps with the decision to initiate lipid-lowering therapy. For high-risk category ($\geq$20%) initiation of high-intensity statin is advised [1]. Lipid-lowering therapy is a key component to a comprehensive approach for primary ASCVD prevention as outlined in a separate guideline [9]. The 2019 European lipid guideline has much more aggressive goals of lipid-lowering therapy than the 2018 ACC/AHA/Multisociety guideline, aiming for an LDL-C of $\leq$55 mg/dL for many patients and an LDL-C goal of $\leq$40 mg/dL for patients with recurrent events [10]. It should be kept in mind that there is not such thing as an LDL-C level being "too low," as the safety of very low LDL-C is well established and there is not an LDL-C level beyond which further reduction is not beneficial [11].

Moderate hypertriglyceridemia is an independent risk factor for ASCVD, while severe hypertriglyceridemia (fasting triglycerides $\geq$500 mg/) can lead to pancreatitis [12]. The 2018 ACC/AHA/Multisociety guideline emphasizes that in adults with severe hypertriglyceridemia and especially fasting triglycerides $\geq$1000 mg/dL, it is reasonable to identify and address other causes of hypertriglyceridemia and, if triglycerides are persistently elevated or increasing, to further reduce triglycerides by implementation of a very low-fat diet, avoidance of refined carbohydrates and alcohol, consumption of omega-3 fatty

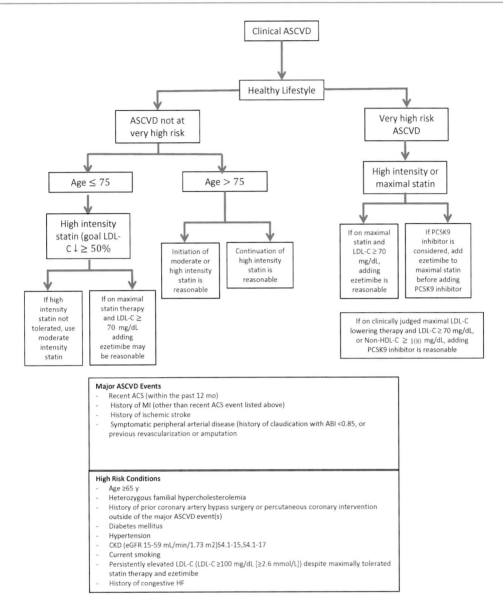

Fig. 1 Algorithm of major recommendations for lipid-lowering therapy for secondary ASCVD prevention based on 2018 ACC/AHA/Multisociety guideline. Heart-healthy lifestyle is the foundation for secondary prevention. In individuals not at very high risk, high-intensity statin therapy should be used, with addition of ezetimibe, if LDL-C remains above the 70 mg/dL threshold. In patients at very high risk, PCSK9 inhibitors should be added if LDL-C remains above the 70 mg/dL threshold and/or 100 mg/dL non-HDL-C threshold despite maximally tolerated statin±ezetimibe therapy. To determine whether a patient is at very high risk, they need to have a history of multiple major ASCVD events or one major ASCVD event and multiple high-risk conditions as listed in the table at the bottom of the figure

acids, and, if necessary to prevent acute pancreatitis, fibrate therapy. No recommendations are made to treat moderate hypertriglyceridemia (175–499 mg/dL), which is considered as a risk-enhancing factor alone and as part of the metabolic syndrome [1]. Recent data have shown treatment of patients with moderate hypertriglyceridemia and ASCVD or type 2 diabetes and several cardiovascular risk factors with 4 g daily of icosapent ethyl (pure EPA omega-3

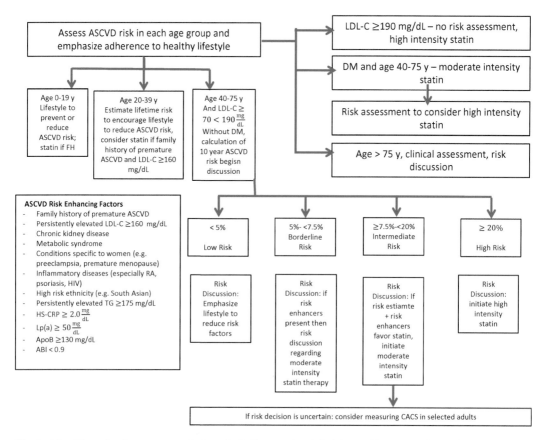

Fig. 2 **Algorithm of major recommendations for lipid-lowering therapy for primary ASCVD prevention based on 2018 ACC/AHA/Multisociety guideline**. Heart-healthy lifestyle is the foundation for prevention across all ages. Statin therapy should be initiated through a shared decision-making process in a patient-centric manner. Inclusion of risk-enhancing factors allows for an individualized approach therapy. CACS allows for detection of subclinical coronary artery disease to help guide clinical decisions

preparation) leads to a 25% reduction of cardiovascular events with a NNT of 21 [13]. This recommendation has been incorporated into the newest European guideline [10]. In contrast to high TG, low HDL-C should be used only as a marker of cardiovascular risk but not as a target of therapy [1].

Medications

There are various classes of drugs used to treat dyslipidemias (Table 1), with several new drugs in development [14]. LDL-C lowering by each 38.4 mg/dL (1 mmol/L) leads to a roughly 23% reduction in cardiovascular events for both primary and secondary prevention as demonstrated in many clinical trials, mostly involving statin therapy but also other interventions including PCSK9 inhibitors and ezetimibe. Statins inhibit hydroxymethylglutaryl-coenzyme A (HMG-CoA) reductase, the rate-limiting enzyme of cholesterol synthesis. This leads to increased removal of LDL-P from plasma by LDLr upregulation in the liver. Statins decrease LDL-C (18–55% reduction), non-HDL-C (15–51%), and TG (7–30%) while increasing HDL-C (5–15%). Bempedoic acid reduces LDL-C by ~18% through inhibiting ATP citrate lyase, an enzyme upstream of HMG-CoA reductase. However, its place in therapy remains unclear, until results of the cardiovascular outcome trial become available. Removing PCSK9 by the use of monoclonal antibodies (evolocumab and alirocumab) allows recycling

Table 1 Lipid-lowering medications

Medication	Dose range	LDL reduction (%)	Cost	Side effects and special considerations	Pregnancy category
Statins (HMG-CoA reductase inhibitors)					
Atorvastatin (Lipitor)	10 mg qd min 80 mg qd max	31–35 50–60	$	CYP3A4 metabolized, long half-life, avoid erythromycin, azoles, protease inhibitors, cyclosporine, and grapefruit juice	X
Rosuvastatin (Crestor)	5 mg qd min 40 mg qd max	40–48 58–64	$–$$	Minimal CYP2C9, long half-life	X
Fluvastatin (Lescol)	20 mg qhs min 80 mg XL max	20–25 27–32	$$	CYP2C9, least chance of myopathy, short half-life	X
Lovastatin (Mevacor)	10 mg qhs min 80 mg qhs or 40 mg bid max	25–30 35–40	$	CYP3A4 metabolized, short half-life, avoid erythromycin, azoles, protease inhibitors, cyclosporine, and grapefruit juice. Best absorbed with food	X
Pitavastatin (Livalo, Zypitamag)	1 mg qd 4 mg qd	32–46	$$$	Minimal CYP2C9 and 2C8, long half-life	X
Pravastatin (Pravachol)	10 mg qhs min 80 mg qhs max	25–32 17–32	$	Minimal CYP metabolism, short half-life, avoid erythromycin	X
Simvastatin (Zocor)	10 mg qhs min 40 mg qhs max	27–32 38–43	$	CYP3A4 metabolized, short half-life, avoid erythromycin, azoles, protease inhibitors, cyclosporine, and grapefruit juice. Decrease dosing of diltiazem, verapamil, amlodipine, and amiodarone	X
Cholesterol absorption inhibitors					
Ezetimibe (Zetia)	10 mg qd	17–22	$–$$	Well tolerated; when combined with statin, it can raise LFTs and contribute to myalgia/myopathy. Available in combination with simvastatin (Vytorin) and atorvastatin (Liptruzet)	C
ATP citrate lyase inhibitors					
Bempedoic acid (Nexletol)	180 mg qd	15–24	$$$	Well tolerated in statin-intolerant patients, can induce gout and tendon rupture, in combination with ezetimibe lowers LDL-C by 48%	?
Bile acid sequestrants					
Colestipol (Colestid)	2–16 g qd or divided (start low and titrate up)	10–25	$$	Do not use when TG >300; constipation; decreased absorption of many drugs and vitamins. Contraindicated when hx of bowel obstruction	B
Cholestyramine (Questran)	4–16 g divided bid (start low and titrate up)	10–25	$$	Do not use when TG >300; constipation; decreased absorption of many drugs and vitamins. Contraindicated when hx of bowel obstruction	C

(continued)

Table 1 (continued)

Medication	Dose range	LDL reduction (%)	Cost	Side effects and special considerations	Pregnancy category
Colesevelam (Welchol)	3.75 g qd or divided bid	10–25	$$$	Easier to use, less interactions. Do not use when TG >300; constipation; decreased absorption of many drugs and vitamins. Lowers A1C 0.5%. Contraindicated when hx of bowel obstruction	B
Niacin (nicotinic acid – not nicotinamide)					
Niacin immediate release, crystalline (Niacor, etc.)	100–3,000 mg initial dose qd, then divided bid/tid, titrate up slowly	5–25	$	Flushing, dry skin, rash, glucose intolerance/new-onset type 2 DM, hyperuricemia, dyspepsia/PUD, afib, infections. May enhance side effects of statins	C
Niacin sustained release (Endur-Acin, etc.)	500–2,000 mg qhs, titrate up slowly	5–25	$	Flushing, dry skin, rash, glucose intolerance/new-onset type 2 DM, hyperuricemia, dyspepsia/PUD, afib, infections. May enhance side effects of statins. Monitor LFTs due to potential hepatotoxicity	C
Niacin extended release (Niaspan)	500–2,000 mg qhs, titrate up slowly	5–25	$$–$$$	Flushing, dry skin, rash, glucose intolerance/new-onset type 2 DM, hyperuricemia, dyspepsia/PUD, afib, infections. May enhance side effects of statins. Monitor LFTs due to potential hepatotoxicity	C
Fibrates					
Gemfibrozil (Lopid)	600 mg bid	6–20 when TF <400, increase when TG >400	$$	Avoid combination with statins due to increased risk of myalgia/myopathy	C
Fenofibrate (Tricor, Trilipix, Lofibra, Fenoglide, Lipofen, Triglide, etc.)	43–200 mg qd	6–20 when TF <400, increase when TG >400	$–$$$	May be combined with statins. Avoid in kidney disease. Multiple formulations make dosing confusing	C
Pemafibrate (Parmodia)	0.1–0.2 mg BID	Lowers TG, raises HDL-C and LDL-C	$$$?	Approved in Japan, awaiting US approval	
ω3 polyunsaturated fatty acids					
DHA/EPA (Lovaza)	4 g qd or 2 g BID	Increase up to 40%	$–$$	Well tolerated,, may increase bleeding time, no cardiovascualr outcomes	C
EPA (Vascepa)	2 g BID	0	$$$$	25% of MACE RRR with 21 NNT Well tolerated, may increase bleeding time	C

(continued)

Table 1 (continued)

Medication	Dose range	LDL reduction (%)	Cost	Side effects and special considerations	Pregnancy category
Microsomal triglyceride transfer protein inhibitors					
Lomitapide (Juxtapid)	Start 5 mg qd, titrate up as tolerated up to 60 mg qd	40–50	$$$$$$$	Use restricted to HoFH, REMS required; risk of hepatotoxicity. Requires strict low-fat diet. GI side effects	X
ApoB antisense oligonucleotide					
Mipomersen (Kynamro)	200 mg Subq injection, q week	40–50	$$$$$$$	Use restricted to HoFH, REMS required; risk of hepatotoxicity; currently not available on the market	B
PCSK9 inhibitor antibodies					
Alirocumab (Praluent)	75 or 150 mg Q14 days or 300 mg q 30 days; sc injection	45–50%	$$–$$$	Very well tolerated, ~15% RRR of cardiovascular events (ODYSSEY OUTCOMES) Can lower Lp(a) 20–30%	Not assigned
Evolocumab (Repatha)	140 mg Q14 days or 420 mg Q30 days; sc injection	59–63%	$$–$$$	Very well tolerated, ~15% RRR of cardiovascular events (FOURIER) Can lower Lp (a) 20–30%	Not assigned
PCSK9 RNA interfering nucleic acid					
Inclisiran	300 mg Q 6 months; sc injection	53–58%	$$$$?	Very well tolerated, no significant side effects; convenience of 2 × year administration in clinician's office	?

of more LDLr to hepatocyte surface and thus for more efficient LDL-P removal from circulation, leading to a dramatic 50–60% LDL-C reduction on top of statins. Finally, ezetimibe blocks both intestinal and biliary cholesterol absorption and thus delivery to hepatocytes, leading to LDLr upregulation in the liver and a modest ~20% LDL-C decrease.

Statins are well tolerated, but up to 10% of patients may show statin intolerance, with many more showing statin aversion due to negative social media profile of this drug category. Myalgias and myopathy are the main reason of switching statin, nonadherence, and discontinuation of therapy. Severe rhabdomyolysis is very rare (1:100,000). However, patients initiating statins should be warned of signs and symptoms of this adverse reaction (tea-colored urine, oliguria, severe muscle pain, nausea, vomiting,

confusion). Following liver function tests (LFTs) is no longer recommended in asymptomatic patients after the initiation of statin therapy. Mild elevation of LFTs ($<3 \times$ upper limit of normal) is observed in 1–2% of patients taking statins and should not lead to discontinuation of therapy. Statins confer a small, dose-dependent risk of developing type 2 DM in predisposed individuals (up to 9–12%). However, CV benefits from their use greatly outweigh this risk. While data from RCTs do not show any adverse effects of statins on cognition, several observational studies reported memory problems and cognitive impairments with statin use, which lead to their discontinuation. Ezetimibe is very well tolerated without major side effects. The same is true for injectable PCSK9 inhibitors, whose main side effects are injection site reactions and short-lasting flu-like symptoms seen in a minority of patients [11].

LDL Apheresis

In severe FH multiple drugs are often used to achieve the therapeutic LDL-C goal. When maximally tolerated pharmacotherapy fails in selected patients (HoFH with LDL-C >500 mg/dL, HeFH and LDL-C >300 mg/dL, HeFH with LDL-C ≥100 mg/dL, and coronary artery disease), they can be treated with LDL apheresis. The procedure lasts 2–4 h and it is performed every 2–4 weeks in special facilities. Each apheresis session leads to a 49–75% decrease in LDL-C levels [15].

Nutraceuticals

Nutraceuticals are very useful in statin-intolerant patients and in patients preferring natural therapies. A combination of nutraceuticals may lead to a significant up to 50% LDL-C lowering. Red yeast rice contains natural lovastatin (2–10 mg), lowers LDL-C by ~27%, and decreases cardiovascular and total mortality by 30% and 33%, respectively. Other agents with significant LDL-C lowering but unproven cardiovascular outcomes include phytosterols, soluble dietary fiber, berberine, bergamot, artichoke, and soy products. There is no solid evidence supporting the use of garlic, guggulipid, policosanol, or tocotrienols in lowering LDL-C. Over-the-counter fish oil (ω3PUFA) lowers TG and LDL-P while raising HDL-C and LDL-C [16]. Statins lower CoQ10 levels; therefore, CoQ10 supplementation may prevent myalgias associated with statin use. However, CoQ10 use is not endorsed by the 2018 ACC/AHA/Multisociety guideline [1].

Referrals

Difficult-to-manage patients with dyslipidemias, especially patients with extreme LDL-C and TG elevations, requiring drugs beyond statins and ezetimibe, and those who do not respond appropriately to therapy should be referred to lipid specialists often practicing within specialized lipid clinics or preventive cardiology groups. Clinical lipidology is an emerging subspecialty open to family physicians [17].

Prevention

Therapeutic lifestyle modifications constitute the foundation of management of dyslipidemias. Adults should engage in at least 150 min per week of accumulated moderate-intensity or 75 min per week of vigorous-intensity aerobic physical activity (or an equivalent combination of moderate and vigorous activity) to reduce ASCVD risk. Diets high in saturated fats raise LDL-C and HDL-C. In addition, trans fats increase Lp(a) levels. High-carbohydrate low-fat diets lower LDL-C and HDL-C but increase TG and LDL-P and therefore should be avoided by patients with metabolic syndrome/type 2 DM. Mediterranean diet decreases LDL-C and raises HDL-C. Nut consumption decreases LDL-C and TG. Alcohol consumption raises TG and HDL-C. Patients with severe hypertriglyceridemia require very low-fat diets to prevent recurrent pancreatitis [1, 9].

Family and Community Issues

Cascade screening of family members is advised, especially in the case of FH and elevated Lp (a) [1]. Prevalence of FH is elevated in some ethnic groups (French Canadians, Ashkenazi Jews, Afrikaners, Lebanese Christians). The FH Foundation provides resources, support, and cascade registry [18]. The Lipoprotein (a) Foundation provides resources and support for patients with high Lp(a) [19]. Patients with FCS can find support and resources with the FCS Foundation [20].

References

1. Grundy SM, Stone NJ, Bailey AL, et al. AHA/ACC/ AACVPR/AAPA/ABC/ACPM/ADA/AGS/APhA/AS PC/NLA/PCNA Guideline on the Management of Blood Cholesterol: a report of the American College of Cardiology/American Heart Association Task Force

on Clinical Practice Guidelines. J Am Coll Cardiol. 2019;24(73):3168–3209.

2. In: Ballantyne C, editor. Clinical lipidology. 2nd ed. Philadelphia: Elsevier Saunders; 2015.

3. Sniderman AD, Thanassoulis G, Glavinovic T, et al. Apolipoprotein B particles and cardiovascular disease: a narrative review. JAMA Cardiol. 2019;(4)12:1287–1295.

4. Benjamin EJ, Muntner P, Alonso A, et al. Heart disease and stroke Statistics-2019 update: a report from the American Heart Association. Circulation. 2019;139 (10):e56–e528.

5. Force USPST, Bibbins-Domingo K, Grossman DC, et al. Statin use for the primary prevention of cardiovascular disease in adults: US preventive services task force recommendation statement. JAMA. 2016;316(19):1997–2007.

6. Force USPST, Bibbins-Domingo K, Grossman DC, et al. Screening for lipid disorders in children and adolescents: US preventive services task force recommendation statement. JAMA. 2016;316(6):625–33.

7. Gidding SS, Champagne MA, de Ferranti SD, et al. The agenda for familial hypercholesterolemia: a scientific statement from the American Heart Association. Circulation. 2015;132(22):2167–92.

8. https://www.acc.org/tools-and-practice-support/mobile-resources/features/2013-prevention-guidelines-ascvd-risk-estimator. 01/16//2020.

9. Arnett DK, Blumenthal RS, Albert MA, et al. 2019 ACC/AHA guideline on the primary prevention of cardiovascular disease: executive summary: a report of the American College of Cardiology/American Heart Association Task Force on Clinical Practice Guidelines. J Am Coll Cardiol. 2019;74(10):1376–414.

10. Mach F, Baigent C, Catapano AL, et al. ESC/EAS Guidelines for the management of dyslipidaemias: lipid modification to reduce cardiovascular risk. Eur Heart J. 2019.

11. Rosenson RS, Hegele RA, Fazio S, et al. The evolving future of PCSK9 inhibitors. J Am Coll Cardiol. 2018;72(3):314–29.

12. Laufs U, Parhofer KG, Ginsberg HN, et al. Clinical review on triglycerides. Eur Heart J. 2019.

13. Bhatt DL, Steg PG, Miller M, et al. Cardiovascular risk reduction with icosapent ethyl for hypertriglyceridemia. N Engl J Med. 2019;380(1):11–22.

14. Hegele RA, Tsimikas S. Lipid-lowering agents. Circ Res. 2019;124(3):386–404.

15. Wang A, Richhariya A, Gandra SR, et al. Systematic review of low-density lipoprotein cholesterol apheresis for the treatment of familial hypercholesterolemia. J Am Heart Assoc. 2016;5(7):e003294.

16. Banach M, Patti AM, Giglio RV, et al. The role of nutraceuticals in statin intolerant patients. J Am Coll Cardiol. 2018;72(1):96–118.

17. https://www.lipidboard.org. 01/16/2020.

18. https://thefhfoundation.org. 01/16/2020.

19. https://www.lipoproteinafoundation.org. 01/16/2020.

20. https://livingwithfcs.org. 01/16/2020.

Nadine El Asmar, Baha M. Arafah, and Charles Kent Smith

Contents

N. El Asmar (✉) · B. M. Arafah
Division of Clinical and Molecular Endocrinology,
University Hospitals-Cleveland Medical Center, Case
Western Reserve University School of Medicine,
Cleveland, OH, USA
e-mail: nadine.elasmar@uhhospitals.org;
baha.arafah@case.edu

C. K. Smith
University Hospitals-Cleveland Medical Center, Case
Western Reserve University School of Medicine,
Cleveland, OH, USA
e-mail: cks@case.edu

© Springer Nature Switzerland AG 2022
P. M. Paulman et al. (eds.), *Family Medicine*,
https://doi.org/10.1007/978-3-030-54441-6_186

Definition

Diabetes mellitus is a group of diseases characterized by hyperglycemia and other metabolic abnormalities resulting from impaired insulin secretion and/or its action at the cellular level.

Epidemiology

Data from 2018 estimated that 10.5% of the US population or 34.2 million Americans had diabetes. Nearly 1.6 million have type 1 diabetes. A total of 1.5 million Americans are diagnosed with diabetes every year. In 2015, 88 million Americans age 18 and older had prediabetes. As the epidemic of obesity in the USA continues to be on the rise, diabetes in youth younger than 20 has followed. In 2014–2015, the annual incidence of diagnosed diabetes in youth was estimated at 18,200 with type 1 diabetes, 5800 with type 2 diabetes [1, 2]. Diabetes is a major risk factor for kidney failure as well as cardiovascular and cerebrovascular disease.

Classification

- Type 1 diabetes mellitus (insulin-dependent DM) is characterized by deficiency of insulin secretion due to autoimmune pancreatic beta-cell destruction.
- Type 2 diabetes mellitus (noninsulin-dependent DM) is usually part of the metabolic syndrome, which is associated with hypertension, dyslipidemia, and obesity. It is characterized by insulin resistance in addition to relative insulin deficiency.
- Latent autoimmune diabetes of adulthood (LADA) has a similar pathophysiology to type 1 DM but occurs in adults.

- Maturity onset diabetes of the young (MODY) is a monogenic diabetes which is characterized by the onset of hyperglycemia at an early age but is not characteristic of type 1 diabetes. It is autosomal dominant in inheritance.
- Gestational diabetes is the development of new onset diabetes during pregnancy, usually during the third trimester.
- Secondary diabetes occurs as a result of either medications such as glucocorticoids, diseases of the pancreas such as cystic fibrosis or pancreatitis, or as a result of a surgical intervention such as a pancreatectomy. Secondary diabetes can also be frequently observed in patients with specific illnesses such as acromegaly, Cushing's syndrome, and pheochromocytoma.

On the other hand, type 2 diabetes accounts for 90–95% of all diabetes. The risk of developing type 2 diabetes mellitus increases with age typically >45. However, given the increased incidence of obesity, there has been an increasing incidence of type 2 diabetes at an age < 45. In type 2 diabetes, there is a progressive loss of adequate B-cell insulin secretion frequently on the background of insulin resistance [3]. Patients with type 2 diabetes mellitus are typically obese. They often present with polyuria, polydipsia, polyphagia, and at times unexplained weight loss. They are also often diagnosed on routine lab testing and screening employed to detect type 2 diabetes onset in patients with risk factors.

Diagnosis of Diabetes Mellitus

The biochemical diagnosis of diabetes mellitus is based on criteria established by the American Diabetes Association. These are listed in Table 1. Patients with type 1 diabetes can also present in an incidental manner on routine testing. Clues to diagnosis include age of onset and the presence of positive antibodies. Table 2 depicts the stages prior to the clinical development of type 1 diabetes.

LADA is characterized by slowly progressive autoimmune diabetes with an adult onset usually above 35 years of age. There is slow autoimmune B-cell destruction that indicates there may be a long duration of marginal and insufficient insulin secretion.

Table 1 Diagnostic criteria for diabetes mellitus and prediabetes

Diabetes mellitus	Prediabetes
1. Fasting blood glucose ≥126 mg/dl	1. Fasting blood glucose 100–125 mg/dl
2. 2 h post prandial glucose ≥200 mg/dl during an OGTT (using 75 g of an oral glucose load)	2. 2 h post prandial glucose 140–199 mg/dl during an OGTT
3. HbA1c of ≥6.5%	3. HbA1c of 5.7–6.4%
4. Random glucose of ≥200 mg/dl along with classic symptoms of hyperglycemia	
Diagnosis requires 2 abnormal test results from the same sample or in 2 separate test samples	

Adapted from the ADA 2020 guidelines

Table 2 Stages of type 1 diabetes

Stages of type 1 diabetes	Stage 1	Stage 2	Stage 3
Characteristics	– Autoimmunity – Normoglycemia – Presymptomatic	– Autoimmunity – Dysglycemia – Presymptomatic	– New-onset hyperglycemia – Symptomatic
Diagnostic criteria	– Antibody Positivity – No IFG or IGT	– Antibody positivity – Dysglycemia: IFG, IGT, and/or elevated HbA1c	– Clinical symptoms – Diabetes by standard criteria

IFG (impaired fasting glucose): Fasting plasma glucose 100–125 mg/dl
IGT (impaired glucose tolerance): 2 h postprandial glucose 140–199 mg/dl
HbA1c: 5.7–6.4%

Adapted from the ADA 2020 guidelines

Of note, the traditional paradigms of type 2 diabetes occurring only in adults and type 1 diabetes only in children are no longer accurate, as both diseases occur in most age groups.

Diabetes is usually preceded by the prediabetes stage which is characterized by impaired fasting glucose (IFG) or impaired glucose tolerance (IGT). Prediabetes should not be viewed as an independent clinical entity but rather as an increased risk for diabetes and cardiovascular disease (CVD). Prediabetes is also associated with obesity (especially abdominal or visceral obesity), dyslipidemia with high triglycerides and/or low HDL cholesterol, and hypertension [3].

Important Aspects in Managing Patients with Type 1 DM

Optimal management of patients with type 1 DM requires a comprehensive and detailed overview of many aspects of the disease process. These include the following: insulin therapy, nutritional guidance, education, prevention of diabetic ketoacidosis (DKA), addressing other comorbidities such as smoking, hyperlipidemia, and hypertension. These will be addressed in some detail in the following sections. It is important to emphasize that insulin therapy is essential for the survival of patients with type 1 DM since this is an insulin-deficient state. That is, insulin therapy should never be interrupted and should be offered in different formulation that ensures the presence of insulin in the body at all times.

Management of Type 1 Diabetes: Insulin Considerations

The Diabetes Control and Complications Trial (DCCT) which was one of the biggest diabetes trials conducted on thousands of type 1 diabetics, demonstrated that intensive therapy with multiple daily injections or continuous subcutaneous insulin infusion (CSII) reduced A1C and was associated with improved long-term outcomes [4]. Lower A1C with intensive control (HbA1c of 7%) led to 50% reductions in microvascular complications

over 6 years of treatment. At the time of its publication, the DCCT study did not show any macrovascular benefit nor any impact on mortality. Importantly, however, when patients enrolled in the DCCT study were followed for longer periods of time (EDIC study), the initial microvascular disease benefit persisted while there was also a demonstration of subsequent macrovascular benefit [5]. The UKPDS study (performed on thousands of type 2 diabetic patients) along with many other large trials also showed a consistent reduction in microvascular complications with implementation of intensive control; but failed to show a significant reduction in macrovascular complications or mortality (Table 1) [6]. Other studies that examined the impact of intensive insulin therapy in patients with type 1 diabetes showed a reduction in microvascular disease complications. The latter studies include the ACCORD, ADVANCE, and the VADT. It is of interest to note that none of the latter studies demonstrated reductions in macrovascular disease. As one can predict, there was an increase in the incidence of hypoglycemia among patients receiving more intensive insulin therapy.

Of note, the DCCT study was carried with human insulins (NPH and Regular) which result in greater incidence of hypoglycemia due to their pharmacokinetics [4]. Over the last 25 years, rapid-acting and long-acting insulin analogs have been developed that have distinct pharmacokinetics compared with recombinant human insulin: basal insulin analogs have longer duration of action with flatter, more constant plasma concentrations than NPH insulin; rapid-acting analogs (RAA) have a quicker onset and peak and shorter duration of action than regular human insulin.

For individuals with type 1 diabetes, intensive flexible insulin therapy education programs using the carbohydrate counting meal planning approach results in improved glycemic control [7]. Patients should be trained to match prandial insulin doses to carbohydrate intake, premeal blood glucose, and anticipated physical activity. Typical multidose regimens for patients with type 1 diabetes combine premeal use of shorter-acting insulins with a longer acting formulation, usually at night.

Table 3   Insulin pharmacokinetics

Insulin	Name	Onset of action	Peak	Duration
Rapid acting analogs	Lispro Glulisine Aspart	5–15 min	1 h	3–4 h
Short acting	Human regular	30 min	2–4 h	6–8 h
Intermediate acting	Human NPH	1–3 h	4–8 h	12–16 h
Concentrated human regular insulin	U-500 human regular insulin	1–3 h	4–8 h	Up to 24 h
Basal analogs	Glargine Detemir Degludec	2 h 2 h 1 h	No distinct peak No distinct peak No peak	20–24 h 12–24 h 42 h
Premixed insulin products	NPH/regular 70/30 NPH/Lispro 75/25 NPH/Aspart 70/30	Kinetics reflect individual components		

The pharmacokinetics of different types of insulin preparations are shown in Table 3 [8].

The rational for having a long-acting insulin is to ensure that insulin is available throughout the day and night. This can be achieved by using a single dose of glargine insulin, for example, or two doses of NPH insulin. Long-acting basal dose is titrated to regulate overnight, fasting glucose. Postprandial glucose excursions are best controlled by a well-timed injection of prandial insulin. The optimal time to administer prandial insulin varies, based on the pharmacokinetics of the formulation (regular, RAA, inhaled). Recommendations for prandial insulin dose administration should therefore be individualized. Typically, RAA should be injected up to 10 min before meals, while regular insulin should be administered 30 min prior to meals to optimize post prandial glycemic control. In general, patients with type 1 diabetes require 50% of their daily insulin as basal and 50% as prandial. Total daily insulin requirements can be estimated based on weight, with typical doses ranging from 0.4 to 1.0 units/kg/day. Higher amounts are required during puberty, pregnancy, and medical illness [7].

An example of a typical type 1 diabetes regimen is the following:

Lantus (glargine) 10 units at bedtime and Humalog (lispro) before meals according to a 1:15 g carb ratio. If 45 g of carbs are consumed with a meal, then 3 units of Humalog must be administered prior to the meal, in addition to a correction factor (or sensitivity factor). For example, one unit must be added for every 50 mg/dl above 150. So, if the premeal blood sugar is 162 mg/dl, the patient should administer $3 + 1 = 4$ units of Humalog prior to that meal. The correction factor (also commonly known as sliding scale) can be modified based on insulin sensitivity, individualized glucose goals, and hypoglycemia risk.

Insulin Delivery Systems

Most patients with diabetes use insulin in the form of vials or pens. Inhaled insulin is also available. Certain insulins, however, are available in strictly vial or pen forms. When choosing the best delivery method, factors such as patient preference and cost should be taken into consideration. The typical syringe sizes used to draw insulin from the vials are 1 ml which allows up to 100 units, 0.5 ml (50 units), and 0.3 ml (30 units) of U-100 insulin at a concentration of 100 unit/ml. U-500 insulin vials and pens are also available at a concentration of 500 units per ml. Syringes are typically used once. In patients with dexterity issues or vision impairment, insulin pens should be considered for the administration of accurate doses. Pens are available with prefilled cartridges or reusable insulin pens with replaceable cartridges. Pens also vary with respect to dosing increment which can range from half-unit doses to 2-unit dose increments. Needles thickness and length should also be taken into consideration with higher gauge indicating thinner needles (22–33) which typically cause less pain. Length varies from 4 mm to 12.7 mm with shorter needles decreasing the risk of intramuscular injections.

Insulin pumps or automated insulin delivery are also available and should be reserved for use for competent patients with good self-management capabilities. These have integrated dose calculators which aid in decision-making with regards to titrating insulin doses. Another available delivery system is a patch-like disposable device which is changed on a daily basis and provides a continuous infusion of rapid acting as basal insulin and, at the same time, allows bolus increments for meals by simply pressing a button [9].

Insulin Injection Technique

While administering insulin, care must be taken to inject into subcutaneous tissue, not intramuscularly. The recommended sites for insulin injection include the abdomen, thigh, buttock, and upper arm.

Lipohypertrophy, which is an accumulation of subcutaneous fat in response to the adipogenic actions of insulin, can occur at a site of multiple injections. Therefore, it is necessary to remind patients to rotate injection sites to avoid this complication which can result in erratic insulin absorption. On exam, lipohypertrophy appears as soft, smooth raised areas which can potentially result in unexplained hypoglycemic episodes.

Patients and/or caregivers should receive education about proper injection site rotation. Finally, health-care providers must also routinely examine the injection sites and evaluate injection techniques as part of a comprehensive diabetes evaluation.

Diabetes Education and Self-Management

This is certainly one of the cornerstones of the management of diabetes. Patients with diabetes 1 or type 2 require education on making the proper food choices and identifying carbohydrate-containing foods. It is crucial to have an initial nutrition visit and regular nutrition follow-up to learn how to read food labels and assess carbohydrate content especially when insulin is required for blood glucose control, as inappropriate administration may result in hypoglycemia. In addition, patients need to be educated on self-monitoring of blood glucose. Instruction of patients in self-titration of insulin doses based on self-monitoring of blood glucose improves glycemic control in patients with type 2 diabetes initiating insulin. In patients with type 1 or 2 diabetes on multiple daily injections, home blood glucose levels should be checked prior to meals and snacks and at bedtime, prior to exercise, when hypoglycemia is suspected, after hypoglycemia treatment and prior to driving, in patients on multiple daily injections or subcutaneous insulin pump.

Another important aspect of self-monitoring of type 1 diabetes is ketone testing. Ketone testing is also important in the management of pregnant patients with diabetes since they are at higher risk to develop ketonemia and diabetic ketoacidosis. Patients should use these strips during illness, when the blood glucose is persistently >300 mg/dl, or when symptoms of nausea, vomiting, or abdominal pain are present. Their presence may indicate DKA and which can in some mild cases be managed at home with increased water intake, administration of insulin every 4 h, and monitoring of symptoms. Medical attention should be sought when symptoms do not improve. Of note, widely available urine home ketone testing strips do not detect beta-hydroxybutyrate, which is the predominant ketone, and may miss cases of DKA. Home blood beta-hydroxybutyrate strips are also available [10].

Glucose Monitoring Devices/Diabetes Technology

Technological advances over the past 25 years had a major impact on diabetes management. The advances introduced newer methods to monitor glucose and others to synchronize insulin administration as illustrated in Fig. 1. Glucose meters

Fig. 1 Historical advancement of glucose monitoring and insulin delivery

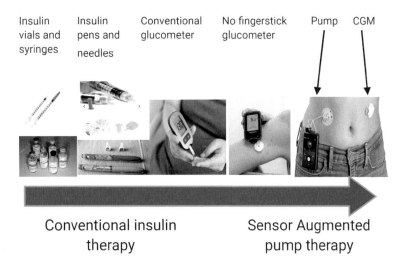

Insulin vials and syringes

Insulin pens and needles

Conventional glucometer

No fingerstick glucometer

Pump   CGM

Conventional insulin therapy

Sensor Augmented pump therapy

Next: Artificial Pancreas?

that meet the FDA requirements for meter accuracy provide the most accurate data for diabetes management. These meters utilize an enzymatic reaction linked to an electrochemical reaction, either glucose oxidase or glucose dehydrogenase. The ones based on glucose oxidase can be falsely low in the setting of high oxygen tension and falsely high in the setting of hypoxia. If there is a discordance between the meter reading and clinical reality, then the reading must be retested in a lab. The FDA standards expects glucose meters for home use to have a 95% accuracy within 15% for all blood glucose in the usable range (numeric readings other than low, high, or error) and a 99% accuracy within 20%. According to the international Organization for Standardization (ISO) which is the reference organization in Europe, readings should be 95% within 15% for blood glucose of ≥ 100 mg/dl or 95% within 15 mg/dl for blood glucose of <100 mg/dl. The Diabetes Technology Society Blood Glucose Monitoring System Surveillance Program provides information on the performance of devices used for self-monitoring of blood glucose.

The meter supplies include strips and lancets. Patients should wash their hands before every blood glucose check. The lancet is then used to prick at the side of the fingertips and a drop of blood should be placed on a strip which is then inserted in the glucose monitor. In few seconds, a glucose reading should appear on the meter. A liquid control solution may be used to check for the glucometer's accuracy. Patients should be advised to purchase meters from pharmacies and avoid purchasing strips or supplies not authorized for sale in the USA. Patients should be advised against purchasing or reselling second-hand test strips, or using expired strips as these may give incorrect results [9]. In addition, strips must be stored in their sealed containers, away from direct light or humidity, and at room temperature.

Diabetes technology involves the devices, software, and hardware used to manage diabetes. It includes delivery systems such as insulin pumps, pens, and syringes as well as continuous glucose monitors (CGM) devices and glucose meters. Newer forms of diabetes technology include hybrid devices that both deliver insulin and monitor glucose levels and software that provides diabetes self-management support. Patients' interest in the use of diabetes technology in the primary care setting has greatly increased. The use of this technology should be individualized based on a patient's needs, desires, skill level, cost, and availability of devices.

There are two types of CGMs: real-time CGMs (for example, Dexcom G6 and Medtronic Guardian Sensor) measure glucose continuously and provide the user-automated alarms and alerts at specific glucose levels, for example, when high or low;

while intermittently scanned CGMs (such as the freestyle libre device) only display glucose when swiped by a reader or a smart phone. Real-time and intermittently scanned CGM in conjunction with insulin therapy are useful tools to lower A1C and/or reduce hypoglycemia in adults with type 2 diabetes who are not meeting glycemic targets. The use of real-time CGM in adults with type 1 diabetes on either subcutaneous pump therapy or multiple daily injections is supported by data showing reduction in both hypoglycemia and A1C [9].

Insulin pump therapy should be considered in all adults and children with type 1 diabetes as long as they are able to manage the pump safely. It may also be considered in certain type 2 diabetic patients. Previous trials have demonstrated modest HbA1c lowering benefits when compared to multiple daily injection regimens in addition to reducing severe hypoglycemia episodes. In addition, in the last few years, the advent of sensor-augmented pump therapy has shown a significant reduction in hypoglycemia. Their use also may be considered to improve glycemic control. These systems increase and decrease insulin delivery based on sensor-derived glucose levels. They also have the ability to suspend insulin delivery if the blood glucose is low or predicted to become low in the next 30 min [9]. These systems, which fall under the artificial pancreas technology, are considered hybrid closed loop systems where basal insulin delivery is automated based on sensor glucose readings. However, the user would still need to manually input carbohydrates for meal boluses. The future of this technology might be a fully automated closed loop system with insulin only or with insulin and glucagon, which does not require any programming by the user.

Sick Day Management of Insulin

Improved education regarding sick day management is paramount, which includes the following:

1. Early contact with the health care provider.
2. Emphasizing the importance of continuing insulin therapy during an illness and the

reasons not to discontinue without contacting the health-care team.
3. Periodic and frequent checking of blood glucose and review of goals and the use of supplemental short- or rapid-acting insulin.
4. Having medications and supplies at home to treat and monitor fever.
5. Increase intake of fluids and promoting ingestion of an easily digestible liquid diet containing carbohydrates and salt when nauseated.
6. Education of family members to help with following up on temperature, blood glucose, and urine/blood ketone testing; insulin administration; oral intake; and weight monitoring.

The use of home ketone testing along with glucose monitoring may allow early recognition of impending ketoacidosis, which may help to guide insulin therapy at home and, possibly, may prevent hospitalization for DKA.

Dawn Phenomenon

The dawn phenomenon is marked early morning elevation in blood glucose levels which results from a surge in counterregulatory hormone concentrations (growth hormone, cortisol, and catecholamines) in the absence of nocturnal hypoglycemia [8]. Delaying nighttime basal insulin might help with these early morning rises, however, continuous sensor-augmented pump therapy might offer a particular benefit since the nighttime/early am insulin rates can be adjusted to control the hyperglycemia.

Somogyi Phenomenon

The Somogyi phenomenon is post hypoglycemia (resulting from insulin therapy) hyperglycemia due to a surge in counterregulatory hormones, rather than overtreatment of hypoglycemia with excess carbohydrates [8]. Glucose sensor trends can provide insight into this phenomenon. Avoidance of hypoglycemia is important.

Hypoglycemia

Hypoglycemia is typically precipitated in patients on secretagogues and patients on insulin therapy. According to the American Diabetes Association (ADA) , the definition of hypoglycemia in the diabetic patient is a glucose level of less than 70 mg/dl, which is considered a level 1. A level 2 hypoglycemia is <54 mg/dl. Level 3 is a severe event characterized by altered mental and/or physical status requiring assistance for treatment of hypoglycemia. Patients should be assessed at every visit for symptomatic and asymptomatic hypoglycemia including assessment of frequency of occurrence. Hypoglycemia unawareness must always be taken into consideration. Patient who develop this condition should be advised to raise their glycemic targets in order to reverse hypoglycemia unawareness. Glucose (15–20 g) in the form of chewable tablets is the preferred treatment for the conscious individual with blood glucose <70 mg/dL [3.9 mmol/L]), although any form of carbohydrate that contains glucose may be used (4 oz. of orange juice). Fifteen minutes after treatment, if blood glucose shows continued hypoglycemia, the treatment should be repeated until blood glucose is normalized. Glucagon, in an injectable form, should also be prescribed for all individuals at increased risk of level 2 hypoglycemia, so it is available should it be needed. Caregivers, school personnel, or family members of these individuals should know where it is and when and how to administer it. Recently, the FDA has approved intranasal glucagon (Baqsimi) which has facilitated the administration of this medication.

Pregnancy Planning

The majority of cases of diabetes in pregnancy are caused by gestational diabetes which typically develops during the third trimester of pregnancy. The remaining cases are attributed to preexisting diabetes type 1 or 2. Preconception counseling of women with diabetes in the reproductive age group should include the employment of effective contraceptive methods until the woman is ready to become pregnant. Tight control if safely possible with a goal HbA1c of <6.5% should be attempted to reduce the risk of congenital anomalies, preeclampsia, macrosomia, and other complications [11].

DM Management During Pregnancy

In early pregnancy, there is increased glucose uptake by the placenta which is not insulin dependent; hence, fasting blood glucose readings are lower in women with normal glucose homeostasis. However, placental hormones are diabetogenic and this results is mild post prandial hyperglycemia. Many women with type 1 diabetes will have a decrease in their insulin requirements early in the pregnancy; which eventually reverses as the pregnancy progresses by about 16 weeks and insulin requirements may reach 2–3 times the pre-pregnancy requirements.

Fasting and postprandial blood sugars must be monitored during pregnancy in preexisting diabetes 1 or 2 in pregnancy and in gestational diabetes. Since HbA1c in pregnant women is slightly lower than in that of a non-pregnant women due to increase RBC turnover, the HbA1c goal is <6% if it can be achieved safely without hypoglycemia but may be relaxed to <7%. Fasting sugars should be <95 mg/dl and post-prandial sugars must be <140 mg/dl, or < 120 mg/dl for 1 h and 2 h respectively [12].

Most women who develop gestational diabetes can be managed by lifestyle modifications. If lifestyle measures are not sufficient, insulin is the first-line therapy. Metformin and glyburide may be used as second-line agents only as both cross the placenta to the fetus. In general, all oral medications lack long term safety data in pregnancy. Women who develop gestational diabetes should be tested at 4–12 weeks post-partum for the development of type 2 diabetes with an oral glucose tolerance test.

In the case of preexisting diabetes 1 or 2, insulin is again, the first-line therapy. Insulin requirements fluctuate during pregnancy but during the third trimester there is an increase in post prandial insulin requirements >50% when compared to basal insulin requirements. In the immediate postpartum state, insulin requirements decrease by about 50% and caution must be implemented to avoid hypoglycemia. Regular insulin, Aspart, Lispro, NPH, and Detemir are all pregnancy category B and may be safely used in pregnancy.

During pregnancy, women should be counseled about the risk of the development/progression of diabetic retinopathy. Close monitoring with a dilated eye exam should take place prior to pregnancy and every trimester if needed.

Diabetes during pregnancy often requires a multidisciplinary approach involving an endocrinologist, maternal-fetal medicine specialist, registered dietitian nutritionist, and diabetes educator, when available.

Dietary Considerations

All patients with type 1 or type 2 diabetes must be referred to medical nutrition therapy (MNT). Nutrition education should emphasize the consumption of nonstarchy vegetables, minimizing added sugars and refined grains, and choosing whole foods over processed foods to the extent possible. In addition, reducing overall carbohydrate intake for individuals with diabetes has shown evidence for improving glycemia. MNT visits should occur frequently, about 3–6 visits in the first 6 months after diagnosis and annually after that. People with prediabetes and obesity should be referred to intensive lifestyle intervention programs for weight loss. A weight loss of 7–10% is needed to prevent the progression to type 2 diabetes [13].

Exercise Considerations

Moderate exercise is recommended for about 30 min per day most days of the week for all patients with diabetes and is a cornerstone of intensive lifestyle modifications. Patients on insulin therapy must check blood sugar prior to onset of physical activity and snack if needed to avoid the development of hypoglycemia.

Other Routine Care for Patients with Type 1 Diabetes

Hypertension Management: Patients with hypertension and diabetes should monitor their blood pressure at home and their blood pressure should be measured at every clinic visit. For patients with type 1 diabetes who have a high cardiovascular risk (existing atherosclerotic cardiovascular disease or 10-year atherosclerotic cardiovascular disease risk >15%), a blood pressure target of <130/80 mmHg may be appropriate, if it can be safely achieved. If the cardiovascular risk is <15% a blood pressure goal of <140/90 is acceptable [14].

Dyslipidemia: Lipid profile should be measured at diagnosis of diabetes and every 5 years if younger than age of 40 and more frequently above the age of 40. Patients with type 1 or 2 diabetes of all ages who have an atherosclerotic cardiovascular disease risk of more than 20%, should be started on high intensity statin. Any patient between 40 and 75 years of age with diabetes should be at least on a moderate intensity statin.

Diabetic Retinopathy: Patients with type 1 diabetes should start getting comprehensive eye exams 5 years after diabetes diagnosis.

Diabetic Nephropathy: Microalbuminuria screening should also be initiated 5 years after the diagnosis of type 1 diabetes.

Diabetic Neuropathy: Screening with monofilament testing should be initiated 5 years after type 1 diagnosis.

Vaccines: All adults with diabetes must receive the Tdap, pneumococcal vaccine, zoster vaccine, hepB vaccine, and influenza.

Foot Care: All patients with diabetes should be instructed to inspect feet regularly and seek podiatry care if needed.

Smoking Cessation: Smoking cessation must be addressed at least annually in all patients with diabetes.

Transplantation Consideration: Patients with type 1 diabetes who have received kidney transplantation or who are candidates for one, are also considered candidates for pancreatic transplantation in centers dedicated to performing these procedures.

Management of Type 2 Diabetes Mellitus

Type 2 DM was previously called noninsulin-dependent or adult onset diabetes. Patients with this disease account for over 90% of all patients diagnosed with diabetes. Classically, the disease initially begins as an insulin resistance state with higher levels of insulin secretion and at times a post-prandial reactive hypoglycemia. Over time, however, relative insulin deficiency leads to hyperglycemia. Patients with type 2 DM are often obese, have prior evidence for glucose intolerance. Women often have a prior history of gestational diabetes. Patients at higher risk for this disease include those who are African Americans, Hispanic/Latinos, Native American, and some who are Asian American. Although the disease is traditionally seen in older adults, it is being more recognized in children and adolescents as well as young men and women. Although infrequent, patients with type 2 DM can present with diabetic keto acidosis (DKA). Type 2 DM is a progressive disease that is initially characterized by being primarily an insulin-resistant state whereby glucose levels are normal while insulin levels are increased to maintain euglycemia. Over time, however, evidence for β cell function gradual failure emerges while the state of insulin resistance persists. The latter combination results in elevation in glucose levels initially post-prandial and subsequently in the fasting state. At the time of presentations for medical care, most patients with type 2 DM have already have evidence for microvascular complications of diabetes. As discussed earlier, a unique form of diabetes is what is described as maturity onset diabetes of the young (MODY). This is an auto-somal dominant disease associated with β cell dysfunction leading initially to mild hypergly-cemia often reaching the diagnostic criteria for diabetes and is usually diagnosed during ado-lescence or early adulthood.

Clinical Features in Patients with Type 2 Diabetes Mellitus

Risk factors for type 2 diabetes include the following: Age $\geq$ 45, Positive family history in a first degree relative, hypertension, dyslipidemia, sedentary lifestyle, history of gestational diabetes, overweight (BMI $\geq$ 25 kg/m^2), high risk ethnic group, prediabetes, polycystic ovarian syndrome.

Physical Exam findings include skin dryness, acanthosis nigericans (Fig. 2), central fat distribution, retinal hemorrhage or exudates, muscle atrophy, decreased sensation, loss of proprioception, foot ulcers.

In young patients who do not fit the typical findings, MODY should be considered, while in older patients who also do not fit these typical findings, LADA should be considered.

There are several pathophysiologic mechanisms that contribute to the development of hyperglycemia in patients with type 2 DM. These include at least the following mechanism;

1. Insulin resistance.
2. Impaired insulin secretion.
3. Decreased incretin effect.

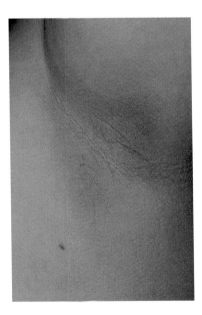

Fig. 2 Acanthosis nigricans, which is dark discoloration and velvety texture of the skin present at skin folds such as neck and underarms

4. Increased hepatic glucose production, decreased skeletal uptake, and questionable increase in its renal reabsorption.

Management of patients with type 2 DM involves a comprehensive approach that is aimed at addressing the basic pathophysiologic mechanisms for the disease itself as well as its known sequalae, such as the microvascular and macrovascular complications. While controlling glycemia is extremely important, it is by no means sufficient. Thus the management should address other aspects of the patients such as ensuring normal blood pressure, lipid levels, smoking cessation as well proper dietary intake and adequate appropriate exercise activity.

Pharmacologic Therapy of Type 2 Diabetes Mellitus

There are several classes of drugs used in the pharmacologic therapy of patients with type 2 DM. These drugs represent attempts to address specific pathophysiologic mechanisms involved in patients with type 2 DM. These are listed below:

1. Insulin sensitizers such as thiozolidinediones and metformin.
2. Insulin secretagouges such as sulfonylureas and glinides.
3. GLP-1 receptor agonists and DPP-4 inhibitors that decrease appetite and decrease GI motility, decrease glucagon and stimulate insulin secretion.
4. SGLT-2 inhibitors which increases glucosuria.
5. Insulin therapy.
6. Alpha glucosidase inhibitors which decrease glucose absorption.

There are important major concepts which should guide the pharmacologic management of type 2 diabetes. These include the following:

1. Metformin should always be a first-line therapy and should be continued unless its use becomes contraindicated.

2. Other agents can be added to metformin, including insulin.
3. Stepwise addition of medications should be performed until HbA1c is at goal.
4. Avoid combining medications which have a similar mechanism of action (such as DPP-IV inhibitors and GLP-1 RA).
5. It is recommended to start insulin therapy in the presence of symptomatic hyperglycemia BG > 300 mg/dl, if HbA1c is >10%, or there is ongoing catabolism and weight loss.
6. In the presence of risk factors such as heart disease, kidney disease, or heart failure, an SGLT2 inhibitor or a GLP1-RA with demonstrated cardiac or renal benefit are recommended for use regardless of HbA1c.
7. Careful considerations need to be made for patients with ESRD (end stage renal disease) or liver cirrhosis since very few of these drugs have been studied for safety. Insulin (with particular attention to pharmacokinetics) is likely to be the safest option in these high risk patients.
8. Careful consideration should be made to cost, side effect profile of medications, hypoglycemia risk, impact on weight, and patient preference.
9. Reassessment of therapy should be made every 3–6 months until HbA1c is at goal.

Specific Pharmacologic Therapy for Type 2 DM

- **Metformin**: This medication is considered first-line therapy in patients with type 2 diabetes. It works by decreasing hepatic glucose production and improves insulin sensitivity by increasing peripheral glucose uptake. It has a favorable metabolic profile, promotes modest weight loss, and can lower the HbA1c by about 1.5%. It is safe, effective and inexpensive and may reduce risk of cardiovascular events and death [7]. Importantly, it does not typically cause hypoglycemia. It is renally cleared and in the event of renal failure, it can be associated with lactic acidosis which is a rare occurrence. Hence, the FDA revised the label for use in patients with moderate kidney dysfunction as long as eGFR is >45 ml/min/1.73 m^2 and advised use with caution in patients with eGFR of 30–45 ml/min/1.73 m^2. Metformin is contraindicated in the setting of acute decompensated heart failure and liver cirrhosis. Principle side effects of metformin include bloating, abdominal discomfort and diarrhea that can be mitigated by gradual dose up titration. Extended release preparations have less gastrointestinal side effects. Metformin should be held prior to IV contrast administration given risk of kidney injury. In addition, long term use (>5 years) has been associated with vitamin B 12 deficiency, hence the need for periodic monitoring of vitamin B12 levels.

- **Thiazolidinediones**: The Thiazolidinediones increase insulin sensitivity by acting on adipose tissue and muscle to increase glucose utilization. To a lesser degree, they decrease glucose production by the liver. These agents are used as second line, or even more commonly, third-line therapy. The main side effects include fluid retention and peripheral edema and therefore they are contraindicated for use in patients with a history of congestive heart failure. They are also contraindicated for use in patients with active liver disease. There is also substantial evidence that they decrease bone density and increase the risk of fractures especially in women; therefore their use should be avoided in older individuals with risk for fractures. Additionally, there have been conflicting reports about use of pioglitazone and an increased risk of bladder cancer; therefore, they should be avoided in patients with a history of active bladder cancer. The main 2 medications in this class are pioglitazone and rosiglitazone. Rosiglitazone is no longer widely available and much more rarely used given some controversial concern for a potential increased risk of cardiovascular events. Pioglitazone may still offer an advantage in certain clinical settings; for example, in the context of high risk for hypoglycemia, severe insulin resistance, coexisting nonalcoholic steatohepatitis (NASH), or recent stroke. In fact, clinical trials have demonstrated a particular benefit in insulin resistant patients with a history of stroke and another benefit in improving fibrosis and inflammation in patients with non-alcoholic steatohepatitis (NASH) [15].

- **Sulfonylureas**: This class of medications falls under the secretagogue class, which act by stimulating insulin release from the pancreas. They have been available since the 1950s. They are highly effective in lowering blood glucose and can lower HbA1c by up to 1–2%. They are typically dosed once or twice a day. They have a neutral cardiovascular profile; however, their main side effect is that they can precipitate hypoglycemia and their use is cautioned especially in the elderly population. Another side effect is weight gain which results from increased endogenous insulin production. Glyburide is falling out of favor given increased risk of hypoglycemia; however, glipizide and glimepiride continue to be used especially given their low cost. They should be used in caution in patients with kidney disease given the augmented hypoglycemia effect. With the development of newer glucose lowering therapies that have a safer side effect profile, these medications are starting to fall out of favor overall.

- **Glinides**: This is another class of secretagogues which has a shorter half-life than sulfonylureas. It provides a faster and briefer stimulus to insulin secretion in comparison to sulfonylureas. It is typically taken with each meal and provides better postprandial control and has very little effect on fasting sugar control. The main available medications are repaglinide and nateglinide. Their main disadvantages are the need for multiple daily doses and their comparably higher cost.

- **DPP-IV inhibitors**: This class of medications are considered incretin-related therapies along with GLP-1 receptor agonists. These drugs inhibit the DPP-IV enzyme which is involved in the degradation of glucagon-like peptide-1 which results in a twofold increase in GLP-1 and GIP levels. This subsequently results in a reduction of pancreatic hypersecretion of glucagon and augmentation of glucose-dependent insulin secretion. These drugs are generally well tolerated with low risk of hypoglycemia and are dosed once daily. HbA1c reduction is intermediate up to 0.7% [7]. They are weight neutral and are not commonly associated with GI side effects. They have a potential risk of causing acute pancreatitis and are contraindicated in the setting of a known history of pancreatitis. They also can potentially cause joint pains. Examples of these medications include linagliptin, sitgaliptin, alogliptin, and saxagliptin. All are renally cleared except linagliptin, therefore require renal adjustment according to GFR.

- **GLP-1 receptor agonists (GLP-RA)**: This is another form of incretin based therapy. Due to their effectiveness, these medications should be attempted in the obese type 2 diabetic patients especially those who are overweight prior to the initiation of insulin. Often, they are used as second line agents in addition to metformin. The main difference when compared to DPP-IV inhibitors is that they achieve pharmacologic levels of levels of GLP-1 as compared to near the physiologic concentrations of GLP-1 when DPP-IV inhibitors are used. Figure 3 shows the physiologic mechanisms of incretin-based therapies. GLP-RA are known to delay gastric motility. This class of medications are highly efficacious drugs in terms of HbA1c lowering (1%). They do not

result in hypoglycemia and have a significant weight loss benefit. Importantly, large randomized controlled trials have demonstrated an added benefit in terms of cardiovascular risk reduction in patients with known cardiovascular disease, with most of these medications (liraglutide, semaglutide, and dulaglutide) [16–18]; which makes them indicated for use in that setting. In addition, these drugs have also been found to potentially be beneficial in patients with CKD primarily by improving microalbuminuria [19]. These medications are safely used as long as the GFR > 30 ml/min/1.73 m^2. There has been some suggestion in the literature that liragulatide is safe in the setting of a GFR of $15 - 30$ ml/min/1.73 m^2, however, in general, they are not well studied in patients with ESRD and therefore use is not recommended. Commonly, these drugs are also very effective when added to basal insulin therapy to help with postprandial blood glucose spikes and to offset the weight gain resulting from the anabolic effect of insulin. Most formulations are administered via subcutaneous injection on a daily, twice daily, or weekly basis which creates a limitation for their use in patients with fear of injections. However, the once weekly formulation of these drugs (semaglutide, dulaglutide, exenatide) can perhaps offset this concern. The main side effects include nausea and vomiting; hence the recommendation for slow uptitration of dose such as

Fig. 3 Physiologic mechanisms behind incretin-based therapies

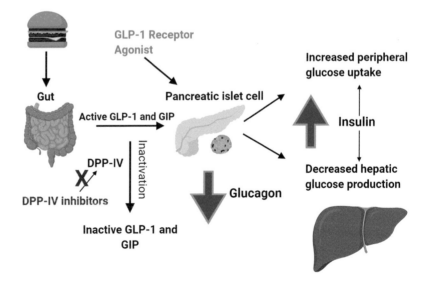

with liraglutide. More recently, an oral GLP-1RA formulation (semaglutide) has been FDA approved for use in type 2 diabetes. It is important to note that these drugs have an FDA black box warning for risk of thyroid C-cell tumors and are contraindicated in the setting of history of medullary thyroid carcinoma. In addition, they do carry a risk of acute pancreatitis. The cost of these medications though is known to be very high.

- **SGLT2 inhibitors**: Sodium glucose cotransporter type 2 is expressed in the proximal renal tubule and mediates reabsorption of approximately 90% of the filtered glucose load. SGLT2 inhibitors promote the renal excretion of glucose by promoting osmotic diuresis. The ability to lower blood glucose is limited by the filtered load of glucose and the osmotic diuresis that is caused by this therapy. Therefore, their efficacy in lowering HbA1c is limited. They are dosed once per day and their risk for precipitating hypoglycemia is extremely low. Due to osmotic diuresis, they can result in blood pressure lowering and potentially AKI due fluid losses. However, they have emerged as a promising therapy for patients with type 2 diabetes with coexisting cardiovascular or renal disease for reduction of CV events, decreased hospitalizations for heart failure, and delaying the progression of kidney disease based on multiple large randomized controlled trials [20–22]. The mechanism of that benefit is quite yet to be fully elucidated, but is thought to be related to their diuretic effect, reduction in hyperfiltration at the kidney level, and potentially being a source of cardiac fuel. The main side effects include risk of acute kidney injury (typically transient) requiring monitoring of kidney function. It is certainly prudent to take into consideration co-therapy with other diuretic therapies and adjustment of doses as needed to avoid volume depletion. Importantly, there is an increased risk of urinary tract infections and genital mycotic infections in females and in males. The FDA has received reports of fatal urosepsis and incidence of Fournier's gangrene. The cost of these medications is considerably high.

Other noninsulin therapies used for the treatment of type 2 diabetes include pramlintide and alpha glucosidase inhibitors which are not very commonly used. Pramlintide is an analogue of amylin that is cosecreted by the pancreatic beta cells in response to food intake. It delays gastric emptying and suppresses glucagon secretion and reduces food intake by centrally suppressing the appetite. It has been studied in both patients with type 1 and type 2 diabetes. However, it requires injections with each meal in the setting of type 1 diabetes and at least twice daily in type 2 diabetes. It cannot be mixed in a syringe with insulin. Pramlintide therapy requires careful patient education and monitoring to avoid severe hypoglycemia. Due to these reasons it has fallen out of favor. Acarbose, which is an alpha glucosidase inhibitor, interferes with digestion and absorption of dietary carbohydrate and mainly influences postprandial blood glucose readings. Their frequent dosing with meals and their significant side effect profile such as nausea, flatus, and diarrhea have significantly limited their use in the diabetic population [7].

Insulin in Type 2 Diabetes: As mentioned prior, it is acceptable to initiate insulin at any time in the course of the disease, particularly if the HbA1c is significantly elevated >10%, if patients are symptomatic, or if there are contraindications for use of oral or injectable therapies. Careful consideration for insulin pharmacokinetics must be observed.

Patients who fail to achieve goal HbA1c on maximal therapy with oral and injectable agents should be started on insulin. Medications with proven cardiovascular benefits such as GLP-RA and SGLT2 inhibitors and pioglitazone must be continued along with insulin regardless of HbA1c, unless use is contraindicated.

Once the need for insulin therapy is ascertained, basal insulin must be started first at a dose of 10 units per day or 0.1–0.2 IU/kg. The next step would be setting a fasting glucose target which is 80–130 mg/dl [23]. Patients can be given instructions to up titrate the dose; for example, increase dose by 2 units every 3 days until fasting goal is achieved without hypoglycemia. For any unexplained hypoglycemia, insulin dose must be reduced by 10–20%. If using NPH as basal insulin, the dose can be split with 2/3 of the dose to be given during the day and 1/3 to be given at bedtime.

Glargine insulin is usually administered at bedtime to provide fasting blood glucose control but can also be administered in the morning especially if patients tend to forget administering nighttime basal insulin. Degludec insulin can be administered any time of the day due to its peakless action. Long acting basal analogues such as U100 glargine and detemir have been demonstrated to reduce the risk of symptomatic and nocturnal hypoglycemia compared with NPH insulin; although these advantages are modest. U300 glargine (300 units/ml) or degludec may convey a lower hypoglycemia risk when compared with U100 glargine when used in combination with oral agents. If the HbA1c continues to be above target despite achieving target fasting glucose or once the basal dose is >0.5 IU/kg, then prandial insulin is the reasonable next step. However, if the patient is not on GLP-1 RA at this time, one can be added to basal insulin prior to adding prandial insulin. This combination can be very potent and provides less weight gain and hypoglycemia when compared with intensified insulin regimens. When adding prandial insulin, it should first be started with the largest meal. It

can be started at 4 units per day or 10% of basal dose and this dose can be increased by 1–2 units every 3 days. Consideration should be given to decreasing the basal insulin dose especially after adding prandial insulin with the evening meal. If the HbA1c continues to be above target then more injections can be added gradually up to 3 injections per day with meals, which is a full basal-bolus regimen i.e. basal insulin and prandial insulin before each meal. Prandial insulin may be administered immediately after a meal in the event a patient has unpredictable oral intake. One can also consider twice daily premixed insulin regimen (NPH/regular or NPH/aspart) starting off from the same total daily dose, especially in patients with compliance issues provided they have fixed meal routines. A basal-bolus regimen offers greater flexibility for patients who eat on an irregular basis. Once a full basal and prandial insulin has been started it would be logical to stop medications such as secretagogues but continue medications such as metformin or medications with proven cardiovascular or renal benefits (Table 4).

Table 4 Oral agents for the treatment of type 2 diabetes

Class	Medication	Dosage strength	Dosing frequency	Maximum dosage
Biguanides	Metformin	500, 850, 1000 mg (also available in extended release form)	QD or BID AC	2000 mg
Sulfonylureas (second generation)	Glimepiride Glipizide Glyburide	1 mg, 2 mg, 4 mg 5 mg, 10 mg 2.5 mg, 5 mg	QD or BID before meals	8 mg 40 mg (IR), 20 mg(XL)
Thiazolidinediones	Pioglitazone	30 mg, 45 mg	QD	45 mg
Meglitinides	Nateglinide Repaglinide	60 mg, 120 mg 0.5 mg, 1 mg, 2 mg	TID before meals	360 mg 16 mg
DPP-IV inhibitors	Alogliptin Saxagliptin Sitagliptin Linagliptin	25 mg 2.5, 5 mg 25, 50 mg, 100 mg 5 mg	QD QD QD QD	25 mg 5 mg 100 mg 5 mg
GLP1-RA	Exenatide Dulaglutide Semaglutide Liraglutide	2 mg 0.75 mg, 1.5 mg 0.5 mg, 1 mg 1.8 mg	Weekly Weekly Weekly QD	2 mg 1.5 mg 1 mg 1.8 mg
SGLT2 inhibitors	Ertugliflozin Dapagliflozin Canagliflozin Empagliflozin	5 mg, 15 mg 5 mg, 10 mg 100 mg, 300 mg 10 mg, 25 mg	QD QD QD QD	15 mg 10 mg 300 mg 25 mg
A-glucosidase inhibitors	Acarbose Miglitol	25 mg, 50 mg, 100 mg 25 mg, 50 mg, 100 mg	TID AC TID AC	300 mg 300 mg
Amylin mimetic	Pramlintide	120 ug pen	Weekly	120 ug
Bile acid sequestrant	Colesevelam	625 mg	QD or BID	3.75 g

Of note, the cost of insulin has been steadily rising over the last few decades at a high pace which poses a significant burden for patients and contributes to medication non-adherence. Consideration of cost is an important component of effective management. In these situations, human insulin (NPH and Regular insulin) may be the appropriate choice of therapy since they can be purchased at considerably lower prices.

Concentrated Insulin: U-500 regular insulin is 5 times more concentrated than U100. It has delayed onset and longer duration of action and acts more like NPH; it can be given as 2 or 3 injections per day. U-300 glargine and U-200 degludec and more recently U-200 lispro allow more units to be administered per volume. These are, for the most part, present in pen forms to decrease the chance of dosing errors.

Inhaled Insulin: This formulation of insulin is not commonly used. It is available in a limited dosing range for prandial use. Larger studies on inhaled insulin are needed. It is contraindicated for use in patients with chronic lung disease or patients who smoke.

Bariatric Surgery: Weight loss results in dramatic improvement in glycemic control and in some cases reversal of diabetes type 2. It may be indicated in the patient with type 2 diabetes who has a BMI >30 if glycemic control is poor. Above a BMI of 40, it is recommended regardless of control. The best results are seen with Roux-en-Y gastric bypass; however, it has the most side effects such as dumping syndrome, hypoglycemia, and vitamin deficiencies.

Glycemic Targets

The main test for assessing glycemic management is the HbA1c, it should be used in addition to self-monitoring of blood glucose (SMBG). HbA1c should be checked every 6 months in patients with adequate control and quarterly in patients not meeting glycemic targets. Point of care HbA1c testing is helpful in making timely adjustments. An HbA1c goal for many non-pregnant adults of <7% is appropriate. Achieving an HbA1c of <6.5% in the appropriate patient population (young, healthy, without comorbidities) is appropriate if it can be achieved safely. In pregnant patients, tight control <6.5% is required to decrease maternal and fetal morbidity. Less stringent goals <8%, might also be appropriate in patients with severe hypoglycemia, limited life expectancy, advanced microvascular or macrovascular complications, extensive comorbid conditions, or long-standing diabetes in whom the goal is difficult to achieve despite appropriate glucose monitoring, and effective doses of multiple glucose-lowering agents including insulin [24]. Fig. 4 depicts a framework for individualizing glucose targets based on multiple factors.

Step-Wise Introduction of Therapeutic Agents

While it is clear that metformin should be the first drug to be used in the initial management of type 2 diabetes, the sequence of additional drugs when metformin fails can vary from one patient to another. A summary of potential sequential use of drugs is illustrated in Fig. 5.

Other Routine Medical Care in Type 2 Diabetes Patients

Eye Exam: All patients must obtain a dilated eye exam at diabetes diagnosis and at least yearly depending on initial findings.

Smoking: All patients with diabetes must be counseled about smoking cessation to decrease the risk of atherosclerotic CVD.

Hypertension: Goal BP must be individualized based on comorbidities. ACE inhibitors are first line especially if there is microalbuminuria.

Dyslipidemia: All diabetic patients above the age of 40–75 must be on a moderate to high intensity statin.

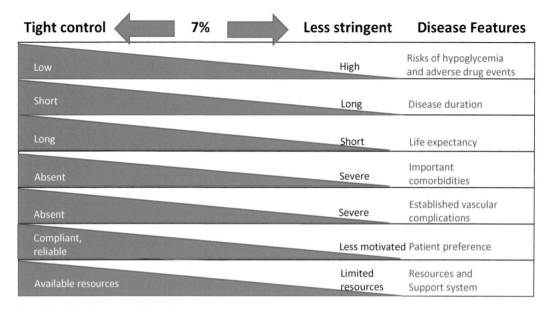

Fig. 4 Individualization of blood glucose targets

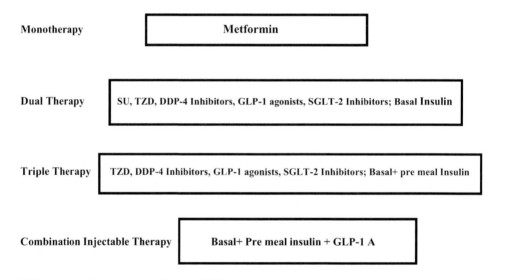

Fig. 5 Management of hyperglycemia in type 2 DM

Alcohol: Patients must be cautioned about risk of hypoglycemia with alcohol use especially if they are on insulin therapy.

Foot Care: Patients should be instructed to inspect and wash but not soak feet, daily; keep nails trimmed, and seek podiatric care if needed.

Vaccines: All adults with diabetes must receive the Tdap, pneumococcal vaccine, zoster vaccine, hepB vaccine, and influenza.

Complications of Diabetes Mellitus

Microvascular Complications

1-Diabetic Retinopathy: Diabetic retinopathy is the most frequent cause of new cases of blindness among adults aged 20–74 years in developed countries. It is a highly specific vascular complication of both type 1 and type 2 diabetes, with prevalence strongly related to both the duration of diabetes and the level of glycemic control. Factors that increase the risk of retinopathy include chronic hyperglycemia, nephropathy, hypertension, and dyslipidemia. Intensive diabetes management with the goal of achieving near-normoglycemia has been shown in large prospective randomized studies to prevent and/or delay the onset and progression of diabetic retinopathy. Blood pressure and lipid control are also important in slowing the progression [25]. Pregnancy is associated with a rapid progression of diabetic retinopathy. Women with preexisting type 1 or type 2 diabetes who are planning pregnancy or who are pregnant should be counseled on the risk of development and/or progression of diabetic retinopathy.

Diabetic Nephropathy: Diabetic kidney disease occurs in 20–40% of patients with diabetes. CKD can progress to end-stage renal disease (ESRD) requiring dialysis or kidney transplantation. The diagnosis is made based on the presence of albuminuria and/or reduced eGFR. Therefore, it is recommended to assess urinary albumin (e.g., spot urinary albumin to creatinine ratio) and eGFR in patients with type 1 diabetes with duration of 5 or more years, in all patients with type 2 diabetes and in all patients with comorbid hypertension. Optimizing glucose control is crucial to reduce the risk or slow the progression of chronic kidney disease [25]. The ADA has added new guidelines involving the use of SGLT2 inhibitors and GLP-1-Receptor Agonists. For patients with type 2 diabetes and chronic kidney disease, the use of an SGLT 2 inhibitor or glucagon-like peptide 1 receptor agonist shown to reduce risk of chronic kidney disease progression, cardiovascular events, or both; should be considered unless the risk outweighs the benefit [14]. BP control is also of paramount importance. In nonpregnant patients with diabetes and hypertension, either an ACE inhibitor or an ARB is recommended for use in those with modestly elevated urinary albumin–creatinine ratio (30–299 mg/g creatinine) and strongly recommended with a ratio of more than 300 mg/g creatinine and/or eGFR <60 ml/min/1.73 m^2. For patients with CKD,

dietary protein intake should be approximately 0.8 g/kg body weight per day. Periodic monitoring of serum creatinine and potassium must be performed. Patients should be referred for consideration of renal replacement therapy if GFR <30 ml/min/1.73 m^2, or if there is concern about another etiology for kidney disease, or for rapidly progressing disease [25].

Diabetic Neuropathy

Patients with type 1 diabetes for 5 or more years and all patients with type 2 diabetes should be assessed annually for the development of diabetic neuropathy. Patients should have an annual foot exam including a 10-g monofilament testing to identify feet at risk for ulceration and amputation. Patients with evidence of sensory loss or prior ulceration or amputation should have their feet inspected at every visit. Symptoms and signs of autonomic neuropathy should also be assessed in patients with microvascular complications. The treatment involves optimizing glucose control to prevent or delay the development of neuropathy in patients with type 1 diabetes and to slow the progression of neuropathy in patients with type 2 diabetes. The ADA recommends the use of duloxetine, pregabalin, and gabapentin as pharmacologic therapy for painful diabetic neuropathy. Both duloxetine and pregabalin are FDA approved for this indication. The use of specialized therapeutic footwear is recommended for high-risk patients with diabetes including those with severe neuropathy, foot deformities, or history of amputation [25].

Other Considerations

As mentioned previously, diabetes is considered an independent risk factor for the development of ASCVD (atherosclerotic cardiovascular disease). Coexisting conditions that are clear risk factors include hypertension, dyslipidemia, and smoking. Benefits are seen when multiple risk factors are addressed simultaneously. Heart failure is also another cause of morbidity and mortality from

CVD. In addition, heart failure hospitalizations are two fold higher in patients with diabetes compared to patients without diabetes. Recent data has shown that SGLT2 inhibitors improve the rates of heart failure hospitalizations in patients with type 2 diabetes [21]. Treatment for HTN should include drug classes to reduce cardiovascular events such as ACE inhibitors and ARBs particularly if they have concomitant albuminuria.

As far as lipid management, patients with diabetes aged 40–75 should be initiated on a moderate intensity statin in addition to lifestyle therapy. High-intensity statin should be initiated for patients with diabetes and concomitant ASCVD. PCSK9 inhibitors should be used in patients with ASCVD and diabetes whose LDL is>70 mg/dl on maximal statin and LDL lowering therapy. In addition, recent studies have shown that in patients with ASCVD or other cardiovascular risk factors on a statin with a controlled LDL but elevated Triglyceride levels 135–499, the addition of icosapent ethyl can be considered to reduce vascular risk [26]. Aspirin therapy is effective in secondary prevention in patients with diabetes and ASCVD. However, it may be considered in patients with diabetes as primary prevention after weighing the risks (mainly GI bleeding) versus the benefits.

Diabetic Emergencies

Diabetic ketoacidosis (DKA) and the hyperosmolar hyperglycemic state (HHS) are the two most serious acute metabolic complications of diabetes.

Most patients with DKA have type 1 diabetes and can develop this complication in the setting of a minor illness such as an upper respiratory tract infection and/or noncompliance with insulin intake. However, patients with type 2 diabetes are also at risk of developing DKA during the catabolic stress of acute illness such as trauma, surgery, or infections. DKA results in death 1–5% of patients. DKA is characterized by severe hyperglycemia, metabolic acidosis, and increased total body ketone concentration. The state of insulin deficiency results in free fatty acid oxidation and the formation of ketones, which results in

ketonemia, high anion gap ketoacidosis, and ketonuria. Typically symptoms are acute and patients present within few days with polyuria and polydipsia, along with a constellation of malaise, abdominal pain, nausea, and vomiting. Patients are profoundly dehydrated and can present with hemodynamic instability. In severe cases, patients have altered mental status and obtundation which is life threatening if not managed promptly.

HHS is characterized by severe hyperglycemia, hyperosmolality, and dehydration in the absence of significant ketoacidosis. HHS symptoms can develop over a period of days to weeks due to typically continued though insufficient insulin secretion. These metabolic derangements result from the combination of absolute or relative insulin deficiency and an increase in counterregulatory hormones (glucagon, catecholamines, cortisol, and growth hormone). Mortality attributed to HHS is considerably higher than that attributed to DKA, with recent mortality rates of 5–20% [27].

Diagnostic Testing for DKA and HHS

Typical physical exam findings include poor skin turgor, Kussmaul respirations (in DKA), tachycardia, and hypotension. Mental status can vary from full alertness to profound lethargy or coma, with the latter more frequent in HHS. Lab testing reveals hyperglycemia. In cases of DKA, blood glucose levels are >250 mg/dl and typically higher in HHS. Electrolyte abnormalities are also common and include hyponatremia and hyperkalemia. The admission serum sodium is usually low because of the osmotic flux of water from the intracellular to the extracellular space in the presence of hyperglycemia. An increased or even normal serum sodium concentration in the presence of hyperglycemia indicates a rather profound degree of free water loss. To assess the severity of sodium and water deficit, serum sodium may be corrected by adding 1.6 meq/L to the measured serum sodium for each 100 mg/dl of glucose above 100 mg/dl.

Hyperkalemia often occurs because of an extracellular shift of potassium caused by insulin deficiency along with acidemia since insulin promotes the intracellular flux of potassium. Patients with low normal or low serum potassium concentration on admission have severe total-body potassium deficiency and require careful cardiac monitoring and more vigorous potassium replacement. Acute kidney injury is common and is caused by dehydration and usually reverses with fluid resuscitation.

The key diagnostic feature between DKA and HHS is elevated total blood ketone concentration. Accumulation of ketoacids results in an increased anion gap metabolic acidosis. The anion gap is calculated by subtracting the sum of chloride and bicarbonate concentration from the sodium concentration: [Na - (Cl + HCO3)]. A normal anion gap is between 7 and 9 mEq/l, and an anion gap 10–12 mEq/l indicates the presence of increased anion gap metabolic acidosis.

Management: DKA management involves aggressive fluid resuscitation and the co-administration of intravenous insulin, which serves to metabolize the ketones and alleviate the acidosis.

Fluid and Insulin Therapy: Initial fluid therapy is directed toward expansion of the intravascular, interstitial, and intracellular volume and restoration of renal perfusion; all of which are reduced in hyperglycemic crises. In the absence of cardiac compromise, isotonic saline (0.9% NaCl) is infused at a rate of 15–20 ml kg body weight in the first hour or 1–1.5 l during the first hour. Subsequent choice for fluid replacement depends on hemodynamics, the state of hydration, serum electrolyte levels, and urinary output. Fluid replacement should correct estimated deficits within the first 24 h.

The mainstay in the treatment of DKA involves the administration of regular insulin via continuous intravenous infusion or by frequent subcutaneous injections. The administration of continuous intravenous infusion of regular insulin is the preferred route because of its short half-life and easy titration as compared to the delayed onset of action and prolonged half-life of subcutaneous regular insulin. Typically an initial bolus of 0.1 u/kg is given followed by an infusion rate of 0.1 u/kg/h. Once blood glucose levels drop below 200 mg/dl, the infusion rate can be reduced by around 50% and 5% dextrose should be added to replacement fluids to allow continued insulin administration until ketonemia is controlled while at the same time avoiding hypoglycemia.

Despite total-body potassium depletion, mild-to-moderate hyperkalemia is common in patients with hyperglycemic crises. Insulin therapy, correction of acidosis, and volume expansion decrease serum potassium concentration. To prevent hypokalemia, potassium replacement is initiated after serum levels fall below the upper level of normal for the particular laboratory (5.0–5.2 mEq/l). Generally, 20–30 mEq potassium in each liter of infusion fluid is sufficient to maintain a serum potassium concentration within the normal range.

Patients with DKA and HHS should be treated with continuous intravenous insulin until the hyperglycemic crisis resolves. Criteria for resolution of ketoacidosis include a blood glucose less than 200 mg/dl and two of the following criteria: a serum bicarbonate level 15 mEq/l, a venous pH 7.3, and a calculated anion gap less than 12 mEq/l. When this occurs, subcutaneous insulin therapy can be started. To prevent recurrence of hyperglycemia or ketoacidosis during the transition period to subcutaneous insulin, it is important to allow an overlap of 1–2 h between discontinuation of intravenous insulin and the administration of subcutaneous insulin. In insulin-naïve patients, a multidose insulin regimen should be started at a dose of 0.5–0.8 units per kg per day.

Inpatient Diabetes Care

It is well known that inpatient hypoglycemia and hyperglycemia are associated with adverse outcomes. Hence, it is rather important to control hyperglycemia prior to admission for elective procedures, have inpatient protocols for management, and prepare an outpatient discharge plan for management and transition of care. Consulting with a diabetes management team should be done when possible. All patients admitted who have preexisting diabetes must get an HbA1c test if it has not been performed in the last 3 months. The use of validated computerized protocols that allow set adjustments in insulin dosage is recommended for use in the hospital to help with blood glucose fluctuations. In addition, a set hypoglycemia protocol must be ordered on all patients with diabetes regardless of insulin use. Factors such as the quantity of oral intake, route of nutrition (enteral vs. parenteral nutrition), NPO status, kidney function, and hypoglycemia risk must be taken into consideration. In patients with new onset hyperglycemia, treatment with insulin must start at a threshold of 180 mg/dl. A target glucose of 140–180 mg/dl is the goal for the majority of patients (noncritically ill and critically ill patients) based on a large randomized controlled trial which was done on critically ill patients, the NICE-SUGAR trial which showed no advantage of tightly controlled glycemia (110–140 mg/dl) but rather increased hypoglycemia rates and perhaps slightly increased mortality. A goal of 110–140 mg/dl may be appropriate for certain patients such as post-surgical patients and patients post cardiac surgery, if this can be achieved safely. Less stringent targets >180 mg/dl are acceptable in terminally ill patients or patients with severe comorbidities.

For patients who are noncritically ill with poor PO intake or NPO, the preferred regimen is basal insulin with bolus correction scale. For patients with good oral intake, basal, prandial plus correction scale regimen is the preferred treatment. In patients who are well controlled on their outpatient insulin regimen, a reduction of 25–50% of their home insulin requirements must be done on admission. Using a sliding scale alone during hospital stay is discouraged. Premixed insulin regimens are generally avoided in the inpatient setting. In some cases with type 2 diabetes, patients' oral home regimens may be continued if oral intake is adequate. A reduction in home oral sulfonylureas dosage is advised if those are continued. Metformin may be continued if no procedures are planned including those involving IV contrast and if kidney function allows the safe continuation of this medication. If oral medications are held on admission, it is recommended to restart them 1–2 days prior to discharge. Dipeptidyl peptidase 4 inhibitors may be initiated in specific groups of hospitalized patients to manage hyperglycemia; however, some (saxagliptin) should be avoided in patient with heart failure.

In the critically ill setting, intravenous insulin use is the most effective method for achieving glycemic targets when used according to set protocols.

In type 1 diabetes patients, caution must be taken to ensure basal insulin is administered regularly at all times. Patients on insulin pump therapy may in certain situations continue using their pumps if they are deemed proficient in counting their carbohydrates and managing their glycemic fluctuations through using their pumps. These patients should be advised to reduce their basal rates by at least 20% during hospital admissions or NPO status.

In patients on parenteral nutrition (TPN), ideally the insulin requirements can be calculated by using an IV insulin infusion and then converting 80% of that amount and adding that to the TPN solution over 24 h. In patients on enteral nutrition, long-acting insulin daily or intermediate acting twice daily may be used along with sliding scale. In patients on cycled tube feeds, for example, overnight, the ideal insulin might be NPH which has an activity that lasts a similar duration of time.

Inpatients on Glucocorticoids (GC): Patients on GC therapy develop GC-induced hyperglycemia. They commonly have high insulin requirements particularly in the prandial form. The effect of hyperglycemia when GC are administered is related to their duration of action but typically their effect will last throughout the day when given in the morning. Long acting GC such as dexamethasone have an effect which will last >24 h and long acting insulin along with prandial insulin is often required for adequate control. Caution must be taken when GC therapy is abruptly discontinued (such as with chemotherapy protocols), as continued insulin therapy may result in profound hypoglycemia.

Inpatient new insulin start: In patients who develop hyperglycemia in-house or who are diagnosed with diabetes in the hospital, basal insulin may be started at a 0.2–0.3 u/kg and prandial insulin at 0.05–0.1 u/kg/meal for patients who have adequate PO intake.

Inpatient glucose monitoring: Blood glucose monitoring must be performed every 4–6 h via finger stick in patients who are NPO or on continuous tube feeding or parenteral feeding and before meals and at bedtime for patients who are not NPO. There is currently insufficient data for recommending CGM use in hospitalized patients.

Finally, discharge planning should begin on admission. Patients who are admitted to the hospital and who develop new onset hyperglycemia or diabetes should be given diabetes education while admitted and the proper transition of care to the outpatient provider must be performed prior to discharge [28].

References

1. https://www.diabetes.org/resources/statistics/statistics-about-diabetes. 20 Apr 2020.
2. https://www.cdc.gov/diabetes/data/statistics/statistics-report.html. 20 Apr 2020.
3. American Diabetes Association. Classification and diagnosis of diabetes: standards of medical care in diabetes-2020. Diabetes Care. 2020;43(Suppl 1):S14–31. https://doi.org/10.2337/dc20-S002.
4. The Diabetes Control and Complications Trial Research Group. The effect of intensive treatment of diabetes on the development and progression of long term complications in insulin dependent diabetes mellitus. N Engl J Med. 1993;329:977–86.
5. Epidemiology of Diabetes Interventions and Complications (EDIC). Design, implementation, and preliminary results of a long-term follow-up of the diabetes control and complications trial cohort. Diabetes Care. 1999;22(1):99–111.
6. UK Prospective Diabetes Study (UKPDS) Group. Intensive blood-glucose control with sulfonylureas or insulin compared with conventional treatment and risk of complications in patients with type 2 diabetes (UKPDS 33). Lancet. 1998;352:837–53.
7. Pharmacologic Approaches to Glycemic Treatments. Standards of medical care in diabetes-2020. Diabetes Care. 2020;43(Suppl 1):S98–S110.
8. Melmed S, Polonsky K, Larsen PR, Kronenberg H. Williams textbook of endocrinology. 12th ed. Philadelphia: Elsevier Saunders; 2011.
9. American Diabetes Association. Diabetes technology: standards of medical Care in Diabetes – 2020. Diabetes Care. 2020;43(Suppl 1):S77–88. https://doi.org/10.2337/dc20-S007.
10. American Diabetes Association. Tests of glycemia in diabetes. Diabetes Care. 2004;27(Suppl 1):s91–3. https://doi.org/10.2337/diacare.27.2007.S91.
11. American Diabetes Association. Standards of medical care in diabetes-2020 abridged for primary care providers. Clinical Diabetes. 2020;38(1):10–38.
12. American Diabetes Association. Management of Diabetes in pregnancy: standards of medical Care in Diabetes – 2019. Diabetes Care. 2019;42(Suppl 1):S165–72.
13. American Diabetes Association. Lifestyle management: standards of medical care in diabetes-2019. Diabetes Care. 2019;42(Suppl 1):S46–60.
14. American Diabetes Association. Cardiovascular disease and risk management: standards of medical care in diabetes-2019. Diabetes Care. 2019;42(Suppl 1):S103–23.
15. Kernan W, Viscoli CM, Furie K, Young L, Inzucchi S, Gorman M. Pioglitazone after ischemic stroke or transient ischemic attack. N Engl J Med. 2016;374:1321–31.
16. Marso S, Daniels G, Brown-Frandsen K, Kristensen P, Mann J, Nauck M, et al. Liraglutide and cardiovascular outcomes in type 2 diabetes. N Engl J Med. 2016;375:311–22.
17. Marso S, Bain S, Consoli A, Eliaschewitz F, Jodar E, Leiter L, et al. Semaglutide and cardiovascular outcomes in patients with type 2 diabetes. N Engl J Med. 2016;375:1834–44.
18. Gesrtein H, Colhoun H, Dagenais G, Diaz R, Lakshmanan M, Pais P, et al. Dulaglutide and cardiovascular outcomes in type 2 diabetes (REWIND): a double blind, randomized placebo-controlled trial. Lancet. 2019;394:121–30.
19. Mann J, Orsted D, Brown-Frandsen K, Steven M, Poulter N, Rasmussen S, et al. Liraglutide and renal outcomes in type 2 diabetes. N Engl J Med. 2017;377:839–48.
20. Zinman B, Wanner C, Lachin J, Fitchett D, Bluhmki E, Hantel S, et al. Empagliflozin, cardiovascular outcomes and mortality in type 2 diabetes. N Engl J Med. 2015;373:2117–28.
21. Mcmurray J, Solomon S, Inzucchi S, Kober L, Kosiborod M, Martinez F, et al. Dapgliflozin in patients with heart failure and reduced ejection fraction. N Engl J Med. 2019;381:1995–2008.
22. Perkovic V, Jardine M, Neal B, Bompoint S, Heerspink H, Charytan DM, et al. Canagliflozin and renal outcomes in type 2 diabetes and nephropathy. N Engl J Med. 2019;380:2295–306.
23. American Diabetes Association. Glycemic targets: standards of medical care in diabetes-2020. Diabetes Care. 2020;43(Suppl 1):S66–76.
24. Beigi I, et al. Individualizing glycemic targets in type 2 diabetes mellitus: implications of recent clinical trials. Ann Intern Med. 2011;154:554–9.
25. American Diabetes Association. Microvascular complications and foot care: standards of medical care in diabetes-2020. Diabetes Care. 2020;43(Suppl 1):S135–51.
26. Bhatt D, Steg G, Miller M, Brinton E, Jacobson T, Ketchum S. Cardiovascular risk reduction with Icosapent ethyl for hypertriglyceridemia. N Engl J Med. 2019;380:11–22.
27. Kitabchi A, Umpierrez G, Miles J, Fisher J. Hyperglycemic crisis in adult patients with diabetes. Diabetes Care. 2009;32(7):1335–43.
28. Diabetes Care in the Hospital: Standards of Medical Care in Diabetes 2020. Diabetes care 2020. Diabetes Care. 2020;43(Suppl 1):S193–202.

Melanie Menning

Contents

M. Menning (✉)
Department of Family Medicine, University of Nebraska
Medical Center, Omaha, NE, USA
e-mail: melanie.menning@unmc.edu

© Springer Nature Switzerland AG 2022
P. M. Paulman et al. (eds.), *Family Medicine*,
https://doi.org/10.1007/978-3-030-54441-6_142

Overview

The thyroid is a 15–20 g gland located in the anterior neck whose role is to primarily make thyroxine (T4), as well as small amounts of tri-iodothyronine (T3). The majority of T3 is formed through extra-thyroidal conversion of T4. Thyroid hormone production is controlled through negative feedback regulation through the release of thyroid-stimulating hormones (TSH) by the pituitary gland which is regulated by thyrotropin-releasing hormone (TRH) from the hypothalamus [1].

Thyroid hormone is key in the regulation of protein, carbohydrate, and lipid metabolism, thermogenesis, and the development of the brain, intestine, bone, skeletal muscle, and auditory system [2, 3].

Thyroid Lab Testing

The most sensitive measure of thyroid hormone levels is TSH with subsequent confirmation with free T4 and T3. The TSH assay, however, can be affected by heterophilic antibodies and biotin intake. Samples in which heterophilic antibodies are suspected should be repeated in another assay or with serial dilutions. Biotin intake should be stopped at least 2 days prior to testing as to not interfere with the assay [3].

Hypothyroidism

A deficiency in circulating thyroid hormone results in hypothyroidism. Patients with overt hypothyroidism will have an elevated TSH with low or undetectable levels of T3 and T4. Patients with subclinical hypothyroidism have elevated TSH levels with normal levels of T3 and T4. Within the USA the prevalence of overt hypothyroidism is 0.3–0.4% with subclinical hypothyroidism prevalence between 4.3% and 8.5% [1, 4]. Worldwide, the most common cause of hypothyroidism is iodine insufficiency, with patients presenting with a large goiter. Iodine deficiency; however, is very rare in the USA [2, 4]. Other etiologies of hypothyroidism include Hashimoto's thyroiditis, iatrogenic from thyroidectomy or radioactive iodine treatment, congenital, infiltrative disease, and in rare cases decreased TSH production from the pituitary gland [1, 2]. Hypothyroidism is eight to nine times more common in women than men with an increased prevalence with age. It is more prevalent in white individuals than black or Hispanic [2, 4]. TSH naturally increases with age; however, these increases are usually asymptomatic and subclinical [2].

Clinical Presentation

Patients with hypothyroidism have variable presentations with symptoms often not appearing until late in the disease process. Symptoms are often nonspecific and have a low sensitivity and positive predictive value for hypothyroidism. Patients may note fatigue, lethargy, poor concentration, impaired memory, weight gain, tinnitus, vertigo, polyneuropathy, tremor, obstructive sleep apnea, depressed or anxious mood, menstrual irregularities, impotence, decreased libido, constipation, cool and dry skin, hair loss, non-pitting edema (myxedema), enlarged tongue, husky, low-pitched voice with slowed speech, brittle and thickened nails, muscle cramps, and proximal muscle weakness [2, 4]. Hypothyroidism has been associated with decreased quality of life, increased sick leave, and increased mortality [4]. Prolonged hypothyroidism can result in severe complications including atrial fibrillation, coronary artery disease, and increased fracture risk due to osteoporosis. If hypothyroidism occurs during the fetal and neonatal stages, more profound effects can be seen including severe intellectual deficits, impaired fine motor skills, spasticity, impaired balance, and deafness [2].

Diagnostic Evaluation

Workup for hypothyroidism begins with TSH, T4 and T3 levels. Elevated TSH with depressed T4 and T3 levels is consistent with primary hypothyroidism or hypothyroidism originating from the thyroid gland itself. Low or inappropriately normal levels of TSH with depressed T4 and T3 levels are consistent with central hypothyroidism or hypothyroidism originating from the pituitary or hypothalamus gland with an otherwise normal thyroid gland [2].

Hypothyroidism is also associated with other lab abnormalities. Hypothyroidism has been associated with increased insulin resistance, but decreased insulin degradation resulting in a higher risk of hypoglycemia in diabetics. It additionally affects lipid metabolism resulting in increased low-density lipoprotein (LDL), high-density lipoprotein (HDL), and triglycerides. Liver enzymes and creatinine kinase may also be elevated. Patients may have a depressed GFR and hyponatremia. Anemia may be present in up to 30% of adults and 60% of kids. EKG and echocardiogram may reveal evidence of cardiomegaly, depressed diastolic and systolic function, and prolonged QTC [2].

Treatment

The mainstay treatment for hypothyroidism is thyroid hormone replacement with levothyroxine (LT4), which is identical to T4. A synthetic version of thyroid hormone first became available in the 1950s and is now the mostly commonly prescribed medication in the USA. Levothyroxine is initiated using weight-based dosing of 1.6 µg/kg/day with females requiring 75–125 µg daily and males requiring 100–150 µg daily [2, 4]. Lower doses should be utilized in the elderly and individuals with coronary artery disease, often starting at a dose of 25–50 µg [4]. It take 6–8 weeks to reach a steady state, and TSH should be checked at that time. Most guidelines recommend against the addition of L-triiodothyronine (LT3) to levothyroxine as it has not consistently proven beneficial in trials [2, 4]. Furthermore, desiccated thyroid supplementation is not recommended due to large variations in levels of thyroid hormones between batches [2].

Thyroid hormone is primarily absorbed in the small intestine and has higher absorption levels if taken fasting and separate from other medications. Other comorbid conditions and medications that affect gastric acid secretion or small bowel absorption, such as celiac disease or prior bowel surgery, result in decreased absorption of levothyroxine and need for increased dosing. The liquid formulation is better absorbed than the tablet formulation. Many medications also affect levothyroxine absorption (Table 1) [2]. Levothyroxine has a half-life of 1 week. This allows for thyroid hormone to be given in daily or weekly dosing. Levothyroxine should be taken 30 min prior to the first meal of the day and separate from other medications [2, 4].

Additionally, certain medical conditions can affect thyroid hormone levels including

Table 1 Medication effects on thyroid hormone levels [2]

Medication	Effect
Bile acid sequestrants	Decreases absorption. Take 4–5 h apart
Sucralfate	Decreases absorption
Ferrous sulfate	Decreases absorption
Calcium carbonate	Decreases bioavailability
Phosphate binders	Decrease bioavailability
Raloxifene, orlistat	Decrease absorption
Estrogen	Increase thyroid-binding globulin decreasing clearance
Selective estrogen receptor modifiers	Decreases clearance
Antiepileptics	Decrease absorption, increase clearance
Tuberculosis medications	Decrease absorption, increase clearance
Tyrosine kinase inhibitors	Alter thyroid regulation

pregnancy, Addison's disease, and pernicious anemia. Pregnancy results in increased levels of thyroid-binding globulin resulting in decreased availability of thyroid hormone and the need to increase dosing by 25–50%. If a patient is experiencing severe morning sickness, dosing can be taken at night. In Addison's disease thyroid levels will often be low due to decreased glucocorticoids; however, glucocorticoid replacement alone often corrects the thyroid dysfunction. In fact, replacing thyroid hormone before correcting the glucocorticoid deficiency can precipitate adrenal crisis. Pernicious anemia also decreases thyroid hormone absorption and increases the dosing needed for replacement [2].

Myxedema Coma

Myxedema coma is a life-threatening systemic decompensation as a result of severe hypothyroidism. It is most common in elderly women. It can be triggered by cold temperatures, infections, medications, nonadherence to thyroid replacement and other serious comorbidities such as stroke and heart failure. Patients present with extreme lethargy and in severe cases coma. They are often hypothermic, bradycardic, hypercapnic, and hyponatremic and have renal impairment.

Failing to recognize and treat myxedema coma in a timely fashion can result in death with a mortality rate of 25–60% despite appropriate treatment. Lab work will reveal severely low of undetectable levels of T4. TSH may be low or normal in patients with central hypothyroidism or elevated in patients with primary hypothyroidism. Patients suffering from myxedema coma should be cared for by a multidisciplinary team in the intensive care unit. Treatment consists of aggressive thyroid hormone replacement with a loading dose of 200–400 μg of levothyroxine given intravenously followed by a maintenance dose of 1.6 μg/kg/day orally. Patients also require supportive care including intravenous fluids, electrolytes, warming blankets, and stress-dose steroids [1].

Hashimoto's Thyroiditis

Hashimoto's thyroiditis was first described in 1912 and is the most common autoimmune disorder with a prevalence of 10–12% [2]. Hashimoto's thyroiditis results in a lymphocytic infiltration of the thyroid resulting in destruction, atrophy, and fibrosis [2, 5]. Hashimoto's thyroiditis is the most common cause of hypothyroidism in iodine-rich areas accounting for 20–30% of hypothyroid patients. Hashimoto's thyroiditis has an incidence rate of 0.3–1.5 per 1000 subjects per year [5]. It is found in females at a rate ten times higher than the rate in males [2, 5]. Its prevalence increases with age. It is most common in white individuals at a prevalence of 14.3% and least common in African Americans with a prevalence of 5.3% [2]. Hashimoto's thyroiditis is more common in individuals who have other autoimmune disorders and those with a family history of Hashimoto's with a 29–55% monozygotic twin concordance rate. Up to 50% of the siblings of patients with Hashimoto's thyroiditis will also have circulating antithyroid antibodies [5].

Diagnostic Workup

Physical exam may reveal a firm, enlarged thyroid or a non-palpable atrophic thyroid. Some patients may have a goiter. The diagnosis of Hashimoto's thyroiditis is made based on the presence of hypothyroidism (elevated TSH with low T4 and T3) and the presence of thyroid peroxidase (TPO) antibodies, which are present in 80–90% of patients and/or the presence of antithyroglobin antibodies, which are present in 60–80% of patients. Of note, patients with other thyroid dysfunction can also have these antibodies present. About 40–60% of patients with Graves' disease will have antithyroglobin antibodies present, and 50–60% will have TPO antibodies [2, 5]. Additionally, women with postpartum thyroiditis may have TPO antibodies present, and this is predictive of progression to permanent hypothyroidism. In patients with subclinical hypothyroidism, the presence of TPO antibodies predicts progression to overt hypothyroidism [5]. If thyroid ultrasound is obtained, it will reveal a hypoechogenic, dyshomogenous parenchyma [2, 5]. The hypoechogenic appearance on ultrasound may be present even before TPO antibody development [2]. Cytology and radioactive iodine uptake are not needed to make the diagnosis [5].

Treatment

Hashimoto's thyroiditis cannot be cured. Thyroid hormone replacement will however alleviate symptoms. Start levothyroxine at 1.5–1.7 μg/kg daily. Hashimoto's thyroiditis has been associated with papillary thyroid cancer. Due to this there should be a low threshold for thyroidectomy if there are any suspicious lesions [5].

Iatrogenic Hypothyroidism

Another common cause of hypothyroidism is iatrogenic. This includes hypothyroidism secondary to thyroidectomy, iodine ablation, external irradiation, antithyroid drugs, and other medications such as lithium, ethionamide, sulfonamides, iodine, tyrosine kinase inhibitors, and cytokines which can have destructive effects on the thyroid.

These conditions are often permanent and require thyroid hormone replacement [2].

Painless Thyroiditis, Postpartum Thyroiditis, and Subacute Thyroiditis

Painless thyroiditis, postpartum thyroiditis, and subacute thyroiditis have a triphasic course which may include a hypothyroid period. The hypothyroid phase is often self-limited and only requires treatment if patients are symptomatic [2]. These conditions are discussed further in detail in the section on "Hyperthyroidism."

Riedel's Thyroiditis

Riedel's thyroiditis is a very rare chronic sclerosing replacement of the thyroid gland with connective tissue overgrowth into adjacent structures. This rare condition requires specialist assistance in diagnosis and treatment [6].

Thyroid Infiltration

Certain systemic conditions such as amyloidosis, hemochromatosis, sarcoidosis, cystinosis, and scleroderma can have local, destructive effects on the thyroid resulting in hypothyroidism [2]. These conditions are beyond the scope of this chapter, but further information can be found in other chapters on these conditions.

Congenital Hypothyroidism

Congenital hypothyroidism is the most frequent congenital endocrine disorder occurring in 1 out of every 3000–4000 of all live births. It is most commonly seen in Hispanic and Asian individuals. It occurs due to congenital TSH deficiency or TRH defect. Congenital hypothyroidism is now included on newborn screening, which allows for early identification and treatment to avoid the previous severe consequences of this disease [2].

most frequently found in the Caucasian individuals [7].

Central Hypothyroidism

Central hypothyroidism is a rare cause of hypothyroidism with a prevalence of 1 in 20,000 to 1 in 80,000 individuals. Central hypothyroidism occurs due to pituitary or hypothalamic dysfunction resulting in insufficient TSH stimulation of a normal thyroid gland. Unlike other causes of hypothyroidism, central hypothyroidism has equal prevalence regardless of gender and age. It can occur for many reasons including pituitary invasion by benign or malignant tumors or aneurysms, iatrogenic dysfunction due to prior surgery, radiation or medications, injury, pituitary infarction, infiltrative disease such as hemochromatosis, sarcoidosis, or histiocytosis or infectious causes such as tuberculosis, syphilis, and mycoses. Identification of central hypothyroidism requires further evaluation of the other pituitary hormones and pituitary imaging with MRI. Central hypothyroidism is treated with hormone replacement often under the direction of endocrinology. Free T4 is monitored for treatment efficacy instead of TSH [2].

Clinical Presentation

Symptoms of thyrotoxicosis can vary by patient and do not strongly correlate with levels of free T4 and T3. Additionally, older patients often have fewer symptoms then their younger counterparts [3]. Symptoms may include weight loss, atrial fibrillation, tachycardia, anxiety, muscle weakness, fatigue, tremor, polydipsia, menstrual irregularities, infertility, sleep disturbance, heat intolerance, fatigue, diaphoresis, confusion, and edema [1–3, 7]. Long-standing thyrotoxicosis can result in osteoporosis, embolic events, cardiovascular collapse, and even death [3]. Thyrotoxicosis can also result in thyrotoxic periodic paralysis, a rare condition most common in the Asian population, which results in muscle paralysis, acute hypokalemia, and thyrotoxicosis [2, 7]. Older patients tend to have fewer symptoms but are at higher risk for major complications [7]. Individuals over the age of 60 have a three times increased risk of developing atrial fibrillation resulting in increased risk of embolic stroke as well [7].

Hyperthyroidism

An excess in circulating thyroid hormone results in thyrotoxicosis. It is referred to as hyperthyroidism when it is the result of excess hormone synthesis or excretion. Thyrotoxicosis without hyperthyroidism occurs when preformed thyroid hormone is released from damaged follicles in the thyroid or through the introduction of thyroid hormone from extrathyroidal sources [7]. In the USA, the overall prevalence of hyperthyroidism is 1.2% with 0.5% of patients having overt hyperthyroidism (low TSH with elevated T3 and/or T4) and 0.7% having subclinical hyperthyroidism (low TSH with normal T3 and T4) [3]. The incidence of hyperthyroidism is higher in women than men. Rates of hyperthyroidism increase with age. It is

Diagnostic Workup

Workup for thyrotoxicosis should not delay treatment especially in severe cases. Initial workup for thyrotoxicosis should include a comprehensive history and physical exam. A patient with thyrotoxicosis may be found to be tachycardic, hypertensive, and tachypneic. The thyroid may be diffusely enlarged or nodular and may be tender depending on the cause [3]. Additional possible signs include exophthalmos, tremor, hyperreflexia, and thyroid dermopathy, which are slightly thickened, discrete violaceous plaques on the shins and dorsum of feet, pretibial myxedema, and peripheral edema with or without acropachy [1, 3, 7]. Initial lab workup includes TSH, free T4, and total T3. In cases of overt hyperthyroidism, TSH will be undetectable with elevated T4 and/or T3 [7]. In subclinical hyperthyroidism, TSH is elevated but still detectable with normal levels of T4 and T3 [7] In elderly patients or patients with multiple comorbidities an EKG, Holter monitor and echocardiogram should be considered given high risk of cardiovascular complications [3].

Once a patient has been identified as being hyperthyroid, workup should include a thyroid radioiodine uptake scan and serum testing for antibodies including thyrotropin (TSH-R) receptor antibodies and thyroid-stimulating immunoglobulin (TSI) [7]. TSH-R and TSI will be present in Grave's disease but not in other conditions resulting in hyperthyroidism [3, 7]. Radioiodine uptake scan will reveal diffuse increased uptake in Graves' disease, localized increased uptake in toxic adenoma, and normal or decreased uptake in subacute thyroiditis, postpartum thyroiditis, painless thyroiditis, excess iodine intake, and factitious ingestion of thyroid hormone [3]. Thyroid ultrasound may help in treatment planning, for example, by identifying a nodule suspicious of malignancy, but offers little additional benefit in the workup of hyperthyroidism in comparison to antibody and radioactive iodine uptake testing [3, 7].

Thyroid Storm

In severe cases, thyrotoxicosis can result in a rare, but emergent condition known as thyroid storm. Thyroid storm is hyperthyroidism with severe life-threatening manifestations that is triggered by trauma, surgery, infection, inappropriate medication use, excessive iodine exposure, or severe health conditions [1, 7]. In 70% of cases, a trigger can be identified with the most common reason being nonadherence to antithyroid drugs followed by infection [7]. Patients present with fever, cardiac arrhythmia, vomiting, and altered mental status [1]. Burch and Wartofsky have a predictive scoring system that predicts the likelihood of thyroid storm based on symptoms including fever, altered mental status, gastrointestinal and hepatic dysfunction, tachycardia, heart failure, atrial fibrillation, and a precipitating event. The utility of this scale, however, is limited by its validation

in a small population [3, 7]. Thyroid storm has a 10–20% mortality rate and requires rapid identification and treatment [1]. Treatment of thyroid storm should take place in the intensive care unit with a multidisciplinary team and involves inorganic iodine, high-dose corticosteroids, antithyroid drugs, beta-blockers, Tylenol, and external cooling [1, 3, 7].

Graves' Disease

Graves' disease is the most common cause of hyperthyroidism accounting for over 80% of cases with 20–30 cases per 100,000 people [2, 7]. It is six to seven times more common in females than in males with a lifetime prevalence of 3% in females compared to 0.5% in males. While Graves' disease can occur at any age, it is most common in the third and fourth decade of life. It is also commonly triggered after pregnancy [2]. Graves' disease is thought to occur in genetically susceptible individuals following an environmental trigger, which leads to the development of antibodies against the thyroid-stimulating hormone receptor [2, 7]. These antibodies activate the thyrocytes stimulating thyroid hormone production and thus resulting in elevated levels of thyroid hormone (Fig. 1) [2]. Environmental triggers include smoking, pregnancy, immune reconstitution, increased iodine intake, allergic rhinitis,

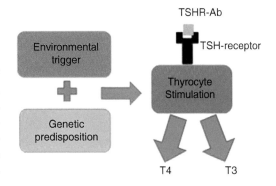

Fig. 1 Pathophysiology of Graves' disease. An environmental trigger in a genetically predisposed individual results in the formation of TSH receptor antibodies which stimulate the TSH receptor resulting in production of T4 and T3 by the thyrocyte

vitamin D deficiency, and infections, in particular *Yersinia enterocolitica* which mimics the TSH receptor [2, 7].

Clinical Presentation

While symptom onset is gradual, 80% of patients will be symptomatic at presentation. Common symptoms include weight loss, fatigue, anxiety, restlessness, heat intolerance, palpitations, shortness of breath, insomnia, menstrual irregularities, hair loss, hyperreflexia, hypertension, and edema. Some patients will also have signs and symptoms associated with Graves' ophthalmology, which is discussed in further detail below [2].

Diagnostic Workup

Patients with Graves' disease will have undetectable TSH levels in conjunction with elevated T4 and/or T3 levels. TSH receptor antibodies can be detected in several ways; however, many utilize a TPO antibody assay which is over 90% sensitive [2]. Radionuclide uptake scan will show diffuse increased uptake [3]. Thyroid ultrasound has little utility in the workup of Graves' disease. Workup should also include a pregnancy test if applicable and EKG. For treatment planning, one should consider checking a CBC. If a CMP is obtained, individual may note a mildly elevated alkaline phosphate and other liver function tests as well as hypercalcemia [2].

Treatment

The goal in the treatment of Graves' disease is to revert to a euthyroid state as quickly as possible while controlling the symptoms associated with thyrotoxicosis. Beta-adrenergic blockade can be used to decrease conversion of T4 to T3 resulting in lower heart rate, decreased shortness of breath, decreased fatigue, and improved overall functioning. If a patient is unable to tolerate a beta-blocker, verapamil or diltiazem can be utilized [3]. There are three different modalities that can be utilized

to revert to a euthyroid state: antithyroid drugs (ATDs), radioiodine, and surgery.

Antithyroid Drugs

Antithyroid drugs (ATDs) are gradually gaining popularity in the USA and are the treatment of choice outside of the USA. ATDS are most likely to be successful in achieving long-term remission in women, those with mild disease, and small goiter. It is the preferred treatment in elderly and high-risk patients, pregnancy, those needing rapid disease control, and those with moderate to severe Graves' orbitopathy. The most common reason for ATD treatment failure is nonadherence [3].

There are two options of ATDs available within the USA, methimazole and propylthiouracil (PTU). Methimazole and PTU act as a substrate for thyroid peroxidase thereby inhibiting the metabolism of iodine and iodination of tyrosine residues needed to make thyroid hormone. They have no effect on T4 or T3 that has already been released from the thyroid, although PTU does decrease conversion of T4 to T3 in the periphery [7]. Methimazole is usually the agent of choice given its better efficacy, longer half-life and duration of action resulting in fewer daily doses, and more favorable side effect profile [3, 7]. The exception to this is in first trimester pregnancy, when PTU is the preferred agent [7]. This is discussed in further depth in the special populations section below.

Initially, a dose of 10–30 mg daily of methimazole is often needed to render a patient euthyroid with continued 5–10 mg thereafter for maintenance dosing. In severe cases twice daily dosing may be needed initially. Higher doses are often needed for more elevated levels of free T4. PTU dosing usually starts between 50 and 150 mg two to three times daily with maintenance dosing 50 mg two to three times daily [3]. Free T4 and total T3 should be monitored every 2–6 weeks after initiation and dose adjustment of ATDs. TSH is not a reliable marker of treatment efficacy as it can remain suppressed for months despite normalization of free T4 and T3. Once a patient is rendered, euthyroid dosing may be decreased 30–50% with continued lab monitoring every 4 to 6 weeks then 2–3 months once stable. Once a patient has been stable on treatment for 12–18 months, TSH and TRAb may be checked, and if normal, treatment may be discontinued. If not normal continued low-dose ATD vs. radioactive iodine or thyroidectomy should be considered. Remission is defined as persistent normal TSH, free T4, and total T3 1 year after discontinuing ATD therapy. Following remission TSH should be monitored annually. Remission rates are lower in males, smokers, patients with large goiters, and patients with elevated TRAb levels [3].

In general, ATDs are well tolerated with 5–13% of patients reporting minor side effects such as pruritus, minor rash, arthralgia, and gastrointestinal distress [3, 7]. At low doses 17% of patients discontinue methimazole therapy, whereas 29% discontinue on high-dose methimazole and 34% discontinue on PTU [3]. In rare cases, severe side effects may develop including agranulocytosis, hepatotoxicity, and vasculitis. The vasculitis is an ANCA antibody associated small vessel vasculitis, which while rare is most commonly seen with PTU and presents with fever, arthralgia, and vasculitis with potential renal or pulmonary involvement [3, 7]. The vasculitis usually resolves with drug discontinuation [3].

Agranulocytosis, defined as an absolute granulocyte count less than 500 cells per mm^3, is a rare but potentially life-threatening complication. It has an annual incidence of 0.1–0.3% annually but a 4% mortality rate. It manifests with fever and sore throat and sometimes chills, diarrhea, or myalgia often within the first 90 days of ATD initiation. Any patient on ATDs who develops these symptoms should immediately stop their ATD and obtain a CBC with differential. If their white blood cell count is less than 1000, treatment should be discontinued. Current guidelines recommend a CBC prior to initiation of ATDs, but do not recommend routine surveillance after initiation unless symptomatic [3, 7].

Hepatotoxicity, defined as elevation in liver transaminases more than three times the upper limit of normal, is a rare complication occurring in 0.4–2.7% of patients. It can occur with both methimazole and PTU but is more common and more severe with PTU [3, 7]. Methimazole most often causes a cholestatic pattern of hepatocellular injury, whereas PTU can result in fulminant hepatic necrosis. Higher rates of fulminant liver failure due to PTU are seen in pediatric patients resulting in an FDA warning against its use in this population [3]. Liver failure most commonly occurs within the first 3 months of treatment initiation and peaks within 30 days [7]. It occurs at an average daily dose of 25 mg for methimazole and 217 mg for PTU [3]. Guidelines recommend checking liver function tests at baseline and thereafter if patients show signs of liver failure such as pruritic rash, jaundice, light-colored stools, or dark urine [3, 7].

Radioactive Iodine

Radioactive iodine (RAI) has historically been the treatment of choice for Graves' disease within the USA although it is less often used in other countries [3]. It is contraindicated in pregnant and breastfeeding mothers or women desiring pregnancy in the next 6 months, those with nodules suspicious for malignancy, those unable to comply with safety recommendations, and those individuals with moderate to severe Grave's orbitopathy [3, 7]. In general, radioactive iodine is a safe treatment; however, it can result in a transient exacerbation of hyperthyroidism or in rare cases thyroid storm due to the release of preformed hormone [3]. Some studies have additionally suggested RAI can worsen Graves' orbitopathy. Patients with mild to moderate Graves' orbitopathy can still be treated with radioactive iodine, but should be pretreated with steroids. Individuals with moderate to severe Graves' orbitopathy should avoid radioactive iodine. Additionally, radioactive iodine rarely can precipitate acute thyroiditis. This occurs in less than 1% of cases and can usually be managed with nonsteroidal anti-inflammatories alone or steroids if severe [7].

Consider beta-adrenergic blockade prior to radioactive iodine to help prevent a transient exacerbation [3]. In elderly individuals or individuals with severe symptoms, consider pretreatment with ATDs. Methimazole is the preferred agent and should be held 3–5 days prior to radioiodine treatment and restarted 3–7 days posttreatment. ATDs should be continued until thyroid function normalizes [3, 7]. Beta-blockade can be discontinued when free T4 reaches a normal level [3].

Following RAI it is recommended to check a TSH at 4–8 weeks and continue repeating every 4–6 weeks until normalized [3, 7]. About 48–77% of patients are rendered hypothyroid after RAI and should be initiated on thyroid replacement [8, 9]. Once rendered euthyroid patients should continue annual thyroid screening for their lifetime [3]. Radioactive iodine can be repeated at 3–6 months if patients fail to respond completely or relapse [3, 7].

Thyroidectomy

While often not utilized as first line treatment, in certain situations, such as patients with a large goiter, greater than 80 g, or large nodules, greater than 4 cm, patients with low radioiodine uptake, patients with suspected cancer, coexisting hyperparathyroidism, moderate to severe Graves' ophthalmopathy or patient preference, thyroidectomy can be the preferred treatment for hyperthyroidism. Prior to surgery, patients should be rendered euthyroid with ATDs and started on beta-blockers to reduce the risk of thyroid storm. Postoperatively patients should be initiated on levothyroxine with weight-based dosing (1.6 μg/kg daily with lower dosing in the elderly). TSH levels should be rechecked 6–8 weeks postoperatively [3, 7]. When performed by a high volume surgeon, complications of surgery are rare at 1–3% with the most common complications being hypocalcemia secondary to permanent hypoparathyroidism and permanent recurrent laryngeal nerve injury [7].

Special Populations

Pregnancy

Graves' disease is the most common cause of hyperthyroidism in pregnancy affecting 5.9 per 1000 pregnancies annually. Risk of Graves' disease is highest in the first trimester and decreases throughout pregnancy. Women see a second peak in Graves' disease 7–9 months postpartum. A diagnosis of Graves' disease in pregnancy is made based on thyrotoxicosis and the presence of TPO antibodies. TSH receptor antibodies can cross the placenta and affect fetal thyroid

function. Antibody levels should be assessed at 18–24 weeks and 30–34 weeks. If high levels of antibody are detected the neonate should be monitored for hyperthyroidism [3, 7].

Other causes of hyperthyroidism in pregnancy include gestational thyrotoxicosis and transient subclinical hyperthyroidism. Gestational thyrotoxicosis is a benign, transient condition in which human chorionic gonadotropin affects thyroid production, but no thyroid antibodies are present. This conditions is usually self-limited and only requires treatment if the patient becomes symptomatic [3, 7]. A small percentage of pregnant women will also have subclinical hyperthyroidism (elevated TSH with normal T4 and T3). This is thought to be secondary to changes in pregnancy and does not require treatment [7].

PTU is the preferred agent in the first trimester of pregnancy followed by methimazole in the second and third trimester. In the first trimester, methimazole has been associated with increased risk of aplasia cutis, choanal atresia, esophageal atresia, and omphalocele. While PTU is also associated with birth defects such as preauricular sinuses and cysts and urinary tract abnormalities, these are less severe than the defects associated with methimazole, and thus it is the preferred agent. Following the first trimester, methimazole has been shown to be safe and becomes the preferred agent secondary to the hepatotoxic risk associated with PTU. In pregnancy PTU is often started at a 50–300 mg daily dose and methimazole at 5–15 mg daily dose. PTU dosing can be converted to methimazole using a 10–15 mg PTU to 1 mg methimazole ratio. TSH should be monitored 2 weeks after dosing changes and every 2–6 weeks throughout pregnancy. Pregnancy adjusted TSH, and T4 levels should be utilized as levels in pregnancy can be 150% higher than nonpregnancy levels. As radioactive iodine is contraindicated in pregnancy, if ATDs do not adequately control thyroid levels, thyroidectomy is the preferred treatment modality and is usually completed in the second trimester [3, 7, 10].

Lactating Mothers

Both methimazole and PTU are found in small amounts in breast milk. For lactating mothers, methimazole and PTU are both safe to be taken up to 20 and 300 mg daily, respectively; however, methimazole is the preferred agent [3, 7]. Medication should be dosed immediately after feeding [7]. Beta-blockers can be utilized to help manage symptoms with metoprolol and propranolol being the preferred agents in lactating mothers [3].

Pediatrics

Methimazole is the treatment of choice for pediatric patients with Graves' disease. PTU is not routinely used due to the high risk of hepatotoxicity (1 in 2000 to 4000 patients). RAI may be considered in patients over the age of 5 as well as thyroidectomy; however, these treatments are associated with high risk of permanent hypothyroidism [3].

Graves' Ophthalmopathy

Graves' ophthalmopathy is a unique finding found only in patients with hyperthyroidism secondary to Graves' disease [2]. Up to 40–50% of patients with Graves' disease will have some evidence of Graves' ophthalmopathy with 5% having moderate to severe disease. Risk factors for Graves' ophthalmopathy include smoking, untreated or delayed treatment of hyperthyroidism, high thyroid receptor antibody levels, and radioiodine therapy [2, 3]. TSH receptor antibodies stimulate orbital fibroblasts resulting in the production of inflammatory cytokines, hyaluronan, and glycosaminoglycans resulting in muscle and connective tissue volume expansion within the orbit [2].

Clinical Presentation

Graves' ophthalmopathy can result in ocular discomfort and irritation, dry eyes, photophobia, diplopia, reduced color perception, visual field loss, restricted eye movement, and anterior proptosis of the eye. Prolonged exposure can result in keratitis and corneal ulcers. Symptoms usually occur bilaterally; however, severity can be asymmetric. Physical exam may reveal eyelid retraction with bright-eyed stare, periorbital edema, conjunctival erythema, proptosis, chemosis, and restricted eye movements [2].

Diagnosis and Treatment

If the diagnosis of Graves' ophthalmopathy is uncertain or if findings are not symmetric consider CT or MRI for further evaluation to rule out an orbital tumor, CT or MRI will demonstrate enlarged extraocular muscle and increased orbital fibroadipose tissue. Treatment of Graves' disease can improve Graves' ophthalmopathy, but once present, it is not curable. Treatment is best managed in conjunction with endocrinology and ophthalmology and includes prompt restoration to a euthyroid state usually through the use of antithyroid drugs and sometimes steroids, smoking cessation, and symptomatic treatment including utilizing sunglasses, artificial tears, and taping the eyes shut in the evening [2, 3].

Toxic Adenoma

Another cause of hyperthyroidism is toxic adenoma. Toxic adenomas are well-encapsulated, homogenous neoplasia, which secrete thyroid hormone independent of TSH and the rest of the thyroid gland. In iodine-rich areas, toxic adenomas are relatively rare, but they are a leading cause of hyperthyroidism in iodine-deficient areas. Toxic adenomas are more common in women. They can occur at any age but are most common between the age of 30 and 60 years. While usually there is a single hyperfunctioning nodule, at times individuals may have multinodular goiters with multiple functioning nodules. This most commonly occurs in older individuals who are iodine deficient. Exam will often reveal a palpable nodule and possibly a goiter. A radioiodine uptake scan will reveal avid uptake within the nodules with decreased uptake in the surrounding tissue [7]. Treatment of choice is ablative surgery or radioiodine ablation [3, 7]. Lobectomy results in a less than 1% treatment failure rate and a 2–3% risk of permanent hypothyroidism, whereas RAI has a 6–18% treatment failure rate and a 7.6% risk of permanent hypothyroidism at 1 year and a 46% risk of hypothyroidism at 10 years [3].

Thyroiditis

Thyroiditis is inflammation of the thyroid that results in thyrotoxicosis without hyperthyroidism as thyroid hormone levels are elevated due to the release of preformed thyroid hormone rather than increased production and release [2, 7]. It can be characterized by its time course as acute or subacute. Causes of acute thyroiditis include infectious thyroiditis, radiation thyroiditis, and traumatic thyroiditis. Causes of subacute thyroiditis include subacute thyroiditis, silent thyroiditis, and drug-induced thyroiditis [2].

Causes of Acute Thyroiditis

Infectious Thyroiditis

Infectious thyroiditis is a very rare condition accounting for only 0.1–0.7% of thyroid disease, which results in an acute painful neck swelling, fever, sore throat, dysphagia, dysphonia, desire to keep head flexed, and potentially systemic symptoms of infection due to a bacterial or fungal infection of the thyroid. Rapid identification and treatment is essential as infectious thyroiditis can have severe complications including sepsis, neck compression, necrotizing mediastinitis or pericarditis and even death. While infection of the thyroid is rare, the following conditions put individuals at increased risk: piriform sinus tract fistula, third and fourth brachial arch abnormalities, operative manipulation (thyroid lobectomy or biopsy, central line placement), intravenous drug use, immunocompromised states, endocarditis, tooth abscess, and esophageal perforation or rupture [2, 6].

The infection is usually polymicrobial with both gram-positive bacteria, most commonly *Staph. aureus or Streptococcus pyogenes, Streptococcus epidermidis, or Streptococcus pneumoniae*, and gram-negative aerobes, most commonly *E. coli*, and anaerobes, most commonly *Clostridium septicum*, Gram-negative bacilli, and peptostreptococcus, present. Rarely fungi or parasitic infections may also be present. In patients with a more subacute or chronic presentation that may mimic carcinoma or a multinodular goiter, mycobacterium tuberculosis should be suspected [2, 6].

Workup for infectious thyroiditis should include CBC, inflammatory blood markers, TSH, and evaluation for sepsis if warranted. HIV testing should also be considered. Patients may be euthyroid or hyperthyroid due to release of preformed hormone on presentation. Ultrasound should be obtained to evaluate for abscess or aggressive cancer mimicking infection. A CAT scan with intravenous contrast can also be considered to better evaluate the extent of the infection. A barium swallow can be obtained if a fistula is suspected. An FNA should be utilized to obtain a culture to direct antibiotic therapy [2, 6].

The patient should initially be started on broad-spectrum intravenous antibiotics and deescalated based on culture. Percutaneous drainage should also be considered if an abscess is present. If a fistula is present, individuals are at risk of recurrence and the fistula should be surgically removed once stable. Infectious thyroiditis has a 12% mortality rate if untreated. For those who survive, their prognosis is excellent with only a small number developing permanent hypothyroidism [2, 6].

Radiation Thyroiditis

Radiation exposure to the anterior neck can result in inflammation of the thyroid and release of preformed hormone. Radiation thyroiditis is seen in 1–5% of patient who undergo radioactive iodine, with those being treated with higher doses for cancer more susceptible than those treated for hyperthyroidism. Patients may experience anterior neck pain and swelling within a few days or up to 2 weeks following radiation. In severe cases thyroid storm may be elicited. Treatment is usually symptomatic with NSAIDs or steroids if symptoms are severe [2].

Traumatic Thyroiditis

Traumatic thyroiditis is direct anterior neck pressure or manipulation that results in the release of preformed thyroid hormone resulting in thyrotoxicosis. It often is self-limited and goes unrecognized and unreported. It most often occurs after parathyroidectomy. It usually does not result in pain. If patients are symptomatic, they can be treated with corticosteroids [2].

Causes of Subacute Thyroiditis

Silent Thyroiditis

Silent or sporadic painless thyroiditis is a painless, subacute lymphocytic inflammation of the thyroid in nonpregnant patients that results in the release of preformed hormone resulting in thyrotoxicosis [3]. Silent thyroiditis has an incidence rate of 1–10%. It is most commonly seen in females between the age of 30 and 50 years of age. Often patients have no known preexisting thyroid disease [2]. It is triggered by medications such as lithium, interferon-α, tyrosine kinase inhibitors, monoclonal antibodies, interleukin therapy, and amiodarone. Trauma, autoimmune triggers, and hormone fluctuations such as those that occur after adrenalectomy, steroid cessation, or in Addison's disease or hypopituitarism can also trigger silent thyroiditis. For some patients, no cause or trigger can be identified [2, 3].

Silent thyroiditis often follows a similar triphasic course as seen in postpartum thyroiditis with a hyperthyroid phase followed by a hypothyroid phase and finally resolution to a euthyroid state. About 5–20% will be thyrotoxic at diagnosis with symptoms such as palpitations, anxiety, and tremor. Symptoms are usually relatively limited and less severe than those seen in Graves' disease. The thyrotoxic phase lasts approximately 3 months and is often followed by a hypothyroid phase for 3–6 months before returning to a euthyroid state usually within 1 year of disease onset. About 10–20% of patients with silent thyroiditis will go on to develop permanent hypothyroidism. Ultrasound of the thyroid will reveal a hypoechogenic appearance with low radioiodine uptake on uptake scan.

Treatment during the thyrotoxic phase is symptomatic only with beta-blockers. As the thyrotoxic phase is due to release or preformed hormone and not ongoing production, ATDs have no role in treatment. The hypothyroid phase can be monitored if symptoms are mild. If symptoms increase in severity patients should be treated with levothyroxine for 6–12 months after which it can be discontinued and monitored for recovery to a euthyroid state. About 5–10% of patients will have a recurrent episode of silent thyroiditis [2].

Postpartum Thyroiditis

Postpartum thyroiditis is an autoimmune, destructive thyroiditis that occurs within 1 year postpartum or following a miscarriage. It has been proposed that postpartum thyroiditis occurs due to postpartum hormonal and immunological rebound [2]. Up to 10% of women will experience postpartum thyroid dysfunction [3].

It is important to differentiate the thyrotoxic phase of postpartum thyroiditis, a transient condition, from Graves' disease, a permanent condition. Postpartum thyroiditis is 20 times more common than Graves' disease in this population [2]. Postpartum thyroiditis is usually painless. It is more common in individuals with a personal or family history of autoimmune disorders, smoking, and individuals with antithyroid peroxidase antibodies [3].

Postpartum thyroiditis classically has a triphasic course with a transient hyperthyroid phase followed by a 1- to 6-month hypothyroid phase and resolution to euthyroid. While this is the classic presentation, only 24–28% of patients experience all three phases with 43–50% only experiencing hypothyroidism and 24–32% only experiencing hyperthyroidism [2, 3].

Diagnostic Evaluation

Antithyroid peroxidase antibodies and thyroglobulin antibodies may be elevated [2, 3]. The ratio of T4 to T3 is usually less than 20 ng/μg, whereas Graves' disease results in a ratio greater than 20 ng/μg [3]. Radioactive iodine uptake scan will show decreased uptake. Ultrasound will show hypoechogenicity [2].

Treatment

ATDs are usually not indicated as the hyperthyroidism is transient. Beta-blockers can be utilized for symptomatic management with metoprolol and propranolol being the preferred agents if breastfeeding [2, 3]. The hypothyroid state can be treated with thyroid hormone replacement if patients are symptomatic, planning pregnancy or breastfeeding. Treatment can usually be withdrawn at 1 year. TSH should continue to be monitored. Some women will have persistent hypothyroidism. Women who are multiparous, older have higher TPO antibodies, higher TSH at diagnosis, and increased hypoechogenicity on ultrasound are at increased risk of permanent hypothyroidism [2]. Women who have experienced postpartum thyroiditis are at increased risk of experiencing it again following subsequent deliveries with some studies showing up to a 70% recurrence rate [2, 3]. Patients are also at increased risk of developing Graves' disease in the future [3].

Subacute Painful Thyroiditis

Subacute thyroiditis, also known as De Quervain thyroiditis or subacute granulomatous thyroiditis, results in fever and moderate to severe pain over the thyroid that radiates to the ears, jaw, and throat. Patients may also complain of fatigue and malaise, anorexia, arthralgia, and myalgia. The thyroid may be enlarged and firm [2, 3, 6]. Initially the inflammation results in damage to follicles resulting in the release of preformed thyroid hormone. In response to the influx of thyroid hormone, TSH inhibition decreases production of new thyroid hormone. As the inflammation resides, the thyroid regenerates, and the patient returns to a euthryoid state [2]. Subacute thyroiditis has an incidence of 1.8% and is more common in females [6]. Incidence peaks in the fifth decade of life. Subacute thyroiditis has a strong association with HLA-B35 and HLA-B67 [2]. It is often triggered by a virus, and patients often have upper respiratory symptoms prior to onset [3, 6]. Several viruses have been linked to subacute painful thyroiditis including mumps, influenza, adenovirus, measles, mononucleosis, coxsackievirus, enterovirus, echovirus, Epstein-Barr virus, cytomegalovirus, hepatitis E, dengue fever, rubella, HIV, and cat scratch fever [2, 6]. Inflammatory markers such as ESR and CRP may be elevated. Patient may also have a mild leukocytosis. Up to 25% may have mild elevation in antithyroid antibodies. Ultrasound if obtained will demonstrated diffuse heterogenicity with focal hypoechoic areas and decreased or normal color flow on Doppler. Radioiodine uptake scan will show diffuse low uptake levels. Most cases are transient with a 3- to 6-month thyrotoxic phase followed by hypothyroidism in 30%. Only 60% are symptomatic in the hyperthyroid phase at presentation. For the majority of patients, the hypothyroid phase is mild and asymptomatic. Most return to a euthyroid state over 6–12 months, but up to 5–15% will have persistent hypothyroidism [2, 3]. Patients who have experienced subacute thyroiditis are at increased risk for late-onset permanent hypothyroidism and Graves' disease in the future [2]. Treatment is supportive with NSAIDs and beta-blockers. If not well controlled with these measures, a corticosteroid taper over 4–6 weeks can be utilized [2, 3, 6].

Drug-Induced Thyrotoxicosis

Medications can result in thyroid dysfunction. One medication commonly associated with this is amiodarone, which results in thyrotoxicosis in up to 5–10% of users [3, 7]. Amiodarone can result in an overproduction and release of thyroid hormone due to the high iodine content or it can have a direct toxic effect on thyrocytes resulting in release of preformed thyroid hormone [7]. If this occurs amiodarone should be discontinued. Corticosteroids can also be considered. Because of the high risk of thyrotoxicosis, it is recommended that all patients started on amiodarone be screened with TSH for thyroid dysfunction within 3 months of treatment initiation and every 3–6 months thereafter [3]. Other medications associated with thyroid dysfunction include lithium, tyrosine kinase inhibitors, and interferon [2].

Secondary Hyperthyroidism

Secondary hyperthyroidism is rare but occurs when elevated or inappropriately normal levels of TSH result in overproduction of thyroid hormones. This is most often the result of a TSH producing pituitary adenoma and can be further evaluated with an MRI of the pituitary gland [3].

Factious Ingestion

At times, individual may take thyroid hormone replacement unbeknownst to their provider. This results in low TSH levels with elevated T3 and T4 levels with a ratio less than 20 and nearly no radioiodine uptake on radioiodine uptake scan [3].

Rare Causes

Rare causes of hyperthyroidism include thyrotropin-induced thyrotoxicosis, euthyroid hyperthyroxinemia secondary to thyroid-binding protein disorders, and trophoblastic tumors [3, 7]. These conditions are beyond the scope of this review and patients should be referred to endocrinology if they are suspected.

Subclinical Hyperthyroidism

Up to 1.8% of the population will have evidence of subclinical hypothyroidism defined as a TSH below the lower limits of normal with normal T3 and T4 levels. The majority of patients will revert to normal levels without intervention within 5 years; however, 0.5–7% will progress to overt hyperthyroidism. Guidelines recommend rechecking TSH at 2–6 weeks and if persistently low repeat every 3–6 months. If TSH is persistently low greater than 6 months and the patient is elderly, at increased cardiac risk, diagnosed with osteoporosis or symptomatic consider treatment with thyroid hormone replacement. If they do not meet any of these criteria, continued observation is warranted [3].

Summary (Table 2)

Thyroid Nodule

Thyroid nodules are exceedingly common in the general population with 4–7% of the population with palpable nodules identified on physical exam [11] and up to 50–76% of the population having nodules identified on clinical imaging or autopsy [10, 11]. With an annual incidence rate of 0.1%, there will be over 350,000 new nodules identified in the USA over the next year. The risk of having a thyroid nodule increases with age and is four

times more common in women than men [11]. Fortunately, the vast majority of these nodules are benign and asymptomatic [10]. Nodules have an increased likelihood of being malignant in individuals with a history of head and neck radiation, a personal or family history of thyroid cancer, and in particular medullary thyroid cancer or multiple endocrine neoplasia (MEN) syndrome, age less than 14 years or greater than 70 years, males, and if symptoms are present [10, 11]. When nodules are symptomatic, they may result in a choking sensation, cervical tenderness, dysphagia, or dysphonia, although, the presence of these symptoms does not necessarily indicate the presence of a thyroid nodule as these most often are the results of a different etiology [10]. Routine suppression of thyroid nodules with thyroid hormone replacement is not warranted given the high risk of side effects and limited efficacy in trials [10].

Evaluation

Laboratory Studies

A TSH level should be evaluated in all individuals with a thyroid nodule. If TSH levels are normal, no further testing is needed. If TSH levels are elevated, a free T4 and TPO antibodies should be obtained to evaluate for Hashimoto's thyroiditis. If TSH levels are low, a patient should be further evaluated with free T4, total T3, and thyroid scintigraphy. Thyroid scintigraphy can also be helpful in multinodular goiter as hyperfunctioning nodules have a very low risk of malignancy [11] and do not warrant fine needle aspiration (FNA) unless they have suspicious features [10]. If the above criteria are not met, thyroid scintigraphy has little utility in the evaluation of a thyroid nodule [10].

Imaging

Any palpable nodule or nodule visualized on other imaging modalities (CT scan, MRI, or PET scan) should be further evaluated with a dedicated thyroid ultrasound [10]. Nodules detected on PET scan have a high risk of malignancy with over 82% of nodules being malignant [11]. Nodules identified on PET scan should be further evaluated with

Table 2 Summary of etiology of thyrotoxicosis, cause, diagnostic findings, and treatment

Etiology	Cause	Diagnostic findings	Treatment
Graves' disease	TSH-R Ab	TSH-R AB	ATDS, thyroidectomy or radioactive iodine
		TPO-AB	
		TG-AB	
		T4:T3 >20 ng/μg	
		Increased radioactive iodine uptake	
Toxic adenoma	TSH-independent hyperfunctioning nodule(s)	Palpable nodule or goiter on exam	Surgical excision or radioactive iodine ablation
		Avid, localized uptake with decreased uptake in the surrounding tissue on radioiodine uptake scan	
Infectious thyroiditis	Bacteria or fungal infection	Fever + painful thyroid + systemic symptoms	Broad-spectrum antibiotics. Percutaneous drainage if abscess. Remove fistula if present
		Leukocytosis, elevated ESR, CRP	
		Ultrasound or CT scan may demonstrate abscess	
		Barium swallow may demonstrate fistula	
		FNA culture for infectious agent	
Traumatic thyroiditis	Trauma, neck surgery, or pressure	Non-tender self-limited thyrotoxicosis	Usually self-limited
			Steroids if symptomatic
Silent thyroiditis	Medications, autoimmune, trauma, idiopathic	Painless thyroid Thyroid antibodies may be present Triphasic course Ultrasound hypoechogenic Low radioiodine uptake	Thyrotoxic phase-symptomatic treatment Hypothyroid phase-levothyroxine if moderate to severe symptoms
Postpartum thyroiditis	Postpartum (within 1 year) immunological rebound	Triphasic course APO-AB TG-AB T4:T3 <20 ng/μg Ultrasound hypoechogenic Low radioiodine uptake	Thyrotoxic phase-symptomatic treatment Hypothyroid phase-levothyroxine if symptomatic, planning pregnancy or breastfeeding
Subacute painful thyroiditis	Viral trigger	Fever + pain over thyroid Elevated ESR, CRP, leukocytosis Ultrasound diffuse heterogenicity with focal hypoechoic areas Diffuse decreased uptake on radioiodine uptake scan	Mild to moderate-beta-blocker and NSAID Severe corticosteroids
Drug induced	Lithium, interferon, amiodarone, monoclonal antibodies, tyrosine kinase inhibitors	Painless thyrotoxicosis	Discontinue offending agent
Radiation induced	Radiation within last 2 weeks	Anterior neck pain or swelling	Mild-NSAIDS
			Severe corticosteroids
Factious thyrotoxicosis	Inappropriate ingestion thyroid hormone	Low TSH, elevated T4 and T3	Discontinue ingestion of thyroid hormone
		No uptake on radioiodine uptake scan	
Secondary hyperthyroidism	Pituitary adenoma	Inappropriately normal or elevated TSH in setting of elevated T4 and T3 levels	Referral

both a dedicated thyroid ultrasound and FNA [10]. While there are several classification schemes based on ultrasound findings, the American Association of Clinical Endocrinologists (AACE), American College of Endocrinology (ACE), and the Associazione Medici Endocrinologi (AME) recommend categorizing thyroid nodules as low, intermediate, or high risk for malignancy [10, 11] with further workup based on these classifications (Table 3, Fig. 2).

If an FNA is warranted, it should be performed by an experienced clinician as this increases

Table 3 Thyroid nodule characterization and treatment and follow-up recommendation based on risk categorization by ultrasound [10, 11]

Risk categorization	Ultrasound characteristics	Malignancy risk	Obtain FNA if size
Low risk	Thyroid cysts	<1%	>20 mm or growing
	Mostly cystic (>50%)		
	Isoechoic spongiform nodule		
Intermediate risk	Slightly hypoechoic	5–15%	>10 mm
	Central vascularity		
	Macrocalcifications		
	Indeterminate hyperechoic spots		
	Ovoid to round		
	Smooth or ill-defined margins		
	Elevated stiffness		
High risk	Markedly hypoechoic	50–90%	>5 mm
	Microcalcifications		
	Irregular speculated, microlobulated margins		
	Taller than wide		
	Extracapsular/thyroidal extension		
	Pathologic adenopathy		

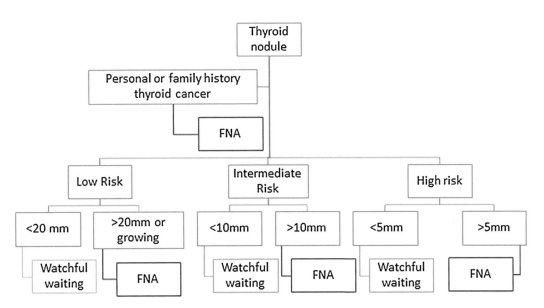

Fig. 2 Summary of thyroid nodule diagnostic workup based on risk categorization as outlined by the American Association of Clinical Endocrinologists (AACE), American College of Endocrinology (ACE), and the Associazione Medici Endocrinologi (AME) guidelines

sensitivity to 97.0%, specificity to 50.5%, and diagnostic accuracy to 68.8% and decreases the risk of false-negative and nondiagnostic results [10]. False negatives can further be reduced to 1–6% through the use of ultrasound to guide biopsy location, the aspiration of at least two sites within the nodule, and evaluation and interpretation by an experienced cytopathologist [10, 11]. If a suspicious lymph node is identified on ultrasound, it should also be biopsied. A sample is considered diagnostic if greater than six groups of well-preserved thyroid epithelial cells with at least ten cells per group [10]. AACE/ACE/AME categorize thyroid nodules into five distinct cytological classifications which are heavily based on the Bethesda System for Reporting Thyroid Cytopathology: nondiagnostic, benign, indeterminate, suspicious, and malignant [10, 11] (Table 4).

A sample is considered to be nondiagnostic when the sample contains fewer than six groups of well-preserved thyroid epithelial cells with at least ten cells per group. If a sample is nondiagnostic but appears cystic and there are no concerning clinical or ultrasound features, the nodule can be followed conservatively with follow-up in 1 year for clinical exam and ultrasound. If it is stable, ultrasound and clinical exam should be repeated after 24 months. If a nodule appears solid and is nondiagnostic, an FNA biopsy should be repeated at least 1 month from the original biopsy [10]. Up to 50% of repeat FNA biopsies will remain nondiagnostic [11], and as there is a 2–16% malignancy rate, surgical excision should be considered at that time [10].

The most common cytopathology classification is benign. These nodules have a low risk of malignancy. If clinical and ultrasound findings are favorable and the patient is asymptomatic, no further workup is necessary. If the nodule is benign with favorable clinical and ultrasound findings, but symptomatic, it can be followed conservatively as described above. Finally, if biopsy results return as benign; however, the ultrasound shows concerning features, the nodules increases its volume by more than 50% in 1 year, or it becomes symptomatic a repeat FNA biopsy should be obtained. If symptoms persist surgical intervention, image-guided thermal ablation or percutaneous ethanol injections can be considered [10]. Furthermore, all nodules greater than 3–4 cm should be evaluated for surgical excision regardless of FNA findings as there is an increased risk of false-negative results [10, 11].

About 10–25% of FNA biopsies will return as indeterminate. This is a difficult group to manage given high variability in malignancy rates. Due to these complicating factors, referral to a specialist should be considered. The AACE/ACE/AME have recommended subdividing this group into low-intermediate and high-risk groups to better

Table 4 AACE/ACE/AME cytopathology classification of thyroid nodules, risk of malignancy, and diagnostic workup [10]

Cytopathology classification	Rate of result	Malignancy risk	Workup
Nondiagnostic	<10%	2–16%	If cystic or predominantly cystic and no suspicious US features conservative management[a]
			If solid repeat FNA. Surgical excision if persistently nondiagnostic unless favorable US and clinical factors
Benign	54–54%	0–3.7%, expertise centers <1%	If no suspicious US features and asymptomatic no further workup
			If no suspicious US features but symptomatic conservative management
			If suspicious US or increase in volume >50% in 1 year, or becomes symptomatic repeat FNA
Indeterminate	10–25%	Low risk 5 15%	Conservative management, consider elastography
		High risk 15–30%	Lobectomy plus isthmectomy or total thyroidectomy
Suspicious	2.5–5%	70–75%	Total thyroidectomy or lobectomy plus isthmectomy
Malignant	2.7–5.4%	>95%	Total thyroidectomy

[a]Conservative management: clinical exam and US at 12 months and if unchanged repeat at 24 months

convey the malignancy risk. Nodules in the low-intermediate risk group may be followed with conservative management. Nodules in the high-risk group should be removed with a thyroid lobectomy and isthmectomy. A total thyroidectomy can also be considered but is not required unless malignancy is confirmed. Additionally, all nodules suspicious or confirmed malignant should be removed with surgical excision [10].

Special Populations

There are two special populations in which the above evaluation and treatment scheme for thyroid nodules do not apply. The first is children, in whom the risk of malignancy, diagnosis, and treatment vary widely and thus should be managed if possible in conjunction with a pediatric endocrinologist. In addition, women who are pregnant are at higher risk for developing new thyroid nodules or having an increase in size in a known nodule. Diagnostic workup and treatment, however, are the same as in nonpregnant individuals with the caveat that if surgical excision is needed, it should be performed in the second trimester if possible [10].

References

1. Leung AM. Thyroid emergencies. J Infus Nurs. 2016;39(5):281–6.
2. Vitti P, Hegedus L, editors. Thyroid diseases: pathogenesis, diagnosis and treatment. Cham: Springer International Publishing; 2018.
3. Ross DS, Burch HB, Cooper DS, Greenlee MC, Laurberg P, Maia AL, et al. 2016 American Thyroid Association guidelines for diagnosis and management of hyperthyroidism and other causes of thyrotoxicosis. Thyroid. 2016;26(10):1343–421.
4. Chiovato L, Magri F, Carle A. Hypothyroidism in context: where we've been and where we're going. Adv Ther. 2019;36(Suppl 2):47–58.
5. Ragusa F, Fallahi P, Elia G, Gonnella D, Paparo SR, Giusti C, et al. Hashimoto's thyroiditis: epidemiology, pathogenesis, clinic and therapy. Best Pract Res Clin Endocrinol Metab. 2019;33(6):101367.
6. Shrestha RT, Hennessey J. Acute and subacute, and Riedel's thyroiditis. In: Feingold KR, Anawalt B, Boyce A, Chrousos G, Dungan K, Grossman A, et al., editors. Endotext. South Dartmouth: MDText.com; 2000.
7. De Leo S, Lee SY, Braverman LE. Hyperthyroidism. Lancet. 2016;388(10047):906–18.
8. Aung ET, Zammitt NN, Dover AR, Strachan MWJ, Seckl JR, Gibb FW. Predicting outcomes and complications following radioiodine therapy in graves' thyrotoxicosis. Clin Endocrinol. 2019;90(1):192–9.
9. Husseni MA. The incidence of hypothyroidism following the radioactive iodine treatment of Graves' disease and the predictive factors influencing its development. World J Nucl Med. 2016;15(1):30–7.
10. Gharib H, Papini E, Garber JR, Duick DS, Harrell RM, Hegedus L, et al. American Association of Clinical Endocrinologists, American College of Endocrinology, and Associazione Medici Endocrinologi medical guidelines for clinical practice for the diagnosis and management of thyroid nodules – 2016 update. Endocr Pract. 2016;22(5):622–39.
11. Fisher SB, Perrier ND. The incidental thyroid nodule. CA Cancer J Clin. 2018;68(2):97–105.

Katherine Reeve, Anna Meola, and Ryan West

Contents

K. Reeve (✉)
Yale New Haven Health Northeast Medical Group,
Uncasville, CT, USA

A. Meola
Eastern Connecticut Health Network Family Medicine
Residency, Manchester, CT, USA
e-mail: AMeola@echn.org

R. West
Nellis Family Medicine Residency, Nellis AFB, Las Vegas,
NV, USA
e-mail: Ryan.west.7@us.af.mil

Osteoporosis is a major health concern worldwide and within the United States. Approximately 9% of US adults over the age of 50 have osteoporosis, and up to 50% have some degree of low bone density [1]. Osteoporosis causes more than two million fractures per year with $19 billion in associated costs in the United States alone [2]. The clinical costs of an osteoporotic fracture are equally great and include increased mortality, increased disability, and an increased need for long-term nursing care. The most common sites of fracture are the hip, vertebrae, and wrist. Hip fractures are particularly deadly, carrying a 26%

© This is a U.S. Government work and not under copyright protection in the U.S.; foreign copyright protection
may apply 2022
P. M. Paulman et al. (eds.), *Family Medicine*,
https://doi.org/10.1007/978-3-030-54441-6_129

1-year mortality rate for patients over the age of 69. Of those who survive, functional skills are significantly decreased with decreased fine motor and mobility scores [3]. Vertebral fractures lead to chronic back pain and deformity in up to 30% of patients. These fractures may have a long-term impact on overall quality of life and the ability to carry out activities of daily living (ADL).

Osteoporosis is defined as decreased bone mineral density leading to increased fragility and an increased risk of fractures. Symptoms are usually not present early on, and an osteoporotic fracture is often the first sign of disease. The lifetime risk of an osteoporotic fracture is 44% [4].

Osteoporosis can be primary or secondary. Primary osteoporosis is bone loss as a result of aging alone. Secondary osteoporosis refers to bone loss as a result of chronic conditions that lead to accelerated bone loss. It can be caused by endocrine disorders such as hyperparathyroidism or hyperthyroidism. Other causes include malignancy, renal failure, and nutritional deficiencies [5].

Risk Factor Assessment

Risk factor assessment begins with taking a detailed history and performing a physical exam. Risk factors for developing osteoporosis include family history, lifestyle, and contributing medical conditions (Table 1).

Lifestyle

Lifestyle choices can affect bone density. Excessive use of alcohol and cigarette smoking are both associated with increased fracture risk [4]. Regular physical activity early in life is associated with

higher peak bone mass, and continued activity leads to lower rates of hip fractures in postmenopausal women [5]. Maintaining healthy eating habits is necessary to obtain the required nutrients to build healthy bone mass. Calcium and Vitamin D are two of these essential nutrients.

Genetics

Several genetic factors can increase the risk of developing osteoporosis. Those of northern European or Asian descent have higher rates of osteoporosis and osteopenia. Women are at a much higher risk of developing osteoporosis than men due to accelerated bone loss after menopause. Certain genetic conditions such as Turner's syndrome increase risk of osteoporosis due to decreased estrogen production.

Endocrine Factors

There are several endocrine disorders that can increase risk of osteoporosis. Any disorder that decreases estrogen production will increase risk. This includes early menopause, surgical menopause, or premature ovarian failure. Risk is also increased by endocrine disorders that disrupt normal bone metabolism, such as hyperthyroidism, hyperparathyroidism, Addison's disease, and Cushing's syndrome.

Medications

Certain medications can have a negative effect on bone metabolism, including anticoagulants, corticosteroids, thyroid hormone, chemotherapeutic agents, anticonvulsants, loop diuretics, proton pump inhibitors, antidepressants, and

Table 1 Risk factors for osteoporosis

Lifestyle	Family history	Genetic/Medical
Poor diet	History of osteoporosis	Menopause
Low activity level	History of fractures	Caucasian or Asian ethnicity
Tobacco use		Endocrine disorders
Alcohol use		Certain medications
Low body weight < 128 lb		

medroxyprogesterone acetate (MDA). Chronic use of any of these medications may increase the risk of developing osteoporosis and suffering osteoporotic fractures.

There are a few medications associated with increased bone mass and decreased rate of factures, including thiazide diuretics, statins, and beta blockers [6].

Laboratory Assessment

If the history and physical exam suggests secondary causes of osteoporosis, laboratory testing should be considered and must be guided by the patient presentation. Useful initial testing may include thyroid-stimulating hormone (TSH), parathyroid hormone (PTH), calcium, vitamin D, complete blood count (CBC), complete metabolic panel, 24 h urinary calcium, and testosterone in men. To measure vitamin D levels, 25(OH)D should be used, not 1,25-dihydroxyvitamin D (4).

Bone Densitometry Assessment

The most important evaluation for osteoporosis is determining the bone mineral density (BMD). The diagnosis of osteoporosis it made primarily based on the BMD and is defined as a BMD 2.5 standard deviations (SD) below the mean for young Caucasian females.

It is important to determine the BMD of patients who are at increased risk of osteoporosis to identify, prevent, and treat osteoporosis. Using the BMD we can estimate future fracture risk, guide treatment decisions, and monitor response to treatment. Both the US Preventive Services Task Force (USPSTF) and the International Society for Clinical Densitometry (ISCD) have issued recommendations on who should be screened for osteoporosis with BMD testing (see Table 2).

The mostly widely used and universally accepted method of measuring BMD is the dual-energy x-ray absorptiometry (DXA) scan. It has been accepted as the gold standard for determining the BMD of the hip and spine. It has replaced the quantitative computed tomography (CT) scan,

which requires significantly greater radiation exposure. The DXA report includes both a T score and a Z score. The T score is defined as the number of standard deviations above or below the mean BMD for a young Caucasian female. The Z score is similar but uses a mean BMD that is adjusted for age, gender, and race.

Although there has been some disagreement in the past, currently both the World Health Organization (WHO) and the ISCD recommend using T-scores as the standard to evaluate all postmenopausal women and men older than 50 [7]. Based on their T-score, patients can be classified into three categories: normal BMD, osteopenia, or osteoporosis. A different classification is recommended for premenopausal women, men under 50, and children. In these cases the Z score should be used instead [8]. Based on their Z score, patients can be classified into two categories: below expected range or within expected range for chronological age with a Z score below or above -2.0 respectively.

Alternative studies exist to evaluate for fracture risk, including quantitative ultrasonography (QUS) and peripheral DXA (pDXA). These modalities are generally less expensive and more portable and may be used in settings where DXA is not available. Both of these may help predict future fractures. However, they cannot be used to reliably determine BMD and should not be used for diagnosis or tracking disease progression if DXA or quantitative CT is available.

FRAX Score

The Fracture Risk Assessment tool (FRAX) was developed in 2008 by the WHO to estimate 10-year probability of hip fracture and major osteoporotic fracture. These estimates are based on untreated patients between 40 and 90 years of age. The calculation uses several risk factors including age, fracture history, steroid use, body mass, smoking, alcohol use, rheumatoid arthritis, parental history of hip fracture, and having secondary causes of osteoporosis. Femoral neck bone mineral density (BMD) can also be factored in if available but is not needed to generate the 10-year

Table 2 Indications for bone mineral density (BMD) screening

US Preventive Services Task Force[a]	International Society for Clinical Densitometry[b]
Women ≥65	Women ≥65
Women <65 with fracture risk equal to or greater than 65-year-old white female	Women 60–64 with fracture risk equal to or greater than 65-year-old white female
Men: insufficient evidence to determine benefit vs harm	Women on prolonged hormone replacement therapy
	Men ≥70
	Anyone with a fragility fracture
	Anyone receiving or considering treatment for osteoporosis

[a]United States Preventive Services Task Force. Osteoporosis: Screening, 2018
[b]International Society for Clinical Densitometry. Osteoporosis Screening Guidelines, 2012

Table 3 World Health Organization (WHO) Diagnostic criteria for osteoporosis

Diagnosis	Bone Mineral Density (BMD) T score [a]
Normal	≤1
Osteopenia	1–2.5
Osteoporosis	≥2.5

Source: WHO Assessment of Osteoporosis at the primary care level (2004)
[a]Standard deviation (SD) below the mean in healthy young females

risk. There is a calculator available online at www.shef.ac.uk/FRAX. It is often included on DXA reports [11]. This information can help guide management and may indicate the need for earlier treatment in patients with osteopenia (see section "Pharmacological Treatment" below).

Diagnosis

The diagnosis of osteoporosis is made primarily from bone mineral density using DXA as the gold standard for assessment. Osteoporosis in postmenopausal women and in men greater than 50 is defined as bone mineral density 2.5 standard deviations below normal as reflected by a T score of −2.5. Osteopenia is defined as a bone mineral density of 1–2.5 standard deviations below normal with a T score of −1 to −2.5. In premenopausal women and men less than 50 they are considered to be below the expected range for age if the bone mineral density is more than 2.0 standard deviations below normal adjusted for age as reflected by a Z score of −2.0. Alternatively, a clinical diagnosis of osteoporosis can be

made in any adult based on the presence of a fragility (low trauma) fracture [9] (Table 3).

Prevention and Treatment

Nonpharmacological

There are several nonpharmacological measures that can be taken to help prevent and treat osteoporosis. These measures include an active lifestyle with weight bearing exercises, fall precautions, avoidance of tobacco and excessive alcohol use, and adequate intake of calcium and vitamin D. These measures should be started early in life and continued. BMD peaks around age 35 and then is slowly lost. This loss is accelerated in women after menopause when estrogen levels drop.

Calcium

The recommended daily intake of calcium for postmenopausal women is 1200 mg/day. For adult men, it is slightly lower at 1000 mg/day [10]. Calcium supplementation is recommended if a sufficient amount cannot be obtained by diet alone. There are different formulations of calcium supplements, citrate and carbonate. Calcium citrate is best absorbed when taken between meals. Conversely, calcium carbonate is best absorbed when taken with meals. No form of calcium should be taken with iron as iron decreases intestinal absorption of calcium. Studies have shown that calcium in combination with Vitamin D can increase BMD and may or may not decrease fracture risk in postmenopausal women

[11]. Given its mild effect on BMD and fracture risk, supplementation alone is not recommended as monotherapy for osteoporosis.

Vitamin D

Vitamin D assists with calcium absorption. The recommended daily intake of vitamin D needed for adequate calcium absorption is 600–800 IU according to the National Institutes of Health (see Table 4). The National Osteoporosis Foundation (NOF) differs slightly. NOF recommends 400–800 IU for those under age 50 and a higher intake of 800–1000 IU for those over age 50 [12]. Patients with a documented Vitamin D deficiency (<20 ng/mL) or insufficiency (20-29 ng/mL) should be treated with 5000 IU of Vitamin D3 (cholecalciferol) daily for 8–12 weeks followed by a maintenance dose of 1000 IU of Vitamin D3 daily. Supplementation with D3 rather than D2 (ergocalciferol) may be preferable because many laboratory assays do not measure D2 as accurately. The treatment goal is a serum 25(OH)D level greater than 30 ng/mL. Rarely, higher doses (up to 10,000 IU weekly) may be required to achieve adequate levels of vitamin D.

Table 4 Optimal calcium[a] and vitamin D intake[b]

Population	Calcium	Vitamin D
Infants, children, and young adults		
0–6 months	200	400
6–12 months	260	400
1–13 years	700–1300	400–600
14–18 years	1300	600
Adult women		
Pregnant or lactating		
14–18 years	1300	600
19–50 years	1200	600
Other		
51–70 years	1200	600
71+ years	1200	800
Adult men		
19–70 years	1000	600
71+ years	1200	800

Adapted from the National Institutes of Health Recommendations on Calcium and Vitamin D 2019

[a]Calcium recommendations in mg/day

[b]Vitamin D recommendations in IU/day

Physical Activity

Maintaining an active lifestyle with adequate physical activity, particularly weight-bearing exercise is important in maintaining musculoskeletal health. Exercise has been shown to slightly increase BMD and slightly reduce the risk of having a fracture. Weight-bearing activities include but are not limited to walking, climbing stairs, elliptical machines, and resistance training with weights. Maintaining a healthy and active lifestyle may also reduce the risk of falls, which in turn may reduce the risk of fractures [13].

Fall Prevention

Falls cause the majority of osteoporotic fractures. Risk factors for falls are numerous and include visual or hearing impairments, musculoskeletal disorders, cognitive disorders, and advanced age. Many medications can also increase the risk of falls. These include antidepressants, antipsychotics, benzodiazepines, diuretics, beta blockers, and antihypertensives. A detailed history should be obtained on each patient to document fall risks and identify any potentially concerning medications. It may be appropriate to start patients in an exercise program or physical therapy to improve balance and strength or adjust medications to prevent future falls.

Pharmacological Treatment

Pharmacological treatment is the mainstay of osteoporosis management. Available agents for prevention and treatment of osteoporosis include bisphosphonates, calcitonin, hormone therapy, estrogen agonists/antagonists, parathyroid hormone (PTH), the RANK Ligand inhibitor Denosumab, and Romosozumab.

Indications for treatment:

- Diagnosis of osteoporosis
- Diagnosis of osteopenia plus >3% risk of hip fracture or >20% risk of major osteoporotic fracture in 10 years based on FRAX score
- A history of vertebral or hip fractures

The optimal duration of treatment has not been determined. The decision of when to stop treatment or consider a drug holiday remains controversial and will depend on the agent used and the severity of disease.

Bisphosphonates

Bisphosphonates are considered first-line therapy for the treatment and prevention of osteoporosis due to high efficacy, low side effects, and reasonable cost [9]. They are available in both oral and intravenous preparations. All of the agents listed below are FDA approved for both the prevention and treatment of postmenopausal osteoporosis except Ibandronate, which is approved for treatment only. The most common side effect from the oral preparations is acid reflux. Therefore patients should be advised to take the medication with a full glass of water on an empty stomach and remain upright for 30–60 min. Osteonecrosis of the jaw is a rare but serious side effect, affecting 1/10,000 to 1/100,000 people each year. This risk is higher with IV than oral bisphosphonates.

Alendronate (Fosamax)

Alendronate reduces the incidence of spine and hip fractures by about 50% over 3 years with or without a history of previous fracture. It is an oral medication. The recommended starting dose for postmenopausal osteoporosis prevention is 5 mg/day or 35 mg/week. Treatment dose is 10 mg/day or 70 mg/week. Weekly dosing may increase adherence as it is simpler and causes less esophageal irritation from acid reflux.

Risedronate (Actonel)

Risedronate reduces the incidence of vertebral fractures by 41–49% and nonvertebral fractures by 36% over 3 years. It is an oral medication and has fewer gastrointestinal side effects than alendronate. Dosing options include 5 mg daily, 35 mg weekly, 75 mg twice monthly, and 150 mg monthly.

Ibandronate (Boniva)

Ibandronate has been shown to decrease the incidence of vertebral fractures by about 50%. However, it has not been shown to significantly reduce nonvertebral fractures. It is available oral or IV. The recommended dose is 150 mg every month by mouth or 3 mg IV every 3 months.

Zoledronic Acid (Reclast)

Zoledronic acid is the only exclusively IV preparation among the bisphosphonates. It has been shown to decrease vertebral fractures by 70%, hip fractures by 41%, and other nonvertebral fractures by 25% over 3 years in those with osteoporosis. Zoledronic acid is given as 5 mg IV once a year for osteoporosis treatment. For prevention in postmenopausal women, the same dose is given but every 2 years.

Hormonal

Hormone Replacement Therapy (HRT)

Hormone replacement therapy is FDA approved for the prevention of osteoporosis in women. However, it should not be used unless there are no viable alternatives due to safety issues. HRT has been shown to decrease vertebral and hip fractures by 34% but may increase risk of myocardial infarction, stroke, breast cancer, pulmonary embolus, and deep vein thrombosis [14]. These risks increase with higher doses and longer duration of use.

Estrogen Agonist/Antagonists

Estrogen Agonist/Antagonists work by acting on estrogen receptors within the bone to prevent resorption and have been shown to increase BMD and decrease vertebral fractures in postmenopausal women. However, they are less effective than bisphosphonates and carry a risk of venous thromboembolism similar to HRT. They may also cause menopausal symptoms during use. They are therefore considered second-line treatments. Raloxifine is the preferred agent in this category and has been shown to decrease the risk of breast cancer. It may be a reasonable alternative for postmenopausal women who cannot tolerate bisphosphonates or are at increased risk of invasive breast cancer. Premenopausal women should not be treated with estrogen agonist/antagonist as they may actually decrease BMD in this population [15].

Calcitonin

Calcitonin is an alternative treatment for osteoporosis. It inhibits bone resorption by binding to osteoclasts. It is available in several forms including intranasal, intramuscular, and subcutaneous. The nasal dosing is usually preferred due to ease of use and lower side effect profile. Though not as effective, calcitonin may be a reasonable alternative for patients unable to tolerate bisphosphonates [16]. It can also be used for short-term analgesia following a vertebral fracture [17].

Parathyroid Hormone (PTH)

PTH works as an anabolic agent by stimulating osteoblastic activity rather than reducing bone resorption. It is the only anabolic agent FDA approved for the prevention and treatment of osteoporosis. Two formulations are available, teriparatide (Forteo) and abaloparatide (Tymlos). It is administered in a daily subcutaneous injection and has been shown to significantly increase BMD and decrease fractures. PTH is not a first-line treatment because it can have more side effects than other agents. It can cause hypercalcemia, hyperuricemia, and increased risk of osteosarcoma, though this has not been confirmed in any human trials [18]. The FDA recommends limiting PTH therapy to 2 years until further longitudinal studies have been completed. The benefits of PTH fade quickly after discontinuation unless followed by antiresorptive therapy such as a bisphosphonate.

RANK Ligand Inhibitor

Denosumab (Prolia) is FDA approved for the treatment of osteoporosis in postmenopausal women with high risk of fracture. It has been shown to decrease vertebral and hip fractures at similar rates to bisphosphonates. It is given as subcutaneous injection every 6 months. It can decrease serum calcium levels, so any underlying hypocalcemia should be corrected prior to starting treatment [19]. Benefit fades quickly with discontinuation of denosumab and there may be an increased risk of multiple vertebral fractures. Because of this, patients should be counseled on the risks of missed doses and transitioned to an oral bisphosphonate after discontinuation.

Romosozumab (Evenity)

Romosozumab is FDA approved for the treatment of osteoporosis in women at high risk of fracture.

It works by both anabolic and antiresorptive mechanisms. It is given as a subcutaneous injection of 210 mg each month for 12 months. After 1 year of treatment, patients must be transitioned to another antiresorptive therapy such as a bisphosphonate to maintain clinical benefits, much like PTH and denosumab. Romosozumab may increase the risk of serious cardiovascular events, limiting its use in those with high risk of such events, recent MI, or recent stroke. It is not currently recommended as a first line agent [4].

Monitoring and Duration of Treatment

DXA scans should not be repeated less than 2 years apart for most patients [7]. Optimal frequency of bone density monitoring is unknown, but evidence does not support routine monitoring with DXA every 2 years. For example, a study of women with normal or mildly osteopenic BMD found that 90% will remain in that range at 15 years. Only 10% will progress to osteoporosis [9]. Thus, intervals of up to 10–15 years may be appropriate for these patients. Among women with moderate or severe osteopenia, 10% developed osteoporosis at 5 years and 1 year, respectively [9]. DXA should be repeated when results will change management or rapid changes are expected [4].

For those on pharmacologic therapy, American College of Physicians (ACP) guidelines recommend against monitoring in the first five years of treatment based on evidence that treatment reduces fracture risk even in the absence of improvements in measured bone density [9]. Duration of treatment is commonly 5–10 years. It is reasonable to consider discontinuation after 5 years of treatment with an oral bisphosphonate. Patients at high risk of fracture may benefit from continuation beyond 5 years.

Conclusion

Osteoporosis is a common condition that greatly increases the risk of fracture with subsequent increases in morbidity and mortality. Measures should be taken early in life to prevent the development of osteoporosis including exercise, adequate calcium and vitamin D intake, and avoidance of tobacco and excessive alcohol use. A detailed history is essential to identify patients at increased risk of developing osteoporosis. Universal screening is recommended for all women at age 65 and above and should be considered in other patients at risk. DXA is the gold standard for screening and diagnosis of osteoporosis. Bisphosphonates are first-line therapy for both prevention and treatment of osteoporosis. The optimal interval for repeating DXA is unclear but up to 5 years for those being started on treatment with bisphosphonates and up to 10–15 years for those with normal or mildly low bone density may be appropriate. Patients with high risk of fracture may require monitoring as frequently as every 2 years. Routine monitoring with DXA every 1–2 years is likely unnecessary for most patients.

References

1. Looker AC, Borrud LG, Dawson-Hughes B, Shepherd JA, Wright NC. Osteoporosis or low bone mass at the femur neck or lumbar spine in older adults: United States, 2005–2008. NCHS Data Brief. 2012;93:1–8.
2. National Osteoporosis Foundation. What is osteoporosis? http://www.nof.org/osteoporosis/articles/7. Accessed 19 Feb 2014
3. Bentler SE, Liu L, Obrizan M, Cook EA, Wright KB, Geweke JF, Chrischilles EA, Pavlik CE, Wallace RB, Ohsfeldt RL, Jones MP, Rosenthal GE, Wolinsky FD. The aftermath of hip fracture: discharge placement, functional status change, and mortality. Am J Epidemiol. 2009;170(10):1290.
4. Camacho P, Petak S, Binkley N, Diab D, Eldeiry L, Farooki A, et al. American Association of Clinical Endocrinologists/American College of Endocrinology Clinical Practice Guidelines for the diagnosis and treatment of postmenopausal osteoporosis. Endocr Pract. 2020;26(5):564–70.
5. Feskanich D, Willett W, Colditz G. Walking and leisure-time activity and risk of hip fracture in postmenopausal women. JAMA. 2002;288(18):2300.
6. Wang PS, Solomon DH, Mogun H, Avorn J. HMG-CoA reductase inhibitors and the risk of hip fractures in elderly patients. JAMA. 2000;283:3211.
7. The International Society for Densitometry. ISCD official positions – adult. Middletown: The International Society for Densitometry; 2013. http://www.iscd.org/official-positions/2013-iscd-official-positions-adult/. Accessed 3 Jan 2015.
8. Kanis JA, on behalf of the World Health Organization Scientific Group. Assessment of osteoporosis at the primary health-care level. Technical report. World Health Organization Collaborating Centre for Metabolic Bone Diseases, University of Sheffield. http://www.shef.ac.uk/FRAX/pdfs/WHO_Technical_Report.pdf. Accessed 22 Dec 2014.
9. Qaseem A, Forciea M, McLean R, Denberg T. Treatment of low bone density or osteoporosis to prevent fractures in men and women: a clinical practice guideline update from the American College of Physicians. Ann Intern Med. 2017;166(11):818.
10. New recommended daily amounts of Calcium and Vitamin D. NIH Medline Plus. Winter 2011;5(4):12. http://www.nlm.nih.gov/medlineplus/magazine/issues/winter11/articles/winter11pg12.html. Accessed 19 Feb 2015.
11. Jackson RD, LaCroix AZ, Gass M, Wallace RB, Robbins J, Lewis CE, et al. Calcium plus vitamin D supplementation and the risk of fractures. N Engl J Med. 2006;354(7):669.
12. National Osteoporosis Foundation. Calcium and Vitamin D: what you need to know. http://nof.org/articles/10#howmuchvitamind. Accessed 23 Dec 2014.
13. Howe TE, Shea B, Dawson LJ, Downie F, Murray A, Ross C, et al. Exercise for preventing and treating osteoporosis in postmenopausal women. Cochrane Database Syst Rev. 2011;7:CD000333.
14. Rossouw JE, Anderson GL, Prentice RL, et al. Risks and benefits of estrogen plus progestin in healthy postmenopausal women: principle results from the Women's Health Initiative randomized controlled trial. JAMA. 2002;288(3):321–33.
15. Eng-Wong J, Reynolds JC, Venzon D, Liewehr D, Gantz S, Danforth D, et al. Effect of raloxifene on bone mineral density in premenopausal women at increased risk of breast cancer. J Clin Endocrinol Metab. 2006;91(10):3941.
16. Downs RW Jr, Bell NH, Ettinger MP, Walsh BW, Favus MJ, Mako B, Wang L, Smith ME, Gormley GJ, Melton ME. Comparison of alendronate and intranasal calcitonin for treatment of osteoporosis in postmenopausal women. J Clin Endocrinol Metab. 2000;85(5):1783.
17. Knopp-Sihota JA, Newburn-Cook CV, Homik J, Cummings GG, Voaklander D. 1-calcitonin for treating acute and chronic pain of recent and remote osteoporotic vertebral compression fractures: a systematic review and meta-analysis. Osteoporos Int. 2012;23(1):17.
18. Vahle JL, Sato M, Long GG, et al. Skeletal changes in rats given daily subcutaneous injections of recombinant human parathyroid hormone (1–34) for 2 years and relevance to human safety. Toxicol Pathol. 2002;30(3):312.
19. Cummings SR, San Martin J, McClung MR, et al. Denosumab for prevention of fractures in postmenopausal women with osteoporosis. N Engl J Med. 2009;361(8):756–65.

Douglas J. Inciarte and Susan Evans

Contents

Introduction

Nutrition disorders seen in primary care are common in the daily medical practice, either in the inpatient or outpatient setting. The assessment and management of nutritional disorders are linked to intestinal and liver disorders that interfere with the nutrient metabolism, affecting the overall care of the patient. Malabsorption of nutrients in the human body causes multiple symptoms and signs such as diarrhea, musculoskeletal, neurological, skin, and mucous membrane pathology resulting in weight loss, weakness, malnutrition, and electrolyte abnormalities.

This chapter will discuss the most common nutritional disorders by mineral or vitamin deficiency causing neurological disorders and other symptoms.

Vitamin and Mineral Deficiencies

Vitamin D Deficiency

Vitamin D deficiency continues to be fairly common in children and adults. In recent years, significant proportions of the populations in North America and global populations are affected with Vitamin D deficiency, although it is not consider

D. J. Inciarte (✉)
West Kendall Baptist Health/Florida International University, Herbert Wertheim, College of Medicine, Family Medicine Residency Program, Florida, SW, USA
e-mail: douglasi@baptisthealth.net

S. Evans
Department of Family Medicine, University of Nebraska College of Medicine, Omaha, NE, USA
e-mail: susan.evans@unmc.edu

© Springer Nature Switzerland AG 2022
P. M. Paulman et al. (eds.), *Family Medicine*,
https://doi.org/10.1007/978-3-030-54441-6_130

as a pandemic. A consequence of low vitamin D levels resulted in rickets which was considered a disease that was essentially eliminated years ago after milk was fortified with vitamin D, we now know that even in utero and during childhood, vitamin D deficiency can cause growth retardation and skeletal deformities.

Applying the correct method to data from the National Health and Nutrition Examination Survey (NHANES) for 2007 through 2010 reveals that 13% of Americans 1 to 70 years of age are "at risk" for vitamin D inadequacy. Less than 6% are deficient in vitamin D [serum 25(OH)D levels <12.5 ng per milliliter.

Vitamin D deficiency in adults can increase the risk of osteopenia and osteoporosis and can cause osteomalacia and muscle weakness, thereby increasing the risk of fracture.

The discovery that most tissues and cells in the body have a vitamin D receptor and that several possess the enzymatic machinery to convert the primary circulating form of vitamin D, 25-hydroxyvitamin D, to the active form, 1,25-dihydroxyvitamin D, has provided new insights into the function of this vitamin. Of great interest is the role it can play in decreasing the risk of many chronic illnesses, including common cancers, autoimmune diseases, infectious diseases, and cardiovascular disease [1].

Vitamin D is not a vitamin. It is a prohormone that is synthesized in the skin simplistic from a metabolite of cholesterol.

It is further metabolized to a family of molecules that principally function in the regulation of intestinal calcium absorption [2].

Solar ultraviolet B radiation (wavelength, 290–315 nm) penetrates the skin and converts 7-dehydrocholesterol to previtamin D3, which is rapidly converted to vitamin D3. Because any excess previtamin D3 or vitamin D3 is destroyed by sunlight, excessive exposure to sunlight does not cause vitamin D3 intoxication.

Few foods naturally contain or are fortified with vitamin D. Vitamin D2 is manufactured through ultraviolet irradiation of ergosterol from yeast and vitamin D3 through the ultraviolet irradiation of 7-dehydrocholesterol from lanolin. Both are used in over-the-counter vitamin D supplements, but the form available by prescription in

the United States is vitamin D2. Vitamin D from the skin and diet is metabolized in the liver to 25-hydroxyvitamin D, which is used to determine a patient's vitamin D status, and 25-hydroxyvitamin D is metabolized in the kidneys by the enzyme 25-hydroxyvitamin D-1α- hydroxylase (CYP27B1) to its active form, 1,25-dihydroxyvitamin D. The renal production of 1,25-dihydroxyvitamin D is tightly regulated by plasma parathyroid hormone levels and serum calcium and phosphorus levels. The efficiency of the absorption of renal calcium and of intestinal calcium and phosphorus is increased in the presence of 1,25-dihydroxyvitamin D [1].

Patients with chronic kidney disease (CKD) are at a higher risk of vitamin D deficiency due to either renal losses or decreased synthesis of 1,25-dihydroxyvitamin D. Measuring parathyroid hormone (PTH) levels to identify optimal levels of Vitamin D 25(OH) remains controversial as the relationship between both is inconsistent.

Because vitamin D is produced by the actions of sunlight on the skin, its deficiency does not usually represent a dietary deficiency, but is seen in those whose skin exposure to ultraviolet light is inadequate; this group includes individuals who, as a result of illness or frailty, seldom venture outdoors, who live at high latitude (particularly if they have dark skin), and who habitually completely cover their skin (e.g., veiled women). The melanin in pigmented skin absorbs ultraviolet light and reduces vitamin D synthesis. This is a valuable protective mechanism in those living in intensely sunny climates, but becomes a liability when these individuals move to relatively sunless environments, such as the cities of Northern Europe and North America. Low 25-hydroxyvitamin D levels are found in the exclusively breastfed infants of vitamin D-deficient mothers, so supplementation of pregnant women and their infants in high-risk groups is advised [3].

Although there is no consensus on optimal levels of 25-hydroxyvitamin D as measured in serum, vitamin D deficiency is defined by most experts as a 25-hydroxyvitamin D level of less than 20 ng per milliliter (50 nmol per liter) [4–6].

Serum 25-hydroxyvitamin D level is the best indicator to assess overall vitamin D levels due to that this measurement reflects total vitamin D from dietary intake and sunlight exposure, as well as the conversion of vitamin D from adipose stores in the liver.

Symptoms of vitamin D deficiency are related to rickets in children and osteomalacia in adults. It is very common that patients with vitamin D deficiency can present with bone pain, fatigue fractures, muscular cramps, muscle pain, and gait disorders, with an increased incidence of falls in the elderly [7].

Vitamin D deficiency is treated with vitamin D oral supplementation, and the recommended dose of vitamin D depends upon the nature and severity of the vitamin D deficiency.

In patients who do not have problems absorbing vitamin D:

- If 25-hydroxyvitamin (25-OH-D) is less than 20 ng/mL (50 nmol/L), treatment includes 50,000 international units of vitamin D2 or D3 by mouth once per week for 6–8 weeks, and then 800–1,000 (or more) international units of vitamin D3 daily thereafter. The vitamin D levels should be retested in 6 weeks after the treatment was started.
- In patients with a level between 20 and 30 ng/mL (50–75 nmol/L), treatment usually includes 800–1,000 international units of vitamin D3 by mouth daily, usually for a 3-month period. However, many individuals will need higher doses.
- Once a normal level is achieved, continued therapy with 800 international units of vitamin D per day is usually recommended.
- In infants and children whose 25-OH-D is less than 20 ng/mL (50 nmol/L), treatment usually includes 1,000–5,000 international units of vitamin D2 by mouth per day (depending on the age of the child) for 2–3 months.
- In patients who have diseases or conditions that prevent them from absorbing vitamin D normally (e.g., kidney or liver disease), the recommended dose of vitamin D will be determined on an individual basis. When vitamin D level is normal (>30 ng/mL [≥75 nmol/L]), a dose of 800 international units of vitamin D per day is usually recommended [8].
- Vitamin D dosing represents the safe boundary at the high end of the scale and should not be misunderstood as amounts people need or should strive to consume. While these values

vary somewhat by age, intakes of vitamin D should not surpass 4,000 IUs per day, due to increased risk for harm. Once intakes surpass 2,000 IU per day for calcium, the risk for harm also increases. As Americans take more supplements and eat more of foods that have been fortified with vitamin D and calcium, it becomes more likely that people consume high amounts of these nutrients. Kidney stones have been associated with taking too much calcium from dietary supplements. Very high levels of vitamin D (above 10,000 IUs per day) are known to cause kidney and tissue damage [9].

Vitamin B12 Deficiency

Vitamin B_{12} (cobalamin) deficiency was recognized as a health concern nearly 100 years ago and continues to have clinical significance.

It is particularly common in the elderly (>65 years of age), but is often unrecognized because of its subtle clinical manifestations, although they can be potentially serious, particularly from a neuropsychiatric and hematological perspective. In the general population, the main causes of cobalamin deficiency are pernicious anemia and food-cobalamin malabsorption.

Food-cobalamin malabsorption syndrome, which has only recently been identified, is a disorder characterized by the inability to release cobalamin from food or its binding proteins.

Cobalamin malabsorption syndrome is usually caused by atrophic gastritis, related or unrelated to *Helicobacter pylori* infection, and long-term ingestion of antacids and biguanides [10].

Both the clinical recognition of vitamin B12 deficiency and confirmation of the diagnosis by means of testing can be difficult. The patient's history may include symptoms of anemia, underlying disorders causing malabsorption, and neurologic symptoms.

The most common neurologic symptoms are symmetric paresthesia or numbness and gait problems [11, 12].

Physical examination may reveal pallor, edema, pigmentary disorders in the skin, jaundice, or neurologic defects such as impaired vibration sense, impaired position and cutaneous sensation, ataxia, and general weakness.

The first test performed to confirm the diagnosis of vitamin B12 deficiency is generally measurement of the serum vitamin B12 level. Both false negative and false positive values are common (occurring in up to 50% of tests) with the use of the laboratory-reported lower limit of the normal range as a cutoff point for deficiency [11].

Given the limitations of available assays, clinicians should not use a laboratory's reported lower limit of the normal range to rule out the diagnosis of vitamin B12 deficiency in patients with compatible clinical abnormalities; because of this concern, obtaining a methylmalonic acid (MMA) level, total homocysteine, or both is useful in making the diagnosis of vitamin B12 deficiency in patients who have not received treatment. The levels of both methylmalonic acid and total homocysteine are markedly elevated in the vast majority (>98%) of patients with clinical B12 deficiency [13].

Elevated levels of MMA and total homocysteine decrease immediately after treatment, and the levels can be remeasured to document adequate vitamin B12 replacement.

The level of serum total homocysteine is less specific, since it is also elevated in folate deficiency [13], classic homocystinuria, and renal failure.

If the patient consumes sufficient amounts of vitamin B12 and has clinically confirmed B12 deficiency, then malabsorption (pernicious anemia) must be present. Chronic atrophic gastritis and intestinal vitamin B12 malabsorption should be investigated. A positive test for anti-intrinsic factor or antiparietal cell (both highly specific 100% and 50–100%) antibodies is indicative of pernicious anemia; surveillance for autoimmune thyroid disease is reasonable in patients with positive antibody tests.

Chronic atrophic gastritis can be diagnosed on the basis of an elevated fasting serum gastrin level and a low level of serum pepsinogen I [14]. Some experts recommend endoscopy to confirm gastritis and rule out gastric carcinoid and other gastric cancers, since patients with pernicious anemia are at increased risk for such cancers [14].

For the treatment of vitamin B12 deficiency, oral replacement must be considered. Healthy older adults should consider taking supplemental crystalline vitamin B12 as recommended by the Food and Nutrition Board. Unfortunately, most patients with clinical vitamin B12 deficiency have malabsorption and will require parenteral or high-dose oral replacement. Adequate supplementation results in resolution of megaloblastic anemia and resolution of or improvement in myelopathy.

The most recommended treatment is schedules for injections of vitamin B12 (called cyanocobalamin in the United States and hydroxocobalamin in Europe) [15, 16].

Patients with severe disease should receive injections of 1,000 μg at least several times per week for 1–2 weeks, then weekly until clear improvement is shown, followed by monthly injections. Hematologic response is rapid, with an increase in the reticulocyte count in 1 week and correction of megaloblastic anemia in 6–8 weeks. Patients with severe anemia and cardiac symptoms should be treated with transfusion and diuretic agents, and electrolytes should be monitored. Neurologic symptoms may worsen transiently and then subside over weeks to months [12].

The treatment for pernicious anemia is lifelong, and in patients in whom vitamin B12 supplementation is discontinued after clinical recovery, past neurologic symptoms will recur within as short a period as 6 months, and megaloblastic anemia recurs in several years [15].

Folic Acid Deficiency

Folic acid or folate refers to a family of compounds that belongs to the group of vitamin B cofactors that participate in the methylation of homocysteine to methionine and to the conversion of S-adenosylmethionine (SAM), the universal methyl donor, to processes involving DNA, RNA, hormones, neurotransmitters, membrane lipids, and proteins. Food folates are present in animal products as well as green leafy vegetables, fruits, cereals and grains, nuts, and meats.

The most common cause of folic acid or folate deficiency is nutritional, either due to poor diet and/or alcoholism. Normal body stores are small (5–10 mg), and individuals on a folate-deficient diet and/or alcoholics can develop megaloblastic anemia within 4–5 months, even sooner if they have a low folate intake (5–10 weeks) [17].

In child-bearing women, a high dose of folic acid supplement reduces the incidence of recurrent neural tube defects by 70% [18].

Folate deficiency is also common in elderly older adults. In one study the age-specific prevalence of folate deficiency was approximately 5–10% in those ages 65–74 years [19].

Alcohol abuse produces a sharp fall in serum folate within 2–4 days by impairing its enterohepatic cycle and inhibiting its absorption. Alcoholics can develop megaloblastosis within 5–10 weeks. Folate depletion is quicker than the 4–5 months required in normal patients in part because alcoholics often have lower folate stores due to previous dietary habits.

Several drugs interfere with folic acid metabolism including trimethoprim, pyrimethamine, methotrexate, and phenytoin.

The classic clinical presentation of folate deficiency is quite different from that of B12 deficiency; in folic acid deficiency, it is rare to see neurological changes or symptoms.

Exceptions to this general rule are the rare cases of hereditary folate malabsorption and/or metabolism, which are associated with progressive neurologic deterioration early in life [20]. For the diagnosis of folate deficiency, one must obtain assays of serum or red cell folate, serum B12, methylmalonate, and homocysteine to distinguish between folate and vitamin B12 deficiency.

The treatment of folic acid deficiency is 1–5 mg per day of oral folate supplementation, and the duration of the treatment should be for 1–4 months or until complete hematologic recovery occurs.

A dose of 1 mg per day of folic acid is usually sufficient and recommended for disease prevention in normal adults, alcoholics, the elderly, and prevention of neural tube defects in female patients of child-bearing age.

Iron Deficiency

Iron deficiency is the most prevalent nutritional deficiency worldwide affecting people in both developing and developed countries. Globally, iron deficiency anemia caused 34.7 million years lived with disability between 2000 and 2016 which puts in in the top five causes of disability globally (GDB 2016) [21]. Iron deficiency is prevalent in pediatric patients and in premenopausal women in both low-income and developed countries [21].

Symptoms of iron deficiency can include pallor, fatigue, cheilosis, and atrophy of the lingual papillae. In developing countries, the most common causes of iron deficiency are poor dietary intake and chronic blood loss due to parasitic infections. In developed countries, those at risk include children up to age 5 due to their rapid growth and menstruating and pregnant women. Gastrointestinal conditions resulting in malabsorption, a history of weight loss surgery, gastrointestinal bleed, gastrointestinal cancer, or the use of antiacid medicines can cause iron deficiency. The elderly are also at risk due to increased prevalence of chronic disease and medication use such as aspirin, NSAIDs, and anticoagulants. (Lopez) [22].

While a low hemoglobin level diagnoses anemia, it is not a good screening test for iron deficiency because many people are iron deficient while their hemoglobin remains normal. A low ferritin <15 μg is diagnostic of iron deficiency, but a normal ferritin does not rule out iron deficiency in the context of inflammation. A higher cutoff for ferritin such as 30 μg has been recommended to increase the sensitivity of ferritin for iron deficiency. In iron deficiency, serum iron will be reduced and total iron-binding capacity will be increased. This results in a decrease in transferrin saturation to less than 16% or less than 20% in the context of inflammation. (Lopez) [22].

Iron replacement therapy can be administered orally or parenterally. The recommended dose for adults is 100–200 mg elemental iron in divided daily doses taken without food. Children are recommended to take 3–6 mg per kg body weight of liquid iron daily. While this should lead to rapid improvement, ongoing therapy for several months may be needed to replete iron stores. Long-term use of oral iron is limited by side effects including nausea, vomiting, constipation, and metallic taste. Parenteral replacement of iron has become more common with newer and safer intravenous iron and is indicated when blood loss is too rapid for oral replacement, the patient is not able to absorb oral iron or is unable to tolerate the side effects. The dose of iron needed is calculated with the following formula: body weight in kg × 2.3 × hemoglobin deficiency. Hemoglobin deficiency is the target hemoglobin level – patient hemoglobin level. Another 500–1000 mg iron can be added to replace iron stores. There are several forms of IV iron available in the USA including iron sucrose which is often given at a dose of 200 mg IV over 2–5 min and repeated until the target dose is reached. (Camaschella) [23].

Malnutrition

Malnutrition is a very important problem that is encountered more often than expected in medical practice and results from inadequate or poor-quality food intake or from diseases that alter food intake or nutrient requirements, metabolism, or absorption.

Malnutrition can be classified via primary and secondary causes. Primary malnutrition presents in third-world or developing countries where social or political conditions have deteriorated. Secondary malnutrition is seen in first-world or industrialized countries. It presents in populations with adequate food supplies which can become malnourished as a result of acute or chronic diseases that alter nutrient intake or metabolism, particularly diseases that cause acute or chronic inflammation.

In terms of primary malnutrition, the most common diseases are *marasmus* and *kwashiorkor*. Marasmus results from long-term deficit of dietary energy. Kwashiorkor is the result of a poor protein intake diet. Energy-poor diets with minimal inflammation cause gradual erosion of body mass, resulting in classic marasmus. By contrast, inflammation from acute illnesses such as injury

or sepsis or from chronic illnesses such as cancer, lung or heart disease, or HIV infection can erode lean body mass even in the presence of relatively sufficient dietary intake, leading to a kwashiorkor-like state. Quite often, inflammatory illnesses impair appetite and dietary intake, producing combinations of the two conditions [24].

The difference between marasmus and cachexia is that marasmus is a starvation-related malnutrition where all available body fat stores have been exhausted due to starvation without systemic inflammation. Cachexia is related to chronic disease malnutrition with loss of lean body mass due to chronic systemic inflammation. The diagnosis is based on fat and muscle wastage resulting from prolonged calorie deficiency and/or inflammation. Diminished skinfold thickness reflects the loss of fat reserves; reduced arm muscle circumference with temporal and interosseous muscle wasting reflects the catabolism of protein throughout the body, including in vital organs such as the heart, liver, and kidneys [24].

Routine laboratory findings in cachexia/marasmus are relatively unremarkable. The creatinine-height index (24-h urinary creatinine excretion compared with normal values based on height) is low, reflecting the loss of muscle mass. Occasionally, the serum albumin level is reduced, but it remains above 2.8 g/dL when systemic inflammation is absent. In kwashiorkor there is a connection with acute, life-threatening conditions such as trauma and sepsis. The physiologic stress produced by these illnesses increases protein and energy requirements at a time when intake is often limited. Physical exam and laboratory findings include increased hair pluckability, edema, skin breakdown, and poor wound healing with severe decrease of albumin (<2.8 g/dL) and transferrin (<150 mg/dL). Lymphocytopenia (<1,500 lymphocytes/μL) can be also encountered.

Other mineral deficiencies such as vitamin C and zinc are relatively common in sick patients. Scurvy is rare in developed countries. Signs of corkscrew hairs on the lower extremities are found frequently in chronically ill and/or alcoholic patients. Scurvy can be diagnosed by determination of plasma vitamin C levels. Low zinc levels are common in patients with malabsorption syndromes such as inflammatory bowel disease, and they present with poor wound healing, pressure ulcer formation, and impaired immunity.

Thiamine deficiency is a common problem of alcoholism and is replaced with oral formulations.

The treatment of vitamin C deficiency is 250–500 mg/d of oral formulations. Patients with zinc deficiencies will need oral supplementation with 220 mg of zinc sulfate one to three times daily.

In the inpatient setting, hypophosphatemia results from rapid intracellular shifts of phosphate in underweight or alcoholic patients receiving intravenous glucose, with numerous complications such as acute cardiopulmonary failure, collectively called refeeding syndrome, and can be life-threatening; in these situations, consulting a clinical nutritionist is necessary.

Nutritional Requirements for Health Maintenance, Gender/Age/Disease, or Activity

Data from the 2007 to 2008 National Health and Nutrition Examination Survey (NHANES) suggested that nearly half of US adults aged 20–69 reported taking at least one dietary supplement in the past month. The factors that were independently associated with a greater likelihood of supplement use are as follows: being female, older, white race, having higher level of education, nonsupplemental nutrition access program (SNAP) participation, and living in a food-secure household. When considering nutrients from food, supplement users tended to consume greater amounts of vitamin A, vitamin C, vitamin E, folic acid, calcium, and iron. There was no association between supplement use and daily intakes of vitamin B12 and zinc from food sources only. Including nutrients from daily supplement use, supplement users consumed greater amounts of all eight nutrients [25].

One research study regarding the use of vitamins did show additional support for the conclusion that the vast majority of consumers recognize that multivitamins and other supplements can be helpful in filling nutrient gaps in the diet but should not be viewed as replacements for a healthy diet or healthy lifestyle habits. This finding suggests that policy makers and health professionals could feel comfortable recommending rational dietary supplementation as one means of improving nutrient intakes, without being unduly concerned that such a recommendation would lead consumers to discount the importance of good dietary habits.

The online tool at http://fnic.nal.usda.gov/interactiveDRI/ allows health professionals to calculate individualized daily nutrient recommendations for dietary planning based on the DRIs for persons of a given age, sex, and weight. To provide guidance for food education, a good reference is the U.S. Department of Agriculture (USDA) MyPlate Food Guide for individuals (www.supertracker.usda.gov/default.aspx), to create food-exchange lists for therapeutic diet planning, and as a standard for describing the nutritional content of foods and nutrient-containing dietary supplements [26].

The authors conclude that a well-balanced lifestyle along with exercise should never be replaced by the use of vitamins; however, the use of daily calcium, vitamin D, and folic acid in child-bearing women has been proven to prevent diseases.

References

1. Hoick MF. Medical progress vitamin D deficiency. N Engl J Med. 2007;357:266–81.
2. Reid IR. What diseases are causally linked to vitamin D deficiency. Arch Dis Child. 2014. https://doi.org/10.1136/archdischild-2014-307961.
3. Holick MF. High prevalence of vitamin D inadequacy and implications for health. Mayo Clin Proc. 2006;81:353–73.
4. Bischoff-Ferrari HA, Giovannucci E, Willett WC, Dietrich T, Dawson-Hughes B. Estimation of optimal serum concentrations of 25-hydroxyvitamin D for multiple health outcomes. Am J Clin Nutr. 2006;84:18–28. [Erratum, Am J Clin Nutr 2006;84:1253.]
5. Malabanan A, Veronikis IE, Holick MF. Redefining vitamin D insufficiency. Lancet. 1998;351:805–6.
6. Thomas KK, Lloyd Jones DM, Thadhani RI, et al. Hypovitaminosis D in medical inpatients. N Engl J Med. 1998;338:777–83.
7. Rader, et al. Osteomalacia and vitamin D deficiency. Orthopade. 2015;44(9):695–702. https://doi.org/10.1007/s00132-015-3141-9. German
8. Drezner, et al. Uptodate patient information: vitamin D deficiency (Beyond the Basics) literature review current through. June 2015.

9. Institute of Medicine. Dietary reference intakes for calcium and vitamin D report brief. Nov 2010. For more information visit www.iom.edu/vitamind

10. Dali-Youcef N, Andrès E. An update on cobalamin deficiency in adults. Q J Med. 2009;102:17–28.

11. Lindenbaum J, Healton EB, Savage DG, et al. Neuropsychiatric disorders caused by cobalamin deficiency in the absence of anemia or macrocytosis. N Engl J Med. 1988;318:1720–8.

12. Healton EB, Savage DG, Brust JC, Garrett TJ, Lindenbaum J. Neurologic aspects of cobalamin deficiency. Medicine. 1991;70:229–45.

13. Savage DG, Lindenbaum J, Stabler SP, Allen RH. Sensitivity of serum methylmalonic acid and total homocysteine determinations for diagnosing cobalamin and folate deficiencies. Am J Med. 1994;96:239–46.

14. Toh BH, Chan J, Kyaw T, Alderuccio F. Cutting edge issues in autoimmune gastritis. Clin Rev Allergy Immunol. 2012;42:269–78.

15. Stabler SP. Megaloblastic anemias: pernicious anemia and folate deficiency. In: Young NS, Gerson SL, High KA, editors. Clinical hematology. Philadelphia: Mosby; 2006. p. 242–51.

16. Carmel R. How I treat cobalamin (vitamin B12) deficiency. Blood. 2008;112:2214–21.

17. MRC Vitamin Study Research Group. Prevention of neural tube defects: results of the Medical Research Council vitamin study. Lancet. 1991;338:131–7.

18. Anthony CA. Megaloblastic anemias. In: Hoffman R, Benz EJ, Shattil SJ, et al., editors. Hematology: basic principles and practice. 2nd ed. New York: Churchill Livingston; 1995. p. 552.

19. Clarke R, Grimley Evans J, Schneede J, et al. Vitamin B12 and folate deficiency in later life. Age Ageing. 2004;33:34.

20. Clayton PT, Smith I, Harding B, et al. Subacute combined degeneration of the cord, dementia and parkinsonism due to an inborn error of folate metabolism. J Neurol Neurosurg Psychiatry. 1986;49:920.

21. GBD 2017 Disease and Injury Incidence and Prevalence Collaborators. Global, regional, and national incidence, prevalence, and years lived with disability for 354 diseases and injuries for 195 countries and territories, 1990–2017: a systematic analysis for the Global Burden of Disease Study 2017 [published correction appears in Lancet. 2019 Jun 22;393(10190):e44]. Lancet. 2018;392(10159): 1789–858. https://doi.org/10.1016/S0140-6736(18) 32279-7.

22. Lopez A, Cacoub P, Macdougall IC, Peyrin-Biroulet L. Iron deficiency anaemia. Lancet. 2016;387 (10021):907–16. https://doi.org/10.1016/S0140-6736 (15)60865-0.

23. Camaschella C. Iron-deficiency anemia. N Engl J Med. 2015;372(19):1832–43. https://doi.org/10.1056/ NEJMra1401038.

24. Heimburger DC. Malnutrition and nutritional assessment. In: Kasper D, Fauci A, Hauser S, Longo D, Jameson J, Loscalzo J, editors. Harrison's principles of internal medicine, vol. 19e. New York: McGraw-Hill; 2015.

25. Kennedy, et al. Dietary supplement use pattern of U.S. adult population in the 2007–2008 National Health and Nutrition Examination Survey (NHANES). Ecol Food Nutr. 2013;52(1):76–84.

26. Dickinson A, MacKay D, Wong A. Consumer attitudes about the role of multivitamins and other dietary supplements: report of a survey. Nutr J. 2015;14:66.

Selected Disorders of the Endocrine and Metabolic System

129

Ashley Falk, Scott G. Garland, Nathan P. Falk, Dianna Pham, and Trevor Owens

Contents

A. Falk · S. G. Garland (✉) · N. P. Falk · D. Pham ·
T. Owens
Florida State University College of Medicine Family
Medicine Residency at BayCare Health System,
Winter Haven, FL, USA
e-mail: scott.garland@baycare.org;
nathan.falk@med.fsu.edu; Dianna.Pham@baycare.org;
Trevor.Owens@baycare.org

© Springer Nature Switzerland AG 2022
P. M. Paulman et al. (eds.), *Family Medicine*,
https://doi.org/10.1007/978-3-030-54441-6_188

The endocrine system governs the metabolic activities of the body, affects tissue growth, and regulates the functioning of many organ systems that influence behavior and cognition. Because the endocrine system is involved in an extraordinary range of physiological processes, it is important to consider an endocrine disorder in many clinical situations, especially when a patient presents with vague multisystem complaints.

The Pituitary

The pituitary is often called the master gland as it controls most of the other endocrine glands' function. The hypothalamus regulates most of the pituitary gland's hormone secretion in response to target gland stimulation requirements. The pituitary has two functional parts the anterior lobe (adenohypophysis) and the posterior lobe (neurohypophysis). The pituitary also has a vestigial intermediate lobe. The hypothalamus secretes oxytocin and vasopressin (also known as arginine vasopressin, antidiuretic hormone [ADH], and argipressin) through the posterior pituitary. The hypothalamus secretes regulatory hormones (e.g., gonadotropin-releasing hormone [GnRH]) which control the secretion of anterior pituitary hormones in a pulsatile pattern every 1–3 h. The anterior pituitary secretes six main hormones which are the following: growth hormone (GH), adrenocorticotropic hormone (ACTH), thyroid-stimulating hormone (TSH), follicle-stimulating hormone (FSH), luteinizing hormone (LH), and prolactin (see Table 1 for more details). Pituitary gland disorders usually originate from adenomas that either overproduce hormones

Table 1 Hormones of the anterior pituitary

Pituitary cell type (staining characteristic)	Hormones secreted	Target site	Clinical excess	Clinical deficiency
Somatotrophs (eosinophilic)	GH	Bones	Gigantism; acromegaly	Dwarfism
		Glucose metabolism	Glucose intolerance	Fasting hypoglycemia
Lactotrophs (eosinophilic)	Prolactin	Breasts	Galactorrhea	Inability to lactate
Corticotrophs (basophilic)	ACTH	Adrenal cortex	Cushing's syndrome	Adrenal insufficiency
	B-Lipoprotein	Skin	Hyperpigmentation	Hypopigmentation
Thyrotrophs (chromophobic)	TSH	Thyroid	Hyperthyroidism	Hypothyroidism
Gonadotrophs (chromophobic)	FSH, LH	Females: ovaries Males: testes	Precocious puberty	Delayed puberty; infertility; loss of secondary sexual characteristics

ACTH, adrenocorticotropic hormone; FSH, follicle-stimulating hormone; GH, growth hormone; LH, luteinizing hormone; TSH, thyroid stimulating hormone

or cause underproduction by obstructing portal veins. Hormone-secreting adenomas usually produce a single hormone which is typically prolactin, GH, or ACTH.

Hyperprolactinemia and Galactorrhea

Overview

Prolactin is synthesized and secreted by the anterior lobe of the pituitary gland [1]. Its two main functions are the development of mammary glands within breast tissue and milk production. It also maintains lactation of the primed breast. The hypothalamus secretes dopamine which inhibits prolactin release, and thyrotropin-releasing hormone (TRH) stimulates prolactin release. Estrogen, epidermal growth factor, and dopamine receptor antagonists also induce prolactin release.

Hyperprolactinemia can develop from pituitary tumors, pharmacotherapy, external stimulation, or pathological interruption of the hypothalamic-pituitary dopaminergic pathways (see Table 2 for a more complete list). Chronic conditions such as renal failure, cirrhosis, and hypothyroidism can also cause hyperprolactinemia. Hyperprolactinemia may be

asymptomatic or result in hypogonadism, infertility, galactorrhea, and bone loss. Decrease in bone density from hyperprolactinemia occurs secondary to sex steroid attenuation. The population prevalence of prolactinomas peaks between ages 25 and 34 years with an estimated prevalence between 6 and 50 cases per 100,000 [2, 3].

Clinical Presentation

Women with hyperprolactinemia typically present with symptoms ranging from shortened luteal phases, vaginal dryness, infertility, decreased libido, and oligomenorrhea to hypogonadism, galactorrhea, amenorrhea, and osteopenia [1, 4]. Higher levels of prolactin are associated with worsening symptoms. Men can present with decreased libido, impotence, decreased sperm production, infertility, gynecomastia, erectile dysfunction, and rarely galactorrhea. Patients with macroadenomas may also present with headaches or changes in vision.

Diagnosis

The diagnosis of hyperprolactinemia is generally confirmed with a single measurement of serum

Table 2 Selected causes of hypopituitarism [7]

Neoplastic	Pharmacologic
Pituitary adenoma	Anesthetics
Craniopharyngioma	Anticonvulsants
Meningioma	Antidepressants
Cysts (Rathke's cleft, arachnoid, epidermoid, dermoid)	Antihistamines
Germinoma	Antihypertensives
Glioma	Cholinergic agonists
Astrocytoma	Drug-induced hypersecretion
Ganglioneuroma	Catecholamine depletory
Paraganglioma	Dopamine receptor blockers
Teratoma	Dopamine synthesis inhibitors
Chordoma	Estrogen
Pituicytoma	Neuroleptics/antipsychotics
Ependymoma	Neuropeptides
Pituitary carcinoma	Opiates and opiate antagonists
Metastases	
Treatment of sellar, parasellar, and hypothalamic disease	**Traumatic**
Surgery	Head injury
Radiotherapy	
Infectious	**Vascular**
Bacterial	Pituitary tumor apoplexy
Fungal	Sheehan's syndrome
Parasites	Intrasellar carotid artery aneurysm
Tuberculosis	Subarachnoid hemorrhage
Syphilis	
Infiltrative/inflammatory disease	**Miscellaneous causes**
Autoimmune disease	Pituitary apoplexy
Hemochromatosis	Cavernous sinus thrombosis
Granulomatous	Primary empty sella syndrome
Langerhans cell histiocytosis	Immunologic
Giant cell granuloma	Idiopathic
Xanthomatous hypophysitis	

prolactin above the upper limit of normal (25 mcg/L); however, morning prolactin levels (4 to 6 a.m.) can peak to 30 mcg/L [4]. Borderline elevated values can be confirmed by measuring prolactin levels every 15 to 20 min to identify possible prolactin pulsatility [1]. Marked serum prolactin levels >100 mcg/L are associated with hypogonadism, galactorrhea, and amenorrhea. Osteopenia presents mainly with hypogonadism. Serum prolactin levels between 51 and 75 mcg/L are associated with oligomenorrhea. Mild prolactin excess with levels between 31 and 50 mcg/L is associated with short luteal phases and decreased libido. Men typically present with decreased libido, impotence, decreased sperm production, infertility, and rarely gynecomastia and galactorrhea. Serum prolactin levels above 200 mcg/L indicate the presence of a lactotroph adenoma.

Diagnosis of suspected drug-induced symptomatic hyperprolactinemia involves discontinuation of the offending agent followed by measurement of serum prolactin 3 days later [1]. An alternative medication should be used if possible and antipsychotic agents should be substituted or discontinued cautiously. A pituitary MRI can identify pituitary or hypothalamic masses if the offending agent cannot be discontinued. Additionally, visual field testing can identify macroadenomas along with aid from pituitary MRI.

Management

The management of hyperprolactinemia changes depending on the etiology [1]. Drug-induced hypogonadism treatment involves discontinuation of the offending agent if possible. An alternative medication not known to cause hyperprolactinemia should be used instead. If substitution is not possible, a dopamine agonist can cautiously be used to attenuate hyperprolactinemia symptoms. Dopamine agonists are also used in the treatment of symptomatic prolactinomas (both micro- and macroadenomas) to lower serum prolactin, decrease tumor size, and restore gonadal function.

Cabergoline is the first-line dopamine agonist as it normalizes prolactin levels and shrinks pituitary tumors more effectively than bromocriptine. The initial cabergoline dose is 0.25 mg twice weekly and can be titrated up to 1 mg twice weekly (every 4 weeks) to normalize prolactin levels. Cabergoline use is associated with valvular regurgitation, and high doses should be used cautiously [5]. Bromocriptine, a dopamine agonist, may be used second line and can be administered intravaginally if patients are intolerant to oral administration [1]. Dopamine agonists may be tapered and discontinued after 2 years minimum treatment if serum prolactin has normalized and previous tumors are no longer visible on MRI.

Patients with amenorrhea secondary to microadenomas can be treated with either dopamine agonists or oral contraceptives [1]. Patients that develop long-term hypogonadism or low bone mass should be treated with estrogen or testosterone. Asymptomatic patients should not be treated. Transsphenoidal surgery in patients with prolactinomas is considered if patients either cannot tolerate high doses of cabergoline or are unresponsive to dopamine therapy. Radiation is an alternative if surgery fails or in situations with malignant prolactinomas.

Hypopituitarism

Overview

Hypofunction of the pituitary presents as either partial or complete (panhypopituitarism) reduction in pituitary hormones. It is a rare disorder with an estimated prevalence of 45 cases per 100,000 [6]. The disorder includes adrenal insufficiency, hypothyroidism, hypogonadism, GH deficiency, and diabetes insipidus (DI) [7]. Causes of hypopituitarism are varied and include both disturbances of the gland directly (primary hypopituitarism) or the hypothalamus (secondary hypopituitarism) (see Table 2).

Clinical Presentation

Hypopituitarism typically presents as progressive hormone deficiencies starting with GH followed by gonadotropins, TSH, and ACTH [7]. However, exceptions exist to the order which makes identifying a specific hormone deficiency challenging as partial function loss may mimic primary failure of the target site. Symptoms may develop abruptly (as in Sheehan's syndrome) or slowly (as with a slow-growing nonsecretory adenoma). Children may present with growth failure and delayed puberty. Adults typically present with a confusing array of psychological problems, family or social difficulties, and multisystem somatic complaints that are due to hormonal deficiencies and the underlying disease that causes the hypopituitarism. Common complaints include fatigue, weight loss, dry skin, menstrual abnormalities, and sexual dysfunction; however, a wide range of manifestations are possible [7].

Panhypopituitarism is ultimately fatal. Patients appear pale and chronically ill with a loss of secondary sexual characteristics. Galactorrhea can occur in secondary hypopituitarism (e.g., hypothalamic sarcoidosis) because the hypothalamus inhibits pituitary prolactin. Lack of vasopressin produces polydipsia and polyuria of central DI.

Diagnosis

The diagnosis of hypopituitarism begins with a full clinical history and physical examination [7]. Hypopituitarism manifests as reduction in target gland hormone levels such as GH, prolactin, ACTH, TSH, LH, and FSH. Reduction in vasopressin may occur if the posterior pituitary is affected. Obtaining a hormonal assay and knowing the characteristics and limitations are essential when confirming the diagnosis.

Management

Treatment involves the hormonal replacement of panhypopituitarism [7]. A specialist consult should be obtained to oversee treatment as target gland hormonal replacement should attempt to mimic normal physiologic patterns. A deficiency of glucocorticoids is corrected before thyroid hormone replacement to prevent precipitating an adrenal crisis. Because aldosterone secretion is unaffected, mineralocorticoids are not necessary. Sex hormones can be started once the patient is euthyroid, but gonadotropins are required to restore fertility. In children, GH is required. In adults, replacement of GH reduces body fat, increases muscle mass and bone density, and improves exercise tolerance in the short term; the long-term benefits have not been evaluated. At least one study has suggested that patients affected by traumatic brain injury may demonstrate a higher percentage of abnormality in GH production, which may improve after 1 year [8]. Patients with hypopituitarism should wear a medical identification bracelet or necklace.

Neuroendocrine Disorders of Water Balance

Endocrine diseases may manifest as disorders of water balance such as hypernatremia, hyponatremia, polydipsia, or polyuria. Osmotic homeostasis is regulated by a complex coordination between the endocrine system, brain, heart, and kidneys. Plasma tonicity and blood volume are the two factors that affect this homeostasis. Blood volume is detected by baroreceptors and the pressure exerted on the renal blood vessels. The plasma tonicity is monitored by the hypothalamus' osmoreceptors; when there is hypernatremia, the thirst mechanism and the release of ADH are concurrently stimulated.

Polydipsia

Primary Polydipsia

Primary polydipsia (PP) means excessive fluid intake that is not secondary to deficient ADH production or response. Excessive volume expansion can cause hyponatremia and inhibit ADH release. A central defect in thirst regulation is presumed to play a significant role in primary polydipsia, but the mechanism is still unknown; the disorder itself is known as dipsogenic DI. PP can be induced by hypothalamic lesions, caused by infiltrative diseases like sarcoidosis, that affect the thirst center. It is important to perform a cranial MRI to observe the hypothalamus before idiopathic or psychogenic polydipsia is presumed. An iatrogenic source should also be considered as certain drugs (e.g., anticholinergics) can cause dry mouth. PP can also be seen in anxious patients preparing for imaging or attempting to dilute their urine to avoid a positive urine drug screening [9].

Secondary Polydipsia

Secondary polydipsia is a protective measure against polyuria of any etiology. Dehydration can otherwise result in hypernatremia and possible death. For psychiatric patients with polyuria or hyponatremia, it should not be automatically assumed that psychogenic polydipsia is the cause. A water deprivation test can be helpful in evaluating for central or nephrogenic DI versus PP. The clinician should use imaging and lab values to assess for hypopituitarism. Assessment of thyroid, adrenal, and renal function can help rule out other causes.

Polyuria and Central Diabetes Insipidus

Polyuria can be due to osmotic (solute) diuresis or water diuresis. Osmotic diuresis includes glucosuria, urea diuresis, administration of high amounts of protein orally (or via IV or feeding tube), mannitol diuresis, and sodium diuresis (e.g., large volumes of IV saline or after resolution of bilateral urinary tract obstruction). Common causes of glucosuria are uncontrolled diabetes mellitus, excess IV dextrose and water, or administration of sodium-glucose transport 2 inhibitors. Examples of urea diuresis include acute kidney injury and tissue catabolism (which can be secondary to glucocorticoid therapy). Water diuresis includes PP (seen mainly in adults and adolescents), nephrogenic DI, and central DI. Central DI is due to ADH deficiency which can be caused by destruction of the posterior pituitary's capillary beds or loss of the hypothalamic neurons that produce vasopressin [10]. Acquired central DI generally is caused by head trauma or transsphenoidal surgery. Central DI can be complete or partial, permanent or temporary, and the solely presenting condition or associated with other pituitary abnormalities. It can be inherited as an X-linked or autosomal dominant disease. Pregnancy can produce transient central DI.

and urine are measured hourly. At the conclusion of the test, a urine concentration >750 mosmol/kg is normal, whereas a concentration <300 mosmol/kg indicates either central or nephrogenic DI. Desmopressin is administered after the dehydration test; if the urine concentrates to >750 mosmol/kg, the patient likely has central DI, and if the urine fails to concentrate, that indicates nephrogenic DI. The water restriction test should be performed by a specialist as there are safety concerns associated with the test.

Copeptin assays are a developing diagnostic tool for DI. Copeptin is the C-terminal locus of the vasopressin prohormone, prepro-vasopressin, and a surrogate marker for endogenous ADH. It is easier to monitor than serum ADH and has a high diagnostic specificity [11]. Distinction between central DI and primary polydipsia can also be aided by T1-weighted MRI studies of the posterior pituitary and hypothalamus [10].

Clinical Presentation

Polyuria and polydipsia are the main findings in idiopathic central DI [10]. Acquired central DI may additionally present with associated pituitary lesion symptoms. The onset of central DI may be abrupt or gradual depending on the etiology. Patients with central DI present with polyuria (>3 L/day in adults and >2 L/m^2 in children) that should be differentiated from urinary frequency and nocturia. A dilute urine osmolality <300 mosmol/kg suggests nephrogenic or complete central DI, but a urine osmolality between 300 and 600 mosmol/kg indicates osmotic diuresis, PP, or partial central DI. Nocturia may be present in either case.

Diagnosis

A two-step water restriction test is commonly used to diagnose different types of DI [10]. The test is performed over 8 h. It is designed to dehydrate the patient, causing stimulation ADH which should concentrate urine osmolality. During the test weight and sodium osmolarity of the plasma

Management

Treatment of central DI requires identification and treatment of the underlying cause [10]. Treatment includes replacement of free water deficit and replacement of ADH. Desmopressin acetate given intranasally is the first-line treatment for ADH-deficient DI. Desmopressin nasal may cause rhinitis or conjunctivitis, so oral desmopressin may be considered instead. Oral desmopressin is initiated at 0.05 mg twice daily and, if needed, increased to a maximum of 0.4 mg every 8 h. With the oral route, gastrointestinal symptoms, asthenia, and mild elevation in hepatic enzymes may occur. Other therapeutic agents for central DI are hydrochlorothiazide, clofibrate, and ADH-releasing drugs (e.g., carbamazepine, chlorpropamide). The patient should also wear a medical alert bracelet.

Disorders of Secondary Sexual Characteristics

Secondary sexual characteristics are initially expressed at puberty and are maintained in adults by the sex hormones.

Normal Puberty

The cognitive, physical, and psychological transformation that occurs during adolescence is referred to as puberty. It occurs in two unique stages known as adrenarche and gonadarche. The results of normal puberty are most notable for the development of secondary sexual characteristics. Adrenarche results from increased production of androgens by the adrenal cortex. This normally occurs between the ages of 6 and 8. Physical manifestations of adrenarche include skeletal bone growth and further development of the pilosebaceous units and apocrine sweat glands. Gonadarche is driven by the hypothalamic-pituitary-gonadal axis. Increased pulsatile release of GnRH from the hypothalamus stimulates pulsatile secretion of FSH and LH from the pituitary gland. These hormonal pulsations have different impacts on the development of boys and girls, respectively.

In girls, FSH stimulates development of the ovarian follicles and granulosa cells, whereas LH stimulates ovarian theca cells. Together this leads to the production of estrogens, primarily estradiol. Estradiol is responsible for breast development (thelarche), growth acceleration, and skeletal maturation. The developing ovarian follicles eventually results in ovulation and development of the corpus luteum. Progesterone produced by the corpus luteum along with the effects of estradiol leads to menstruation (menarche). The median age at menarche in the USA decreased from 12.1 in 1995 to 11.9 in 2013–2017 [12]. This is thought to be secondary to the rising rates of childhood obesity as a higher body mass index correlates with an earlier onset of puberty [13].

In boys, LH stimulates the production of testosterone by the Leydig cells of the testes. Testosterone has multiple impacts including development of the seminiferous tubules and spermarche. Testosterone also drives increases in muscular mass, growth of the penis, and deepening of the voice. The impact of FSH is seen through the development of spermatozoa and enlargement of the testes.

Precocious Puberty

Precocious puberty is defined as the development of secondary sexual characteristics prior to the age of 8 years in girls and 9 years in boys [14]. This age distribution is 2–2.5 standard deviations from the norm which is considered 10.5 years of age in girls and 11.5 years of age in boys. Precocious puberty is caused by central or peripheral factors as seen below:

- Central precocious puberty
  - True precocious puberty
  - Central nervous system lesions
  - Gonadotropin-secreting tumor
  - Profound hypothyroidism
  - Chronic adrenal insufficiency
- Peripheral (pseudo) precocious puberty
  - Ovarian tumor
  - Follicular cysts
  - Exogenous estrogens
  - Testicular tumor
  - Autonomous Leydig cell formation
  - Exogenous androgens
  - Polyostotic fibrous dysplasia
  - Adrenal tumor
  - Adrenal hyperplasia

Central precocious puberty is driven by early activation of the hypothalamic-pituitary-gonadal axis resulting in the early production of gonadotropins. It can be separated from peripheral causes in that while pubertal development is early, it progresses in the normal sequence of development. Central precocious puberty is more common in girls, and most cases, especially in girls, are idiopathic. If central precocious puberty begins before the age of 6, a pathologic process such as a CNS tumor is more likely. As central precocious puberty is driven by GnRH, long-acting analogs of GnRH are the mainstay of treatment [15]. For many years, the most common treatment in the United States was monthly intramuscular (IM) depot leuprolide. During the past decades, there has been a substantial increase in the number of extended-release formulations of GnRH agonists including 3- and 6-month IM depot preparations and a subcutaneous implant that is marketed for annual use [16].

Peripheral precocious puberty is caused by early secretion of sex hormones. These sex hormones can be derived from the gonads, adrenal glands, or exogenous sources. Examples of peripheral sources of precocious puberty in girls would be ovarian cysts or tumor. In boys, sources of peripheral precocious puberty include Leydig cell and human chorionic gonadotropin-secreting germ cell tumors. Other sources can be seen in either sex and include primary hypothyroidism, exogenous sex steroids (from exposure to estrogen- or testosterone-containing creams, ointments, or sprays), adrenal tumors, congenital adrenal hyperplasia, and McCune-Albright syndrome.

Delayed Puberty

Delayed puberty is defined as the absence or incomplete development of secondary sexual characteristics by an age that is considered appropriate for 95% of the children of that sex and culture. In the United States, boys who have not had testicular enlargement by age 14 or girls who have not developed breast buds by age 12 are considered to have delayed puberty. Passage of more than 5 years from initial onset of puberty to completion is also considered delayed puberty. Delayed puberty can be caused by constitutional pubertal delay, primary hypogonadism (high circulating levels of LH and FSH), or secondary hypogonadism (low or normal levels of LH and FSH). Appropriate evaluation of a child with suspected pubertal delay includes a complete history including timing of any development of secondary sexual characteristics, physical exam, and growth chart review. Laboratory evaluation should include measurements of LH, FSH, and estradiol (in girls) or testosterone (in boys) and GnRH stimulation test. A radiograph of the left wrist for bone age is also indicated. A magnetic resonance imaging (MRI) of the brain should be performed if a central nervous system lesion is suspected. Causes of primary hypogonadism

include Turner's and Klinefelter's syndrome. Examples of secondary hypogonadism are constitutional delay of growth and puberty, GnRH deficiency, disorders of the pituitary or hypothalamus, and functional causes from poor nutrition or chronic disease.

Hypogonadism in Adults

Hypogonadism can occur in both sexes and result in infertility and loss of secondary sexual characteristics. The most common cause in women is menopause which is the natural process of loss of ovarian (gonadal) function. If this process occurs before the age of 40, it is considered premature ovarian failure. Surgical procedures such as oophorectomy can also result in loss of gonadal function. In men, the most causes of gonadal failure are medications, radiation, alcohol, infection, and trauma. Symptoms of hypogonadism include malaise, decrease libido, infertility, loss of secondary sexual characteristics, and depressed mood. In both men and women, FSH and LH levels will be elevated. If secondary hypogonadism is suspected, MRI should be obtained to evaluate for pituitary or hypothalamic mass.

Hirsutism and Virilization

Both hirsutism and virilization are the result of androgen excess. Hirsutism is the excessive growth of hair in a male pattern on the face, axilla, chest, and suprapubic areas. Development of acne can also be seen with hirsutism. Hirsutism affects between 5% and 10% of women of reproductive age [17]. Hirsutism can range from a minor cosmetic issue to the early sign of an adrenal adenocarcinoma. Virilization is defined as androgen-dependent masculinization of women and is characterized by frontal balding, clitoromegaly, increased muscle mass, and deepening of the voice. When virilization occurs with defeminization (decreased breast size and vaginal atrophy), it is always pathological.

Diagnosis

A thorough history is the first step to determining the cause of hirsutism and virilization [17]. This should include age of onset, symptoms, medications, weight changes, menstrual history, ethnicity, and family history. Physical examination should focus on areas of hair growth, body mass index, signs of virilization, and evidence of defeminization. The skin should be examined for acne, seborrhea, acanthosis nigricans, and striae. The Ferriman-Gallwey score is an evaluation tool which identifies hair growth in 11 areas. A score of 8 or greater confirms hirsutism. An abdominal and pelvic exam shoulder be performed to evaluate for masses that could indicate an androgen-secreting tumor. Laboratory evaluation should include serum total testosterone level. If the level is greater than 200 ng/dL, MRI should be performed to evaluate the adrenal glands and pelvis for mass. If the serum testosterone level is mildly elevated, an ACTH stimulation test can help to differentiate adrenal causes such as 21-hydroxylase deficiency from other causes such as obesity or insulin resistance.

Management

Management of hirsutism and virilization is based on the patient's goals or more emergent treatment of malignant causes [17]. Cosmetic treatments may include shaving, plucking, waxing, or bleaching of unwanted hair growth. Electrolysis and laser therapies are available too but at a higher cost. Eflornithine is a topical medication that may slow hair growth over a period of 4 to 8 weeks. Once stopped, however, the hair growth returns. For women who do not plan to become pregnant, a combined estrogen-progestin oral contraceptive is considered first-line oral medication therapy. The antiandrogen spironolactone maybe added if desired results are not achieved. Insulin-lowering agents are not an effective therapy for hirsutism but maybe used for their other benefits. Flutamide is a nonsteroidal androgen receptor antagonist which has been used off-label for managing hirsutism. Long-acting GnRH agonists may also be used to suppress the hypothalamic-pituitary-ovarian axis.

Calcium Metabolism and Parathyroid Glands

Calcium metabolism is regulated largely by two hormones: parathyroid hormone (PTH) and vitamin D. Calcitonin is another hormone which is produced in response to hypercalcemia by perifollicular cells in the thyroid to inhibit osteoclastic activity. Calcitonin release infrequently leads to hypocalcemia with the rare exception of medullary thyroid tumors. PTH is released by the parathyroid glands which are four small glands located in the neck adjacent to the thyroid. PTH modulates calcium in response to low serum calcium by stimulating osteoclastic activity in bones to free calcium stores, increase calcium resorption in the renal tubules to decrease renal calcium loss, and increase intestinal calcium absorption directly and through renal production of calcitriol. Additionally, PTH is involved in phosphate renal reabsorption inhibition which increases serum calcium.

Hypercalcemia and Hyperparathyroidism

Hypercalcemia is most commonly caused by hyperparathyroidism from benign hyperfunctioning parathyroid adenomas leading to increased bone resorption. While these adenomas account for approximately 80% of primary hyperparathyroidism, idiopathic and familial parathyroid hyperplasia also occur. Other causes include malignancy (including parathyroid carcinomas), hyperthyroidism, prolonged immobilization, Paget's disease, medications (e.g., thiazide diuretics and lithium), sarcoidosis, and vitamin D intoxication.

Clinical Presentation

Hyperparathyroidism and hypercalcemia are commonly identified through routine laboratory testing when an elevated serum calcium is noted.

Patients may also exhibit symptoms leading to the suspicion of hypercalcemia such as nausea, vomiting, abdominal pain, recurrent nephrolithiasis, bradycardia, polyuria, polydipsia, or muscle atrophy.

Diagnosis

The first step in investigating an elevated serum calcium (usually defined as a serum calcium greater than 10.5 mg/dL) is to confirm through repeat testing with correction for albumin level (0.8 mg/dL of calcium for each 1 g/dL of albumin). Alternatively, ionized calcium levels may be obtained. Once hypercalcemia is confirmed, PTH and 25-OH vitamin D levels should be obtained. Patient history and clinical presentation may also necessitate evaluation for malignancy, particularly if PTH and vitamin D levels are normal. This evaluation could include prostate-specific antigen (PSA) testing, alkaline phosphatase levels, TSH, urinary calcium excretion (particularly if PTH is normal or only minimally elevated), and imaging (e.g., radiographs for sarcoidosis or bone scan if malignancy is highly suspected). The patient's medication list should be reviewed, but one should not assume medication as the primary cause without other negative evaluation.

Management

It is critical to identify the cause of hypercalcemia to institute effective therapy. Consideration for discontinuing offending medications should be given. Vitamin D toxic individuals should have supplement dosages lowered. If hyperparathyroidism is confirmed as the cause, symptomatic patients should have parathyroid surgery [18]. Asymptomatic patients may be considered for surgical evaluation if they meet guidelines from the Fourth International Workshop on Asymptomatic Primary Hyperparathyroidism [19]. These include patients whose serum calcium is 1.0 mg/dL or greater than the upper limit of normal, bone density in the osteoporotic range

(T-score < -2.5), previous vertebral compression fracture, age less than 50, renal impairment with an estimated GFR of <60 mL/min, recurrent nephrolithiasis or nephrocalcinosis, or 24-h urinary calcium >400 mg/day. Patients not meeting these criteria may reasonably be managed non-operatively but should have serum calcium, renal function, and bone mineral density monitored every 1 to 2 years as up to one-third of patients may show disease progression and develop one of the previously mentioned indications for surgery [20].

Hypocalcemia and Hypoparathyroidism

While hyperparathyroidism causes hypercalcemia, hypoparathyroidism leads to hypocalcemia and hyperphosphatemia. The most common cause for hypoparathyroidism is iatrogenic parathyroidectomy [21]. Other causes of hypocalcemia which may or may not be associated with hypoparathyroidism include gastrointestinal diseases which limit calcium absorption, poor dietary calcium intake, autoimmune disorders, DiGeorge syndrome, vitamin D deficiency, hypomagnesemia, renal disease, and pancreatitis. Rarely infiltrative diseases (Wilson's disease or hemochromatosis) and metastatic cancer can lead to parathyroid destruction and subsequent hypocalcemia. As with hypercalcemia, identifying the underlying cause is paramount to appropriately treating hypocalcemia.

Clinical Presentation

The signs and symptoms of hypocalcemia generally correlate to the severity and are most often neurologic in nature. Mild hypocalcemia may produce no symptoms or produce depression or other psychiatric symptoms. More severe hypocalcemia may produce tetany, paresthesia, carpopedal spasm, delirium, or seizures. Carpopedal spasm may be elicited using a blood pressure cuff pumped up to the patient's systolic blood pressure (Trousseau's sign), and facial muscle hypercontractility (Chvostek's sign) may be elicited with tapping on the ipsilateral facial nerve. Hypocalcemia may also be suspected in patients with a prolonged QT interval on ECG.

Diagnosis

As with hypercalcemia, hypocalcemia must be confirmed after correction for serum albumin, which is commonly low in the elderly population. Once confirmed, PTH levels should be checked to assist in determining the underlying cause. Low PTH is most likely from removal or destruction of the parathyroid glands [21]. Magnesium levels should also be checked as hypomagnesemia, or significant hypermagnesemia may cause a functional hypoparathyroid state. Hypocalcemia in the setting of hypomagnesemia can be very difficult to correct. Elevated PTH levels in the setting of low calcium may be associated with vitamin D deficiency, pancreatitis, chronic kidney disease, severe illness or sepsis, or metastasis.

Management

As per hypercalcemia and hyperparathyroidism, treatment should target the underlying cause [22]. In acute, severe hypocalcemia with severe symptoms or ECG changes, intravenous calcium replacement is often indicated with an initial starting dose of 1 to 2 g of calcium gluconate infused over 10 to 20 min. Caution should be used when using IV calcium in patients with impaired renal function. Concomitant hypomagnesemia should be corrected. Management of chronic hypocalcemia or non-severe acute hypocalcemia should be done orally, and vitamin D supplementation implemented if low. Generally, 1.5–2 g of elemental calcium daily can be safely administered and levels monitored, adjusting the dosage as necessary.

Adrenal Dysfunction

The adrenal gland is comprised of the adrenal medulla, 10% of the gland, and the adrenal cortex, 90% of the gland, which is further divided into the zona glomerulosa, zona fasciculata, and zona reticularis. The adrenal medulla secretes the catecholamines epinephrine and norepinephrine. The medulla is linked to the autonomic nervous system.

The zona glomerulosa is 15% of the adrenal cortex and produces mineralocorticoids which are part of the renin-angiotensin system. The primary product of the zona glomerulosa is aldosterone which regulates electrolyte and fluid volume through potassium and magnesium secretion and sodium reabsorption. The zona fasciculata makes up 60% of the cortex and produces glucocorticoids, primarily cortisol, which regulate fat, carbohydrate, and protein metabolism. The zona reticularis makes up the remaining 25% of the cortex and produces sex hormones, e.g., testosterone and estradiol.

Adrenocortical Insufficiency

Primary adrenal insufficiency (Addison's disease) occurs when the adrenal cortex does not produce enough cortisol or aldosterone [23]. The most common etiology is idiopathic autoimmune adrenalitis. Other causes are damage to the adrenal glands, tuberculosis, fungal infections, neoplasia, or amyloidosis. Addison's disease is rare with a prevalence of 100 to 140 cases per million in the Western society, most commonly at ages 30 to 50 years [23].

Secondary adrenal insufficiency is classified as hyposecretion of ACTH from the pituitary which causes reduced cortisol levels. The most common etiology of secondary insufficiency is exogenous steroid use which leads to the suppression of the hypothalamic-pituitary-adrenal axis (HPA axis).

Clinical Presentation

The onset of Addison's disease is typically chronic, and patients may not seek medical attention in early disease [23]. Signs and symptoms are the results of gluco- and mineralocorticoid deficiency. Signs include weight loss, orthostatic hypotension due to dehydration, hyponatremia, hyperkalemia, anemia, and hypoglycemia. Nonspecific symptoms of Addison's disease are weakness, fatigue, musculoskeletal pain, weight loss, abdominal pain, depression, and anxiety. Some patients may have salt craving. Increased secretion of ACTH may lead to hyperpigmentation of the skin and mucous membranes; patients with pale skin generally have associated hypopituitarism.

Due to delay in treatment, the initial clinical presentation may occur when a patient is in acute life-threatening adrenal crisis. Signs and symptoms of adrenal crisis include severe weakness, syncope, acute abdominal pain, and hypotension leading to shock, renal failure, and death. Secondary adrenal insufficiency can present as moderate symptoms to severe adrenal crisis [24]. Abrupt discontinuation of corticosteroids after long-term treatment (e.g., Cushing's syndrome, sarcoidosis, rheumatoid arthritis) can also lead to adrenal insufficiency.

Diagnosis

Patients who present with symptoms suggestive of adrenal insufficiency (e.g., volume depletion, hypotension, hyponatremia, hyperkalemia, fever, abdominal pain, hyperpigmentation, and hypoglycemia) should be tested for primary adrenal insufficiency [23]. A low 8:00 AM serum cortisol (less than 5 mcg/dL) with mentioned symptoms suggests adrenal insufficiency. Plasma ACTH can be measured at the same time as serum cortisol to aid diagnosis. Lack of cortisol production from the adrenal cortex should be confirmed with an ACTH stimulation test. To confirm decreased adrenal cortisol production, patients are administered 0.25 mg ACTH intravenously, and serum cortisol levels are measured at baseline, 30, 60, and 90 min. Peak cortisol levels less than 18 mcg/dL at 30 or 60 min are indicative of adrenal insufficiency. Addison's disease presents with low cortisol levels and persistently elevated plasma ACTH (more than twofold the upper limit of normal). A specialist referral should be considered to aid in the etiology or diagnosis of Addison's disease.

Management

The first-line treatment for Addison's disease is hydrocortisone (15–25 mg in two or three divided doses orally) as it has both glucocorticoid and mineralocorticoid effects [23]. Oral cortisone acetate is another first-line option. Hydrocortisone should be given at awakening and either 2 h after lunch (2 daily doses) or at lunch and in the afternoon (3 daily doses). For noncompliant patients, prednisolone may be given either once or twice daily. All patients with confirmed aldosterone deficiency should have mineralocorticoid replacement with fludrocortisone (50–100 mcg daily) and no restriction on salt intake. If patients develop hypertension on fludrocortisone, the dose should be decreased, and antihypertensives initiated if necessary.

Monitoring involves clinical assessment with body weight, blood pressure, and energy levels. Patients with suspect adrenal crisis should be immediately treated with parenteral hydrocortisone followed by fluid resuscitation and a continuous IV hydrocortisone infusion over 24 h. Treatment of suspected adrenal crisis should not be delayed by diagnostic confirmation. Every patient should have an emergency glucocorticoid injection kit (injection or per rectum) and wear medical identification.

Adrenocortical Excess

Adrenocortical excess (Cushing's syndrome) symptoms result from either endogenous or, more commonly, exogenous increases in glucocorticoids [25]. Exogenous Cushing's syndrome occurs with the administration of glucocorticoids. Endogenous etiologies can be caused by ACTH overproduction (ACTH-dependent) by a pituitary adenoma (Cushing's syndrome), a glucocorticoid-producing adrenal adenoma or carcinoma, or other neoplasm (usually lung, thyroid, or pancreas). Less common causes are independent of ACTH usually with adrenal adenoma or carcinoma etiologies.

Clinical Presentation

Cushing's syndrome is primarily characterized by facial rounding (moon faces) and truncal obesity with a prominent dorsal cervical fat pad (buffalo hump) [25]. Other characteristics include hypertension, hirsutism, osteoporosis, glucose intolerance, hypokalemia, abdominal striae (reddish purple color greater than 1 cm), and psychiatric disturbances. Symptoms include proximal muscle weakness, menstrual abnormalities, and sexual dysfunction.

Diagnosis

Diagnosis of adrenocortical excess, or Cushing's syndrome, involves establishing hypercortisolism and then determining the etiology [25]. Patients who have unusual features for their age have multiple progressive features or have adrenal incidentaloma; suspect of adenoma should have a clinical workup for Cushing's syndrome. The primary care physician should first confirm hypercortisolism with lab work; however, iatrogenic causes of hypercortisolism (e.g., administration of glucocorticoids) should be excluded before lab work is obtained. Typical tests are the measurement of 24-h free urine cortisol (UFC) or a low-dose dexamethasone test (DST); other options include measuring late-night salivary cortisol, midnight plasma cortisol, or a longer low-dose DST. For the low-dose DST, patients are instructed to take 1 mg of dexamethasone between 11:00 PM and midnight; a serum cortisol level is then obtained at 8:00 AM the next morning. A normal response to DST is a serum cortisol less than 1.8 mcg/dL; some use a threshold of less than 5 mcg/dL, but it has a lower test sensitivity.

Once hypercortisolism is established, physiologic causes should be excluded including pregnancy, depression, alcohol dependence, glucocorticoid resistance, obesity, or diabetes mellitus. An endocrinology consult should be obtained for further evaluation to confirm or exclude diagnosis and determine the etiology.

Management

Once the diagnosis is confirmed, treatment of Cushing's syndrome involves normalizing cortisol levels to eliminate signs and symptoms and treating comorbidities [25]. If possible, resection of the primary lesion is the preferred treatment option; radiation and chemotherapy can also be used. If surgery is not possible or if patients decline, glucocorticoid antagonists can be used as second line to normalize cortisol levels. Different pharmacotherapy options are available for ectopic ACTH syndrome, pituitary-dependent, and adrenal adenomas or carcinomas.

Hyperaldosteronism

Primary hyperaldosteronism, or Conn syndrome, is a rare condition caused by an aldosterone-secreting neoplasia or hyperplasia of the adrenal gland [26]. Secondary hyperaldosteronism is associated with renin hypersecretion (e.g., renal artery stenosis). Primary hyperaldosteronism is a common secondary form of arterial hypertension with a particularly high prevalence among patients with resistant hypertension.

Consensus guidelines recommend a workup for primary aldosteronism in patients with resistant hypertension (sustained elevated blood pressure while on the maximum dose of three antihypertensives of which one is a diuretic); controlled hypertension but on four or more antihypertensives; hypertension and diuretic-induced hypokalemia, adrenal incidentaloma, sleep apnea, or a family history of cerebrovascular accident at a young age (less than 40 years); hypertension and a first-degree relative with primary aldosteronism. The plasma aldosterone/renin ratio (ARR) is used to detect possible cases. Patients should be referred to endocrinology for confirmatory testing and imaging after a positive ARR test; however, confirmatory testing is not needed with spontaneous hypokalemia or plasma renin below detection levels with plasma aldosterone concentration (PAC) >20 ng/dL. Adrenal computed tomography scan and adrenal venous sampling (AVS) can distinguish between unilateral and bilateral primary aldosteronism and adrenal hyperplasia.

First-line treatment for unilateral primary aldosteronism is surgery. In bilateral pulmonary aldosteronism, or if patients decline surgery, mineralocorticoid receptor antagonists (e.g., spironolactone or eplerenone) are used for treatment. Mineralocorticoid receptor antagonists should be used at the lowest effective dose with low sodium diets to normalize blood pressure and potassium [27].

Hypoglycemia

Overview

Hypoglycemia in adults is usually caused by medications used to treat diabetes mellitus. Other causes include critical illness, hormone deficiency (e.g., cortisol), nonislet cell tumor, or endogenous hyperinsulinism. In the absence of diabetes mellitus treatment, hypoglycemia must be confirmed with the presence of Whipple's triad: symptoms, signs, or both consistent with hypoglycemia, a low plasma glucose concentration, and resolution of those symptoms or signs after the plasma glucose concentration is raised [28]. Confirmation with Whipple's triad prevents expensive and unnecessary evaluation. Hypoglycemia is generally defined as a plasma glucose concentration of less than 70 mg/dL, severe if less than 55 mg/dL. However, individuals will have varied physiologic responses to low plasma glucose concentrations. Symptoms of hypoglycemia are either neurogenic (autonomic nervous system response) or neuroglycopenic (result of low brain blood glucose concentrations). Neurogenic symptoms include palpitations, tremor, anxiety, sweating, and hunger. Neuroglycopenic symptoms are behavioral changes, fatigue, confusion, diplopia, seizure, and loss of consciousness which can lead to death.

Diagnosis

A thorough workup should be completed for patients with Whipple's triad-confirmed hypoglycemia in the absence of diabetes mellitus [28]. The general differential should include a careful medication history as drugs are the most common cause of hypoglycemia. The most common drug culprits are insulin, insulin secretagogues, and alcohol. Some uncommon medication causes of hypoglycemia are angiotensin-converting enzyme inhibitors or angiotensin receptor antagonists, beta blockers, and fluoroquinolones. Acute illness

such as sepsis and renal or hepatic failure should be ruled out. Cortisol deficiency-associated hypoglycemia is rare. In symptomatic patients, plasma measurements of glucose, insulin, C-peptide, proinsulin, β-hydroxybutyrate, and insulin antibodies can help distinguish between endogenous and exogenous causes of hypoglycemia. An increase in plasma glucose in response to administered glucagon 1.0 mg IV can help identify insulin-mediated hypoglycemia. Endogenous hyperinsulinism presents as high levels of insulin, C-peptide, and proinsulin at low fasting plasma glucose concentrations.

A diagnostic approach involves a supervised 72-h fast where all medications are stopped and plasma glucose, insulin, C-peptide, and proinsulin are measured at specified intervals. The fast is completed once the patient develops symptoms of hypoglycemia with corresponding hypoglycemic plasma glucose. An endocrine consult should be obtained after confirmation of postprandial endogenous hyperinsulinemic hypoglycemia without endogenous agents or circulating insulin antibodies to help identify the insulinoma.

Management

Treatment is dependent on the specific hypoglycemia disorder. Offending exogenous causes (e.g., alcohol, medications known to cause hypoglycemia) of hypoglycemia should be limited as appropriate [28]. Patients with a history of gastric surgery or gastric bypass are prone to hypoglycemia secondary to hyperinsulin response; eating smaller but more frequent meals can alleviate hypoglycemia. Exercise-induced hypoglycemia may be treated by carbohydrate loading before and during exercise. Insulinomas are extremely rare and may require surgical treatment. The severity of hypoglycemia should be considered before invasive treatment.

Gout

Gout is the most common form of inflammatory arthritis with a prevalence of approximately 9.2 million adults in the United States [29]. It is caused by a deposition of monosodium urate crystals in tissue and joints; however, visualization of these crystals is not required for diagnosis. Risk factors include cardiovascular disease, diabetes mellitus, hyperlipidemia, chronic kidney disease, as well as specific dietary and demographic factors. Treatment is available for acute attacks as well as urate-lowering therapy for long-term management. Lifestyle changes, especially reduction in purine-rich foods such as organ and glandular meat, are important for a good prognosis.

Clinical Presentation

Gout is a form of arthritis which presents as acute or chronic. Acute gout, referred to as a "gout flare," presents as a sudden onset of severe pain, swelling, warmth, and erythema of synovitis. The most commonly affected joint is the first metatarsophalangeal joint, the podagra. Gout flares are self-limiting, peak within 12 to 24 h, and resolve over 1 to 2 weeks even without treatment. Chronic tophaceous gout occurs if gout flares occur at short intervals without complete resolution of symptoms that cause joint destruction. Common signs of chronic gout are uric acid tophi which are deposits of uric acid in periarticular fibrous tissue and in the cartilage of the ear and kidneys. Patients may have asymptomatic hyperuricemia; no treatment is recommended for these patients.

Diagnosis

Synovial fluid analysis for detection of monosodium urate crystals is the gold standard in confirming the diagnosis [30]. However, it should be reserved for patients who are suspected of having a septic joint, in which a culture and gram stain of the aspirate should be performed, in addition to analysis of monosodium urate crystals. Serum uric acid levels may be normal in patients with acute gout. There are several algorithms that can aid in the diagnosis of gout clinically without invasive joint aspirations. These algorithms include the Rome and New York Criteria, ARA Criteria, Janssens Diagnostic Rule, Clinical Gout Diagnosis Criteria, Monoarthritis of the First Metatarsophalangeal Joint, Study for Updated Gout Classification Criteria (SUGAR), and the 2015 ACR/European League Against Rheumatism Gout Classification Criteria. Another method of diagnosis is imaging such as sonography and dual-energy computerized tomography.

Management

First-line treatment for acute gout flares includes nonsteroidal anti-inflammatory drugs (NSAIDs) and colchicine [29]. Oral colchicine or glucocorticoids may be used when NSAIDs are contraindicated such as in comorbid cardiovascular disease, chronic kidney disorder, or cerebrovascular disease. A typical NSAID and dose are naproxen 500 mg twice daily which is equivalent to prednisolone 35 mg orally daily. Low-dose colchicine should be administered within 24 h (less efficacy if within 36 h) of symptom onset at a dose of 1.2 mg followed 0.6 mg 6 h later. Colchicine 0.6 mg daily should be continued until resolution of gout flare. High-dose colchicine should not be used as it has similar efficacy to low-dose colchicine but with increased adverse effects such as diarrhea. When oral administration is not feasible, glucocorticoids may be given via the intramuscular, intravenous, or intraarticular route. Topical ice may be used as an adjuvant to pharmacologic therapy of a gout flare.

Urate-lowering therapy is recommended for patients who have ≥1 subcutaneous tophi, evidence of radiographic damage related to gout, or ≥2 gout flares annually. Urate-lowering therapy may be considered in patients with a history of more than one gout flare. Urate-lowering therapy should not be initiated during a gout flare as it can lead to worsening of symptoms. Allopurinol with a starting dose of 100 mg daily is the preferred first-line treatment even for patients with moderate-to-severe chronic kidney disease. Allopurinol should be titrated weekly by 100 mg increments to a serum uric acid level <6 mg/dL. Some experts prefer treating serum uric acid to <5 mg/dL [31]. Slow titration of allopurinol helps to avoid gout flares [29]. In addition, concomitant anti-inflammatory prophylaxis with NSAIDs, colchicine, or corticosteroids to avoid flares is recommended for 3 to 6 months after starting urate-lowering therapy. Before starting allopurinol, patient of Southeast Asian descent (e.g., Han Chinese, Korean, Thai) and African Americans should be tested for HLA-B*5801 allele. Allopurinol is contraindicated in patients carrying the allele. Febuxostat is an alternative to allopurinol-intolerant patients, but it should be avoided in patients with a history of cardiovascular disease or with a new cardiovascular event. Pegloticase has been approved as an alternative in patients with refractory gout.

References

1. Melmed S, Casanueva FF, Hoffman AR, et al. Diagnosis and treatment of hyperprolactinemia: an Endocrine Society clinical practice guideline. J Clin Endocrinol Metabol. 2011;96(2):273–88.
2. Fernandez A, Karavitaki N, Wass JA. Prevalence of pituitary adenomas: a community-based, cross-sectional study in Banbury (Oxfordshire, UK). Clin Endocrinol. 2010;72(3):377–82.
3. Daly AF, Rixhon M, Adam C, et al. High prevalence of pituitary adenomas: a cross-sectional study in the province of Liege, Belgium. J Clin Endocrinol Metabol. 2006;91(12):4769–75.
4. Serri O, Chik CL, Ur E, Ezzat S. Diagnosis and management of hyperprolactinemia. CMAJ. 2003;169(6): 575–81.
5. Budayr A, Tan TC, Lo JC, et al. Cardiac valvular abnormalities associated with use and cumulative exposure of cabergoline for hyperprolactinemia: the CATCH study. BMC Endocr Disord. 2020;20(1):1–9.
6. Regal M, Páramo C, Sierra SM, Garcia-Mayor RV. Prevalence and incidence of hypopituitarism in an adult Caucasian population in northwestern Spain. Clin Endocrinol. 2001;55:735–40.
7. Fleseriu M, Hashim IA, Karavitaki N, et al. Hormonal replacement in hypopituitarism in adults: an endocrine society clinical practice guideline. J Clin Endocrinol Metabol. 2016;101(11):3888–921.
8. Tanriverdi F, Senyurek H, Unluhizarci K. High risk of hypopituitarism after traumatic brain injury: a prospective investigation of anterior pituitary function in the acute phase and 12 months after trauma. J Clin Endocrinol Metab. 2006;91(6):2105–11.
9. Klonoff DC, Jurow AH. Acute water intoxication as a complication of urine drug testing in the workplace. JAMA. 1991;265(1):84–5.
10. Garrahy A, Moran C, Thompson CJ. Diagnosis and management of central diabetes insipidus in adults. Clin Endocrinol. 2019;90(1):23–30.
11. Timper K, Fenske W, Kühn F, et al. Diagnostic accuracy of copeptin in the differential diagnosis of the polyuria-polydipsia syndrome: a prospective multicenter study. J Clin Endocrinol Metabol. 2015;100(6): 2268–74.
12. Martinez GM. Centers for Disease Control and Prevention National Center for Health Statistics Trends and Patterns in Menarche in the United States: 1995 through 2013–2017. National Health Statistics Reports. 2020;146.
13. Kaplowitz PB, Slora EJ, Wasserman RC, et al. Earlier onset of puberty in girls: relation to increased body mass index and race. Pediatrics. 2001;108(2):347–53.
14. Boepple PA, Crowley WF Jr. Precocious puberty. In: Adashi EY, Rock JA, Rosenwaks Z, editors. Reproductive endocrinology, surgery, and technology, vol. 1. Philadelphia: Lippincott-Raven; 1996. p. 989.
15. Brown DB, Loomba-Albrecht LA, Bremer AA. Sexual precocity and its treatment. World J Pediatr. 2013;9(2):103–11.
16. Aguirre RS, Eugster EA. Central precocious puberty; from genetics to treatment. Best Pract Res Clin Endocrinol Metab. 2018;32(4):343–54.
17. Ferriman D, Gallwey JD. Clinical assessment of body hair growth in women. J Clin Endocrinol Metab. 1961;21:1400.
18. Mack LA, Pasieka JL. Asymptomatic primary hyperparathyroidism: a surgical perspective. Surg Clin Borth Am. 2004;84(3):803.
19. Bilezikian JP, Brandi ML, Eastell R, et al. Guidelines for the management of asymptomatic primary hyperparathyroidism: summary statement from the fourth international workshop. J Clin Endocrinol Metab. 2014;99:3561.
20. Rubin MR, McMahon DJ, Jacobs T, et al. The natural history of primary hyperparathyroidism with or without parathyroid surgery after 15 years. J Clin Endocrinol Metab. 2008;93(9):3462.
21. Lopes MP, Klieman BS, Bini IB, et al. Hypoparathyroidism and pseudohypoparathyroidism: etiology, laboratory features and complications. Arch Endocrinol Metab. 2016;60:532.
22. Cooper MS, Gittoes NJ. Diagnosis and Management of Hypocalcemia. BMJ. 2008;336:1298.
23. Bornstein SR, Allolio B, Arlt W, et al. Diagnosis and treatment of primary adrenal insufficiency: an endocrine society clinical practice guideline. J Clin Endocrinol Metabol. 2016;101(2):364–89.
24. Charmandari E, Nicolaides NC, Chrousos GP. Adrenal insufficiency. Lancet. 2014;383(9935):2152–67.
25. Nieman LK, Biller BM, Findling JW, et al. The diagnosis of Cushing's syndrome: an Endocrine Society clinical practice guideline. J Clin Endocrinol Metab. 2008;93:1526–40.
26. Funder JW, Carey RM, Mantero F, et al. The management of primary aldosteronism: case detection, diagnosis, and treatment: an endocrine society clinical practice guideline. J Clin Endocrinol Metab. 2016;101:1889–916.

27. Young WF Jr. Diagnosis and treatment of primary aldosteronism: practical clinical perspectives. J Intern Med. 2019;285(2):126–48.

28. Cryer PE, Axelrod L, Grossman AB, et al. Evaluation and management of adult hypoglycemic disorders: an Endocrine Society clinical practice guideline. J Clin Endocrinol Metabol. 2009;94(3):709–28.

29. FitzGerald JD, Dalbeth N, Mikuls T, et al. American College of Rheumatology guideline for the management of gout. Arthritis Care Res. 2020;72:744.

30. Newberry SJ, FitzGerald JD, Motala A, et al. Diagnosis of gout: a systematic review in support of an American College of Physicians clinical practice guideline. Ann Intern Med. 2017;166(1):27–36.

31. Hui M, Carr A, Cameron S, British Society for Rheumatology Standards, Audit and Guidelines Working Group. The British Society for Rheumatology guideline for the management of gout [published correction appears in Rheumatology (Oxford). 2017; 56 (7): 1246]. Rheumatology (Oxford). 2017;56(7):e1–20.

Part XXV

The Blood and Hematopoietic System

Anemia

130

Daniel T. Lee and Monica L. Plesa

Contents

D. T. Lee (✉) · M. L. Plesa (✉)
Department of Family Medicine, David Geffen School of
Medicine at UCLA Health System, Santa Monica, CA,
USA
e-mail: dtlee@mednet.ucla.edu; mplesa@mednet.ucla.edu

© Springer Nature Switzerland AG 2022
P. M. Paulman et al. (eds.), *Family Medicine*,
https://doi.org/10.1007/978-3-030-54441-6_132

Background and Introduction

Anemia is a reduction in blood hemoglobin (Hgb) concentration or hematocrit (Hct). Normal values of Hgb and Hct vary based on age, gender, ethnicity, and other special considerations and have been widely studied over the years. Data from large samples selected to represent the population of the United States suggests that the lower limit of normal hemoglobin concentrations be 13.7 g/dL in young white men (ages 20–59 years) and

12.9 g/dL in young black men; 13.2 g/dL in white and 12.7 g/dL in black men ages 60 years and over; and 12.2 g/dL in white women and 11.5 g/dL in black women 20 years and over, including elderly women [1]. The lower limit of normal for children age 1–3 years is 11 g/dL, with the cutoff rising to approach adult values by age 15–19 years. Between 2003 and 2012 data from five National Health and Nutrition Examination Surveys estimated that 5.6% of the United States' population had anemia based on the World Health Organization's criteria, with pregnant women, women of reproductive age, the elderly, non-Hispanic blacks, and Hispanics at highest risk [2].

It can be particularly difficult to diagnose the cause of anemia in the elderly population, and between 30% and 50% of anemia in this age group can be considered "undiagnosed anemia of the elderly" after extensive workup [3]. People residing at higher altitudes have higher baseline Hgb and Hct levels than residents at sea level. Smokers and patients exposed to significant secondhand smoke may have higher Hgb and Hct levels as well [4]. Endurance athletes can have a "sports anemia" as a result of increased plasma volume that lowers hematocrit despite stimulated erythropoiesis and higher red blood cells counts (RBCs) compared to sedentary individuals [5]. Gastrointestinal (GI) bleeds, anemia of chronic inflammation (ACI) due to increased cytokine release with exercise, hemolysis of senescent RBCs in contracting or compressed muscles, hematuria, and sweating can further contribute to this "sports anemia," especially in long distance runners [5, 6]. Additionally, it is always important to evaluate results in the context of previous data. For example, a low "normal" Hgb may be significant if a recent value was higher.

On occasion, the Hgb and Hct may not accurately reflect red cell mass as they are concentrations and depend on the plasma volume. For example, patients with expanded plasma volume, as in pregnancy or congestive heart failure, may have falsely low values while patients with plasma contraction, as in burns or dehydration, may have falsely elevated values. In the setting of acute blood loss, both RBCs and plasma are lost equally, and the true degree of anemia may not be appreciated until plasma volume has time to expand.

Anemia may be categorized by the RBC size (microcytic, normocytic, or macrocytic) or by cause (RBC underproduction, RBC destruction, or RBC loss). A patient's history, physical exam, and laboratory studies are integral to determine the etiology of the anemia regardless of the diagnostic approach taken.

Clinical Presentation

Symptoms

Symptoms of anemia are highly variable, and depend on the degree of anemia and the rapidity of its development. They arise from the effects of decreased oxygen delivery to end organs and can be exacerbated by hypovolemia. In response to a decrease in Hct, the body increases oxygen extraction by its tissues as well as increases the delivery of oxygen to these tissues by augmenting cardiac output with a faster heart rate and larger stroke volume. Those with mild or gradually developing anemias may be seemingly asymptomatic, although these patients may also demonstrate symptoms that are not yet recognized by the patient and/or physician [7]. Others may present with a range of symptoms including fatigue, weakness, decreased exercise tolerance, dizziness, headache, tinnitus, palpitations, syncope, impaired concentration, and restless leg syndrome (RLS). Some patients experience abdominal discomfort, nausea, and bowel irregularity as blood is shunted from the splanchnic bed. Children with anemia may present with impaired cognitive or psychomotor development. Decreased blood flow to the skin may result in cold intolerance. Patients with preexisting vascular disease are prone to exacerbations of angina, claudication, or cerebral ischemia.

History

Historical clues assist in determining the cause of anemia. Family history of anemia or onset of anemia in childhood suggests an inherited etiology. Chronic medical conditions such as hepatic, renal, endocrine, or inflammatory disorders can lead to anemia of chronic disease (ACD). Malignancies and infections may also cause anemia. Exposure to some medications, alcohol, and toxins (e.g., lead) can lead to anemia due to bone marrow suppression or interference with vitamin absorption. Chronic diarrhea or a history of GI conditions associated with malabsorption suggests a nutritional deficiency anemia. Obesity or a history of bariatric surgery or other GI surgeries can predispose to iron deficiency anemia (IDA). Dietary intake of iron, folate, and vitamin B12 (cobalamin) should be obtained. Paresthesias of the extremities or alteration in mental status may point to vitamin B12 deficiency. A history of gallstones or jaundice points to hemolysis. Pica is the craving for nonfood items frequently seen with iron deficiency. Patients will often crave ice, or earthy items such as clay or soil, or raw starches such as corn starch or raw rice among multiple other substances. Potential blood loss from the GI tract or heavy uterine bleeding must be ascertained. Frequent blood donations or blood draws in hospitalized patients may lead to an induced anemia.

Physical Examination

Tachycardia and wide pulse pressure may be present in the anemic patient as a result of increased cardiac output. The skin and conjunctiva may demonstrate pallor. In very severe anemias, retinal hemorrhages may be seen. Jaundice may suggest hemolysis or liver disease. Glossitis can be present in vitamin B12 and iron deficiency. Lymphadenopathy may occur in the presence of hematologic malignancies and infections such as HIV and tuberculosis. A systolic ejection murmur and venous hum may be heard. Signs of liver disease and splenomegaly should be sought. Proprioception and balance deficits may occur in vitamin B12 deficiency. The stool may be examined for blood.

Laboratory Data

Complete Blood Count. Once a patient is determined to be anemic by Hgb and/or Hct, a complete blood count (CBC) with differential should be obtained for the RBC indices as well as the platelet and white blood cell (WBC) values. Mean corpuscular volume (MCV) reflects the size of the RBC. The normal MCV for adults is debatable, with the lower limit of normal defined as 80–82 fl and the upper limit of normal as 98–100 fl. MCV in children is lower, starting at 70 fl at 1 year of age and increasing 1 fl/year until adult values are reached at puberty. Table 1 divides common causes of anemia into microcytic (<82 fl), normocytic (82–98 fl), and macrocytic (>98 fl).

The red cell distribution width (RDW) quantitates the variation in size of the RBCs. Normal RDW is less than 14.5%. An elevation of the RDW may make the MCV by itself less reliable. An example is a patient who has both iron and B12 deficiencies. In this case, the MCV may be normocytic, but the RDW will be elevated [8]. Data obtained from ICU and cardiac patients suggests a possible correlation between increased RDW and increased inflammation, oxidant damage, or vascular trauma that may be predictive of poor outcomes irrespective of the presence of anemia [9].

Mean corpuscular hemoglobin (MCH) and mean corpuscular hemoglobin concentration (MCHC) generally mirror the MCV (i.e., smaller RBCs tend to have lower MCHs and MCHCs, such as in iron deficiency and thalassemias). Larger RBCs tend to have greater MCH and MCHC values, such as in spherocytosis or sickle cell anemia.

The presence of hypochromic and hyperchromic RBCs is also important in evaluating anemia. Hypochromic erythrocytes (MCHC <28 g/dL) tend to be more prevalent in IDA than in thalassemias while hyperchromic erythrocytes (MCHC >41 g/dL) can easily identify hereditary spherocytosis [9].

Platelet and WBC counts should be noted. Among other things, decreased platelet levels (thrombocytopenia) and/or decreased WBCs (leukopenia) suggest bone marrow suppression, aplastic anemia, hypersplenism, vitamin B12 deficiencies, infections, or malignancies. Elevated platelet counts (thrombocytosis) are often seen in IDA, trauma, and infections. Increased WBC counts (leukocytosis) can also be seen in infections and malignancies. Severe pancytopenia should prompt a workup for aplastic anemia, hematologic malignancy, or chemotherapy and/or radiation side effects, among other causes.

Table 1 Classification of Anemia Based on MCV

Microcytic	Macrocytic
Iron deficiency	Non-megaloblastic
Thalassemia	Alcoholism
Anemia of chronic disease*	Chronic liver disease
Hemoglobin E*	Bone marrow disorders
Sideroblastic anemia*	Hypothyroidism*
Lead poisoning*	Sideroblastic anemias*
Hereditary*	Marked reticulocytosis
Myelodysplastic syndrome*	Spurious*
Severe alcoholism*	Normal variant*
Medications*	Neonatal period
Normocytic	Megaloblastic
	Folate deficiency
Elevated reticulocyte count	Poor intake
Acute blood loss	Malabsorption
Hemolysis	Ethanol
Pregnancy	Medications
Decreased reticulocyte count	Pregnancy
Anemia of chronic disease	Infancy
Chronic kidney disease	High folate requirement
Chronic liver failure	B12 (cobalamin) deficiency
Endocrine disease	Pernicious anemia
Iron deficiency	Gastric or ileal surgery*
Myelodysplastic syndromes	Ileal disease*
Aplastic anemia*	Strict veganism*
Pure red cell aplasia*	Fish tapeworm infection*
Myelophthisic anemia*	Bacterial overgrowth*
Sideroblastic anemia*	Pancreatic insufficiency*
	Medications* (anticonvulsants, chemotherapy, zidovudine)
	Congenital disorders*

*less common

Reticulocyte Count. Reticulocytes, which are newly formed RBCs, normally account for about 1% of circulating RBCs. Reticulocyte formation is increased in a normal individual who loses blood, with the degree of reticulocytosis increasing as anemia becomes more severe. Therefore, a patient's reported reticulocyte percentage should be adjusted for the degree of anemia to determine if the bone marrow response is appropriate:

$$\text{corrected reticulocyte\%} = \text{reticulocyte\%} \times$$
$$\text{patient's Hct/normal Hct.}$$

A corrected reticulocyte percentage (also known as reticulocyte index) greater than 1% indicates appropriate bone marrow response to anemia. If the value is less than 1%, causes of hypoproliferative bone marrow should be sought. Increased reticulocyte counts are present in hemolysis, acute hemorrhage, and response to treatment in anemias from other causes. An alternative to corrected reticulocyte percentage is the absolute reticulocyte count, which equals the reported reticulocyte percentage multiplied by the RBC count. The absolute reticulocyte count is normally 50,000–75,000/mm^3.

Peripheral Smear. Abnormalities in the peripheral smear, such as burr cells seen in renal failure or tear drop cells found in myelofibrosis, can assist in determining the etiology of anemia.

Other Laboratory Tests. Further laboratory testing may be warranted, depending on the above RBC indices and peripheral smear. Bone marrow biopsy is reserved for situations in which anemia remains unexplained or is suspected to arise from marrow dysfunction. Algorithms for evaluation of microcytic, normocytic, and macrocytic anemias are provided in Figs. 1, 2, and 3.

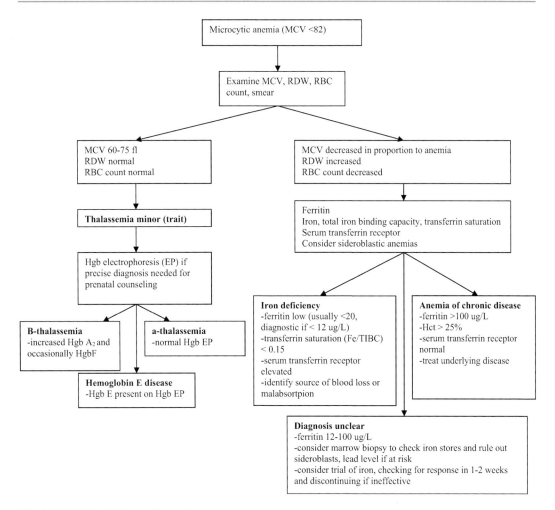

Fig. 1 Evaluation of microcytic anemia

Microcytic Anemias (Fig. 1)

Iron Deficiency Anemia

IDA is probably the most common cause of anemia in the world, accounting for about half of all cases [10]. The recommended dietary allowance (RDA) for iron is 8 mg daily for men and 18 mg daily for women [11]. Daily requirements increase during pregnancy, lactation, and adolescence. Meats, eggs, vegetables, legumes, and cereals are principal sources of iron in the American diet, with iron from meats being much more available for absorption than iron from other dietary sources.

In the United States, approximately 4% of children aged 5 months to 4 years old were found to be anemic between 2003 and 2012, with prevalence varying based on race/ethnicity. IDA accounts for approximately 40% of anemia in children, with Hispanic children ages 1–3 years old twice as likely to have IDA compared to black and white children in this age group [2]. Term, healthy infants have sufficient iron stores for at least the first 4 months of life. However, breast milk does not contain as much iron as does formula, so full term infants who are exclusively or mostly breastfed may become iron deficient around 4–6 months of age until they receive sufficient iron through solid food sources. Therefore, iron supplementation of 1 mg/kg/day may be

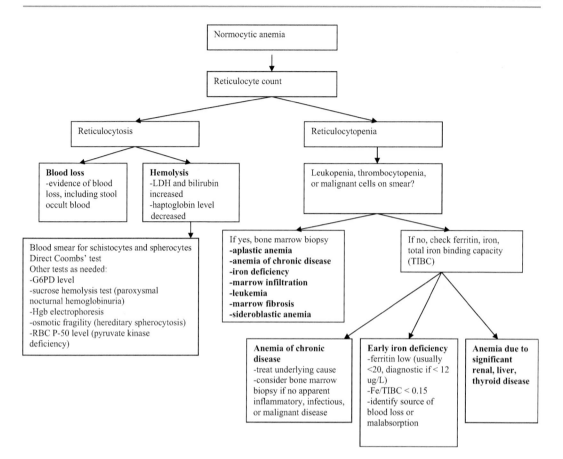

Fig. 2 Evaluation of normocytic anemia

considered in these infants starting at 4 months of age until appropriate iron-containing complementary foods (including iron-fortified cereals) are introduced into the diet.

IDA may also be seen in older infants fed primarily cow's milk because the iron content is low and cow's milk may displace other sources of iron in these infants' diets. Furthermore, the high levels of calcium and phosphorous in cow's milk can decrease iron absorption. Thus, the American Academy of Pediatrics recommends screening for anemia in all infants around 12 months of age [12]. A serum ferritin and C-reactive protein level (CRP) should be checked if patient is anemic. Elevations of both ferritin and CRP can occur in the setting of inflammation. On the other hand, a low serum ferritin (<12 ug/L) confirms IDA, and these infants should be treated appropriately. Alternatively, infants with mild anemia (10–11 dL/g)

can undergo a trial of iron supplementation for 1 month, and a repeat Hgb showing an appropriate rise of 1 dL/g would confirm IDA [12].

Other populations that may develop IDA include children and adolescents whose iron needs are increased due to their rapidly growing bodies in conjunction with poor iron intake. Females lose iron in menstrual blood and can become iron deficient if their bleeding outpaces their iron intake. Pregnancy places additional demands on a woman's iron stores as the placenta and fetus require iron and blood is lost during childbirth. Obesity can predispose to IDA due to increased inflammation from adipose tissue and subsequent increased production of hepcidin, which directly impairs absorption of iron and iron availability for erythropoiesis. Patients with a history of bariatric surgery are at risk of IDA given their history of obesity and possible

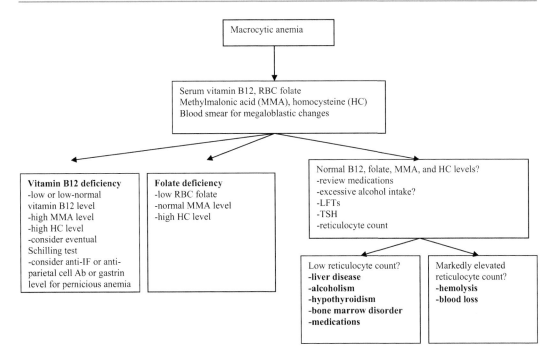

Fig. 3 Evaluation of macrocytic anemia

malabsorption resulting from the surgery itself [13]. IDA is also seen in decreased absorption states such as celiac disease and prior bariatric or other GI surgeries.

In men and postmenopausal women, GI blood loss is the most likely cause of IDA. In these patients, a diligent search for occult GI bleeding is imperative when another source of bleeding is not readily appreciated. This should include upper and lower endoscopy with small bowel biopsy. Radiologic tests may substitute if endoscopy is not practical. In over one-third of patients with IDA, no source of blood loss will be found despite this evaluation [14]. In these patients, prognosis is good, with anemia resolving in more than two-thirds without recurrence [15]. Further search for source of GI blood loss is required only for persistent bleeding or severe anemia.

Physician examination may reveal glossitis and angular stomatitis. Esophageal webs, spleno-megaly, and koilonychias (spoon-shaped nails) rarely occur. Patients may complain of RLS. Although the relationship is unclear, one study showed 24% of patients with IDA also had RLS [16].

The most sensitive and specific laboratory test for IDA is serum ferritin, which reflects iron stores. While a ferritin below 12 ug/L is diagnostic, a workup for IDA should be considered in patients with ferritins of 13–20 ug/L since a significant number of these patients will have IDA. Since ferritin is an acute phase reactant, falsely normal levels may occur with coexisting inflammatory conditions. Normal ferritin values also increase with age and must be considered when evaluating anemia in an older adult. Nonetheless, a ferritin level above 100 ug/L practically rules out IDA [17]. A decreased serum iron and increased total iron binding capacity (TIBC) are helpful but less reliable indicators of IDA. The transferrin saturation (iron/TIBC) should be less than 0.15, but this ratio may be reduced in ACD as well. The MCV is usually normal in early iron deficiency and typically decreases after the Hct drops. The MCV then changes in proportion to the severity of anemia. The RDW is often increased. Although not as widely available, soluble serum transferrin receptor (TfR) rises in IDA and may assist diagnosis in difficult cases, although an increase in

TfR may also be seen in increased or ineffective erythropoiesis [18, 19]. The transferrin receptor-ferritin index (ratio of TfR to the logarithm of serum ferritin) may also play a role in these difficult cases, with a value >2 suggesting IDA and a value <1.0 indicating ACD [20].

Occasionally, ferritin values fall in the indeterminate range of 12–100 ug/L and the diagnosis remains uncertain. Bone marrow biopsy is the gold standard to determine iron stores but is rarely necessary. An alternative is a several week trial of iron replacement. Reticulocytosis should peak after 1 week and the Hct should normalize in about a month. If no response to therapy occurs, iron should be discontinued to prevent potential iron overload and iron therapy side effects.

Oral iron replacement is available in ferrous and ferric forms. Ferrous forms are preferred due to superior absorption and include ferrous sulfate, gluconate, and fumarate. Although most patients with IDA may not need this much, ferrous sulfate 325 mg TID (65 mg of which is elemental iron) is the cheapest and provides the theoretically needed 150–200 mg of elemental iron per day in patients with IDA. Some studies suggest that much less iron supplementation is needed in patients with IDA as their GI tracts absorb more iron after becoming iron deficient. Thus, as little as 60 mg elemental iron once or twice a week may suffice if the patient is unable to tolerate daily dosing [20]. Although Hct should normalize in a few weeks, iron replacement should continue until ferritin reaches 50 ug/L or at least 4–6 months. Many patients experience side effects of nausea, constipation, diarrhea, or abdominal pain as a result of activated hydroxyl radicals released during the oxidation of ferrous compounds within the lumen of the gut or the mucosa [7]. Enteric-coated iron preparations are meant to decrease these symptoms but are not well absorbed and should be avoided. To minimize these effects, iron may be started once a day and titrated up. In addition, iron may be taken with food, although this can decrease absorption by 40–66% [21]. Taking iron with vitamin C may help increase absorption [22]. Liquid iron preparations may be tried. Despite these measures, 10–20% of patients will not tolerate oral iron replacement [23]. Bran, eggs,

milk, tea, caffeine, calcium-rich antacids, H_2-blockers, proton pump inhibitors, and tetracycline can interfere with iron absorption and should not be taken at the same time. Also, iron supplementation can interfere with the absorption of other medications, including quinolones, tetracycline, thyroid hormone, levodopa, methyldopa, and penicillamine.

Most patients respond well to oral replacement of iron. Treatment failures may result from poor adherence, continued blood loss, interfering substances listed above, or gastrointestinal disturbances limiting absorption. In the rare case where poor absorption or severe intolerance to iron cannot be overcome, parenteral replacement may be needed. Iron dextran may be given IV or as a painful IM injection. The total dose (mg) required to replenish stores equals:

$$0.3 \times \text{body weight (lb)} \times (100 - \text{Hgb [g/dL]} \times 100)/14.8$$

Adverse reactions include headache, flushing, dyspnea, nausea, vomiting, fever, hypotension, seizures, and chest, back, and abdominal pain. Urticaria and anaphylaxis can occur. A test dose (0.5 ml = 12.5 mg) should be given to determine whether anaphylaxis will occur. If tolerated, the remainder of the dose may be given up to a maximum daily dose of 100 mg over 2 min or more. If possible, intravenous iron is preferred over intramuscular due to a lower incidence of local reactions and more consistent absorption.

Thalassemia

The thalassemias are inherited disorders of hemoglobin synthesis that are more common in people from the Mediterranean, Asia, and Africa. The rare thalassemia majors cause severe anemia and are discovered early in life. Family physicians are more likely to encounter thalassemia trait (thalassemia minor) occurring in individuals heterozygous for alpha or beta globin chain mutations.

Thalassemia trait should be suspected in an asymptomatic patient with mild anemia and a disproportionately low MCV (56–74 fl). The

RDW is usually normal and the RBC count is normal or increased by 10–20%. Iron studies are normal unless concomitant IDA is present. Blood smear may show target cells, ovalocytes, and basophilic stippling. If a precise diagnosis is required (for prenatal counseling, for example), hemoglobin electrophoresis may be performed. In beta thalassemia trait, elevated levels of Hgb A2 and occasionally Hgb F will be seen. In alpha thalassemia trait, the hemoglobin electrophoresis will be normal, and the diagnosis is made by exclusion. It is important to determine the etiology of anemia in these patients as treatment with iron therapy is unnecessary and potentially harmful in patients with thalassemia trait who do not have IDA.

Hemoglobin E

Hgb E has a prevalence of 5–30% in certain groups from Southeast Asia. The heterozygote has mild microcytosis and normal Hct. Homozygotes have marked microcytosis (MCV 60–70 fl) and mild anemia. Target cells may be present on peripheral smear. Hgb electrophoresis reveals the presence of Hgb E, establishing the diagnosis. Patients who have both Hgb E and beta thalassemia develop severe transfusion-dependent anemias.

Sideroblastic Anemia

Sideroblastic anemias are a heterogeneous group of disorders in which ringed sideroblasts are found on bone marrow staining. Sideroblastic anemia may be X linked or due to toxins or medications (lead, alcohol, isoniazid, chloramphenicol, chemotherapy). It may be related to neoplastic, endocrine, or inflammatory diseases or a part of myelodysplastic syndrome. The MCV is usually low but may range from low to high. Iron saturation and ferritin are normal to high. Marrow examination is diagnostic and treatment is aimed at the underlying cause. In the case of lead poisoning, anemia is microcytic and basophilic stippling may be seen on peripheral smear.

This diagnosis should be suspected and serum lead level tested in high-risk groups such as children ingesting paint, soil, and dust, and adults with occupational exposure.

Normocytic Anemias (Fig. 2)

The absolute reticulocyte count or corrected reticulocyte percentage is important in determining the cause of a normocytic anemia.

Normocytic Anemia with Elevated Reticulocytes

Acute Blood Loss. Acute blood loss is usually obvious but can be missed in cases such as hip fractures and retroperitoneal or pulmonary hemorrhages. The true degree of anemia may not be revealed in the Hct at first, since RBCs and plasma are lost equally. It may take several days for equilibration of blood volume and Hct to fully reflect the degree of bleeding.

Hemolysis. There are many causes of hemolytic anemia (Table 2). Laboratory values consistent with hemolysis include elevated serum lactate dehydrogenase (LDH) and indirect bilirubin. Haptoglobin, a plasma protein that binds and clears Hgb, drops precipitously in the presence of hemolysis. If hemolysis is suspected, the peripheral smear should be examined for schistocytes (mechanical hemolysis) and spherocytes (autoimmune hemolysis or hereditary spherocytosis). A direct Coombs' test will reveal an autoimmune basis for hemolysis. Further confirmatory testing may be performed as appropriate (Fig. 2), usually with the guidance of a hematologist. Treatment of hemolytic anemia is directed at the underlying cause and providing supportive care. Corticosteroids and splenectomy may be indicated for specific causes.

Pregnancy. Pregnancy can result in a physiologic anemia as a woman's blood volume expands by approximately 50% while her red blood cell mass increases by only 25%. As a result pregnant women require approximately 1 additional gram of iron daily. Because IDA during pregnancy has

Table 2 Causes of hemolysis

Intrinsic (defect in RBCs)	Extrinsic (defect external to RBCs)

Hemoglobinopathies
  sickle syndromes
  unstable hemoglobins
  methemoglobinemia
	Immune
	  autoimmune
	  lymphoproliferative
	  malignancy
	  collagen vascular disorders
	  drug induced (methyldopa, procainamide, quinidine, levodopa, sulfas, penicillin, NSAIDS)

Membrane disorders
  paroxysmal nocturnal hemoglobinuria
  hereditary spherocytosis
  elliptocytosis
  pyropoikilocytosis
  stomatocytosis
	Mechanical
	  disseminated intravascular coagulation (DIC)
	  thrombotic thrombocytopenia purpura (TTP)
	  hemolytic uremic syndrome (HUS)
	  prosthetic heart valves
	  disseminated neoplasms
	  burns
	  malignant hypertension
	  vasculitis
	  severe hypophosphatemia
	  physical activity ("march" hemoglobinuria)
	  strenuous exercise

Enzyme deficiencies
  glucose-6-phosphate dehydrogenase (G-6-PD)
  pyruvate kinase
  glucose phosphate isomerase
  congenital erythropoietic porphyria	

	Hypersplenism
	Infections Clostridium, Plasmodium, Borrelia, Mycoplasma, Babesia, Hemophilus, Bartonella

	Bites
	  snakes
	  spiders

been associated with adverse maternal-fetal outcomes including an increased risk of low birth weight, preterm delivery, and perinatal mortality, pregnant women found to have IDA should be treated with supplemental iron. Those who do not respond to iron supplementation should be further evaluated [24].

Normocytic Anemias with Decreased Reticulocytes

Anemia of Chronic Disease. ACD, also called anemia of chronic inflammation (ACI), results from chronic inflammatory disorders, infections, and malignancies. ACD is the second most common cause of anemia after iron deficiency. It is probably the most common form of anemia in the elderly [25]. The pathogenesis of ACD is multifactorial and not fully understood. Proposed mechanisms include reduction in RBC life span, impaired utilization of iron stores, and a relative erythropoietin deficiency. Although the anemia is

customarily normocytic, it can be microcytic in 30–50% of cases [26]. The degree of anemia is usually mild, with Hgb between 7 and 11 g/dl. The serum iron, TIBC, and transferrin saturation are usually low and not helpful in distinguishing ACD from IDA. More useful is the ferritin level, which is normal or high in ACD. Ferritin greater than 100 ug/L essentially rules out IDA, whereas levels less than 12 ug/L are diagnostic of IDA. In cases of uncertain ferritin levels (12–100 ug/L), a brief therapeutic trial of iron or a bone marrow biopsy may help with the diagnosis. Normal TfR levels may be useful in diagnosing ACD due to the suppression of TfR by inflammatory cytokines [17].

Treatment of ACD is directed toward management of the underlying disorder. Erythropoietin plus iron supplementation is effective in raising Hct in certain cases. Iron treatment by itself is not indicated for ACD since iron stores are adequate. However, if the anemia is more severe than expected, one should search for a coexisting cause. For example, a patient with rheumatoid arthritis may develop concomitant IDA from GI blood loss due to chronic NSAID use.

Chronic Kidney Disease. Anemia occurs frequently in chronic kidney disease (CKD) due primarily to the kidney's inability to secrete erythropoietin. Generally, the creatinine is above 3 mg/dl or the estimated glomerular filtration rate (eGFR) is less than 30 ml/min/1.73 m^2. The peripheral smear is usually normal, but burr cells can be seen. The ferritin is typically increased. If a low to low-normal ferritin is noted, concomitant IDA should be entertained. In fact, many patients with end stage kidney disease may suffer from "functional iron deficiency." The Kidney Disease: Improving Global Outcomes guidelines recommends considering iron repletion in patients with CKD with anemia and serum transferrin saturation ≤30% and ferritin ≤500 μg/L. [27]

Therapy consists of ameliorating the renal disease and administering erythropoiesis-stimulating agents (ESAs), namely erythropoietin and darbapoietin. ESA should be considered for non-hemodialysis patients with CKD and Hgb < 10 g/dl, with a goal Hgb of 10–11.5 g/dl. Initial dosing of ESA is based on the patient's Hgb concentration, body weight, and clinical circumstances, and it is adjusted based on the patient's response to treatment. The FDA recommends starting Epoetin alfa at 50–100 units/kg three times per week; however, more commonly it is dosed at 10,000 units weekly or 20,000 units every other week. Patients with concomitant IDA should have iron repleted prior to and during ESA therapy in order to prevent worsening IDA and enhance erythropoiesis. Iron stores should be assessed at least every 3 months during treatment [27]. The treatment and dosing of ESA with iron supplementation may be performed in consultation with a hematologist and/or nephrologist. Hemodialysis may improve RBC production, but ESA is the mainstay of treatment, even before dialysis is required. Blood transfusions should be minimized. Complications of ESAs include increased blood pressure.

Chronic Liver Disease. Chronic liver disease causes a normocytic or occasionally macrocytic anemia. Target cells can be seen on peripheral smear. Spur cells are seen in severe liver failure.

Treatment is directed at improving liver function. Alcoholics with liver disease have additional causes for anemia that are discussed under non-megaloblastic macrocytic anemias.

Endocrine Disease. Various endocrine diseases such as hypothyroidism, hyperthyroidism, hypogonadism, hypopituitarism, hyperparathyroidism, and Addison's disease are associated with anemia. The anemia is corrected with treatment of the underlying endocrine problem.

Aplastic Anemia. Aplastic anemia is due to an injury or destruction of a common pluripotential stem cell resulting in pancytopenia. Bone marrow biopsy reveals severe hypoplasia and fatty infiltration. In the United States, approximately half the cases are idiopathic. Other causes include viral infections (HIV, hepatitis, EBV), drugs and chemicals (chemotherapy, benzene, chloramphenicol), radiation, pregnancy, immune diseases (eosinophilic fasciitis, hypoimmunoglobulinemia, thymoma, thymic carcinoma, graft-versus-host disease), paroxysmal nocturnal hemoglobinuria, systemic lupus erythematosus, and inherited disorders.

Treatment includes managing the underlying cause and supportive care in conjunction with a hematologist. Judicious use of transfusions may be needed if the anemia is severe. Immunosuppressive therapy and bone marrow transplantation are indicated in certain cases.

Myelophthisic Anemia. Myelophthisic anemias result from bone marrow infiltration by invading tumor cells (hematologic malignancies or solid tumor metastases), infectious agents (tuberculosis, fungal infections), or granulomas (sarcoidosis). Less common causes include lipid storage diseases, osteopetrosis, and myelofibrosis. Treatment is directed at the underlying cause.

Red Cell Dysplasia. Pure red cell dysplasias involve a selective failure of erythropoiesis. The granulocyte and platelet counts are normal. Red cell dysplasias share many causes with aplastic and myelophthisic anemia, including malignancies, connective tissue disorders, infections, and drugs. There is an idiopathic form and a congenital form. One infection that specifically targets red cell production is parvovirus B19. This virus also causes erythema infectiosum ("fifth" disease), an acute polyarthropathy syndrome, and hydrops fetalis. Anemia results from parvovirus B19 infection mostly in those with chronic hemolysis, by suppressing erythropoiesis and disrupting a tenuous balance needed to keep up with RBC destruction. In this situation, anemia can be profound but is usually self-limited. Parvovirus B19 infections may become chronic in immunosuppressed individuals who cannot form antibodies to the virus. Treatment concepts for red cell aplasia are similar to treatments for aplastic anemia.

Myelodysplastic Syndromes. The myelodysplastic syndromes (MDS) are a group of clonal hematologic diseases of unknown etiology that result in the inability of bone marrow to produce adequate erythrocytes, leukocytes, platelets, or some combination of these. Patients are usually over 60 years of age and have an increased risk for leukemia. MDS may account for as much as 15–20% of anemia in the elderly [3]. Bone marrow biopsy is diagnostic, revealing characteristic dysplastic blood precursor cells. Treatment is largely supportive.

Macrocytic Anemias (Fig. 3)

Macrocytic anemias may be separated into megaloblastic and non-megaloblastic types, based on peripheral smear findings (Table 1). A sensitive and specific sign of megaloblastic anemia is hypersegmented neutrophils, in which neutrophils contain nuclei with more than five lobes. A marked elevation of MCV (>120 fl) is also highly suggestive of megaloblastosis. RBCs of megaloblastic anemias, in addition to being increased in size, are often oval in shape (macroovalocytes).

Most macrocytosis, however, results from non-megaloblastic causes. Drug therapy and alcoholism may account for $>50\%$ of macrocytosis, whereas vitamin B12 and folate deficiencies may be responsible for only 6% of cases [28].

Megaloblastic Anemias

Vitamin B12 Deficiency. Vitamin B12 (cobalamin) is ingested from primarily animal sources,

including meats, eggs, and dairy products. The US RDA of vitamin B12 increases with age and is 2.4 ug daily for adults. A typical Western diet provides 5–30 ug/day. After ingestion, B12 is bound by intrinsic factor, which is produced by gastric parietal cells. Bound vitamin is absorbed in the terminal ileum. Body stores of vitamin B12 total 2,000–5,000 ug. Thus, B12 deficiency takes years to develop and rarely occurs from dietary insufficiency except in strict vegans. The majority of B12 deficiency is due to pernicious anemia, which occurs primarily in the elderly and is most often due to autoimmune atrophy of the gastric mucosa and intrinsic factor deficiency. Less often, pernicious anemia can be due to *H. pylori* infections or Zollinger-Ellison syndrome. Other causes of B12 deficiency include gastric and ileal surgeries, including gastric bypass surgery and ileal absorption problems such as Crohn's disease, sprue, tapeworm infection, and medications such as metformin, proton pump inhibitors, H2-blockers, and antacids.

Signs and symptoms of B12 deficiency include glossitis, sore mouth, and GI disturbances such as constipation, diarrhea, and indigestion. Neurologic symptoms such as paresthesias of the extremities and subacute combined degeneration (loss of lower extremity vibration and position sense) may occur. Dementia and subtle neuropsychiatric changes may be present. Importantly, anemia or macrocytosis are absent in 28% of patients with neurologic abnormalities due to B12 deficiency [29].

In addition to peripheral smear changes of hypersegmented neutrophils and macroovalocytes, laboratory findings include a low B12 level (<200 pg/ml) and reticulocyte count. However, low normal B12 levels (<350 pg/ml) are present in many patients with neurologic disease or anemia, so further workup may be indicated if the diagnosis is still suspected. Falsely low B12 levels may be found in folate deficiency, pregnancy, and myeloma. Elevated serum methylmalonic acid (MMA) levels are highly sensitive and essentially rule out B12 deficiency if normal. In one study, elevated MMA levels occurred in 98% of cases of clinically defined B12 deficiency. Falsely elevated levels occur in kidney disease and hypovolemia, and spot urine MMA levels may be superior in this setting. Homocysteine level rises with B12 deficiency (96% of cases in one study) but are less specific, occurring in folate deficiency and kidney disease as well [30–32]. Occasionally, a mild thrombocytopenia and leukopenia, along with an elevated LDH and indirect bilirubin from ineffective erythropoiesis, are present.

Traditionally, the Schilling test was performed to determine the etiology of B12 deficiency. It measures 24-h urinary excretion of radiolabeled B12 given orally and distinguishes pernicious anemia from bacterial overgrowth and other absorption problems. This test is not commonly utilized as it is expensive, difficult to perform properly, and no longer available in many centers. Antibodies to intrinsic factor may be measured and are the preferred test for diagnosing pernicious anemia. These antibodies are highly specific for pernicious anemia but present in only about 50% of cases. Antibodies to gastric parietal cells are found in about 85% of cases of pernicious anemia but also in 3–10% of healthy persons [32]. Extremely elevated serum gastrin levels and low pepsinogen 1 levels also suggest pernicious anemia.

B12 replacement regimens vary. One common method is 1,000 ug vitamin B12 IM daily for 1 week, then weekly for 1 month, and then every 1–3 months. The Hct should return to normal in 2 months. Failure to normalize should trigger a search for coexisting iron deficiency, which occurs in up to one-third of patients. Six months or more may be needed for neurologic improvement and up to 80% of patients will have at least partial resolution of neurologic manifestations. An alternative to parenteral B12 is high dose oral therapy. Patients with pernicious anemia can absorb 1–2% of oral B12 without the addition of intrinsic factor, so treatment with daily oral B12 1,000–2,000 ug can be considered in adherent patients [33]. B12 maintenance can also be accomplished with an intranasal gel preparation 500 ug once weekly, although this form is more costly than parenteral and oral forms. Treatment should continue indefinitely as the deficiency will likely return unless a reversible cause is identified and addressed.

Folate Deficiency. Folate is found in a wide variety of unprocessed foods. Especially rich sources include green leafy vegetables, citrus fruits, liver, and certain beans and nuts. The RDA for folate is about 200 ug daily and is increased to 400 ug in pregnancy. In contrast to vitamin B12, folate stores remain adequate for only 2–4 months, so folate deficiency anemia is often the result of inadequate dietary intake. The typical Western diet provides only 200–300 ug of folate daily. Persons at risk for folate deficiency include malnourished alcoholics, neglected elderly, and the homeless. Patients who are pregnant or have certain malabsorption disorders are also at risk. Impaired absorption may occur in patients taking oral contraceptives, metformin, methotrexate, or antibiotics such as trimethoprim or pyrimethamine or anticonvulsants, such as phenytoin, valproate, and carbamazepine. Cirrhosis can lead to deficiency through decreased storage and metabolism capabilities of the liver. Dialysis can cause loss of folate and deficiency.

The clinical findings of folate deficiency are similar to B12 deficiency except neurologic symptoms are generally absent. The laboratory findings are similar except that the homocysteine level alone is elevated while MMA remains normal. The serum folate can rise to normal after a recent folate rich meal, vitamin ingestion, or hemolysis, so serum folate should not be used for diagnosis. Although expensive, RBC folate level is felt to be more accurate. Confirmation with homocysteine levels should be obtained if the diagnosis is suspected.

Treatment is aimed at the underlying problem. Replacement is usually 1 mg orally daily. If present, concurrent vitamin B12 deficiency must be treated as well, because folate replacement can resolve hematologic abnormalities while permitting neurologic damage from vitamin B12 deficiency to progress.

Drugs. Certain drugs cause megaloblastic anemia. Most common causes are chemotherapy agents. Infrequent causes are phenytoin, sulfasalazine, zidovudine, trimethoprim, pyrimethamine, methotrexate, triamterene, sulfa compounds, and oral contraceptives.

Non-megaloblastic Anemias

Alcoholism. The most common cause of non-megaloblastic macrocytic anemia is alcoholism. Anemia in alcoholics may arise from multiple causes. Alcohol suppresses erythropoiesis and decreases folate absorption in patients whose diets are often poor. Alcoholics can lose blood from varices and ulcers. Anemia is worsened if liver failure occurs. Moreover, alcoholics are prone to develop sideroblastic or hemolytic anemia. They are also at increased risk for developing infections that can lead to ACD. Comprehensive therapy includes reduction of alcohol intake, folate supplementation, and treatment of complications.

Miscellaneous. The anemia of hypothyroidism, chronic liver disease, post-splenectomy, and primary bone marrow disorders may be macrocytic instead of normocytic. Hemolytic anemia or hemorrhage can result in macrocytosis when reticulocytes, which are larger than normal RBCs, are markedly increased. Certain drugs occasionally cause non-megaloblastic macrocytic anemia. Spurious macrocytosis, although rare, must also be considered due to cold agglutinins causing the RBCs to clump and appear larger to automated counters. Other causes include hyperglycemia causing RBCs to swell when diluted during blood processing or leukocytosis leading to increased blood sample turbidity with a subsequent overestimation in cell size by the machine [34].

Summary

Discovery of anemia should lead the physician to investigate its underlying cause. Conversely, it may be reasonable to check for anemia in patients who develop certain acute or chronic medical conditions. The history and physical examination combined with the CBC, peripheral smear, and reticulocyte count reveal the etiology in most cases. However, it is not uncommon to find multifactorial causes for a patient's anemia. If the type of anemia remains unclear or there is additional evidence of marrow dysfunction (pancytopenia), a bone marrow biopsy and hematology consultation may be indicated.

References

1. Beutler E, Waalen J. The definition of anemia: what is the lower limit of normal of the blood hemoglobin concentration? Blood. 2006;107(5):1747–50.
2. Le CHH. The prevalence of anemia and moderate-severe anemia in the US population (NHANES 2003-2012). PLoS One. 2016;11(11):e0166635. https://doi.org/10.1371/journal.pone.0166635.
3. Pang WW, Schrier S. Anemia in the elderly. Curr Opin in Hematol. 2012;19(3):133–40. https://doi.org/10.1097/MOH.0b013e3283522471. Accessed 10 Dec 2014.
4. Ruíz-Argüelles GJ. Altitude above sea level as a variable for definition of anemia. Blood. 2006;108(6):2131. author reply 2131–2
5. Mairbäurl H. Red blood cells in sports: effects of exercise and training on oxygen supply by red blood cells. Front Physiol. 2013;4:332. https://doi.org/10.3389/fphys.2013.00332. Accessed 10 Dec 2014.
6. Peeling P, Dawson B, Goodman C, Landers G, Trinder D. Athletic induced iron deficiency: new insights into the role of inflammation, cytokines and hormones. Eur J Appl Physiol. 2008;103(4):381–91. https://doi.org/10.1007/s00421-008-0726-6. Accessed 3 Dec 2014.
7. Gasche C, Lomer MC, Cavill I, Weiss G. Iron, anaemia, and inflammatory bowel diseases. Gut. 2004;53(8):1190–7.
8. Bessman JD, Gilmer PR Jr, Gardner FH. Improved classification of anemias by MCV and RDW. Am J Clin Pathol. 1983;80(3):322–6.
9. Brugnara C, Mohandas N. Red cell indices in classification and treatment of anemias: from M.M. Wintrobe's original 1934 classification to the third millennium. Curr Opin Hematol. 2013;20(3):222–30. https://doi.org/10.1097/MOH.0b013e32835f5933. Accessed 10 Dec 2014.
10. World Health Organization. The global prevalence of anaemia in 2011. http://apps.who.int/iris/bitstream/10665/177094/1/9789241564960_eng.pdf?ua=1. Accessed 10 June 2020.
11. Office of Dietary Supplements (US). Iron dietary supplement fact sheet. U.S. Department of Health and Human Services, National Institutes of Health; 2014 Apr 8. Available from: http://ods.od.nih.gov/factsheets/Iron-HealthProfessional/
12. Baker RD, Greer FR. Committee on Nutrition American Academy of Pediatrics. Diagnosis and prevention of iron deficiency and iron-deficiency anemia in infants and young children (0–3 years of age). Pediatrics. 2010;126(5):040–50. https://doi.org/10.1542/peds.2010-2576. Accessed 3 Dec 2014.
13. Aigner E, Feldman A, Datz C. Obesity as an emerging risk factor for iron deficiency. Nutrients. 2014;6

(9):3587–600. https://doi.org/10.3390/nu6093587. Accessed 1 Dec 2014.

14. Rockey DC, Cello JP. Evaluation of the gastrointestinal tract in patients with iron-deficiency anemia. New Engl J Med. 1993;329(23):1691–5.

15. Fireman Z, Kopelman Y, Editorial SA. Endoscopic evaluation of iron deficiency anemia and follow-up in patients older than 50. J Clin Gastroenterol. 1998;26 (1):7–10.

16. Allen RP, Auerbach S, Bahrain H, Auerbach M, Earley CJ. The prevalence and impact of restless legs syndrome on patients with iron deficiency anemia. Am J Hematol. 2013;88(4):261–4. https://doi.org/10.1002/ajh.23397. Accessed 1 Dec 2014.

17. Punnonen K, Irjala K, Rajamaki A. Serum transferrin receptor and its ratio to serum ferritin in the diagnosis of iron deficiency. Blood. 1997;89(3):1052–7.

18. Guyatt GH, Oxman AD, Ali M, Willan A, McIlroy W, Patterson C. Laboratory diagnosis of iron-deficiency anemia: an overview. J Gen Intern Med. 1992;7 (2):145–53.

19. Knovich MA, Storey JA, Coffman LG, Torti SV, Torti FM. Ferritin for the clinician. Blood Rev. 2009;23 (3):95–104. https://doi.org/10.1016/j.blre.2008.08.001. Accessed 1 Dec 2014.

20. Gross R, Schultink W, Juliawati. Treatment of anemia with weekly iron supplementation [letter]. Lancet. 1994;344(8925):821.

21. Ritey MR. Iron-containing products. In: Drug facts and comparisons staff, editor. Drug facts and comparisons. St. Louis: Facts and comparisons; 2000. p. 31–41.

22. Hallberg L, Brune M, Rossander-Hulthén L. Is there a physiological role of vitamin C in iron absorption? Ann N Y Acad Sci. 1987;498:324–32.

23. Little DR. Ambulatory management of common forms of anemia. Am Fam Physician. 1999;59(6):1598–604.

24. Obstet Gynecol 2008; 112(1):201–7. https://doi.org/10.1097/AOG.0b013e3181809c0d.

25. Joosten E, Pelemans W, Hiele M, Noyen J, Verghaeghe R, Boogaerts MA. Prevalence and causes of anaemia in a geriatric hospitalized population. Gerontology. 1992;38(1–2):111–7.

26. Krantz SB. Pathogenesis and treatment of the anemia of chronic disease. Am J Med Sci. 1994;307:353–9.

27. Kidney Disease: Improving Global Outcomes KDIGO) Anemia Work Group. KDIGO clinical practice guideline for anemia in chronic kidney disease. Kidney Int Suppl 2012;2:279–335.

28. Savage DG, Ogundipe A, Allen R, Stabler S, Lindenbaum J. Etiology and diagnostic evaluation of macrocytosis. Am J Med Sci. 2000;319(6):343–52.

29. Lindenbaum J, Healton EB, Savage DG, Brust JC, Garrett TJ, Podell ER, et al. Neuropsychiatric disorders caused by cobalamin deficiency in the absence of anemia or macrocytosis. New Engl J Med. 1988;318 (26):1720–8.

30. Savage DJ, Lindenbaum J, Stabler SP, Allen RH. Sensitivity of serum methylmalonic acid and total homocysteine determinations for diagnosing cobalamin and folate deficiencies. Am J Med. 1994;96(3):239–46.

31. Klee GG. Cobalamin and folate evaluation: measurement of methylmalonic acid and homocysteine vs. vitamin B(12) and folate. Clin Chem. 2000;46 (8 Pt 2):1277–83.

32. Snow CF. Laboratory diagnosis of vitamin B12 and folate deficiency: a guide for the primary care physician. Arch Intern Med. 1999;159(12):1289–98.

33. Elia M. Oral or parenteral therapy for B12 deficiency. Lancet. 1998;352:1721–2.

34. Kaferle J, Strzoda CE. Evaluation of macrocytosis. Am Fam Physician. 2009;79(3):203–8.

Selected Disorders of the Blood and Hematopoietic System

Emily Emmet, Anusha Jagadish, Rajat Malik, and Raj Mehta

Contents

E. Emmet · A. Jagadish · R. Malik · R. Mehta (✉)
AdventHealth Family Medicine Residency, Winter Park,
FL, USA
e-mail: emily.emmet.do@adventhealth.com;
anusha.jagadish.do@adventhealth.com;
rajat.malik.do@adventhealth.com;
raj.mehta.md@adventhealth.com

© Springer Nature Switzerland AG 2022
P. M. Paulman et al. (eds.), *Family Medicine*,
https://doi.org/10.1007/978-3-030-54441-6_158

Bleeding Disorders

Bleeding disorders can be present in both adult and pediatric populations. Diagnosing a suspected bleeding can be a difficult task in hematology. However, with the combination of a good history, diagnostic approach and understanding of various disorders, a diagnosis and management plan can be made [1].

Patients can present in many waves, ranging from easy bruising to excessive bleeding. As stated before, a family history is key in identifying bleeding disorders. A positive family history is a good indicator warranting further work-up. Additional history like diet and medications can also lead a physician to a correct diagnosis, ruling out iatrogenic causes [2].

Once the suspicion is high, blood work should be done to either confirm or dismiss the diagnosis. Labs include complete blood count (CBC), prothrombin time (PT), partial thromboplastin time (PTT), bleeding time, and platelet function assay. Patients can also be referred to a hematologist for further work-up and management, especially if lab findings are normal but there is a high clinical concern.

Management of bleeding disorders is based on the comfort level of both the physician and the patient. It can become complex, and referral to Hematology at the time of diagnosis is appropriate. Ultimately, a patient-centered approach is important and associated with improvement in level of functioning and compliance.

Congenital Coagulation Disorders

Von Willebrand's Disease

One of the most common bleeding disorders, Von willebrand's Disease (vWD), has a prevalence as high as 1.5%. It is defined by a deficiency of von Willebrand factor (vWF), a glycoprotein that mediates adhesion of platelets to sites of vascular damage [2]. It is inherited in an autosomal dominant pattern, affecting males and females equally. It is also common to have low levels of Factor VIII with vWD [3].

Symptoms of hemorrhage include epistaxis, gastrointestinal bleeding, easy bruising, menorrhagia, postpartum bleeding, Gastrointestinal (GI) bleeds, hemarthrosis, and bleeding after trauma or procedures like dental extraction. Type III is usually much more severe compared to Type I and II. Most individuals never come to get medical attention for bleeding because the disease is often mild.

Complete blood count with platelet PT and PTT are usually normal. vWD can be confirmed with the laboratory findings of decreased Factor VIII levels and activity, decreased vWF activity, and decreased vW antigen. Bleeding time is no longer used due to its time-consuming nature and that it does not correlate with bleeding risk. vWF Ristocetin cofactor assay is the gold standard for platelet-binding activity. vWWF activity to vWF antigen ratios are then used to further characterize the type and severity of von Willebrand disease [4].

When treating vWD, the goal is to prevent bleeding and correct coagulation abnormalities. There are different methods of treating based on severity and contact of bleeding. vWF concentrates and recombinant vWF can be used for major life-threatening bleeding. DDAVP (desamino-D-arginine vasopressin) is a medication that works by increasing plasma levels of vWF, Factor VIII, and tissue plasminogen activator (t-PA) [5]. Patients with mild vWD can be treated with DDAVP 0.2–0.3 mcg/kg administered intravenously or 150–300 mcg intranasally. Antifibrinolytic agents and Factor VIII can be used in adjunct to these treatments. Platelet transfusion for those with thrombocytopenias is also a consideration. Oral contraception can also be used in females who have menorrhagia due to vWD, it causes increased levels of Factor VIII and vWF. Surgical and dental procedures can be performed in most patients, starting treatment 1 h prior and up to 2–3 days after. vWD can be preventable through genetic counseling; there is a 50% chance of children with a parent with vWD at risk of developing it [3].

Hemophilia A

Hemophilia A is a bleeding disorder caused by a deficiency in Factor VIII. It's mode of transmission and gene expression is X-linked recessive; therefore, males have Hemophilia A and females are asymptomatic carriers. All daughters of fathers with the disorder will be carriers and all their sons will be normal, where male children of a mother who carries the gene have a 50% chance of having the disease. Hemophilia A affects approximately 1/10,0000–20,000 males in the United States [6]. Initial presentations in children include easy bruising, hemarthrosis, oral bleeding, and post-procedural bleeding within the first year of life.

Factor VIII is involved in the clotting pathway. Its deficiency results in larger sites of bleeding like hemorrhage into muscles or joints. Severe hemophilia will present within a year and a half of life. Common bleeding also includes genitourinary tract, central nervous system, gastrointestinal tract, and oral cavity. Unlike platelet disorders, excessive bleeding after minor cuts or abrasions is not common. When screening bleeding disorder, there is a prolonged activated aPTT. Other coagulation tests like platelet count, bleeding time, and PT are all normal. To confirm the diagnosis, a serum Factor VIII activity level <40% or 0.40 IU/mL [7].

It is important to institute integrated care once a diagnosis is made, as this disease can be complex, routine, and comprehensive care is important [6]. Newborns should follow normal immunization schedules. Dental care is important to prevent gum and tooth disease, which increase the chances of bleeding. Anticoagulants, Aspirin, and NSAIDs should be avoided. Special considerations must be taken when a patient with hemophilia has any surgery or procedure done: done at a facility with an adequate blood bank and transfusion services, experienced surgeons in treating those with coagulopathies, discussion with hematologist and anesthesiologist, no intramuscular medications, avoidance of salicylate, and maintenance of Factor VIII levels.

The goal of treatment is to increase levels of Factor VIII. Hemorrhage is prevented by infusion of recombinant or human-derived Factor VIII. Serum Factor VIII level is targeted based on symptoms: 0.3 U/mL for patients with minor hemorrhage, 0.5 U/mL with severe hemorrhage, and 0.8–1.0 U/mL. However, treatment of choice is intravenous desamino-D-arginine vasopressin (DDAVP) (Desmopressin acetate 0.3 ug/kg) for patients with mild hemophilia [8]. E-Aminocaproic acid (EACA), a potent inhibitor of fibrinolysis, can also be used as a single or adjunctive postoperative dose (4 g PO q4–6hrs for 2–8 days for dental procedures [9]).Ultimately, genetic counseling and testing women who are at risk for carriers can help prevent future generations with Hemophilia A.

Hemophilia B

Hemophilia B is a bleeding disorder caused by a deficiency in Factor IX. It is an X-linked recessive inheritance pattern. This disorder has an incidence of about 1/30,0000 males. It is diagnosed via a Factor IX assay.

Clinically, Hemophilia B is almost indistinguishable from Hemophilia A, the same clotting cascade is affected. Diagnosis is based on Factor IX activity. Treatment includes intravenous human-derived or recombinant Factor IX concentrate. You can also treat the disorder with Fibrinolytic factors. Unlike Hemophilia A, DDAVP has no value in treatment [5].

Easy Bruising

Ecchymosis, or a bruise, is a collection of blood beneath the skin resulting from extravasation from surrounding vessels. Easy bruising is reported in about 18% of the population, predominantly affecting women [8]. It can be considered mostly normal when other life-threatening or pathological causes have been ruled out. There are some characteristic lesions however that can be identified.

For example, senile purpura is a lesion of the elderly caused by progressive loss of collagen in vessels and skin likely due to sun exposure. These lesions occur on the upper extremities, especially on the dorsal aspect. They are described as large, dark purple, and well-demarcated. Senile purpuras is a clinical diagnosis. Coagulation studies are usually normal. There is no specific treatment, lesions usually resolve slowly. Counseling the patient and limiting sun exposure may minimize skin changes of aging.

Etiology of bruising is classified into disorders of blood vessels and tissue, platelet abnormalities, and coagulation disorders [8]. These disorders are discussed in this chapter. When evaluating easy bruising, a thorough history, physical exam, and associated trauma are important to know. If warranted, laboratory tests include CBC, PT, aPTT, platelet function. When abnormalities are found, further testing can be done to explore avenues that explain lab findings.

Acquired Coagulation Disorders

Vitamin K Deficiency

Vitamin K is an essential part of the clotting pathway, involved in the synthesis of Factors II, VII, IX, and X. It is a fat-soluble compound that comes from our diet (Especially green leafy vegetables) and is also synthesized by intestinal bacteria [10]. Daily adult requirement of Vitamin K is 100–200 ug/day. Newborns are born with a deficiency because they lack intestinal bacteria to synthesize it. The elderly, those with liver disease, cystic fibrosis, malabsorption syndromes, patients on warfarin, and other long-term medications that disrupt flora can become deficient too.

Vitamin K deficiency presents with bleeding from mucosal surfaces or skin, internal bleeding is less likely. Work-up will be significant for prolonged PT, with a normal bleeding time and platelet count; sometimes aPTT can be prolonged.

Usually correcting Vitamin K deficiency can be diagnostic as well. A direct laboratory assay for Vitamin K available as well [10].

Treatment includes replenishing Vitamin K, can be given IV, IM, or PO. If there is life-threatening hemorrhage, fresh frozen plasma is given. The goal of therapy is to prevent further bleeding and correct PT. A diet with adequate Vitamin K and careful use of long-term antibiotics can prevent a deficiency. Newborns are given Vitamin K 0.5–0.1 mg IM to prevent hemorrhagic disease of the newborn. Supplementation can be useful when on anticonvulsant therapy or prolonged treatment with antibiotics. It is important to remember that for the elderly, Vitamin K deficiency can be a sign of neglect or poor diet [10].

Thrombocytopenia

Thrombocytopenia is identified by a low-platelet count below 50,000/µL [11]. It typically occurs due to decreased platelet production or increased platelet destruction. Common causes include liver disease and medication-induced thrombocytopenia. Redistribution and hypersplenism are also possible culprits. Heparin-induced thrombocytopenia (HIT) should be suspected for anyone with falling platelet counts while on heparin. Two forms often presenting with rash and spontaneous bruising include immune thrombocytopenic purpura and thrombotic thrombocytopenic purpura. Disseminated intravascular coagulation is a more severe cause of thrombocytopenia associated with sepsis, trauma, cancer, etc. Treatment of thrombocytopenia depends on identifying the underlying cause and severity of the disease [11].

Hereditary Hemorrhagic Telangiectasia (HHT)

Hereditary Hemorrhagic Telangiectasia (HHT), formerly known as Osler-Weber-Rendu Disease, is a congenital disorder that results in small vessel malformations in the skin and mucosa, creating telangiectasias. It is an autosomal dominant disorder that affects males and females equally [12]. The most common presentations are GI bleeds or epistaxis. The lesions become apparent in the second and third decade of life; lesions would be visible in the mouth, face, hands, and feet. They are described as spider-like, round, red-purple, and about 1–3 mm in diameter. Lesions can also occur in almost any organ, however, mostly found in the lungs. Diagnosis is usually made with history and physical exam, there is usually a positive family history. Coagulation studies are usually normal. Treatment is applying pressure to the bleeding sites, or cautery and surgery therapy of lesions if need be. GI bleeding can be stopped by either resection or embolectomy. Unfortunately, HHT is not preventable [13].

Neutropenia

Neutropenia is defined by an absolute neutrophil count less than 1500/mm^3. Absolute neutrophil count (ANC) can be calculated by the following: ANC = WBC × (%bands + %mature neutrophils) × 0.01 [14]. This definition holds true for males, females, and many ethnicities with the exception of children less than 12 months of age, in which case neutropenia is defined by ANC <1000/mm^3. Certain nationalities, including those of African descent, Jewish Yemenites, and some Arab populations, typically have lower ANC counts than the general population (around 1400/mm^3), but will rarely fall below 1000/mm^3. The diagnosis should be confirmed by repeating complete blood count with manual differential and peripheral smear. There are three major causes of neutropenia: decreased production, increased destruction, and margination of neutrophils from blood to tissue. If neutropenia coexists with thrombocytopenia, anemia, and/or abnormalities noted on peripheral smear, further investigation should be pursued in the form of bone marrow aspiration to determine if there are any underlying blood cell line disorder or bone marrow pathology [15].

Neutropenic patients should be referred to hematology for further management after the diagnosis is confirmed. If a neutropenic patient develops fever, broad-spectrum antibiotics must be initiated while awaiting culture results and antibiotic sensitivity. There are certain situations that warrant immediate evaluation in the inpatient setting for a patient with neutropenia, such as signs of sepsis, hemodynamic instability, and respiratory compromise. Patients with ANC <500/mm^3 and/or worrisome findings on peripheral smear (blasts, schistocytes) should also be evaluated in the inpatient setting for prompt diagnosis and treatment. If the patient has moderate (>500 but <1000) neutropenia, is asymptomatic, and has no worrisome findings on peripheral smear, CBC may be repeated in 1–2 weeks to confirm and verify that the neutropenia is true. If the patient has mild >1000 neutropenia and is asymptomatic, CBC may be repeated in 2–6 weeks in the outpatient setting. Granulocyte colony-stimulating factor can be given to stimulate the production of neutrophils in order to reduce the duration of neutropenic fever. It may also be given chronically for the long-term treatment of primary neutropenia.

Acquired Neutropenia

Postinfectious Neutropenia

The most common cause of acquired neutropenia is postinfectious neutropenia [16]. The underlying mechanism of why infections cause neutropenia can be explained by the macrophage activation syndrome (MAS). This occurs when macrophages become activated in response to certain stimuli and the degree by which this happens may be sufficient enough to cause splenomegaly and cytopenias. This occurs after either bacterial or viral infections. Two common bacteria that are associated with neutropenia are *Staphylococcus aureus* and *Escherichia coli*. Additional bacterial infections known to cause neutropenia rather than leukocytosis in some instances are typhoid fever (may also cause pancytopenia), Shigella enteritis, Brucellosis (coexisting anemia is common), Tularemia, and Tuberculosis. Viral infections that are commonly known to cause neutropenia are Epstein–Barr virus, Hepatitis B, cytomegalovirus, and influenza. Neutropenia is common among those patients with HIV/AIDS. The degree of neutropenia can be directly correlated to the severity of infection, for example. in sepsis, the neutropenia may be more severe. ANC will typically normalize as the infection resolves.

Drug-Induced Neutropenia

Drug-induced neutropenia is the second most common cause of acquired neutropenia (Table 1). The estimated incidence of idiosyncratic drug reactions is 1/10,000 to 1/100,000. The drugs that are known to commonly cause agranulocytosis are clozapine, thionamides (methimazole), sulfasalazine, and ticlopidine.Treatment of drug-induced neutropenia involves removing the offending drug and consulting a hematologist if the neutropenia does not resolve [17].

Congenital Neutropenia

Congenital neutropenia, also known as "Severe congenital neutropenia" refers to neutropenia that is present at or near the time of birth and is due to a primary bone marrow failure syndrome involving primarily the myeloid series [15]. The incidence is rare, occurring in 2–3 cases per million. There are a variety of mutations that cause SCN and inheritance may be recessive, dominant, or X-linked depending on the mutation.

Kostmann syndrome results from mutations in the *HAX1* gene and has an autosomal recessive inheritance. The *HAX1* gene is responsible for maintaining the inner mitochondrial membrane potential and protecting against apoptosis in myeloid cells.

About 50–60% of patients with SCN have mutations in the gene for neutrophil elastase which is an autosomal dominant condition. Cyclic neutropenia is a subtype of inherited neutropenia which is also associated with mutations in this gene (ELANE). Patients will typically present with fever, malaise, and mucosal ulcerations every 3 weeks, with otherwise good health in between episodes. The incidence is 1 case per million in the general population.

The mechanism of neutropenia is due to activation of excessive apoptosis in myeloid precursors. The expression of neutropenia in SCN may be either homogeneous or variable, suggesting different pathogenetic mechanisms and effects of interacting genes. Patients will clinically present with oropharyngeal problems, otitis media, respiratory infections, and skin infections. Oral ulcerations and painful gingivitis are very common in 2 years of age. Diagnosis of SCN is made in an infant with an average absolute neutrophil count of $<200/\mu L$ with elevated monocytes. Treatment includes granulocyte-colony stimulating factor or hematopoietic stem cell transplantation if severe. The introduction of G-CSF has allowed these patients to live into adulthood but with additional consequences. Patients with SCN have a

Table 1 Drugs that can cause neutropenia

Nonchemotherapy	Chemotherapy
Clozapine	Alkylating agents
Dapsone	Anthracyclines
Hydroxychloroquine	Antimetabolites
Infliximab	Camptothecins
Lamotrigine	Epipodophyllotoxins
Methimazole	Hydroxyurea
Oxacillin	Mitomycin C
Penicillin G	Taxanes
Procainamide	Vinblastine
Quinidine/Quinine	
Rituximab	
Sulfasalazine	
Trimethoprim-sulfamethoxazole	
Vancomycin	

predisposition to myelodysplastic syndrome and leukemia. The development of these conditions appears to be a complication of the underlying disease rather than a side effect of treatment with G-CSF [18].

Autoimmune Neutropenia

Autoimmune neutropenia is thought to be caused by granulocyte-specific antibodies and has been associated with various underlying disease including infection, collagen vascular disease, or other primary abnormalities of the immune system [15]. Most cases of autoimmune neutropenia are not associated with underlying disease and referred to as Chronic Benign Neutropenia (CBN). In children, this commonly occurs between ages of 5 and 15 months, but the range extends from 1 month to adulthood. The disease is characterized by the inability to increase WBC count when ill. The majority of pediatric cases will recover by adulthood without intervention. Antineutrophil antibodies are detected in 98–100% of patients with autoimmune neutropenia. Diagnosis can be assumed if a patient has isolated neutropenia, no dysmorphic features, no hepatosplenomegaly, no bone pain, no chronic diarrhea, no severe or unusual infections, and no other signs of significant underlying disorders. Treatment of the neutropenia is not typically required as it is usually mild and not associated with severe infections [19].

Chronic Idiopathic Neutropenia

Chronic idiopathic neutropenia (CIN), also known as benign chronic neutropenia, is a term which describes patients with chronic neutropenia for which there is no underlying cause. This condition tends to occur in late childhood or adulthood and does not usually undergo spontaneous remission. The ANC ranges from 500 to 1000/μL and often accompanied by monocytosis. The clinical course is typically benign despite the degree of neutropenia, possibly because there is usually marrow reserve. Treatment directed at increasing the neutrophil count should be reserved for those with significant and recurrent infectious complications.

Alloimmune (Isoimmune Neutropenia)

The incidence of alloimmune neutropenia has been estimated at 2 per 1000 live births. The neutropenia occurs due to transplacental passage of maternal IgG antibodies to neutrophil specific antigens inherited from the father. The pathogenesis is similar to that of Rh hemolytic disease. Infants may present with sepsis or be asymptomatic. It may be difficult to discern if the sepsis was caused by neutropenia or if the neutropenia is a result of sepsis. Antinuclear antibodies can be detected in infant and maternal serum and may show specificity for father's neutrophils. This is typically noted in an otherwise normal infant and the course is usually benign. Neutropenia resolves within 12–15 weeks although prolonged cases have occurred. If necessary, infants who are severely septic may be treated with G-CSF and complete evaluation can occur after the course of illness to determine if the neutropenia is alloimmune or a subtype of congenital neutropenia.

Nutritional Neutropenia

Neutropenia may be caused by deficiencies in vitamin B12, folate and copper, all of which are common in those who abuse alcohol. The neutropenia will typically resolve with appropriate supplementation of the deficient vitamins but may take 2–4 weeks to resolve. Deficiencies of folate and B12 may also result in a concomitant macrocytic anemia.

Other Hematologic Disorders

Hemochromatosis

Hereditary hemochromatosis (HH) is an autosomal recessive inherited disorder with low penetrance, meaning that biallelic mutations are usually required for clinically significant disease but many individuals with biallelic mutations will

Table 2 Screening thresholds for Hereditary Hemochromatosis molecular and genetic testing

	TSAT (transferrin saturation)	Ferritin
British Society for Hematology (2018)	>40% for women and >50% for men	>300 ng/mL (>300 mcg/L) for men or >200 ng/mL (>300 mcg/L) for women
American Association for the Study of Liver Disease (2011)	>45%	>200 ng/mL for men and >150 ng/mL for women or above the upper limit of normal for the testing laboratory
American College of Physicians (2005)	>55%	>300 ng/mL (>300 mcg/L) for men or >200 ng/mL (>300 mcg/L) for women

not be affected [20]. It is considered one of the most common genetic disorders in Caucasians in the United States and Europe. Mutations in the HFE gene are seen in most individuals with HH. The two common mutations include the C282Y allele and the H63D allele. Homozygosity for C282Y accounts for 90% of HH cases and is more commonly associated with clinical disease. The likelihood of clinically significant iron overload resulting in organ damage is most common in homozygous C282Y/C282Y, resulting in 10% of patients or higher. Compound heterozygous C282Y/H63D and homozygous H63D/H63D have significantly less propensity to iron-overload states. Clinical manifestations of HH typically occur after age 40 in males and even later in females due to blood loss from menstruation. Symptoms generally occur after decades of organ iron deposition and total body accumulation as high as 20 g. These symptoms may include cardiomyopathy, dysrhythmias, cirrhosis, hepatocellular carcinoma, bronzing of the skin, diabetes, arthralgias, generalized cognitive impairment, secondary hypothyroidism, susceptibility to certain infections, osteoporosis and hypogonadism. Routine availability of iron studies and identification of the HFE gene have converted the typical presentation of HH from end-stage disease to a laboratory diagnosis typically made in asymptomatic individuals.

There should be a low threshold to perform laboratory testing if the diagnosis is suspected. This may be the case in individuals with unexplained fatigue, clinical symptoms of iron overload, porphyria cutanea tarda, a first- or second-degree relative diagnosed with HH or found to have an HFE mutation or the following laboratory test results: unexplained liver function test abnormalities, high serum ferritin (>300 ng/ml in men or postmenopausal women; >200 ng/ml in premenopausal women), high transferrin saturation (TSAT; >45% for men or >55% for women) or the HFE gene mutation. Iron studies are the initial test used to determine whether there is clinical evidence of iron overload. Routine studies include serum iron, serum transferrin (also reported as total iron-binding capacity), TSAT, and serum ferritin level. There are varying values that are considered concerning for excess iron stores depending on the institution's guidelines. The table below details the thresholds for the British Society for Hematology, the American Association for the Study of Liver Disease and the American College of Physicians (Table 2).

Diagnosis is made in an individual with iron overload and homozygous or compound heterozygous HFE mutations. Diagnosis based on laboratory values may be challenging due to ferritin being an acute phase reactant as well as the iron storage protein. If there is any question about interpretation of high ferritin level/presence of excess iron deposition, MRI should be used to further assess. MRI of the liver should be performed in individuals with elevated LFTs, hepatomegaly or clinical findings suggestive of cirrhosis, or ferritin >1000 ng/mL. Cardiac MRI should be performed in individuals with signs of heart failure on history or echocardiography, unexplained conduction abnormalities on electrocardiography, or significant liver iron deposition. Liver biopsy is not required for the diagnosis for HH and has been replaced by MRI for estimation of iron stores in the majority of patients. It may be useful, however, to obtain information regarding the extent of fibrosis, presence of cirrhosis, and ruling out alternative causes of advanced liver disease.

Treatment should include regular phlebotomy (typically start at once-weekly sessions) to reduce the amount of circulating iron. The amount of phlebotomy needed to maintain appropriate circulating iron varies by patient and degree of overload. The degree of response is typically assessed by the serum ferritin level. Some guidelines (AASLD) target a ferritin level in the normal range, which is variably defined as 50 ng/mL, 30–100 ng/mL, or 50–150 ng/mL. Other guidelines (BSH) use a target ferritin level in the low-normal or iron-deficient range of approximately 5–10 ng/mL or 20–30 ng/mL. Individuals with advanced hepatic fibrosis are at risk for development of hepatocellular carcinoma and should have surveillance as per guidelines for any cirrhotic patient, including biannual ultrasonography or biannual AFP levels.

Polycythemia

Polycythemia Vera is one of the chronic myeloproliferative neoplasms which is distinguished clinically from other MPNs by the presence of an elevated red blood cell mass, although this alone is insufficient to make the diagnosis [21]. The 2016 World Health Organization Major criteria for diagnosis is as follows: Hemoglobin >16.5 g/dL in men or >16.0 g/dL in women, hematocrit >49% in men or >48% in women, or other evidence of increased red cell volume, bone marrow biopsy showing hypercellularity for age with trilineage growth including prominent erythroid, granulocytic and megakaryocytic proliferation with pleomorphic, mature megakaryocytes, and JAK2 V617F or JAK2 exon 12 mutation. Minor criteria include serum erythropoietin level below the reference range for normal. Diagnosis is made when all three major criteria are met or when two major and one minor criteria is met. PV occurs in all populations and in all ages, with median age at diagnosis being approximately 60 years. Incidence is slightly higher in men than women (2.8 vs. 1.3 cases/100,000 per year). Most patients are discovered incidentally with elevated hemoglobin or hematocrit found on routine blood work.

Classic clinical symptoms of patients with PV include headache, dizziness, visual disturbances, pruritus, erythromelalgia (burning pain in hands or feet accompanied by erythema, pallor, or cyanosis), early satiety, splenomegaly, and vasomotor symptoms [22]. Aquagenic pruritus is often the chief complaint in patients with PV, characterized by pruritus following a warm bath or shower.

The goals of treatment are to reduce the risk of thrombosis, prevent bleeding events, alleviate symptom burden, and minimize the risk of evolution to other myelodysplastic syndromes. Patients are categorized as high risk or low risk based on age (<60 years old vs. >60 years old) and history of prior thrombosis. Low-risk patients (those less than 60 and with no history of thrombosis) may be treated with serial phlebotomy to maintain HCT <45% in men and <42% in women, low-dose aspirin, and optimal medical management of cardiovascular risk factors. High-risk patients (those older than 60 years old or have a history of thrombosis) should be treated with phlebotomy, low-dose aspirin, cytoreductive therapy with hydroxyurea (interferon alfa or busulfan may be used as alternatives), treatment of symptoms, and assessment of cardiovascular risk factors.

Secondary polycythemia can arise from underlying lung or heart disease, living at high altitudes, or smoking. If hypoxia is associated with lung or heart disease, RBC counts should improve with the addition of supplemental oxygen.

Sickle-Cell Disease

Sickle-Cell Disease (SCD) is an autosomal recessive inherited disease caused by a defect in the beta chain of the normal hemoglobin molecule, hemoglobin A, resulting in sickle hemoglobin molecule, hemoglobin S [23]. Hemoglobin S is less soluble than hemoglobin A and when it is deoxygenated, it becomes dysfunctional. Those who are homozygous for the sickle-cell gene have sickle-cell anemia (Hb SS), while those who are heterozygous have sickle-cell trait (Hb S trait). The clinical manifestations of SCD are related to hemolytic anemia and vaso-occlusion, which may lead to acute/chronic pain, as well as tissue ischemia or infarction. Splenic infarction leads to functional hyposplenism early which predisposes these patients to infection. Sickle-cell disease affects 70,000–100,000 people in the United States, of predominantly African and Hispanic descent.

The morbidity and mortality associated with sickle-cell disease primarily stems from complications of chronic hemolysis, tissue infarction, and acute pain crises. The vaso-occlusion results from the reduction in deformability, increased adhesion to vascular endothelial cells, inflammation, and activation of hemostatic mechanisms. This typically results in severe pain, which may be superimposed on underlying chronic pain. Pain may be accompanied by tissue ischemia and inflammation. There are certain triggers such as cold temperatures, wind, low humidity, dehydration, stress, alcohol, and menses. Over 90% of patients will have experienced a pain crisis by the age of 6. Patients with Hb SS have significant clinical manifestations compared to Hb S trait patients who typically are asymptomatic.

Sickle-cell patients are susceptible to infection due to functional asplenia that develops early in life, but preventive measures including vaccination (particularly against pneumococcal organisms) and prophylactic penicillin (from age 2 months to 5 years) have decreased the mortality associated with these infections. Administration of both the conjugate (PCV13) and polysaccharide (PPSV23) pneumococcal vaccine provides protection at the earliest possible age and broadens protection against most of the invasive pneumococcal serotypes. A fever should be considered a medical emergency and should prompt evaluation by a healthcare provider, blood cultures, and broad-spectrum antibiotics.

Acute manifestations of SCD include painful crises, acute chest syndrome (ACS), and multi-organ failure syndrome. Pain crises should be managed with opiates, and patient-controlled analgesia should be considered in those that are difficult to manage. Ketorolac may be used adjunctively. Oxygen supplementation should be reserved for patients who are hypoxic and incentive spirometry should be used to prevent the progression to acute chest syndrome. Acute chest syndrome typically presents with shortness of breath, cough, chest pain, fever, and infiltrate on chest x-ray. Antibiotics should be administered when fever or infection is present. Hydration with hypotonic fluids is indicated after appropriate volume resuscitation. Multi-organ failure may manifest with rhabdomyolysis, altered mental status, decreased urine output, worsening anemia, and decreasing platelet counts. Preventative measures include prophylactic antibiotics and immunizations, hydroxyurea, and transfusions. Stem cell transplant may be indicated in young patients with multiple sickle-cell disease-related complications.

Red blood cell transfusion should be reserved for clinical scenarios in which they may reduce morbidity, including stroke prevention, reduction of acute chest syndrome and pain crises, given that the pain is occurring in the setting of severe anemia. Other transfusion indications include acute multi-organ failure, acute symptomatic anemia, a drop in baseline reticulocyte count, and hepatic or splenic sequestration. Prophylactic transfusion should be considered preoperatively to achieve a hemoglobin level of 10 g/dL to reduce complications. Side effects of recurrent transfusion include iron overload which may be treated with deferoxamine. Routine transfusions carry the same risk as in the normal population, including acute transfusion reactions and delayed hemolytic reactions.

There are significant psychosocial factors associated with sickle-cell disease, including the management of chronic pain which may be stigmatized. This may cause patient's significant psychological distress, caregiver burnout, and/or secondary gain. It is imperative for physicians to take into account these factors when caring for patients with chronic and undertreated pain. Families of patients should also be educated extensively on the course of this disease and how to manage the complications that may arise.

Hematologic Malignancies

Multiple Myeloma

Multiple myeloma (MM) is the most common bone malignancy characterized by the neoplastic proliferation of plasma cells producing a monoclonal immunoglobulin, or M proteins (IgG, IgM, or IgA or rarely IgE or IgD). These clonal plasma cells proliferate in the bone marrow and can cause skeletal destruction with osteolytic lesions, osteopenia, and/or pathologic fractures [24]. The number of new cases diagnosed in the U.S. is 4–5 per 100,000 men and women per year [25]. Median age at diagnosis is66 years old, and incidence increases with age [26]. The diagnosis is more common among males than females (approximately 1.4:1) and two to three times more common in African Americans than Caucasians [24]. Clinical symptoms include bone pain, malaise/generalized weakness, weight loss, anemia, recurrent infections, renal insufficiency, and hypercalcemia. As routine blood work has become more common, patients are being diagnosed earlier in the disease course. Initial workup when diagnosis is suspected includes CBC, CMP, ESR, and serum and urine protein electrophoresis in addition to cross-sectional imaging. MM is sometimes suspected based on an increased serum protein level along with signs and symptoms that suggest myeloma. However, patients with light chain myeloma may have a normal total serum protein level as the free light chains may not rise to a level that affects total protein [24].

Among patients with MM, 97% will have a monoclonal M protein produced and secreted by plasma cells. This can be detected by protein electrophoresis of the serum (SPEP), or an aliquot of urine (UPEP) from a 24-h collection, combined with immunofixation of the serum and urine [26], in addition to end-organ impairment (hypercalcemia, renal insufficiency/elevated creatinine, anemia, and bone lesions). Peripheral smear will most frequently show rouleaux formation (>50%), where red blood cells take on the appearance of a stack of coins, leukopenia (20%), or thrombocytopenia (5%) [26].Cross-sectional imaging is preferred for diagnosing myeloma for the increased sensitivity in detecting bone involvement compared to plain radiographs [24]. A whole-body low dose CT is used initially as a baseline assessment for bone involvement; if these results are inconclusive and MM is the leading diagnostic differential, a whole-body MRI, or MRI of spine and pelvis is used to confirm the absence of bone lesions as MRI is more sensitive

in detecting focal bone marrow lesions. MRI is also preferred if there is a concern for spinal cord compression or soft tissue plasmacytomas. PET/CT is used to detect extramedullary disease outside the spine.

The diagnosis of MM requires biopsy-proven bony or soft tissue plasmacytoma, or clonal bone marrow plasma cells greater than or equal to 10% estimated by a core biopsy specimen or aspirate, plus either the presence of end-organ damage or a biomarker indicating inevitable progression to end-organ damage (i.e. greater than or equal to 60% clonal plasma cells in the bone marrow) [24].

A premalignant disorder known as monoclonal gammopathy of undetermined significance (MGUS) carries a risk of progressing to MM at about 1% per year. The criteria of diagnosing MM include <10% of clonal bone marrow plasma cells, the absence of end-organ damage, and serum M protein <3 g/dL [24]. Waldenstrom macroglobulinemia is demonstrated by lymphoplasmacytic lymphoma in the bone marrow and IgM monoclonal gammopathy in the blood.

All patients with symptomatic MM are evaluated for hematopoietic stem cell transplant (HCT) eligibility, which can prolong overall survival compared to chemotherapy alone [26]. Bisphosphates should be prescribed to prevent vertebral fractures, as well as opiates for bone pain management. Vertebral compression fractures can benefit from percutaneous vertebroplasty and kyphoplasty for stabilization. Almost all patients will eventually relapse after initial treatment and will require additional therapy in the form of HCT or chemotherapy [26].

Myelodysplastic Syndromes

Myelodysplastic syndromes (MDS) are a group of malignant disorders involving hematopoietic stem cells that lead to dysplastic and ineffective production of red blood cells (RBC), platelets, and mature granulocytes, with a risk of progression to acute leukemia [27]. The defects of RBC, platelets, and neutrophils can result in symptomatic anemia (most common), bleeding, and increased risk of infection, respectively. Approximately 10,000 cases are diagnosed annually in the U.S, although this is likely an underestimate as patients with early, nonspecific symptoms may evade testing due to comorbidities. The median age of diagnosis is 65 years, with a male predominance [28]. The age-adjusted 3-year survival rate for MDS is approximately 60%. Environmental factors (including exposure to benzene, radiation, or chemotherapy), genetic abnormalities (Fanconi anemia, trisomy 21, Bloom syndrome, ataxia telangiectasias), and benign hematologic disorders (paroxysmal nocturnal hemoglobinuria, congenital neutropenia) can predispose one to develop MDS [27].

Signs and symptoms of MDS are nonspecific, and many patients at presentation are asymptomatic or may present with fatigue or infection from a previously unrecognized cytopenia (ref2). MDS is commonly diagnosed based on anemia (hgb < 10 g/dL), neutropenia (absolute neutrophil count <1.8109/L), and thrombocytopenia (<100 109/L) (ref1). Peripheral blood smears usually reveal dysplasia in the red and white blood cell lines, whereas platelets are morphologically normal (ref1). Bone marrow aspirate will reveal a shift towards more immature precursors, with a blast percentage of less than 20% on aspirate as well as peripheral blood indicating MDS (ref2). Bone marrow biopsy will reveal specific histological features associated with MDS (fibrosis) and can help determine the stage of MDS [28].

Immediate treatment is warranted for those with symptomatic anemia, recurrent episodes of bleeding, or recurrent infections secondary to neutropenia [28]. Treatment of asymptomatic patients does not improve long-term survival, but these patients can be monitored with serial lab work. Allogeneic hematopoietic cell transplantation is the only cure.

Therapy including hematopoietic growth factors and immunosuppressive therapy can improve quality of life but are not curative. Chemotherapy can quickly improve blood counts and alter the disease course, reducing the risk of death [28].

Leukemias

Leukemias are a group of blood cell cancers that result from uncontrolled clonal proliferation of hematopoietic stem cells in the bone marrow [29]. These cells disrupt the normal expansion of blood cells causing symptoms such as weakness, infection, bleeding, and other complications [29]. Classification of leukemias is based on acute versus chronic, and lymphoblastic versus myelogenous.

The age-adjusted incidence rate of leukemia within the United States was 14.1 per 100,000 persons between 2012 and 2016 (for all races and both sexes) [30]. Roughly 1.6% of people will develop leukemia in their lifetime based on data from 2014–2016. Disease incidence increases with age with the median age of diagnosis around 65 years, and white males have a higher predominance than females or other ethnicities [30].

Acute lymphoblastic leukemia (ALL) is the most common childhood cancer accounting for about 25% of childhood malignancies, and acute myelogenous leukemia (AML) accounts for 80% of acute leukemias in adults [29]. Chronic lymphocytic leukemia (CLL) occurs most commonly in people over the age of 50 and affects males more often than females. Chronic myelogenous leukemia (CML) accounts for 20% of all adult leukemias, with median age of diagnosis at age 65.

Predisposing risk factors include genetic abnormalities (Down syndrome, Neurofibromatosis, Fanconi anemia), genetic familial mutations, exposure to ionizing radiation, industrial chemical exposure (benzene), myelodysplastic syndrome, and prior chemotherapy or radiation therapy.

Common presenting signs of leukemia in children are persistent fever, anorexia, pallor, fatigue, abnormal bleeding or bruising, or petechial rash [31]. Hepatosplenomegaly is also a common finding and is a manifestation of anorexia or abdominal pain. Patients with lymphadenopathy unresponsive to antibiotics should be evaluated for ALL. One-third of all children can have bone pain that is usually presented with a limp or inability to weight bear. Priapism is a red flag for childhood leukemia. Adults will have the common presenting signs detailed above in addition to weight loss and anemia-related symptoms such as dyspnea or chest pain. Palpable lymphadenopathy and organomegaly are not as common in adults.

If diagnosis is suspected, an initial CBC and differential is drawn which, at presentation, may show normocytic, normochromic anemia, thrombocytopenia, but a varying leukocyte count with about 25–40% of patients having less than 5000 cells/μL, and 20% of patients having a count above 100,000 cells/μL. Reticulocyte count will be normal or decreased [32]. A complete metabolic panel and coagulation panel may be assessed for any concurrent abnormalities and will give the hematologist/oncologist baseline liver functions.

Hyperphosphatemia, hypocalcemia, hyperuricemia, and/or hyperkalemia is indicative of tumor lysis syndrome and is an oncologic emergency [33]. A peripheral smear and bone marrow exam are required to detect characteristic morphology and immunophenotypic of cells for diagnosis. Excisional or needle core biopsy is pertinent to evaluate any suspicious lymph node. Any positive lab findings in light of symptoms require prompt referral to a hematology/oncology specialist.

The optimal treatment for children with ALL is a multidrug regimen with a protocol taking up to 3 years to complete [32]. Most patients require transfusion support at the time of diagnosis as well as antibiotic therapy. Rarely, exchange transfusion may be required in cases of extreme leukocytosis. Treatment for AML is based on medical fitness, prognostic features of cytology, and goals of care [33]. Chemotherapy is the mainstay of treatment, and supportive care includes transfusions and antibiotics as needed. Treatment for CLL is indicated if the patient has certain disease-related complications, including progressive bone marrow failure indicated by worsening anemia/thrombocytopenia, extranodal involvement, splenomegaly extending to greater than or equal to 6 cm below the costal margin, lymphadenopathy greater than or equal to 10 cm in length, constitutional symptoms, or progressive lymphocytosis because patients with CLL without treatment can have survival rates comparable to the normal population [34]. Treatment options for patients with CML include tyrosine kinase inhibitors, allogeneic hematopoietic stem-cell transplantation, or cytotoxic agents.

As more and more children with leukemia are surviving postchemotherapy, it is important for the family physician to provide routine care for these patients. In addition to any age-appropriate USPSTF cancer screening guidelines, a leukemia survivor should have follow-up with oncology every month for the first year after completion of therapy, then less frequently for the next 2–4 years, with yearly follow-up being appropriate after 3–5 years [32]. The primary care physician should be vigilant in regards to relapse with symptom monitoring, which are similar to those at initial presentation, as well as paying close attention to abnormal blood counts at follow-up, as 2–3% of ALL survivors can develop a second malignancy and many are at risk of developing a primary brain tumor [35]. Long-term effects of leukemia and its treatment are becoming more common as more patients survive these cancers.

Late adverse effects include CNS impairment, impaired linear growth, cardiotoxicity, endocrinopathies, higher likelihood of a secondary cancer, neurocognitive dysfunction, and depression. There is additionally an increased risk of late-occurring stroke in survivors of ALL. A decline in cognitive function is a common finding, especially in patients who received cranial radiation or triple intrathecal chemotherapy. These patients should receive neuroimaging and intermittent cognitive testing. Endocrinopathies include gonadal dysfunction, thyroid disorders, obesity, and low-growth hormone levels, although "catch-up" growth can be attained after completing chemotherapy. Patients that have been treated with anthrayclines (such as doxorubicin) need to be monitored for cardiotoxicity, including fatal cardiomyopathy. Since high-dose steroids are often used with chemotherapeutic regimens, monitoring for osteonecrosis of joints and osteoporosis must be undertaken. All patients having had a hematopoietic stem-cell transplant must have an initial bone scan 1 year after transplantation and then serially repeated based on clinical picture [35].

References

1. Ballas M, Kraut EH. Bleeding and bruising: a diagnostic work-up. Am Fam Physician. 2008;77(8):1117–24.
2. Biochemistry and genetics of Von Willebrand factor. Annu Rev Biochem [Internet]. [Cited 2020 Jun 3]. Available from: https://www.annualreviews.org/doi/10.1146/annurev.biochem.67.1.395

3. Swami A, Kaur V. von Willebrand disease: a concise review and update for the practicing physician. Clin Appl Thromb Off J Int Acad Clin Appl Thromb. 2017;23(8):900–10.

4. Nichols WL, Hultin MB, James AH, Manco-Johnson MJ, Montgomery RR, Ortel TL, et al. von Willebrand disease (VWD): evidence-based diagnosis and management guidelines, the National Heart, Lung, and Blood Institute (NHLBI) Expert Panel report (USA). Haemophilia. 2008;14(2):171–232.

5. Kaufmann JE, Vischer UM. Cellular mechanisms of the hemostatic effects of desmopressin (DDAVP). J Thromb Haemost. 2003;1(4):682–9.

6. Bolton-Maggs PHB. Optimal haemophilia care versus the reality. Br J Haematol. 2006;132(6):671–82.

7. Hoots W, Shapiro A. Clinical manifestations and diagnosis of hemophilia. In: Post TW, Rutgeerts P, Grover S, editors. 2020. Available from https://www.uptodate.com/contents/clinical-manifestations-and-diagnosis-of-hemophilia

8. Valente MJ, Abramson N. Easy bruisability. South Med J. 2006;99(4):366–70.

9. Rick ME. Diagnosis and management of von Willebrand's syndrome. Med Clin North Am. 1994;78(3):609–23.

10. Mihatsch WA, Braegger C, Bronsky J, Campoy C, Domellöf M, Fewtrell M, et al. Prevention of vitamin K deficiency bleeding in newborn infants: a position paper by the ESPGHAN Committee on Nutrition. J Pediatr Gastroenterol Nutr. 2016;63(1):123–9.

11. Achterbergh R, Vermeer HJ, Curtis BR, Porcelijn L, Aster RH, Deenik W, et al. Thrombocytopenia in a nutshell. Lancet Lond Engl. 2012;379(9817):776.

12. Kühnel T, Wirsching K, Wohlgemuth W, Chavan A, Evert K, Vielsmeier V. Hereditary hemorrhagic telangiectasia. Otolaryngol Clin N Am. 2018;51(1):237–54.

13. Jackson SB, Villano NP, Benhammou JN, Lewis M, Pisegna JR, Padua D. Gastrointestinal manifestations of hereditary hemorrhagic telangiectasia (HHT): a systematic review of the literature. Dig Dis Sci. 2017;62 (10):2623–30.

14. Boxer LA. How to approach neutropenia. Hematol Am Soc Hematol Educ Program. 2012;2012:174–82.

15. Rezaei N, Moazzami K, Aghamohammadi A, Klein C. Neutropenia and primary immunodeficiency diseases. Int Rev Immunol. 2009;28(5):335–66.

16. Hsieh MM, Everhart JE, Byrd-Holt DD, Tisdale JF, Rodgers GP. Prevalence of neutropenia in the U.S. population: age, sex, smoking status, and ethnic differences. Ann Intern Med. 2007;146(7):486.

17. Moore DC. Drug-induced neutropenia: a focus on rituximab-induced late-onset neutropenia. P T Peer-Rev J Formul Manag. 2016;41(12):765–8.

18. Coates T. Congenital neutropenia. In: Post TW, Rutgeerts P, Grover S, editors. 2020. Available from https://www.uptodate.com/contents/congenital-neutropenia

19. Coates T. Immune neutropenia. In: Post TW, Rutgeerts P, Grover S, editors. 2020. Available from https://www.uptodate.com/contents/immune-neutropenia

20. Bardou-Jacquet E, Brissot P. Diagnostic evaluation of hereditary hemochromatosis (HFE and non-HFE). Hematol Oncol Clin North Am. 2014;28(4):625–35, v.

21. Pillai AA, Fazal S, Babiker HM. Polycythemia. In: StatPearls [Internet]. Treasure Island: StatPearls Publishing; 2020 [cited 2020 Jun 5]. Available from: http://www.ncbi.nlm.nih.gov/books/NBK526081/

22. Raedler LA. Diagnosis and Management of Polycythemia Vera. Am Health Drug Benefits. 2014;7(7 suppl 3): S36–47.

23. Kavanagh PL, Sprinz PG, Vinci SR, Bauchner H, Wang CJ. Management of children with sickle cell disease: a comprehensive review of the literature. Pediatrics. 2011;128(6):e1552–74.

24. Kyle RA, Gertz MA, Witzig TE, Lust JA, Lacy MQ, Dispenzieri A, et al. Review of 1027 patients with newly diagnosed multiple myeloma. Mayo Clin Proc. 2003;78(1):21–33.

25. Kyle RA, Therneau TM, Rajkumar SV, Larson DR, Plevak MF, Melton LJ. Incidence of multiple myeloma in Olmsted County, Minnesota: trend over 6 decades. Cancer. 2004;101(11):2667–74.

26. Rajkumar S. Multiple myeloma: overview of management. In: Post TW, Rutgeerts P, Grover S, editors. 2020. Available from https://www.uptodate.com/contents/multiple-myeloma-overview-of-management

27. Aster C, Stone R. Clinical manifestations and diagnosis of myelodysplastic syndromes. In: Post TW, Rutgeerts P, Grover S, editors. 2020. Available from https://www.uptodate.com/contents/clinical-manifestations-and-diagnosis-of-the-myelodysplastic-syndromes

28. Estey E, Sekeres M. Overview of the treatment of myelodysplastic syndromes. In: Post TW, Rutgeerts P, Grover S, editors. 2020. Available from https://www.uptodate.com/contents/overview-of-the-treatment-of-myelodysplastic-syndromes

29. Arber DA, Orazi A, Hasserjian R, Thiele J, Borowitz MJ, Le Beau MM, et al. The 2016 revision to the World Health Organization classification of myeloid neoplasms and acute leukemia. Blood. 2016;127 (20):2391–405.

30. Siegel RL, Miller KD, Jemal A. Cancer statistics, 2017. CA Cancer J Clin. 2017;67(1):7–30.

31. Clarke RT, den BAV, Bankhead C, Mitchell CD, Phillips B, Thompson MJ. Clinical presentation of childhood leukaemia: a systematic review and meta-analysis. Arch Dis Child. 2016;101(10):894–901.

32. Horton T, Steuber P, Aster M. Overview of the clinical presentation and diagnosis of acute lymphoblastic leukemia/lymphoma in children. In: Post TW, Rutgeerts P, Grover S, editors. 2020. Available from https://www.uptodate.com/contents/overview-of-the-clinical-presentation-and-diagnosis-of-acute-lymphoblastic-leukemia-lymphoma-in-children

33. Kolitz J, MD. Overview of acute myeloid leukemia in adults. In: Post TW, Rutgeerts P, Grover S, editors.

2020. Available from https://www.uptodate.com/contents/overview-of-acute-myeloid-leukemia-in-adults

34. Rai K, Stilgenbauer S. Overview of the treatment of chronic lymphocytic leukemia. In: Post TW, Rutgeerts P, Grover S, editors. 2020. Available from https://www.uptodate.com/contents/overview-of-the-treatment-of-chronic-lymphocytic-leukemia

35. Horton T, Steuber P. Overview of the outcome of acute lymphoblastic leukemia/lymphoma in children and adolescents. In: Post TW, Rutgeerts P, Grover S, editors. 2020. Available from https://www.uptodate.com/contents/overview-of-the-outcome-of-acute-lymphoblastic-leukemia-lymphoma-in-children-and-adolescents

Part XXVI

Family Medicine Applications

Michael D. Hagen

Contents

History of Medical Informatics

General purpose electronic computers appeared in 1946 with the creation of ENIAC and were first theorized as potentially useful for medical diagnosis by Ledley and Lusted in the 1950s [1].

In the 1970s, Dr. Octo Barnett developed an electronic record system at Massachusetts General Hospital using a computer language (MUMPS) created for the purpose [2]. The term "medical informatics" appears to have arisen in France in the 1960s ("Informatique Medicale") [3] and came into common use in the 1980s as the preferred terminology to describe information technology applications in healthcare [4].

Healthcare applications exploded with the development of the World Wide Web by Tim Berners-Lee in the early 1990s, which enabled the development of information exchanges, online libraries and healthcare computer applications [2]. As health informatics applications became more prevalent, informatics practitioners began to form organizations to support their professional

M. D. Hagen (✉)
Department of Family and Community Medicine,
University of Kentucky College of Medicine, Lexington,
KY, USA
e-mail: hagenmd@twc.com; michael.hagen@uky.edu

© Springer Nature Switzerland AG 2022
P. M. Paulman et al. (eds.), *Family Medicine*,
https://doi.org/10.1007/978-3-030-54441-6_51

efforts. The first annual meeting of the Symposium on Computer Applications in Medical Care (SCAMC) occurred in 1977 and included tutorials on computer technology as well as presentations regarding use of computers in diagnosis and decision-making and laboratory analyses [5]. SCAMC ultimately evolved into the American Medical Informatics Association (AMIA), which continues to serve as a convening organization for informaticists of all disciplines and supports efforts in the following missions: Translational Informatics, Clinical Research Informatics, Clinical Informatics, Consumer Health Informatics, and Public Health Informatics [6].

The American Board of Medical Specialties (ABMS) approved Clinical Informatics as a new subspecialty sponsored by the American Board of Preventive Medicine and the American Board of Pathology. In creating the specialty, AMIA defined the content and a proposed curriculum for clinical informatics training programs (the specialty approval included a practice-eligibility pathway that will expire at the end of 2022) [7–10].

The Role of Clinical Informaticists

So what roles do these board-certified clinical informaticists assume in their professional contexts? A recent survey of clinical informaticists identified five principal domains: fundamental knowledge and skills, improving care delivery and outcomes, enterprise information systems, data governance and data analytics, and leadership and professionalism [11]. According to this survey, respondents spent the largest percentage of their time, 32%, in the improving clinical care domain [11]. Leadership and professionalism consumed 26%; they spent 18% of their efforts in the Enterprise Information systems and data governance/analytics domains [11]. The authors of this survey indicated that evolution of the subspecialty, particularly in response to nearly universal use of electronic health records and the data they generate, has led to greater emphasis on data governance and

analytics than identified in the original core content specification [8, 11].

Starting in 2023, clinical informatics certification will require formal fellowship training. As of this writing, 35 Accreditation Council for Graduate Medical Education (ACGME)-accredited training programs exist in primarily academic health centers across the country. AMIA maintains a listing of currently available training programs and their contact information [12]. Specific information regarding application for the Clinical Informatics Subspecialty certificate can be found at the American Board of Preventive Medicine website, https://www.theabpm.org/become-certified/subspecialties/clinical-informatics/ (note that pathologists must apply through the American Board of Pathology, https://www.abpath.org/index.php/taking-an-examination/subspecialty-certificate-examinations).

Artificial Intelligence (AI) and Machine Learning

Since the previous edition of this textbook, advances in computing power and access to greatly enhanced storage capacity (i.e., through cloud computing) have enabled AI and machine learning algorithms to assume a larger role in creating knowledge from vast quantities of information [13]. AI systems have found successful application in "data-intensive specialties like radiology, pathology, and ophthalmology" [14]. However, evidence for safety and effectiveness in actual patient care and outcomes remains elusive [15].

Early AI systems relied primarily on rule-based algorithms and tended not to function well when presented with information outside their intended range [15]. As noted, increasingly powerful computing technology and availability of large data repositories have promoted the use of statistical and computational reasoning methodologies (such as neural networks) not feasible just a few decades ago. These powerful technologies do, however, present new challenges in clinical application. For many of these systems, their "black

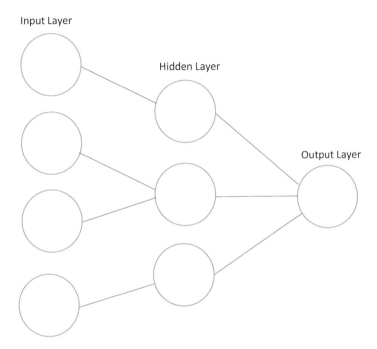

Input Layer

Hidden Layer

Output Layer

Fig. 1 Simple neural network with four input nodes, three hidden nodes, and a single output node. The input nodes represent the clinical characteristics the modeler wishes to use for predicting outcomes (e.g., demographics, clinical findings such as blood pressure). The hidden nodes evolve automatically as the network trains on a data training set. The output layer represents the outcome the modeler wishes to predict (e.g., mortality.) The lines between the nodes represent mathematical functions that change as the network trains. These functions serve as weights which combine mathematically with the node values to generate an output value. This output value compares to the true value; the difference generates a correction value that propagates back through the network iteratively until the network output values match the true values within a prespecified range

box" nature can present discomfort for patient and clinician alike if the developers haven't provided sufficient detail (such as the demographic and contextual characteristics of the data used to train the system, and problems identified in system creation) about the system's development, validation, and implementation [15]. Figure 1 displays a simple prototypical neural network. For those who might wish to explore machine learning techniques further, researchers at the University of Waikato in New Zealand have created an open-source platform (Weka) for learning about and using these tools [16]. This platform includes multiple machine learning methods (such as neural networks, Bayesian networks, linear regression, and others) and provides access to example datasets and tutorials that facilitate learning about these techniques.

Medical Informatics and Electronic Health/Medical Record Systems

The previous edition of this chapter included substantial information regarding vetting and selecting electronic health/medical record systems. Information from the Robert Graham Center for Policy Studies in Family Medicine indicates that at least 80% of new Family Medicine residency graduates enter employed positions after completing training [17]. This suggests that recent graduates will likely enter settings with already established information and electronic record systems (as of 2017 nearly 90% of office-based practices and 96% of non-federal hospitals had adopted electronic record systems [18]). Indeed, family physicians seeking employed status might want to consider characteristics of organizations' electronic information systems in their position decisions. A consensus statement from the American Academy of Family Physicians (AAFP), the American Board of Family Medicine (ABFM), the American Academy of Pediatrics (ABPeds), and the North American Primary Care Research Group (NAPCRG) examined functionality of existing electronic record systems and identified characteristics needed to enable electronic record systems to better support primary care: enhanced extraction, prioritization, and interpretation of information for individual patients and patient panels; advanced information exchange to support coordination, integration, and collaboration across providers and healthcare contexts (i.e., interoperability); greater facility for patient engagement; and reduced documentation burden [19].

The characteristic of interoperability remains a major challenge and shortcoming among currently available electronic medical record (EMR)/electronic health record (EHR) systems, particularly for small- and medium-sized practices [19]. The US federal government addressed interoperability in the twenty-first Century Cures Act [20]. The Act tasked the Office of the National Coordinator for Health Information Technology (ONCHIT) and the National Institute of Standards and Technology (NIST) to develop and promote standards "to ensure full network to network exchange of health information." [20] The ONCHIT released its final rule in March 2020 [21]. This rule establishes several requirements for electronic health records (EHRs): EHR providers must enable an individual patient's access to her data to qualify for EHR certification; providers must not block access to information (the rule does include exceptions for security and privacy); and EHR vendors have 3 years to bring their systems into compliance. Rather than have the vendors modify their proprietary data structures and interfaces to accomplish this interoperability, the ONCHIT has adopted the Health Level 7® (HL7) Fast Healthcare Interoperability Resources® (FHIR, pronounced "fire") standard for creating Application Programming Interfaces (APIs) to access individual products [22]. According to the rule, "this certification criterion will align industry efforts around FHIR Release 4 and advance interoperability of API-enabled 'read' services for single and multiple patients" [23]. Detailed discussion of the FHIR® standard is beyond the scope of this chapter, but suffice it to say that implementation of FHIR® promises to hasten access to disparate vendors' and systems' information for providers and patients alike.

Another technology related to FHIR and that can promote interoperability is the Substitutable Medical Applications and Reusable Technologies (SMART) specification [24]. SMART can be viewed as analogous to the apps developed for mobile devices. Using the SMART on FHIR approach, one can view the FHIR as the application programming interface (API) to a particular EHR product, while the SMART application serves as the app that performs a desired task (e.g., creating a graph) on the data extracted by the FHIR interface.

These interoperability developments should facilitate the progress of health information exchange (HIE). New payment models (e.g., value-based payment) and focus on patient-centered medical homes require coordination between multiple providers and organizations, and this coordination requires access to patients' data [25]. HIEs have demonstrated benefit in multiple outcomes: reduced hospital readmissions, reduced total costs, improved medication reconciliation, and improved immunization rates represent several of the benefits attained with effective HIE networks [25].

The Internet

The Internet developed as the Advanced Research Projects Agency Network (ARPANET) in the 1960s and served to support collaboration among defense researchers [26]. In 1983, ARPANET adopted the Transmission Control Protocol and Internet Protocol (TCP/IP) as the standard for data transmission, which enabled the Internet as a "network of networks" [26]. Subsequently, Tim Berners-Lee in 1990 created the components needed to enable the World Wide Web: hypertext transfer protocol (http), the universal resource identifier (URI), and the hypertext markup language (html) that enabled creation of web "pages" [27].

The World Wide Web (WWW) has provided clinicians access to myriad healthcare sites that provide medical decision support, access to the medical literature, and options for communicating directly with patients (e.g., through secure patient portals). (The large number of WWW citations in the reference list attest to the Web's impact on healthcare delivery!)

Clinical Decision Support

Numerous decision support resources exist on the Web, both subscription and open access. Several examples of subscription services include UpToDate® [28], DynaMed® [29], and Essential Evidence Plus® [30]. UpToDate® provides access to medical calculators, current medical management information and links to full-text articles, drug-drug interactions, and patient education. DynaMed® similarly provides calculators and specialty-specific (including Family Medicine) medical information. Essential Evidence Plus also provides calculators and evidence-based decision aids and adds access to Patient-Oriented Evidence that Matters (POEMs), Cochrane Systematic Reviews, and Evaluation and Management (E/M) coding support.

A number of open-access resources also provide valuable decision aids. The Mayo Clinic provides access to multiple sources for clinical guidelines (such as the American College of Physicians, United States Preventive Services Task Force, and the Centers for Disease Control and Prevention) [31]. Until recently, the Agency for Healthcare Research and Quality (AHRQ) supported the National Guidelines Clearinghouse, which provided access to clinical guidelines from multiple sources [32]. Funding has ended for this resource, but the ECRI Institute Guidelines Trust® now provides a similar tool [33]. The ECRI site does require a no-charge registration for access to the resources. Once registered, the user can browse/search for information by topic, specialty (interestingly they don't include Family Medicine in the specialty list!), care setting, or role.

Epocrates® (see https://www.epocrates.com/ for a detailed description of features) represents another point-of-care resource that includes drug information, clinical guidelines, formulary information, medical calculators, and information on multiple specialty topics. Epocrates® comes in both free and subscription versions and supports both online and smart device (e.g., iPad®, iPhone®, and Android®) access.

The National Institute for Health and Care Excellence (NICE) in the United Kingdom provides access to rigorously developed evidence-based guidelines [34]. Additionally each technology appraisal created by the NICE includes a cost-effectiveness analysis which serves as the basis for service coverage by the National Health Service (NHS) in the United Kingdom. For example, the NICE guidance for naltrexone-bupropion concludes that this treatment is not recommended for weight loss, based largely on a cost-effectiveness analysis that was "highly uncertain because of uncertainties in the modeling assumptions." The NHS concluded that "more certainty is needed" that this treatment would provide value in managing obesity in the United Kingdom.

The National Library of Medicin (NLM) in the United States has created and provides free access to multiple online resources for providers, patients, and researchers [35]. PubMed provides access to all of the peer-reviewed literature that the NLM has indexed and provides tools for facilitating search strategies. MedlinePlus provides patients access to useful health information; the Open-I Tool provides a means to search multimedia such as images. TOXNET enables searches for hazardous substances and chemicals. ClinicalTrials.gov includes a database of private and publicly funded research trials around the world [36].

The PubMed Clinical Queries tool represents a particularly useful resource for searchers who wish to fine-tune their literature searches [37]. Using this tool, searchers can limit their queries to specific literature categories, such as systematic reviews or original clinical studies. The tool includes filters that the user can utilize to further tweak the search. Additionally, the site includes tutorials and training materials to help users maximize their results. The NLM has recently introduced a new interface to the PubMed tool, which provides somewhat more streamlined access to these tools [38].

The World Wide Web also includes voluminous resources for patients, more than can be listed here. The American Academy of Family Physicians (AAFP) provides a large number of patient resources at https://familydoctor.org/. WebMD® provides another source of information for patients, including resources regarding drugs, illness symptoms, and finding a doctor [39]. The Mayo Clinic also makes available a site that provides patient-oriented information regarding diseases and conditions, as well as a "symptom checker" and first aid recommendations (available at: https://www.mayoclinic.org/diseases-conditions).

Generalized search engines, such as Google® (www.google.com) and Yahoo® (www.yahoo.com), also provide access to legions of health information. However, users should be aware that some authors have questioned the reliability of recommendations obtained using these tools [40, 41] and that concerns about authorship, conflict of interest, and quality of evidence may affect the quality of the information obtained [42].

Emerging Internet Technologies

Blockchain

Several emerging technologies hold promise for healthcare contexts. Blockchain represents one of those technologies. Blockchain is essentially a digital ledger that maintains a nearly tamper-proof history of transactions related to the information in a chain of events. The blockchains are maintained in series of computer networks; each new transaction or "block" gets added to an existing chain, and the result (or "blockchain") becomes "sealed" through cryptographic techniques. In the healthcare realm, the technology theoretically could facilitate patient access to electronic record data, in that blockchains could maintain a record of all the various systems in which their data reside. The actual health information would remain in the respective record systems, but the blockchain would maintain a permanent record of how to access those data (see: https://munkschool.utoronto.ca/mowatcentre/inside-the-black-blocks/).

Additionally, a blockchain-based system could facilitate professional credentialing (e.g., hospital privileging) by consolidating the record of a physician's educational, training. and certification history [43]. As of this writing, these remain potential blockchain applications.

The Internet of Things (IoT)

Multiple devices (appliances, monitors, sensors, etc.) increasingly include Internet access among their features. These devices promise to improve the quality of life for aging populations. Ambient Assisted Living devices (such as smart thermometers/thermostats that can automatically respond to extreme heat events) and fall detectors can help maintain frail patients in their homes and facilitate daily activities of living [44].

According to the International Electrotechnical Commission/Systems Committees, Active Assisted Living (AAL) "has been shown to increase general health and quality of life measures" (more details available at: https://www.iec.ch/dyn/www/f?p=103:186:16692527879311::::FSP_ORG_ID,FSP_LANG_ID:11827,25). Indeed, remote patient monitoring (RPM), defined as "the delivery of healthcare to patients outside conventional settings enabled by a technological application or device," promises to connect patients to providers and services from the comfort of their homes [45, 46]. As an example, monitoring an asthmatic for acute attacks can alert providers and facilities to the need for urgent services and intervention [47].

Telemedicine/Telehealth

As this chapter goes to press, the United States finds itself in the throes of the worldwide novel coronavirus pandemic. The pandemic has placed a strain on traditional patient-facing healthcare services, emphasizing the need for patient interactions that don't involve face-to-face visits with a provider. Enter telemedicine/telehealth.

Just what is telemedicine/telehealth? The American Telemedicine Association (ATA) advocates using the term "telehealth" rather than "telemedicine" to indicate the broad nature of current applications. ATA defines telehealth as "technology-enabled health and care management and delivery systems that extend capacity and access" (available from: https://www.americantelemed. org/resource/why-telemedicine/). The landscape for telemedicine/telehealth has changed quite substantially since this textbook's previous edition, particularly for video interactions. The ATA defines several examples of telehealth approaches: "mobile health," which uses the Internet and/or cellular telephone network to provide health information and peer-peer interactions; "live videoconferencing" (in a synchronous mode) which can include live consultations between primary care physicians and sub-specialists regarding specific patient care issues; "store and forward" (in asynchronous mode), which can include forwarding and storing images, laboratory, and other patient information for later review (email represents an asynchronous store-and-forward process); and "remote patient monitoring" that can include devices that measure vital signs, blood glucose, blood pressure, and other clinical parameters for use in managing patients' healthcare needs in their home environments (details available at: https://www.americantelemed.org/ resource/why-telemedicine/) (Table 1).

So what sorts of patient care scenarios best lend themselves to telehealth approaches? Table 2 identifies a number of potential candidates.

How does a practice or organization get started with telehealth? The American Health Information Management Association has created a comprehensive tool kit for guiding providers through the process [48]. The AHIMA tool kit identifies three fundamental steps: "assess and define," "develop and plan," and "implement and monitor" [48].

Let's look at these steps in further detail. The AHIMA guidance indicates that the "assess and define" step includes the following components: identify and document the need and rationale for a telemedicine/telehealth program; define the services the telehealth/telemedicine program will provide; define the delivery mechanisms for the program; perform an environmental scan to determine the need and payment options for the services; determine who will own the record/s created in delivering the services; define responsibility for changes to the services, release of information, and data breaches; and identify possible jurisdictional issues (e.g., licensure) if the service/s cross state lines [48]. The "develop and plan" includes the following: define a plan using all the information gleaned in Step 1; define the steps needed to create and deploy the identified services; estimate the work effort required to create and deploy the services; create a timeline for system development; identify staff needs for the development effort; and create a plan for monitoring and evaluating the program's progress [48]. Step 3, "implement and monitor" includes actual deployment of the plans developed in Step 2 and monitoring the results [48].

In developing and deploying the services, the provider needs to involve the program's potential stakeholders. Table 3 illustrates those stakeholders telehealth developers might wish to consider.

Table 1 Features that clinicians should investigate when encountering a new electronic health/medical record system (After Kennell et al. [51])

Features to look for in a modern EHR	
Capture of adverse events (e.g., medication errors)	Capture of medication list information
Support for Clinicians' Cognitive Processes (i.e., medical decision support)	Support for identifying and documenting patient preferences
Standardized data format (e.g., HL-7 or C-CDA[a])	Support for capturing patient-reported outcomes data
Support for genomic information	Support for identifying phenotypic information (e.g., specific physical characteristics)

[a]Consolidated Clinical Data Architecture. Description available at: https://www.healthit.gov/topic/standards-technology/consolidated-cda-overview

Table 2 Patient care services particularly amenable to telehealth/telemedicine approaches. (After Texas Medical Association [52])

Services most amenable to telehealth approaches	
Acute, uncomplicated clinical conditions	Surgical follow-up
Review of laboratory results	Urgent care conditions
Mental health sessions	Coverage for after-hours needs
Medication management	Triage for the need for additional care
Follow-up of chronic care conditions	Nutrition consultation and services

Table 3 Stakeholders to consider in developing telehealth/telemedicine services. After Anderson et al. [48]

Potential telemedicine/telehealth stakeholders	
Organizational executives and leaders	Risk management
Providers (e.g., nurses and physicians)	Marketing
Organizational information technology/informatics representatives	Patient safety/QI leadership
Department heads	Patient representatives
Education and training personnel	Program consumers
Human resources representative/s	Regulatory and Compliance representatives

What about reimbursement for telehealth/telemedicine services? As of this writing, the US Department of Health and Human Services (HHS) has relaxed HIPAA-related regulations, and CMS has liberalized reimbursement policies for telehealth/telemedicine services. These changes might not persist beyond the passing of the coronavirus pandemic; family physicians should check with all of their payors regarding reimbursement and coding requirements for telehealth/telemedicine visits (see https://www.ama-assn.org/delivering-care/public-health/key-changes-made-telehealth-guidelines-boost-covid-19-care for more detail).

What equipment will a practice need for delivering telehealth/telemedicine services? This could be as simple as a telephone (note that many payors will not reimburse for telephone-only services); video "virtual visits" will require a computer with video camera and broadband Internet access or a smart device as described earlier. For best audio quality, the physician should consider using a headset with microphone for higher fidelity than usually afforded by built-in computer microphones. Under current circumstances, HHS has relaxed security requirements for virtual visits, which means that physicians can use free services such as Skype® and FaceTime®, and subscription services such as Zoom® and GoToMeeting®, to deliver these services (more detail available at: https://www.ama-assn.org/delivering-care/public-health/key-changes-made-telehealth-guidelines-boost-covid-19-care). Again, these requirements could change once the pandemic has receded.

Patient portals represent a secure, HIPAA-compliant option for patient-physician interaction. Through a patient portal, individuals can access EHR records such as recent doctor visits, hospital discharge summaries, immunizations, medication lists, and laboratory results (see https://www.healthit.gov/faq/what-patient-portal for more detail). Many organizations' portals also support direct secure email interactions between patient and physician, as well as prescription refill requests.

In providing direct clinical care via telemedicine/telehealth, physicians have ethical obligations to ensure that they provide accurate information and perform competently. This includes proficiency in managing the technology used and understanding possible limitations of the modality [49]. Telehealth/telemedicine isn't appropriate for circumstances that require in-person, "hands on" interaction with a patient (e.g., auscultating the lungs in a patient with cough and fever). Physicians delivering these services need to remain mindful of the need for patients' informed consent, including determining whether or not patients and/or their surrogates have proficiency with the technology used [49]. Likewise, clinicians must practice the same privacy and confidentiality policies that they would in a hospital or outpatient setting; patients should be apprised of the potential security issues associated with care delivered electronically (e.g., potential for "hacking" of personal health information). Additionally, clinicians must document the encounter either through their electronic health record or a written note to assure continuity of care and appropriate follow-up [49].

Individual healthcare organizations might have their own specific guidelines/protocols for conducting telemedicine/telehealth services. For example, the University of Kentucky healthcare system has created documentation guidelines for use in its ambulatory electronic health record (Allscripts®) (details available at: https://covid-19.ukhc.org/wp-content/uploads/sites/121/2020/03/Enterprise-Tele health-Documentation-AEHR.pdf). The templates provided include recommendations for verifying patient identity, assuring that the patient resides in the state, authorizations and consent for telemedicine services, and instructions for creating customized macros.

Conclusion

In conclusion, biomedical/clinical informatics represents a dynamic and rapidly evolving discipline. The family physician can keep abreast of new developments by accessing several general clinically oriented resources. Hoyt and Hersh's *Health Informatics: Practical Guide* (seventh edition) represents a useful single resource and is endorsed by the American Medical Informatics Association [50]. The *Journal of the American Medical Informatics Association* (JAMIA) and *Applied Clinical Informatics* (ACI) Journal provide cutting edge informatics developments but do require subscriptions. Finally, ACI Open represents a relatively new open-access, free source of informatics information (available at https://www.thieme.com/books-main/clinical-informatics/product/4339-aci-open).

References

1. Ledley RS, Lusted LB. Reasoning foundations of medical diagnosis; symbolic logic, probability, and value theory aid our understanding of how physicians reason. Science. 1959;130(3366):9–21.
2. Hoyt RE, Hersh WR. Overview of health informatics, in Health Informatics. Practical Guide. Hersh WR, Hoyt RE, editors. Informatics Education; 2018. p. 1–27.
3. Collen MF, Ball MJ. The history of medical informatics in the United States. 2nd ed. London: Springer; 2015.
4. Shortliffe EH, Cimino JJ. Biomedical informatics: the science and the pragmatics. In: Shortliffe EH, Cimino JJ, editors. Biomedical informatics. Computer applications in health care and biomedicine. New York: Springer; 2014.
5. IEEE. The first annual symposium on computer applications in medical care. 1977. [cited 2020 February 5]; 2018: Available from: https://www.computer.org/csdl/magazine/co/1977/08/01646597/13rRUxC0SK6.
6. AMIA Mission. Improve health through informatics education, science and practice. 2020 [cited 2020 February 5]; Available from: https://www.amia.org/about-amia/mission-and-history
7. Detmer DE, Lumpkin JR, Williamson JJ. Defining the medical subspecialty of clinical informatics. JAMIA. 2009;16:167–168.8.
8. Gardner RM, Overhage JM, Steen EB, Munger BS, Holmes JH, Williamson JJ, Detmer DE. AMIA Board white paper: core content for the subspecialty of clinical informatics. JAMIA. 2009;16:153–7.
9. Safran C, Shabot MM, Munger BS, Holmes JH, Steen EB, Lumpkin JR, Detmer DE. AMIA board white paper: program requirements for fellowship education in the subspecialty of Clinical Informatics. JAMIA. 2009;16:158–66.
10. Clinical Informatics. 2020. [cited 2020 February 5]; Available from: https://www.theabpm.org/become-certified/subspecialties/clinical-informatics/
11. Silverman HD, et al. Domains, tasks, and knowledge for clinical informatics subspecialty practice: results of a practice analysis. J Am Med Inform Assoc. 2019;26(7):586–93.
12. AMIA. Clinical informatics fellowship programs. 2020 [cited 2020 February 5]; Available from: https://www.amia.org/membership/academic-forum/clinical-informatics-fellowships.
13. Liyanage H, et al. Artificial intelligence in primary health care: perceptions, issues, and challenges. Yearb Med Inform. 2019;28(1):41–6.
14. Yu KH, Kohane IS. Framing the challenge of artificial intelligence in medicine. BMJ Qual Saf. 2019;28:238–41.
15. Magrabi F, et al. Artificial intelligence in clinical decision support: challenges for evaluating AI and practical implications. Yearb Med Inform. 2019;28(1):128–34.
16. Weka. The workbench for machine learning. 2020 [cited 2020 March 11]; Available from: https://www.cs.waikato.ac.nz/ml/weka/index.html.

17. Robert Graham Center. Shrinking scope of practice reflects trends in family physician employment, hospital privileges. 2019 [cited February 11 2020]; Available from: https://www.graham-center.org/rgc/press-events/press/all-releases/111219-shrinking-scope-practice-reflects-trends-fp-employment-hosp-priv.html.

18. Office of the National Coordinator for Health Information Technology. Health IT Dashboard. 2017 [cited 2020 February 11]; Available from: https://dashboard.healthit.gov/quickstats/quickstats.php.

19. Krist AH, Beasley JW, Crosson JC, et al. Electronic health record functionality needed to better support primary care. J Am Med Inform Assoc. 2014;21:764–71.

20. Lengyel-Gomez B. 21st century cures act-a summary. 2017 [cited 2020 March 12]; Available from: https://www.himss.org/resources/21st-century-cures-act-summary.

21. ONCHIT. Download ONC's cures act final rule. 2020 [cited 2020 March 12]; Available from: https://www.healthit.gov/cerus/sites/cerus/files/2020-03/ONC_Cures_Act_Final_Rule_03092020.pdf.

22. HL-7. Welcome to FHIR. 2019 [cited 2020 March 12]; Available from: https://www.hl7.org/fhir/index.html.

23. Office of the National Coordinator for Health Information Technology. 21st century cures act: interoperability, information blocking, and the ONC Health IT. Washington, DC: Health and Human Services.a.H. Services; 2020.

24. Mandel JC, Kreda DA, Mandl KD, Kohane IS, Ramoni RB. SMART on FHIR: a standards-based interoperable apps platform for electronic health records. JAMIA. 2016;23:899–908.

25. Menachemi N, Rahurkar S, Harle CA, Vest JR. The benefits of health information exchange: an updated systematic review. JAMIA. 2018;25(9):1259–65.

26. Andrews, E. Who invented the internet? 2019 October 28, 2019 [cited 2020 February 6]; Available from: https://www.history.com/news/who-invented-the-internet.

27. World Wide Web Foundation. History of the web. 2020 [cited 2020 March 20]; Available from: https://webfoundation.org/about/vision/history-of-the-web/

28. UpToDate 2020 [cited 2020 February 6]; Available from: https://www.uptodate.com/home.

29. Dynamed. 2020 [cited 2020 February 6]; Available from: https://www.dynamed.com/.

30. Essential Evidence Plus. 2020. [cited 2020 February 6]; Available from: https://www.essentialevidenceplus.com/.

31. Mayo Clinic. Clinicians: guidelines and manuals. December 19, 2019 [cited 2020 February 6]; Available from: https://libraryguides.mayo.edu/clinicians.

32. Agency for Healthcare Research and Quality (AHRQ) Guidelines and measures. [cited 2020 February 6]; Available from: https://www.ahrq.gov/gam/index.html.

33. ECRI Guidelines Trust. Guided by Rigor. Grounded in truth. 2020 [cited 2020 February 6]; Available from: https://guidelines.ecri.org/.

34. National Institute for Health and Care Excellence (NICE). Improving health and social care through evidence-based guidance. 2020 [cited 2020 February 6]; Available from: https://www.nice.org.uk/.

35. National Library of Medicine (NLM). National library of medicine. Accelerating biomedical discovery and data-powered health. 2020 [cited 2020 February 10]; Available from: https://www.nlm.nih.gov/.

36. National Library of Medicine (NLM). New Pubmed! 2020 [cited 2020 February 10]; Available from: https://www.ncbi.nlm.nih.gov/pubmed/.

37. National Library of Medicine (NLM). PubMed Clinical queries. 2020 [cited 2020 February 10]; Available from: https://www.ncbi.nlm.nih.gov/pubmed/clinical.

38. National Library of Medicine (NLM) PubMed.Gov. 2020 [cited 2020 February 10]; Available from: https://pubmed.ncbi.nlm.nih.gov/.

39. WebMD. 2020 [cited 2020 February 10]; Available from: https://www.webmd.com/.

40. Kothari M, Moolani S. Reliability of "Google" for obtaining medical information. Indian J Opthalmol. 2015;63(3):267–9.

41. Sharma V, Holmes JH, Sarkar IN. Identifying complementary and alternative medicine usage information from internet resources. A systematic review. Methods Inf Med. 2016;55(4):322–32.

42. Ma Y, Yang AC, Duan Y, Dong M, Yeung AS. Quality and readability of online information resources on insomnia. Front Med. 2017;11(3):423–31.

43. Urban MC, Pineda D. Inside the black blocks. A policymaker's introduction blockchain, distributed ledger technology and the "internet of value". 2019 June 27, 2019 [cited 2020 March 11]; Available from: https://munkschool.utoronto.ca/mowatcentre/inside-the-black-blocks/.

44. Bublitz FM, Oetomo A, Sahu KS, Kuang A, Fadrique LX, Velmovitsky PE, Nobrega RM, Morita PP. Disruptive technologies for environment and health research: an overview of artificial intelligence, Blockchain, and internet of things. Int J Environ Res Public Health. 2019;16(20):3847–71.

45. Chronaki CE, Vardas P. Remote monitoring : costs, benefits, and reimbursement. A European perspective. Europace. 2013;15:i59–64.

46. Infoway CH. Connecting patients with providers: A Pan-Canadian study on remote patient monitoring. Executive summary. In: Technical report. Toronto: Canada Health Infoway; 2014.

47. Canadian Health Infoway. Canadian physicians can improve patient care with advanced EMR use. Toronto: Canada Health Infoway; 2016.

48. Anderson R, Beckett B, Fahy K, et al. Telemedicine toolkit. Chicago: American Health Information Management Association (AHIMA); 2017.

49. Chaet D, Clearfield R, Sabin JE, Skimming K. Ethical practice in Telehealth and telemedicine. J Gen Intern Med. 2017;32(10):1136–40.

50. Hoyt RE, Hersh WR. Health informatics. Practical guide. 7th ed: Informatics Education; 2018.

51. Kennell TI, Willig JH, Cimino JJ. Clinical informatics researcher's desiderata for the data content of the next generation electronic health record. Appl Clin Inform. 2017;8:1159–72.

52. Texas Medical Association. Telemedicine 101 for practices. Austin. 2019. Accessible at: https://www.texmed.org/Telemedicine/

Complementary and Alternative Medicine

William Hay, Laurey Steinke, and Louisa Foster

Contents

W. Hay (✉)
Department of Family Medicine, University of Nebraska
Medical Center, Omaha, NE, USA
e-mail: whay@unmc.edu

L. Steinke
Department of Biochemistry and Molecular Biology,
University of Nebraska Medical Center, Omaha, NE, USA
e-mail: lsteinke@unmc.edu

L. Foster
The Center for Mindful Living, Omaha, NE, USA

© Springer Nature Switzerland AG 2022
P. M. Paulman et al. (eds.), *Family Medicine*,
https://doi.org/10.1007/978-3-030-54441-6_143

A family physician guided by evidence finds themselves in a difficult position regarding complementary and alternative medicine (CAM). There is little evidence for the efficacy of these methods, and sometimes no evidence for their safety. On the other hand, patients are likely to use them. In 2007, 38% of adults in the USA used some form of complementary or alternative medicine according to the CDC National Health Statistics Report #12 [1]. It is important for a physician to maintain a welcoming atmosphere, in which a patient is comfortable discussing any and all forms of CAM they might be using, so they may provide important information to the patient about the possible benefits, limitations and risks of these methods [2].

Biological Based Therapies

Supplements

Supplements are by far the most used CAM in the USA, with 17,7% of adults reporting the use of a non-vitamin supplement in 2012; if vitamins are included the number goes up to 52%. While patient's think of these as distinct from their prescription medications, it should be made clear that, just as with prescription medications, these

entities can have side effects and drug interactions. Additional confusion can arise because many of these supplements are known by several names [3] (Table 1).

It is important to remember that dietary supplements do not require FDA approval before marketing and will only be withdrawn for the market if complaints are made [4]. The Dietary Supplement Health and Education Act of 1994 limited the FDA's ability to oversee supplements, and thus there is no guarantee of quality, safety, or effectiveness. Only products that make specific claims about disease treatments must be proven safe and effective for their intended use via clinical trials, thus most products on the market make vague claims, and so are not required to undergo testing. Even the claims made in advertising are not scrutinized by the FDA; rather they are investigated by the FTC, which regulates truth in advertising, only when complaints are made.

Adulteration of supplements, meaning they contain unauthorized FDA regulated pharmaceuticals, is a frequent problem and the most common reason for the FDA to recall these products. The most commonly adulterated classes include supplements marketed for weight-loss (diuretics and stimulants), bodybuilding (anabolic steroids) and "male enhancement" (sildenafil). Microbial and heavy metal contaminants have also been found

Table 1 Resources on supplements

Using Dietary Supplements; Wisely National Center for Complementary and Integrative Medicine (NCCIM)	https://www.nccih.nih.gov/health/using-dietary-supplements-wisely
Herbs at a glance (NCCIM)	https://www.nccih.nih.gov/health/herbsataglance
Office of Dietary Supplements	https://ods.od.nih.gov/
MedlinePlus	https://medlineplus.gov/druginformation.html
Cochrane library	https://www.cochranelibrary.com
Agency for Healthcare Research and Quality	https://www.ahrq.gov/topics/m.htm
FDA dietary supplement ingredient advisory list	https://www.fda.gov/food/dietary-supplement-products-ingredients/dietary-supplement-ingredient-advisory-list
National Institutes of Health, Office of Dietary Supplements (NIH ODS): health professionals	https://ods.od.nih.gov/HealthInformation/healthprofessional.aspx

in a variety of supplements at levels unsafe for consumption [5]. In one study, 20% of 193 Ayurvedic medicines (a traditional health care system from India) tested, contained excessive levels of heavy metals [6]. This is also a frequent problem with imported traditional Chinese and Mexican herbs. Supplements have also been found to be to contain unlisted natural or synthetic ingredients, while others contained no DNA of the herbs listed on the label [5].

There are companies that independently evaluate products for quality (Fig. 1), certifying that products contain only the listed ingredients in the stated quantities and that they contain no contaminants or ingredients known to be unsafe. While these certifications do not indicate effectiveness or protect patients against issues such as drug interactions and side effects, this analysis does reduce the risk of using supplements and it is highly recommended to use products displaying the seals of these laboratories.

Multivitamins

Multivitamins, which can contain as many as two dozen vitamins and minerals, without standard dosages, are the most used of the supplements in the USA. While erroneously thought to be needed routinely, their use can lead to over supplementation when taken by those already consuming a nutrient-rich diet. There is evidence that use of a multivitamin/multimineral supplement is associated with an increase in total mortality [7]. Iron supplementation is the most detrimental, while calcium and Vitamin D supplementation were associated with decreased total mortality. The takeaway message seems to be that supplementation is only needed in response to identified deficiencies.

Megavitamin Therapy

Megavitamin therapy, defined as the use of vitamins at dose at many times the usually

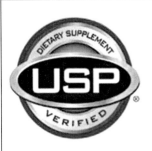

United States Pharmacopeia

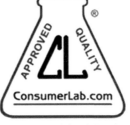

Consumer labs (also has subscription service which lists products they've reviewed)

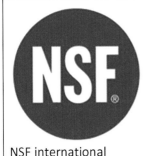

NSF international

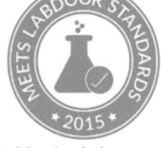

Labdoor Standard

Fig. 1 Product seals of companies that certify supplements

recommended dosing, has not been proven an effective treatment for any condition except those involving malabsorption or vitamin metabolism issues. On the other hand, many vitamins, most famously pyridoxine, can cause toxicity when excessively dosed. Although some supplements contain such excessive doses, this issue arises more commonly in patient ingesting multiple supplements containing the same nutrient.

Probiotics

Ingesting various solutions of "beneficial" bacteria is currently a common practice and has been investigated for a number of conditions. Common organisms included are *Bacillus* spp., *Bifidobacterium* spp., *Clostridium butyricum*, *Lactobacilli* spp., *Lactococcus* spp., *Leuconostoc cremoris*, *Saccharomyces* spp., and *Streptococcus* spp., alone or in combination. Keep in mind that because one probiotic helps a condition, it doesn't mean another probiotic will have a similar effect.

Probiotics have been shown to assist pediatric patients with IBS [8]. These studies were short term, and stool-samples showed that the gut microbiome rapidly returned to its normal state after supplementation ceased, so this intervention may need to be long term. No clear evidence of benefit exists for adults. For the more serious IBD, there is a lack of randomized-controlled trials [9]. Probiotics also have a moderate effect when used to prevent and treat antibiotic associated diarrhea in children [10] and in the prevention of *Clostridium difficile*-associated diarrhea in adults and children [11]. Caution is indicated when using these agents in the severely debilitated and immunocompromised since adverse events have been reported [10]. There are reports of inclusion of bacteria other than those on the label [12], which can put those suffering from chronic disease or the immunocompromised at risk of infection.

Herbal Medicines

Safety and efficacy of herbal medicines will be dependent in a large part on the expertise of those gathering the plants. This process is not regulated and for the most part not standardized. The active ingredients will vary with the batch and are generally not measured. Also, the number of active compounds in an herbal medicine varies, and can be large, making drug interactions and side effects more likely. The top botanicals sold in the USA in 2011–2012 are included in Table 2, while Table 3 lists supplements that are particularly dangerous.

Diet-Based Therapies

While there are many dietary modifications overseen by nutritionists and dieticians that are appropriate treatments for disease (examples are keto-diets for epilepsy and diabetes) it must be noted that the most common comment in meta-analysis and reviews for diet-based therapies is "paucity of evidence." In addition to this, there is not long-term evidence regarding the possible health benefits or dangers of the numerous fad diets that circulate. Some of the most common dietary interventions are dealt with in more detail below.

All of these fad diets can result in short-term weight loss resulting from caloric restriction, but none produce better results long-term than calorie restriction.

FODMAP

The low-FODMAP diet restricts foods with highly fermentable oligo-, di-, and monosaccharides, and polyols -, which purportedly trigger and/or exacerbate IBS. Although a low FODMAP diet was found to have a favorable impact on abdominal pain, bloating and diarrhea [14] this diet is not clearly superior to conventional IBS diets. A low FODMAP diet, administered by a dietician, is recommended by the British Dietetic Association and the NIDDK for management of IBS.

Keto- and Paleo-Diets

Keto diets are low-carbohydrate and high-fat diets that are claimed to produce weight-loss and provide benefits against diabetes, epilepsy, cancer and Alzheimer disease. A ketogenic diet results in the metabolism of fat for energy, with production of ketosis. The Paleo (or paleolithic) diet

Table 2 Common supplements [45]

Supplement	Suggested use	Evidence	Contraindications and side effects
Alfalfa	Lower LDL cholesterol and numerous other conditions	Insufficient evidence to rate benefit	Safe in dietary amounts, Interferes with warfarin and other medications
Black Elderberry	Colds and flu, pain relief	No evidence of benefit	Parts of the plant and unripe berries are stomach irritants
Bilberry (European blueberry, whortleberry, huckleberry)	Poor circulation, menstrual cramps, eyestrain, skin problems or diarrhea	No support for use to treat any condition	Interacts with warfarin
Cannabidiol (CBD)	Nausea and vomiting, chronic pain, epilepsy	Low-quality evidence for efficacy, currently under active study	Diarrhea, sleeplessness, or abnormal liver function. Interacts with many medications including warfarin [46]. Not legal (federal)
Cranberry	Prevent or treat UTI	Some low-quality evidence of decreased risk of UTI. Not effective at treating UTI	In large amounts may cause stomach upset and diarrhea. May interact with warfarin
Echinacea (purple coneflower, coneflower, American coneflower)	Common cold	Does not decrease the length of the common cold, low-quality evidence it may reduce occurrence of colds	Digestive upsets, possibility of allergies, interacts with warfarin and other medications
Evening Primrose oil (EPO)	Eczema, rheumatoid arthritis, premenstrual syndrome, breast pain, and menopause symptoms	No evidence of efficacy	Digestive upsets, complications of pregnancy, interacts with warfarin to increase bleeding
Garlic	Lower cholesterol, prevent cancer, hypertension	Conflicting and weak evidence for all claims	Digestive upsets, interacts with warfarin and other medications
Ginger	Nausea	Moderate evidence of efficacy	Safe as a spice. Caution with large doses in pregnancy and with gallstones. Large doses can interact with warfarin, antihyperglycemics and other medications
Gingko biloba (fossil tree, maidenhair tree, Japanese silver apricot, baiguo, yinhsing)	Dementia, eye problems, intermittent claudication	No evidence that it is helpful for any condition	Seeds are poisonous. Possible increased liver and thyroid cancer risk, interacts with warfarin and other medications
Polyunsaturated fatty acids (Fish oil, Omega-3 Fatty acids)	Heart disease, high cholesterol, eye diseases, eczema, neurologic disorders	In statin treated patients, improves cardiovascular outcomes but not all-cause mortality [47]. All other conditions inconclusive or no benefit	Generally considered safe, can interfere with coagulation. Do not use some forms if allergic to seafood
Saw Palmetto (American dwarf palm tree, cabbage palm)	Benign Prostate Hyperplasia, chronic pelvic pain, migraine, hair loss	No more effective than placebo for BPH, no evidence of efficacy other conditions	May be unsafe during pregnancy or while breastfeeding
Soy	Menopausal symptoms, bone health, improving	Small effect on LDL when replaces other proteins. Low quality evidence for small	Dietary amounts safe. Supplements may cause Endometrial hyperplasia.

(continued)

Table 2 (continued)

Supplement	Suggested use	Evidence	Contraindications and side effects
	memory, hypertension and hyperlipidemia,	effects on menopause. Other conditions, no evidence	Safety not established for those with or at risk for breast cancer
St. John's Wort (hypericum, Klamath weed, goatweed, Tipton's weed, rosin rose, chase-devil)	Depression, ADHD, menopausal symptoms, IBS,	Inconclusive data for depression, no positive data for any other conditions	Interacts with many medications in a severe and often life -threatening way
Tumeric/Curcumin	Arthritis, diabetes, digestive disorders, respiratory infections, allergies, liver disease, depression, and others	Low quality evidence with no clear benefits. Currently under active study	Safe used as a spice, large amounts may be unsafe for use during pregnancy or while breastfeeding
Zinc [48]	COVID-19, common cold, viral infections, immune support	Poor quality evidence for reduction in length of common cold	Large doses produce digestive upset or, over the long term, reduced immune function. Interferes with absorption of some antibiotics

attempts to replicate the diet of ancient hunter-gatherers. While not as restrictive as the keto diet, and mimicking mainstream nutritional advice about avoiding processed food, it eliminates dairy, which can result in low calcium intake.

Juicing and Detoxification Diets

Juicing and detoxification diets promote very low-calorie intake for a short period of time (two to 21 days). Diarrhea is a frequent side effect. Herbs in these mixtures can cause difficulties as previously discussed. Such severely restricted diets can increase cortisol levels and lead to rebound weight gain.

Intermittent Fasting Diets

Intermittent fasting diets involve fasting for 16–48 h, followed by a period of unrestricted eating.

Gluten-free Diets

While necessary for those with Celiac Disease (1% of the population), gluten-free diets are also suggested for a variety of conditions in the popular press, including mood disorders and autism. There are no high-quality studies in favor of treating any disorder, other than celiac disease, with a gluten-free diet. Nonceliac gluten sensitivity is considered

to be common (1–6% of the population). Food challenge studies indicate that in half the cases where nonceliac gluten sensitivity is reported, the symptoms were not replicated. Once on a gluten-free diet, reintroduction of gluten can provoke bloating and gas until an equilibrium is reached in the gut bacteria, so determining the efficacy of a gluten-elimination trial is difficult There is no scientific evidence of general contribution to a healthier life-style or effect on weight-loss [14]. Additionally, gluten-free foods are approximately three-times more expensive and may lack nutrients added to enriched grain products.

Mind-Body Medicine

This category includes practices that are based on the human mind, but that have an effect on the human body and physical health, such as meditation, prayer, and mental healing.

Deep Breathing

Deep breathing and breathing exercises are the second most commonly used CAM after supplements and are useful in focusing a patient's

Table 3 Dangerous supplements [49, 50]

Supplement	Suggested uses	Toxicities
Aconite (helmet flower, monkshood, devil's helmet, and wolfsbane)	Fever, pain, cough, asthma	Nausea, vomiting, weakness, paralysis, breathing and heart problems, possibly death
Bitter Orange (aurantii fructus, Citrus aurantium, zhi shi)	Weight loss, nasal congestion, allergies	Fainting, heart-rhythm disorders, heart attack, stroke, death
Caffeine Powder (1,3,7-trimethylxanthine)	Improves attention, enhances athletic performance, weight loss	Seizures, heart arrhythmia, cardiac arrest, possibly death; particularly dangerous when combined with other stimulants
Chaparral (Creosote bush, greasewood, larrea divaricata, larrea tridentata, larreastat)	Weight loss, improves inflammation. Treating infections, skin rashes, cancer	Kidney problems, liver damage, possibly death
Colloidal Silver	COVID-19, sinus infections, pain, bacterial infection, daily health.	Argyria (bluish-gray discoloration of skin, usually permanent), interferes with absorption of thyroxine and some antibiotics
Coltsfoot (Coughwort, farfarae folium leaf, foalswort, tussilago farfara)	Cough, sore throat, laryngitis, bronchitis, asthma	Liver damage, possible carcinogen
Comfrey (Blackwort, bruisewort, slippery root, symphytum officinaleh)	Cough, heavy menstrual periods, stomach problems, chest pain; treats cancer	Liver damage, cancer, possibly death
Country Mallow (heartleaf, Sida cordifolia, silky white mallow)	Nasal congestion, allergies, asthma, weight loss, bronchitis.	Heart attack, heart arrhythmia, stroke, death.
Germander (Teucrium chamaedrys, viscidum)	Weight loss; alleviates fever, arthritis, gout, stomach problems	Liver damage, hepatitis, possibly death
Germanium	Pain, infections, glaucoma, liver problems, arthritis, osteoporosis, heart disease, HIV/AIDS, cancer.	Nephrotoxicity and death
Greater Celandine (Celandine, chelidonium majus, chelidonii herba)	Alleviates stomachache	Liver damage
Green Tea Extract Powder (Camellia sinensis and many others)	Weight loss	Dizziness, tinnitus, decreased iron absorption, and glaucoma; elevates blood pressure and heart rate; liver damage; possibly death
Kava kava (Ava pepper, piper methysticum)	Anxiety, insomnia, premenstrual symptoms, and stress	Hepatotoxicity and liver failure [22], Parkinson's and depression, impairs driving, possibly death
Lobelia (Asthma weed, lobelia inflata, vomit wort, wild tobacco)	Respiratory problems, aids smoking cessation	Nausea, vomiting, diarrhea, tremors, rapid heartbeat, confusion, seizures, hypothermia, coma, possibly death
Methylsynephrine (Oxilofrine, p-hydroxyephedrine, oxyephedrine, 4-HMP)	Weight loss, increases energy, improves athletic performance	Causes heart rate and rhythm abnormalities, cardiac arrest; particularly risky when taken with other stimulants
Pennyroyal Oil (Hedeoma pulegioides, mentha pulegium)	Breathing problems, digestive disorders	Liver and kidney failure, nerve damage, convulsions, possibly death
Red Yeast Rice (Monascus purpureus)	Lowers LDL, prevents heart disease	Kidney, muscle and liver problems, hair loss; duplicates effect of statin drugs, increasing the risk of side effects
Usnic Acid (Beard moss, tree moss, usnea)	Weight loss, pain relief	Liver injury

(continued)

Table 3 (continued)

Supplement	Suggested uses	Toxicities
Yohimbine (Johimbi, pausinystalia yohimbe, corynanthe johimbi)	Treats low libido and erectile dysfunction, depression, obesity	Raises blood pressure; causes rapid heart rate, headaches, seizures, liver and kidney problems, heart problems, panic attacks, possibly death

attention on the process of inhalation and exhalation. For patients who suffer panic disorder and anxiety, this exercise gives a focus to the thought process. It can improve lung function and exercise capacity in lung disease, the symptoms of GERD, and speed post-anesthesia recovery.

Meditation

Drawing from Buddhist practices and philosophy, meditation promotes healing by helping patients cultivate mindfulness skills and helping them to change their relationship with their own experience. Meditation is the formal discipline used to develop mindfulness, through awareness of the breath, use of a mantra or a passage in a sacred text, loving-kindness meditation or compassion practices, among others. Contrary to popular belief, it is not an attempt to "empty one's mind," rather it is a skill-based means of redirecting watchful attention to one's own cognition and affective reactions, without engagement or judgment. Cultivating these practices helps patients to shift focus from unconscious, automatic patterns of thought to present moment, non-judgmental awareness. As a result, patients experience a host of physiological benefits, including greater affect regulation, an increased capacity to tolerate distress, and decreased sympathetic nervous system arousal [15]. Ongoing mindfulness training engenders the development of "equanimity," a nonreactive posture to life events.

The development of mindfulness skills has significant implications in primary care populations as it promotes increased treatment compliance and engagement in preventative health care behaviors, as well as decreased subjective experiences of pain, yielding less reliance on opioids and narcotic interventions [16]. It has

also been shown to decrease relapse of major depression and substance abuse [17]. Furthermore, mindfulness skills have positive implications for the clinician as well as the patient, by improving patient-centered communication skills, and increasing the personal well-being of the physician [18].

The availability of mindfulness training through a multitude of venues such as meditation centers, yoga studios, gyms and churches, and online training, makes it an affordable and accessible alternative to patients who have limited resources. In cases where stigma exists around accessing mental health treatment, mindfulness can offer resiliency training, allowing isolated patients to become connected in like-minded, health promoting settings.

Yoga

Yoga can be traced back to early civilizations in India. It focuses on the following principles: proper breathing (pranayama), proper relaxation (savasana), proper exercise (asanas), meditation (dhyana), and proper diet (vegetarian). There are many different styles of yoga, and none of them have been found to be superior over the other. Yoga was introduced to the USA in the late nineteenth century, but its popularity has rapidly increased since the 1960s. Randomized controlled studies have only been done on Yoga for a limited number of conditions. Beneficial effects are supported for depression, anxiety, LBP (equal to physical therapy) [19], and asthma. It has a small but consistent effect on hypertension (similar to other exercises). There is limited evidence of effect on sleep in patient's receiving chemotherapy. Studies show no effect on menopausal symptoms [20]. Minor MSK injuries are not uncommon. Relative contraindications include hypermobility and osteoporosis or other conditions with increased fracture risk. Patients with severe cardiac conditions, a predisposition to syncope, and pregnant women should avoid hot yoga (Bikram).

Biofeedback

Biofeedback is a technique a patient can use to learn to control some of their body's functions by using electrical sensors that help them receive information about their body. This feedback is used to achieve physiologic changes, such as relaxing muscles or reducing heart rate, to obtain a desired result such as reducing anxiety or pain. There are two types of biofeedback: physiological biofeedback and biomechanical biofeedback. Most evidence of effectiveness is in the areas of musculoskeletal and neurologic rehabilitation, anxiety, depression, and sports performance. There is no evidence of effectiveness in hypertension.

Hypnosis

Hypnosis is defined as "a trance-like state that resembles sleep but is induced by a person whose suggestions are readily accepted by the subject" (Merriam-Webster Medical Dictionary). Hypnosis is used for chronic pain, mental distress, smoking cessation, and sexual dysfunction, as well as changing other habits. While it is sometimes considered part of standard medical practice, and numerous workshops and schools offering certification in hypnotherapy are available, there is at best low-quality evidence for its efficacy in treatment of chronic pain and adverse outcome data in trials and clinical interventions does not seem appropriately documented. Controls vary widely in trials. Some studies compare hypnosis to other psychological interventions, some to patients maintained on a waiting list, some provide education and still others include an attention-equivalent empathic intervention. For adults, a meta-analysis [21] found hypnosis moderately effective for chronic pain in fibromyalgia,

Multiple Sclerosis, phantom limbs, cancer and disability. The results in general are encouraging but no more so than other psychological interventions such as autogenic training, guided imagery and progressive muscle relaxation. Hypnosis is somewhat effective in reducing mental distress, but not pain, in adults undergoing dental procedures. Repeated studies have failed to find hypnosis effective for smoking cessation. In children, hypnotherapy (including guided imagery) was found effective in children presenting with recurrent abdominal pain in studies lasting up to 5 years. Side effects are infrequently evaluated in hypnosis studies, but when documented, minor, usually transient, effects such as dizziness, panic attacks, drowsiness, confusion, headaches, and fear occur at high rates [22].

Manual Medicine

The philosophies of manual medicine involve therapies that consist of movement or manipulation of the body. When considered together they represent the second most common class of CAM.

Osteopathic Manipulation

Osteopathy was started in 1874 by Andrew Taylor Still, MD, DO. His term "osteopathy" was based on the hypothesis that the pathology of most conditions stems from the bones themselves. Though this theory proved not to be true, osteopathic manipulative techniques (OMT) are still a part of osteopathic practice, albeit in a much-reduced role, primarily for treatment of musculoskeletal conditions and pain. Using OMT, an osteopathic physician (DO) moves a patient's muscles and joints using techniques that include stretching, gentle pressure and resistance. Treatments most commonly involve the spine, but OMT is used all over the body; common areas include the pelvis, shoulders, knees, ribs, and the paranasal sinuses. Today, OMT is most commonly used by primary care physicians and a smaller group of DOs who practice it full time. Courses and curricula are available to teach MDs these techniques and principles. Many studies show the effectiveness of OMT in low back pain with additional evidence for other musculoskeletal issues such as shoulder and neck pain, and headaches. Studies of non-MSK problems are limited but specifically do not support OMT for respiratory conditions [23]. Contraindications include local infection, fracture, herniated vertebral disc, inflammatory arthritis of the spine, cauda equina syndrome, and cancer. Serious complications are rare.

Chiropractic Therapy

Chiropractic was founded in 1895 by DD Palmer, a 'magnetic healer'. The chiropractic health model posits that most illness arises from chiropractic vertebral subluxations – improper juxtaposition of the vertebrae - which interfere with the flow of energy, originally called "Innate Intelligence," down the spine, through the nerves and into the body. This is considered the cause of most bodily dysfunction and disease; as opposed to the medical model in which diseases are caused by germs or pathophysiology (e.g., cancer). Traditional chiropractic treatment involves "adjustments", which correct these subluxations allowing proper flow of energy and natural healing. Practitioners may additionally manipulate other parts of the musculoskeletal system. Many Chiropractors today also use other techniques, frequently alternative ones as described elsewhere in this chapter, which is controversial within the chiropractic community. Indeed, the use of routine X-rays and even the concept of the subluxation are currently sources of controversy in the Chiropractic community.

Chiropractors are the only alternative practitioners licensed in all USA and Canadian provinces. Many Chiropractors focus adjustments on musculoskeletal disorders, particularly those of the spine. Studies show effectiveness for low back pain and neck pain; its effectiveness in headaches is more mixed. Chiropractic treatment of non-musculoskeletal conditions is controversial, but most chiropractors and their professional organizations consider adjustments appropriate for a wide variety of problems, from otitis media, asthma, and gastrointestinal symptoms to HIV and ADHD. There are, however, no high-quality studies show efficacy of chiropractic adjustments for these or any other non-musculoskeletal condition [24].

Minor side effects, such as muscular soreness, are common, occurring in up to a quarter of patients. Rare severe complications include fracture, vertebral disc herniation and cervical artery dissection [25, 26]. Contraindications to chiropractic manipulation include conditions where bony structures are susceptible to trauma such as fractures, bone tumors, severe rheumatoid arthritis, and osteoporosis. Manipulation should also be avoided in patients with a progressive neurologic deficit and in those who have a deteriorating condition without a clear diagnosis. Pediatric chiropractic care remains controversial. Given the lack of any published studies showing the benefits of chiropractic treatment in pediatric patients and the documented reports of serious complications, the treatment of infants and children cannot be recommended.

Massage Therapy

Massage therapy involves manipulating the soft tissues of the body. Massage has been practiced in most cultures, both Eastern and Western, throughout human history, and was one of the earliest tools that people used to try to relieve pain. Swedish massage is the most commonly used technique in the USA, but deep tissue, hot stone, aromatherapy, sports, pregnancy, Thai, and Shiatsu methods are also widely used.

There is surprisingly little evidence of benefits in MSK disorders and low back pain other than very short-term improvements. In athletes, there is no evidence of performance enhancement but some evidence of small improvements in flexibility and duration of soreness. There is positive evidence of improvement of QOL in fibromyalgia patients. There is mixed evidence of improvement in constipation, post-operative pain and labor pain. In cancer patients there is mixed evidence of improvements in pain, anxiety and depression but there are no studies to show any effects on cancer progression. Massage is a common intervention in infant nurseries with some evidence of benefits in feeding, weight-gain and hyperbilirubinemia, but study interventions are highly variable and firm conclusions are elusive. There is no evidence of benefits in COPD, non-cancer related depression or pressure ulcers.

Alternative Medicine Systems

Alternative medical systems refer to an entire system of theory and practice that developed separately from conventional medicine.

Homeopathy

Created in 1796 by Samuel Hahnemann, homeopathy is based on the prescientific principle of "like treats like," the belief that a substance that causes symptoms of a disease in healthy people would cure similar symptoms in sick people; for example, the aconite plant, which increases the pulse and elevates the temperature, is used for fever. However, many of these substances are very toxic so Hahnemann diluted them, eventually concluding that the remedies became more effective with increasing dilution, now called the "law of infinitesimal doses." Homeopathic remedies are diluted with alcohol or water either 1:10 (noted as "X" or "D") or 1:100 ("C"). So, a 6X product has been diluted 1:10 six times. a dilution of 10^6. Potencies of 30C or lower are called low-potency remedies or medicines, and potencies of 200C or higher are considered high-potency medicines. However, modern chemistry informs us that by a 12C dilution there is only a 60% chance of a single molecule being present in a solution, a chance that drops nearly to zero with an additional 1:100 dilution. The lack of any of the original compound in most homeopathic remedies has led to the concept of "water memory,, according to which water "remembers" the substances mixed in it and transmits the effect of those substances when consumed – a theory incompatible with modern chemistry.

As of 2020, all 12 Cochrane reports involving homeopathy failed to document any effects. Five large meta-analyses of homeopathy reached the conclusion, after excluding methodologically inadequate trials and accounting for publication bias and likely random statistical variation, that homeopathy produced no statistically significant effect over placebo" [27]. While such dilute solutions would appear to pose no risk, in addition to the possible delay or avoidance of effective treatments for serious conditions and preventative care, contaminated and inadequately diluted product have resulted in illness and even death [28]. As of 2020, no homeopathic products have ever been approved by the FDA

Traditional Chinese Medicine (TCM)

Traditional Chinese Medicine is based on the concept of Qi (pronounced "chee"), believed to be a vital force forming part of any living entity and circulating through 12 primary and 8 accessory channels. These channels (also known as meridians) are described as having branches connected to bodily organs and functions. In this belief, if the flow of qi along these meridians is blocked or unbalanced, illness can occur. Another important concept in traditional Chinese medicine is the concept that all things, including the body, are composed of opposing forces called yin and yang. Traditional Chinese medicine doctors look at the balance of body, mind, and spirit to determine how to restore qi, the yin-yang balance, and good health.

Diagnosis in TCM is focused on the "Four pillars": Inspection, focusing on the face and particularly the tongue; Auscultation (of voice, breathing and cough) and Olfaction (attending to breath and body odors); Inquiry, focusing on the "seven inquiries" - chills and fever, perspiration, appetite, thirst and taste, defecation and urination, pain, sleep, and menses and leukorrhea; and Palpation of the body for tender "Ashi" points, of pulses with special attention to the wrist, and of the abdomen.

TCM therapies include: acupuncture, acupressure, Chinese herbs, cupping (uses warm air in glass jars to create suction), diet (foods being either yin or yang), massage (tui na), moxibustion (uses heated Chinese mugwort), and exercises (tai chi and qigong). Evaluation of effectiveness is made more difficult as the basis concepts of TCM are radically different from "Western" scientific medication. However, reviews of TCM have found little evidence of effectiveness, often due to the low quality of the available studies. In addition to safety concerns with TCM reviewed elsewhere in this article. concerns exist over the illegal trade and transport of endangered species including rhinoceroses and tigers, and the welfare of specially farmed animals including bears

Acupuncture

Acupuncture is an alternative practice that involves stimulation of superficial points on the body for a medical effect. This is generally done using needles but pressure, electricity, lasers, and even bee stings are alternatively used. In TCM, qi is felt to flow through the body along paths called meridians and stimulation at acupuncture points corrects or balances this flow. In TCM, acupuncture is frequently combined with other TCM techniques. In the United States and Europe, acupuncturists frequently practice Western Medical acupuncture, which links acupuncture to medical diagnoses and frequently rejects qi-based theories in favor of those involving nerve or endorphin stimulation. Western Medical acupuncture focuses primarily on the relief of pain and other somatic symptoms while TCM is considered applicable to a wide variety of conditions as diverse as pain, infertility, allergies, and cancer. Practitioners who seek to refer a patient for acupuncture should understand the philosophy and techniques used by the consultant.

While acupuncture is often viewed as homogeneous, in fact there are many different forms of acupuncture [29]. Even within traditional needle acupuncture there are many variations involving differences in types of needles, depth of insertion, insertion techniques, how the needles are manipulated and most significantly the location of acupoints. Additionally, a 2009 review found

"considerable variation" in localization of acupoints among qualified medical "acupuncturists" [30].

Overall, the effectiveness of acupuncture in randomized controlled trials has been disappointing; moderate evidence of effectiveness was found for acupuncture on prostatitis and fibromyalgia pain (but not fatigue), but not for the vast majority of other indications studied, including asthma, smoking, autism, depression, osteoarthritis, and neuropathic pain. In most of these studies either true acupuncture did not prove more effective than sham acupuncture (often using toothpicks or placebos that don't puncture the skin) or were too low in quality to allow a conclusion of effectiveness [31]. Recent reviews of acupuncture for pain, the most common indication in the USA, are conflicting on its effectiveness [32, 33].

Although most patients will not experience any complications from acupuncture, adverse events are not rare. Discomfort is by far the most common side effect; however, serious side effects include syncope, pneumothorax, infection, subarachnoid hemorrhage, and, rarely, death.

Naturopathy

Naturopathy is "a system of alternative medicine based on the theory that diseases can be successfully treated or prevented without the use of drugs, by techniques such as control of diet, exercise, and massage." While the stated goal of naturopathy, "to treat the whole person," is laudable, and addressing the root causes of illness using stress-management, exercise, and lifestyle changes are all appropriate goals, studies of naturopathic treatments are generally lacking in rigor and appropriate controls [34]. It is difficult to include a double-blind randomized control for an intervention such as naturopathy, and individual counseling by nutritionist and exercise therapists is not normally used as a control. There are 13 trials described in the Cochrane Library, but no reviews. The Doctor of Naturopathic Medicine (ND) is a 4-year degree. The curriculum includes approximately 60% of the clinical hours required for a Doctorate in Medicine or Osteopathy, with principles of homeopathy and other types of alternative medical treatments comprising most of the academic training [35]. Only a small minority of NDs complete anything akin to a residency. Twenty-five jurisdictions within the United States offer licensure to NDs although scope of practice varies from state to state. While there are some NDs practicing evidence-based medicine, in general naturopathy is based on the principle of vitalism, the idea there is a unique "life force."

Energy Medicine

These techniques involve the manipulation and application of energy fields to the body. In addition to electromagnetic fields outside of the body, it is hypothesized that energy fields exist within the body. The existence of these biofields has not been experimentally proven

Therapeutic Touch

Therapeutic (or Healing) Touch (TT) is an energy medicine intervention developed in the early 1970s by Deloris Krieger, a professor of nursing and Dora Kunz, a psychic and natural healer. TT posits that the body, mind, and emotions form a complex Human Energy Field (HEF) and that illness represents a disruption in this. TT practitioners claim to be able to sense this HEF, which extends several inches beyond the skin. The practitioner starts by "centering" or focusing themselves mentally, then assesses the patient by examining the patient's HEF using "the hands as sensors." They then can intervene using a series of hand "movements" to facilitate the symmetric flow of energy through the HEF in a process called "unruffling" and rebalance the field by transferring energy with in the field and by giving the patient some of the provider's own energy [36].

TT practitioners report treating a wide variety of conditions from pain, fever, and decubiti up to improving hemiplegia due to a stroke [37] and saving newborns who have failed conventional resuscitation [38]. Published studies of TT have focused almost exclusively on subjective symptoms such as pain, fatigue, and quality of life but results are mixed, generally showing little effect when compared to sham controls [39]. Studies on wound healing [40] and radiation dermatitis [41] have found no effect. Significantly, studies have shown that TT practitioners have been unable to sense HEFs when tested under controlled conditions [42]. While complications of TT are probably minimal, considerations should be given to unnecessary patient exposure (e.g., in the recent COVID-19 epidemic), delay of definitive therapies and distraction of the provider from other duties [43].

Reiki

Reiki was developed in the early twentieth century by Mikao Usui, a Buddhist spiritualist. The therapeutic aspects of this practice were emphasized by his students and their successors resulting in the healing practice used today. Reiki is felt to affect the vibrations arising from nondual primordial chi, or Tao, as distinguished from the bioenergetic level of chi stimulated by therapeutic acupuncture, allowing the practitioner to rebalance this energy field, removing the causes of illness and restoring overall resilience. Hands-on Reiki treatment involves light touch on a fully clothed recipient who is seated or reclining. If touch is contraindicated, Reiki may be performed with the hands several inches off the body and advanced practitioners are felt to be able to perform Reiki from a distance. A typical treatment involves placing the hands on 12 positions on the head and torso. A typical session lasts 45–75 minutes but may be shorter or longer. The patient need not be conscious [44]. In the USA, there is no central authority regulating the training or practice of Reiki

Reiki treatments are generally directed toward reducing stress, enhancing mood and quality of life, and improving pain. It is recommended for patients with a wide variety of conditions, from diabetics to cancer patients, but is generally felt to help with these previously mentioned areas rather than function as a direct treatment of the medical condition. Although studies frequently show improvement in these areas compared to no treatment, there is very little evidence of Reiki causing more improvement than sham Reiki treatments. This implies that these effects may come primarily from the use of a soothing treatment and the attention of a caring professional.

References

1. Barnes PM, Bloom B. Complementary and alternative medicine use among adults and children: United States, 2007. National Health Statistics Report 2008;12. https://www.cdc.gov/nchs/data/nhsr/nhsr012.pdf. Accessed 29 Aug 2020
2. Strewler A, Conroy R, Kao H. Approach to overuse of herbal and dietary supplements: a teachable moment. JAMA Intern Med. 2014;174(7):1033–4.
3. Wu C-H, Wang C-C, Tsai M-T, Huang W-T, Kennedy J. Trend and pattern of herb and supplement use in the United States: results from the 2002, 2007, and 2012 national health interview surveys. Evid Based Complement Alternat Med. 2014;2014:872320.
4. Thompson ME, Noel MB. Issues in nutrition: dietary supplements. FP Essent. 2017;452:18–25.
5. White CM. Dietary supplements pose real dangers to patients. Ann Pharmacother. 2020;54(8):729–41.
6. Saper RB, Phillips RS, Sehgal A, et al. Lead, mercury, and arsenic in US- and Indian-manufactured Ayurvedic medicines sold via the Internet. JAMA. 2008;300(8):915–23.
7. Mursu J, Robien K, Harnack LJ, Park K, Jacobs DR Jr. Dietary supplements and mortality rate in older women: the Iowa Women's Health Study. Arch Intern Med. 2011;171(18):1625–33.
8. Gordon M, Farrell M, Thomas AG, Akobeng AK, Wallace C. Probiotics for management of functional abdominal pain disorders in children. Cochrane Database Syst Rev. 2017;11:CD012849.
9. Knox NC, Forbes JD, Van Domselaar G, Bernstein CN. The gut microbiome as a target for IBD treatment: are we there yet? Curr Treat Options Gastroenterol. 2019;17(1):115–26.
10. Guo Q, Goldenberg JZ, Humphrey C, El Dib R, Johnston BC. Probiotics for the prevention of pediatric antibiotic-associated diarrhea. Cochrane Database Syst Rev. 2019;(4):CD004827.
11. Goldenberg JZ, Yap C, Lytvyn L, Lo CKF, Beardsley J, Mertz D, Johnston BC. Probiotics for the prevention of Clostridium difficile-associated diarrhea in adults and children. Cochrane Database Syst Rev. 2017;12: CD006095.
12. Kolaček S, Hojsak I, Berni Canani R, Guarino A, Indrio F, Orelet R, et al. Commercial probiotic products: a call for improved quality control. A position paper by the ESPGHAN working group for probiotics and prebiotics. J Pediatr Gastroenterol Nutr. 2017;65(1):117–24.
13. Altobelli R, Del Negro V, Angeletti PM, Latella G. Low-FODMAP diet improves irritable bowel syndrome symptoms: a meta-analysis. Nutrients. 2017;9(9):940–59.
14. Leonard MM, Sapone A, Catassi C, Fasano A. Celiac disease and nonceliac gluten sensitivity: a review. JAMA. 2017;318(7):647–56.
15. Simon R, Engström M. The default mode network as a biomarker for monitoring the therapeutic effects of meditation. Front Psychol. 2015;6:776.
16. Garland EL, Brintz CE, Hanley AW, et al. Mind-body therapies for opioid-treated pain: a systematic review and meta-analysis. JAMA Intern Med. 2020;180(1):91–105.
17. Cavicchioli M, Movalli M, Maffei C. The clinical efficacy of mindfulness-based treatments for alcohol and drugs use disorders: a meta-analytic review of randomized and nonrandomized controlled trials. Eur Addict Res. 2018;24(3):137–62.
18. Beach MC, Roter D, Korthuis PT, et al. A multicenter study of physician mindfulness and health care quality. Ann Fam Med. 2013;11(5):421–8.
19. Saper RB, Lemaster C, Delitto A, et al. Yoga, physical therapy, or education for chronic low back pain: a randomized noninferiority trial. Ann Intern Med. 2017;167(2):85–94.
20. Guthrie KA, LaCroix AZ, Ensrud KE, et al. Pooled analysis of six pharmacologic and nonpharmacologic interventions for vasomotor symptoms. Obstet Gynecol. 2015;126(2):413–22.
21. Adachi T, Fujino H, Nakae A, Mashimo T, Sasaki J. A meta-analysis of hypnosis for chronic pain problems: a comparison between hypnosis, standard care, and other psychological interventions. Int J Clin Exp Hypn. 2014;62(1):1–28.
22. Bollinger JW. The rate of adverse events related to hypnosis during clinical trials. Am J Clin Hypn. 2018;60(4):357–66.
23. Slattengren AH, Nissly T, Blustin J, Bader A, Westfall E. Best uses of osteopathic manipulation. J Fam Pract. 2017;66(12):743–7.
24. Ernst E. Chiropractic: a critical evaluation. J Pain Symptom Manag. 2008;35(5):544–62.
25. Nielsen SM, Tarp S, Christensen R, Bliddal H, Klokker L, Henriksen M. The risk associated with spinal manipulation: an overview of reviews. Syst Rev. 2017;6(1):64.
26. Stevinson C, Ernst E. Risks associated with spinal manipulation. Am J Med. 2002;112(7):566–71.
27. Goldacre B. Benefits and risks of homoeopathy. Lancet (London, England). 2007;370(9600):1672–3.
28. Novella S. FDA warns about homeopathic teething products. Science-Based Medicine website. October 5, 2016. https://sciencebasedmedicine.org/fda-warns-about-homeopathic-teething-products/. Accessed 24 Aug 2020

29. Crislip M. Infinite variety? So many styles of acupuncture. Science-Based Medicine website. October 21, 2014. https://sciencebasedmedicine.org/infinitevariety/. Accessed 25 Aug 2020.

30. Godson DR, Wardle JL. Accuracy and precision in acupuncture point location: a critical systematic review. J Acupunct Meridian Stud. 2019;12(2):52–66.

31. Colquhoun D, Novella SP. Acupuncture is theatrical placebo. Anesth Analg. 2013;116(6):1360–3.

32. Xiang Y, He J-Y, Tian H-H, Cao B-Y, Li R. Evidence of efficacy of acupuncture in the management of low back pain: a systematic review and meta-analysis of randomized placebo- or sham-controlled trials. Acupunct Med J Br Med Acupunct Soc. 2020;38(1):15–24.

33. Paley CA, Johnson MI. Acupuncture for the relief of chronic pain: a synthesis of systematic reviews. Medicina (Kaunas, Lithuania). 2019;56(1):6.

34. Logan AC, Goldenberg JZ, Guiltinan J, Seely D, Katz DL. North American naturopathic medicine in the 21st century: time for a seventh guiding principle – Scientia Critica. Explore (New York, NY). 2018;14(5):367–72.

35. Nelson DH, Perchaluk JM, Logan AC, Katzman MA. The Bell Tolls for Homeopathy: time for change in the training and practice of North American naturopathic physicians. J Evid Based Integ Med. 2019;24:2515690X18823696. https://doi.org/10.1177/2515690X18823696.

36. The Process of Therapeutic Touch. Therapeutic Touch International Association website. 2012. https://therapeutictouch.org/what-is-tt/history-of-tt/. Accessed 25 Aug 2020.

37. Glickman R, Gracely EJ. Therapeutic touch: investigation of a practitioner. Sci Rev Altern Med. 1998;2(1):43–7.

38. Krieger D. Therapeutic touch inner workbook. Santa Fe: Bear; 1997. p. 7.

39. Anderson JG, Taylor AG. Effects of healing touch in clinical practice: a systematic review of randomized clinical trials. J Holist Nurs. 2011;29(3):221–8.

40. O'Mathúna DP. Therapeutic touch for healing acute wounds. Cochrane Database Syst Rev. 2016;(8): CD002766.

41. Younus J, Lock M, Vujovic O, et al. A case-control, mono-center, open-label, pilot study to evaluate the feasibility of therapeutic touch in preventing radiation dermatitis in women with breast cancer receiving adjuvant radiation therapy. Complement Ther Med. 2015;23(4):612–6.

42. Rosa L, Rosa E, Sarner L, Barrett S. A close look at therapeutic touch. JAMA. 1998;279(13):1005–10.

43. O'Mathúna DP. Therapeutic touch: what could be the harm? Sci Rev Alter Med. 1998;2(1):56–62.

44. Miles P, True G. Reiki – review of a biofield therapy history, theory, practice, and research. Altern Ther Health Med. 2003;9(2):62–72. http://search.ebscohost.com. Accessed 1 Sept 2020.; Miles P, True G. Reiki – review of a biofield therapy history, theory, practice, and research. Altern Ther Health Med [Internet]. 2003 Mar [cited 2020 Sept 8];9(2):62–72. Available from http://search.ebscohost.com/login.aspx?direct=true&db=cmedm&AN=12652885&login.asp%3fcustid%3ds5794986&site=ehost-live&scope=site

45. Herbs at a Glance. National Center for Complementary and Integrative Health website. https://www.nccih.nih.gov/health/herbsataglance. Accessed 31 July 2020

46. Antoniou T, Bodkin J, JM-W H. Drug interactions with cannabinoids. CMAJ. 2020;192(9):E206. https://doi.org/10.1503/cmaj.19109.

47. bdelhamid AS, Martin N, Bridges C, Brainard JS, Wang X, Brown TJ, et al. Polyunsaturated fatty acids for the primary and secondary prevention of cardiovascular disease. Cochrane Database Syst Rev [Internet]. 2018 Nov 27 [cited 2020 Sep 8];11: CD012345.

48. Hemilä H. Duration of the common cold and similar continuous outcome should be analyzed on the relative scale: a case study of two zinc lozenge trials. BMC Med Res Methodol. 2017;17(1):82.

49. The Dangers of Dietary and Nutritional Supplements Investigated. Consumer reports website. Updated September 2010. http://www.consumerreports.org/cro/2012/05/dangerous-supplements/index.htm. Accessed 7 July 2020.

50. Supplements Ingredients to Always Avoid. Consumer reports Website. Consumer Reports website. Updated October 30, 2019. https://www.consumerreports.org/vitamins-supplements/15-supplement-ingredients-to-always-avoid/. Accessed 7 July 2020.

Jumana Al-Deek, Leslie Bruce, Bianca Stewart, and Raj Mehta

Contents

Definition of the Medical Home

The Patient-Centered Medical Home (PCMH) has various titles including, but not limited to, "medical home model," "medical home," "person-centered medical home," and "health home" [1]. For simplicity, PCMH will be used and understood to represent all titles throughout this chapter.

A Patient-Centered Medical Home is not a physical location but a theoretical home whose objective is to integrate various aspects of patient care by utilizing a diverse set of healthcare professionals with a range of expertise. The objective is to develop an individualized model that provides quality, comprehensive, efficient, and effective care [2].

There is no single definition for a PCMH. Various states have developed their own definition as it pertains to their unique patient population [1]. A PCMH should incorporate certain core fundamentals including access, continuity, planned care, population health, care management, patient and caregiver engagement, comprehensiveness, and coordination [3]. The primary

J. Al-Deek · L. Bruce · B. Stewart · R. Mehta (✉)
AdventHealth Family Medicine Residency, Winter Park, FL, USA
e-mail: jumana.al-deek.do@adventhealth.com;
leslie.bruce.md@adventhealth.com;
bianca.stewart.md@adventhealth.com;
raj.mehta.md@adventhealth.com

© Springer Nature Switzerland AG 2022
P. M. Paulman et al. (eds.), *Family Medicine*,
https://doi.org/10.1007/978-3-030-54441-6_154

care collaborative, endorsed by AAFP, does, however, offer a specific definition:

PCMH includes the identification of a personal physician in the context of a physician-directed medical practice, enhanced access to coordinated and/or integrated medical care with a whole person orientation, high standards of quality and safety, and payment that appropriately recognizes the added value provided to patients within the model [4].

History of the Medical Home

The PCMH is not a new design; however, it has gained a renewed sense of popularity in the past decade. The concept was first described by the AAP and later adopted and revised by numerous colleges and academies. Below is an outline of the history of the medical home.

- 1967: The American Academy of Pediatrics (AAP) introduces the concept of a medical home as a centralized location for children's medical records with a focus on patients with specialized healthcare needs [5].
- 1978: The Declaration of Alma-Alta calls for urgent development and implementation of primary healthcare both nationally and internationally – the first international announcement of the necessity of primary care for the health of all people [6].
- 1996: The Institute of Medicine (IOM) defines primary as "the provision of integrated, accessible health care services by clinicians who are accountable for addressing a large majority of personal health needs, developing a sustained partnership with patients, and practicing in the context of family and community" [7].
- 2001: The IOM recognizes that patients and families are at the center of the medical team and should be partners in making medical decisions by defining "patient-centered care" as "health care that establishes a partnership among practitioners, patients, and their families (when appropriate) to ensure that decisions respect patients' wants, needs, and preferences and that patients have the education and

support they require to make decisions and participate in their own care" [8].

- 2002: As a solution to the fragmented US healthcare system, the Future of Family Medicine (FFM) project was initiated which emphasized the need for all patients to establish a medical home and create a model for compensation that sustains primary care [9].
- 2005: Dr. Barbara Starfield describes six primary care mechanisms that benefit health in the article "Contribution of primary care to health systems and health": (1) greater access to needed services, (2) better quality of care, (3) a greater focus on prevention, (4) early management of health problems, (5) the cumulative effect of the main primary care delivery characteristics, and (6) the role of primary care in reducing unnecessary and potentially harmful specialist care [10].
- 2007: The American Academy of Family Physicians, the American College of Physicians, the American Osteopathic Association, and the AAP published "The Joint Principles of the Patient-Centered Medical Home" to create a standardization of the PCMH [11].
- 2010: President Barack Obama signs the Patient Protection and Affordable Care Act which highlights the application and promotion of the medical home model for patients of all ages [12].
- 2011: The Center for Medicare & Medicaid services (CMS) began programs to test changes in primary care delivery and payment [13].
- 2013: State Innovation Models Initiative via CMS promoted state-led delivery transformations to improve quality of care and lower costs, with a majority of focus on primary care [13].
- 2015: The Medicare Access and CHIP Reauthorization Act (MACRA) streamlined multiple quality programs under a new Merit-Based Incentive Payment System (MIPS) [14].
- 2019: After much planning, CMS implemented the first MIPS performance period in 2019. MIPS contain improvement activities similar to the function of Patient-Centered Medical Home model [15].

Principles and Characteristics of Medical Homes

PCMH can be described as three different conceptual categories: characteristics of primary care practices, patterns of care that patients experience, and interventions applied to primary care practices [16]. "PCMH characteristics" describe how close a practice might be (with greater or lesser degree of success) to the ideal of our PCMH model. "PCMH patterns of care" describe patient experiences such as health outcomes or resource utilization. "PCMH interventions" are empirically testable approaches to improve "characteristics" and "patterns of care" and can be used to inform policy decisions.

The "PCMH characteristics" have been described in various ways throughout its history. In 2007 the American Academy of Family Physicians, the American College of Physicians (AAP), the American Osteopathic Association (AOA), and the AAP published "The Joint Principles of the Patient-Centered Medical Home" outlining essential elements of the PCMH as evidenced by the following [11].

Principles

Personal physician – Each patient has an ongoing relationship with a personal physician trained to provide first-contact, continuous, and comprehensive care.

Physician-directed medical practice – The personal physician leads a team of individuals at the practice level who collectively take responsibility for the ongoing care of patients.

Whole person orientation – The personal physician is responsible for providing for all the patient's healthcare needs or taking responsibility for appropriately arranging care with other qualified professionals. This includes care for all stages of life: acute care, chronic care, preventive services, and end-of-life care.

Care is coordinated and/or integrated across all elements of the complex healthcare system (e.g., subspecialty care, hospitals, home health agencies, nursing homes) and the patient's community (e.g., family, public, and private community-based services). Care is facilitated by registries, information technology, health information exchange, and other means to assure that patients get the indicated care when and where they need and want it in a culturally and linguistically appropriate manner.

Quality and safety are hallmarks of the medical home:

- Practices advocate for their patients to support the attainment of optimal, patient-centered outcomes that are defined by a care planning process driven by a compassionate, robust partnership between physicians, patients, and the patient's family.
- Evidence-based medicine and clinical decision support tools guide decision-making.
- Physicians in the practice accept accountability for continuous quality improvement through voluntary engagement in performance measurement and improvement.
- Patients actively participate in decision-making, and feedback is sought to ensure patients' expectations are being met.
- Information technology is utilized appropriately to support optimal patient care, performance measurement, patient education, and enhanced communication.
- Practices go through a voluntary recognition process by an appropriate nongovernmental entity to demonstrate that they have the capabilities to provide patient-centered services consistent with the medical home model.
- Patients and families participate in quality improvement activities at the practice level.

Enhanced access to care is available through systems such as open scheduling, expanded hours and new options for communication between patients, their personal physician, and practice staff.

Payment appropriately recognizes the added value provided to patients who have a Patient-Centered Medical Home. The payment structure should be based on the following framework:

- It should reflect the value of physician and nonphysician staff patient-centered care management work that falls outside of the face-to-face visit.
- It should pay for services associated with coordination of care both within a given practice and between consultants, ancillary providers, and community resources.
- It should support adoption and use of health information technology for quality improvement.
- It should support provision of enhanced communication access such as secure e-mail and telephone consultation.
- It should recognize the value of physician work associated with remote monitoring of clinical data using technology.
- It should allow for separate fee-for-service payments for face-to-face visits. (Payments for care management services that fall outside of the face-to-face visit, as described above, should not result in a reduction in the payments for face-to-face visits.)
- It should recognize case mix differences in the patient population being treated within the practice.

In summary, the Agency for Healthcare Research and Quality explains the five functions and attributes of a PCMH as a model of the organization of primary care [17].

- Provides comprehensive care that is accountable for meeting the *majority* of healthcare needs including prevention and wellness, acute care, and chronic care with a team of providers that includes physicians, advanced practice nurses, physician assistants, nurses, pharmacists, nutritionists, social workers, educators, and care coordinators.
- *Provides* patient-centered care that is *cultivated* through partnering with patients and their families and respecting each patient's unique needs, culture, values, and preferences.
- Supports patients in coordinating care across all elements of the broader healthcare system, including specialty care, hospitals, home health care, and community services and

supports – particularly critical during transitions between sites of care.
- Delivers accessible services with shorter waiting times for urgent needs, enhanced in-person hours, around-the-clock telephone or electronic access to a member of the care team, and alternative methods of communication such as e-mail and telephone care.
- Is committed to using evidence-based medicine and clinical decision support tools to guide shared decision-making with patients and families, engaging in performance measurement and improvement, measuring and responding to patient experiences and patient satisfaction, and practicing population health management. Sharing robust quality and safety data and improvement activities publicly is also an important marker of a system-level commitment to quality [17].

The Role of Family Medicine in the Medical Home

The "PCMH characteristics" and goals are largely consistent with the skillset of the family medicine physicians. Family physicians are comprehensively trained in screening/prevention, pediatrics, women's health, obstetrics, geriatrics, and behavioral health. Family medicine is a key team leader for the design and implementation of PCMH models.

Studies have shown that the presence of primary care physicians reduces mortality, has better health outcomes and lower costs, and is more impactful than specialists for all-cause mortality. These themes are recurrent when discussing the PCMH. For every dollar put into primary care, the healthcare system saves $13 [18].

The training and goals of the family medicine physician also places them in a position to represent their community to local government as an advocate for improved health policies. Local policies impact how PCMH are able to operate and best impact their community. It will also serve to address barriers to PCMH implementation which include low resources and inadequate staffing or ancillary support.

Role of the PCMH in the Health System

The PCMH model is being implemented all throughout the country. The goals of the PCMH align well, if not seamlessly, with many healthcare organizations including Centers for Medicare & Medicaid which serve a large portion of our society.

In an ideal PCMH model, patients have improved access, and this tends to be especially important in vulnerable populations. It also avoids duplication of services, helps avoid unnecessary and costly services, reduces medical errors, and keeps patients engaged in their medical care.

A further expansion of the ideal PCMH model includes that of the "medical neighborhood." This concept expands the PCMH model to include all forms of ambulatory care, diagnostic services, pharmacy, and acute and post-acute care facilities. Even more, it further enlists the community and social services available to the population that it serves. The medical neighborhood would serve as another mechanism for improving outcomes, safety, and patient experience, lowering costs, and decreasing medical errors. Medical homes that exist within this structure become critical points of contact and coordination of services to aid patients as they navigate this growing network.

Results and Evidence

The Patient-Centered Medical Home model has been widely implemented in many different patient populations over the last two decades. The cumulative available data offers a mixed picture that suggests a broad failure to deliver large transformative changes, but smaller successes in specific patient populations and disease processes. The confusing state of the PCMH literature underlies the importance of carefully reviewing the methodology of each paper and subdividing based on differences between studying "characteristics" vs "interventions" [19].

Discussing evidence for PCMH should start with studies on "PCMH characteristics." Research findings have shown that healthcare systems with greater "PCMH characteristics" tend to have a more positive impact on utilization, costs, quality of patient care, patient satisfaction, and patient access. For example, a large VA study looked at a pool of 1,650,976 patients who were seen at their PCMH clinics and found that they had fewer ED visits [20]. Another study showed that patients with diabetes who received care from a practice with more PCMH characteristics had 19% greater odds of having well-controlled HbA1c values [21]. The same study also found African Americans had less benefit from efforts to improve blood pressure and HbA1C control, suggesting a persistence in social disparities that needs to consider community factors when implementing PCMH [21].

Unfortunately, despite the positive association between "PCMH characteristics" and healthcare outcomes, the studies on "PCMH interventions" have been much less successful. A prospective cohort study in 2016 with 438 primary care providers and 136,480 patients compared PCMH to non-PCMH practices over a 5-year period. Overall, they found patterns of quality were similar across groups, with some modest changes in utilization [22]. The Maryland Multipayor Patient-centered Medical Home Program which involved 52 PCMH practices had mixed results, with lower costs among Medicaid beneficiaries, but no sustained lower costs in privately insured beneficiaries, no change in provider or patient satisfaction, and higher administrative burden [23]. The strongest null evidence comes from an RCT on healthcare hotspotting. This study on 800 hospitalized patients with very high use of healthcare services found 6-month interventions with intensive case management and coordination of outpatient care did not reduce emergency or hospital utilization. The study questions one key hypothesis of the PCMH model (practice changes can reduce healthcare utilization and costs) and suggests that if PCMH interventions are to be successful, they may require monitoring over a long period of time and with greater community involvement [24].

Overall, the accumulation of disappointing or modest findings highlight the difficulty of implementing PCMH. Practices with greater success at transformation may require support over years to complete necessary structural and cultural changes. Providing team and non-visit-based care is also difficult in fee-for-service models, and at least one study has suggested it may require a shift in reimbursement practices to higher levels of capitation payments [25].

Certification, Recognition, and Accreditation

Since its release in 2007, the Patient-Centered Medical Home has provided primary care practices a model to improve the quality, efficiency, and effectiveness of patient care by redesigning their practice. In order to streamline this process, several entities began offering medical home recognition or accreditation for Patient-Centered Medical Homes. The AAFP, AAP, ACP, and AOA developed the "Guidelines for Patient-centered Medical Home Recognition and Accreditation Programs" [23] to help create a standard for accreditation. These guidelines specify that accreditation programs should:

- Incorporate the Joint Principles of the Patient-Centered Medical Home
- Address the complete scope of primary care services
- Ensure the incorporation of patient- and family-centered care emphasizing engagement of patients and their caregivers
- Engage multiple stakeholders in the development and implementation of the program
- Align standards, elements, characteristics, and/or measures with meaningful use requirements
- Identify essential standards, elements, and characteristics
- Address the core concept of continuous improvement that is central to the PCMH model
- Allow for innovative ideas
- Care coordination within the medical neighborhood
- Clearly identify PCMH recognition or accreditation requirements for training programs
- Ensure transparency in program structure and scoring

- Apply reasonable documentation/data collection requirements
- Conduct evaluations of the program's effectiveness and implement improvements over time

Currently, there are four individual certifying agencies that exist and comply with the "Guidelines for Patient-Centered Medical Home Recognition and Accreditation Programs." The agencies include the National Committee for Quality Assurance (NCQA), URAC, the joint commission, and Accreditation Association for Ambulatory Health Care (AAAHC).

Although formal accreditation is not always required to be considered a Patient-Centered Medical Home, some circumstances may require completion of an accredited or recognized program. This is an important factor to keep in mind when establishing an agreement between a practice and another entity like a federal grant, major practice payer agreements, etc.

In Context

The concept of the medical home was first introduced by the American Academy of Pediatrics in 1967 to refer to a central location for archiving a child's medical record. The AAFP and AACP have since developed their own models for improving patient care called the "Patient-Centered Medical Home." The medical home's focus is the patient, and it is important not to lose sight of this among all the metrics. The most important aspect of primary care is the patient-physician relationship. It is important to keep in mind that, while the medical home is valued for its focus on this aspect, physicians should remind themselves of the importance of keeping that concept at the forefront of their minds.

References

1. State Definitions of the Medical Home. https://www.aafp.org/dam/AAFP/documents/advocacy/coverage/pcmh/ES-StateDefinitionsofMedicalHome-032912.pdf
2. The Patient Centered Medical Home [Internet]. [cited 2020 May 21]. https://www.aafp.org/practice-management/transformation/pcmh.html

3. Medical Home [Internet]. [cited 2020 May 21]. https://www.aafp.org/about/policies/all/medical-home.html

4. Medical homes with the patient at the center [Internet]. Primary Care Collaborative. [cited 2020 May 21]. https://www.pcpcc.org/2013/05/06/medical-homes-patient-center

5. Sia C, Tonniges TF, Osterhus E, Taba S. History of the medical home concept. Pediatrics. 2004;113 (5 Suppl):1473–8.

6. Declaration of Alma-Ata. International conference on primary health care, Alma-Ata, USSR, 6–12 Sept 1978. Development. 2004;47(2):159–61.

7. Institute of Medicine (US) Committee on the Future of Primary Care. Primary care: America's health in a new era [Internet]. Donaldson MS, Yordy KD, Lohr KN, Vanselow NA, editors. Washington, DC: National Academies Press; 1996 [cited 2020 May 21]. http://www.ncbi.nlm.nih.gov/books/NBK232643/

8. Institute of Medicine (US) Committee on the National Quality Report on Health Care Delivery. Envisioning the National Health Care Quality Report [Internet]. Hurtado MP, Swift EK, Corrigan JM, editors. Washington, DC: National Academies Press; 2001 [cited 2020 May 21]. http://www.ncbi.nlm.nih.gov/books/NBK223318/

9. Martin JC, Avant RF, Bowman MA, Bucholtz JR, Dickinson JR, Evans KL, et al. The future of family medicine: a collaborative project of the family medicine community. Ann Fam Med. 2004;2(Suppl 1): S3–32.

10. Starfield B, Shi L, Macinko J. Contribution of primary care to health systems and health. Milbank Q. 2005;83 (3):457–502.

11. Joint Principles of the Patient-Centered Medical Home. [Internet]. [cited 2020 May 21]. https://www.aafp.org/dam/AAFP/documents/practice_management/pcmh/initiatives/PCMHJoint.pdf

12. What is Medical Home? [Internet]. [cited 2020 May 21]. https://medicalhomeinfo.aap.org/overview/Pages/Whatisthemedicalhome.aspx

13. Sessums LL, Conway PH. Saving primary care. JAMA Intern Med. 2017;177(11):1560–2.

14. MACRA: MIPS & APMs|CMS [Internet]. [cited 2020 Jun 2]. https://www.cms.gov/Medicare/Quality-Initiatives-Patient-Assessment-Instruments/Value-Based-Programs/MACRA-MIPS-and-APMs/MACRA-MIPS-and-APMs

15. MIPS: Explaining the improvement activities performance category [Internet]. [cited 2020 Jun 2]. https://www.aafp.org/practice-management/payment/medicare-payment/mips/ia.html

16. Friedberg MW. What do you mean by medical home? Ann Intern Med. 2016;164(6):444–5.

17. Defining the PCMH|PCMH Resource Center [Internet]. [cited 2020 May 21]. https://pcmh.ahrq.gov/page/defining-pcmh

18. Bujold E. The impending death of the patient-centered medical home. JAMA Intern Med. 2017;177 (11):1559–60.

19. Martsolf GR, Kandrack R, Baird M, Friedberg MW. Estimating associations between medical home adoption, utilization, and quality: a comparison of evaluation approaches. Med Care. 2018;56(1):25–30.

20. Aysola J, Schapira MM, Huo H, Werner RM. Organizational processes and patient experiences in the patient-centered medical home. Med Care. 2018;56(6):497–504.

21. Kinsell HS, Hall AG, Harman JS, Tewary S, Brickman A. Impacts of initial transformation to a patient-centered medical home on diabetes outcomes in federally qualified health centers in Florida. J Prim Care Community Health. 2017;8(4):192–7.

22. Kern LM, Edwards A, Kaushal R. The patient-centered medical home and associations with health care quality and utilization: a 5-year cohort study. Ann Intern Med. 2016;164(6):395–405.

23. Marsteller JA, Hsu Y-J, Gill C, Kiptanui Z, Fakeye OA, Engineer LD, et al. Maryland multipayor patient-centered medical home program: a 4-year quasi-experimental evaluation of quality, utilization, patient satisfaction, and provider perceptions. Med Care. 2018;56(4):308–20.

24. Finkelstein A, Zhou A, Taubman S, Doyle J. Health care hotspotting – a randomized, controlled trial. N Engl J Med [Internet]. 2020 Jan 8 [cited 2020 May 21]; https://www.nejm.org/doi/pdf/10.1056/NEJMsa1906848?articleTools=true

25. Basu S, Phillips RS, Song Z, Bitton A, Landon BE. High levels of capitation payments needed to shift primary care toward proactive team and nonvisit care. Health Aff Proj Hope. 2017;36(9):1599–605.

Robert B. Taylor and Paul M. Paulman

Year	Event	Significance
1900	At least 80% of American physicians were general practitioners: one general practitioner for every 600 persons	General practice was the predominant model of medical care
1910	Publication of the *Flexner Report* by the Carnegie Foundation, with cooperation of the American Medical Association (AMA)	Prompted changes in methods and quality of medical education: premedical education, biomedical research, and postgraduate training
1940	General practitioners (GPs) comprised 76% of private physicians:	Decline of generalism paralleled the rise of specialty practice
	1950–62% of physicians were general practitioners	
	1960–45% of physicians were general practitioners	

(continued)

Year	Event	Significance
	1970–21% of physicians were general practitioners	
1941	General Practice Certifying Board proposed in AMA House of Delegates	First call for a certifying board for general practitioners; not passed
1946	Section on General Practice of the AMA organized	An early organization of general practitioners with nationwide representation
1947	American Academy of General Practice (AAGP) founded by a small group (no more than 150) of general practitioners meeting in Atlantic City, New Jersey	First major medical organization to require continuing medical education as a condition of membership
1950	First residency training programs in general practice established	Signified need for postgraduate generalist training beyond the internship year
	Publication of journal *GP*	First scientific journal for GPs
1958	Family Health Foundation of America incorporated	Early funding for conferences on generalist education
1960	American Board of General Practice formed	First successful effort to obtain general practice board status

(continued)

R. B. Taylor (✉)
Department of Family and Community Medicine, Eastern Virginia Medical School, Norfolk, VA, USA

Oregon Health Science University, Portland, OR, USA
e-mail: taylorr@ohsu.edu

P. M. Paulman
Department of Family Medicine, University of Nebraska Medical Center, Omaha, NE, USA
e-mail: ppaulman@unmc.edu

© Springer Nature Switzerland AG 2022
P. M. Paulman et al. (eds.), *Family Medicine*,
https://doi.org/10.1007/978-3-030-54441-6_50

Year	Event	Significance
1964	19% of US medical graduates entered general practice	Continued decline in numbers of general practitioners
	American Board of Family Practice Advisory Group formed	Developed objectives for the American Board of Family Practice (see 1969)
1965	National Family Health Conference sponsored by Family Health Foundation of America	Studied unmet needs of Americans for comprehensive health care, what practitioner can meet this need, and how he or she can best be trained
1966	Report of Citizens' Commission on Graduate Medical Education: *The Graduate Education of Physicians* (Millis Commission Report)	Identified fragmentation in health care and proposed concept of a "primary physician"
	Report of the Ad Hoc Committee on Education for Family Practice of the Council on Medical Education: *Meeting the Challenge of Family Practice* (Willard Commission Report)	Recommended training of a "family physician"
1967	Formation of Society of Teachers of Family Medicine (STFM)	First organization of family medicine educators
1969	STFM published *Family Medicine Times* (FMT)	First publication (newsletter) for family medicine educators
	American Board of Family Practice (ABFP) founded	Organized as official certifying board for the new specialty
	Recognition of family practice as a specialty on February 6, 1969, based upon approval of the Liaison Committee for specialty boards	The 20th American medical specialty
	Fifteen approved family practice residencies in the USA	Model graduate training programs established
1970	First examination by ABFP	Successful candidates sitting for 1970 and 1971 examinations became Charter Diplomates

(continued)

Year	Event	Significance
1971	American Academy of General Practice changed its name to American Academy of Family Physicians (AAFP)	The academy recognized shift in emphasis to family practice
1972	AAFP fellowships first awarded	Recognized "interest and participation in special educational programs designed to enhance professional competence and the quality of health care provided to the people of America"
	First meeting of North American Primary Care Research Group (NAPCRG)	Forum for presentation of family practice research results
	WONCA (World Organization of Family Doctors) formed	Worldwide organization begins with member organizations in 18 countries
1973	Publication of *Family Practice* (Conn, Rakel, Johnson, editors)	First major family practice textbook
	First National Conference of Family Practice Residents and Student Members	First national meeting of family practice trainees
1974	*Journal of Family Practice* began publication	First family practice peer-reviewed journal
	Medical students and residents gain seats in AAFP Congress of Delegates	First major specialty to recognize medical student and resident delegates
1975	Residency Assistance Program (RAP) initiated	Family medicine educators develop guidelines and offer consultation to family practice residency training programs
	STFM Foundation formed	The charitable arm of STFM established
1976	First recertification examination by ABFP	First recertification examination by any medical specialty
	Publication of the Virginia Study in the Journal of Family Practice	First major report of doctor-patient contacts in family practice

(continued)

Year	Event	Significance
1977	Doctors Ought to Care (DOC) founded	Championed positive health strategies for the clinic, classroom, and community
1978	Publication of *Family Medicine: Principles and Practice,* 1st edition (Taylor, editor; Buckingham, Donatelle, Jacott, Rosen, associate editors)	First edition of the second major family practice textbook
	Practice eligible route to ABFP certification expired	Candidates for the ABFP certification examination subsequently must have satisfactorily completed a 3-year approved family practice residency
	Association of Departments of Family Medicine (ADFM) established	First organization of family medicine academic units
1979	End of first decade as a specialty: Residency training programs: 364. FP residents in training: 6531. Members of AAFP: 43,956 Diplomates of ABFP: 22,246	Continuing growth of the specialty
	Family Medicine Teacher established	Official journal of STFM
1980	Graduate Medical Education National Advisory Committee (GMENAC) report published	"Near balance" of general practitioners/ family physicians vs. need was predicted for 1990; no change recommended for family practice residencies
1981	*Family Medicine Teacher* became *Family Medicine*	Society's publication becomes an academic peer-reviewed journal
	Family Practice Research Journal began publication	Third peer-reviewed journal in family practice
1982	Report of the Study Group on Family Medicine Research: *Meeting the Challenge of Research in Family Medicine*	Documented past achievements and current status; indicated future directions in family medicine research

Year	Event	Significance
1983	Publication of *Family Medicine: Principles and Practice,* 2nd edition (Taylor, editor; Buckingham, Donatelle, Jacott, Rosen, associate editors)	Principles and practice of discipline integrated as "Family Medicine Content"
1984	Conjoint meeting of STFM and NAPCRG	First joint assembly of family medicine educators and researchers
	Keystone I Conference held at Keystone, Colorado	A time for family practice leaders to meditate and reflect
1985	Liaison Committee on Medical Education (LCME) report *Functions and Structure of a Medical School* called for predoctoral training "necessary to enter graduate medical education programs in family medicine…"	Official recognition of need for medical schools to present family medicine knowledge, skills, attitudes, and behaviors
	FM student interest groups established at US medical schools	Emphasis on recruitment of medical students to careers in family practice
1986	Family Practice redefined by AAFP and ABFP	New definition affirms independence from other specialties
	More than 20,000 physicians were graduates of 3-year family practice residencies	Record number of residency-trained family physicians
	"Michigan lawsuit" won in United States Supreme Court after 10-year battle	Successful challenge of a Medicare statute that discriminated against family physicians on basis of different fees for the same procedure
1987	First Leadership Skills Development Conference held by the AAFP	Emphasis on enhancing the skills of family physician leaders
1988	*Journal of the American Board of Family Practice* began publication	Fourth US peer-reviewed journal in the specialty
	More than half of all AAFP members were	Most general practitioners had

(continued)

(continued)

Year	Event	Significance
	certified by ABFP (26,500 ABFP diplomates)	become board-certified family physicians
	Keystone II Conference held in Keystone, Colorado	FP leaders meet to reflect and plan for the future
	First examination for Certificate of Added Qualifications (CAQ) in Geriatric Medicine	Joint venture of American Board of Family Practice and American Board of Internal Medicine
	Publication of *Family Medicine: Principles and Practice,* 3rd edition. (Taylor, editor; Buckingham, Donatelle, Johnson, Scherger, associate editors)	Core problems and procedures in family medicine identified
1989	Anniversary of 20 years as a specialty: 384 residency training programs. 7,392 FP residents in training	Family medicine entered third decade as residency-trained physicians began to assume leadership roles
	New active members of AAFP required to be residency-trained family physicians	Affirmed the distinction between family physicians vs. general practitioners and others
	Association of Family Practice Residency Directors (AFPRD) formed	First organization of directors of family practice residency programs
1990	President George Bush signed into law Medicare Physician Payment Reform based on Resource-Based Relative Value Scale (RBRVS)	Projected Medicare payment to be based on resource costs integral to providing a service
	AMA adopted policy that every US medical school should have a family practice department	Recognition of need for medical student exposure to family medicine content and family physician role models
1991	AMA resolved "to develop recommendations for adequate reimbursement of primary care physicians, improved	Evidence of AMA support of family practice and primary care

(continued)

Year	Event	Significance
	recruitment of medical school graduates, and training a sufficient number of primary care physicians to meet projected national needs"	
1992	Medicare physician payment reform began	Beginning phase-in of Medicare fee schedule, eliminating specialty differentials
	Council on Graduate Medical Education (COGME) recommended that half of all medical school graduates enter primary care careers	Recognition that medical schools must meet health care needs of the nation
	Archives of Family Practice began publication	American Medical Association affirmed value of family medicine research through support of a new specialty journal
1993	First examination for CAQ in Sports Medicine for primary care physicians	Joint venture of the American Boards of Family Practice, Emergency Medicine, Internal Medicine, and Pediatrics
	Liaison Committee on Medical Education document, *Functions and Structure of a Medical School,* changed to read: "Clinical education programs involving patients should include disciplines such as family medicine, internal medicine, obstetrics and gynecology, pediatrics, psychiatry, and surgery"	Family medicine achieved parity with other specialties in requirements for the medical school curriculum
	Number of family practice residencies exceeded 400	New residencies included inner city, rural, and health maintenance organizations
1994	Publication of *Family Medicine: Principles and Practice,* 4th edition (Taylor,	Emphasis on core problems in clinical family medicine

(continued)

Year	Event	Significance	Year	Event	Significance
	editor; David, Johnson, Phillips, Scherger, associate editors)				family practice research
	End of practice pathway to CAQ in Geriatric Medicine	Candidates must complete formal accredited geriatric fellowship program		Center for Policy Studies in Family Practice and Primary Care begun in Washington, DC	AAFP initiative intended to bring a family practice and primary care perspective to national health policy deliberations
1995	American Boards of Family Practice and Internal Medicine called for educational resource sharing and collaborative training	Indicated trend for family physicians to teach our knowledge and skills to other specialists	1999	Anniversary of 30 years as a specialty: Residency training programs: 474 FP residents in training: 10,632 Graduates of FP residency programs: 56,859	Family medicine continues to prosper as it enters the new millennium
1996	Publication of *Fundamentals of Family Medicine* (Taylor, editor; David, Johnson, Phillips, Scherger, associate editors)	First predoctoral clerkship textbook based on health problems of a single extended family		AAFP begins national practice-based network for primary care research	The network's mission will be to "conduct, support, promote, and advocate primary care research in practice-based settings that (1) addresses questions of importance to the discipline of family medicine and (2) improves the health care delivery to and health status of patients, their families, and communities"
	Alaska's first graduate medical education program was a family practice residency	Family practice became the first specialty to have residency programs established in all 50 states			
1997	Fiftieth anniversary of the AAGP/AAFP	Fifty years since 1947 founding of AAGP in Kansas City Missouri			
	Revised Program Requirements for Residency Education in Family Practice	Changes reflect the evolution of the discipline by no longer defining training elements as derivatives of other specialties and emphasizing the role of family physicians as teachers		Practice pathway to CAQ in Sports Medicine ends	One-year sports medicine fellowship required for eligibility
	Graduates of US family practice residency programs top 50,000	AAFP annual survey confirms that 50,002 physicians have graduated from FP residencies since the 1960s	2000	112 departments of family medicine in US medical schools	Continued success of family practice at the beginning of the new millennium
				476 US family practice residency programs	
1998	Publication of *Family Medicine: Principles and Practice,* 5th edition (Taylor, editor; David, Johnson, Phillips, Scherger, associate editors)	Expanded emphasis on clinical problems in generalist health care		61,000 board-certified family physicians	
				Keystone III Conference held in Colorado Springs, Colorado	A forum for family physicians to share ideas and advance the specialty
	AAFP Research Initiative begun	AAFP commits $7.7 million to support	2001	Certificate of Added Qualifications in Adolescent Medicine begun	Collaborative effort of ABFP, the American Board of Pediatrics, and the American

(continued)   (continued)

Year	Event	Significance
		Board of Internal Medicine
2002	Thirtieth anniversary of the founding of WONCA, which comprises 58 member organizations in 53 countries	World organization of family doctors has total membership exceeding 150,000 general practitioners/family physicians
2003	*Annals* of *Family Medicine* begins publication	New research journal cosponsored by the AAFP, ABFP, AFPRD, NAPCRG, ADFM, and STFM
	Publication of *Family Medicine: Principles and Practice,* 6th edition (Taylor, editor; David, Fields, Phillips, Scherger, associate editors)	Emphasis on evidence-based health care and patient/community-centered practice in the new millennium
2004	AAFP-WONCA combined meeting in Orlando, Florida, USA	Largest meeting in the history of family and general physicians worldwide
2005	American Board of Family Practice changes its name to the American Board of Family Medicine (ABFM)	A new name for the specialty, and the *family practitioner* became the family *physician*
2006	*Preparing the Personal Physician for Practice (P4)* project developed	Fourteen family medicine residency programs to put training innovations into practice
2007	Joint Principles of the Patient-Centered Medical Home developed and endorsed by the major primary care physician associations	A health care setting that facilitates partnerships between individual patients and their personal physicians, and when appropriate, the patient's family
2008	The World Health Organization (WHO) publishes *The World Health Report 2008*	Report titled *Primary Health Care: Now More Than Ever* calls for renewal of primary health care as a response to the issues created by globalization
2009	Family medicine celebrates its 40th anniversary as a specialty	Four decades since the specialty was created in 1969

Year	Event	Significance
2010	The Patient Protection and Affordable Care Act, commonly called the Affordable Care Act (ACA), signed into law	Most comprehensive overhaul of the United States health care system since the passage of Medicare and Medicaid in 1965
2011	Family medicine residencies achieve a record 94% enrollment rate and add 100 new positions to accommodate the applicant demand	Health system changes seen spurring the increased student interest in family medicine as a career
2012	WONCA celebrates its 40th anniversary	Originally founded in 1972 by member organizations in 18 countries, WONCA grows to 97 member organizations in 79 countries, with a total membership in the member organizations of over 200,000 general practitioners/family physicians
2013	ABFM sponsors pilot of program of 4-year residency training programs	New programs to allow more flexibility in family medicine residency training curriculum
	Family Medicine Working Party launches the *Family Medicine for America's Health* initiative	Multiyear strategic program to define the role of the 21st century family physician
2014	AAFP report *Family Physician Workforce Reform* calls for 65 new family medicine training positions yearly over the next 10 years	Proposal calls for adding 4,475 family medicine training positions by 2025, projected to end the shortage of family physicians in the United States
2015	AAFP Foundation begins the Family Medicine Leads Program and sponsors the First Emerging Leader Institute for medical students	New medical student program offers tracks in policy and public health leadership, personal and practice leadership, and philanthropy and mission-driven leadership

(continued)   (continued)

Year	Event	Significance
2016	Publication of *Family Medicine: Principles and Practice,* 7th edition (P. Paulman, R. Taylor, editors; L. Nasir, A. Paulman, associate editors)	A new editorial team for the book "by family physicians for family physicians," and the new edition published both in digital and print media
2017	Fiftieth anniversary of the founding of STFM	The STFM mission: Advancing family medicine to improve health through a community of teachers and scholars
2018	Fortieth anniversary of ADFM	The ADFM mission supports academic departments of family medicine to lead and achieve their full potential in care, education, scholarship, and advocacy to

(continued)

Year	Event	Significance
		promote health and health equity
2019	Fiftieth anniversary of founding of Family Medicine as a specialty	A third generation of leaders for the specialty
2020	Family Medicine Advocacy Summit held in Washington, DC, USA	An opportunity for family physicians to get practical, hands-on experience in advocacy within the legislative process
2022	Publication of the 8th edition of *Family Medicine: Principles and Practice* (editors: P. Paulman, R. Taylor, L. Nasir, A. Paulman	The latest edition of the reference book compiled by family physicians for family physicians. First published in 1976
	Fiftieth anniversary of the founding of NAPCRG	The world's largest organization devoted to research in family medicine, primary care, and related fields

Engaging the Future of Family Medicine and Healthcare

Warren P. Newton

Contents

Introduction

In the late fourteenth century, Florence had survived the Black Death and begun its transformation to a center of cloth making, international banking, and the revival of classical learning. Unfortunately, the greatest statesman of the age, the Milanese leader, Giangaleazzo, came to power and began a series of military and political campaigns to take control of what is now northern Italy. By 1402, Florence stood alone with Milan's armies on the boarder and about to invade again. Remarkably, however, the plague spread through the countryside and killed the Milanese leader, lifting the immediate threat to the city. Having survived the most serious crisis of their history, the Florentines explored why they came so close to extinction. Their answer, in part, was their system of education, an arid scholasticism which emphasized the importance of scholars being detached from society. In its place, they put in place a new approach to education, once that put scholars in service to the needs of society. This new approach to education, civic humanism, is now known as the liberal arts [1].

Family Medicine and the US healthcare system face such a challenge today. As a child of the 1960s' demand for access to community physicians, Family Medicine grew to hundreds of residencies in a decade, and family physicians are now the largest and most widely distributed group of personal physicians. Family Physician scope of practice remains the broadest of clinicians, and, in

W. P. Newton (✉)
Department of Family Medicine, University of North Carolina, Chapel Hill, NC, USA

American Board of Family Medicine, Lexington, KY, USA
e-mail: WNewton@theabfm.org

© Springer Nature Switzerland AG 2022
P. M. Paulman et al. (eds.), *Family Medicine*,
https://doi.org/10.1007/978-3-030-54441-6_171

many regions, family physicians continue to be critical for access to health care across the continuum of care [2]. At the same time, however, despite the demands of the Affordable Care Act and huge demand in the market, the numbers of students from allopathic medical schools interested in Family Medicine has begun to drop, burnout is widespread, and scope of practice is diminishing.

The broader health care system is similarly coming to a crisis. American healthcare has always been dynamic, with a parade of new drugs and devices, but the amplitude and speed of recent changes have not been seen in two generations: they represent *transformation*. A major component of the transformation is the rapid consolidation of hospitals and health systems, driven by health care reform, the promise of payment for population health, and market and regulatory forces. In parallel are the rapid spread of integrated electronic health records and employment of physicians. The majority of US physicians are now employed, as are almost 70% of family physicians [3]. A second phase of

transformation is just starting. Changes in genomics are revolutionizing cancer and autoimmune disease treatment and promise more. Augmented intelligence promises to change health care as much as has already happened in banking and retail businesses. Attracted by the opportunity for profit, new business models are coming into medicine – CVS and Aetna, Humana and Walmart, Amazon, JP Morgan and Berkshire Hathaway along with many others. And the COVID pandemic will have long term effects on health care, including likely widespread adoption of telehealth and lasting changes in the organization and financing of health care.

Unfortunately, despite transformation of care, and despite health care reform, the population outcomes of health care in the USA are the worst among developed countries, and getting worse. As the National Research Council demonstrated [4], Americans are sicker and die earlier than citizens of comparable countries. This is true at all ages and for almost all diseases – and at a health care cost much greater than comparable countries. As examples, Figs. 1 and 2 depict the

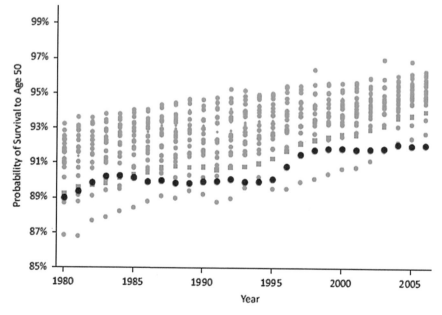

Fig. 1 Probability of survival to age 50 for males in 21 high-income countries, 1980–2006. (Notes: Red circles show the probability of newborn male in the United States will live to age 50. Grey circles show the probability of survival to age 50 in Australia, Austria, Belgium, Canada, Denmark, Finland, France, Iceland, Ireland, Italy, Japan, Luxembourg, the Netherlands, New Zealand, Norway, Portugal, Spain, Sweden, Switzerland, the United Kingdom, and West Germany. Source: National Research Council (2011, Figs. 1–5))

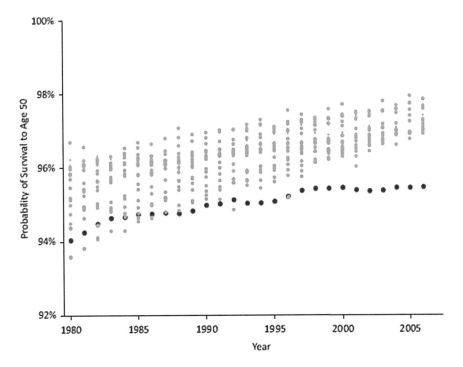

Fig. 2 Probability of survival to age 50 for females in 21 high-income countries, 1980–2006. (Notes: Red circles show the probability a newborn female in the United States will live to age 50. Grey circles show the probability of survival to age 50 in Australia, Austria, Belgium, Canada, Denmark, Finland, France, Iceland, Ireland, Italy, Japan, Luxembourg, the Netherlands, New Zealand, Norway, Portugal, Spain, Sweden, Switzerland, the United Kingdom, and West Germany

likelihood of survival beyond the age of 50 [4], and Fig. 3 compares US public and private health care expenditure to other countries [5]. More recently, it has become clear that US life expectancy has begun to decline, as the result of increased mortality from many diseases [6]. This was apparent even before the COVID pandemic highlighted dramatic disparities of incidence and mortality for Blacks, Hispanics, and Native Americans.

The premise of this chapter is that both Family Medicine and the broader health care system are in a phase of dramatic change. Family Physicians, as the most common and widely distributed personal physicians, currently play a major role in health and health care across the country. At the same time, as the needs of society are changing, family medicine must change to meet society's needs and help lead the health care changes necessary to improve health and health care. What follows summarizes the origin and current role of family physicians, the drivers of primary care's population benefits, the challenges health care faces, and how family medicine must evolve to meet the needs of society and the broader healthcare system.

The Origins and Current Role of Family Medicine

In 1960, in a classic article in Lancet [7], Fox argued the health care needed a new kind of doctor, a personal doctor with additional training and support who could address the large majority of a patient's problems and, if necessary, accompany the patient through an ever more complex health care system. Combining the heritage of general practitioners with the sixties' call for access to care, and with impetus from the Folsom, Millard, and Willis reports [8], the new specialty was born with the creation of the American Board of Family

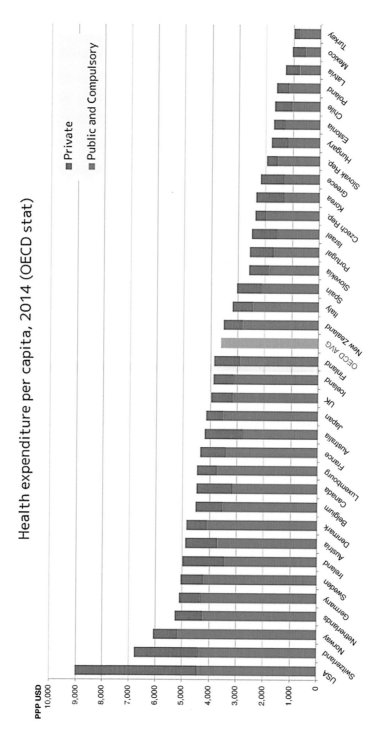

Fig. 3 OECD.Stat: Health Expenditure and Financing. Organisation for Economic Co-Operation and Development

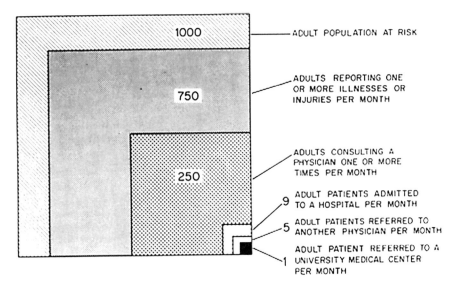

Fig. 4 Ecology of Care. (Monthly prevalence estimates of illness in the community and the roles of physicians, hospitals, and university medical centers in the provision of medical care (adults sixteen years of age and over). White et al. [11])

Medicine in 1969. The new specialty was marked by a commitment to 50 hours of CME a year, the importance of ongoing and independent assessment of cognitive expertise, and the conviction that both knowledge and performance in practice were important. Powered by the social movement of the 1960s, the specialty grew very rapidly, with hundreds of residencies beginning over the next decade.

Family physicians now constitute the largest population of personal physicians in the USA, growing rapidly even as many fewer go into general medicine and general pediatrics [2]. For all common chronic diseases, the large majority of Americans who name a personal physician name a family physician [2, 9]. Family physicians also have a broad scope of care, providing substantial amounts of inpatient care, obstetric care, and emergency room care, especially in rural areas. Maps of the USA without family physicians demonstrate dramatic number of physician shortage areas [10]. Large numbers of nurse practitioners and physicians' assistants are being trained, and many go into primary care, often with family physicians or but many more go into subspecialty practice [2].

It is important to put primary care into the context of the broader health care system. Kerr

White in a classic study of the ecology of medical care in 1961 [11] used current evidence to describe what happens to patients are seen in average month. As Fig. 4 depicts, of 1000 adults over a month, 750 will develop symptoms, 250 will go to a primary care doctor, 9 will be hospitalized, and 1 will be hospitalized in an academic medical center. Interestingly, 40 years later, Green demonstrated that the proportions were still approximately the same [12]. The figure demonstrates the major role of primary care in health care as well as the need for medical education outside of academic hospitals.

The Primary Care Advantage

In considering the future of Family Medicine, an important first step is to explore the core functions of primary care. At this stage, there is a deep and broad literature on the impact of primary care. Starting with Starfield's classic article in the Lancet [13], there has been ample demonstration that countries with robust primary care have increased quality of care, decreased cost, and better patient satisfaction. While Starfield and others' work is largely ecologic in nature, the findings have been replicated across states and other levels of organization [14].

What about primary care provides such a robust health benefit? The key elements have been termed the "four Cs": first contact, continuity, comprehensiveness, and coordination. First contact care means access to care, along many dimensions including location, hours, cost, and trust. Especially after the COVID pandemic, access does not necessary mean *in person*, but in happening some way for ongoing care and improvement of health. Continuity of care makes possible trusting relationships and the knowledge of patient context that drives trust, medication adherence, behavior change, and shared decision making. Comprehensiveness is taking care of the whole person, supporting prevention and well as diagnosis and treatment and mental as well as physical problems. Comprehensiveness is often operationalized as a clinician being able to care for almost all of the problems that patients coming in have in a given day. Finally, coordination is necessary as patients travel through the health care system and is especially important as they age and have multiple medical problems.

Of course, these core functions are interrelated – for example, continuity of care makes comprehensiveness of care and coordination more feasible. What Starfield and others have demonstrated is that the better these functions are achieved by primary care in a particular country or region, the greater the benefit to the health of the population. It is important to recognize that these are functions, not specific kinds of providers, and that support of primary care through data exchange, connections to communities and public health and robust connections with hospital care is critical. Importantly for the policy discussions, there is little in the literature that says that primary care must be provided by family physicians as opposed to other specialties or professions. In addition, primary care in the USA and Canada is distinguished by its breadth of scope. Family physicians practice not just in continuity of care in the community but also often in the hospital, the labor deck, in nursing homes, and many other community settings.

The Challenges of the Future

The crisis facing health care is complex, including fundamental changes in the clinical problems we are facing, growing complexity of the health care system, continuing increases in the cost of care and an increasing loss of trust in health care systems and in doctors. Clinically, and very different from the time of the founding of family medicine, multimorbidity drives the vast majority of cost, mortality, morbidity, and cost [15]. Health care – and family physicians – must thus be able to address the challenges of patients with many clinical problems. There are also new clinical problems. In addition to the threat of emerging infectious disease made clear by COVID, there has also been epidemic opiate and other substance abuse. Opiates now kill more than automobile accidents. More broadly, deaths due to behavioral problems have grown greatly and suicide attempts among adolescents have increased dramatically [16, 17], while social issues such as isolation, poor health literacy, and lack of access have common and important clinical implications.

Contemporary organization of health care has not kept up with the dramatic changes in disease and in society. The Center for Medicare and Medicaid services has emphasized that poor transitions of care remain a major cause of unnecessary cost and poor quality [18]. To what extent has the growing separation of hospital care from primary care contributed to this problem? Vast "obstetrical deserts [19]" have been created with the accelerating closure of rural hospitals and the lack of family physicians to deliver babies in rural communities. The lack of integration of behavioral health and physical health has greatly increased the cost and dyscoordination of care, even as the COVID pandemic has underscored the importance of a robust link between primary care and public health [20]. Finally, both COVID and the new civil rights movement have again underscored the presence of shameful disparities of health outcomes across race, ethnicity, and socioeconomic status.

Family Medicine faces its own crisis, with decreasing scope of practice and, like other specialties and professions, epidemic burnout. Phillips underscored the risks of the current trajectories of Family Medicine. If not addressed, they portend a dystopic future:

> The role of the US family physician is to provide episodic outpatient care in 15-minute blocks with coincidental continuity and a reducing scope of care. The family physicians surrender care coordination of care to care management functions divorced from practices and works in small ill-defined teams whose members have little training and few in depth relationships with the physicians and with patients. The family physician serves as the agent of a larger system whose role is to feed patients to subspecialty services and hospital beds. The family physician is not responsible for patient panel management, community health or collaboration with public health. [21]

On the other hand, by taking advantage of technology and other advances, Phillips paints a different and more positive vision for the future of Family Medicine based on greater use of technology and other advances:

> Family physicians are personal doctors for people of all ages and health conditions. They are a reliable first contact for health concerns and directly address most health care needs. Through enduring partnerships, family physicians help patients prevent, understand, and manage illness, navigate the health system, and set health goals. Family physicians and their staff adapt their care to the unique needs of their patients and communities. They use data to monitor and manage their patient population and use best science to prioritize services most likely to benefit health. They are ideal leaders of health care systems and partners for public health. [21]

The Way Forward for Family Medicine

The first step is to commit to the goal of improving health and healthcare. In 2013, Don Berwick and his colleagues set out for the nation a triple aim – improving health, patient experience and reducing the cost of care [22]. At the same time, as burnout across medicine and other health professions has increased, we have realized that resilience and wellness of health care workers is a necessary foundation for the triple aim. The preventable deaths of health care workers in the COVID pandemic as the result of the lack of personal protective equipment have underscored this issue.

Within this overall goal, what is the special role for family medicine and primary care? Primary care, re-envisioned robustly, and implemented by personal physicians and their teams, can play an important role but it is necessary to reconsider the core functions of primary care and adapt them to the 2020s. Post COVID, both first contact care and continuity of care will likely include telehealth and often team based care; the innovation challenge will be to organize care to support continuity of care, patient engagement, and the shared decision making so critical for managing critical clinical decisions. Although family physician scope of practice has declined in recent years [23], the COVID Pandemic has highlighted the value of flexibility of family physicians to take care of patients across the continuum of care – on the wards, in the ICU, in the diagnostic tent, or by a hybrid in person/telehealth role. Can new models of care with family physicians rotating through both the office and the hospital address the cost and quality problem of transitions of care, while preventing as many hospitalizations as possible? Can family physicians providing more emergency care, prenatal care, and deliveries with caesarian section capability help rural communities survive, helping to reverse recent increases in rural mortality? In an age of multimorbidity, when large proportions of Medicare patients see over 15 doctors a year or are on over 10 medications, can better continuity and comprehensiveness, supplemented by smart care coordination, improve care? Finally, can family physicians working and engaging in communities help improve disparities and increase social capital?

A key priority at the health system and payer level will be developing, testing, and spreading innovations of care that improve population health. Population health has had increasing attention over the last decade but means different things to different people. Population health is more than a killer app or an EHR or just having an integrated clinical system! A major challenge will be combining innovation in delivery models with payment reforms which focus on defined populations and have primary care at their foundation and all both growth and sustainability. Family physicians have played major roles in large scale practice demonstration projects; given family physicians' clinical breadth, interpersonal skills, and pragmatism, it is not surprising that there is a growing interest in development of family physicians in leadership roles in large systems [24].

At the individual and community level, family physicians must adjust to being employees in increasingly large health care systems. The large majority of family physicians are now employed, with increasing numbers in large multispecialty practices or clinically integrated systems. Post COVID, it is likely that this trend will accelerate. For a specialty and culture born of small group independent practices, this has major ramifications. Learning how to navigate a large system clinically takes time and practice, as does effective advocacy for both individual patients and system changes. The intrinsic professionalism we bring to our work must be adjusted to the new context.

At the level of clinical care, the most important challenge will be learning to manage panels and populations of patients. Most family physicians are well trained in the care of individual patients but have not been trained in the skills for managing panels. But panels/denominators are fundamental for improving access, effectiveness, and patient experience. Thinking at both the population and the individual level requires both training and practice.

Another key challenge will be adopting new technology thoughtfully. Virtually all of primary care in the USA switched to telehealth in the course of a few weeks in March 2020 – a stunning achievement that demonstrates the professionalism and flexibility of our health care profession. The technology challenge will be much greater than telehealth – it is making sense of the plethora of devices and tests that will allow family physicians to broaden their scope across the continuum of care. It is making cost-effective use of new pharmaceutical agents that cost thousands of dollars a month: it is making genomics useful beyond cancer treatment and autoimmune diseases; it is building AI into patient care systems. American healthcare is awash with technology and data, from new tests to new apps to new drugs and devices: all will sound good, almost all will increase costs, and a few will improve health outcomes. The challenge of thoughtful cost-effective

adoption of technology is one of the most important roles of personal physicians.

Where does team-based care fit in? A large proportion of family physician currently practice with NPs (55.9%), PAs (42.5%), Pharmacists (25.8%), and Social Workers (26.3%) but how to work together optimally over time is still evolving [25]. The doctor patient relationship is key to the shared decision making and the behavioral changes necessary to address chronic disease, but it is also clear that much of the care perceived by patients is provided by team members. Our models for team-based care come from the inpatient setting, where patients were in the hospital for a very long time and different professionals work together over weeks. In the primary care setting, however, teams function very differently. A large office can see 300 patients in a day; teams evolve, start, and stop hour by hour. In primary care, moreover, patients are vertical rather than horizontal – to a much greater extent than patients in the hospital, patients can choose to comply or not with recommendations. It is thus critical to involve patients and family in the team of care. Improving team-based care is thus important, but who should be on the team and how to best deploy teams remains one of the most exciting challenges in the specialty.

Addressing these problems will require a new kind of ongoing professional development. In 1947, the American Association of General Practice made a remarkable commitment to lifelong learning through 50 hours a year of continuing medical education (CME) [26]. At the time it was, and still is, a major commitment – by the biggest commitment of any specialty. In the three generations since that commitment, however, there has been a stunning shift in pedagogy. We now understand that active learning is vastly better than the passive learning typical of "butts in the seats" CME, that physicians like other experts are not good at assessing their own knowledge, and that the right kind of assessment drives learning [27]. All of these mean that the continuing professional education system for family physicians must change dramatically.

Perhaps the most challenging task for the family physicians of the future will be maintaining connection with their patients through many channels and multiple priorities. The goal remains both care and cure – providing treatment and counsel, improving quality of live, and promoting empowerment through shared decision making, keeping up to date, while balancing the needs of the individual and the population, keeping up to date and engaging in one's own community. Such a complex task requires the most able of physicians and the professionalism to commit to ongoing self-assessment and improvement.

Conclusion

Since its founding as a specialty in 1969, Family Medicine has met the need of society for access to community-based physicians. The specialty has grown to become the largest and most widely distributed group of personal physicians, and family physicians play a huge role delivering care for patients and communities across the country. Now, however, as the progress of health and health care falters, family medicine must evolve to meet the evolving needs of society. Personal physicians can and must contribute to improving health and healthcare, one patient at a time, one community at a time, and one health system at a time. After recognizing the time in history, the first step, the most practical step, is to change our educational systems across the continuum, from undergraduate to graduate to continuing medical education. Like the Florentines did more than 600 years ago, like the AAGP and the ABFP did 50 years ago, we must start with education, in service to society' needs.

References

1. Baron H. The crisis of the early Italian renaissance. Princeton: Princeton University Press; 1966.
2. Willis J, Antonio B, Bazemore A, Jetty A, Petterson S. The state of primary care in the United States: a chartbook of facts and statistics. IBM: Washington, DC; 2020.
3. JAMA Career Center – Practice Arrangements. Employment Trends Report. 2019. https://careers.jamanetwork.com/article/employment-trends-report-practice-arrangements. Accessed 9 Apr 2020.
4. U.S. Health in International Perspective: Shorter Lives, Poorer Health. Washington, DC: National Research Council: Institute of Medicine of the National Academies; 2013.
5. OECD.Stat: Health Expenditure and Financing. Organisation for Economic Co-Operation and Development. https://upload.wikimedia.org/wikipedia/commons/thumb/0/0b/OECD_health_expenditure_per_capita_by_country.svg/800px-OECD_health_expenditure_per_capita_by_country.svg.png. Accessed 19 Sept 2020.
6. Woolf SH, Schoomaker H. Life expectancy and mortality rates in the United States, 1959–2017. JAMA. 2019;322(20):1996–2016.
7. Fox TF, Cantab MD, Glasg LLD. The personal doctor and his relation to the hospital observations and reflections on some American experiments in general practice by groups. Lancet. 1960;1(7127): 743–60.
8. Gutierrez C, Scheid P. The history of family medicine and its impact in US Health Care Delivery. https://www.aafpfoundation.org/content/dam/foundation/documents/who-we-are/cfhm/FMImpactGutierrezScheid.pdf. Accessed 17 Sept 2020.
9. Martin JC, Avant RF, Bowman MA, et al. The future of family medicine: a collaborative project of the family medicine community. Ann Fam Med. 2004;2(Suppl 1): S3–32.
10. Crowley C, Proser M, Bazemore A. High demand, low supply: health centers and the recruitment of family physicians. https://www.aafp.org/afp/2018/0801/afp20180801p146.pdf. Accessed 14 Sept 2020.
11. White KL, Williams TF, Greenberg BC. The ecology of medical care. Reprinted from NEJM. 1961; 265:885–92.
12. Green LA. The ecology of medical care revisited. NEJM. 2001;344(26):2021–5.
13. Starfield B. Is primary care essential? Lancet. 1994;344(8930):1129–34.
14. Macinko J, Starfield B, Shi L. Contribution of primary care systems to health outcomes within Organization for Economic Cooperation and Development (OECD) countries, 1970–1998. Milbank Memorial Fund Q. 2005;83(3):457–502.
15. McPhail SM. Multimorbidity in chronic disease: impact on health care resources and costs. Risk Manag Healthc Policy. 2016;9:143–56.
16. Opiod Overdose. https://www.cdc.gov/drugoverdose/index.html. Accessed 17 Sept 2020.
17. Bilsen J. Suicide and youth: risk factors. Front Psychol. 2018;9:1–5.
18. Community-Based Care Transitions Program. https://innovation.cms.gov/innovation-models/cctp. Accessed 19 Sept 2020.
19. Cullen J. New AAFP initiative addresses rural health care crisis. Ann Fam Med. 2019;17:471–2.
20. Committee on Integrating Primary Care and Public Health, In. Primary care and public health: exploring integration to improve population health. Washington, DC: National Academies Press (US); 2012.
21. Phillips RL, Brungardt S, Lesko SE, et al. The future role of the family physician in the United States: a

Rigorus exercise in definition. Ann Fam Med. 2014;12(3):250–5.

22. Berwick DM, Nolan TW. Whittington. The triple aim: care, health, and cost. Health Aff. 2008;27: 759–69.

23. Coutinho AJ, Phillips RL, Peterson LE. Intended vs reported scope of practice. JAMA. 2016;315(20): 2234–5.

24. Changing the Face of Medicine. 2003. https://cfmedicine.nlm.nih.gov/physicians/biography_304.html. Accessed 14 Sept 2020.

25. Jabbarpour Y, Jetty A, Dai M, Magill M, Bazemore A. The evolving family medicine team. JABFM. 2020;33:499–501.

26. The American Academy of Family Physicians. Significant Events in AAFP History 1947–2017. https://www.aafpfoundation.org/content/dam/foundation/documents/who-we-are/cfhm/factsonfile/AAFPChronology.pdf. Accessed 17 Sept 2020.

27. McMahon GT, Newton WP. Continuing board certification: seeing our way forward. JABFM. 2020; 33:S10–4.

Normal Laboratory Values/Adult Patients

Clinical Chemistry Tests

Alanine aminotransferase (ALT, SGPT)	13–48 U/L
Albumin	3.6–5.2 g/dL
Alkaline phosphatase (ALP)	35–120 U/L
Amylase, serum	44–128 U/L
Aspartate aminotransferase (AST, SGOT)	15–41 U/L
Bilirubin, conjugated	0–0.2 mg/dL
Bilirubin, total	0.2–1.2 mg/dL
Calcium	8.5–10.5 mg/dL
Carbon dioxide (CO_2), total	23–30 mEq/L
Chloride	98–109 mEq/L
Creatine kinase (CK, CPK)	40–260 U/L
Creatinine	0.7–1.2 mg/dL
Gamma glutamyltransferase (GGT)	5–40 U/L
Glucose, fasting	65–110 mg/dL
Hemoglobin A_{1C}	5.0–7.0% of total Hb
Iron, serum	50–170 µg/dL
Iron-binding capacity, total (TIBC)	270–390 µg/dL
Lactate, serum (venous)	5.0–20.0 mg/dL
Lactate dehydrogenase (LDH)	110–260 U/L
Lipase	10–140 U/L
Magnesium	1.5–2.5 mg/dL
Potassium	3.5–5.1 mEq/L
Prostate-specific antigen	0–4 ng/mL
Protein, total	6.1–7.9 g/dL
Sodium	136–147 mEq/L
Troponin I	<2.5 ng/mL
Troponin T	<0.2 ng/mL
Urea nitrogen	6.0–20.0 mg/dL
Uric acid	2.6–7.2 mg/dL

Lipid Panel

Cholesterol, total	160–240 mg/dL
HDL cholesterol	>40 mg/dL
LDL cholesterol	<130 mg/dL
Triglycerides	55–200 mg/dL

Thyroid Function Tests

Thyroid stimulating hormone (TSH)	2–11 µU/mL
Thyroxine, free (FT_4)	0.8–2.4 ng/dL
Thyroxine, total (T_4)	4.0–12.0 µg/dL
Triiodothyronine (T_3)	70–200 ng/dL
Triiodothyronine (T_3) resin uptake (T_3RU)	25–38%

Blood Gases

	Arterial	Venous
Base excess	−3.0 to +3.0 mEq/L	−5.0 to +5.0 mEq/L
Bicarbonate (HCO_3)	18–25 mEq/L	18–25 mEq/L
pO_2	80–95 mm Hg	30–48 mm Hg
O_2 saturation	95–98%	60–85%
pCO_2	34–45 mm Hg	35–52 mm Hg
Total CO_2	23–30 mEq/L	24–31 mEq/L
pH	7.35–7.45	7.32–7.42

© Springer Nature Switzerland AG 2022
P. M. Paulman et al. (eds.), *Family Medicine*,
https://doi.org/10.1007/978-3-030-54441-6

Hematology and Coagulation Tests

White blood cell (WBC) count	4.4–11.0 K/mm^3
Hemoglobin	12.2–15.0 g/dL
Hematocrit	37.0–54.0%
Red blood cell (RBC) count	3.80–5.20 million/mm^3
Mean corpuscular volume (MCV)	85.0–95.0 μm^3
Mean corpuscular hemoglobin (MCH)	26.0–34.0 pg/cell
MCH concentration (MCHC)	32.6–36.0 g/dL
Red cell distribution width (RDW)	11.5–15.0%
Platelet count	150.0–420.0 K/mm^3
Reticulocyte count	0.5–1.5% of RBCs
WBC differential	
Neutrophils	38–70%

(continued)

Lymphocytes	16–49%
Monocytes	2–9%
Eosinophils	0–5%
Basophils	0–2%
Sedimentation rate	
Adult male	≤15 mm/h
Adult female	≤20 mm/h
Coagulation tests	
Fibrinogen	200–400 mg/dL
Partial thromboplastin time (PTT)	60–85 s
Activated PTT	25–35 s
Prothrombin time (PT)	11–14 s

Note: The reference intervals shown are for adults and may vary according to technique or laboratory, or as new methods are introduced. Always consult the reference range for your own laboratory.

Index

© Springer Nature Switzerland AG 2022
P. M. Paulman et al. (eds.), *Family Medicine*,
https://doi.org/10.1007/978-3-030-54441-6

Printed by Printforce, the Netherlands